# Nutrient Requirements of Dairy Cattle

## Seventh Revised Edition, 2001

Subcommittee on Dairy Cattle Nutrition
Committee on Animal Nutrition
Board on Agriculture and Natural Resources
National Research Council

NATIONAL ACADEMY PRESS
Washington, D.C.

**NATIONAL ACADEMY PRESS • 2101 Constitution Avenue, NW • Washington, D.C. 20418**

NOTICE: The project that is the subject of this report was approved by the Governing Board of the National Research Council, whose members are drawn from the councils of the National Academy of Sciences, the National Academy of Engineering, and the Institute of Medicine. The members of the committee responsible for the report were chosen for their special competences and with regard for appropriate balance.

This study was supported by the Agricultural Research Service of the U.S. Department of Agriculture under Agreement No. 59-32U4-5-6, the Center for Veterinary Medicine of the U.S. Department of Health and Human Services under Agreement No. R-13-FD01495, and the American Feed Industry Association.

**Library of Congress Cataloging-in-Publication Data**

Nutrient requirements of dairy cattle / Subcommittee on Dairy Cattle Nutrition, Committee on Animal Nutrition, Board on Agriculture, National Research Council. — 7th rev. ed.

p. cm.

Includes bibliographical references (p. ).

ISBN 0-309-06997-1

1. Dairy cattle—Nutrition—Requirements. 2. Dairy cattle—Feeding and feeds. I. National Research Council (U.S.). Subcommittee on Dairy Cattle Nutrition.

SF203 .N883 2001

636.2′13—dc21 00-012828

Additional copies of this report are available from the National Academy Press, 2101 Constitution Avenue, N.W., Lockbox 285, Washington, D.C. 20055; (800) 624-6242 or (202) 334-3313 (in the Washington metropolitan area); Internet, http://www.nap.edu.



Printed in the United States of America.

# THE NATIONAL ACADEMIES

National Academy of Sciences
National Academy of Engineering
Institute of Medicine
National Research Council

The **National Academy of Sciences** is a private, nonprofit, self-perpetuating society of distinguished scholars engaged in scientific and engineering research, dedicated to the furtherance of science and technology and to their use for the general welfare. Upon the authority of the charter granted to it by the Congress in 1863, the Academy has a mandate that requires it to advise the federal government on scientific and technical matters. Dr. Bruce M. Alberts is president of the National Academy of Sciences.

The **National Academy of Engineering** was established in 1964, under the charter of the National Academy of Sciences, as a parallel organization of outstanding engineers. It is autonomous in its administration and in the selection of its members, sharing with the National Academy of Sciences the responsibility for advising the federal government. The National Academy of Engineering also sponsors engineering programs aimed at meeting national needs, encourages education and research, and recognizes the superior achievements of engineers. Dr. William A. Wulf is president of the National Academy of Engineering.

The **Institute of Medicine** was established in 1970 by the National Academy of Sciences to secure the services of eminent members of appropriate professions in the examination of policy matters pertaining to the health of the public. The Institute acts under the responsibility given to the National Academy of Sciences by its congressional charter to be an adviser to the federal government and, upon its own initiative, to identify issues of medical care, research, and education. Dr. Kenneth I. Shine is president of the Institute of Medicine.

The **National Research Council** was organized by the National Academy of Sciences in 1916 to associate the broad community of science and technology with the Academy's purposes of furthering knowledge and advising the federal government. Functioning in accordance with general policies determined by the Academy, the Council has become the principal operating agency of both the National Academy of Sciences and the National Academy of Engineering in providing services to the government, the public, and the scientific and engineering communities. The Council is administered jointly by both Academies and the Institute of Medicine. Dr. Bruce M. Alberts and Dr. William A. Wulf are chairman and vice chairman, respectively, of the National Research Council.

## SUBCOMMITTEE ON DAIRY CATTLE NUTRITION

JIMMY H. CLARK, *Chair*, University of Illinois
DAVID K. BEEDE, Michigan State University
RICHARD A. ERDMAN, University of Maryland
JESSE P. GOFF, USDA/ARS/NSDC, Ames, Iowa
RIC R. GRUMMER, University of Wisconsin
JAMES G. LINN, University of Minnesota
ALICE N. PELL, Cornell University
CHARLES G. SCHWAB, University of New Hampshire
TREVOR TOMKINS, Milk Specialties Company
GABRIELLA A. VARGA, Pennsylvania State University
WILLIAM P. WEISS, The Ohio State University

## COMMITTEE ON ANIMAL NUTRITION

GARY L. CROMWELL, *Chair*, University of Kentucky
MARY E. ALLEN, National Zoological Park
MICHAEL L. GALYEAN, Texas Tech University
RONALD W. HARDY, University of Idaho
BRIAN W. McBRIDE, University of Guelph
KEITH E. RINEHART, Perdue Farms Inc.
L. LEE SOUTHERN, Louisiana State University
JERRY W. SPEARS, North Carolina State University
DONALD R. TOPLIFF, West Texas A&M University
WILLIAM P. WEISS, The Ohio State University

*Staff*

CHARLOTTE KIRK BAER, *Program Director*
NORMAN GROSSBLATT, *Editor*
STEPHANIE PADGHAM, *Project Assistant*
MELINDA SIMONS, *Project Assistant**

* through January 1999

# Preface

Dairy cattle production is an important component of the food industry. Nutrition is a key factor in the performance, health, and welfare of dairy cattle. Given the large variation in dairy cattle types and the various environments in which they are maintained, producers must increasingly concern themselves with optimizing feeding programs.

To that end, the Subcommittee on Dairy Cattle Nutrition, which was appointed in 1997 under the guidance of the Committee on Animal Nutrition in the National Research Council's Board on Agriculture and Natural Resources, embarked on a monumental task in the development of a new edition of *Nutrient Requirements of Dairy Cattle*. As we conducted our work, it was our desire to provide users of this volume an accurate, comprehensive, and useful review of the scientific literature and practical experiences that have shaped our knowledge of dairy cattle nutrition over the past decade.

We chose to provide both a written description of the biologic basis for predicting nutrient requirements and a computer model on a compact disk to use for estimating requirements of lactating, nonlactating, growing, and young dairy animals. The subcommittee recognizes that some users of this revision will prefer to apply tables of requirements for an average situation, and we have attempted to provide those tables. Although there is often uncertainty using a modeling approach to estimate nutrient requirements, we believed that we had a responsibility to move the science forward, so we included a model that was constructed on a substantial amount of data. We believe that the model builds on the work of previous Research Council committees and moves the science forward without reaching so far that estimates cannot be validated. We found that an abundance of new science-based knowledge had surfaced since the last edition, but we also found that our knowledge of many aspects of dairy cattle nutrition is incomplete; we chose not to venture too far from what our knowledge base would allow.

In developing this report, the subcommittee considered current issues in dairy cattle production inasmuch as they affect nutrient requirements and animal feeding management, including new emphasis on environmental considerations in the feeding of dairy cattle. We have attempted in this new edition to focus more than in the past on considerations and criteria for establishing nutrient requirements.

This study was conducted through the concerted efforts of the members of the Subcommittee on Dairy Cattle Nutrition. We began our 3-year task in 1997 and completed this volume in 2000. We hope that it will be used with the same passion and enthusiasm with which it was developed.

JIMMY H. CLARK, *Chair*
Subcommittee on Dairy Cattle Nutrition

# Acknowledgments

A volume of this magnitude represents the combined efforts of many individuals. The subcommittee thanks all those who shared their insights and knowledge to bring this document to fruition. We would first like to thank everyone who participated in our public sessions and the special sessions that were organized for our benefit during the American Dairy Science Association meetings over the past several years.

During the course of its deliberations, the subcommittee sought advice and special assistance from several people who gave generously of their time to help us complete our task. Very special thanks are due to Carl Davis, University of Illinois; Jim Drackley, University of Illinois; Gale Bateman, University of Illinois; Danny Fox, Cornell University; Brian Garthwaite, Food and Drug Administration; and Normand St. Pierre, Ohio State University. We are extremely indebted to them. In addition, we sought and received guidance early on from R. Lee Baldwin, University of California, Davis; Mark Hanigan, Purina Mills, Inc.; Rick Kohn, University of Maryland; and Dale Waldo, U. S. Department of Agriculture (retired).

The expertise of Vajesh Durbal, Cornell University, is gratefully acknowledged. He was instrumental in programming the computer model, and we could not have accomplished what we did without his skill and patience.

The subcommittee is grateful to members of the National Research Council staff who worked diligently to maintain progress and quality in our work. Through her dedication, guidance, and skill, Charlotte Kirk Baer transformed our spirited verbal pondering and imperfect written drafts into a comprehensive report. Stephanie Padgham provided able assistance and much-needed momentum during the final stages of our study. Melinda Simons supported all of us cheerfully and effectively during the early phases of the study and Laura Boschini shared her skills in preparing the report for publication.

This report has been reviewed in draft form by individuals chosen for their diverse perspectives and technical expertise, in accordance with procedures approved by the NRC's Report Review Committee. The purpose of this independent review is to provide candid and critical comments that will assist the institution in making its published report as sound as possible and to ensure that the report meets institutional standards for objectivity, evidence, and responsiveness to the study charge. The review comments and draft manuscript remain confidential to protect the integrity of the deliberative process. We wish to thank the following individuals for their review of this report: R. Lee Baldwin, University of California, Davis; Paul Chandler, Chandler Associates; Larry Chase, Cornell University; Jud Heinrichs, Pennsylvania State University; Roger Hemken, University of Kentucky; Alois Kertz, Agri Brands International; David Mertens, U.S. Department of Agriculture Dairy Forage Research Center; Jerry Olson, University of Minnesota; Leo Timms, Iowa State University; Michael Van Amburgh, Cornell University; Harold Van Horn, University of Florida; and Michael VandeHaar, Michigan State University. Although the reviewers listed above have provided many constructive comments and suggestions, they were not asked to endorse the conclusions or recommendations nor did they see the final draft of the report before its release. The review of this report was overseen by Michael Galyean, Texas Tech University, appointed by the Committee on Animal Nutrition, and Robert Wilson, Mississippi State University, appointed by the Board on Agriculture and Natural Resources. These individuals were responsible for making certain that an independent examination of this report was carried out in accordance with institutional procedures and that all review comments were carefully considered. Responsibility for the final content of this report rests entirely with the authoring subcommittee and the institution.

# Contents

# Tables and Figures

## TABLES

## FIGURES

# Nutrient Requirements of Dairy Cattle

## Seventh Revised Edition, 2001

# Overview

Since 1944, the National Research Council has published six editions of *Nutrient Requirements of Dairy Cattle*. This seventh revised edition, *Nutrient Requirements of Dairy Cattle 2001*, applies new information and technology to current issues in the field of dairy cattle production. Reflecting the rapidly changing face of dairy cattle production and dairy science, it includes more comprehensive descriptions of management and environmental factors that affect nutrient requirements and provides expanded discussions of nutrient needs for various life stages and levels of production. A revised approach to predicting nutrient requirements increases the user's responsibility for accurately defining animals, diet, and management conditions to estimate nutrient requirements. A benefit associated with the increased responsibility is the ability of the user to make more-informed decisions in the field.

A substantial part of the increase in decision-making power comes from the presentation of requirements with a computer model. Computer models are the only effective means of taking animal variation into account. Unlike static tabular values, computer models such as the one provided in this edition can describe animals in different states with differing needs. A model can accommodate fluctuations caused by the effect of feed ingredients on nutrient absorption and consequently on the animal's performance potential, which affects its nutrient requirements. The model prepared in this publication was designed to provide practical, situation-specific information in a user-friendly format.

Chapter 1 presents a discussion of dry matter intake, including factors that affect intake and methods of predicting it. Characteristics of the animal's diet, environment, and physiologic makeup are considered, as are relevant management issues. After a brief description of available equations for predicting dry matter intake, the chapter discusses the dry matter intake equations included in this edition and closes with tables and graphs of intake across a lactation.

Chapter 2 addresses energy, defining energy units and expressing methods of obtaining, estimating, and expressing energy values of feeds. The chapter discusses energy requirements for maintenance, lactation, activity, and pregnancy. Tissue mobilization and repletion and the effects of environment are discussed. The chapter concludes with a section on body condition scoring, which is accompanied by a reference chart.

Chapter 3 covers digestibility and energy values of fat. It contains information on effects of fat on rumen fermentation and the use of fat in lactation diets. A table of fatty acid composition of fats and oils is presented.

A comprehensive review of carbohydrates is provided in Chapter 4. Nonstructural and structural carbohydrates are discussed, with special attention to requirements for neutral detergent fiber (NDF) and acid detergent fiber (ADF).

Chapter 5 covers all aspects of protein and amino acid nutrition. This chapter documents an extensive literature base used in the development of equations and provides detailed explanations for estimating metabolizable-protein requirements for maintenance, pregnancy, lactation, and growth. The amino acid section is a substantial advance over the previous edition and provides readers with a discussion of predicting passage to the small intestine and equations for estimating lysine and methionine requirements.

Requirements for macrominerals and trace minerals, and information on toxic minerals appear in Chapter 6. Each category includes an extensive list of minerals and covers their function, bioavailability, requirements by different classes of dairy animals, toxicity, and symptoms of mineral deficiency.

Chapter 7 covers vitamins in a similar fashion, dividing them into fat-soluble and water-soluble categories. Like the minerals in Chapter 6, the vitamins in Chapter 7 are discussed in the context of the animals that will be ingesting them. Sources and bioavailability of vitamins are provided, followed by a discussion of the functions of each vitamin, animal response to it, requirements for it, and factors that affect the requirements.

Metabolism and requirements open the discussion of water in Chapter 8. This chapter furnishes information on factors in the environment and the water itself that affect intake. Among the factors considered are nutrients in the water and the presence of bacteria and algae.

Chapter 9 addresses important issues peculiar to dairy nutrition. It considers the feeding of the transition cow, metabolic disorders (such as udder edema and milk fever), and performance modifiers (such as buffering agents and directly fed microbials).

Chapter 10 offers information specifically on the nutrient requirements of the young calf and Chapter 11 on the heifer, and aspects of growth, maturity, and body reserves.

One of the most important features of this revision is the inclusion of a discussion on the effect of dairy cattle feeding on the environment. Chapter 12 provides an overview of nutrients of concern and applies science to the challenges faced by managers in reducing nutrient excretion.

Chapter 13 provides a discussion of feed chemistry and processing. Analytic procedures are described, and the effects of processing on energy in feed are reviewed.

Nutrient requirement tables are presented in Chapter 14. These tables were generated with the accompanying computer model. Tables are provided for small- and large-breed cows at various stages of lactation.

Chapter 15 provides a greatly expanded set of feed composition tables and an explanation of their use. The tables include nutrient breakdowns for a comprehensive list of feedstuffs commonly present in dairy cattle diets and some feeds that are less common.

Chapter 16 presents an evaluation of the computer model. Data from experiments in which 100 different diets were fed in continuous feeding trials and published in the *Journal of Dairy Science* were used in the evaluation. After the evaluation, the anatomy and use of prediction equations in the computer program are presented. An introduction to this edition's computer model is present in a user's guide.

Finally, a glossary of terms used in this edition is provided to increase readers' ease of use and comprehension.

Although the science base for predicting nutrient requirements summarized here has greatly expanded since the previous edition of this report, there are still gaps in our knowledge, particularly for specific animals of different ages and levels of production. The users of this volume are encouraged to seek a firm understanding of the principles and assumptions described here, because this understanding is essential for proper use of the tables and text and of the computer model and its output.

The estimates of nutrient requirements that are presented in this report for different classes of animals were generated as examples and are intended for use as guidelines by professionals in diet formulation. Because there are many factors that affect requirements of animals under various conditions, the values presented here cannot be considered all encompassing and should not be interpreted as accurate or applicable in all situations.

# 1 Dry Matter Intake

Dry matter intake (DMI) is fundamentally important in nutrition because it establishes the amount of nutrients available to an animal for health and production. Actual or accurately estimated DMI is important for the formulation of diets to prevent underfeeding or overfeeding of nutrients and to promote efficient nutrient use. Underfeeding of nutrients restricts production and can affect the health of an animal; overfeeding of nutrients increases feed costs, can result in excessive excretion of nutrients into the environment, and at excessively high amounts may be toxic or cause adverse health effects.

Many factors affect voluntary DMI. Individual theories based on physical fill of the reticulorumen (Allen, 1996; Mertens, 1994), metabolic-feedback factors (Illius and Jessop, 1996; Mertens, 1994), or oxygen consumption (Ketelaars and Tolkamp, 1996) have been proposed to determine and predict voluntary DMI. Each theory might be applicable under some conditions, but it is most likely the additive effect of several stimuli that regulate DMI (Forbes, 1996).

Feeds low in digestibility are thought to place constraints on DMI because of their slow clearance from the rumen and passage through the digestive tract. The reticulorumen and possibly the abomasum have stretch and touch receptors in their walls that negatively impact DMI as the weight and volume of digesta accumulate (Allen, 1996). The neutral detergent fiber (NDF) fraction, because of generally low rates of digestion, is considered the primary dietary constituent associated with the fill effect.

The conceptual framework for the metabolic-feedback theory contends that an animal has a maximal productive capacity and maximal rate at which nutrients can be used to meet productive requirements (Illius and Jessop, 1996). When absorption of nutrients, principally protein and energy, exceeds requirements or when the ratio of nutrients absorbed is incorrect, negative metabolic-feedback impacts DMI.

An alternative to the metabolic theory is the theory Ketelaars and Tolkamp (1996) proposed based on oxygen consumption. This theory suggests that animals consume net energy at a rate that optimizes the use of oxygen and minimizes production of free radicals that lead to aging.

In addition to the complexity and interaction of the physical, metabolic, and chemostatic factors that regulate DMI is the psychologic and sensory ability of animals (Baumont, 1996). Consistently accurate prediction of DMI in ruminants has been difficult to achieve because a complicated, diffuse, and poorly understood set of stimuli regulate DMI. For additional discussions and reviews on intake, see Baile and McLaughlin (1987); Forbes (1995); Ketelaars and Tolkamp (1992a,b); Mertens (1994); National Research Council (1987).

In lactating dairy cattle, milk production (energy expenditure) usually peaks 4 to 8 weeks postpartum, and peak DMI (energy intake) lags until 10 to 14 weeks postpartum (National Research Council, 1989). It has been debated whether milk production is driven by intake or intake is driven by milk production. On the basis of energy intake regulation theory and others (Baile and Forbes, 1974; Conrad et al., 1964; Mertens, 1987; National Research Council, 1989), cows appear to consume feed to meet energy needs, so intake is driven by milk production.

This increase in energy intake in response to energy expenditure has been clearly shown in the numerous lactation studies with bovine somatotropin where DMI follows milk production (Bauman, 1992; Etherton and Bauman, 1998).

## EQUATIONS FOR PREDICTING DMI

### *Lactating Cows*

Earlier editions of *Nutrient Requirements of Dairy Cattle* used various approaches to predict DMI. The 1971 edition (National Research Council, 1971) simply recommended feeding ad libitum during the first 6 to 8 weeks of lactation, and then feeding to energy requirements after that for lactating dairy cows. In 1978 (National Research

Council, 1978), DMI guidelines were established by using a set of selected studies to create an interpolation table. Body weight and 4 percent fat-corrected milk were factors used to estimate DMI, which ranged from 2 to 4 percent of body weight. The 1989 edition (National Research Council, 1989) predicted DMI on the basis of energy requirement theory and expressed it simply as

$$\text{DMI (kg)} = \frac{\text{NE}_\text{L}\text{ required (Mcal)}}{\text{NE}_\text{L}\text{ concentration of diet (Mcal/kg)}} \qquad (1\text{-}1)$$

where net energy of lactation ($NE_L$) included requirements for maintenance, milk yield, and replenishment of lost weight. Suggested modifications for expected DMI were an 18 percent reduction during the first 3 weeks of lactation and DMI reduction of 0.02 kg per 100 kg of body weight for each 1 percent increase in moisture content of the diet above 50 percent when fermented feeds were being fed. The DMI guidelines in the 1989 publication were based entirely on energy balance (that is, over the long term, energy intake must equal energy expenditure). The method was not designed to estimate daily DMI in the short term. It required accurate estimates of changes in body tissue mass (although the equation was based on changes in body weight, it assumed that body weight changes equaled changes in body tissue mass) and accurate estimates of the concentration of $NE_L$ in the diet. Because of changes in gut fill and inaccurate measurements, short-term changes in body tissue mass and the energy needed or provided because of those changes are difficult to measure accurately, as is the concentration of $NE_L$ in the diet. To improve the utility of this report, the present subcommittee decided to include an empirical equation to estimate short-term DMI.

Several DMI prediction equations have been developed for use in the field, but only a few have been published in the scientific literature and tested for accuracy (Fuentes-Pila et al., 1996; Roseler et al., 1997a). The equations reported in the literature are based on the principle that animals consume dry matter to meet energy requirements or are developed by regression of various factors against observed DMI. DMI prediction equations that include animal, dietary, or environmental factors have been developed by Holter and Urban (1992) and Holter et al. (1997).

In the approach used to develop DMI prediction equations in this edition, DMI prediction is based on actual data with the inclusion of only animal factors, which would be easily measured or known. Dietary components were not included in models for lactating cows, because the approach most commonly used in formulating dairy cattle diets is to establish requirements and a DMI estimate before dietary ingredients are considered. Equations containing dietary factors are best used to evaluate postconsumption rather than to predict what will be consumed.

DMI data published in the *Journal of Dairy Science* from 1988 to 1998 (see Chapter 16 for references) and data from Ohio State University and the University of Minnesota (May, 1994) were used in evaluating and developing an equation for lactating Holstein dairy cows. The data set included 17,087 cow weeks (5962 first lactation and 11,125 second lactation or greater cow weeks), a diverse set of diets, and studies with and without bovine somatotropin and encompassed a 10-year period from 1988 to 1997. Weeks of lactation ranged from 1 to 80; most data were from 1 to 40 weeks. Equations evaluated were those of Roseler et al. (1997b) and May (1994) and an equation reported by Rayburn and Fox (1993) based on DMI values in the 1989 *Nutrient Requirements of Dairy Cattle* (National Research Council, 1989). The best overall prediction equation, based on bias (−0.27 kg/day) and mean square prediction error (3.31 $kg^2$/day) was a combined equation of Rayburn and Fox (1993) and an adjustment for week of lactation developed by Roseler et al. (1997b). The equation for predicting DMI of lactating Holstein cows is

$$\begin{aligned}\text{DMI (kg/d)} &= (0.372 \times \text{FCM} \\ &\quad + 0.0968 \times \text{BW}^{0.75}) \\ &\quad \times (1 - e^{(-0.192 \times (\text{WOL}+3.67))}) \qquad (1\text{-}2)\end{aligned}$$

where FCM = 4 percent fat corrected milk (kg/day), BW = body weight (kg), and WOL = week of lactation. The term $1 - e^{(-0.192 \times (\text{WOL}+3.67))}$ adjusts for depressed DMI during early lactation. For early lactation cows, Equation 1-2 was compared to those developed by Kertz et al. (1991) using the validation data from Kertz et al. (1991). Dry matter intake predictions for the first 14 weeks of lactation are shown in Figure 1-1. Equation 1-2 predicts DMI very closely to the actual DMI for the first 10 weeks of lactation and then slightly under predicts DMI thereafter compared to the general overall predictions of Kertz et al. (1991).

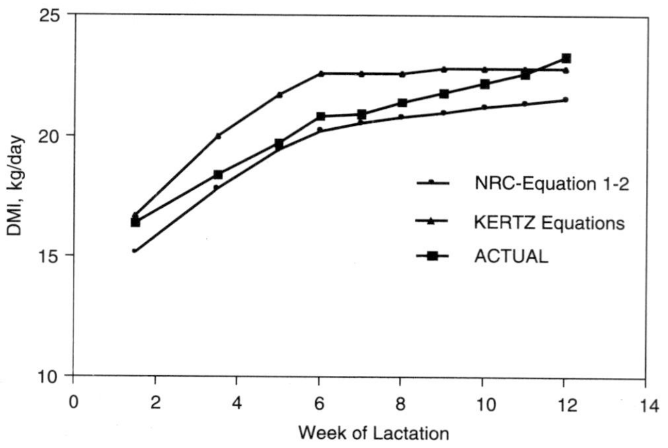


FIGURE 1-1 Dry matter intake prediction of early lactation cows using Equation 1-2 and Kertz et al. (1991) equations.

Equation 1-2 is based entirely on Holstein cows. No published DMI data were available for developing or modifying the current equation for use with breeds other than Holstein. For DMI of Jersey cattle, readers are referred to Holter et al. (1996).

No adjustment to the DMI equation for parity is needed. The bias and mean square prediction error for primiparous (−0.16 kg/day and 3.05 $kg^2$/day) and multiparous (0.12 kg/day and 3.20 $kg^2$/day) were similar and were not different from the overall combined prediction equation statistics. However, body weight and milk production data appropriate for first and second lactation animals must be used in the equation to estimate DMI accurately for these animals.

The actual DMI, FCM, and body weight data from animals used to develop and validate the lactating cow DMI prediction equation are shown in Figure 1-2. Body weight change is based on animals becoming pregnant by week 17 of lactation, so later weights reflect cow and conceptus gain during the lactation.

The DMI of lactating cows is affected by environmental conditions outside the thermal neutral zone (5 to 20°C). Both Eastridge et al. (1998) and Holter et al. (1997) have shown DMI decreases with temperatures above 20°C. The equation used for predicting DMI of lactating cows (Equation 1-2) in this edition does not include a temperature or humidity adjustment factor because of insufficient DMI data outside of the thermal neutral zone to validate equation modifiers. However, use of lowered milk production in Equation 1-2 during heat stress periods will reflect the reduction in DMI commonly observed during heat stress periods. Eastridge et al. (1998) suggested the following changes occur in DMI when temperatures are outside of

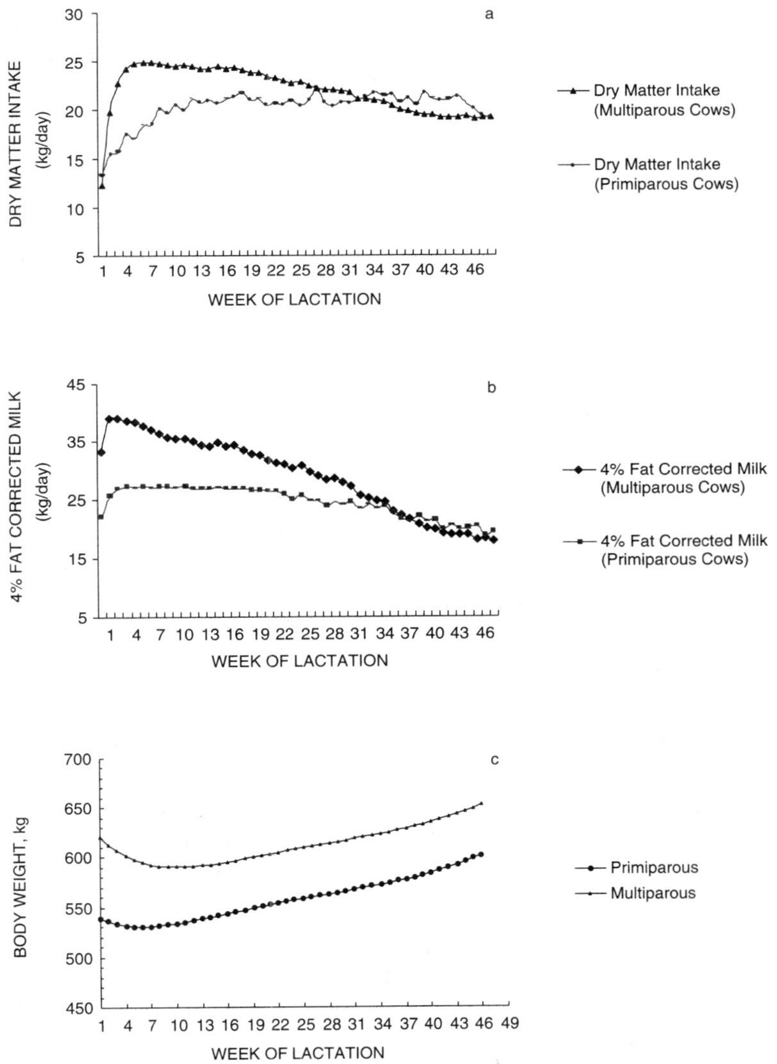


FIGURE 1-2 a) Dry matter intake, b) 4 percent fat corrected milk production, and c) body weight change of primiparous and multiparous cows during 48 weeks of lactation.

the thermal neutral zone; temperatures >20°C, DMI × (1 − ((°C − 20) × 0.005922)) and temperatures <5°C, DMI/(1 − ((5 − °C) × 0.004644)). Application of the Eastridge et al. (1998) adjustment factors to a DMI prediction from Equation 1-2 based on lowered milk production during periods of heat stress may result in an excessively low prediction of DMI.

### *Growing Heifers*

Published data on DMI of growing heifers weighing from 60 to 625 kg are sparse. Most research studies used fewer than 40 animals with a narrow weight range and limited experimental observation period. Dry matter intake equations from Quigley et al. (1986) and Stallings et al. (1985) and calf equation from the *Nutrient Requirements of Beef Cattle* (National Research Council, 1996) were selected for initial evaluation using data from New Hampshire and Minnesota where dietary composition, heifer growth, and DMI were measured over several months. The equation of Quigley et al. (1986) and the *Nutrient Requirements of Beef Cattle* equation (National Research Council, 1996) include dietary energy content and body weight. An equation based only on animal parameters was preferred to one including dietary components, however, the only published heifer DMI equation without dietary components found was from Stallings et al. (1985). On evaluation, the limited animal parameter equation of Stallings et al. (1985) was found to have a much larger prediction error, especially for heifers above 350 kg, than either the Quigley et al. (1986) or the National Research Council's *Nutrient Requirements of Beef Cattle* (1996) equation, which had similar predictive accuracy (Table 1-1).

Because of more current evaluation and a much larger validation data set than Quigley et al. (1986), the equation for beef calves from the 1996 *Nutrient Requirements of Beef Cattle* (National Research Council, 1996) was further validated using a data set from Purina Mills, St. Louis, Missouri. This data set included 2727 observations on growing heifers ranging from 58 to 588 kg and dietary net energy-maintenance concentrations from 1.24 to 1.55 Mcal/kg. Based on the fit of the data from the initial evaluation and the validation (Figure 1-3), the National Research Council equation for beef cattle is recommended for predicting DMI of growing, nonlactating Holstein heifers.

$$\text{DMI (kg/d)} = (\text{BW}^{0.75} \times (0.2435 \times \text{NE}_M - 0.0466 \times \text{NE}_M^2 - 0.1128)/\text{NE}_M) \quad (1\text{-}3)$$

where BW = body weight (kg) and $NE_M$ is net energy of diet for maintenance (Mcal/kg).

No adjustments for breed, empty body fat, feed additives, or anabolic implant were made. There is a considerable difference in the DMI predicted from the growing heifer equation (Eq. 1-3) during late gestation and the equation used to predict DMI of heifers the last 21 days of gestation (Eq. 9-1, Chapter 9). To avoid a large disconnect in DMI between days 260 and 261 in the model, the following adjustment factor for Equation 1-3 based on days of gestation is applied to Equation 1-3: [1 + ((210 − DG) × 0.0025)]; where DG = day of gestation. The adjustment is applied for utility in model usage and is not validated. Reported information on DMI of growing heifers during the last trimester of pregnancy is nonexistent.

Data for predicting DMI of growing heifers for breeds other than Holstein or adjusting Equation 1-3 to fit other breeds was not found. Likewise, there is a dearth of information for developing adjustments to Equation 1-3 for temperature and other environmental factors. Fox and Tylutki (1998) modified the temperature and mud adjustments listed in the *Nutrient Requirements of Beef Cattle* (National Research Council, 1996) for growing dairy heifers, but did not validate the adjustments because of the lack of data. Hoffman et al. (1994) have shown that season, type of housing, muddy conditions, length of hair, and body condition all affect average daily gain; and adjustments to energy requirements for gain were suggested, but effects on DMI were not evaluated.

TABLE 1-1 Validation Statistics for Prediction of Dry Matter Intake by Heifers

| Equation source | Bias, kg/d | MSPE,[a] kg$^2$/d |
|---|---|---|
| Quigley et al. (1986) | −0.32 | 1.47 |
| Stallings et al. (1985) | −1.32 | 1.90 |
| National Research Council[b] (1996) Calves | −0.51 | 1.48 |

[a] Mean square prediction error.
[b] *Nutrient Requirements of Beef Cattle* (National Research Council, 1996).

## NUTRIENTS AND FEEDING MANAGEMENT RELATED TO DMI OF LACTATING DAIRY COWS

### *Moisture*

Studies reviewed by Chase (1979) and included in the 1989 *Nutrient Requirements of Dairy Cattle* (National Research Council, 1989) indicate a negative relationship between DMI and diets high in moisture content. A decrease in total DMI of 0.02 percent of body weight for each 1 percent increase in moisture content of the diet above 50 percent was indicated when fermented feeds were included in the ration. In a study using alfalfa silage to vary dietary DM, Kellems et al. (1991) found a trend of reduction in DMI with increasing moisture in the diet. Holter and Urban (1992) summarized data on 329 lactating

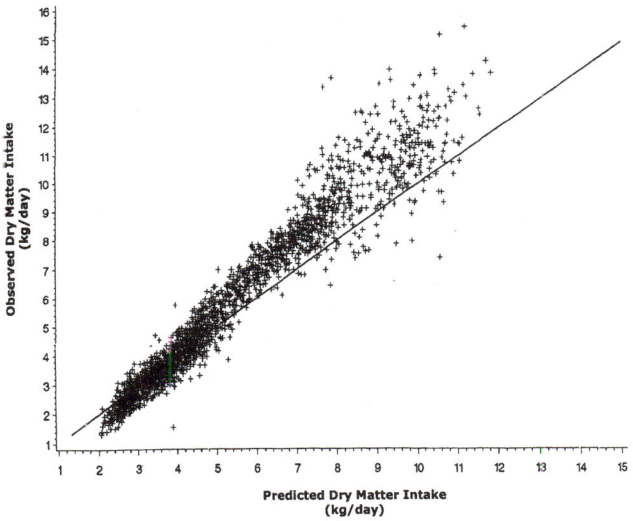


FIGURE 1-3 Observed versus predicted dry matter intake of growing dairy heifers using beef calf equation from *Nutrient Requirements of Beef Cattle* (National Research Council, 1996).

cows fed diets ranging from 30 to 70 percent DM and found that DMI was not decreased when dietary DM decreased to below 50 percent. Most high moisture feeds are fermented, and the decrease in DMI when they are fed is generally thought to result from fermentation end products and not water itself. When cows were given diets identical in composition except for the addition of water (78, 64, 52, or 40 percent DM in diets), DMI of cows increased linearly ($P < 0.01$) as percentage DM in the ration increased (Lahr et al., 1983). However, DMI was not affected by soaking grain mixes in water to achieve a dietary DM of 35, 45, or 60 percent (Robinson et al., 1990). Published reports on the relationship between dietary DM content and DMI are conflicting and no optimum DM content of the diet for maximum DMI is apparent.

### *Neutral Detergent Fiber*

Mertens (1994) suggested that NDF be used to define the upper and lower bounds of DMI. At high NDF concentrations in diets, rumen fill limits DMI whereas, at low NDF concentrations energy intake feedback inhibitors limit DMI. Dado and Allen (1995) demonstrated the fill relationship in cows during early lactation: 35 percent NDF diets restrict DMI because of feed bulkiness and rumen fill, but DMI was not limited when 25 percent NDF diets were fed with or without inert bulk in the rumen. In a review on feed characteristics affecting DMI of lactating cattle, Allen (2000) summarized 15 studies and showed a general decline in DMI with increasing NDF concentrations in diets when diets exceeded 25 percent NDF. At any particular NDF concentration in the diet, however, a considerable range in DMI was observed suggesting the source or sources of NDF in the diet as affected by particle size, digestibility, and rate of passage from the reticulorumen affect DMI.

The use of NDF as a variable in DMI prediction models has been reviewed in two studies. Rayburn and Fox (1993) concluded that DMI prediction was most accurate and least biased when dietary NDF, particularly from forages, was included in a model with BW, FCM, and days in milk. However, in models for predicting DMI of lactating cows fed high energy diets ranging in NDF from 25 to 42 percent of DM, less than 1 percent of the variation in DMI was accounted for by dietary NDF (Roseler et al., 1997a).

### *Forage to Concentrate Ratio*

The ratio of forage to concentrate (F:C) in lactating dairy cow diets has been reported to affect DMI. Many of the study results are probably associated with the amount and digestibility of forage fiber and a propionate limiting effect on DMI as discussed by Allen (2000), rather than a specific ratio of forage to concentrate. In alfalfa or orchardgrass based diets, cows fed concentrate as 20 percent of the dietary DM produced less milk ($P < 0.01$) than cows fed diets that contained 40 or 60 percent concentrate (Weiss and Shockey, 1991). The DMI increased linearly ($P < 0.01$) with increasing concentrate in diets regardless of forage type. Digestible DM also increased linearly ($P < 0.01$) with increasing concentrate in the diet. Because intake of undigested DM was not affected by the amount of concentrate, rates of passage and digestion and physical characteristics of the feedstuffs are probable causes of differences in DMI.

Llamas-Lamas and Combs (1991) fed diets with three ratios of forage (alfalfa silage) to concentrate (86:14, 71:29, and 56:44). DMI was greatest for the diet highest in concentrate but similar for the other two diets. Petit and Veira (1991) fed concentrate at either 1.3 or 1.8 percent of BW and alfalfa silage ad libitum (F:C, 63:37 and 54:46) to Holstein cows during early lactation. Both groups of cows ate similar amounts of silage, but cows consuming the high-concentrate diet gained weight, and animals consuming the low-concentrate diet lost weight. Similar results were observed by Johnson and Combs (1992): cows fed a 74 percent forage diet (2:1 alfalfa silage to corn silage) consumed 2.7 kg less DM per day than cows fed a diet containing 50 percent forage. In general, increasing concentrate in diets up to about 60 percent of the DM increased DMI.

### *Fat*

Assuming that cows consume DM to meet their energy requirements (Baile and Forbes, 1974; Mertens, 1987; National Research Council, 1989), often less DM is consumed when fat replaces carbohydrates as an energy source in diets (Gagliostro and Chilliard, 1991). Fats may also decrease ruminal fermentation and digestibility of fiber (Palmquist and Jenkins, 1980; Chalupa et al., 1984, 1986) and so contribute to rumen fill and decrease the rate of passage. Allen (2000) also indicated fats may contribute to decreased DMI through actions on gut hormones, oxidation of fat in the liver and the general acceptability of fat sources by cattle.

The response in DMI to the addition of fatty acids in lactating dairy cattle diets is dependent on the fatty acid content of the basal diet and source of added fatty acids (Allen, 2000). For the diets containing 5 to 6 percent total fatty acids, the addition of oilseeds and hydrogenated fatty acids to diets resulted in a quadratic effect on DMI with minimums occurring at 3 and 2.3 percent added fatty acids, respectively. Additions of tallow, grease, and calcium salts of palm fatty acids to diets resulted in a general negative linear decrease in DMI. Smith et al. (1993) reported ruminally active fats have a greater negative effect on DMI, ruminal fermentation, and digestibility of NDF when diets are high in corn silage than when they are high in alfalfa hay.

Palmquist and Jenkins (1980) indicated that increased saturation of fatty acids usually reduces the negative ruminal effects associated with fats. However, Allen (2000) found that as the proportion of unsaturated fatty acids in the fat source increased, DMI generally decreased. Most all of the studies that Allen (2000) cited fed the calcium salts of palm fatty acids. However, total digestible energy intake in many of the studies was not reduced, as digestibility of the calcium salts of palm fatty acids was high and greater than hydrogenated palm fatty acid comparisons.

While the trend is for a reduction in DMI with the addition of fatty acids to diets (Allen, 2000; Chan et al., 1997; Elliot et al., 1996; Garcia-Bojalil et al., 1998; Jenkins and Jenny, 1989; Rodriguez et al., 1997), some studies (Pantoja et al., 1996; Skaar et al., 1989) have reported increases in DMI. Potential reasons for increased DMI with fat addition is a lower heat increment during periods of heat stress and/or a reduction in propionate inhibition on DMI when fat is substituted for grain (Allen, 2000).

## COW BEHAVIOR, MANAGEMENT, AND ENVIRONMENTAL FACTORS AFFECTING FEED INTAKE

### *Eating Habits and Cow Behavior*

Dado and Allen (1994) studied eating habits of lactating dairy cows housed in a tie-stall barn. Twelve Holstein cows ranging in milk production from 22 to 45 kg/d were monitored during the ninth week of lactation. The six highest-producing cows averaged 11 kg more milk per day and consumed about 6 kg more DM per day than the lowest-producing six cows. The time spent eating (average, 300 minutes/day) and the number of meals (average, 11/day) did not differ between the two groups, but the high-producing cows consumed more DM per meal than did the low-producing cows (2.3 vs. 1.7 kg). High-producing cows ruminate fewer times per day (13 vs. 14.5 times/day) but ruminate an average of 5 min more per rumination period than low-producing cows.

Grouping cows according to their nutrient requirements can decrease the variation in DMI among cows within the group. The DMI shown in Figure 1-2 illustrates the difference between primiparous and multiparous cows in total DMI and pattern of DMI during lactation. Primiparous cows do not peak in DMI as early in lactation, but they are more persistent in DMI after peak than are multiparous cows. Thus, primiparous and multiparous cows should be grouped separately because of differences in DMI and social hierarchy. Primiparous cows are usually more timid and of lower social rank in the herd initially, but they gradually rise in social rank as more cows enter the herd or as older cows leave (Wierenga, 1990). Phelps and Drew (1992) reported an increase of 725 kg in milk over a 305-day lactation for first-lactation animals when grouped separately instead of being mixed in with older cows.

Behavior at the feed bunk is often affected by social dominance. Dominant cows, usually older and larger, tend to spend more time eating than do cows with a lower social rank in a competitive situation , such as when bunk space is restricted (Albright, 1993). Socially dominant animals, not necessarily the highest producers, tend to consume more feed at the bunk in these situations (Friend and Polan, 1974). In a situation of competition for feed, cows consume slightly more feed but do it in less time per day than when there is no competition and access to feed is ample (Olofsson, 1999).

In 1993, Albright (1993) recommended at least 46 cm of bunk space per cow. Friend et al. (1977) evaluated bunk spaces of 50, 40, 30, 20, and 10 cm per cow, for early lactation cows with mature equivalent productions of 7,700 to 10,000 kg/year. Average time spent at the feed bunk (3.7 hours/day) did not decrease until only 10 cm of space per cow was available (Table 1-2). When there was 20 or 10 cm per cow, the correlation of dominance to duration of eating periods increased. The optimal or critical feed bunk space needed is probably not a constant number and will depend on competition between cows, the total number of cows having access to the feed space, and the availability of feed over a 24-hour period.

For growing dairy heifers, feed-bunk space requirement varies with age. Longenbach et al. (1999) found that rapid growth in growing heifers fed a total mixed diet could be maintained in young heifers (4 to 8 months old) with 15 cm of bunk space. But, by the age of 17 to 21 months,

TABLE 1-2 Effect of Bunk Space Per Cow on Feeding Behavior and Intake of Early Lactation Cows[a]

| | Feed Bunk Length Per Cow (cm) | | | | |
|---|---|---|---|---|---|
| | 50 | 40 | 30 | 20 | 10 |
| Time at feed bunk h | 3.82 | 3.73 | 3.73 | 3.76 | 2.57[b] |
| Correlation of time with social dominance | 0.46 | 0.32 | 0.30 | 0.67[c] | 0.71[d] |
| Percentage of time at feed bunk, % | 21.5 | 26.9 | 34.6 | 51.9 | 70.6 |
| Daily feed intake, kg of DM | 17.5 | 17.6 | 17.8 | 16.9 | 15.7 |

[a]From Friend et al. (1977).
[b]Differs from 50 cm feed bunk/cow.
[c]Differs from zero ($P < 0.05$).
[d]Differs from zero ($P < 0.01$).

feed bunk space needed to be similar (47 cm) to that recommended for lactating cows.

Cattle prefer mangers that allow them to eat off a smooth surface in a natural grazing position. Albright (1993) cited evidence showing cows eating with their heads down produce 17 percent more saliva than cows eating with their heads in a horizontal position. Feed-wasting activities associated with elevated bunks, such as feed tossing, are eliminated when cows eat with their heads down (Albright, 1993).

*Weather*

The thermal neutral zone of dairy cattle is about 5 to 20°C, but it varies among animals. Temperatures below or above the thermal neutral range alter intake and metabolic activity. Young (1983) stated ruminants adapt to chronic cold stress conditions by increasing thermal insulation, basal metabolic intensity, and DMI. Rumination activity, reticulo-rumen motility, and rate of passage are also increased (Young, 1983). However, in extreme cold, DMI does not increase at the same rate as metabolism, so animals are in a negative energy balance and shift energy use from productive purposes to heat production.

A rise in ambient temperature above the thermal neutral zone decreases milk production because of reduced DMI. Holter et al. (1997) found pregnant multiparous middle- to late-lactation Holstein cows decreased DMI more (22 percent) than primiparous cows (9 percent) at the same stage of lactation and pregnancy when subjected to heat stress. A decrease in DMI up to 55 percent of that eaten in the thermal neutral zone along with an increase of 7 to 25 percent in maintenance requirement has been reported for cows subjected to heat stress (National Research Council, 1981). Water consumption of cattle increases as ambient temperature increases up to 35°C, but further temperature increases decrease water consumption because of inactivity and low DMI. Similar effects as those observed under high temperature conditions can be seen in cattle at temperatures as low as 24°C with high humidity (Coppock, 1978).

*Feeding Method—Total Mixed Ration vs. Individual Ingredient*

The goal of any feeding system or method is to provide the opportunity for cows to consume the amount of feed specified in a formulated diet. Considerations in the choosing of a feeding system should include housing facilities, equipment necessities, herd size, labor availability, and cost. Nutrients can be effectively supplied by feeding either a total mixed ration (TMR) or individual ingredients. A TMR allows for the mixing of all feed ingredients together based on a prescribed amount of each ingredient. When consumed as a TMR without sorting of ingredients, more even rumen fermentation and a better use of nutrients should occur than feeding of separate ingredients. Computerized or electronic feeders reduce the labor involved in individual-concentrate feeding and provide an opportunity to control and regulate concentrate feeding to cows through several small amount feedings each day. Limitations to feeding forages and concentrates separately are the forages as they are usually provided free-choice and the amount fed is usually unknown or individual cow amounts are calculated from a group average intake. Maltz et al. (1992) reported that cows fed a TMR or concentrate by computer feeders did not differ in milk production (32.7 vs. 32.7 kg/d) or differ much in DMI (19.7 vs. 20.4 kg/d) during the first 20 weeks of lactation. Allocation of concentrates through a computer feeder based on milk yield per unit of body weight was more successful in economizing on concentrate feeding without losses in milk production and management of body weight than allocation only by milk yield.

*Feeding Frequency*

It has been suggested that increasing the frequency of offering feed to cows increases milk production and results in fewer health problems. Gibson (1981) concluded in a review on feeding frequency that changing from one or two offerings of feed per day to four increased average daily gain of cattle by 16 percent and increased feed use by 19 percent. Improvements in gain or feed use were greatest when cattle were fed high-concentrate diets. In a review of 35 experiments on feeding frequency in lactating dairy cows, Gibson (1984) reported that increasing feedings to four or more times per day compared to once or twice increased milk fat percentage by an average of 7.3 percent and milk production 2.7 percent. Higher milk fat concentration with increased feeding frequency also was reported by Sniffen and Robinson (1984). The benefit of increased feeding frequency might be more stable and consistent ruminal fermentation. When Robinson and McQueen (1994) fed a basal diet two times per day and then a protein supplement two or five times per day, production and composition of milk were not affected by the frequency of feeding protein supplement, but both pH and propionate concentration in the rumen were higher with five than with two feedings per day. Klusmeyer et al. (1990) reported that ruminal fermentation pattern and production of milk and milk components were not improved by increasing feedings from two to four times per day. Similar results were found with the feeding of concentrate two or six times per day as milk production, milk-component yield, DMI, or ruminal fermentation characteristics were not affected (Macleod et al., 1994). Fluctuations in diurnal patterns of ruminal metabolites probably have to affect microbial growth and fermentation adversely before a benefit of increasing feedings to more than two times per day will be seen.

All of the studies reviewed for feeding frequency involved the actual offering of new feed to cattle and not the pushing in of existing feed to the manger. Whether the act of pushing feed in stimulates the same effects as the offering of new feed is unknown. In the study of Macleod et al. (1994), whenever fresh concentrate was offered to the cows fed concentrate six times per day, cows fed concentrate only twice per day would begin eating also, suggesting the act of feeding, or maybe pushing in feed, has a stimulating affect on eating.

### *Sequence of Feeding*

Sniffen and Robinson (1984) hypothesized the following reasons for feeding forages as the first feed offered in the morning before concentrates. The feeding of highly fermentable carbohydrates to cows that have been without feed for over 6 hours could cause acidotic conditions in the rumen depressing feed intake and fiber digestion. Feeding forage(s) as the first feed in the morning before other feedstuffs would allow for the formation of a fiber mat in the rumen and provide buffering capacity in the rumen from both the forage and the increased salivation associated with forage consumption. Forages of medium to long chop length were advocated as they should prolong eating and thereby increase salivation and reduce particle passage from the rumen. However, evidence to support this hypothesis is lacking. In two studies (Macleod et al., 1994; Nocek, 1992) where legume forages were fed before concentrates, no effects on rumen fermentation characteristics, rumen pH or milk production were found. In both studies, feeding forage after concentrates resulted in a numerical increase in DMI compared to feeding forage before concentrate.

### *Access to Feed*

Maximal DMI can only be achieved when cows have adequate time for eating. Data from Dado and Allen (1994) indicated early lactation cows (63 days in milk) producing 23 to 44 kg of milk per day fed a TMR ad libitum ate an average of 5 hours per day. Feed intake occurred during 9 to 13 (average of 11) eating bouts per day that averaged 29 minutes per bout. Mean DMI at each eating bout was about 10 percent of the total daily DMI, which ranged from 15 to 27 kg/day. Cows in this study (Dado and Allen, 1994) were housed in tie-stalls and had access to feed 22 of 24 hours per day. This study demonstrates there is a considerable difference in eating behavior between cows in a non-competitive feed environment and that the accessibility of feed must be considerably more than the 5 hours of actual eating time per day. Martinsson (1992) and Martinsson and Burstedt (1990) found that limiting the access of feed to 8 hours a day decreased milk production of cows averaging about 25 kg/day by 5 to 7 percent compared with cows that had free-choice access to feed.

## REFERENCES


Albright, J.L. 1993. Feeding behavior of dairy cattle. J. Dairy Sci. 76:485–498.

Allen, M. S. 2000. Effects of diet on short-term regulation of feed intake by lactating dairy cows. J. Dairy Sci. 83:1598–1624.

Allen, M. S. 1996. Physical constrains on voluntary intake of forages by ruminants. J. Anim. Sci. 74:3063–3075.

Baile, C. A., and J. M. Forbes. 1974. Control of feed intake and regulation of energy balance in ruminants. Physiol. Rev. 54:160–214.

Baile, C. A., and C. L. McLaughlin. 1987. Mechanisms controlling feed intake in ruminants: A review. J. Anim. Sci. 64:915–922.

Bauman, D. E. 1992. Bovine somatotropin: Review of an emerging animal technology. J. Dairy Sci. 75:3432–3451.

Baumont, R. 1996. Palatability and feeding behavior in ruminants. A review. Ann. Zootech. 45:385–400.

Chalupa, W., B. Rickabaugh, D. S. Kronfeld, and D. Sklan. 1984. Rumen fermentation in vitro as influenced by long-chain fatty acids. J. Dairy Sci. 67:1439–1444.

Chalupa, W., B. Vecchiarelli, A. E. Elser, D. S. Kronfeld, D. Sklan, and D.L. Palmquist. 1986. Ruminal fermentation in vivo as influenced by long-chain fatty acids. J. Dairy Sci. 69:1293–1301.

Chan, S. C., J. T. Huber, K. H. Chen, J. M. Simas, and Z. Wu. 1997. Effects of ruminally inert fat and evaporative cooling on dairy cows in hot environmental temperatures. J. Dairy Sci. 80:1172–1178.

Chase, L. E. 1979. Effect of high moisture feeds on feed intake and milk production in dairy cattle. Proc., Cornell Nutr. Conf. Feed Manu. p. 52–56.

Conrad, H. R., A. D. Pratt, and J. W. Hibbs. 1964. Regulation of feed intake in dairy cows. I. Change in importance of physical and physiological factors with increasing digestibility. J. Dairy Sci. 47:54–62.

Coppock, C. E. 1978. Nutrient considerations in feeding. C. J. Wilcox, H. H. Van Horn, B. Harris, Jr., H. H. Head, S. P. Marshall. W. W. Thatcher, D. W. Webb, and J. M. Wing (eds.). *In* Proc., Large Dairy Herd Management. Gainesville. Univ. Presses of Florida.

Dado, R. G., and M. S. Allen. 1994. Variation in and relationships among feeding, chewing and drinking variables for lactating dairy cows. J. Dairy Sci. 77:132–144.

Dado, R. G., and M. S. Allen. 1995. Intake limitations, feeding behavior, and rumen function of cows challenged with rumen fill from dietary fiber of inert bulk. J. Dairy Sci. 78:118–133.

Eastridge, M. L., H. F. Bucholtz, A. L. Slater, and C. S. Hall. 1998. Nutrient requirements for dairy cattle of the national research council versus some commonly used software. J. Dairy Sci. 81:3049–3062.

Elliott, J. P., J. K. Drackley, and D. J. Weigel. 1996. Digestibility and effects of hydrogenated palm fatty acid distillate in lactating dairy cows. J. Dairy Sci. 79:1031–1039.

Etherton, T. D., and D. E. Bauman. 1998. Biology of somatotropin in growth and lactation of domestic animals. Physiol. Reviews 78:745–761.

Forbes, J. M. 1995. Voluntary Food Intake and Diet Selection in Farm Animals. CAB International, Wallingford, U.K.

Forbes, J. M. 1996 Integration of regulatory signals controlling forage intake in ruminants. J. Anim. Sci. 74:3029–3035.

Fox, D. G., and T. F. Tylutki. 1998. Accounting for the effects of environment on the nutrient requirements of dairy cattle. J. Dairy Sci. 81:3085–3095.

Friend, T. H., and C. E. Polan. 1974. Social rank, feeding behavior, and free stall utilization by dairy cattle. J. Dairy Sci. 57:1214–1220.

Friend, T. H., C. E. Polan, and M. L. McGilliard. 1977. Free stall and feed bunk requirements relative to behavior, production and individual feed intake in dairy cows. J. Dairy Sci. 60:108–116.

Fuentes-Pila, J., M. A. DeLorenzo, D. K. Beede, C. R. Staples, and J. B. Holter. 1996. Evaluation of equations based on animal factors to predict intake of lactating Holstein cows. J. Dairy Sci. 79:1562–1571.

Gagliostro, G., and Y. Chilliard. 1991. Duodenal rapeseed oil infusion in early and midlactation cows. 2. Voluntary intake, milk production, and composition. J. Dairy Sci. 74:499–509.

Garcia-Bojalil, C. M., C. R. Staples, C. A. Risco, J. D. Savio, and W. W. Thatcher. 1998. Protein degradability and calcium salts of long-chain fatty acids in the diets of lactating dairy cows: productive responses. J. Dairy Sci. 81:1374–1384.

Gibson, J. P. 1981. The effects of feeding frequency on the growth and efficiency of food utilization of ruminants: an analysis of published results. Anim. Prod. 32:275–283.

Gibson, J. P. 1984. The effects of feeding frequency on milk production of dairy cattle: an analysis of published results. Anim. Prod. 38:181–189.

Hoffman, P. C., N. M. Brehm, W. T. Howard, and D. A. Funk. 1994. The influence of nutrition and environment on growth of Holstein replacement heifers in commercial dairy herds. The Prof. Anim. Sci. 10:59–65.

Holter, J. B., and W. E. Urban, Jr. 1992. Water partitioning and intake predicition in dry and lactating Holstein cows. J. Dairy Sci. 75:1472–1479.

Holter, J. B., J. W. West, M. L. McGillard, and A. N. Pell. 1996. Predicating ad libitum dry matter intake and yields of Jersey cows. J. Dairy Sci. 79:912–921.

Holter, J. B., J. W. West, and M. L. McGillard. 1997. Predicting ad libitum dry matter intake and yield of Holstein cows. J. Dairy Sci. 80:2188–2199.

Illius, A. W., and N. S. Jessop. 1996. Metabolic constraints on voluntary intake in ruminants. J. Anim Sci. 74:3052–3062.

Jenkins, T. C., and B. F. Jenny. 1989. Effect of hydrogenated fat on feed intake, nutrient digestion, and lactational performance of dairy cows. J. Dairy Sci. 72:2316–2324.

Johnson, T. R., and D. K. Combs. 1992. Effects of inert rumen bulk on dry matter intake in early and midlactation cows fed diets differing in forage content. J. Dairy Sci. 75:508–519.

Kellems, R. O., R. Jones, D. Andrus, and M. V. Wallentine. 1991. Effect of moisture in total mixed rations on feed consumption and milk production and composition in Holstein cows. J. Dairy Sci. 74:929–932.

Kertz, A. F., L. F. Reutzel, and G. M. Thomson. 1991. Dry matter intake from parturition to midlactation. J. Dairy Sci. 74:2290–2295.

Ketelaars, J. J. M. H., and B. J. Tolkamp. 1992a. Toward a new theory of feed intake regulation in ruminants 1. Causes of differences in voluntary feed intake: Critique of current views. Livestock Prod. Sci. 30:269–296.

Ketelaars, J. J. M. H., and B. J. Tolkamp. 1992b. Toward a new theory of feed intake regulation in ruminants 3. Optimum feed intake: In search of a physiological background. Livest. Prod. Sci. 31:235–258.

Ketelaars, J. J. M. H., and B. J. Tolkamp. 1996. Oxygen efficiency and the control of energy flow in animals and humans. J. Anim Sci. 74:3036–3051.

Klusmeyer, T. H., M. R. Cameron, G. C. McCoy, and J. H. Clark. 1990. Effects of feed processing and frequency of feeding on ruminal fermentation, milk production, and milk composition. J. Dairy Sci. 73:3538–3543.

Lahr, D. A., D. E. Otterby, D. G. Johnson, J. G. Linn, and R. G. Lundquist. 1983. Effects of moisture content of complete diets on feed intake and milk production by cows. J. Dairy Sci. 66:1891–1900.

Llamas-Lamas, G., and D. K. Combs. 1991. Effect of forage to concentrate ratio and intake level on utilization of early vegetative alfalfa silage by dairy cows. J. Dairy Sci. 74:526–536.

Longenbach, J. I., A. J. Henrichs, and R. E. Graves. 1999. Feed bunk length requirements for Holstein dairy heifers. J. Dairy Sci. 82:99–109.

Macleod, G. K., P. E. Colucci, A. D. Moore, D. G. Grieve, and N. Lewis. 1994. The effects of feeding frequency of concentrates and feeding sequence of hay on eating behavior, ruminal environment and milk production in dairy cows. Can. J. Anim. Sci. 74:103–113.

Maltz, E., S. Devir, O. Kroll, B. Zur, S. L. Spahr, and R. D. Shanks. 1992. Comparative responses of lactating cows to total mixed rations or computerized individual concentrates feeding. J. Dairy Sci. 75:1588–1603.

Martinsson, K. 1992. Effects of conservation method and access time on silage intake and milk production in dairy cows. Grass and Forage Sci. 47:161–168.

Martinsson, K., and E. Burstedt. 1990. Effects of length of access time to feed and allotment of hay on grass silage intake and production in lactating dairy cows. Swed. J. Agric. Res. 20:169–176.

May, M. G. 1994. Factors affecting and the prediction of dry matter intake for Holstein dairy cows. Ph.D. thesis. University of Minnesota.

Mertens, D. R. 1987. Predicting intake and digestibility using mathematical models of ruminal function. J. Dairy Sci. 64:1548–1558.

Mertens, D. R. 1994. Regulation of forage intake. *In*: Forage Quality, evaluation and Utilization. G. C. Fahey, *ed.* Am. Soc. Agron., Crop Sci. Soc Amer., Soil Sci. Soc. Amer. Madison, WI. pp. 450–493.

National Research Council. 1971. Nutrient Requirements of Dairy Cattle., 4th rev. ed. Washington D.C.: National Academy of Sciences.

National Research Council. 1978. Nutrient Requirements of Dairy Cattle., 5th rev. ed. Washington D.C.: National Academy of Sciences.

National Research Council. 1981. Effect of Environment on Nutrient Requirements of Domestic Animals. Washington D.C. National Academy Press.

National Research Council. 1987. Predicting Feed Intake of Food-Producing Animals. Washington, D.C.: National Academy Press.

National Research Council. 1989. Nutrient Requirements of Dairy Cattle., 6th rev. ed. Update 1989. Washington D.C.: National Academy Press.

National Research Council. 1996. Nutrient Requirements of Beef Cattle, 7th rev. ed. 1996. Washington D.C.: National Academy of Sciences.

Nocek, J. E. 1992. Feeding sequence and strategy effects on ruminal environment and production performance in first lactation cows. J. Dairy Sci. 75:3100–3108.

Olofsson, J. 1999. Competition for total mixed diets fed for ad libitum intake using one or four cows per feeding station. J. Dairy Sci. 82:69–79.

Palmquist, D. L., and T. C. Jenkins. 1980. Fat in lactation rations: Review. J. Dairy Sci. 63:1–14.

Pantoja, J., J. L. Firkins, and M. L. Eastridge. 1996. Fatty acid digestibility and lactation performance by dairy cows fed fats varying in degree of saturation. J. Dairy Sci. 79:429–437.

Petit, H. V., and D. M. Veira. 1991. Effects of grain level and protein source on yield, feed intake, and blood traits of lactating cows fed alfalfa silage. J. Dairy Sci. 74:1923–1932.

Phelps, A., and B. Drew. 1992. Vastly superior first lactations when heifers fed separately. Feedstuffs. 64(19):11.

Quigley, J., III, R. E. James, and M. L. McGilliard. 1986. Dry matter intake in dairy heifers. 2. Equations to predict intake of heifers under intensive management. J. Dairy Sci. 69:2863–2867.

Rayburn, E. B., and D. G. Fox. 1993. Variation in neutral detergent fiber intake of Holstein cows. J. Dairy Sci. 76:544–554.

Roseler, D. K., D. G. Fox, A. N. Pell, and L. E. Chase. 1997a. Evaluation of alternative equations for prediction of intake for Holstein dairy cows. J. Dairy Sci. 80:864–877.

Roseler, D. K., D. G. Fox, L. E. Chase, A. N. Pell, and W. C. Stone. 1997b. Development and evaluation of equations for the prediction of feed intake for lactating Holstein dairy cows. J. Dairy Sci. 80:878–893.

Robinson, P. H., P. L. Burgess, and R. E. McQueen. 1990. Influence of moisture content of mixed rations on feed intake and milk production of dairy cows. J. Dairy Sci. 73:2916–2921.

Robinson, P. H., and R. E. McQueen. 1994. Influence of supplemental protein source and feeding frequency on rumen fermentation and performance in dairy cows. J. Dairy Sci. 77:1340–1353.

Rodriguez, L. A., C. C. Stallings, J. H. Herbein, and M. L. McGilliard. 1997. Diurnal variation in milk and plasma urea nitrogen in Holstein and Jersey cows in response to degradable dietary protein and added fat. J. Dairy Sci. 80:3368–3376.

Skaar, T. C., R. R. Grummer, M. R. Dentine, and R. H. Stauffacher. 1989. Seasonal effects of prepartum and postpartum fat and niacin feeding on lactation performance and lipid metabolism. J. Dairy Sci. 72:2028–2038.

Smith, W. A., B. Harris, Jr., H. H. Van Horn, and C. J. Wilcox. 1993. Effects of forage type on production of dairy cows supplemented with whole cottonseed, tallow and yeast. J. Dairy Sci. 76:205–215.

Sniffen, C. J., and P. H. Robinson. 1984. Nutritional strategy. Can. J. Anim. Sci. 64:529–542.

Stallings, C. C., G. Kroll, J. C. Kelley, M. L. McGilliard. 1985 A computer ration evaluation program for heifers, dry cows and lactating cows. J. Dairy Sci. 68:1015–1019.

Weiss, W. P., and W. L. Shockey. 1991. Value of orchardgrass and alfalfa silages fed with varying amounts of concentrate to dairy cows. J. Dairy Sci. 74:1933–1943.

Wierenga, H. K. 1990. Social dominance in dairy cattle and the influences of housing and management. Appl. Anim. Behav. Sci. 27:201–229.

Young, B. A. 1983. Ruminant cold stress: Effect on production. J. Anim. Sci. 57:1601–1607.

# 2 Energy

## ENERGY REQUIREMENTS OF LACTATING AND PREGNANT COWS

### *Energy Units*

Energy requirements for maintenance and milk production are expressed in net energy for lactation ($NE_L$) units. The net energy for lactation system (Moe and Tyrrell, 1972) uses a single energy unit ($NE_L$) for both maintenance and milk production because metabolizable energy (ME) was used with similar efficiencies for maintenance (0.62) and milk production (0.64) (Moe and Tyrrell, 1972) when compared with directly measured fasting heat production (Flatt et al., 1965). The energy values of feed are also expressed in $NE_L$ units. Thus in the tables in Chapter 14 and in the computer model, one feed value ($NE_L$) is used to express the requirements for maintenance, pregnancy, milk production, and changes in body reserves (not growth) of adult cows.

## ENERGY VALUES OF FEEDS

The method used to obtain and express feed energy values in this edition is substantially different from that used in previous versions. In the 6th revised edition of the *Nutrient Requirements of Dairy Cattle* (National Research Council, 1989) feedstuffs were assigned total digestible nutrient (TDN) values that had been determined experimentally using similar feeds. The concentrations of digestible energy (DE), ME, and $NE_L$ for each feedstuff were then calculated from the TDN value using Equations 2-1, 2-2, and 2-3. Equations 2-1 and 2-2 assume intake is the same for the independent and dependent variables (e.g., both at one times maintenance or 1X). Equation 2-2 was derived with cows fed at 3 times maintenance (3X), and questions have been raised (Vermorel and Coulon, 1998) about its accuracy when used to convert $DE_{1X}$ to $ME_{1X}$. Equation 2-3 converts $TDN_{1X}$ to $NE_{L3X}$ assuming an 8 percent reduction in digestibility at 3X maintenance.

$$\text{DE (Mcal/kg)} = 0.04409 \times \text{TDN(\%)} \quad (2\text{-}1)$$

$$\text{ME (Mcal/kg)} = 1.01 \times \text{DE (Mcal/kg)} - 0.45 \quad (2\text{-}2)$$

$$NE_L \text{ (Mcal/kg)} = 0.0245 \times \text{TDN(\%)} - 0.12 \quad (2\text{-}3)$$

The problems with this approach are:

- Most of the experimentally determined TDN values currently available in feed composition tables are from experiments conducted many years ago; however, other composition data have been updated. The TDN values in the table may not correspond to the feed with the nutrient composition given in Table 15-1.
- A published TDN value is only appropriate when the nutrient composition of the feed is essentially the same as that for the feed used in the digestibility trial.
- For many feeds, TDN cannot be measured directly because the feed cannot comprise a major portion of the diet. Calculating TDN using the difference method can lead to inaccurate (because of associative effects) and imprecise estimates of TDN.
- Very few ME and $NE_L$ values of individual feedstuffs are available; rather ME and $NE_L$ values of mixed diets are measured. The equations used to convert TDN to ME and $NE_L$ were derived for complete diets, and the TDN for many feedstuffs are outside of the range for TDN values of the diets used to generate the equations, and the equations may not be linear over a wide range of TDN.
- A constant discount of 8 percent as calculated in Equation 2-3 assumes all cows are consuming at 3X maintenance. Based on the normal distribution of milk production among herds, the mean energy intake for a herd may range from 2 to more than 4X maintenance.

Because of these problems, the TDN values at 1X maintenance ($TDX_{1X}$) in Table 15-1 and in the software dictionary were calculated from composition data rather than being experimentally determined. In addition, $NE_L$ values are calculated based on actual intake and the digestibility of the entire diet. In Table 15-1, $NE_L$ values for individual feeds are shown assuming intake at 3 and 4X maintenance and a total diet $TDN_{1X}$ of 74 percent. The $NE_L$ of diets formulated using the $NE_L$ values in Table 15-1 may be different than the $NE_L$ of diets formulated by the computer model because intake and digestibility discount (estimated from total diet $TDX_{1X}$) may be different from those assumed in Table 15-1.

### *Estimating TDN of Feeds at Maintenance*

A summative approach was used to derive the $TDN_{1X}$ values in Table 15-1. In this approach, the concentrations (percent of dry matter) of truly digestible nonfiber carbohydrate (NFC), CP, ether extract (EE), and NDF for each feed are estimated (Weiss et al., 1992) using Equations 2-4a, 2-4b, 2-4c, 2-4d, 2-4e. Ether extract does not represent a nutritionally uniform fraction and therefore does not have a constant digestibility across feedstuffs. Fatty acids (FA) are a uniform fraction with a true digestibility of 95 to100 percent when diets contain 3 percent or less EE (Palmquist, 1991). A value of 100 percent digestibility was chosen. FA content of feed can be estimated as FA = EE − 1 (Allen, 2000). A more accurate approach would be to measure FA directly; however, limited data prevented the inclusion of FA data in Table 15-1. In all equations listed below, measured FA or EE − 1 can be used to represent the FA fraction.

Truly digestible NFC (tdNFC)

$$= 0.98\ (100 - [(NDF - NDICP) + CP + EE + Ash]) \times PAF \qquad (2\text{-}4a)$$

Truly digestible CP for forages (tdCPf)

$$= CP \times \exp[-1.2 \times (ADICP/CP)] \qquad (2\text{-}4b)$$

Truly digestible CP for concentrates (tdCPc)

$$= [1 - (0.4 \times (ADICP/CP))] \times CP \qquad (2\text{-}4c)$$

Truly digestible FA (tdFA)

$$= FA \quad \text{Note: If EE} < 1\text{, then FA} = 0 \qquad (2\text{-}4d)$$

Truly digestible NDF (tdNDF)

$$= 0.75 \times (NDFn - L) \times [1 - (L/NDFn)^{0.667}] \qquad (2\text{-}4e)$$

In Equations 2-4a, 2-4b, 2-4c, 2-4d, 2-4e, NDICP = neutral detergent insoluble N × 6.25, PAF = processing adjustment factor (see below), ADICP = acid detergent insoluble N × 6.25, FA = fatty acids (i.e., EE − 1), L = acid detergent lignin, and NDFn = NDF − NDICP. All values are expressed as a percent of dry matter (DM).

Note: Digestible NDF can be obtained using a 48-hour rumen in vitro assay. The in vitro NDF digestibility is entered into the model when the software is used and that value is used to calculate digestible NDF at maintenance.

Equations 2-4a, 2-4b, 2-4c, 2-4d, and 2-4e are based on true digestibility, but TDN is based on apparent digestibility; therefore, metabolic fecal TDN must be subtracted from the sum of the digestible fractions. Weiss et al. (1992) determined that, on average, metabolic fecal TDN equalled 7. The $TDN_{1X}$ is then calculated using Equation 2-5.

$$TDN_{1X}\ (\%) = tdNFC + tdCP + (tdFA \times 2.25) + tdNDF - 7 \qquad (2\text{-}5)$$

Equations 2-4 and 2-5 were used to calculate $TDN_{1X}$, for most, but not all, feedstuffs in Table 15-1. Different equations are used to estimate TDN for animal protein meals and fat supplements (see below).

#### EFFECT OF PROCESSING ON NFC DIGESTIBILITY

Physical processing, and heat and steam treatment of feeds usually does not greatly change their composition as measured by conventional feed testing assays but often increases the digestibility of starch (see Chapter 13). To account for the effect of processing and some other nonchemical factors on starch digestibility, an empirical approach was used. Based on in vivo digestibility data (see Chapter 13), a processing adjustment factor (PAF) was developed (Table 2-1). Expected true digestibility of NFC at 1X maintenance is about 0.98 and 0.90 at 3X maintenance (approximately the feeding level used in the digestibility studies) (Tyrrell and Moe, 1975; Van Soest, 1982).

TABLE 2-1 Processing Adjustment Factors (PAF) for NFC[a]

| Feedstuff | PAF |
|---|---|
| Bakery waste | 1.04 |
| Barley grain, rolled | 1.04 |
| Bread | 1.04 |
| Cereal meal | 1.04 |
| Chocolate meal | 1.04 |
| Cookie meal | 1.04 |
| Corn grain, cracked dry[b] | 0.95 |
| Corn grain, ground[b] | 1.00 |
| Corn grain, ground high moisture[b] | 1.04 |
| Corn and cob meal, ground high moisture[b] | 1.04 |
| Corn grain, steam flaked[c] | 1.04 |
| Corn silage, normal | 0.94 |
| Corn silage, mature | 0.87 |
| Molasses (beet and cane) | 1.04 |
| Oats grain | 1.04 |
| Sorghum grain, dry rolled | 0.92 |
| Sorghum grain, steam-flaked[d] | 1.04 |
| Wheat grain, rolled | 1.04 |
| All other feeds | 1.00 |

[a] See Chapter 13 for details on how values were calculated. For feeds not shown, PAF = 1.0.

[b] Mean of several experiments, actual PAF depends on particle size. Finer grinding will increase PAF.

[c] Mean density of 0.36 kg/L; PAF should be negatively correlated with density.

[d] Mean density of 0.36 kg/L; PAF should be negatively correlated with density.

The PAF was calculated by dividing in vivo starch digestibility of different feeds by 0.90. The PAF is used only for NFC. The PAF adjustment will result in overestimation of energy values in some feeds when fed at maintenance, but $NE_L$ values when fed at 3 times maintenance should be correct.

ANIMAL PROTEIN MEALS

Animal products contain no structural carbohydrates; however, certain animal products contain substantial amounts of neutral detergent insoluble residue. Because this material is not cellulose, hemicellulose, or lignin, the above equations cannot be used. For those feeds, $TDN_{1X}$ was estimated using Equation 2-6.

$$TDN_{1X} (\%) = CPdigest \times CP + FA \times 2.25 + 0.98(100 - CP - Ash - EE) - 7 \quad (2\text{-}6)$$

Where CPdigest = estimated true digestibility of CP (Table 2-2) and FA = EE − 1. The CPdigest values are from Table 15-2 assuming an intake of 2 percent of body weight (BW). The method used to obtain those values is explained in Chapter 5.

TABLE 2-2 True Digestibility Coefficients of CP Used to Estimate $TDN_{1X}$ Values of Animal-Based Feedstuffs

| Feedstuff | True Digestibility |
|---|---|
| Blood meal, batch dried | 0.75 |
| Blood meal, ring dried | 0.86 |
| Hydrolyzed feather meal | 0.78 |
| Hydrolyzed feather meal with viscera | 0.81 |
| Fish meal (Menhaden) | 0.94 |
| Fish meal (Anchovy) | 0.95 |
| Meat and bone meal | 0.80 |
| Meat meal | 0.92 |
| Whey | 1.00 |

FAT SUPPLEMENTS

The $TDN_{1X}$ values of different fat supplements were calculated from measured fatty acid digestibility. Partial digestion coefficients (Table 2-3) of fatty acids from supplemental fat sources were determined indirectly by difference [(additional fatty acid intake during fat supplementation minus additional fecal fatty acid output during fat supplementation)/(additional fatty acid intake during fat supplementation); Grummer, 1988]. Assumptions associated with this method are that endogenous lipid remains constant, and digestibility of fatty acids in the basal diet does not change when supplemental fat is fed. For fat sources containing triglycerides (tallow, partially hydrogenated tallow, and vegetable oil), ether extract was assumed to contain 90 percent fatty acids and 10 percent glycerol, and the glycerol was assumed to be 100 percent digestible at 1X. In the experiments used to determine fat digestibility, cows were fed at approximately 3X maintenance. Therefore, the original values were divided by 0.92 to adjust values to $TDN_{1X}$. After adjusting digestibility for intake (Table 2-3), digestible fat was multiplied by 2.25 to convert to $TDN_{1X}$ (Equations 2-7a and 2-7b).

TABLE 2-3 True Digestibilities at Maintenance (assumed 8 percent increase in digestibility compared with 3X maintenance) of Fatty Acids from Various Fat Sources

| Fat | Fat type | Mean % | SD | N |
|---|---|---|---|---|
| Calcium salts of fatty acids | Fatty acids | 0.86 | 0.11 | 15 |
| Hydrolyzed tallow fatty acids | Fatty acids | 0.79 | 0.08 | 9 |
| Partially hydrogenated tallow | Fat plus glycerol | 0.43 | 0.13 | 9 |
| Tallow | Fat plus glycerol | 0.68 | 0.13 | 10 |
| Vegetable oil | Fat plus glycerol | 0.86 | — | — |

For fat sources that contain glycerol:

$$TDN_{1X} (\%) = (EE \times 0.1) + [FAdigest \times (EE \times 0.9) \times 2.25] \quad (2\text{-}7a)$$

For fat sources that do not contain glycerol:

$$TDN_{1X} (\%) = (EE \times FAdigest) \times 2.25 \quad (2\text{-}7b)$$

where FAdigest = digestibility coefficients for fatty acids (Table 2-3).

### *Estimating DE of Feeds*

Crampton et al. (1957) and Swift (1957) computed that the gross energy of TDN is 4.409 Mcal/kg. Because nutrients have different heats of combustion (e.g., 4.2 Mcal/kg for carbohydrates, 5.6 Mcal/kg for protein, 9.4 Mcal/kg for long chain fatty acids, and 4.3 Mcal/kg for glycerol; Maynard et al., 1979), the gross energy value of TDN is not constant among feeds. The gross energy of TDN of a feed that has a high proportion of its TDN provided by protein will be greater than 4.409. Conversely the gross energy of TDN of a feed with a high proportion of its TDN provided by carbohydrate or fat will be less than 4.409. Therefore, the calculation of DE as 0.04409 × TDN (percent) as in the previous edition (National Research Council, 1989) was abandoned. Digestible energy was calculated by multiplying the estimated digestible nutrient concentrations (Equations 2-4a through 2-4e) by their heats of combustion, as shown in Equations 2-8a, 2-8b, 2-8c, and 2-8d. Since DE is based on apparent digestibility and Equations 2-4a through 2-4e are based on true digestibility, a correction for metabolic fecal energy is needed. The heat of combustion of metabolic fecal TDN was assumed to be 4.4 Mcal/kg; metabolic fecal DE = 7 × 0.044 = 0.3 Mcal/kg.

For most feeds:

$$DE_{1X}\ (\text{Mcal/kg}) = (\text{tdNFC}/100) \times 4.2 + (\text{tdNDF}/100) \times 4.2 + (\text{tdCP}/100) \times 5.6 + (\text{FA}/100) \times 9.4 - 0.3 \quad (2\text{-}8a)$$

For animal protein meals:

$$DE_{1X}\ (\text{Mcal/kg}) = (\text{tdNFC}/100) \times 4.2 + (\text{tdCP}/100) \times 5.6 + (\text{FA}/100) \times 9.4 - 0.3 \quad (2\text{-}8b)$$

For fat supplements with glycerol:

$$DE_{1X}\ (\text{Mcal/kg}) = 9.4 \times (\text{FAdigest} \times 0.9 \times (\text{EE}/100)) + (4.3 \times 0.1 \times (\text{EE}/100)) \quad (2\text{-}8c)$$

For fat supplements without glycerol:

$$DE_{1X}\ (\text{Mcal/kg}) = 9.4 \times \text{FAdigest} \times (\text{EE}/100) \quad (2\text{-}8d)$$

In the above Equations, 2-8a through 2-8d, tdNFC, tdNDF, tdCP, and FA are expressed as percent of DM.

In Equation 2-8b protein digestibilities are from Table 2-2. For Equations 2-8c and 2-8d, fatty acid digestibilities (FAdigest) are from Table 2-3. Because the method used to estimate those values already accounts for the difference between apparent and true digestibility, the 0.3 adjustment is not needed in Equations 2-8c and 2-8d.

*Estimating DE at Actual Intake*

The digestibility of diets fed to dairy cows is reduced with increasing feed intake (Tyrrell and Moe, 1975). This reduces the energy value of any given diet as feed intake increases. This is particularly important in today's high producing dairy cows where it is not uncommon for feed intake to exceed 4 times maintenance level of intake. The rate of decline in digestibility with level of feeding has been shown to be related to digestibility of the diet at maintenance (Wagner and Loosli, 1967). Diets with high digestibility at maintenance exhibit a greater rate of depression in digestibility with level of feeding than diets with low digestibility fed at maintenance. Previous National Research Council reports (National Research Council, 1978, 1989) used a constant depression of 4 percent per multiple of maintenance to adjust maintenance energy values to 3X maintenance energy values. Using this method of discounting, the percentage unit decline in TDN for a diet containing 75 percent $TDN_{1X}$ would be 3 percentage units per multiple of maintenance, while the depression for a diet containing 60 percent $TDN_{1X}$ would be 2.4 units. The differences in rate of depression in digestibility are generally negligible for diets having maintenance TDN values of 60 percent or less.

Figure 2-1 shows the relationship between digestibility at maintenance and the percentage unit decline in digestibility per multiple of maintenance feeding from literature reports (Brown, 1966; Colucci, et al., 1882; Moe et al., 1965; Tyrrell and Moe, 1972; 1974; 1975; Wagner and Loosli, 1967). It was apparent that the rate of decline in digestibility with level of feeding was a function of the maintenance digestibility of the diets fed: TDN percentage unit decline $= 0.18 \times TDN_{1X} - 10.3$ ($r^2 = 0.85$). Because DE, not TDN, is used to calculate ME and $NE_L$, this equation was converted so that a percent discount, not a TDN percentage unit discount, was calculated:

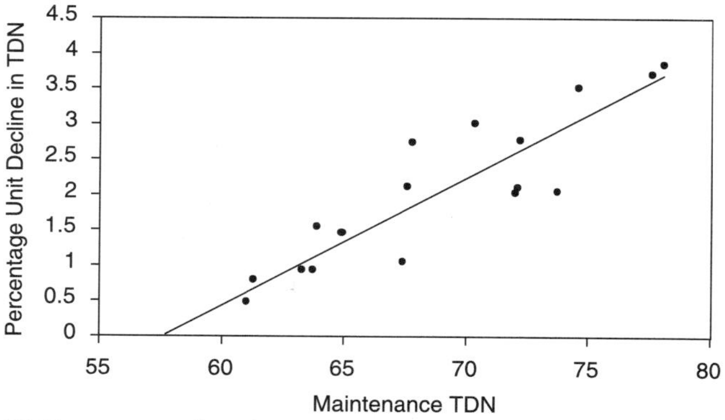


FIGURE 2-1 The relationship between feeding level expressed as multiples of maintenance and the unit decline in diet TDN per multiple of maintenance where TDN percentage unit decline $= 0.18 \times -10.3$, $r^2 = 0.85$.

$$\text{Discount} = [(TDN_{1X} - [(0.18 \times TDN_{1X}) - 10.3]) \times \text{Intake})]/TDN_{1X} \quad (2\text{-}9)$$

where $TDN_{1X}$ is as a percent of dry matter and is for the entire diet, not the individual feed, and intake is expressed as incremental intake above maintenance (e.g., for a cow consuming 3X maintenance, intake above maintenance = 2). For example, for a cow consuming a diet that contains 74 percent $TDN_{1X}$ at 3X intake, digestibility would be expected to be 0.918 times the value obtained at maintenance.

Based on Equation 2-9, a diet with a $TDN_{1X}$ of 57.2 would exhibit no depression in digestibility with level of intake. Based on Figure 2-1, the discount for diets with 60 percent or less $TDN_{1X}$ is negligible; therefore, for diets with 60 percent or less $TDN_{1X}$ the discount was set to 1.0 (i.e., no discount was applied). Furthermore, a maximum discount was set so that discounted diet TDN could not be less than 60 percent. Data on effects of intake much greater than 4X maintenance are lacking. Vandehaar (1998) suggested that the effect of intake on digestibility is not linear, but rather the digestibility discount increases at a decreasing rate as feed intake increases. The possibility of a nonlinear response was one reason the minimum discounted TDN was set at 60 percent. Data are needed on the effects of very high intake on digestibility. The data in Figure 2-1 were generated with diets not containing supplemental fat. It was assumed that increasing $TDN_{1X}$ by increasing dietary fat above 3 percent would not affect the digestibility discount. Therefore the $TDN_{1X}$ value, used only for the discount calculation, does not include TDN provided by dietary fat in excess of 3 percent. Diets with $TDN_{1X}$ of 62, 67, 72, and 77 percent would exhibit a 0.9, 1.8, 2.7, and 3.6 percentage unit decline in TDN, respectively, per multiple of maintenance feeding. The percent decline in digestibility in the respective diets would be 1.5, 1.8, 3.8, and 4.7 percent. This adjustment is used continuously across all levels of feeding as contrasted to constant adjustment to 3X level of feeding used in the 1989 National Research Council report. The $DE_{1X}$ for each feed was determined and then multiplied by the discount factor obtained using Equation 2-9 to calculate DE at productive levels of intake ($DE_p$).

*Estimating ME at Actual Intake*

Equation 2-2 was derived to convert DE into ME when cows were fed at production levels of intake. Therefore ME at production levels of intake ($ME_p$) should be calculated from $DE_p$. Equation 2-2 was developed with diets containing about 3 percent ether extract, but because the efficiency of converting DE from fat into ME is approximately 100 percent (Andrew et al., 1991; Romo et al., 1996), Equation 2-2 underestimates ME of high fat diets. A theoretical approach was used to adjust ME values of feeds with more than 3 percent EE. Assuming a feed with 100 percent EE has ME = DE and subtracting that equation from Equation 2-2 (1.01 × DE − 0.45) and dividing by the change in EE concentration (100 − 3) yields the expression: 0.000103 × DE + 0.00464 change in ME per increase in EE content (percentage unit). The DE term was assumed to be negligible; therefore, $ME_p$ values of feeds with more than 3 percent EE were increased by 0.0046 per percentage unit increase in EE content above 3 percent (Equation 2-10). For feeds with less than 3 percent EE, Equation 2-2 is used to calculate $ME_p$.

$$ME_p\ (\text{Mcal/kg}) = [1.01 \times (DE_p) - 0.45] + 0.0046 \times (EE - 3) \quad (2\text{-}10)$$

where $DE_p$ is Mcal/kg and EE is percent of DM.

For fat supplements, $ME_p$ (Mcal/kg) = $DE_p$ (Mcal/kg).

*Estimating $NE_L$ at Actual Intake*

The use of Equation 2-3 to estimate $NE_L$ has been criticized because it results in essentially equal efficiencies of converting DE to $NE_L$ for all feeds (Vermorel and Coulon, 1998). Using Equation 2-3, a feed with 40 percent TDN (DE = 1.76 Mcal/kg) has an efficiency of converting DE to $NE_{L3X}$ of 0.49 and for a feed with a TDN of 90 percent (DE = 3.97 Mcal/kg), the efficiency is 0.53. That range in efficiencies is less than would be expected among feeds when DE is converted to $NE_L$. To overcome this problem, an equation derived by Moe and Tyrrell (1972) to convert $ME_p$ to $NE_L$ at production levels of intake ($NE_{Lp}$) was chosen to replace the previous TDN-based $NE_L$ equation.

$$NE_{Lp}\ (\text{Mcal/kg}) = [0.703 \times ME_p\ (\text{Mcal/kg})] - 0.19 \quad (2\text{-}11)$$

A modification was made to adjust for improved metabolic efficiency of fat. The average efficiency of converting ME from fat to $NE_L$ is 0.80 [sd = 0.05; N = 3; (Andrew et al., 1991; Romo et al., 1996)]. The same approach as discussed above to adjust $ME_p$ for fat content was used to account for increased efficiency of converting ME from fat to $NE_L$. The resulting term was: (0.097 × $ME_p$ + 0.19)/97 increase in $NE_L$ per percentage unit increase in feed EE content above 3 percent (Equation 2-12). For feeds with less than 3 percent EE, Equation 2-11 is used to calculate $NE_{Lp}$.

$$NE_{Lp}\ (\text{Mcal/kg}) = 0.703 \times ME_p - 0.19 + ([(0.097 \times ME_p + 0.19)/97] \times [EE - 3]) \quad (2\text{-}12)$$

where $ME_p$ is Mcal/kg and EE is percent of DM.

For fat supplements, $NE_{Lp}$ (Mcal/kg) = 0.8 × $ME_p$ (Mcal/kg).

*Estimating Net Energy of Feeds for Maintenance and Gain*

The equations used to estimate the net energy for maintenance ($NE_M$) and net energy for gain ($NE_G$) used for beef cattle (National Research Council, 1996) were retained. The $NE_M$ and $NE_G$ content of feeds assumed dry matter intake at 3 times maintenance and are calculated by multiplying $DE_{1X}$ (described above) by 0.82 to obtain ME (National Research Council, 1996). That ME value is then converted to $NE_M$ and $NE_G$ using the following relationships (Garrett, 1980):

$$NE_M = 1.37\ ME - 0.138\ ME^2 + 0.0105\ ME^3 - 1.12 \quad (2\text{-}13)$$

$$NE_G = 1.42\ ME - 0.174\ ME^2 + 0.0122\ ME^3 - 1.65 \quad (2\text{-}14)$$

where ME, $NE_M$, and $NE_G$ are expressed in Mcal/kg.

Those equations are not appropriate for fat supplements. For those feeds, $ME_p$ = $DE_p$, and the same efficiency (0.80) of converting ME to $NE_L$ was used to convert ME to $NE_M$. The efficiency of converting ME to $NE_G$ was set at 0.55 for fat supplements. The method used to calculate feed energy values for calves weighing less than 100 kg is described in Chapter 10.

### *Comparison of New $NE_L$ Values with Values from 1989 Edition*

For feedstuffs in Table 15-1, $NE_L$ values were calculated using the approach outlined above for cows fed at 3X maintenance and compared with values in Table 7-1 in the previous edition of the *Nutrient Requirements of Dairy Cattle* (National Research Council, 1989). The mean $NE_L$ value for all feeds listed in Table 15-1 is 2 percent lower than the mean $NE_L$ value for the same feeds in the 6th revised edition of *Nutrient Requirements of Dairy Cattle* (National Research Council, 1989). Although on average the values are similar, some marked differences exist. In general, forages, especially lower quality forages, have lower $NE_L$ values, high protein feeds have higher $NE_L$ values, and starchy concentrates have values similar to those in the previous edition (National Research Council, 1989). The $NE_L$ for cottonseeds is about 16 percent lower and the value for roasted soybeans is about 25 percent higher than in the previous edition. In the previous edition, cottonseeds had more $NE_L$ than roasted soybeans; however, cottonseed has much more NDF (50 vs. 22 percent), more lignin (13 vs. 3 percent), and less CP (23 vs. 43 percent). The NDF in cottonseed hulls, which provide most of the NDF in whole cottonseeds, has a low digestibility. These differences in composition and fiber digestibility imply that soybeans should provide more energy than cottonseeds. Because of differences in the ability of soybeans and cottonseeds to stimulate chewing and rumination, in low fiber diets, cottonseed may reduce negative associative effects and appear to have more energy than soybeans. Diets including whole cottonseeds and roasted soybeans were included in the evaluation of the software model (Chapter 16). Although data are very limited, estimated $NE_L$ provided by those diets did not deviate greatly from estimated $NE_L$ expenditures.

Using two different methods, the $NE_L$ values for feeds in the 6th revised edition of the *Nutrient Requirements of Dairy Cattle* (National Research Council, 1989) were found to be about 5 percent (Weiss, 1998) and 5 to 7 percent (Vermorel and Coulon, 1998) too high. When $NE_L$ values were calculated as described above and applied to the data set of Weiss (1998), the overestimation of feed energy was reduced from 5 percent to 1.2 percent. Dhiman et al. (1995) conducted an experiment with cows fed different ratios of alfalfa silage and concentrate (ground high moisture ear corn and soybean meal) for the entire lactation. Based on the nutrient composition of their feeds and calculated energy balance, $NE_L$ values for the diets calculated using Equation 2-12 ranged from +5.6 percent to −7.3 percent with a mean bias of 0 percent. For the four diets used by Tyrrell and Varga (1987), the calculated $NE_L$ values (Equation 2-11) ranged from 1.3 to 5.1 percent higher than measured values (mean bias was 2.8 percent). For the four diets used by Wilkerson and Glenn (1997), the calculated values ranged from 7 percent lower to 1.2 percent higher than measured values (mean bias was 3.5 percent).

### *Precautions*

The energy values for feeds and diets are based mostly on chemical characteristics of the feed and assume that feed characteristics limit energy availability. Composition of the total diet and dry matter intake have marked effects on digestibility and subsequent energy values. Diets that do not promote optimal ruminal fermentation will result in an overestimation of energy values. For example, if digestibility of diets is constrained by a lack of ruminally available protein or by low pH caused by feeding diets with insufficient fiber (or excess NFC), calculated energy values will be overestimated. Positive associative effects are not considered. In a situation where a fibrous feed is added to a diet with insufficient fiber, the energy value of that feed may appear to be higher than values calculated with Equation 2-12 because of overall improved ruminal digestion.

## ENERGY REQUIREMENTS

### *Maintenance Requirements*

Measured fasting heat production (Flatt et al., 1965) in dry non-pregnant dairy cows averaged 0.073 Mcal/kg $BW^{0.75}$, and estimated fasting heat production using regression analysis suggested an identical value. Because these measurements were made with cows housed in tie stalls in metabolic chambers, a 10 percent activity allowance was added to account for normal voluntary activity of cows that would be housed in drylot or free stall systems, such that the maintenance requirement for $NE_L$ is set at 0.080 Mcal/kg $BW^{0.75}$ for mature dairy cows.

Cows of similar size and breed may vary in their maintenance requirements, even under controlled activity conditions, by as much as 8 to 10 percent (Van Es, 1961). The National Research Council (1996) used a net energy maintenance value of 0.077 Mcal/$kg^{0.75}$ empty body weight (EBW) for British beef cattle breeds with adjustments to maintenance requirements based on breed and/or genotype. Assuming an empty body mass of 85 percent of live weight, the implied maintenance requirement on a live weight basis would be 0.065 Mcal/$kg^{0.75}$. A breed adjustment factor of 1.2 was used for Holsteins and Jerseys by the National Research Council (1996), which would then adjust the maintenance requirement to 0.079 Mcal/$kg^{0.75}$, which is nearly identical to the current value of 0.080 Mcal/kg $BW^{0.75}$ used in this report.

It has been suggested that maintenance requirements among beef cattle breeds varies with milk production. Very few direct comparisons have been made of the effect of dairy cattle breed on energy metabolism. Tyrrell et al. (1991) compared nonlactating and lactating Holstein and Jersey cows. Although actual milk yields were greater for Holstein cows than for Jersey cows, energy output in milk as a function of metabolic weight was similar, and there was no evidence to suggest that energy requirements for maintenance or production differed between breeds.

*Lactation Requirements*

The NE required for lactation ($NE_L$) is defined as the energy contained in the milk produced. The $NE_L$ concentration in milk is equivalent to the sum of the heats of combustion of individual milk components (fat, protein, and lactose). Reported heats of combustion of milk fat, protein, and lactose are 9.29, 5.71, and 3.95 Mcal/kg, respectively. Frequently, milk fat and protein but not milk lactose are measured. Milk lactose content is the least variable milk component and is essentially a constant 4.85 percent of milk and varies only slightly with breed and milk protein concentration.

Milk crude protein, when estimated as N times 6.38, contains approximately 7 percent nonprotein nitrogen (NPN) (DePeters et al., 1992). Urea N accounts for about 50 percent of NPN in milk; and ammonia, peptides, creatine, creatinine, hippuric acid, uric acid, and other N-containing components make up the remainder of NPN in milk (DePeters et al., 1992). Based on the average composition and the heats of combustion of individual NPN constituents, the heat of combustion for NPN is 2.21 kcal/g crude protein. Where total and not true protein is determined, the coefficient (weighted average of the different N compounds in milk) for milk crude protein is 5.47 kcal/g. This value is slightly higher than the coefficient of 5.31 determined by regression analysis of milk energy on milk fat, protein, and lactose (Tyrrell and Reid, 1965). Where individual components are measured directly, $NE_L$ concentration in milk is calculated as:

$$NE_L\ (\text{Mcal/kg}) = 0.0929 \times \text{Fat \%} + 0.0547 \times \text{Crude Protein \%} + 0.0395 \times \text{Lactose \%} \quad (2\text{-}15)$$

When only fat and protein in milk are measured and the lactose content of milk is assumed to be 4.85 percent, the $NE_L$ concentration of milk is calculated as:

$$NE_L\ (\text{Mcal/kg}) = 0.0929 \times \text{Fat \%} + 0.0547 \times \text{Crude Protein \%} + 0.192 \quad (2\text{-}16)$$

If milk true protein rather than crude protein is measured, the coefficient in the equation above should be changed from 0.0547 to 0.0563, which reflects the relative proportions of true protein and NPN and their energy values discussed above.

The Gaines formula (Gaines, 1928) for 4 percent fat-corrected milk (4 percent FCM, kg/d = 0.4 × milk, kg/d + 15 × fat, kg/d) has been used for more than 70 years as a means to correct milk yields to a constant energy basis. The Gaines formula is based on an assumed $NE_L$ concentration of 0.749 Mcal/kg of milk when milk contains 4 percent fat. The 1989 National Research Council report used a value of 0.74 Mcal/kg, but based on measured heats of combustion (Moe and Tyrrell, 1972), the actual coefficient is 0.749/kg of FCM when calculated using the Gaines equation. The Gaines formula, which is based on volume of milk and total yield of fat, underestimates the energy value of milk when milk fat content is less than 3 percent. When milk fat is the only milk constituent measured, $NE_L$ concentration can be calculated using the Tyrrell and Reid (1965) formula:

$$NE_L\ (\text{Mcal/kg of milk}) = 0.360 + [0.0969(\text{fat \%})] \quad (2\text{-}17)$$

The feed energy requirements for production of individual milk components have not been defined. The $NE_L$ system in this edition is based on yield of total energy in milk and does not account for many of the differences in metabolic transactions or the substrates required for synthesis of individual milk components. The measured calorimetric inefficiency of use of ME for milk includes losses associated with metabolic transactions for conversion of absorbed nutrients into milk components, the energy required for nutrient absorption, and increased rates of metabolism in visceral tissues required for support of increased milk production. Theoretical calculations of energy requirements for production of individual milk components have been made (Baldwin, 1968; Dado et al., 1993). These estimates only account for energy losses in metabolic transactions associated with production of individual milk components. Theoretical efficiencies for use of ME for milk fat, protein, and lactose synthesis as estimated from Mertens and Dado (1993) were 81, 89, and 77 percent, respectively, each well above the 64 percent measured calorimetric efficiency for use of dietary ME for milk energy production (Moe and Tyrrell, 1972). Metabolic models that incorporate changes in visceral metabolism, transport, resynthesis of metabolites, and other energy costs (Baldwin et al., 1987) account for most of this discrepancy, but it is still difficult to assign these costs to production of individual milk components. It is envisioned that future net energy requirements for milk will be centered more on substrate requirements for production of individual milk components rather than a more general requirement for total milk energy output.

*Activity Requirements*

The energy required for maintenance includes a 10 percent allowance for activity, which should provide sufficient energy for the usual activity of lactating cows that are fed in individual stalls or drylot systems. At similar production, grazing cattle expend more energy than animals fed in confinement because: 1) the distance between the milking center and pasture is usually greater than the distance between the milking center and most confinement housing areas; 2) grazing cattle may have to walk where elevations change; and 3) grazing cattle spend more time eating than do confinement fed cattle. The increase in energy requirement for grazing cattle is largely a function of the distance walked, topography of the pasture, and BW. Heat production increases 0.00045 Mcal/kg BW for every kilometer a cow walks horizontally (Agricultural Research Council, 1980; Bellows et al., 1994; Coulon et al., 1998). Because no net work is actually done, increased energy required for physical activity is reflected in increased heat production and by definition is equivalent to $NE_L$ required for maintenance. Thus in $NE_L$ units, the energy required for excessive walking was set at 0.00045 Mcal/kg per kilometer walked. Excessive walking was defined as the distance a grazing cow travels between the pasture and the milking center. For a grazing 600-kg cow walking 0.5 km to and from the milking parlor 2 times per day (2 km total), the extra $NE_L$ allowance is 0.54 Mcal or about a 5 percent increase in maintenance requirements.

Based on data generated with growing cattle (Holmes et al., 1978; Havstad and Malechek, 1982), the increased eating activity associated with grazing compared with stall-fed cattle required 0.003 Mcal of ME/kg BW per day or approximately 0.002 Mcal of $NE_L$/kg BW. That value was for cattle consuming only pasture and should be reduced to reflect the amount of concentrate fed. In this edition, it is assumed that the diet for grazing lactating cows would be 60 percent pasture (dry basis). Therefore the activity allowance for eating act by grazing lactating cows (Mcal of $NE_L$) is calculated as 0.0012/kg of BW. For good quality, high yielding pastures, we assumed that energy expended walking within a paddock would be similar to that of cows housed in free stall barns. The total increase in the daily energy requirement for maintenance of cows grazing relatively flat, high yielding pasture should be increased 0.00045 Mcal of $NE_L$/kg BW per km of distance between the pasture and milking center plus 0.0012 Mcal per kilogram BW. For example, a 600-kg cow grazing a flat pasture (comprised 60 percent of total diet) approximately 0.5 km from the milking center and milked twice daily will walk 2 km/d to and from the milking center. The maintenance energy requirement should be increased by $2 \times 0.00045 \times 600 = 0.54$ Mcal for walking and $0.0012 \times 600 = 0.7$ Mcal for eating activity or approximately 1.2 Mcal of $NE_L$/day (approximately a 12 percent increase in maintenance requirement).

The energetic cost for cows grazing hilly topography is higher than that for cows grazing relatively flat pastures. The actual cost for a specific situation is difficult to quantify, because the change in elevation usually will not be known, and cows will walk both up and down hills. The Agricultural Research Council (1980) estimated that 0.03 Mcal of $NE_L$ per kg BW is required for a cow to walk 1 vertical km. The committee used a qualitative system to adjust for topography. A 'hilly' pasture system was defined as one in which cows moved a total of 200 m of vertical distance (50 m hill walked 4 times each day). Using the Agricultural Research Council (1980) value, the energy requirement for maintenance of cows grazing a hilly location was increased 0.006 Mcal of $NE_L$/kg BW. That adjustment is in addition to the increases in energy requirements for walking from the pasture to the milking center and for eating. Using the previous example for a cow that is milked twice daily and is grazing a hilly pasture located 0.5 km from the milking center, maintenance requirements would be increased $(0.00045 \times 600 \times 2) + (0.0012 \times 600) + 0.006 \times 600 = 4.9$ Mcal $NE_L$/day or an increase in maintenance of about 50 percent. As milk yield increases, appetite and the amount of energy expended gathering food would also increase, but this effect is not included in activity requirement calculations.

The time spent grazing is dependent on the amount of forage consumed and the relative availability of herbage. Where abundance of herbage is low, cows spend more time to consume the same amount of forage. Forage intake is dependent on milk production of cows and the amount of supplemental grain that is fed with the pasture. In a review (CSIRO, 1990), it was estimated that grazing activity increased energy requirements relative to maintenance by 20 percent on flat terrain and by as much as 50 percent on hilly pasture. They proposed a system to account for increased energy costs associated with grazing based on forage intake and digestibility, terrain, and herbage availability. This system was included in the National Research Council's *Nutrient Requirements of Beef Cattle* (1996); however, the proposed equation has not been evaluated. Evaluation of that equation suggested that a 600-kg milking cow, consuming 15 kg of DM from good quality pasture (65 percent DM digestibility) with moderate to good availability of forage (2 to 3 metric tons/hectare), increased $NE_L$ requirements by 4 to 4.4 Mcal/d.

For growing heifers on pasture, energy requirements should be increased to cover increased eating activity and walking. The same energy costs used for lactating cows were used for heifers ($NE_M$ values assumed to be equivalent to $NE_L$). The energy required for walking by heifers was set at 0.00045 Mcal of $NE_M$/kg BW per kilometer walked. The distance heifers walk each day will vary depending on availability of forage and placement of water. Havstad and Malechek (1982) reported that grazing beef heifers walked 3.9 km per day when forage supply was adequate. The committee assumed the average growing heifer would walk approximately twice as much when grazing as when housed in confinement (an increase of approximately 2 km/d). Therefore, the $NE_M$ requirement for walking for grazing heifers was set at $0.00045 \times 2 = 0.0009$ Mcal/kg BW per day. The energy associated with eating activity was the same as that used for lactating cows except pasture was assumed to provide 80 percent of the diet (0.0016 Mcal $NE_M \times$ BW). The total adjustment for the daily energetic cost ($NE_M$, Mcal/day) of grazing for growing heifers is $(0.0016 \times \text{BW}) + (0.0009 \times \text{BW})$. The same equation as that used to estimate energy required for walking in hilly pasture for lactating cows was used for heifers. For hilly pastures, maintenance requirements should be increased an additional 0.006 Mcal of $NE_M$/kg BW per day. For example a 300-kg heifer grazing a hilly pasture would require $(0.0009 \times 300) + (0.0016 \times 300) + (0.006 \times 300) = 2.6$ Mcal of ME for activity (or an increase in maintenance requirement of about 40 percent).

The energy requirements for activity given above are based on many assumptions and very limited data. Accurate information on walking distances, topography, pasture yields, etc., for a specific situation is very difficult to quantify. The actual energy required for activity under specific circumstances could vary greatly from those calculated with the above equations. The previous edition of the *Nutrient Requirements of Dairy Cattle* (National Research Council, 1989) stated that maintenance energy should be increased by 10 percent with good quality, high yielding pastures. Based on available data, that value is probably too low. The value probably ranges from about 10 (flat pasture located close to the milking center) to more than 50 (hilly pasture located far from the milking center) percent of maintenance energy.

### *Environmental Effects*

For lactating cows in cold environments, the change in energy requirement is probably minimal because of the normally high heat production of cows consuming large amounts of feed. Even with the increased use of naturally ventilated free stall housing systems, it is unlikely that cows will require increased intake of energy to counteract cold environments if they are kept dry and are not exposed directly to wind. Young (1976) summarized experiments with ruminants in which an average reduction in DM digestibility of 1.8 percentage units was observed for each 10°C reduction in ambient temperature below 20°C. Much of this lowered digestibility under cold stress may be related to an increased rate of passage of feed through the digestive tract (Kennedy et al., 1976). Because of the effects of low temperature on digestibility, under extremely cold weather conditions, feed energy values could possibly be lower than expected.

Mild to severe heat stress has been estimated (National Research Council, 1981) to increase maintenance requirements by 7 to 25 percent, respectively (for a 600-kg cow, this equates to between 0.7 and 2.4 Mcal of $NE_L$/day); however, insufficient data are currently available to quantify these effects accurately. Heat stress induces behavioral and metabolic changes in cattle (West, 1994). Some changes, such as panting, increase energy expenditures, while other changes (reduced dry matter intake, selective consumption, reduced activity, and reduced metabolic rate) will reduce heat production. An equation to adjust maintenance requirement based on environmental factors related to heat stress (ambient temperature, relative humidity, radiant energy, and wind speed) has been developed (Fox and Tylutki, 1998), but it has not been sufficiently validated. Because of limited data, no adjustments for heat stress have been included in the calculation of maintenance requirements of adult cattle in this version. Users, however, should be aware of the effects heat stress has on maintenance requirement and may wish to make dietary adjustments to account for those effects.

### *Pregnancy Requirements*

Estimates of the energy requirements for gestation during the last 100 days of pregnancy are from Bell et al. (1995). The energy required for gestation is assumed to be 0 when the day of gestation is less than 190 and the maximum gestation length is set to 279 days (longer gestation periods result in no change in energy requirements). Bell et al. (1995) serially slaughtered Holstein cows at various stages of gestation and generated a quadratic equation to describe the energy content of the gravid uterus. The first derivative of that equation yields the daily change in energy content. The subcommittee assumed that energy requirements for gestation would depend on birth weight of the calf; therefore, an adjustment relative to the mean birth weight of Holstein calves (45 kg) was included in the Bell et al. equation. Efficiency of ME use by the gravid uterus was assumed to be 0.14 (Ferrell et al., 1976). Therefore, the ME requirement for gestation is described as:

$$\text{ME (Mcal/d)} = [(0.00318 \times \text{D} - 0.0352) \times (\text{CBW}/45)]/0.14 \qquad (2\text{-}18)$$

where D = day of gestation between 190 and 279, and CBW is calf birth weight in kilograms. To convert ME to $NE_L$ an efficiency of 0.64 was used; therefore, the $NE_L$ requirement for pregnancy is:

$$NE_L \text{ (Mcal/d)} = [(0.00318 \times \text{D} - 0.0352) \times (\text{CBW}/45)]/0.218 \qquad (2\text{-}19)$$

where D = day of gestation between 190 and 279, and CBW is calf birth weight in kilograms.

*Tissue Mobilization and Repletion During Lactation and the Dry Period*

The growth model (Chapter 11) computes growth requirements until females reach their mature weight. However, changes in body composition during lactation and the dry period primarily reflect depletion and repletion of tissues when diets provide insufficient or excess energy. The body tissues involved (primarily internal and external fat depots) are commonly called body reserves.

Optimum management of energy reserves is critical to economic success with dairy cows. When cows are too fat or thin, they are at risk for metabolic disorders and diseases, decreased milk yield, low conception rates, and difficult calving (Ferguson and Otto, 1989). Overconditioning is expensive and can lead to calving problems and lower dry matter intake during early lactation. Conversely, thin cows may not have sufficient reserves for maximum milk production and often do not conceive in a timely manner.

The dairy cow mobilizes energy from body tissue to support energy requirements for milk production during early lactation and repletes mobilized tissue reserves during mid and late lactation for the subsequent lactation. As this is a normal physiological process that occurs in all mammals, it should be expected that all cows will mobilize energy stores in early lactation. There have been a number of experiments in which amounts of energy mobilized from tissue during early lactation were measured (Andrew et al., 1994, 1995; Komaragiri and Erdman, 1997, 1998; Chillard et al., 1991; Gibb et al., 1992). In addition, experiments with bST (Tyrrell et al., 1988; Brown et al., 1989; McGuffey et al., 1991) clearly demonstrate that the initial increase in milk production associated with bST relies on partial mobilization of energy stores. In both early lactation and during a 4- to 6-week period after bST injection, increases in DMI lag behind the increase in milk production. Under these circumstances body tissue is mobilized as a source of energy and to a lesser extent a source of protein to support nutrient requirements for milk production.

Changes in BW of cows may not reflect true changes in stores of tissue energy. In experiments where stores of body energy were measured by slaughter analysis, stores of energy differed by as much as 40 percent, and there was little or no change in BW from calving to 5 to 12 weeks postpartum (Andrew et al., 1994; Gibb et al., 1992). As feed intake increases, gastrointestinal contents (gut fill) increase. The average gut fill in dairy cows is approximately 15 percent of BW. French workers (Chillard et al., 1991) suggested a 4 kg increase in gut fill for each kilogram increase in DMI. Data from more recent experiments using both direct and indirect measurements of gut fill suggest gut fill increases 2.5 kg for each kilogram increase in dry matter intake (Komaragiri and Erdman, 1997, 1998; Gibb et al., 1992). Because tissue mobilization during early lactation occurs at the same time that feed intake is rapidly increasing, decreases in body tissue weight are masked by increases in gut fill such that changes in BW do not reflect changes in tissue weight. After peak milk production, feed intake declines and gut fill decreases, such that increases in BW underestimate true changes in body tissue weight.

The energy value of a kilogram of true body tissue that is lost or gained is dependent on the relative proportions of fat and protein in the tissue and their respective heat of combustion. On average, fat-free mass contains 72.8 percent water, 21.5 percent protein, and 5.7 percent ash (Andrew et al., 1994, 1995; Komaragiri and Erdman, 1997, 1998; Chilliard et al., 1991; Gibb et al., 1992); nearly identical to the respective values of 72.91, 21.64, and 5.34 percent reported by Reid (1955).

This committee chose to use the National Research Council (1996) body reserves model with modifications by Fox et al. (1999) to predict body composition based on body condition score (BCS; see section below) of cows of different body sizes and amounts of body reserves. Body condition score (BCS) measurements can be made readily on farms, and BCS is correlated with body fat and energy contents.

Equations relating BCS with body composition were developed from data using a nine point BCS scale (1 to 9 scoring system, BCS(9)) on 106 mature cows of diverse breed types, mature weights and BCSs. The resulting equations that describe relationships between BCS(9) and empty body percentage of fat (Equation 2-20, protein; Equation 2-21, water) and ash were linear. The BCS accounted for 65, 52, and 66 percent of the variation in body fat, body protein, and body energy, respectively between individual animals.

$$\text{Proportion of empty body fat} = 0.037683 \times \text{BCS}(9) \qquad (2\text{-}20)$$

$$\text{Proportion of empty body protein} = 0.200886 - 0.0066762 \times \text{BCS}(9) \qquad (2\text{-}21)$$

Equations 2-20 and 2-21 use BCS on a 1 to 9 scale (i.e., BCS(9)); however, a 1 to 5 scale is commonly used for dairy cattle (Wildman et al., 1982; Edmonson et al., 1989; Figure 2-2). In the model, users input BCS on a 1 to 5 scale, and the program internally converts those to the 1 to 9 scale as

$$\text{BCS}(9) = ((\text{Dairy BCS} - 1) \times 2) + 1 \qquad (2\text{-}22)$$

Equations 2-20 and 2-21 are used to estimate the composition of body tissue gain or loss, which is then used to calculate the energy supplied or required for changes in body reserves. Regression analysis on slaughter data from

| | SCORE | 1<br>Spinous processes (SP) (anatomy varies) | 2<br>Spinous to Transverse processes | 3<br>Transverse processes | 4<br>Overhanging shelf (care – rumen fill) | 5<br>Tuber coxae (hooks) & Tuber ischii (pins) | 6<br>Between pins and hooks | 7<br>Between the hooks | 8<br>Tailhead to pins (anatomy varies) |
|---|---|---|---|---|---|---|---|---|---|
| SEVERE UNDERCONDITIONING (emaciated) | 1.00 | individual processes distinct, giving a saw-tooth appearance | deep depression | very prominent, >1/2 length visible | definite shelf, gaunt, tucked | extremely sharp, no tissue cover | severe depression, devoid of flesh | severely depressed | bones very prominent with deep "V" shaped cavity under tail |
| | 1.25 | | | | | | | | |
| | 1.50 | | | | | | | | |
| | 1.75 | | | 1/2 length of process visible | | | | | |
| FRAME OBVIOUS | 2.00 | individual processes evident | obvious depression | | prominent shelf | prominent | very sunken | | bones prominent "U" shaped cavity formed under tail |
| | 2.25 | | | between 1/2 to 1/3 of processes visible | | | | | |
| | 2.50 | sharp, prominent ridge | | 1/3-1/4 visible | moderate shelf | | thin flesh covering | definite depression | first evidence of fat |
| | 2.75 | | | | | | | | |
| FRAME & COVERING WELL BALANCED | 3.00 | | smooth concave curve | <1/4 visible | slight shelf | smooth | depression | moderate depression | bones smooth, cavity under tail shallow & fatty tissue lined |
| | 3.25 | | | appears smooth, TP's just discernable | | | | | |
| | 3.50 | smooth ridge, the SP's not evident | smooth slope | distinct ridge, no individual processes discernable | | covered | slight depression | slight depression | |
| | 3.75 | | | | | | sloping | | |
| FRAME NOT AS VISIBLE AS COVERING | 4.00 | flat, no processes discernable | nearly flat | smooth, rounded edge | none | rounded with fat | | flat | bones rounded with fat and slight fat-filled depression under tail |
| | 4.25 | | | | | | flat | | |
| | 4.50 | | | edge barely discernable | | buried in fat | | | bones buried in fat, cavity filled with fat forming tissue folds |
| | 4.75 | | | | | | | | |
| SEVERE OVERCONDITIONING | 5.00 | buried in fat | rounded (convex) | buried in fat | bulging | | rounded | rounded | |

FIGURE 2-2 Body condition scoring chart adapted from Edmonson et al. (1989).

25 cows at various stages of lactation (Andrew et al., 1991) suggested a heat of combustion for body fat and protein of 9.2 and 5.57 Mcal/kg, respectively. These values are similar to the values of 9.4 and 5.55 Mcal/kg reported for growing steers (Garrett, 1987). The committee chose 9.4 and 5.55 Mcal/kg for body fat and protein. To determine the total energy contained in 1 kg of reserves, the heats of combustion are multiplied by the estimated proportions of fat and protein:

$$\text{Total reserves energy (Mcal/kg)} = \text{Proportion empty body fat} \times 9.4 + \text{proportion of empty body protein} \times 5.55 \quad (2\text{-}23)$$

The amount of energy per kilogram of BW for different BCS are shown in Table 2-4. Reserve energy when used to support milk production has an efficiency of 0.82. Therefore $NE_L$ provided by body reserves is:

$$NE_L \text{ from body reserve loss (Mcal/kg)} = \text{Reserve energy (Equation 2-23)} \times 0.82 \quad (2\text{-}24)$$

The measured efficiency of use of dietary ME for body tissue energy deposition was 0.60 percent in nonlactating cows and 0.75 in lactating cows (Moe et al., 1971). If the efficiencies of ME used for milk production and BW gain by lactating animals are 0.64 and 0.75, respectively, the amount of $NE_L$ required for 1 kg of gain in reserves during lactation is:

$$NE_L \text{ (Mcal/kg gain)} = \text{Reserve energy (Equation 2-23} \times (0.64/0.75)) \quad (2\text{-}25)$$

In nonlactating cows, the efficiency term in the previous equation is (0.64/0.60). Because digestibility is decreased when large amounts of feed are consumed by cows, the feed required for tissue gain during the dry period would be less than projected because of greater digestibility of any given diet when cows are fed at maintenance. The $NE_L$ provided by loss of reserves or needed to replenish reserves is shown in Table 2-4 for cows with different BCS.

To estimate the amount of energy provided by or required for a one-unit change in BCS, change in BW relative to change in BCS must be calculated. The mean change in empty BW (EBW) per one-unit change in BCS (5-point scale) is 13.7 percent (Fox et al., 1999). The EBW is calculated as 0.851 × shrunk BW; shrunk BW = 0.96 × BW; therefore, EBW = 0.817 × BW. The BCS 3 (5-point scale) was set as the base (1.00); the relative EBW (or BW) can be calculated at other BCS (Table 2-4). For example, a 600-kg cow with a BCS of 3 (EBW of 513 kg) would be expected to weigh 518 kg (600 × 0.863; Table 2-4) at a BCS of 2. The amount of tissue energy required per kilogram gain in EBW (Table 2-4) is calculated as the energy provided by fat and protein at the next higher BCS (weighted by EBW at next higher BCS), subtracted from the energy provided by fat and protein at the current BCS (weighted by EBW at the current BCS), divided by EBW at next higher BCS minus EBW at current BCS. To calculate energy provided per kilogram of EBW loss, the same equation is used except values at current BCS are subtracted from values at next lower BCS.

This model was validated with the data of Otto et al. (1991), as described by Fox et al. (1999). In this study, body composition and BCS of 56 Holstein cows selected to represent the range in dairy body condition scores 1 to 5 were determined. Body fat at a particular condition score in Holstein cows was predicted with an $r^2$ of 0.95 and a bias of −1.6 percent. The relationship between BW change and BCS in these Holstein cows was 84.6 kg/BCS ($r^2 = 0.96$). This value of 84.6 kg/BCS compared well to 80 kg predicted by the model and 82 kg in the data previously mentioned

TABLE 2-4 Empty Body (EB) Chemical Composition at Different Body Condition Scores (BCS), Relative EB Weight (EBW), and $NE_L$ Provided by Live Weight (LW) Loss and $NE_L$ Needed for LW Gain[a]

| | % of EB | | | | | | | |
|---|---|---|---|---|---|---|---|---|
| BCS | Fat | Protein | Ash | Water | EBW (% of BCS 3) | Energy, Mcal/kg EBW change[b] | Mcal $NE_L$/kg of LW loss[c] | Mcal $NE_L$/kg of LW gain[c] |
| 1.0 | 3.77 | 19.42 | 7.46 | 69.35 | 72.6 | 5.14 | . . . | 3.60 |
| 1.5 | 7.54 | 18.75 | 7.02 | 66.69 | 79.4 | 5.72 (5.14) | 3.44 | 4.01 |
| 2.0 | 11.30 | 18.09 | 6.58 | 64.03 | 86.3 | 6.41 (5.72) | 3.83 | 4.50 |
| 2.5 | 15.07 | 17.42 | 6.15 | 61.36 | 93.1 | 6.98 (6.41) | 4.29 | 4.90 |
| 3.0 | 18.84 | 16.75 | 5.71 | 58.70 | 100.0 | 7.61 (6.98) | 4.68 | 5.34 |
| 3.5 | 22.61 | 16.08 | 5.27 | 56.04 | 106.9 | 8.32 (7.61) | 5.10 | 5.84 |
| 4.0 | 26.38 | 15.42 | 4.83 | 53.37 | 113.7 | 8.88 (8.32) | 5.57 | 6.23 |
| 4.5 | 30.15 | 14.75 | 4.43 | 50.71 | 120.6 | 9.59 (8.88) | 5.95 | 6.73 |
| 5.0 | 33.91 | 14.08 | 3.96 | 48.05 | 127.4 | (9.59) | 6.43 | . . . |

[a]Empty body weight = 0.817 × live weight.

[b]Tissue energy contained in 1 kg of EBW gain going to next higher 0.5 BCS. Values in parentheses are tissue energy contained in 1 kg of EBW loss going to next lower 0.5 BCS.

[c]Values were calculated by converting tissue energy per kilogram of EBW into tissue energy per kilogram of BW (EBW × 0.855) and then converting to dietary $NE_L$ using an efficiency of 0.82 for converting tissue energy from live weight loss to dietary $NE_L$, and an efficiency of 1.12 for converting dietary $NE_L$ to tissue energy for live weight gain.

TABLE 2-5 Energy Provided by or Needed to Change Body Condition Score (BCS) of Cows of Different Live Weights and BCS

| | Live weight (kg) | | | | | | | |
|---|---|---|---|---|---|---|---|---|
| BCS | 400 | 450 | 500 | 550 | 600 | 650 | 700 | 750 |
| | Mcal of $NE_L$ provided by a loss of one BCS[a] | | | | | | | |
| 2 | 230 | 259 | 288 | 317 | 346 | 375 | 404 | 432 |
| 3 | 245 | 276 | 307 | 338 | 368 | 399 | 430 | 460 |
| 4 | 257 | 289 | 321 | 353 | 385 | 417 | 450 | 482 |
| 5 | 266 | 299 | 332 | 365 | 399 | 432 | 465 | 498 |
| | Mcal of $NE_L$ needed to gain one BCS[b] | | | | | | | |
| 1 | 287 | 323 | 359 | 395 | 431 | 467 | 502 | 535 |
| 2 | 298 | 335 | 372 | 410 | 447 | 484 | 522 | 559 |
| 3 | 306 | 344 | 382 | 421 | 459 | 497 | 535 | 574 |
| 4 | 312 | 351 | 390 | 429 | 468 | 507 | 546 | 585 |

[a]Represents the $NE_L$ provided by mobilization of reserves when moving to next lower score. For example, a 400-kg cow in BCS 3 will provide 245 Mcal of $NE_L$ when BCS decreases one unit.

[b]Represents the $NE_L$ required to replenish reserves when moving to the next higher score. For example a 600-kg cow in BCS 3 will require 459 Mcal of $NE_L$ to increase BCS one unit.

in this chapter. Although the evaluation strongly supports the use of this model, further validation with other data sets should be conducted.

This model predicts energy reserves to be 5.47 Mcal/kg live weight loss from BCS 3.0 to BCS 2.0. The mean value of tissue energy is 6 Mcal/kg (Gibb et al., 1992; Andrew et al., 1994; Komaragiri and Erdman, 1997; Tamminga, 1981) and that is the value used in the 1989 edition (National Research Council, 1989). The predicted energy content of weight loss ranged from 4.36 Mcal/kg at BCS 1.5 to 7.59 Mcal/kg at BCS 4.5 compared to CSIRO (1990) values of 3.0 and 7.1, respectively. Protein in the weight loss from BCS 3 to BCS 2 was predicted to be 68 g/kg, compared to 135, 138, and 160g/kg weight loss for the CSIRO (1990), AFRC (1993), and National Research Council (1989).

### *Body Condition Scoring*

Body condition scoring (BCS), although subjective in nature, is the only practical method of evaluation of body energy stores in dairy cows. In the U.S., the most common systems of BCS use a five-point scale originally proposed by Wildman et al. (1982) with a BCS of 1 being extremely thin and a score of 5 being extremely fat. This system included a combination of both visual appraisal and manual palpation to score individual cows. Edmonson et al. (1989) suggested a BCS chart system using a 5-point scale based on visual appraisal of only 8 separate body locations. Analysis of variation due to cows and to individuals assessing BCS suggested that visual appraisal of two key locations (between the hooks and between the hooks and pins) had the smallest error due to assessor and accounted for the greatest proportion of variation due to individual cows. Figure 2-2 shows the suggested BCS chart based on these two key areas.

Loss of BCS is expected during early lactation when a cow is mobilizing body fat in support of energy needs for lactation. Typical observed changes in BSC range from 0.5 to 1.0 condition score units during the first 60 days postpartum. A 1-unit decrease in BCS for a cow weighing 650 kg at calving (BCS 4) would provide 417 Mcal of $NE_L$ (Table 2-5). That amount of $NE_L$ is sufficient to support 564 kg of 4 percent fat-corrected milk.

## REFERENCES

Agricultural Research Council (ARC). 1980. The Nutrient Requirements of Ruminant Livestock. Technical Review. Farnham Royal U.K. Commonwealth Agricultural Research Bureau.

Agricultural and Food Research Council (AFRC). 1993. Energy and protein requirements of ruminants. Wallingford, U.K., CAB International.

Allen, M. S. 2000. Effects of diet on short-term regulation of feed intake by lactating dairy cattle. J. Dairy Sci. 83:1598–1624.

Andrew, S. M., H. F. Tyrrell, C. K. Reynolds, and R. A. Erdman. 1991. Net energy for lactation of calcium salts of long-chain fatty acids for cows fed silage-based diets. J. Dairy Sci. 74:2588–2600.

Andrew, S. M., R. A. Erdman, and D. R. Waldo. 1995. Prediction of body composition from deuterium oxide and urea dilution in dairy cows at three physiological stages. J. Dairy Sci. 78:1083–1095.

Andrew, S. M., D. R. Waldo, and R. A. Erdman. 1994. Direct analysis of body composition of dairy cows at three physiological stages. J. Dairy Sci. 77:3022–3033.

Baldwin, R. L. 1968. Estimation of theoretical calorific relationships as a teaching technique. J. Dairy Sci. 51: 104.

Baldwin, R. L., J. France, and M. Gill. 1987. Metabolism of the cow 1. Animal elements of a mechanistic model. J. Dairy Res. 54:77–105.

Bell, A. W., R. Slepetis, and R. A. Ehrhardt. 1995. Growth and accretion of energy and protein in the gravid uterus during late pregnancy in Holstein cows. J. Dairy Sci. 78:1954–1961.

Bellows, R. A., R. E. Short, and R. B. Staigmiller. 1994. Exercise and induced-parturition effects on dystocia and rebreeding in beef cattle. J. Anim. Sci. 72:1667–1674.

Brown, L. D. 1966. Influence of intake on feed utilization. J. Dairy Sci. 49:223–230.

Brown, D. L., S. J. Taylor, E. J. DePeters, and R. L. Baldwin. 1989. Influence of sometribove, USAN (recombinant methionyl bovine somatotropin) on body composition of lactating cattle. J. Nutr. 119:633–638.

Chillard, Y., M. Cisse, R. LeFaivre, and B. Remond. 1991. Body composition of dairy cows according to lactation stage, somatotropin treatment, and concentrate supplementation. J. Dairy Sci. 74:3103–3116.

Commonwealth Scientific and Industrial Research Organization (CSIRO). 1990. Feeding Standards for Australian Livestock: Ruminants. East Melbourne, Victoria, Australia. CSIRO Publications.

Colucci, P. E., L. E. Chase, and P. J. Van Soest. 1982. Feed intake, digestibility, and rate of particulate passage in dairy cattle. J. Dairy Sci. 65:1445–1456.

Coulon, J. B., P. Pradel, T. Cochard, and B. Poutrel. 1998. Effect of extreme walking conditions for dairy cows on milk yield, chemical composition, and somatic cell count. J. Dairy Sci. 81:994–1003.

Crampton, E. W., L. E. Lloyd, and V. G. MacKay. 1957. The calorie value of TDN. J. Anim. Sci. 16:541–552.

Dado, R. G., D. R. Mertens, and G. E. Shook. 1993. Metabolizable energy and absorbed protein requirements for milk component production. J. Dairy Sci. 76:1575–1588.

DePeters, E. J., J. D. Ferguson, and L. D. Baker. 1992. Nonprotein nitrogen and protein distribution in the milk of cows. J. Dairy Sci. 75:3192–3209.

Dhiman, T. R., J. Kleinmans, N. J. Tessmann, H. D. Radloff, and L. D. Satter. 1995. Digestion and energy balance in lactating dairy cows fed varying ratios of alfalfa silage and grain. J. Dairy Sci. 78:330–341.

Edmonson, A. J., I. J. Lean, L. D. Weaver, T. Farver, and G. Webster. 1989. A body condition scoring chart for Holstein dairy cows. J. Dairy Sci. 72:68–78.

Ferguson, J. D., and K. A. Otto. 1989. Managing body condition in cows. Proc. Cornell Nutr. Conf. Feed Manuf. Conf. pp. 75–87.

Ferrell, C. L., W. N. Garrett, N. Hinman, and G. Grichting. 1976. Energy utilization by pregnant and nonpregnant heifers. J. Anim. Sci. 42:937–950.

Flatt, W. P., C. E. Coppock, and L. A. Moore. 1965. Energy balance studies with dry, non-pregnant dairy cows consuming pelleted forages. Proc. 3rd Symp. Energy Metab. on Farm Anim. EAAP Publ. 11:131.

Fox, D. G., and T. P. Tylutki. 1998. Accounting for the effects of environment on the nutrient requirements of dairy cattle. J. Dairy Sci. 81:3085–3095.

Fox, D. G., M. E. Van Amburgh, and T. P. Tylutki. 1999. Predicting requirements for growth, maturity, and body reserves in dairy cattle. J. Dairy Sci. 82:1968–1977.

Gaines, 1928.

Garrett, W. N. 1980. Energy utilization by growing cattle as determined by 72 comparative slaughter experiments. Energy Metab. Proc. Symp. 26:3–7.

Garrett, W. N. 1987. Relationship between energy metabolism and the amount of protein and fat deposited in growing cattle. Page 98 *in* Energy Metabolism of Farm Animals. P. W. Moe, H. F. Tyrrell, and P. J. Reynolds, ed. Eur. Assoc. Anim. Prod. Publ. No. 32. Rowman and Littlefield, Totowa, NJ.

Gibb, M. J., W. E. Irvings, M. S. Dhanoa, and J. D. Sutton. 1992. Changes in body components of autumn-calving Holstein Friesian cows over the first 29 weeks of lactation. Anim. Prod. 55:339–360.

Grummer, R. R. 1988. Influence of prilled fat and calcium salt of palm oil fatty acids on ruminal fermentation and nutrient digestibility. J. Dairy Sci. 7111–7123.

Havstad, K. M., and J. C. Malechek. 1982. Energy expenditure by heifers grazing crested wheatgrass of diminishing availability. J. Range Management 35:447–450.

Holmes, C., N. A. McLean, and K. J. Lockyer. 1978. Changes in the rate of heat production of calves during grazing and eating. New Zealand J. Agr. Res. 21:107–112.

Kennedy, P. M., R. J. Christopherson, and L. P. Milligan. 1976. The effect of cold exposure of sheep on digestion, rumen turnover time, and efficiency of microbial synthesis. Br. J. Nutr. 36:231.

Komaragiri, M., and R. A. Erdman. 1997. Factors affecting tissue mobilization in early lactation dairy cows: 1. Effect of dietary protein. J. Dairy Sci. 80:929–937.

Komaragiri, M., and R. A. Erdman. 1998. Factors affecting tissue mobilization in early lactation dairy cows: 2. Effect of dietary fat. J. Dairy Sci. 81:169–175.

Maynard, L. A., J. K. Loosli, H. F. Hintz, and R. G. Warner. 1979. Animal Nutrition. 7th. McGraw-Hill, Inc., New York, NY.

McGuffey, R. K., R. P. Basson, and T. E. Spike. 1991. Lactation response and body composition of cows receiving somatotropin and three ratios of forage to concentrate. J. Dairy Sci. 74:3095–3102.

Mertens, D. R., and R. G. Dado. 1993. System of equations for fulfilling net energy and absorbed protein requirements for milk component production. J. Dairy Sci. 76:3464–3478.

Moe, P. W., J. T. Reid, and H. F. Tyrrell. 1965. Effect of level of intake on digestibility of dietary energy by high producing cows. J. Dairy Sci. 48:1053.

Moe, P. W., and H. F. Tyrrell. 1972. The net energy value of feeds for lactation. J. Dairy Sci. 55:945–958.

Moe, P. W., H. F. Tyrrell, and W. P. Flatt. 1970. Partial efficiency of energy use for maintenance, lactation, body gain, and gestation in the dairy cow. Proc. 4th Symp. Energy Metab. EAAP Publ. 13:65.

Moe, P. W., H. F. Tyrrell, and W. P. Flatt. 1971. Energetics of body tissue mobilization. J. Dairy Sci. 54:548.

National Research Council. 1978. Nutrient Requirements of Dairy Cattle. (5th Rev. Ed.) Washington, D.C.: National Academy Press.

National Research Council. 1981. Effect of Environment on Nutrient Requirements of Domestic Animals. Washington, D.C.: National Academy Press.

National Research Council. 1989. Nutrient Requirements of Dairy Cattle (6th Rev. Ed.) Washington, D.C.: National Academy Press.

National Research Council. 1996. Nutrient Requirement of Beef Cattle (7th Rev. Ed.) Washington, D.C.: National Academy Press.

Otto, K. A., J. D. Ferguson, D. G. Fox, and C. J. Sniffen. 1991. Relationship between body condition score and composition of 9-10-11 rib tissue in Holstein dairy cows. J. Dairy Sci. 74:852–859.

Palmquist, D. L. 1991. Influence of source and amount of dietary fat on digestibility in lactating cows. J. Dairy Sci. 74:1354–1360.

Romo, G. A., D. P. Casper, R. A. Erdman, and B. B. Teter. 1996. Abomasal infusion of cis or trans fatty acid isomers and energy metabolism of lactating dairy cows. J. Dairy Sci. 79:2005–2015.

Swift, B. W. 1957. The caloric value of TDN. J. Anim. Sci. 16:1055–059.

Tamminga, S. S. 1981. Page 123 *in* Nitrogen and Amino Acid Metabolism in Dairy Cows. M.S. Thesis, Wageningen Agric. Univ., Wageningen, The Netherlands.

Tyrrell, H. F., and P. W. Moe. 1972. Net energy values for lactation of a high and low concentrate ration containing corn silage. J. Dairy Sci. 55:1106–1112.

Tyrrell, H. F., and P. W. Moe. 1974. Energy value of a corn and a barley ration for lactation. J. Dairy Sci. 57:451–458.

Tyrrell, H. F., and P. W. Moe. 1975. Effect of intake on digestive efficiency. J. Dairy Sci. 58:1151–1163.

Tyrrell, H. F., and J. T. Reid. 1965. Prediction of the energy value of cow's milk. J. Dairy Sci. 48:1215–1223.

Tyrrell, H. F., A. C. G. Brown, P. J. Reynolds, G. L. Haaland, D. E. Bauman, C. J. Peel, and W. D. Steinhour. 1988. Effect of bovine somatotropin and metabolism of lactating dairy cows: energy and nitrogen utilization as determined by respiration calorimetry. J. Nutr. 118:1024–1030.

Tyrrell, H. F., C. K. Reynolds, and H. D. Baxter. 1991. Utilization of dietary energy by Jersey compared to Holstein cows during the lactation cycle. Proc. 12th Symp. Energy Metab. on Farm Anim. EAAP Publ. 58.

Tyrrell, H. F., and G. A. Varga. 1987. Energy value for lactation of rations containing ground whole ear maize or maize meal both conserved dry or ensiled at high moisture. Eur. Assoc. Anim. Prod. 32:308–309.

Vandehaar, M. 1998. Efficiency of nutrient use and relationship to profitability on dairy farms. J. Dairy Sci. 81:272–282.

Van Es, A. J. H. 1961. Between animal variation in the amount of energy required for the maintenance of cows. Thesis. Wageningen, The Netherlands.

Van Soest, P. J. 1982. Nutritional Ecology of the Ruminant. O & B Books, Inc., Corvalis, OR.

Vermorel, M., and J. B. Coulon. 1998. Comparison of the National Research Council energy system for lactating cows with four European systems. J. Dairy Sci. 81:846–855.

Wagner, D. G., and J. K. Loosli. 1967. Studies on the energy requirements of High-producing cows. Memoir 400, Cornell Univ. Agr. Exp. Sta.

Weiss, W. P. 1998. Estimating the available energy content of feeds for dairy cattle. J. Dairy Sci. 81:830–839.

Weiss, W. P., H. R. Conrad, and N. R. S. Pierre. 1992. A theoretically-based model for predicting total digestible nutrient values of forages and concentrates. Anim. Feed Sci. Technol. 39:95–110.

West, J. W. 1994. Interactions of energy and bovine somatotropin with heat stress. J. Dairy Sci. 77:2091–2102.

Wildman, E. E., G. M. Jones, P. E. Wagner, R. L. Boman, H. F. Troutt, Jr., and T. N. Lesch. 1982. A dairy cow body condition scoring system and its relationship to standard production characteristics. J. Dairy Sci. 65:495–501.

Wilkerson, V. A., and B. P. Glenn. 1997. Energy and nitrogen balance in lactating cows fed diets containing dry or high moisture corn in either rolled or ground form. J. Dairy Sci. 80:2487–2496.

Young, B. W. 1976. Effects of cold environments on nutrient requirements of ruminants. Pp. 491–496 in Proc. 1st Int. Symposium on Feed Composition, Animal Nutrient Requirements, and Computerization of Diets, P. V. Fonnesbeck, L. F. Harris, and L. C. Kearl, eds. Logan: Utah State University.

# 3 Fat

Fat is typically fed to increase the energy density of the diet, but fat supplementation has other potential benefits, such as increased absorption of fat-soluble nutrients and reduced dustiness of feed. Fat is usually used as a generic term to describe compounds that have a high content of long-chain fatty acids (FAs) including triglycerides, phospholipids, nonesterified FAs, and salts of long-chain FAs. Long-chain FAs are the energy-rich moiety of fats. Various forms of fat are fed to dairy cattle, including oilseeds, animal and animal-vegetable blends, dry-granular fats, and "protected" fats. Oilseeds contain mostly triglycerides that are rich in unsaturated FAs. Animal and animal-vegetable blends can be made up of triglycerides, free FAs, or both and have an unsaturated to saturated fatty acid ratio greater than or equal to 1:1. Dry-granular fats are often referred to as ruminally inert fats, because they have been manufactured to have minimal effects on ruminal fermentation. Protected fats have been encapsulated in some manner, so ruminal microorganisms are not affected by them; the types of fat and encapsulation process vary.

## DIGESTION AND ABSORPTION

For an excellent review of lipid digestion and absorption in ruminants see Noble (1981) and Jenkins (1993). Esterified FAs, mainly triglyceride, are rapidly hydrolyzed to the free form by lipolytic microorganisms within the rumen. Following hydrolysis, unsaturated FAs are hydrogenated by ruminal microorganisms, but the extent of hydrogenation is dependent on the degree of unsaturation of FAs and the level and frequency of feeding. Estimates for ruminal hydrogenation of polyunsaturated fatty acids (PUFAs) range from 60 to 90 percent (Bickerstaffe et al., 1972; Mattos and Palmquist, 1977). Biohydrogenation of supplemental unsaturated FAs may be as low as 30 to 40 percent if the FAs are fed as calcium salts (Klusmeyer and Clark, 1991). Because of hydrogenation in the rumen, C18:0 and various isomers of C18:1 are the major FAs leaving the rumen. The generation time for bacteria that are able to degrade long-chain FAs is relatively long precluding substantial inhabitation of the rumen. Consequently, little degradation of long-chain FAs occurs in the rumen. Regression of dietary lipid (measured as fatty acid or ether extract) flow to the duodenum (total lipid flow minus estimate of microbial lipid flow) vs. lipid intake revealed a slope of 0.92 indicating an 8 percent loss of lipid in the rumen (Jenkins, 1993). Digestion coefficients for total FAs within the rumen are negative, which reflects microbial synthesis of FAs. The majority of FAs synthesized by rumen microbes are incorporated into phospholipids. Jenkins (1993) estimated microbial lipid synthesis to be 15 g/kg of lipid-free organic matter digested in the rumen. Approximately 85 to 90 percent of the FAs leaving the rumen are free FAs, and approximately 10 to 15 percent are microbial phospholipids. Since FAs are hydrophobic, they associate with particulate matter and pass to the lower gut.

Although little triglyceride reaches the small intestine of ruminants, bile and pancreatic lipase are required for lipid absorption. If triglycerides are fed at moderate levels in a form that protects them from hydrolysis (e.g., formaldehyde protected casein-fat emulsion), there appears to be sufficient lipase for triglyceride hydrolysis (Noble, 1981). However, pancreatic lipase does not appear to be inducible (Johnson et al., 1974) and may become limiting if large quantities of triglyceride are presented to the small intestine. In the absence of substantial amounts of monoglyceride reaching the small intestine, ruminants are believed to be dependant on lysolecithin and the monounsaturate, oleic acid, for fatty acid emulsification. Lysolecithin is formed by pancreatic phospholipase activity on lecithin that may be of microbial or hepatic origin. Monounsaturated fatty acid is predominantly from digesta leaving the rumen. Therefore, it is critical that a portion of dietary unsaturated fatty acids avoid complete hydrogenation by ruminal organisms. Fatty acid emulsification and micelle formation in the small intestine is essential for the efficient absorption of fat.

## DIGESTIBILITY AND ENERGY VALUE OF FATS

Energy values of the fat supplements listed in Table 2-3 were determined as described in Chapter 2. The variability in $NE_L$ content among fat supplements is a function primarily of the long-chain FA content and the digestibility of the long-chain FAs. Digestibility of FAs can be influenced by dry matter (DM) intake, amount of fat consumed, characteristics of fat in the basal diet, and characteristics of the supplemental fat. Degree of unsaturation is probably the most important characteristic that influences digestion (Grummer, 1995). Fatty acid composition and IV values of selected fat sources are listed in Table 3-1.

Iodine value is an indicator of the degree of unsaturation: the higher the IV, the greater the content of unsaturated fatty acids in the fat. Digestibility may decrease if the iodine value (IV) is below 45 (Firkins and Eastridge, 1994). Maximal digestibility of fats with an IV greater than 40 was 89 percent, compared with 74 percent for fats with an IV less than 40 (Jenkins, 1994). Saturated FAs are less digestible than unsaturated FAs, and the difference is greatest when predominantly saturated fats are supplemented (Børsting et al., 1992). That indicates that unsaturated FAs may have a synergistic effect on the digestibility of saturated FAs.

Increasing FA chain length may also increase digestibility, but the effects appear to be more subtle than the effects of degree of unsaturation (Grummer, 1995). There are probably interactions between degree of unsaturation and chain length. Firkins and Eastridge (1994) reported that increasing the C16:C18 ratio has a greater effect on digestion as IV increases. Digestibility in the intestine is inversely related to the melting point of the FA, which probably influences micelle formation and movement of fatty acids through the unstirred water layer adjacent to the microvilli of the small intestine.

Decreasing particle size of dry granular fats may increase digestibility, but responses have tended to be small and not statistically significant. A summary of trials (Firkins and Eastridge, 1994) indicated that mean FA digestibility of prilled (n = 8) and flaked (n = 5) hydrogenated tallow was 77 and 69 percent, respectively.

Fat structure—the form in which FAs are fed—may have modest effects on digestibility. A review of the literature (Firkins and Eastridge, 1994) indicated that FA digestibility of diets containing triglyceride prills or FA prills was 77 or 73 percent of control diets without added fat. However, effects of fat structure might have been confounded: mean IV and C16:18 ratio were 20.7 and 0.41 for triglyceride prills and 11.2 and 0.45 for FA prills. If FAs are fed as a salt, digestibility will be determined by

TABLE 3-1 Fatty Acid Composition and Iodine Values of Fats and Oils[a]

| Type of Fat | Reference[b] | C14:0 | C16:0 | C16:1 | C18:0 | C18:1 | C18:2 | C18:3 | Other Fatty Acids | Iodine Value |
|---|---|---|---|---|---|---|---|---|---|---|
| *Granular fats:* | | | | | | | | | | |
| Calcium salt palm oil FAs | 1 | 1.3 | 48.6 | 1.1 | 4.1 | 36.5 | 7.8 | 0.3 | 0.2 | 49 |
| Hydrolyzed tallow FAs | 1 | 2.4 | 39.7 | 0.7 | 42.7 | 10.9 | 1.0 | — | 2.6 | 12 |
| Partially hydrogenated tallow[c] | 1 | 1.4–2.4 | 25.4–25.8 | 0.2–0.7 | 37.2–52.6 | 13.8–31.9 | 0–0.9 | 0.1–0.2 | 3.2–4.3 | 14–31 |
| *Animal and animal-vegetable blends:* | | | | | | | | | | |
| Tallow | 1, 2, 3 | 3.0 | 24.5 | 3.7 | 19.3 | 40.9 | 3.2 | 0.7 | 4.9 | 48 |
| Choice white grease | 1, 2 | 1.9 | 23.4 | 4.3 | 13.3 | 43.4 | 10.9 | 1.3 | 1.5 | 62 |
| Yellow grease | 1, 2 | 1.8 | 22.1 | 3.5 | 11.5 | 43.7 | 14.6 | 0.9 | 1.9 | 72 |
| Poultry fat | 1, 2 | 1.0 | 22.1 | 7.2 | 6.5 | 43.0 | 18.5 | 0.9 | 0.7 | 82 |
| Fish oil, menhaden[d] | 3 | 8.0 | 15.1 | 10.5 | 3.8 | 14.5 | 2.2 | 1.5 | 44.5 | 31 |
| Fish oil, herring[d] | 3 | 7.2 | 11.7 | 9.6 | 0.8 | 12.0 | 1.1 | 0.8 | 56.8 | 25 |
| *Vegetable oils:* | | | | | | | | | | |
| Canola (rapeseed) | 3 | — | 4.8 | 0.5 | 1.6 | 53.8 | 22.1 | 11.1 | 6.1 | 119 |
| Corn | 3 | 0.0 | 10.9 | — | 1.8 | 24.2 | 58.0 | 0.7 | 4.4 | 126 |
| Cottonseed | 3 | 0.8 | 22.7 | 0.8 | 2.3 | 17.0 | 51.5 | 0.2 | 4.7 | 107 |
| Linseed | 3 | — | 5.3 | — | 4.1 | 20.2 | 12.7 | 53.3 | 4.4 | 185 |
| Palm | 3 | 1.0 | 43.5 | 0.3 | 4.3 | 36.6 | 9.1 | 0.2 | 5.0 | 50 |
| Peanut | 3 | 0.1 | 9.5 | 0.1 | 2.2 | 44.8 | 32.0 | — | 11.3 | 95 |
| Safflower | 3 | 0.1 | 6.2 | 0.4 | 2.2 | 11.7 | 74.1 | 0.4 | 4.9 | 145 |
| Sesame | 3 | — | 8.9 | 0.2 | 4.8 | 39.3 | 41.3 | 0.3 | 5.2 | 111 |
| Soybean | 3 | 0.1 | 10.3 | 0.2 | 3.8 | 22.8 | 51.0 | 6.8 | 5.0 | 131 |
| Sunflower | 3 | — | 5.4 | 0.2 | 3.5 | 45.3 | 39.8 | 0.2 | 5.6 | 113 |

[a] Selected FAs are expressed as a percent of total FAs (g/100 g × 100).
[b] 1, scientific literature; 2, rendering industry, including Pearl (1995); 3, US Department of Agriculture *Food Composition Standard Release 12* (1998).
[c] Composition of partially hydrogenated tallow is reported as a range because degree of hydrogenation varies considerably among products.
[d] Other fatty acids consist predominantly of polyunsaturated fatty acids greater than 18 carbons in length.

fatty acid profile, because the salts are dissociated in the acidic abomasum and duodenum (Sukhija and Palmquist, 1990).

Concentration of fat in the diet also can affect postruminal fat digestion. FA digestibility decreased by 2.2 percent for each 100 g of FA intake as intake of supplemental fat increased from 200 to 1400 g/d (Palmquist, 1991). True FA digestibility of tallow was curvilinear with diminishing digestibility as FA intake increased from 200 to 900 g/d (Weisbjerg et al., 1992). Apparent digestibility increased when supplemental fat was increased from 0 to 3 percent of (DM) but decreased when fat was increased from 3 to 6 percent of DM (Wu et al., 1991). The increase in digestibility of fat at low intakes might indicate that supplemental fat was more digestible than fat in the basal diet or that endogenous fat was being diluted. A summary of 20 studies indicated that the rate of decline in digestibility of fat as fat intake increases is greater for fats with an IV greater than 40 than for fats with an IV less than 40 (Jenkins, 1994).

## EFFECTS OF FAT ON RUMINAL FERMENTATION

Although increasing the degree of unsaturation increases digestibility of FAs, it also increases the likelihood that ruminal fermentation will be adversely affected (Jenkins, 1993). Fat sources with high amounts of polyunsaturated fatty acids include fish oils and some vegetable oils (Table 3-1). Reductions in DM intake, milk fat percentage, and ruminal fiber digestion are indicators that fermentation has been altered. The rate at which unsaturated FAs are released from feeds and exposed to ruminal microorganisms determines whether rumen fermentation is affected. Ruminal microorganisms hydrogenate unsaturated FAs. If the microbial capacity to saturate FAs is exceeded, unsaturated FAs can accumulate and interfere with fermentation. Feeding polyunsaturated oils as part of a whole-oilseed diet has minimal effects on fermentation (Knapp et al., 1991; DePeters et al., 1987), probably because the oil is released slowly from the seed to ruminal fluid. Extrusion of oilseeds releases some of the oil, so the rate of exposure of microorganisms to oil might be sufficient to influence their metabolism. Polyunsaturated fats can be encapsulated to minimize interaction of fat with microorganism. Mineral salts of long-chain FAs and hydrogenated fatty acids are examples of dry granular fats that inhibit fermentation less than unsaturated FAs, probably because they have lower solubility in an aqueous medium. Tallow and yellow grease might be more likely than oilseeds or dry granular fats to inhibit rumen fermentation. However, up to 3 percent of DM as tallow or yellow grease in totally mixed diets has been fed without altering feed intake, milk fat percentage, or fermentation (DePeters et al., 1987; Knapp et al., 1991). Effects of oilseeds, tallow or yellow grease on fermentation can vary depending on the basal diet. Adverse effects might be more likely when diets based on corn silage (Smith et al., 1993) or low forage (Grant and Weidner, 1992) are fed.

## UTILIZATION OF FAT IN CALF DIETS

See Chapters 10 and 11 on calf and heifer replacement nutrition for discussions of fat in calf and heifer diets.

## FAT IN LACTATION DIETS

Milk-yield response to supplemental fat can be influenced by several factors, including basal diet, stage of lactation, energy balance, fat composition, and amount of supplemental fat. If fat supplementation is begun during the early postpartum period, there can be a lag before a milk response (Jerred et al., 1990; Schingoethe and Casper, 1991). An extensive summary by Chilliard (1993) indicated that the average fat-corrected milk response to fat supplementation (average increase 4.5 percent ether extract) during early lactation (beginning before 4 weeks and ending before 11 weeks postpartum) was 0.31 kg/d and not significantly different from controls. Average fat-corrected milk response to fat supplementation during peak lactation (beginning before 8 weeks and ending at 11–24 weeks postartum; average increase, 3.6 percent ether extract) or middle to late lactation (beginning after 7 weeks postpartum and lasting longer than 5 weeks; average increase, 3.4 percent ether extract) was 0.72 or 0.65 kg/d; the former was significantly different from controls. Another summary (Grummer, 1994) indicated that average fat-corrected milk response to supplementation with dry granular fats (average supplementation 2.3 percent of DM) vs. tallow or vegetable oils (average supplementation 2.65 percent of DM) when diets already contained whole oilseeds was 1.1 vs. 0.1 kg/d, respectively. Average milk production of cows in both summaries was less than 35 kg/d. Milk-yield responses to supplemental fat in cows that produce more than 40 kg/d are not well defined.

Milk-yield response to supplemental fat is curvilinear; the response diminishes as supplemental fat in the diet increases (Palmquist, 1983; Jenkins, 1994). Kronfeld (1976) indicated that milk production reaches its maximal efficiency when FAs constitute 16 percent of metabolizable energy. That equates to about 600–700 g of supplemental fat per day (Jenkins, 1997). A review of the literature indicated that maximal milk-yield responses to dietary fat rarely exceed 3.5 kg of FCM per day. About 700 g of supplemental fat is required to support production of 3.5 kg of FCM, assuming that fat is 80 percent digestible and uptake of absorbed FAs by the mammary gland is 75 percent (Jenkins, 1997). Assuming 23 kg of DM intake, 700 g of supplemental fat equates to about 3 percent of DM.

Supplemental fat has increased milk yield in many studies; however, responses have been variable. Some of the variation may be due to depression of feed intake when feeding supplemental fat. If feed intake is depressed sufficiently, total energy intake by the cow may not be increased. Mechanisms by which fat reduces feed intake are not known. Potential factors were recently reviewed (Allen, 2000) and include effects on feed intake and gut motility, acceptability of diets supplemented with fat, release of gut hormones, and oxidation of fat by the liver. Sanchez et al. (1998) speculated that insufficient metabolizable protein may account for feed intake depression when feeding fat. However, an extensive summary of the literature indicated that crude protein content of the diet does not appear to have any appreciable effect on intake responses to supplemental fat (Allen, 2000). The same review yielded a comparison among oilseeds, unprocessed fat (tallow and grease), hydrogenated FAs and triglycerides, and calcium salts of FAs on their effects on dry matter intake (Allen, 2000). Calcium salts of FAs decreased dry matter intake by 2.5 percent for each percentage unit in the diet above control. Unprocessed fat also decreased intake, but the decrease was approximately 50 percent of that observed with calcium salts of FAs. Added hydrogenated FAs and triglyceride did not decrease dry matter intake. Feeding oilseeds resulted in a quadratic effect with minimum dry matter intake occurring at 2 percent added fatty acid. The magnitude of depression when feeding oilseeds was less than that when feeding calcium salts of FAs. Differences among fat sources could be due to acceptability, fatty acid chain length or degree of saturation, or form (free fatty acid, triglyceride, or salt). Several studies have suggested that unsaturated FAs are more likely to depress feed intake than saturated FAs (Drackley et al., 1992; Christensen et al., 1994; Firkins and Eastridge, 1994; Bremmer et al., 1998). Dietary unsaturated FAs may be hydrogenated in the rumen. Extent of hydrogenation varies among fat sources; therefore, the profile of FAs reaching the duodenum should be better than the profile of FAs consumed for predicting effects on feed intake. Top-dressed calcium salts of palm oil FAs were less acceptable than tallow, sodium alginate encapsulated tallow, or prilled long-chain FAs (Grummer et al., 1990). Differences were no longer significant when fats were mixed with grain or when cows were allowed an adaptation period.

The influence of supplemental fat on milk fat percentage is variable and depends on fat composition and the amount fed. In general, encapsulated fats, FAs fed as calcium salts, and saturated fats either have no effect on or increase milk fat percentage (Sutton, 1989; DePeters, 1993). As the amount of unsaturated FAs fed in free or esterified form increases, the likelihood of milk-fat depression increases. Greater formation of trans-FAs during microbial hydrogenation of polyunsaturated FAs might negatively affect mammary lipid synthesis (See Chapter 9; Davis and Brown, 1970; Gaynor et al., 1994).

Feeding supplemental fat decreases milk protein percentage and the effect diminishes slightly as the amount of supplemental fat increases (for example, $y = 101.1 - 0.6381x + 0.0141x^2$, where y = milk protein concentration [(treated/control, %) × 100] and x = total dietary fat, %); Wu and Huber, 1994). Casein is the milk nitrogen fraction that is most depressed (DePeters and Cant, 1992). Although milk protein percentage is usually depressed, total protein production usually remains constant or is increased. Of 83 treatment comparisons (fat supplementation vs. control) summarized by Wu and Huber (1994), milk protein production was unchanged or increased in 65 comparisons and decreased in 26. However, in 15 of the 26 comparisons in which protein production was decreased, milk production also was decreased. Why milk protein production does not increase at a similar rate as milk volume during fat supplementation has not been determined.

Fat supplementation can positively influence reproductive performance of dairy cows. A summary of 20 studies indicated that first-service conception rate or overall conception rate was increased in 11 of the studies (Staples et al., 1998). The mean increase was 17 percentage units for all studies. Three studies indicated a negative influence of supplemental fat on reproduction, but the effects were confounded by substantial increases in milk production. Feeding fat increases follicle numbers and the size of the dominant follicle. It has not been determined whether those changes in follicular dynamics have a positive effect on reproductive performance. Potential mechanisms by which fat influences reproduction include amelioration of negative energy balance, enhancement of follicular development via changes in insulin status, stimulation of progesterone synthesis, and modification of the production and release of prostaglandin $F_{2a}$, which influences the persistence of the corpus luteum (Staples et al., 1998). In the 20 studies reviewed by Staples et al. (1998), there was little evidence of a relationship between change in energy status and change in conception rate. Likewise, the effects of fat on insulin have not been consistent, although, the trend is toward a reduction. How a reduction in plasma insulin could benefit reproduction has not been determined. Fat supplementation consistently increases plasma progesterone concentration, but the change might be because of depressed clearance rather than increased production (Hawkins et al., 1995). Staples et al. (1998) proposed that feeding fats that are rich in linoleic acid suppresses prostaglandin $F_{2\alpha}$ and prevents regression of the corpus luteum.

In most situations, total dietary fat should not exceed 6–7 percent of dietary DM. Feeding higher concentrations of fat can result in reduced DM intake, even if the fat has minimal effects on ruminal fermentation (Schauff and Clark, 1992). A reduction in DM intake will negate part or all of the advantage of using fat to increase dietary energy density and can limit milk-production responses. Optimal amounts of fat to include in dairy cattle diets will depend on numerous factors, including type of fat, feeds making up the basal diet, stage of lactation, environment, level of milk production, and feeding management. Feeding less than 6 percent total dietary fat might be prudent during early lactation, when feed-intake depression due to fat supplementation has been observed (Jerred et al., 1990; Chilliard, 1993). Mixtures of cereal grains and forages usually contain about 3 percent fat. Therefore, up to 3 or 4 percent of dietary DM can come from supplemental fat. Oilseeds and animal or animal-vegetable blends are acceptable fat supplements; however, partial substitution with ruminally inert fats might be warranted if the previously mentioned fat supplements are adversely affecting ruminal fermentation, milk fat percentage, or DM intake.

Feeding supplemental fat to ruminants has reduced digestibility of calcium, magnesium, or both in some studies (Tillman and Brethour, 1958; Steele, 1983; Palmquist and Conrad, 1978; Rahnema et al., 1994, Zinn and Shen, 1996). FAs can form insoluble soaps with cations in the rumen, distal small intestine, and large intestine. Soap formation is favored as pH increases (Sukhija and Palmquist, 1990). Soap formation can reduce magnesium absorption from the rumen and calcium absorption from the intestine. Consequently, concentrations of dietary calcium and magnesium higher than those listed in tables in Chapter 14 might be warranted when supplemental fat is fed. However, interactions between diet and cation absorption when fat is fed have not been adequately described, and research to identify optimal amounts of dietary calcium and magnesium to feed when supplementing fat to the diet has not been conducted.

## REFERENCES


Allen, M. S. 2000. Effects of diet on short-term regulation of feed intake by lactating dairy cattle. J. Dairy Sci. 83:1958–1624.

Bickerstaffe, R., D. E. Noakes, and E. F. Annison. 1972. Quantitative aspects of fatty acid biohydrogenation, absorption and transfer of milk fat in the lactating goat, with special reference to the cis- and trans-isomers of octadecenoate and linoleate. Biochem. J. 120:607–609.

Borsting, C. F., M. R. Weisbjerg, and T. Hvelplund. 1992. Fatty acid digestibility in lactating cows fed increasing amounts of protected vegetable oil, fish oil, or saturated fat. Acta Agric. Scand., Sect. A, Animal Sci. 42:148–156.

Bremmer, D. R., L. D. Ruppert, J. H. Clark, and J. K. Drackley. 1998. Effects of chain length and unsaturation of fatty acid mixtures infused into the abomasum of lactating dairy cows. J. Dairy Sci. 81:176–188.

Chilliard, Y. 1993. Dietary fat and adipose tissue metabolism in ruminants, pigs, and rodents: a review. J. Dairy Sci. 76:3897–3931.

Christensen, R. A., J. K. Drackley, D. W. LaCount, and J. H. Clark. 1994. Infusion of four long-chain fatty acid mixtures into the abomasum of lactating dairy cows. J. Dairy Sci. 77:1052–1069.

Davis, C. L., and R. E. Brown. 1970. Low-fat milk syndrome. Pp. 545–565 in Physiology of Digestion and Metabolism in the Ruminant. A. T. Phillipson, ed. Newcastle upon Tyne: Oriel Press Limited.

DePeters, E. J. 1993. Influence of feeding fat to dairy cows on milk composition. Pp. 199–215 in Proc. Cornell Nutr. Conf. for Feed Manufacturers. Cornell University, Ithaca, NY.

DePeters, E. J., and J. P. Cant. 1992. Nutritional factors influencing the nitrogen composition of bovine milk: a review. J. Dairy Sci. 75:2043–2070.

DePeters, E. J., S. J. Taylor, C. M. Finley, and T. R. Famula. 1987. Dietary fat and nitrogen composition of milk from lactating cows. J. Dairy Sci. 70:1192–1201.

Drackley, J. K., T. H. Klusemeyer, A. M. Trusk, and J. H. Clark. 1992. Infusion of long-chain fatty acids varying in saturation and chain length into the abomasum of lactating dairy cows. J. Dairy Sci. 75:1517–1526.

Firkins, J. L., and M. L. Eastridge. 1994. Assessment of the effects of iodine value on fatty acid digestibility, feed intake, and milk production. J. Dairy Sci. 77:2357–2366.

Gaynor, P. J., R. A. Erdman, B. B. Teter, J. Sampugna, A. V. Capuco, D. R. Waldo, and M. Hamosh. 1994. Milk fat yield and composition during abomasal infusion of cis or trans octadecenoates in Holstein cows. J. Dairy Sci. 77:157–165.

Grant, R. J., and S. J. Weidner. 1992. Effect of fat from whole soybeans on performance of dairy cows fed rations differing in fiber level and particle size. J. Dairy Sci. 75:2742–2751.

Grummer, R. R. 1994. Fat sources and levels for high milk production. Pp. 130–139 in Proc. Southwest Nutrition and Management Conference. University of Arizona, Tucson, AZ.

Grummer, R. R. 1995. Ruminal inertness vs. intestinal digestibility of fat supplements: can there be harmony. Pp. 13–24 in Proc. Cornell Nutr. Conf. for Feed Manufacturers. Cornell University, Ithaca, NY.

Grummer, R. R., M. L. Hatfield, and M. R. Dentin. 1990. Acceptability of fat supplements in four dairy herds. J. Dairy Sci. 73:852–857.

Hawkins, D. E., K. D. Niswender, G. M. Oss, C. L. Moeller, K. G. Odde, H. R. Sawyer, and G. D. Niswender. 1995. Increase in serum lipids increases luteal lipid content and alters the disappearance rate of progesterone in cows. J. Anim. Sci. 73:541–545.

Jenkins, T. C. 1993. Lipid metabolism in the rumen. J. Dairy Sci. 76:3851–3863.

Jenkins, T. C. 1994. Feeding fat to dairy cattle. Pp. 100–109 in Proc. Dairy Herd Management Conf. University of Georgia, Athens, GA.

Jenkins, T. C. 1997. Success of fat in dairy rations depends on the amount. Feedstuffs 69(2):11–12.

Jerred, M. J., D. J. Carroll, D. K. Combs, and R. R. Grummer. 1990. Effects of fat supplementation and immature alfalfa to concentrate ratio on nutrient utilization and lactation performance of dairy cattle. J. Dairy Sci. 73:2842–2854.

Johnson, T. O., G. E. Mitchell, R. E. Tucker, and O. T. Schelling. 1974. Pancreatic lipase secretion by sheep. J. Anim. Sci. 39:947–951.

Klusmeyer, T. H., and J. H. Clark. 1991. Effects of dietary fat and protein on fatty acid flow to the duodenum and in milk produced by dairy cows. J. Dairy Sci. 74:3055–3067.

Knapp, D. M., R. R. Grummer, and M. R. Dentine. 1991. The response of lactating dairy cows to increasing levels of whole roasted soybeans. J. Dairy Sci. 74:2563–2579.

Kronfeld, D. S. 1976. The potential of the proportions of glucogenic, lipogenic, and aminogenic nutrients in regard to the health and productivity of dairy cows. Adv. Anim. Phys. Anim. Nutr. 7:5–26.

Mattos, W., and D. L. Palmquist. 1977. Biohydrogenation and availability of linoleic acid in lactating cows. J. Nutr. 107:1755–1761

Noble, R. C. (1981). Digestion, absorption, and transport of lipids in ruminant animals. In Lipid metabolism in ruminants, p. 57. (W. W. Christie, Ed.), Pergamon Press, Oxford.

Palmquist, D. L. 1983. Use of fats in diets for lactating dairy cows. Pp. 357–381 in Proc. 37th Easter School in Agriculture, J. Wiseman, ed. London: Butterworth.

Palmquist, D. L. 1991. Influence of source and amount of dietary fat on digestibility in lactating cows. J. Dairy Sci. 74:1354–1360

Palmquist, D. L., and H. R. Conrad. 1978. High fat rations for dairy cows. Effects on feed intake, milk and fat production, and plasma metabolites. J. Dairy Sci. 61:890–901.

Pearl, G. C. 1995. Feeding fats. Fats and Proteins Research Foundation Publication No. 269. Bloomington IL: Fats and Proteins Research Foundation. 23 pp.

Rahnema, S., Z. Wu, O. A. Ohajuruka, W. P. Weiss, and D. L. Palmquist. 1994. Site of mineral absorption in lactation cows fed high-fat diets. J. Anim. Sci. 72:229–235.

Sanchez, W. K, I. P. Moloi, and M. A. McGuire. 1998. Relationship between UIP and inert fat examined. Pages 12–13 in Feedstuffs, July 13, 1998.

Schauff, D. J., and J. H. Clark. 1992. Effects of feeding diets containing calcium salts of long-chain fatty acids to lactating dairy cows. J. Dairy Sci. 75:2990–3002.

Schingoethe, D. J., and D. P. Casper. 1991. Total lactational response to added fat during early lactation. J. Dairy Sci. 74:2617–2622.

Smith, W. A., B. Harris, Jr., H. H. Van Horn, and C. J. Wilcox. 1993. Effects of forage type on production of dairy cows supplemented with whole cottonseed, tallow, and yeast. J. Dairy Sci. 76:205–215.

Staples, C. R., J. M. Burke, and W. W. Thatcher. 1998. Influence of supplemental fats on reproductive tissues and performance of lactating cows. J. Dairy Sci. 81:856–871.

Steele, W. 1983. Intestinal absorption of fatty acids, and blood lipid composition in sheep. J. Dairy Sci. 66:520–527.

Sukhija, P. S., and D. L. Palmquist. 1990. Dissociation of calcium soaps of long-chain fatty acids in rumen fluid. J. Dairy Sci. 73:784–1787.

Sutton, J. D. 1989. Altering milk composition by feeding. J. Dairy Sci. 72:2801–2814.

Tillman, A. D., and J. R. Brethour. 1958. The effect of corn oil upon the metabolism of calcium and phosphorous by sheep. J. Anim. Sci. 17:782–786.

U.S. Department of Agriculture, Agricultural Research Service. 1998. USDA Nutrient Database for Standard Reference, Release 12-1. Nutrient Data Laboratory Homepage, http://www.nal.usda.gov/fnic/foodcomp.

Weisbjerg, M. R., C. Borsting, and T. Hvelplund. 1992. Fatty acid metabolism in the digestive tract of lactating cows fed tallow in increasing amounts at two feed levels. Acta Agric. Scand., Sect. A, Animal Sci. 42:106–114.

Wu, Z., and J. T. Huber. 1994. Relationship between dietary fat supplementation and milk protein concentration in lactating cows: A review. Livest. Prod. Sci. 39:141–155.

Wu, Z., O. A. Ohajuruka, and D. L. Palmquist. 1991. Ruminal synthesis, biohydrogenation, and digestibility of fatty acids by dairy cows. J. Dairy Sci. 74:3025–3034.

Zinn, R. A., and Y. Shen. 1996. Interaction of dietary calcium and supplemental fat on digestive function and growth performance of feedlot steers. J. Anim. Sci. 74:2303–2309.

# 4 Carbohydrates

Carbohydrates are the major source of energy in diets fed to dairy cattle and usually comprise 60 to 70 percent of the total diet. The main function of carbohydrates is to provide energy for rumen microbes and the host animal. A secondary, but essential, function of certain types of carbohydrates is to maintain the health of the gastrointestinal tract. The carbohydrate fraction of feeds is a complex mixture of numerous monomers and polymers that are usually defined according to analytic procedures and availability to the animal. Carbohydrates are broadly classified as either nonstructural or structural. Nonstructural carbohydrates (NSC) are found inside the cells of plants and are usually more digestible than structural carbohydrates that are found in plant cell walls.

## NONSTRUCTURAL CARBOHYDRATES

Sugars, starches, organic acids, and other reserve carbohydrates such as fructans make up the NSC fraction and are major sources of energy for high producing dairy cattle. Nonstructural carbohydrates and pectin are highly digestible and are generally increased in the diet at the expense of neutral detergent fiber (NDF) to meet the energy demands of lactating dairy cows. Ruminal fermentation of NSC varies greatly with type of feed and conservation and processing methods.

Nonfibrous carbohydrate (NFC) as calculated by difference: NFC = 100 − (%NDF + %CP + %Fat + %Ash) and NSC (also referred to as total nonstructural carbohydrates), as measured by enzymatic methods (Smith, 1981) are distinct fractions. Mertens (1988) reported that the concentrations of NFC and NSC are not equal for many feeds and the terms should not be used interchangeably. The difference between NFC and NSC concentrations varies considerably (Table 4-1). Much of the difference is caused by the contribution of pectin and organic acids. Pectin is included in NFC but not in NSC. When using the modified (ferricyanide as the colorimetric indicator) enzymatic method of Smith (1981), starch, sucrose, and fructans are measured as NSC. For forages, particularly grasses, fructans and sucrose are major components of NSC. Sucrose is found in beet and citrus pulp and other byproduct feeds. For many of these feeds, the NSC is likely all sugars. For corn silage, grains, and most byproducts, the NSC is nearly all starch (Miller and Hoover, 1998). Table 4-2 illustrates the differences in the components that make up NFC for selected feedstuffs. Depending on preservation method and grain type the composition of NSC can vary greatly, which can affect the rate and extent of digestion and the overall energy value of the feed for the animal.

TABLE 4-1 Nonstructural (NSC) and Nonfiber (NFC) Analyses of Selected Feedstuffs (adapted from Miller and Hoover, 1998)

| Feedstuff | NDF | NFC[a] | NSC[b] |
|---|---|---|---|
| | % of DM | | |
| Alfalfa silage | 51.4 | 18.4 | 7.5 |
| Alfalfa hay | 43.1 | 22.0 | 12.5 |
| Mixed mainly grass hay | 60.9 | 16.6 | 13.6 |
| Corn silage | 44.2 | 41.0 | 34.7 |
| Ground corn | 13.1 | 67.5 | 68.7 |
| Beet pulp | 47.3 | 36.2 | 19.5 |
| Whole cottonseed | 48.3 | 10.0 | 6.4 |
| High moisture shelled corn | 13.5 | 71.8 | 70.6 |
| Barley | 23.2 | 60.7 | 62.0 |
| Corn gluten meal | 7.0 | 17.3 | 12.0 |
| Soyhulls | 66.6 | 14.1 | 5.3 |
| Soybean meal, 48 % CP | 9.6 | 34.4 | 17.2 |

[a]NFC, % = 100 − (NDF, % + CP, % + fat, % + ash, %).

[b]NSC = nonstructural carbohydrates determined using an enzymatic method (Smith, 1981).

Recently, Hall et al. (1999) developed a method to fractionate the neutral detergent soluble carbohydrates (NDSC) in feedstuffs. Differential solubilities of carbohydrates were used to partition NDSC into organic acids and oligosaccharides soluble in ethanol/water from starch and neutral detergent soluble fiber (NDSF) that are insoluble. The method allows the partitioning of the NDSC on a nutritionally relevant basis into 1) organic acids, 2) total

TABLE 4-2 Composition of the NFC[a] Fraction of Selected Feedstuffs (adapted from Miller and Hoover, 1998)

| Feedstuff | Sugar | Starch | Pectin | Volatile Fatty Acids |
|---|---|---|---|---|
| | % of NFC | | | |
| Alfalfa silage | 0 | 24.5 | 33.0 | 42.5 |
| Grass hay | 35.4 | 15.2 | 49.4 | 0 |
| Corn silage | 0 | 71.3 | 0 | 28.7 |
| Barley | 9.1 | 81.7 | 9.2 | 0 |
| Corn grain | 20.9 | 80.0 | 0 | 0 |
| Beet pulp | 33.7 | 1.8 | 64.5 | 0 |
| Soyhulls | 18.8 | 18.8 | 62.4 | 0 |
| Soybean meal 48% CP | 28.2 | 28.2 | 43.6 | 0 |

[a]NFC calculated by difference as shown in footnote 2, Table 4-1.

ethanol/water-soluble carbohydrate, 3) starch, and 4) neutral detergent soluble fiber.

The optimal concentration of NSC or NFC in diets for lactating cows is not well defined. To avoid acidosis and other metabolic problems, the maximum concentration of NSC should be approximately 30 to 40 percent of the ration dry matter (DM) (Nocek, 1997). The acceptable concentrations for NFC are probably 2 to 3 percentage units higher than for NSC. The optimal concentration of NSC or NFC in diets of high producing cows are related to: 1) the effects of rapidly degradable starch on ruminal digestion of fiber, which can decrease the differences between diets relative to total carbohydrate digestion; 2) the amount of NSC or NFC that replaces NDF in the diet, as this can affect volatile fatty acid production, rumination, and saliva production; 3) site of starch digestion; 4) dry matter intake (DMI) and physiologic state of the animal; and 5) conservation and processing methods used to alter rate and extent of NSC or NFC digestion.

Alteration of dietary NFC influences ruminal fermentation patterns, total tract digestion of fiber and milk fat percentage (Sievert and Shaver, 1993; Sutton and Bines, 1987). Batajoo and Shaver (1994) concluded that for cows producing over 40 kg of milk, the diet should contain more than 30 percent NFC, but found little benefit of 42 percent over 36 percent NFC. Nocek and Russell (1988) suggested that 40 percent NFC was optimal in diets for lactating cows from an evaluation of diets based on alfalfa silage, corn silage, and 50:50 alfalfa:corn silage; dietary NFC ranged from 30 to 46 percent. Hoover and Stokes (1991) regressed data from Nocek and Russell (1988) and found that when dietary NFC was greater than 45 to 50 percent or less than 25 to 30 percent, milk production was decreased. In another study, the percentage and yield of milk protein increased when NFC in the dietary DM was increased from 41.7 to 46.5 percent (Minor et al., 1998).

Starch comprises 50 to 100 percent of the NSC in most feedstuffs. In addition to total starch level, the rate and extent of ruminal starch digestion also may affect the amount of a particular starch source that can safely be added to a diet. Rate of fermentation of starch varies extensively by type of grain and grain processing. Herrera-Saldana et al. (1990) ranked the degradability of starch from various sources as follows: oats > wheat > barley > corn > sorghum. Processing methods, such as fine grinding and steam flaking also may alter ruminal availability of starch. Lykos and Varga (1995) demonstrated that effective degradability of starch in situ for cracked corn, fine ground corn, and steam flaked corn was 44.4, 64.5 and 75.4 percent, respectively. In addition, the effective degradability of starch was increased for ground versus cracked soybeans whether raw or roasted. Most grain processing methods increase both rate of starch fermentation and ruminal starch digestibility. Reducing particle size by cracking and grinding significantly increases rate of starch digestion (Galyean et al., 1981; McAllister et al., 1993) and effects are greater with unprocessed than heat processed grains. Grinding increases both rate of digestion and rate of passage, which have counteractive effects on ruminal digestibility (Galyean et al., 1979). Animal characteristics and DMI affect rate of passage. Therefore, fine grinding may have less effect on ruminal starch digestibility at higher DMI, due to faster rate of passage, such as for high producing dairy cows.

Results of lactation studies that compared starch sources with differing digestibilities have been variable and may be related to the carbohydrate source and how it is processed, level of intake, the basal forage in the ration, and the degradability of the protein source. Herrera-Saldana and Huber (1989) reported higher milk production with a barley-cottonseed meal diet than with a sorghum grain-cottonseed meal diet, while McCarthy et al. (1989) and Casper et al. (1990) reported higher milk production by cows fed diets with corn grain compared with barley. Milk yield was increased for cows in early lactation by increasing ruminally available starch fed as steam flaked sorghum instead of dry rolled corn (Moore et al., 1992; Poore et al., 1993) or fed as ground instead of cracked corn (Knowlton et al., 1996). Wilkerson and Glenn (1997) demonstrated an increase in yield of milk for cows fed high moisture corn versus dry corn (41.7 vs. 39.7 kg/d) and ground corn versus rolled corn (41.8 vs. 39.6 kg/d). Ruminal digestibility of starch was greater for high moisture corn than dry corn whether corn was rolled or ground. Lykos et al. (1997) demonstrated that increasing the rate of NSC digestion from 6 to 7.9 percent/h significantly increased milk yield 2.5 kg/d and protein yield 130 g/d. Aldrich et al. (1993) observed 4 percent lower FCM yields when diets high in rapidly fermentable nonstructural carbohydrates (81 percent ruminal degradable NSC) were fed to lactating cows during early lactation. Diets with increased ruminally degraded starch did not affect milk yield or FCM in other studies (Clark and Harshbarger, 1972; Oliveira et al., 1993, 1995). Varga and Kononoff (1999) evaluated the relationship between dietary concentration or intake of NSC or NFC and milk yield in 16 studies published in the *Journal of Dairy Science* from 1992 through 1998. The relationships between concentration of NSC or NFC and milk yield were poor ($r^2 = 0.04$). The relationship between NFC intake and milk yield was good ($r^2 = 0.40$); a 1 kg increase in NFC intake resulted in a 2.4 kg increase in milk yield. See a more detailed discussion related to starch processing in Chapter 13.

## STRUCTURAL CARBOHYDRATES

Crude fiber, acid detergent fiber, and neutral detergent fiber are the most common measures of fiber used for routine feed analysis, but none of these fractions are chemically uniform. Neutral detergent fiber measures most of the structural components in plant cells (i.e., cellulose, hemicellulose, and lignin). Acid detergent fiber does not include hemicellulose, and crude fiber does not quantitatively recover hemicellulose and lignin. Neutral detergent fiber is the method that best separates structural from nonstructural carbohydrates in plants, and NDF measures most of the chemical compounds generally considered to comprise fiber. Within a specific feedstuff, concentrations of NDF, ADF, and crude fiber are highly correlated, but for mixed diets that contain different fiber sources, the correlations among the different measures of fiber are lower. Neutral detergent fiber is the best expression of fiber available currently, but recommendations are also given for ADF because of its widespread use. Crude fiber will not be discussed because it is considered obsolete.

On average NDF is less digestible than nonfiber carbohydrates; therefore, the concentration of NDF in feeds or diets is negatively correlated with energy concentration. The chemical composition of the NDF (proportions of cellulose, hemicellulose, and lignin) affects the digestibility of the NDF fraction. Therefore, feeds or diets with similar NDF concentrations will not necessarily have similar $NE_L$ concentrations, and certain feeds or diets with high NDF may have more $NE_L$ than another feed or diet with lower concentrations of NDF.

The maximum amount of NDF that should be included in diets is a function of the $NE_L$ requirement of the cow, the minimum amount of NFC needed for good ruminal fermentation, and the potential negative effects of high NDF on feed intake. In most cases, the maximum NDF concentration will be determined by the $NE_L$ requirement of the cow. In a summary of published studies, NDF concentration usually did not constrain DMI when diets were formulated to provide adequate $NE_L$ (Mertens, 1994). Based on Mertens (1994), DMI may have been limited when cows producing approximately 40 kg of milk/d were fed diets with more than about 32 percent NDF. For cows producing 20 kg/d of milk, DMI was not restricted until the diet contained about 44 percent NDF. Source of NDF, especially with respect to rate and extent of NDF digestion, will influence those values (Oba and Allen, 1999).

The minimum amount of dietary NDF needed is based largely on ruminal and cow health. The concentration of NDF is inversely related to ruminal pH because NDF generally ferments slower and is less digestible than NFC (i.e., less acid production in the rumen), and because the majority of dietary NDF in typical diets is from forage with a physical structure that promotes chewing and saliva production (i.e., buffering capacity). Various indices have been used to monitor ruminal conditions including milk fat percentage, ruminal pH, rumen VFA concentrations, and time spent chewing. Those measures respond quickly to dietary changes and can be monitored in short-term studies. Long-term effects of poor ruminal health may include increased prevalence of laminitis (Nocek, 1997) and displaced abomasum (Shaver, 1997), but the literature is extremely limited on long-term health responses to dietary NDF concentration.

Based on several studies with cows fed alfalfa-based diets and corn grain as the primary starch source (Colenbrander et al., 1991; Hansen et al., 1991; Weiss and Shockey, 1991; Clark and Armentano, 1993; Depies and Armentano, 1995), diets with 25 percent total NDF resulted in similar milk production with a similar composition as did diets with higher NDF concentrations. In these studies, dietary DM contained 16 to 20 percent NDF from forage. Forage is defined as feedstuffs that are composed of stems, leaves, and possibly grain and is fed as fresh material, hay, or silage (e.g., corn silage is considered a forage even though it contains corn grain). Diets with less than 25 percent total NDF and less than about 16 percent NDF from forage depressed milk fat percentage (Clark and Armentano, 1993; Depies and Armentano, 1995). Few studies designed to determine the minimum amount of NDF needed with corn silage diets have been conducted. Milk fat percentage for cows fed corn silage-based diets with 24 percent NDF was less than that for cows fed 29 or 35 percent NDF (Cummins, 1992), but in another study (Bal et al., 1997) production of milk fat and milk was not different among cows fed corn silage-based diets with 25 or 29 percent NDF. Corn silage elicits similar or greater chewing activity by cows than does alfalfa silage (Mertens, 1997), and mean NDF digestibility is similar for corn and alfalfa silages (Kung et al., 1992); therefore, the minimum amount of NDF needed to maintain ruminal function when diets are based on corn silage is probably similar to that for diets based on alfalfa silage assuming particle size is adequate. The NDF content of corn silage must be measured using amylase, or NDF values will be inflated and the risk of supplying insufficient dietary NDF is increased (See Chapter 13).

*NDF Recommendations*

Based on the above cited studies, the recommended concentration of total dietary NDF for cows fed diets with alfalfa or corn silage as the predominate forage and dry ground corn grain as the predominant starch source was set at 25 percent of dietary DM with the condition that 19 percent of dietary DM must be NDF from forage (Table 4-3). The minimum recommended NDF concentration is increased as the amount of forage NDF in the diet decreases (discussed below). The NDF concentration in the diet must be higher when the forage is finely chopped, but because of the limited amount of data available we did not quantify this relationship. Diets that are formulated at the minimum concentration of NDF should be based on the actual composition of the feedstuffs, not table values. The potential for errors in mixing and feed delivery should be considered, and when the probability for errors is high, diets should be formulated to be above the minimum NDF concentration.

Although cows appear to be able to tolerate diets with 25 percent NDF and 19 percent NDF from forage, those recommendations are for very specific situations (i.e, the diet contains forage with adequate particle size, dry corn grain is the predominant starch source, and diets are fed as total mixed rations). Diets with small particle forage, diets with starch sources that have higher ruminal availability than corn, diets that have less than about 19 percent NDF from forage, and diets not fed as total mixed rations will require higher minimum concentrations of NDF. Inclusion of supplemental buffers may decrease the amount of NDF required in the diet (Allen, 1991). Furthermore, the minimum recommended concentration of NDF should not be considered the optimal concentration. Lower producing cows require less energy, and diets should contain NDF concentrations greater than the minimum.

TABLE 4-3 Recommended Minimum Concentrations (% of DM) of Total and Forage NDF and Recommended Maximum Concentrations (% of DM) of NFC for Diets of Lactating Cows When the Diet is Fed as a Total Mixed Ration, the Forage has Adequate Particle Size, and Ground Corn is the Predominant Starch Source[a]

| Minimum forage NDF[b] | Minimum dietary NDF | Maximum dietary NFC[c] | Minimum dietary ADF[d] |
|---|---|---|---|
| 19[e] | 25[e] | 44[e] | 17[e] |
| 18 | 27 | 42 | 18 |
| 17 | 29 | 40 | 19 |
| 16 | 31 | 38 | 20 |
| 15[e] | 33 | 36 | 21 |

[a]Values in this table are based on the assumption that actual feed composition has been measured; values may not be appropriate when values from feed tables are used.

[b]All feeds that contain substantial amounts of vegetative matter are considered forage. For example, corn silage is considered a forage, although it contains significant amounts of grain.

[c]Nonfiber carbohydrate is calculated by difference 100 - (%NDF + %CP + %Fat + %Ash).

[d]Minimum dietary ADF recommendations were calculated from NDF concentrations (See text).

[e]Diets that contain less fiber (forage NDF, total NDF or total ADF) than these minimum values and more NFC than 44 percent should not be fed.

The committee decided to adjust NDF recommendations based on the concentration of NDF from forage in the diet. The primary reason was that source of NDF has a major impact on cow response to NDF concentrations, and concentration of forage NDF is easily obtainable under field conditions. Forages that are long or coarsely chopped provide NDF in a form that is distinctly different from NDF in nonforage sources such as soyhulls, wheat midds, beet pulp, and corn gluten feed. The NDF from grain sources are also considered nonforage fiber sources. Many nonforage fiber sources have a relatively large pool of potentially degradable NDF, small particle size, and relatively high specific gravity (Batajoo and Shaver, 1994). Nonforage fiber sources have similar or faster passage rates than many forages (Bhatti and Firkins, 1995), and many have rates of NDF digestion that are similar to or slower than those of forages. A large proportion of the potentially available NDF from nonforages may escape ruminal fermentation resulting in less acid production in the rumen (Firkins, 1997).

Most sources of nonforage NDF are significantly less effective at maintaining milk fat percentage than are forages (Swain and Armentano, 1994; Vaughan et al., 1991; Clark and Armentano, 1993, 1997). Based on an empirical relationship developed by Allen (1997), NDF from nonforage was only 0.35 times as effective at maintaining rumen pH as was NDF from forage. Firkins (1997) concluded that NDF from nonforage was about 0.6 times as effective at maintaining NDF digestibility in the gastrointestional tract as was NDF from forage. Based on chewing activity, Mertens (1997) concluded that NDF from high NDF nonforage sources (i.e., byproducts) was about 0.4 and for other concentrates between 0.3 and 0.8 times as effective as NDF from forage. Based on these three studies, the average effective value of NDF from nonforage was set to 50 percent of that for NDF from forage. For every 1 percentage unit decrease in NDF from forage (as a percentage of dietary DM) below 19 percent, the recommended concentration of total dietary NDF was increased 2 percentage units, and maximum NFC concentration was reduced 2 percentage units (Table 4-3). A possible exception to this relationship is whole linted cottonseed. Whole cottonseeds appear to have significantly more value at maintaining milk fat percentage than do other sources of NDF from nonforage fiber sources (Clark and Armentano, 1993).

Determining whether changes in milk fat percentage, ruminal pH, or chewing activity are caused by altering dietary NDF or NFC is difficult because their concentrations are correlated. On average, dietary concentrations of NDF and NFC have a high negative correlation (Armentano and Pereira, 1997). If all nutrients are held constant except for NDF and NFC, a change in NDF concentration from 33 to 28 percent of dietary DM (a 15 percent decrease) means that NFC must increase from 40 to 45 percent of dietary DM (an 11 percent increase) (Armentano and Pereira, 1997). However, because of variations in dietary concentrations of CP and supplemental fat, the correlation is not perfect. The concentrations of NFC in a diet with 25 percent NDF could vary by 2 to 9 percentage units. Diets with excess NFC can cause ruminal upsets and health problems (Nocek, 1997). Therefore, the minimum NDF required must be considered in conjunction with NFC concentrations. Diets that contain lower concentrations of CP and ether extract should have higher NDF concentrations. Recommended maximum NFC concentrations are presented in Table 4-3. The minimum concentration of NDF should be increased so that the maximum recommended concentrations of NFC are not exceeded.

#### QUALITATIVE ADJUSTMENTS TO NDF RECOMMENDATIONS

*Source of Starch* Milk fat percentage, ruminal pH, and ruminal VFA profile are often altered when starch availability in the rumen is increased (e.g., steam-flaked vs. dry processed grains, high moisture vs. dry grains, or corn vs. barley) even when the concentration of dietary NDF is not altered. These alterations in ruminal fermentation and milk fat percentage suggest that the NDF requirement increases when sources of readily available starch replace dry ground corn in the diet. Ruminal fermentation profiles and milk fat data from Knowlton et al. (1998) suggest that diets that contain high moisture corn should contain at least 27 percent NDF. Cows fed diets based on barley should contain about 34 percent NDF (Beauchemin, 1991). Insufficient information is available to give specific recommendations for diets that contain other starch sources. However, diets with steam-flaked corn, steam-flaked sorghum, or other sources of starch that have a high ruminal availability should contain more than 25 percent NDF and less than 44 percent NFC.

*Particle Size of Forage* Particle size of forage as well as concentration of NDF in the diet has an impact on ruminal pH. Allen (1997) reported that when finely chopped forage was substituted for coarsely chopped forage, salivary buffer flow decreased by nearly 5 percent, but an increase in forage NDF in the diet from 20 to 24 percent increased salivary buffer flow less than 1 percent. The mean particle size of alfalfa hay necessary to maintain rumen pH, chewing activity, and milk fat percentage appears to be about 3 mm (Grant et al., 1990a; Woodford et al., 1986; Shaver et al., 1986). Diets with alfalfa silage that had a mean particle length less than about 3 mm resulted in depressed milk fat, decreased rumen pH, and reduced time spent chewing (Grant et al., 1990b; Beauchemin et al., 1994). Allen (1997) evaluated the relationship between particle length of forage and total time spent chewing using data from 10 dairy cattle experiments and found a clear breakpoint at approximately 3 mm at which point no further increase in particle length affected total chewing time. The concentration of NDF in the diet should be increased by several percentage units when the mean particle size of the forage is less than about 3 mm. Diets that contain finely ground forages and sources of rapidly fermentable starch (e.g., barley or high moisture corn) may require even more dietary NDF to maintain milk fat percentage. Quantitative measures of particle size (i.e., mean particle size, mean standard deviation and/or distribution) rather than qualitative descriptions (e.g., coarsely chopped) are needed to improve the accuracy of assessing fiber requirements of dairy cows.

*Effective Fiber* The effective fiber concept is an attempt to formulate diets not only for NDF but also for the ability of a diet to stimulate chewing (Sudweeks et al., 1981; Mertens, 1992, 1997). The origin of the effective fiber concept was to meet the minimum fiber requirement that would maintain milk fat percentages (Mertens, 1997). Effective fiber values were assigned to feeds based on changes in milk fat. When only milk fat is used as the response variable, the physical effects of NDF on chewing, salivation, and ruminal buffering are confounded with metabolic effects caused by different chemical composition of the feeds (Allen, 1997). For example, the effect of feeding whole cottonseed on milk fat percentage may be a result of both its fiber and fat contribution to the diet. Milk composition of cows during mid to late lactation is more sensitive to changes in ration composition than is milk composition of cows during early lactation. For animals in early lactation, ruminal pH is a more meaningful response variable for determining fiber requirements than are other factors (Allen, 1997). Most of the trials evaluating the effectiveness of NDF lasted only a few weeks. Long-term effects on ruminal health, laminitis, and production are not known.

Several researchers have suggested that chewing response is an important characteristic of feeds (Balch, 1971), and that dairy cows have a minimum requirement for chewing activity (Sudweeks et al., 1981; Norgaard, 1986). Mertens (1997) proposed that two terms should be used to distinguish between the effectiveness of fiber in maintaining milk fat percentage or in stimulating chewing activity. Effective NDF (eNDF) was defined as the sum total ability of the NDF in a feed to replace the NDF in forage or roughage in a ration so that the percentage of milk fat is maintained. Physically effective NDF (peNDF) is related to the physical characteristics of NDF (primarily particle size) that affect chewing activity and the biphasic nature of ruminal contents.

Different systems have been proposed to measure effective NDF. Mertens (1997) developed the peNDF system using regression analysis to assign physical effective factors (PEF) to classes of NDF based on the chewing activity they stimulated. The PEF of feeds is expressed relative to the chewing activity of cows when they are fed long grass hay. The PEF of long grass hay was set to 1; coarsely chopped grass silage, corn silage, and alfalfa silage had PEF values of 0.9 to 0.95; and finely chopped forage had values of 0.7 to 0.85. Diets with 22 percent of the DM as physically effective NDF maintained average rumen pH at 6, and diets with 20 percent physically effective NDF maintained milk fat percentage at 3.4 percent for Holstein cows during early to mid lactation. The proportion of DM (or NDF) retained on a sieve with an aperture of 1.18 mm was proposed by Mertens (1997) as a simple laboratory method that might be applicable to the routine analysis of physically effective NDF in feeds. The *Nutrient Requirements of Beef Cattle* (National Research Council, 1996) defined effective NDF as the percentage of total NDF that is retained on a screen with 1.18 mm or greater openings after dry sieving. Buckmaster et al. (1997) developed an effective fiber intake based on particle size distributions from a three screen (>19 mm, 8 to 19 mm, and <8 mm) sieve (Lammers et al., 1996) and the NDF concentration of each fraction. In that system, average legume and corn silages had similar effectiveness values, and both were about 10 percent less than the average value for grass silage (Kononoff et al., 1999). More information is needed to determine the accuracy of all these systems to measure the effectiveness of forage sources for altering milk fat and chewing time.

At the present time, the lack of standard, validated methods to measure effective fiber of feeds or to establish requirements for effective fiber limits the application of this concept. Mertens (1997) peNDF concept is a step towards the quantification of the chemical and physical attributes of fiber into a single measurement. However, this concept is currently not validated; not enough feeds have values, and requirements have not been determined. Effective NDF should be a measure of the sum total ability of a feed to replace forage or roughage in a ration so that the percentage of fat in milk and rumen pH are maintained (Mertens, 1997). Differences in the rate and extent of digestion of NDF and the difference between ruminal digestibility of NDF and NFC are related to acid production and ultimately the ability of a feed to maintain ruminal pH. These factors can differ among different sources of NDF especially when forage and nonforage sources of NDF are compared. More research is needed to identify other chemical and physical characteristics of feeds that influence their ability to maintain optimal ruminal function and animal health before specific values for effectiveness of various forage and nonforage fiber sources can be determined. Because of these problems, a requirement for effective NDF is not given. Dietary NDF concentrations, however, may have to be altered based on differences in particle size of the forage and source of NDF.

*Supplemental dietary buffers* Supplemental dietary buffers increase buffering capacity in the rumen (Erdman, 1988) and should reduce the NDF requirement. Detailed information on the effects of buffers and recommendations regarding their use are in Chapter 9.

*Feeding method* Essentially all recent experiments on fiber requirements have used total mixed rations (TMR). When cows consume a TMR, rate of NSC consumption is moderated due to simultaneous consumption of fiber. Because forage is consumed at the same time as concentrate, increased chewing and salivation occurs, and rumen buffering capacity is high when the NSC is being fermented. Experiments specifically designed to determine whether NDF requirements are increased when cows are fed concentrate separately from forages have not been conducted.

Feeding forage separately from concentrate alters diurnal patterns for pH and fermentation acids in the rumen. The degree of change depends on feeding frequency of the concentrate and the fermentability of the concentrate. Diurnal changes in ruminal pH and fermentation acids are very pronounced when concentrates that are predominantly NFC are consumed twice daily compared with TMR feeding (Robinson, 1989). These severe changes in ruminal pH may be associated with reduced milk fat percentage and yield. When concentrate is offered more than twice daily (e.g., using a computer-controlled concentrate feeder), fewer effects on production, milk composition, and ruminal conditions have been reported (Cassel et al., 1984; Robinson, 1989; Maltz et al., 1992).

The NDF requirement when concentrates are fed twice daily and separately from forages is unknown but is probably higher, and maximum NFC concentrations are lower than the values in Table 4-3. Increased dietary NDF concentrations may not completely overcome the problem associated with the rapid consumption of large amounts of grain. In such cases, the NDF concentration of the concentrate mixture may have to be increased.

Cows grazing high quality pasture and fed concentrate twice daily, often (Polan et al., 1986; Berzaghi et al., 1996), but not always (Holden et al., 1995), produce milk with reduced fat even when they are fed diets that appear adequate in NDF. Lowered milk fat percentage may be caused by reduced salivation when cows are grazing, the highly digestible nature of the fiber in high quality pasture, and the rapid consumption of grain caused by feeding concentrate only twice daily and separately from forage. When high fiber concentrates (e.g., beet pulp or corn gluten feed) replaced starchy feeds (corn or barley) in diets of grazing cows milk fat percentage was increased (Meijs, 1986; Garnsworthy, 1990). However, when a concentrate based on corn was fed alone, or mixed with corn silage twice daily, to grazing cows no difference was observed in milk fat percentage (Holden et al., 1995). The corn silage did not reduce the intake of corn grain but should have increased the time needed to consume the corn. Because data are not available, specific recommendations for NDF concentrations of diets for grazing cattle are not known; therefore, the guidelines in Table 4-3 may not be adequate for grazing cattle. Limited data (Holden et al., 1995) suggest that cows grazing high quality pasture and fed concentrate twice daily should be fed a ruminal buffer (mixed with the concentrate), or the concentrate should not be comprised solely of starchy feedstuffs.

### *ADF Requirement*

Expressing the fiber requirement as NDF is superior to ADF for many reasons; however, ADF requirements are given because of the widespread use of ADF. The ADF requirements shown in Table 4-3 were derived from the recommended NDF concentrations. Concentrations of NDF and ADF are highly correlated within forage classifications. Regression equations were developed to estimate ADF concentrations from NDF concentrations for corn silage, grass forage, and legume forage:

$$\text{Corn silage ADF, \%} = -1.15 + 0.62 \text{ NDF, \%} \ (r^2 = 0.89, \text{syx} = 1.4, N = 2425)$$

$$\text{Grass forage ADF, \%} = 6.89 + 0.50 \text{ NDF, \%} \ (r^2 = 0.62, \text{syx} = 3.1, N = 722)$$

$$\text{Legume forage ADF, \%} = -0.73 + 0.82 \text{ NDF, \%} \ (r^2 = 0.84, \text{syx} = 2.0, N = 2899)$$

The ADF requirements shown in Table 4-3 were derived by formulating numerous test diets that included a wide variety of feedstuffs. The composition values used for all feeds were from Table 15-1 except the ADF concentration of forages were estimated using the above regression equations. The dietary concentration of ADF that resulted when most diets met NDF requirements was set as the ADF requirement. Factors described previously that increase the NDF requirement will also increase the ADF requirement.

## REFERENCES


Aldrich, M. M., L. D. Muller, G. A. Varga, and L. C. Griel, Jr. 1993. Nonstructural carbohydrate and protein effects on rumen fermentation, nutrient flow, and performance of dairy cows. J. Dairy Sci. 76:1091–1105.

Allen, M. S. 1991. Carbohydrate nutrition. Vet. Clin. North. Am. Food Anim. Prod. 7:327–340.

Allen, M. S. 1997. Relationship between fermentation acid production in the rumen and the requirement for physically effective fiber. J. Dairy Sci. 80:1447–1462.

Armentano, L., and M. Pereira. 1997. Measuring the effectiveness of fiber by animal response trials. J. Dairy Sci. 80:1416–1425.

Bal, M. A., J. G. Coors, and R. D. Shaver. 1997. Impact of the maturity of corn for use as silage in the diets of dairy cows on intake, digestion, and milk production. J. Dairy Sci. 80:2497–2503.

Balch, C. C. 1971. Proposal to use time spent chewing as an index of the extent to which diets for ruminants possess the physical property of fibrousness characteristics of roughages. Br. J. Nutr. 26:383–392.

Batajoo, K. K., and R. D. Shaver. 1994. Impact of nonfiber carbohydrate on intake, digestion, and milk production by dairy cows. J. Dairy Sci. 77:1580–1587.

Beauchemin, K. A. 1991. Effects of dietary neutral detergent fiber concentration and alfalfa hay quality on chewing, rumen function, and milk production of dairy cows. J. Dairy Sci. 74:3140–3151.

Beauchemin, K. A., B. I. Farr, L. M. Rode, and G. B. Schaalje. 1994. Effects of alfalfa silage chop length and supplementary long hay on chewing and milk production of dairy cows. J. Dairy Sci. 77:1326–1339.

Berzaghi, P., J. H. Herbein, and C. E. Polan. 1996. Intake, site, and extent of nutrient digestion of lactating cows grazing pasture. J. Dairy Sci. 79:1581–1589.

Bhatti, S. A., and J. L. Firkins. 1995. Kinetics of hydration and functional specific gravity of fibrous feed by-products. J. Anim. Sci. 73:1449–1458.

Buckmaster, D. R., A. J. Heinrichs, R. A. Ward, and B. P. Lammers. 1997. Characterizing effective fiber with particle size and fiber concentration interactions. Int. Grassland Congress, 18:8–19.

Casper, D. P., D. J. Schingoethe, and W. A. Eisenbeisz. 1990. Response of early lactation dairy cows fed diets varying in source of non-structural carbohydrate and crude protein. J. Dairy Sci. 73:1039–1050.

Cassel, E. K., W. G. Merrill, R. A. Milligan, and R. W. Guest. 1984. Evaluation of systems for feeding supplemental concentrate to cows in groups. J. Dairy Sci. 67:560–568.

Clark, P. W., and L. E. Armentano. 1993. Effectiveness of neutral detergent fiber in whole cottonseed and dried distillers grains compared with alfalfa haylage. J. Dairy Sci. 76:2644–2650.

Clark, P. W., and L. E. Armentano. 1997. Replacement of alfalfa neutral detergent fiber with a combination of nonforage fiber sources. J. Dairy Sci. 80:675–680.

Clark, J. H., and K. E. Harshbarger. 1972. High moisture corn versus dry corn in combination with either corn silage or hay for lactating cows. J. Dairy Sci. 55:1474–1480.

Colenbrander, V. F., C. H. Noller, and R. J. Grant. 1991. Effect of fiber content and particle size of alfalfa silage on performance and chewing behavior. J. Dairy Sci. 74:2681–2690.

Cummins, K. A. 1992. Effect of dietary acid detergent fiber on responses to high environmental temperature. J. Dairy Sci. 75:1465–1471.

Depies, K. K., and L. E. Armentano. 1995. Partial replacement of alfalfa fiber with fiber from ground corn cobs or wheat middlings. J. Dairy Sci. 78:1328–1335.

Erdman, R. A. 1988. Dietary buffering requirements of the lactating dairy cow: A review. J. Dairy Sci. 71:3246–3266.

Firkins, J. L. 1997. Effects of feeding nonforage fiber sources on site of fiber digestion. J. Dairy Sci. 80:1426–1437.

Galyean, M. L., D. G. Wagner, and F. N. Owens. 1979. Corn particle size and site and extent of digestion by steers. J. Anim. Sci. 49:204–210.

Galyean, M. L., D. G. Wagner, and F. N. Owens. 1981. Dry matter and starch disappearance of corn and sorghum as influenced by particle size and processing. J. Dairy Sci. 64:1804–1812.

Garnsworthy, P. C. 1990. Feeding calcium salts of fatty acids in high-starch or high-fibre compound supplements to lactating cows at grass. Anim Prod. 51:441–447.

Grant, R. J., V. F. Colenbrander, and D. R. Mertens. 1990a. Milk fat depression in dairy cows: role of particle size of alfalfa hay. J. Dairy Sci. 73:1823–1833.

Grant, R. J., V. F. Colenbrander, and D. R. Mertens. 1990b. Milk fat depression in dairy cows: role of silage particle size. J. Dairy Sci. 73:1834–1842.

Hall, M. B., W. H. Hoover, J. P. Jennings, and T. K. Miller-Webster. 1999 A method for partitioning neutral detergent soluble carbohydrates. J. Sci. Food Agr. 79:2079–2086.

Hansen, W. P., D. E. Otterby, J. G. Linn, and J. D. Donker. 1991. Influence of forage type, ratio of forage to concentrate, and methionine hydroxy analog on performance of dairy cows. J. Dairy Sci. 74:1361–1369

Herrera-Saldana R., R. Gomez-Alarcon, M. Torabi, and J. T. Huber. 1990. Influence of synchronizing protein and starch degradation in the rumen on nutrient utilization and microbial synthesis. J. Dairy Sci. 73:142–148.

Herrera-Saldana, R. E., and J. T. Huber. 1989. Influence of varying protein and starch degradabilities on performance of lactating cows. J. Dairy Sci. 72:1477–1483.

Holden, L. A., L. D. Muller, T. Lykos, and T. W. Cassidy. 1995. Effect of corn silage supplementation on intake and milk production in cows grazing grass pasture. J. Dairy Sci. 78:154–160.

Hoover, W. H., and S. R. Stokes. 1991. Balancing carbohydrates and proteins for optimum rumen microbial yield. J. Dairy Sci. 74:3630–3644.

Knowlton, K. F., M. S. Allen, and P. S. Erickson. 1996. Lasalocid and particle size of corn grain for dairy cows in early lactation. 1. Effect on performance, serum metabolites, and nutrient digestibility. J. Dairy Sci. 79:557–564.

Knowlton, K. F, B. P. Glenn, and R. A. Erdman. 1998. Performance, ruminal fermentation, and site of starch digestion in early lactation Holstein cows fed corn grain harvested and processed differently. J. Dairy Sci. 81:1972–1985.

Kononoff, P. J., A. J. Heinrichs, D. R. Buckmaster, and K. J. Harvatine. 1999. A characterization of effective fiber: the effective fiber system. J. Dairy Sci. 82 (Suppl. 1):85.

Kung, L., Jr., R. S. Tung, and B. R. Carmean. 1992. Rumen fermentation and nutrient digestion in cattle fed diets varying in forage and energy source. Anim. Feed Sci. Tech. 39:1–12.

Lammers, B. P., D. R. Buckmaster, and A. J. Heinrichs. 1996. A simple method for the analysis of particle sizes of forage and total mixed rations. J. Dairy Sci. 79:922–928.

Lykos, T., and G. A. Varga. 1995. Effects of processing method on degradation characteristics of protein and carbohydrate sources in situ. J. Dairy Sci. 78:1789–1801.

Lykos, T., G. A. Varga, and D. Casper. 1997. Varying degradation rates of total nonstructural carbohydrates: Effects on ruminal fermentation, blood metabolites, and milk production and composition in high producing Holstein cows. J. Dairy Sci. 80:3341–3355.

McAllister, T. A., R. C. Phillippe, L. M. Rode, and K. J. Cheng. 1993. Effect of the protein matrix on the digestion of cereal grains by ruminal microorganisms. J. Anim. Sci. 71:205–212.

McCarthy, R. D., Jr., T. H. Klusmeyer, J. L. Vicini, J. H. Clark, and D. R. Nelson. 1989. Effects of source of protein and carbohydrate on ruminal fermentation and passage of nutrients to the small intestine of lactating cows. J. Dairy Sci. 72:2002–2016.

Maltz, E., S. Devir, O. Kroll, B. Zur, S. L. Spahr, and R. D. Shanks. 1992. Comparative responses of lactating cows to total mixed rations or computerized individual concentrates feeding. J. Dairy Sci. 75:1588–1603.

Meijs, J. A. 1986. Concentrate supplementation of grazing dairy cows. 2. Effect of concentrate composition on herbage intake and milk production. Grass Forage Sci. 41:229–235.

Mertens, D. R. 1988. Balancing carbohydrates in dairy rations. Proc. Large Herd Dairy Mgmt. Conf., Dept. Animal Sci., Cornell Univ., Ithaca, NY. p. 150.

Mertens, D. R. 1992. Nonstructural and structural carbohydrates. Page 219 in Large Dairy Herd Management. H. H. Van Horn and C. J. Wilcox, ed. Am. Dairy Sci. Assoc., Champaign, IL.

Mertens, D. R. 1994. Regulation of feed intake. pp. 450–493 *in* Forage Quality, Evaluation, and Utilization J. G. C. Fahey, ed., Amer. Soc. Agronomy, Inc., Madison WI.

Mertens, D. R. 1997. Creating a system for meeting the fiber requirements of dairy cows. J. Dairy Sci. 80:1463–1481.

Miller, T. K., and W. H. Hoover. 1998. Nutrient analyses of feedstuffs including carbohydrates. Animal Sci. Report #1, West Va. Univ.

Minor, D. J., S. L. Trower, B. D. Strang, R. D. Shaver, and R. R. Grummer. 1998. Effects of nonfiber carbohydrate and niacin on periparturient metabolic status and lactation of dairy cows. J. Dairy Sci. 81:189–200.

Moore, J. A., M. H. Poore, T. P. Eck, R. S. Swingle, J. T. Huber, and M. J. Arana. 1992. Sorghum grain processing and buffer addition for early lactation cows. J. Dairy Sci. 75:3465–3472.

National Research Council. 1996. Nutrient Requirements of Beef Cattle, Seventh Revised Ed. Pp. 75–84. Washington, D.C.: National Academy Press.

Nocek, J. E. 1997. Bovine acidosis: implications on lameness. J. Dairy Sci. 80:1005–1028.

Nocek, J. E., and J. B. Russell. 1988. Protein and energy as an integrated system. Relationship of ruminal protein and carbohydrate availability to microbial synthesis and milk production. J. Dairy Sci. 71:2070–2107.

Norgaard, P. 1986. Physical structure of feeds for dairy cows. Research on Rumen Function. A. Neimann-Sorensen, ed. Comm. Eur. Commun., Luxembourg, Luxembourg.

Oba, M., and M. S. Allen. 1999. Evaluation of the importance of the digestibility of neutral detergent fiber from forage: effects on dry matter intake and milk yield of dairy cows. J. Dairy Sci. 82:589–596.

Oliveira, J. S., J. T. Huber, D. Ben-Ghedalia, R. S. Swingle, C. B. Theurer, and M. Pessarakli. 1993. Influence of sorghum grain processing on performance of lactating dairy cows. J. Dairy Sci. 76:575–581.

Oliveira, J. S., J. T. Huber, J. M. Simas, C. B. Theurer, and R. S. Swingle. 1995. Effect of sorghum grain processing on site and extent of digestion of starch in lactating dairy cows. J. Dairy Sci. 78:1318–1327.

Polan, C. E., R. E. Blaser, C. N. Miller, and D. D. Wolf. 1986. Utilization of pasture by lactating cows. J. Dairy Sci. 69:1604–1612.

Poore, M. H., J. A. Moore, T. P. Eck, R. S. Swingle, and C. B. Theurer. 1993. Effect of fiber source and ruminal starch degradability on site and extent of digestion in dairy cows. J. Dairy Sci. 76:2244–2253.

Robinson, P. H. 1989. Dynamic aspects of feeding management for dairy cows. J. Dairy Sci. 72:1197–1209.

Shaver, R. D. 1997. Nutritional risk factors in the etiology of left displaced abomasum in dairy cows: a review. J. Dairy Sci. 80:2449–2453.

Shaver, R. D., A. J. Nytes, L. D. Satter, and N. A. Jorgensen. 1986. Influence of amount of feed intake and forage physical form on digestion and passage of prebloom alfalfa hay in dairy cows. J. Dairy Sci. 69:1545–1559.

Sievert, S. J., and R. D. Shaver. 1993. Effect of nonfiber carbohydrate level and *Aspergillus oryzae* fermentation extract on intake, digestion, and milk production in lactating dairy cows. J. Anim. Sci. 71:1032–1040.

Smith, D. 1981. Removing and analyzing carbohydrates from plant tissue. Wisconsin Agric. Exp. Stn. Rep. No. R2107, Madison.

Sudweeks, E. M., L. O. Ely, D. R. Mertens, and L. R. Sisk. 1981. Assessing minimum amounts and form of roughages in ruminant diets:roughage value index system. J. Anim. Sci. 53:1406–1411.

Sutton, J. D., and J. A. Bines. 1987. A comparison of starchy and fibrous concentrates for milk production, energy utilization and hay intake by Friesian cows. J. Agric. Sci., Camb. 109:375–385.

Swain, S. M., and L. E. Armentano. 1994. Quantitative evaluation of fiber from nonforage sources used to replace alfalfa silage. J. Dairy Sci. 77:2318–2331.

Varga, G. A., and P. Kononoff. 1999. Dairy rationing using structural and nonstructural carbohydrates: from theory to practice. Pages 77–90 in Proc. Southwest Nutr. Conf. Phoenix, AZ.

Vaughan, K. K., S. M. Swain, and L. E. Armentano. 1991. Effectiveness of NDF from ground corn cobs and wheat middlings compared to alfalfa silage. J. Dairy Sci. 74(Suppl. 1):220 (Abstr.).

Weiss, W. P., and W. L. Shockey. 1991. Value of orchardgrass and alfalfa silages fed with varying amounts of concentrates to dairy cows. J. Dairy Sci. 74:1933–1943.

Wilkerson, V. A., and B. P. Glenn. 1997. Energy balance in early lactation Holstein cows fed corn grains harvested and processed differently. J. Dairy Sci. 80:2487–2496

Woodford, J. A., N. A. Jorgensen, and G. P. Barrington. 1986. Impact of dietary fiber and physical form on performance of lactating dairy cows. J. Dairy Sci. 69:1035–1047.

# 5 Protein and Amino Acids

Dietary protein generally refers to crude protein (CP), which is defined for feedstuffs as the nitrogen (N) content × 6.25. The definition is based on the assumption that the average N content of feedstuffs is 16 g per 100 g of protein. The calculated CP content includes both protein and nonprotein N (NPN). Feedstuffs vary widely in their relative proportions of protein and NPN, in the rate and extent of ruminal degradation of protein, and in the intestinal digestibility and amino acid (AA) composition of ruminally undegraded feed protein. The NPN in feed and supplements such as urea and ammonium salts are considered to be degraded completely in the rumen.

## IMPORTANCE AND GOALS OF PROTEIN AND AMINO ACID NUTRITION

Ruminally synthesized microbial CP (MCP), ruminally undegraded feed CP (RUP), and to a much lesser extent, endogenous CP (ECP) contribute to passage of metabolizable protein (MP) to the small intestine. Metabolizable protein is defined as the true protein that is digested postruminally and the component AA absorbed by the intestine. Amino acids, and not protein per se, are the required nutrients. Absorbed AA, used principally as building blocks for the synthesis of proteins, are vital to the maintenance, growth, reproduction, and lactation of dairy cattle. Presumably, an ideal pattern of absorbed AA exists for each of these physiologic functions. The *Nutrient Requirements of Poultry* (National Research Council, 1994) and the *Nutrient Requirements of Swine* (National Research Council, 1998) indicate that an optimum AA profile exists in MP for each physiologic state of the animal and this is assumed to be true for dairy animals.

The goals of ruminant protein nutrition are to provide adequate amounts of rumen-degradable protein (RDP) for optimal ruminal efficiency and to obtain the desired animal productivity with a minimum amount of dietary CP. Optimizing the efficiency of use of dietary CP requires selection of complementary feed proteins and NPN supplements that will provide the types and amounts of RDP that will meet, but not exceed, the N needs of ruminal microorganisms for maximal synthesis of MCP, and the types and amounts of digestible RUP that will optimize, in so far as possible, the profile and amounts of absorbed AA. As discussed later, research indicates that the nutritive value of MP for dairy cattle is determined by its profile of essential AA (EAA) and probably also by the contribution of total EAA to MP. Improving the efficiency of protein and N usage while striving for optimal productivity is a matter of practical concern. Incentives include reduced feed costs per unit of lean tissue gain or milk protein produced, a desire for greater and more efficient yields of milk protein, creation of space in the diet for other nutrients that will enhance production, and concerns of waste N disposal. Regarding milk protein production, research indicates that content (and thus yield) of milk protein can be increased by improving the profile of AA in MP, by reducing the amount of "surplus" protein in the diet, and by increasing the amount of fermentable carbohydrate in the diet.

### *Major Differences from Previous Edition*

In 1985, the Subcommittee on Nitrogen Usage in Ruminants (National Research Council, 1985) expressed protein requirements in units of absorbed protein. Absorbed protein was defined as the digestible true protein (i.e., digestible total AA) that is provided to the animal by ruminally synthesized MCP and feed protein that escaped ruminal degradation. This approach was adopted for the previous edition of this publication (National Research Council, 1989). The absorbed protein method introduced the concept of degraded intake CP (DIP) and undegraded intake CP (UIP). Mean values of ruminal undegradability for common feeds, derived from in vivo and in situ studies using sheep and cattle, were reported. This factorial approach for estimating protein requirements recognized the three fates of dietary protein (fermentative digestion in the reticulo-rumen, hydrolytic/enzymatic digestion in the intestine, and passage of indigestible protein with feces) and separated the requirements of ruminal microorganisms from those of the host animal. However, a fixed intestinal digestibility of 80 percent for UIP was used, no consideration was given to the contribution of endogenous CP to MP, and no consideration was given to the AA composition of UIP or of absorbed protein.

Some differences exist in terminology. To be consistent with the current edition of *Nutrient Requirements of Beef Cattle* (National Research Council, 1996), and to avoid implications that proteins are absorbed, the term MP replaces absorbed protein. To be consistent with the *Journal of Dairy Science*, the terms DIP and UIP are replaced with RDP and RUP, respectively.

The primary differences between the protein system of this publication and that used in the previous edition relate to predicting nutrient supply. Microbial CP flows are predicted from intake of total tract digestible organic matter (OM) instead of net energy intake. The regression equation considers the variability in efficiency of MCP production associated with apparent adequacy of RDP. A mechanistic system developed from in situ data is used for calculating the RUP content of feedstuffs. Insofar as regression equations allow, the system considers some of the factors (DMI, percentage of concentrate feeds in diet DM, and percentage NDF in diet DM) that affect rates of passage of undigested feed and thus the RUP content of a feedstuff. The system is considered to be applicable to all dairy animals with body weights greater than 100 kg and that are fed for early rumen development. To increase the accuracy of estimating the contribution of the RUP fraction of individual feedstuffs to MP, estimates of intestinal digestibility have been assigned to the RUP fraction of each feedstuff (range = 50 to 100). Endogenous protein and NPN also are considered to contribute to passage of CP to the small intestine. Endogenous CP flows are calculated from intake of DM. And finally, regression equations are included that predict directly the content of each EAA in total EAA of duodenal protein and flows of total EAA. Flows of digestible EAA and their contribution to MP are calculated. Dose-response curves that relate measured milk protein content and yield responses to changes of predicted percentages of digestible Lys and Met in MP are presented. The dose-response relationships provide estimates of model-determined amounts of Lys and Met required in MP for optimal utilization of absorbed AA for milk protein production. The inclusion of equations for predicting passage of EAA to the small intestine along with assignment of RUP digestibility values that are unique to individual feedstuffs brings awareness to differences in nutritive value of RUP from different feedstuffs and should improve the prediction of animal responses to substitution of protein sources.

## PROTEIN

### *Chemistry of Feed Crude Protein*

Feedstuffs contain numerous different proteins and several types of NPN compounds. Proteins are large molecules that differ in size, shape, function, solubility, and AA composition. Proteins have been classified on the basis of their 3-dimensional structure and solubility characteristics. Examples of classifications based on solubility would include globular proteins [albumins (soluble in water and alkali solutions and insoluble in salt and alcohol), globulins (soluble in salt and alkali solutions and sparingly soluble or insoluble in water and insoluble in alcohol), glutelins (soluble only in alkali), prolamines (soluble in 70 to 80 percent ethanol and alkali and insoluble in water, salt, and absolute alcohol), histones (soluble in water and salt solutions and insoluble in ammonium hydroxide)] and fibrous proteins [e.g., collagens, elastins, and keratins (insoluble in water or salt solutions and resistant to digestive enzymes)] (Orten and Neuhaus, 1975; Rodwell, 1985; Van Soest, 1994). Globular proteins are common to all feedstuffs whereas fibrous proteins are limited to feeds of animal and marine origin. Albumins and globular proteins are low molecular weight proteins. Prolamines and glutelins are higher molecular weight proteins and contain more disulfide bonds. Generally, feeds of plant origin contain all of the globular proteins but in differing amounts. For example, cereal grains and by-product feeds derived from cereal grains contain more glutelins and prolamines whereas leaves and stems are rich in albumins (Blethen et al., 1990; Sniffen, 1974; Van Soest, 1994). A sequential extraction of 38 different feeds with water, dilute salt (0.5 percent NaCl), aqueous alcohol (80 percent ethanol), and dilute alkali (0.2 percent NaOH) indicated that the classic protein fractions (albumins, globulins, prolamines, and glutelins) plus NPN accounted for an average of 65 percent of total N (Blethen et al., 1990). The unaccounted for, insoluble N would include protein bound in intact aleurone granules of cereal grains, most of the cell-wall associated proteins, and some of the chloroplasmic and heat-denatured proteins that are associated with NDF (Van Soest, 1994). Among the feeds that were evaluated, those with the highest percentage of insoluble protein (> 40 percent of CP) were forages, beet pulp, soy hulls, sorghum, dried brewers grains, dried distillers grains, fish meal, and meat and bone meal (Blethen et al., 1990).

Feedstuffs also contain variable amounts of low molecular weight NPN compounds. These compounds include peptides, free AA, nucleic acids, amides, amines, and ammonia. Nonprotein N compounds generally are determined as the N remaining in the filtrate after precipitation of the true protein with either tungstic or trichloroacetic acid (Licitra et al., 1996). Grasses and legume forages contain the highest and most variable concentrations of

NPN. Most of the reported concentrations of NPN in CP of grasses and legume forages are within the following ranges: fresh material (10B15%), hay (15B25%), and silage (30B65%) (Fairbairn et al., 1988; Garcia et al., 1989; Grum et al., 1991; Hughes, 1970; Krishnamoorthy et al., 1982; Messman et al., 1994; Van Soest, 1994; Xu et al., 1996). Hays and especially silages contain higher amounts of NPN than the same feed when fresh because of the proteolysis that occurs during wilting and fermentation. The proteolysis that occurs in forages during wilting and ensiling is a result of plant and microbial proteases and peptidases. Plant proteases and peptidases are active in cut forage and are considered to be the principal enzymes responsible for the conversion of true protein to NPN in hays and ensiled feeds (Fairbairn et al., 1988; Van Soest, 1994). Rapid wilting of cut forages and conditions that promote rapid reductions in pH of ensiled feeds slow proteolysis and reduce the conversion of true protein to NPN (Garcia et al., 1989; Van Soest, 1994). The NPN content of fresh forage is composed largely of peptides, free AA, and nitrates (Van Soest, 1994). Fermented forages have a different composition of NPN than fresh forages. Fermented forages have higher proportional concentrations of free AA, ammonia, and amines and lower concentrations of peptides and nitrate (Fairbairn et al., 1988; Van Soest, 1994). The NPN content of most non-forage feeds is 12 percent or less of CP (Krishnamoorthy et al., 1982; Licitra et al., 1996; Van Soest, 1994; Xu et al., 1996).

*Mechanism of Ruminal Protein Degradation*

The potentially fermentable pool of protein includes feed proteins plus the endogenous proteins of saliva, sloughed epithelial cells, and the remains of lysed ruminal microorganisms. The mechanism of ruminal degradation has been reviewed (Broderick et al., 1991; Broderick, 1998; Cotta and Hespell, 1984; Jouany, 1996; Jouany and Ushida, 1999; Wallace, 1996; Wallace et al., 1999). In brief, all of the enzymatic activity of ruminal protein degradation is of microbial origin. Many strains and species of bacteria, protozoa, and anaerobic fungi participate by elaborating a variety of proteases, peptidases, and deaminases (Wallace, 1996). The liberated peptides, AA, and ammonia are nutrients for the growth of ruminal microorganisms. Peptide breakdown to AA must occur before AA are incorporated into microbial protein (Wallace, 1996). When protein degradation exceeds the rate of AA and ammonia assimilation into microbial protein, peptide and AA catabolism leads to excessive ruminal ammonia concentrations. Some of the peptides and AA not incorporated into microbial protein may escape ruminal degradation to ammonia and become sources of absorbed AA to the host animal.

Bacteria are the principal microorganisms involved in protein degradation. Bacteria are the most abundant microorganisms in the rumen ($10^{10-11}$/ml) and 40 percent or more of isolated species exhibit proteolytic activity (Broderick et al., 1991; Cotta and Hespell, 1984; Wallace, 1996). Most bacterial proteases are associated with the cell surface (Kopecny and Wallace, 1982); only about 10 percent of the total proteolytic activity is cell free (Broderick, 1998). Therefore, the initial step in protein degradation by ruminal bacteria is adsorption of soluble proteins to bacteria (Nugent and Mangan, 1981; Wallace, 1985) or adsorption of bacteria to insoluble proteins (Broderick et al., 1991). Extracellular proteolysis gives rise to oligopeptides which are degraded further to small peptides and some free AA. Following bacterial uptake of small peptides and free AA, there are five distinct intracellular events: (1) cleavage of peptides to free AA, (2) utilization of free AA for protein synthesis, (3) catabolism of free AA to ammonia and carbon skeletons (i.e., deamination), (4) utilization of ammonia for resynthesis of AA, and (5) diffusion of ammonia out of the cell (Broderick, 1998).

The bacterial population that is responsible for AA deamination has been of considerable interest. Amino acid catabolism and ammonia production in excess of bacterial need wastes dietary CP and reduces efficiency of use of RDP for ruminant production. For many years it was assumed that deamination was limited to the large number of species of bacteria that had been identified to produce ammonia from protein or protein hydrolyzates (Wallace, 1996). However, this assumption was challenged by Russell and co-workers (Chen and Russell, 1988, 1989; Russell et al., 1988) who concluded that the deaminative activity of these bacteria was too low to account for rates of ammonia production usually observed in vivo or in vitro with mixed cultures. Their efforts led to the eventual isolation of a small group of bacteria that had exceptionally high deaminative activity and that used AA as their main source of carbon and energy (Russell et al., 1988; Paster et al., 1993). As a result of these and other studies, it is now accepted that AA deamination by bacteria is carried out by a combination of numerous bacteria with low deaminative activity and a much smaller number of bacteria with high activity (Wallace, 1996). Of particular interest has been the observation that the growth of some of these bacteria with high deaminating activity is suppressed by the ionophore, monensin (Chen and Russell, 1988, 1989; Russell et al., 1988).

Protozoa also are active and significant participants in ruminal protein degradation. Protozoa are less numerous than bacteria in ruminal contents ($10^{5-6}$/ml) but because of their large size, they comprise a significant portion of the total microbial biomass in the rumen (generally less than 10 percent but sometimes as high as 50 percent) (Jouany, 1996; Jouany and Ushida, 1999). Several differences exist between protozoa and bacteria in their metabolism of protein. First, they differ in feeding behavior. Instead of forming a complex with feeds, protozoa ingest particulate matter (bacteria, fungi, and small feed particles). Bacteria are their principal source of ingested protein (Jouany and Ushida, 1999). As a result of this feeding behavior (i.e., ingestion of food), protozoa are more active in degrading insoluble feed proteins (e.g., soybean meal or fish meal) than more soluble feed proteins (e.g., casein) (Hino and Russell, 1987; Jouany, 1996; Jouany and Ushida, 1999). Ingested proteins are degraded within the cell to yield a mixture of peptides and free AA; the AA are incorporated into protozoal protein. Proteolytic specific activity of protozoa is higher than that of bacteria (Nolan, 1993). A second difference between protozoa and bacteria is that while both actively deaminate AA, protozoa are not able to synthesize AA from ammonia (Jouany and Ushida, 1999). Thus, protozoa are net exporters of ammonia and because of this, defaunation decreases ruminal ammonia concentrations (Jouany and Ushida, 1999). And lastly, protozoa release large amounts of peptides and AA as well as peptidases into ruminal fluid. This is the result of significant secretory processes and significant autolysis and death (Coleman, 1985; Dijkstra, 1994). Jouany and Ushida (1999) suggest that excreted small peptides and AA can represent 50 percent of total protein ingested by protozoa. Other studies indicate that 65 percent or more of protozoal protein recycles within the rumen (Ffoulkes and Leng, 1988; Punia et al., 1992).

Much less is known about the involvement of fungi in ruminal protein catabolism. Currently, anaerobic fungi are considered to have negligible effects on ruminal protein digestion because of their low concentrations in ruminal digesta ($10^{3-4}$/ml) (Jouany and Ushida, 1999; Wallace and Monroe, 1986).

*Kinetics of Ruminal Protein Degradation*

Ruminal degradation of dietary feed CP is an important factor influencing ruminal fermentation and AA supply to dairy cattle. RDP and RUP are two components of dietary feed CP that have separate and distinct functions. Ruminally degraded feed CP provides a mixture of peptides, free AA, and ammonia for microbial growth and synthesis of microbial protein. Ruminally synthesized microbial protein typically supplies most of the AA passing to the small intestine. Ruminally undegraded protein is the second most important source of absorbable AA to the animal. Knowledge of the kinetics of ruminal degradation of feed proteins is fundamental to formulating diets for adequate amounts of RDP for rumen microorganisms and adequate amounts of RUP for the host animal.

Ruminal protein degradation is described most often by first order mass action models. An important feature of these models is that they consider that the CP fraction of feedstuffs consists of multiple fractions that differ widely in rates of degradation, and that ruminal disappearance of protein is the result of two simultaneous activities, degradation and passage. One of the more complex of these models is the Cornell Net Carbohydrate Protein System (CNCPS) (Sniffen et al., 1992). In this model, feed CP is divided into five fractions (A, $B_1$, $B_2$, $B_3$, and C) which sum to unity. The five fractions have different rates of ruminal degradation. Fraction A (NPN) is the percentage of CP that is instantaneously solubilized at time zero, which is assumed to have a degradation rate ($k_d$) of infinity; it is determined chemically as that proportion of CP that is soluble in borate-phosphate buffer but not precipitated with the protein denaturant, trichloroacetic acetic (TCA) (Figure 5-1). Fraction C is determined chemically as the percentage of total CP recovered with ADF (i.e., ADIN) and is considered to be undegradable. Fraction C contains proteins associated with lignin and tannins and heat-damaged proteins such as the Maillard reaction products (Sniffen et al., 1992). The remaining B fractions represent potentially degradable true protein. The amounts of each of these 3 fractions that are degraded in the rumen are determined by their fractional rates of degradation ($k_d$) and passage ($k_p$); a single $k_p$ value is used for all fractions. Fraction $B_1$ is that percentage of total CP that is soluble in borate-phosphate buffer and precipitated with TCA. Fraction $B_3$ is calculated as the difference between the portions of total CP recovered with NDF (i.e., NDIN) and ADF (i.e., fraction C). Fraction $B_2$ is the remaining CP and is calculated as total CP minus the sum of fractions A, $B_1$, $B_3$, and C. Reported ranges for the fractional rates of degradation for the three B fractions are: $B_1$ (120–400 %/h), $B_2$ (3–16 %/h), and $B_3$ (0.06–0.55 %/h). The RDP and RUP values (percent of CP) for a feedstuff using this model are computed using the equations

$$\begin{aligned} RDP = {} & A + B_1\,[k_dB_1 / (k_dB_1 + k_p)] \\ & + B_2\,[k_dB_2 / (k_dB_2 + k_p)] \\ & + B_3\,[k_dB_3 / (k_dB_3 + k_p)] \end{aligned}$$

and

$$\begin{aligned} RUP = {} & B_1\,[k_p / (k_dB_1 + k_p)] \\ & + B_2\,[k_p / (k_dB_2 + k_p)] \\ & + B_3\,[k_p / (k_dB_3 + k_p)] + C. \end{aligned}$$

This model is used in Level II of the *Nutrient Requirements of Beef Cattle* (National Research Council, 1996) report.

The most used model to describe in situ ruminal protein degradation divides feed CP into three fractions (A, B, and C). Fraction A is the percentage of total CP that is NPN (i.e., assumed to be instantly degraded) and a small amount of true protein that rapidly escapes from the in situ bag because of high solubility or very small particle size. Fraction C is the percentage of CP that is completely undegradable; this fraction generally is determined as the feed CP remaining in the bag at a defined end-point of degradation. Fraction B is the rest of the CP and includes the proteins

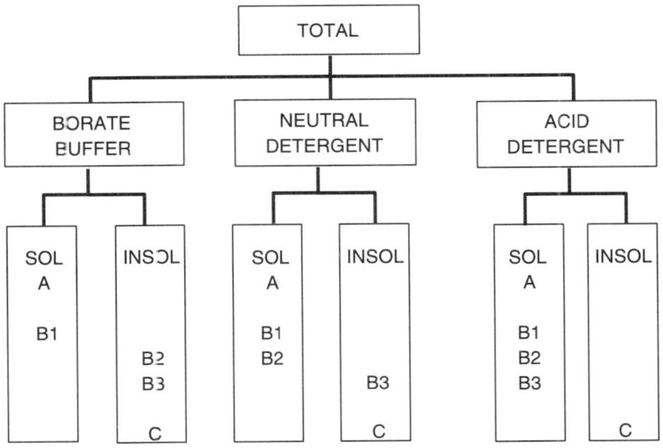


FIGURE 5-1 Analyses of crude protein fractions using borate-phosphate buffer and acid detergent and neutral detergent solutions (Roe et al., 1990; Sniffen et al, 1992).

that are potentially degradable. Only the B fraction is considered to be affected by relative rates of passage; all of fraction A is considered to be degraded and all of fraction C is considered to pass to the small intestine. The amount of fraction B that is degraded in the rumen is determined by the fractional rate of degradation that is determined in the study for fraction B and an estimate of fractional rates of passage. The RDP and RUP values for a feedstuff (percent of CP) using this model are computed using the equations RDP $= A + B [k_d / (k_d + k_p)]$ and RUP $= B [k_p / (k_d + k_p)] + C$. This simple model has been the most widely used model for describing degradation and ruminal escape of feed proteins (e.g., AFRC, 1984; National Research Council, 1985; Ørskov and McDonald, 1979). It is noted that data obtained from in situ, in vitro, and enzymatic digestions generally fit a model that divides feed CP into these fractions (Broderick et al., 1991) and that most of the in situ data used to validate results obtained with cell-free proteases have been obtained using this model (Broderick, 1998). As discussed later, it is this model in conjunction with in situ derived data that is used for predicting ruminal protein degradability in this edition.

Numerous factors affect the amount of CP in feeds that will be degraded in the rumen. The chemistry of feed CP is the single most important factor. The two most important considerations of feed CP chemistry are: (1) the proportional concentrations of NPN and true protein, and (2) the physical and chemical characteristics of the proteins that comprise the true protein fraction of the feedstuff. Nonprotein N compounds are degraded so quickly in the rumen (>300%/h) that degradation is assumed to be 100 percent (Sniffen et al., 1992). However, this is not an entirely correct assumption because degradability is truly related to rate of passage. For example, assuming a $k_p$ of 2.0%/h and a $k_d$ of 300%/h, then degradation $= 3.00/(3.00 + 0.02) = 0.993$ or 99.3 percent, and not 1.00 or 100 percent. Feedstuffs that contain high concentrations of NPN in CP contribute little RUP to the host animal. When dairy cattle are fed all-forage diets, measurements of passage of non-ammonia, non-microbial N (i.e., RUP-N plus endogenous N) often are less than 30 percent of N intake (Beever et al., 1976, 1987; Holden et al., 1994a; Van Vuuren et al., 1992). In contrast to NPN, which is assumed to be completely degraded, the rates of degradation of proteins are highly variable and result in variable amounts of protein being degraded in the rumen. For example, the range in $k_d$ given in Tables 15-2a,b are 1.4 for Menhaden fish meal to 29.2 for sunflower meal. Assuming a $k_p$ for each feed of 7.0 percent, the range in degradabilites of the B fraction would be 16.7 to 80.7 percent. Some characteristics of proteins shown to contribute to differences in rates of degradation are differences in 3-dimensional structure, differences in intra- and inter-molecular bonding, inert barriers such as cell walls, and antinutritional factors.

Differences in 3-dimensional structure and chemical bonding (i.e., cross-links) that occur both within and between protein molecules and between proteins and carbohydrates are functions of source as well as processing. These aspects of structure affect microbial access to the proteins, which apparently is the most important factor affecting the rate and extent of degradation of proteins in the rumen. Proteins that possess extensive cross-linking, such as the disulfide bonding in albumins and immunoglobulins or cross-links caused by chemical or heat treatment, are less accessible to proteolytic enzymes and are degraded more slowly (Ferguson, 1975; Hurrell and Finot, 1985; Mahadevan et al., 1980; Mangan, 1972; Nugent and Mangan, 1978; Nugent et al., 1983; Wallace, 1983). Proteins in feathers and hair are extensively cross-linked with disulfide bonds and largely for that reason, a considerable amount of the protein in feather meal is in fraction C (Tables 15-2a,b). Similarly, a considerable portion of the protein in meat meal and meat and bone meal is in fraction C. Proteins in meat meal and meat and bone meal may contain considerable amounts of collagen that has both intramolecular and intermolecular cross-links (Orten and Neuhaus, 1975). In contrast, a majority of the protein in menhaden fish meal is in fraction B but the fractional rate of degradation of fraction B is slower than in other protein supplements (Tables 15-2a,b). Heat used in the drying of fish protein was shown to induce the formation of disulfide bonds (Opstvedt et al., 1984). Heat processing also coagulates protein in meat products which makes it insoluble (Bendall, 1964; Boehme, 1982), and cooling of the products causes a random relinkage of chemical bonds which shrinks the protein molecules (Bendall, 1964). Collectively, these effects of heating and cooling of proteins decrease microbial access and make the proteins more resistant to ruminal degradation.

Other factors affecting the ruminal degradability of feed protein include ruminal retention time of the protein, microbial proteolytic activity, and ruminal pH. The effect of these factors on the kinetics of ruminal protein degradation have been reviewed (Broderick et al., 1991; National Research Council, 1985).

*Nitrogen Solubility vs. Protein Degradation*

Several commercial feed testing laboratories in the United States provide at least one measurement of N solubility for feedstuffs. Although recognized that N solubility in a single solvent is not synonymous with CP degradation in the rumen, the general absence of alternatives other than using "book values" for RUP (e.g., National Research Council, 1985) left little else to help nutritionists ensure that adequate but not excessive amounts of RDP were fed. Solubility measurements have been useful for ranking feeds of similar types for ruminal CP degradability. This is because of the positive relationship that exists between N solubility and degradation within similar feedstuffs (e.g., Beever et al., 1976; Laycock and Miller, 1981; Madsen and Hvelplund, 1990; Stutts et al., 1988). Many studies have indicated that changing N solubility by adding or removing NPN supplements, by changing method of forage preservation, or processing conditions of protein supplements affects animal response (e.g., Aitchison et al., 1976; Crish et al., 1986; Lundquist et al., 1986). Several different solvents have been used. At present, the most common procedure is incubation in borate-phosphate buffer (Roe et al., 1990). This method has gained in popularity because it is used for determining the A and $B_1$ nitrogen fractions in the CNCPS (Sniffen et al., 1992).

Although a high correlation exists between N solubility in a single solvent and protein degradability for similar feedstuffs, the same does not exist across classes of feedstuffs. For example, Stern and Satter (1984) reported a correlation of 0.26 between N solubility and in vivo protein degradation in the rumen of 34 diets that contained a variety of N sources. Madsen and Hvelplund (1990) also reported a poor relationship between N solubility and in vivo degradation of CP when used over a range of feedstuffs. There appear to be several reasons for these poor relationships. First, as indicated in the section "Chemistry of Feed Crude Protein", the proteins that are extracted by a solvent depend not only on the chemistry of the proteins but also on the composition of the solvent. For that reason, different solvents provide different estimates of CP solubility (Cherney et al., 1992; Crawford et al., 1978; Crooker et al., 1978; Lundquist et al., 1986; Stutts et al., 1988). Second, soluble proteins are not equally susceptible to degradation by rumen enzymes. Among the pure soluble proteins, casein is degraded rapidly whereas serum albumin, ovalbumin, and ribonuclease A are degraded much slower (Annison, 1956; Mahadevan et al., 1980; Mangan, 1972). Mahadevan et al. (1980) also observed that soluble proteins from soybean meal, rapeseed meal, and fish meal were degraded at different rates with rates of degradation for all three supplements being intermediate between those for albumins and casein. Therefore, structure as well as solubility determines degradability. Third, as indicated in the section "Mechanism of Ruminal Protein Degradation", solubility is not a prerequisite to degradation. As an example, Mahadevan et al. (1980) observed that soluble and insoluble proteins of soybean meal were hydrolyzed in vitro at almost identical rates. Because bacteria attach to insoluble proteins and because protozoa engulf feed particles, insoluble proteins need not enter the soluble protein pool before attack by microbial proteases. And last, soluble proteins that are not yet degraded may leave the rumen faster than insoluble proteins. This is because of a more likely association of soluble protein with the liquid fraction of ruminal contents. For example, Hristov and Broderick (1996) observed that although feed NAN in the liquid phase of ruminal contents was only 12 percent of total ruminal feed NAN, 30 percent of the feed NAN that escaped the rumen flowed with the liquids. This indicates a disproportional escape of soluble proteins.

In conclusion, a change in N solubility in a single solvent appears to be a more useful indicator of a change in protein degradation when applied to different samples of the same feedstuff than when used to compare different feedstuffs that differ in chemical and physical properties. Clearly, the relationship between solubility and degradability is the highest when most of the soluble N is NPN (Sniffen et al., 1992).

*Microbial Requirements for N Substrates*

Peptides, AA, and ammonia are nutrients for the growth of ruminal bacteria; protozoa cannot use ammonia. Estimates of the contribution of ammonia versus preformed AA to microbial protein synthesis by the mixed rumen population have been highly variable (Wallace, 1997). Studies using $N^{15}$ ammonia or urea infused into the rumen or added as a single dose demonstrated that values for microbial N derived from ammonia ranged from 18 to 100 percent (Salter et al., 1979). The $N^{15}$ studies of Nolan (1975) and Leng and Nolan (1984) indicated that 50 percent or more of the microbial N was derived from ammonia and the rest from peptides and AA. The mixed ruminal microbial population has essentially no absolute requirement for AA (Virtanen, 1966) as cross-feeding among bacteria can meet individual requirements. However, researchers have observed improved microbial growth or efficiency when peptides or AA replaced ammonia or urea as the sole or major source of N (Cotta and Russell, 1982; Russell and Sniffen, 1984; Griswold et al., 1996). Maeng and Baldwin (1976) reported increased microbial yield and growth rate on 75% urea + 25% AA-N as compared to

100% urea. Microbial requirements for N substrates of ammonia-N, AA, and peptides can also be affected by the basal diet and may explain some of the variability in the above experiments.

There is evidence that AA and especially peptides are stimulatory in terms of both growth rate and growth yield for ruminal microorganisms growing on rapidly degraded energy sources (Argyle and Baldwin, 1989; Chen et al., 1987; Cruz Soto et al., 1994; Russell et al., 1983). However, when energy substrates are fermented slowly, stimulation by peptides and AA does not always occur. Chikunya et al. (1996) demonstrated that when peptides were supplied with rapidly or slowly degraded fiber, microbial growth was enhanced only if the fiber was degraded rapidly. Russell et al. (1992) indicated that microorganisms fermenting structural carbohydrates require only ammonia as their N source while species degrading nonstructural carbohydrate sources will benefit from preformed AA.

Recent experiments (Wallace, 1997) have confirmed the earlier results of Salter et al. (1979) showing that the proportion of microbial N derived from ammonia varies according to the availability of N sources. The minimum contribution to microbial N from ammonia was 26 percent when high concentrations of peptides and AA were present, with a potential maximum of 100 percent when ammonia was the sole N source. Griswold et al. (1996) examined the effect of isolated soy protein, soy peptides, individual AA blended to profile soy protein, and urea on growth of microorganisms in continuous culture. Griswold et al. (1996) demonstrated that N forms other than ammonia are needed not only for maximum microbial growth but also as NPN for adequate ruminal fiber digestion.

Many reports of the uptake of $C^{14}$-AA and peptides have indicated that mixed microbial populations preferentially took up peptides rather than free AA (Cooper and Ling, 1985; Prins et al., 1979). However, Ling and Armstead (1995) found that free AA were the preferred form of AA incorporated by *S. bovis, Selenomonas ruminantium, Fibrobacter succinogenes* and *Anaerovibrio lipolytica*, whereas peptides were preferred only by *P. ruminicola. P. ruminicola* can comprise greater than 60 percent of the total flora in sheep fed grass silage (Van Gylswyk, 1990). In other studies where an AA preference was exhibited, the preference may have been the result of specific dietary conditions where *P. ruminicola* numbers were lower. Wallace (1996) demonstrated that AA deamination is carried out by two distinct bacterial populations, one with low activity and high numbers and the other with high activity and low numbers. *P. ruminicola* occurs in high numbers but has low deaminase activity.

Jones et al. (1998) investigated the effects of peptide concentrations in microbial metabolism in continuous culture fermenters. The basal diet contained 17.8 percent CP, 46.2 percent NSC, and 32.9 percent NDF. Peptides replaced urea as a N source at levels of 0, 10, 20 and 30 percent of total N, a urea-molasses mixture represented 8.6, 7.0, 4.9, and 2.9 percent of DM with increasing peptide and glucose replacement. Digestion of DM and CP and microbial CP production were affected quadratically by peptide addition; the highest values for each variable occurred at 10 percent peptide addition. Fiber digestion decreased linearly with increasing peptide addition. Reduced ammonia-N concentrations appeared to be the cause of reduced microbial CP production and reduced fiber digestion at levels of peptides greater than 10 percent of total N. The efficiency of conversion of peptide N to microbial CP increased with increasing peptides; however, there was no change in grams of microbial N produced per kilogram of OM digested. Jones et al. (1998) suggested that with diets containing high levels of NSC, excessive peptide concentrations relative to that of ammonia can depress protein digestion and ammonia concentrations, limit the growth of fiber-digesting microorganisms, and reduce ruminal fiber digestion and microbial protein production. Microorganisms that ferment NSC produce and utilize peptides at the expense of ammonia production from protein and other N sources (Russell et al., 1992). It should be noted that in continuous culture systems, protozoa can be washed out in the first few days of operation.

### *Animal Responses to CP, RDP, and RUP*

#### LACTATION RESPONSES

*Crude protein.* A data set of 393 means from 82 protein studies was used to evaluate the milk and milk protein yield responses to changes in the concentration of dietary CP (Table 5-1). The descriptive statistics for the data set are presented in Table 5-2. When CP content of diets change, the relative contribution of protein from different sources also change so this evaluation is confounded with source of protein and concentrations of RDP and RUP. Overall, milk yield increased quadratically as diet CP concentrations increased. The regression equation obtained was:

$$\text{Milk yield} = 0.8 \times \text{DMI} + 2.3 \times \text{CP} - 0.05 \times \text{CP}^2 - 9.8 \ (r^2 = 0.29)$$

where milk yield and dry matter intake (DMI) are kilograms/d and CP is percent of diet DM.

Dry matter intake was included in the regression to account indirectly for some of the differences among studies such as basal milk production and BW. Dry matter intake accounted for about 60 percent and CP about 40 percent of non-random variation. Assuming a fixed DMI (there was no correlation between intake and CP percent in this data set), the maximum milk production was obtained at 23 percent CP. The marginal response to

TABLE 5-1 Studies Used to Evaluate Milk and Milk Protein Yield Responses to Changes in the Concentration of Dietary Crude Protein

| | | |
|---|---|---|
| Annexstad et al. (1987) | Henderson et al. (1985) | McCormick et al. (1999) |
| Aharoni et al. (1993) | Henson et al. (1997) | McGuffey et al. (1990) |
| Armentano et al. (1993) | Higginbotham et al. (1989) | Nakamura et al. (1992) |
| Atwal et al. (1995) | Hoffman and Armentano (1988) | Owen and Larson (1991) |
| Baker et al. (1995) | Hoffman et al. (1991) | Palmquist and Weiss (1994) |
| Bertrand et al. (1998) | Holter et al. (1992) | Palmquist et al. (1993) |
| Blauwiekel and Kincaid (1986) | Hongerholt and Muller (1998) | Polan et al. (1997) |
| Blauwiekel et al. (1990) | Howard et al. (1987) | Polan et al. (1985) |
| Bowman et al. (1988) | Huyler et al. (1999) | Powers et al. (1995) |
| Broderick (1992) | Jaquette et al. (1986) | Robinson and Kennelly (1988b) |
| Broderick et al. (1990) | Jaquette et al. (1987) | Robinson et al. (1991b) |
| Bruckental et al. (1989) | Kaim et al. (1983) | Roseler et al. (1993) |
| Canfield et al. (1990) | Kaim et al. (1987) | Santos et al. (1998a,b) |
| Casper et al. (1990) | Kalscheur et al. (1999a,b) | Sloan et al. (1988) |
| Chen et al. (1993) | Kerry and Amos (1993) | Spain et al. (1995) |
| Christensen et al. (1993a, b) | Khorasani et al. (1996a) | Voss et al. (1988) |
| Crawley and Kilmer (1995) | Kim et al. (1991) | Wattiaux et al. (1994) |
| Cunningham et al. (1996) | King et al. (1990) | Weigel et al. (1997) |
| De Gracia et al. (1989) | Klusmeyer et al. (1990) | Wheeler et al. (1995) |
| DePeters and Bath (1986) | Komaragiri and Erdman (1997) | Windschitl (1991) |
| Dhiman and Satter (1993) | Lees et al. (1990) | Wohlt et al. (1991) |
| Garcia-Bojalil et al. (1998a) | Leonard and Block (1988) | Wright (1996) |
| Grant and Haddad (1998) | Lundquist et al. (1986) | Wu et al. (1997) |
| Grings et al. (1991) | Macleod and Cahill (1987) | Wu and Satter (2000) |
| Grings et al. (1992a) | Manson and Leaver (1988) | Zimmerman et al. (1992) |
| Grummer et al. (1996) | Mantysaari et al. (1989) | Zimmerman et al. (1991) |
| Hadsell and Sommerfeldt (1988) | McCarthy et al. (1989) | |

TABLE 5-2 Descriptive Statistics for Data Set Used to Evaluate Animal Responses to CP and RDP

| Variable | N | Mean | Std. Dev. |
|---|---|---|---|
| Milk, kg/d | 393 | 31.4 | 6.1 |
| Milk protein yield, g/d | 360 | 972 | 153 |
| Dry matter intake, kg/d | 393 | 20.2 | 3.4 |
| CP, % of dry matter | 393 | 17.1 | 2.6 |
| RDP, % of dry matter | 172 | 10.7 | 1.8 |
| RUP, % of dry matter | 172 | 6.2 | 1.4 |

increased dietary CP (first derivative of the CP components of the regression equation) is: 2.3 − 0.1 × CP. Therefore, increasing dietary CP one percentage unit from 15 to 16 percent would be expected to increase milk yield an average of 0.75 kg/d and increasing CP one percentage unit from 19 to 20 percent would be expected to increase milk yield by 0.35 kg/d. Although milk production may be increased by feeding diets with extremely high concentrations of CP, the economic and environmental costs must be compared with lower CP diets. The marginal response obtained from this data set was similar to that obtained by Roffler et al. (1986). With their equation, increasing dietary CP from 14 to 18 percent would result in an increase of 2.1 kg/d of milk and with the equation above the expected increase is 2.8 kg/d.

Dietary CP was not correlated (P>0.25) with milk protein percent, but was correlated weakly (r = 0.14; P<0.01) with milk protein yield (because of the relationship of dietary CP with milk yield). The regression equation was: milk protein yield (g/d) = 17.7 × DMI + 55.6 × CP − 1.26 × CP$^2$ + 31.8 ($r^2$ = 0.19) where DMI is kilograms/day and CP is percent of diet DM. Maximum yield of milk protein was obtained at 22 percent CP (essentially the same as for milk yield) and the marginal response is equal to 55.63 − 2.52 × CP where CP is a percent of diet DM.

*Rumen degradable and undegradable protein.* A regression approach also was used to evaluate lactation responses to concentrations of RDP and RUP in the dietary DM. To evaluate lactation responses to RDP in diet DM, 38 studies with 206 treatment means were selected in which diets varied in content of RDP (Table 5-3). All diets were entered into this edition's model for predicted concentrations of RDP and RUP in diet DM. As expected, concentrations of RDP and RUP (as percentages of diet DM) were correlated with concentrations of dietary CP (RDP; r = 0.78, P<0.001; RUP, r = 0.53, P<0.001), therefore it is not possible to separate effects of total CP from those of RDP or RUP. A regression equation for milk yield with RDP and RUP (both as percent of DM) was derived to overcome the problems associated with the correlation between CP and RDP and RUP (the correlation between RDP and RUP was not significant (r = −0.11, P>0.05). Dietary RDP and RUP were calculated using the model described in this publication based on values in the data set described above. The regression equation also included DMI for the reasons explained above. The regression equation (Figure 5-2) was:

$$\text{Milk} = -55.61 + 1.15 \times \text{DMI} + 8.79 \times \text{RDP} - 0.36 \times \text{RDP}^2 + 1.85 \times \text{RUP} \quad (r^2 = 0.52)$$

TABLE 5-3 Studies Used to Evaluate Milk Yield Responses to Changes in the Concentration of Dietary Ruminally Degraded Protein

| | | |
|---|---|---|
| Annexstad et al. (1987) | Grings et al. (1992) | King et al. (1990) |
| Armentano et al. (1993) | Grummer et al. (1996) | Komaragiri and Erdman (1997) |
| Baker et al. (1995) | Ha and Kennelly (1984) | Leonard and Block (1988) |
| Barney et al. (1981) | Harris et al. (1992) | Mantysaari et al. (1989) |
| Bertrand et al. (1998) | Henson et al. (1997) | McGuffey et al. (1990) |
| Blauwiekel et al. (1990) | Higginbotham et al. (1989) | Palmquist and Weiss (1994) |
| Casper et al. (1990) | Hoffman et al. (1991) | Roseler et al. (1993) |
| Christensen et al. (1993a,b) | Holter et al. (1992) | Santos et al. (1998a,b) |
| Cunningham et al. (1996) | Hongerholt and Muller (1998) | Wattiaux et al. (1994) |
| Dhiman and Satter (1993) | Kalscheur et al. (1999a) | Weigel et al. (1997) |
| Garcia-Bojalil et al. (1998a) | Khorasani et al. (1996b) | Windschitl (1991) |
| Grant and Haddad (1998) | Kim et al. (1991) | Wu and Satter (2000) |
| Grings et al. (1991) | | |

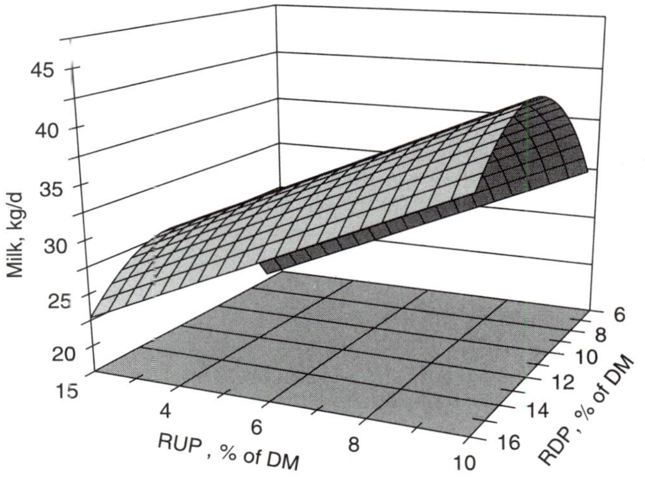


FIGURE 5-2 Response surface for data set described in "Animal Responses to CP, RDP, and RUP" section. Maximum milk yield occurred at 12.2 percent RDP (percent of diet DM). Dry matter intake was held constant at 20.6 kg/day.

where DMI and milk are kilograms/day, and RDP and RUP are percent of diet DM. Based on that equation, maximum milk yield occurred (DMI and RUP held constant) when RDP equaled 12.2 percent of diet DM, and the marginal change in milk to increasing RDP was 8.79 − 0.72 × RDP. The quadratic term for RUP was not significant and was removed from the model. Milk yield increase linearly to RUP at the rate of 1.85 kg for each percentage unit increase in RUP.

In comparison this edition's model estimates an average RDP requirement of 10.2 percent for this data set. Predicted milk yield (using the above regression equation) at 10.2 percent RDP (DMI and RUP held constant mean values of the data set of 20.6 kg/d DMI and 6.2 percent, respectively) is 31.7 kg/d and 33.2 kg/d when RDP is 12.2 percent. A portion of the discrepancy between model predicted requirement for RDP and regression predicted maximal milk production may be caused by the positive correlation between RDP and DM intake (DMI = 14.4 + 0.58 × RDP; r = 0.35, P<0.001). Based on that regression, an increase in 2 percentage units of RDP (i.e., 10.2 to 12.2 percent) would increase DMI by about 1.1 kg/d. Based on this edition's requirements (assumed 72 percent TDN), an increase of about 2 kg/d of milk is expected from that change in DMI. Increasing dietary RDP above model predicted requirements may result in increased DM intake.

A similar shaped function (data not shown) was obtained when milk protein yield was regressed on dietary RDP and RUP:

$$\text{Milk protein} = -1.57 + 0.0275 \times \text{DMI} + 0.223 \times \text{RDP} - 0.0091 \times \text{RDP}^2 + 0.041 \times \text{RUP} \quad (r^2 = 0.51)$$

where milk protein and DMI are kilograms per day and RDP and RUP are percentages of dietary DM. Maximum milk protein yield occurred at 12.2 percent RDP (the same as milk yield). Milk protein yield increased linearly with increasing dietary RUP.

Santos et al. (1998b) published a comprehensive review of the effects of replacing soybean meal with various sources of RUP on protein metabolism (29 published comparisons) and production (127 published comparisons). Santos et al. (1998b) reported that in 76 percent of the metabolism studies, higher RUP decreased MCP flows to the small intestine. Supplementation with RUP usually did not affect flow of total EAA, and RUP supplementation usually did not increase or actually decreased flow of lysine to the duodenum. Supplementation of RUP increased milk production in only 17 percent of the studies and heat-treated or chemically-treated soybean meal or fish meal were the most likely RUP supplements to cause increased milk production (Santos et al., 1998b). When studies were combined, cows fed diets with treated soybean meal (P<0.03) or fish meal (P<0.01) produced statistically more milk than cows fed soybean meal. Cows fed other animal proteins (blood, feather, meat meals) or corn gluten meal produced similar or numerically less milk than cows fed soybean meal (Santos et al., 1998b). See additional discussion in Chapter 16.

The regression equations derived above for milk and milk protein yield responses to dietary CP, RDP, and RUP should be interpreted and used cautiously in view of low $r^2$ values. A more sophisticated statistical analysis (e.g., controlling for trial effects, adjusting for variances within trials, etc.) would probably yield different and more accurate coefficients.

EFFECTS ON REPRODUCTION

Protein in excess of lactation requirements has been shown to have negative effects on reproduction. Several workers have reported that feeding diets containing 19 percent or more CP in diet DM lowered conception rates (Bruckental et al., 1989; Canfield et al., 1990; Jordan and Swanson, 1979; McCormick et al., 1999). Others have observed that cows fed 20–23 percent CP diets (as compared to 12–15 percent CP) had decreased uterine pH, increased blood urea, and altered uterine fluid composition (Jordan et al., 1983; Elrod and Butler, 1993). In a majority of the studies reviewed by Butler (1998), plasma progesterone concentrations in early lactation cows were lower when diets contained 19–20 percent CP vs. lower concentrations of CP.

In a review of protein effects on reproduction, Butler (1998) concluded that excessive amounts of either RDP or RUP could be responsible for lowered reproductive performance. However, intakes of "digestible" RUP in amounts required to adversely affect reproduction without a coinciding surplus of RDP would be uncommon. In most of the studies reviewed by Butler (1998), excessive RDP rather than excessive RUP was associated with decreased conception rates. Canfield et al. (1990) showed that feeding diets containing RUP to meet requirements while feeding RDP in excess of requirements resulted in decreased conception rates. Garcia-Bojalil et al. (1998b) reported that RDP fed in excess (15.7 percent of DM) of recommendations decreased the amount of luteal tissue in ovaries of early lactation cows.

Although most studies have indicated an adverse effect on reproductive performance of feeding high CP diets, others indicate no effect of diet CP on reproduction. Carroll et al. (1988) observed no differences in pregnancy rate or first service conception rates of dairy cows fed 20 percent CP and 13 percent CP diets. Howard et al. (1987) reported no difference in fertility between cows in second and greater lactation fed 15 percent CP or 20 percent CP diets.

There are many theories as to why excess dietary CP decreases reproductive performance (Barton, 1996a, 1996b; Butler, 1998; Ferguson and Chalupa, 1989). The first theory relates to the energy costs associated with metabolic disposal of excess N. To the extent that additional energy may be required for this purpose, this energy may be taken from body reserves in early lactation to support milk production. Delayed ovulation (e.g., Beam and Butler, 1997; Staples et al., 1990) and reduced fertility (Butler, 1998) have been associated with negative energy status. Another effect of negative energy status is decreased plasma progesterone concentrations (Butler, 1998).

Another theory is that excessive blood urea N (BUN) concentrations could have a toxic effect on sperm, ova, or embryos, resulting in a decrease in fertility (Canfield et al., 1990). High BUN concentrations have also been shown to decrease uterine pH and prostaglandin production (Butler, 1998). High BUN may also reduce the binding of leutinizing hormone to ovarian receptors, leading to decreases in serum progesterone concentration and fertility (Barton, 1996a). Ferguson and Chalupa (1989) reported that by-products of N metabolism may alter the function of the hypophysealpituitary-ovarian axis, therefore decreasing reproductive performance. And last, high levels of circulating ammonia may depress the immune system and, therefore, may result in a decline in reproductive performance (Anderson and Barton, 1988).

Milk urea nitrogen (MUN) and blood urea nitrogen (BUN) are both indicators of urea production by the liver. Milk urea N concentrations greater than 19 mg/dl have been associated with decreased fertility (Butler et al., 1995). Likewise, BUN concentrations greater than 20 mg/dl have been linked with reduced conception rates in lactating cows (Ferguson et al., 1988). Bruckental et al. (1989) found that BUN levels increased when diet CP was increased from 17 to 21.6 percent and pregnancy rate decreased by 13 percentage units. In a case study, Ferguson et al. (1988) observed that cows with BUN levels higher than 20 mg/dl were three times less likely to conceive than cows with lower BUN concentrations. Although high BUN concentrations have been associated with decreased reproductive performance, others have reported no adverse effects on pregnancy rate, services per conception, or days open with BUN levels above 20 mg/dl (Oldick and Firkins, 1996).

Studies by Carroll et al. (1987) and Howard et al. (1987) indicate that maintaining a strict reproductive management protocol can reduce the negative effects of excess protein intake on reproduction. Barton (1996a) demonstrated that an intense reproductive program could be used to reach reproductive success regardless of diet CP level or plasma urea N concentrations. These studies highlight the idea that dietary protein is just one of many things that have an effect on reproductive performance. Protein intake, along with other factors such as reproductive management, energy status, milk yield, and health status all have an effect on reproductive performance in dairy cattle.

*Synchronizing Ruminal Protein and Carbohydrate Digestion: Effects on Microbial Protein Synthesis*

Microbial protein synthesis in the rumen depends largely on the availability of carbohydrates and N in the rumen.

Bacteria are capable generally of capturing the majority of ammonia that is released in the rumen from AA deamination and the hydrolysis of NPN compounds. However, dietary conditions often occur in which the rate of ammonia release in the rumen exceeds the rate of uptake by ruminal bacteria. Examples of such conditions would include a surplus of RDP or a lack of available energy (Maeng et al., 1997). This asynchronous release of ammonia and energy in the rumen results in inefficient utilization of fermentable substrates and reduced synthesis of MCP. A variety of studies have focused on increasing the efficiency of microbial protein synthesis by manipulating dietary components (Aldrich et al., 1993a; Hoover and Stokes, 1991; Herrera-Saldana et al., 1990; Maeng et al., 1976). Excellent reviews describe the relationship between ruminal protein and carbohydrate availability and its impact on MCP synthesis in the rumen (Hoover and Stokes, 1991; Clark et al., 1992; Stern et al., 1994; Dewhurst et al., 2000).

Several studies indicate that synchronizing for rapid fermentation with fast degradable starch and protein sources stimulates greater synthesis or efficiency of synthesis of MCP. Herrera-Saldana et al. (1990) reported that MCP passage to the duodenum of lactating cows was highest (3.00 kg/d) when starch and protein degradability were synchronized for fast rates of digestion (barley and cottonseed meal). Flows of MCP were lower when the primary fermentable carbohydrate and protein sources were either synchronized for slow degradability (milo and brewer's dried grains; 2.14 kg/d) or asynchronized (barley and brewer's dried grains or milo and cottonseed meal; 2.64 and 2.36 kg/d, respectively). Efficiency of MCP synthesis (MCP/kg of truly digested OM) followed similar trends as MCP passage to the duodenum. Aldrich et al. (1993b) formulated diets to contain high and low concentrations of rumen-available nonstructural carbohydrates (HRANSC and LRANSC) and high and low concentrations of rumen-available protein (HRAP and LRAP) using high moisture shelled corn vs. coarse ground, dry ear corn and canola meal vs. blood meal, respectively. Flow of MCP to the duodenum was highest (1.64 kg/d) with HRANSC/HRAP and lowest (1.34 kg/d) with HRANSC/LRAP, flows were intermediate (1.46 and 1.48 kg/d) for the two LRANSC diets. Similar to the findings of Herrera-Saldana et al. (1990), efficiencies of synthesis of MCP were highest with the HRANSC/HRAP diet. Stokes et al. (1991a) reported that diets formulated to contain 31 or 39 percent NSC and 11.8 or 13.7 percent RDP in diet DM supported greater MCP synthesis than a diet containing 25 percent NSC and 9 percent RDP. Diets formulated to be synchronous vs. asynchronous in ruminal digestion rates of carbohydrate and protein have also increased flows and efficiency of synthesis of MCP in sheep (Sinclair et al., 1993, 1995). In the study by Sinclair et al. (1995), diets were similar in carbohydrate source (barley) and were either synchronous with rapeseed meal (diet A) or asynchronous with urea (diet B). The efficiency of MCP synthesis was 11–20 percent greater in sheep given diet A vs. diet B.

Numerous other studies have reported higher MCP passage (in vivo or in continuous culture) when either the NSC level was increased or more degradable carbohydrates were substituted for those less degradable (McCarthy et al., 1989; Spicer et al., 1986; Stokes et al., 1991a; Stern et al., 1978) or when RDP in diet DM was increased (Cecava et al., 1991; Hussein et al., 1991; McCarthy et al., 1989; Stokes et al., 1991b). A review of 16 studies indicated that MCP flow to the duodenum was increased by an average of 10 percent when slowly degradable sources of starch (e.g., corn grain) were replaced by more rapidly degraded starch (e.g., barley) (Sauvant and van Milgen, 1995). However, there was no effect of differences in rate of starch degradation on the efficiency of conversion of ruminally digested OM to MCP. Lykos et al. (1997) evaluated diets formulated to have similar rates of RDP with three rates (6.04, 6.98, and 7.94%/h) of NSC degradation in the rumen. Concentrations of RDP and NSC in diet DM were held constant across treatments. Rates of NSC degradation were achieved primarily by replacing cracked corn with ground high moisture corn. Flow of MCP to the duodenum tended to be the highest with the highest rate of NSC degradation. Efficiency of conversion of ruminally digested OM to MCP was increased as ruminal NSC availability increased, demonstrating the importance of timing of available energy to the ruminal microorganisms.

Studies evaluating the importance of providing a gradual or even supply (vs. an uneven supply) of energy and N substrates to ruminal microorganisms are limited. Henning et al. (1993) investigated this issue in cannulated sheep fed both at maintenance and at a higher level of nutrition. Treatments consisted of a soluble carbohydrate mixture (maltose, dextrose and maltotriose) and a soluble N mixture (urea and sodium caseinate). Providing an even supply of energy increased passage of MCP and efficiency of MCP synthesis when the maintenance diet was fed but only tended to increase efficiency of MCP synthesis when the more adequate diet was fed. In contrast, the even supply of N increased passage of MCP only when the more adequate diet was fed. The results indicate that merely improving the degree of synchronization between energy and N release rates in the rumen does not necessarily increase microbial cell yield and that a gradual or even release of energy and possibly N as well are also important.

Synchronizing rates of ruminal degradation of carbohydrates and protein may have a more pronounced effect in animals having high rates of ruminal passage (e.g., high DMI). Newbold and Rust (1992) observed in batch culture that a temporary restriction of supplies of either N or carbohydrate reduced subsequent bacterial growth rate. However, given the same total supply of nutrients, bacterial concentrations recovered after 12 h of incubation to concentrations observed prior to restriction of nutrient supplies. This suggests that microbial cells in the rumen are able to handle periods of nutrient shortage. These results were confirmed by the in vitro studies of Van Kessel and Russell (1997). However, when midlactation dairy cows were provided diets that varied in rumen degradable OM and CP, or fed at different feeding frequencies, no differences were observed in MCP production or microbial efficiency (Shabi et al., 1998).

The importance of providing a synchronized vs. an unsynchronized supply of N substrates to the mixed ruminal microbial population on ruminal protein and carbohydrate synchrony is unclear. Of particular interest is the identification of factors that affect efficiency of bacterial uptake of ammonia and alpha-amino N. Hristov et al. (1997) investigated the effect of different levels of carbohydrates and simultaneous provision of ammonia and alpha-amino N (AA and peptides) on the utilization of ammonia and alpha-amino N by ruminal microorganism in vitro. Rumen inoculum was incubated with five concentrations (0, 1, 5, 15, and 30 g/L) of carbohydrate (75 percent mixed sugars and 25 percent soluble starch) and five N sources (ammonia, free AA, ammonia plus free AA, peptides, and ammonia plus peptides). The ammonia pool in all treatments was labeled with $(^{15}NH_4)_2SO_4$. Observations included: (1) increased uptake and incorporation of ammonia into microbial N from all N treatments with increasing carbohydrate level, (2) a preference for rumen microbes to use alpha-amino N as compared to ammonia N, and (3) increased uptake of AA and peptides with added ammonia. It is concluded that the efficiency of use of ammonia and alpha-amino N by rumen microbes is not constant and is influenced by the availability (or balance) of energy, ammonia, and alpha-amino N.

Others have found that higher NSC or RDP in diet DM does not always support greater microbial growth. The extent to which ammonia is captured as MCP is affected by various factors such as diet type, ruminal fermentation characteristics, and DMI. Therefore, it should not be surprising that several studies conducted to evaluate the effect of synchronizing carbohydrate and protein degradation in the rumen observed no effects on MCP synthesis, efficiency of MCP synthesis, or no carbohydrate by protein interaction effects on MCP passage (Casper et al., 1999; Cecava et al., 1991; Feng et al., 1993; Hussein et al., 1991; McCarthy et al., 1989; Scollan et al., 1996; Stokes et al., 1991b).

The major nutrients required by rumen microbes are carbohydrates and proteins, but the most suitable sources and quantities needed to support maximum growth have not been determined. Although peptides, AA, and ammonia all may serve individually as sources of N for mixed ruminal microbes, the total population achieves the highest growth rate on mixtures of all three sources. Based on data from both in vitro and in vivo studies, there is general agreement that rate of digestion of carbohydrates is the major factor controlling the energy available for microbial growth (Hoover and Stokes, 1991).

It is possible to alter the synchronization of protein and carbohydrate, either by changing dietary ingredients or by altering the relative times of feeding ingredients (Shabi et al., 1998). However it is not possible to identify whether an increase in MCP synthesis by feeding different ingredients (Herrera-Saldana et al., 1990; Aldrich et al., 1993a; Sinclair et al., 1993, 1995) is an effect of synchrony or a factor associated with the manipulation of the ingredients (level and type) themselves (Dewhurst et al., 2000).

In summary, it is well documented that the kinetics of carbohydrate and protein degradation varies widely according to feed source, its chemical composition, and method of processing. The available literature indicates that when rumen fermentation is normal, there is little additional benefit of altering carbohydrate and protein degradation rates, or their level of synchrony, on microbial protein synthesis.

*Ruminally Protected Proteins*

"Rumen protected" has been defined by the Association of American Feed Control Officials (Noel, 2000) as "a nutrient(s) fed in such a form that provides an increase in the flow of that nutrient(s), unchanged, to the abomasum, yet is available to the animal in the intestine." Thus, rumen protected proteins are protein-containing feeds that have been treated or processed in ways to decrease ruminal protein degradability and increase the content of digestible RUP. Most research has focused on oilseeds and oilseed meals. Rumen protected proteins, as well as protein supplements that have an inherent high rate of ruminal escape, are important in dairy cattle nutrition because of the low content of digestible RUP in most feedstuffs. Reliance on feed proteins with a high content of digestible RUP is greatest in high producing cows when most or all of the forage is provided by high quality grasses and legumes. In these situations, the basal diet often contains adequate or more than adequate amounts of RDP but is deficient in RUP. Thus, protein supplementation should be limited to high RUP-containing feedstuffs to avoid large excesses of RDP.

Many methods have been investigated to decrease the rate and extent of ruminal degradation of feed proteins. Most of the methods have involved the use of heat, chemical agents, or a combination of heat and chemical agents (Kaufmann and Lüpping, 1982; Satter, 1986; Broderick et al., 1991; Schwab,1995). The challenge has been to identify treatments or processing conditions that increase digestible RUP to an extent that justifies the cost of the treatment, and in the case of the first three methods, with minimal loss of AA.

Heat processing is the most used treatment in North America. Heat processing decreases rumen protein degradability by denaturation of proteins and by the formation of protein-carbohydrate (Maillard reactions) and protein-protein cross-links. Commercial methods that rely solely on heat (dry or in combination with added moisture) include cooker-expeller processing of oilseeds, additional heat treatment of solvent extracted oilseed meals, roasting, extrusion, pressure toasting, and micronization of legume seeds, and expander treatment of cereal grains and protein supplements. Studies of ruminal degradation of protein of heat processed feedstuffs using the in situ approach indicate reductions in fraction A, increases in fractions B and C, and decreases in the fractional rates of degradation of the B fraction (Goelema et al., 1999; Prestløkken, 1999; Wang et al., 1999).

Careful control of heating conditions is required to optimize the content of digestible RUP (Schwab, 1995a). Under-heating results in only a small increase in digestible RUP. Over-heating of feeds (i.e., heat-damaged protein) reduces the intestinal digestibility of RUP through the formation of indigestible Maillard products and protein complexes (Van Soest, 1994). Over-heating also causes significant absolute losses of lysine, cystine, and arginine (Parsons et al., 1992; Barneveld et al., 1994a; Dale, 1996). Among those AA, lysine is the most sensitive to heat damage and undergoes both destruction and decreased availability (Weiss et al. 1986a,b; Barneveld et al., 1994b,c; Nakamura et al., 1994b). Optimal conditions of heat processing are generally considered to be those which significantly decrease ruminal protein degradability without adverse effects on postruminal digestion or significant losses of AA. However, combined measurements of RUP with measurements (or estimates) of intestinal-available lysine in RUP indicates that some loss of chemically determined available lysine is needed to achieve the heat treatment of oilseeds and oilseed meals that maximizes postruminal available lysine (Broderick and Craig, 1980; Craig and Broderick, 1981; Faldet et al., 1991; Faldet et al., 1992a,b). The relationships between heat input and concentrations of RDP, RUP, indigestible RUP, and digestible RUP have been described (Satter, 1986).

Chemical treatment of feed proteins can be divided into three categories: (1) chemicals that combine with and introduce cross-links in proteins (e.g., aldehydes), (2) chemicals that alter protein structure by denaturation (e.g., acids, alkalis, and ethanol), and (3) chemicals that bind to proteins but with little or no alteration of protein structure (e.g., tannins) (Broderick et al., 1991; Schwab,1995a). For a variety of reasons, often including less than desired levels of effectiveness, use of chemical agents as the sole treatment for increasing the RUP content of feed proteins has not received commercial acceptance. A more effective approach involving "chemical" agents has been to combine chemical and heat treatments. An example of this approach is the addition of lignosulfonate, a byproduct of the wood pulp industry that contains a variety of sugars (mainly xylose), to oilseed meals before heat treatment. The combined treatments enhance nonenzymatic browning (Maillard reactions) because of the enhanced availability of sugar aldehydes that can react with protein (Broderick et al., 1991; Schwab, 1995a).

Successful use of rumen protected proteins and other proteins that have a high ruminal escape requires consideration of AA composition and knowledge of the content and intestinal digestibility of the RUP fraction.

### *Predicting Passage of Microbial Protein*

Ruminally synthesized microbial protein typically supplies a majority of the AA flowing to the small intestine of growing cattle (Titgemeyer and Merchen, 1990b) and dairy cows (Clark et al., 1992). Microbial protein is the protein of the ruminal bacteria, protozoa, and fungi that pass to the small intestine. Bacteria provide most of the microbial protein leaving the rumen. Protozoa contribute significantly to the microbial biomass of ruminal contents. However, because they are more extensively recycled in the rumen than bacteria (Ffoulkes and Leng, 1988; Leng et al., 1986; Punia et al., 1992), protozoa do not contribute to postruminal protein supply in proportion to their contributions to the total microbial biomass in the rumen.

In the 1989 *Nutrient Requirements of Dairy Cattle* publication, bacterial crude protein production (BCP) in lactating dairy cows was predicted from net energy intake using the equation: $BCP = 6.25\,(-30.93 + 11.45\ NE_L)$. For growing animals, BCP was predicted from TDN intake using the equation: $BCP = 6.25\,(-31.86 + 26.12\ TDN)$. These equations were adapted from the 1985 National Research Council's report *Ruminant Nitrogen Usage.*

The most recent *Nutrient Requirements of Beef Cattle* report (National Research Council, 1996) adopted two different strategies in predicting microbial protein production in the rumen. In Level I of the beef model (National Research Council, 1996), BCP was estimated to be 130 grams per kilogram TDN intake with a downward adjustment for diets containing less than 40 percent forage, an unlikely circumstance for growing dairy heifers. Level II of the beef model (National Research Council, 1996) used an adaptation of the Cornell Net Carbohydrate and Protein System to predict BCP in both growing and mature beef cattle.

Using the range in TDN requirements for growing heifers from Table 6-2 in *Nutrient Requirements of Dairy Cattle* (1989), TDN intake would range from 1.82 to 8.80 kg/day. The implied range in BCP production per unit of

TDN would be 53 to 140 g BCP/kg of TDN. The calculated variation in microbial efficiency is due to the negative intercept in the original 1985 National Research Council equation (National Research Council, 1985). The adjustment to a constant 130 g BCP/kg of TDN presented in *Nutrient Requirements of Beef Cattle* (National Research Council, 1996) appears more reasonable. Burroughs et al. (1974) proposed a value of 104.4 for microbial amino acids. Assuming 80 percent microbial amino acids in microbial N, this would correspond to a factor of 130.5 (104.4/0.8) for MCP. However, validation of this was nearly impossible because of the lack of reported data specific to growing dairy heifers in the literature. There are considerable data in the beef cattle literature but unfortunately, most of these reports were in animals fed high concentrate diets that would be atypical of those fed to growing replacement heifers and bulls.

There is a wealth of published data on MCP production, particularly in lactating dairy cows at high feed intakes, which has been published since the 1985 National Research Council's report on *Ruminant Nitrogen Usage*. Several methods were considered for predicting MCP production in the lactating dairy cow. Figure 5-3 shows the relationship between $NE_L$ intake and microbial N flows using a data set (Table 5-4) consisting of 334 treatment means from published literature since 1985 and collected from lactating and dry cows. Superimposed on Figure 5-3 is a prediction line using the 1989 lactating dairy cow equation. Although the previous edition of *Nutrient Requirements of Dairy Cattle* (National Research Council, 1989) equation performed reasonably well at intakes of less than 30 Mcal of $NE_L$, microbial N flow was consistently

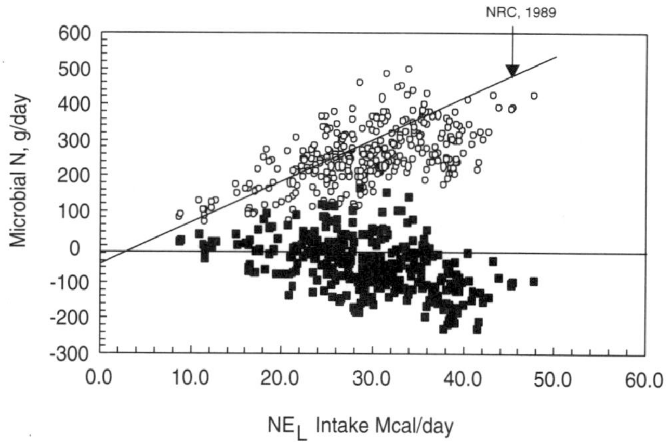


FIGURE 5-3 Plot of observed (open circles) and residuals (squares) for measured microbial N flow (g/day) versus estimated $NE_L$ intake in lactating and dry dairy cows. The National Research Council, 1989, line is the predicted line where microbial N = $-30.93 + 11.45\ NE_L$. At high levels of $NE_L$ intake, microbial N production is over-predicted.

over-predicted at high $NE_L$ intakes which are more common in today's higher producing cows. The 1985 equation was based on cows fed $NE_L$ intakes ranging from 5 to 29 Mcal/day. The maximal $NE_L$ intake in that data set is equivalent to only about 3 times maintenance intake for a 600 kg dairy cow. To overcome this problem, the literature data set (Table 5-4) was used to develop new microbial N prediction equations.

Several different prediction variables were evaluated including both linear and quadratic effects of DM, OM, and $NE_L$ intakes. Although addition of quadratic terms did correct for over prediction at high feed intake, the standard error of prediction for individual treatment means was high (61 g N) and no regression equation had an $r^2$ of more than 0.39. Alternatively, equations used in Level II of the beef model (National Research Council, 1996) were tested on a smaller subset of data with similar results where microbial N flow was again over-predicted at high feed intake with no improvement in overall prediction error. Measured rumen fermentable OM obtained from the literature data set was an even poorer predictor of microbial N with a standard error of prediction of 67 g N.

Within the literature data set (Table 5-4), there was a large range in measured efficiencies of microbial protein synthesis (12-54 g microbial N/kg rumen fermented OM). The wide range in measured efficiencies of microbial protein synthesis explains why fermented OM was a poor predictor of microbial N passage to the duodenum. Because of the variability in efficiency of microbial protein synthesis, it was concluded that systems driven by fermented energy alone or by indirect indicators of fermented energy such as TDN or $NE_L$ would not be accurate enough to predict passage of microbial N to the duodenum unless at least some of the variability was accounted for in efficiency of microbial protein synthesis.

An important factor affecting efficiency of microbial protein synthesis is the relative availability of N for fermentation. Apparent ruminal N balance is an indirect indicator of N availability for microbial protein synthesis. Where balance is positive, N from dietary RDP is in excess of N captured as microbial N and there is a net loss of N from the rumen to the animal tissues. Where apparent ruminal N balance is negative, there is a net gain of N in the rumen indicating inadequate N from RDP for microbial protein synthesis and a net gain from recycling of N from the animal tissues to the rumen. Figure 5-4 shows the relationship between observed microbial efficiency and apparent ruminal N balance using the literature data set where the microbial efficiency (g microbial N/kg truly fermented OM) was equal to 29.74 − 0.30 ARND ($r^2$ = 0.41, SEy = 6.5). The equation suggests a microbial efficiency of 29.74 g N/kg truly fermented OM at an apparent ruminal N digestibility of zero.

TABLE 5-4 Studies Used to Determine the Relationship Between $NE_L$ Intake and Passage of Microbial Protein to the Small Intestine of Lactating Dairy Cows

| | | |
|---|---|---|
| Aldrich et al. (1993b) | Klusmeyer et al. (1991b) | Robinson and Sniffen (1985) |
| Arieli et al. (1993) | Klusmeyer et al. (1990) | Robinson et al. (1991a) |
| Armentano et al. (1986) | Kung et al. (1983) | Robinson et al. (1997) |
| Benchaar et al. (1994a) | Lu et al. (1988) | Robinson et al. (1994) |
| Benchaar et al. (1991) | Lykos et al. (1997) | Robinson et al. (1985) |
| Benchaar et al. (1994b) | Lynch et al. (1991) | Rode and Satter (1988) |
| Blauwiekel et al. (1997) | Mabjeesh et al. (1996) | Rode et al. (1985) |
| Calsamiglia et al. (1995b) | Mabjeesh et al. (1997) | Santos et al. (1984) |
| Cameron et al. (1991) | Madsen (1986) | Sarwar et al. (1991) |
| Chan et al. (1997) | Mansfield and Stern (1994) | Schwab et al. (1992a) |
| Christensen et al. (1993b) | McCarthy et al. (1989) | Schwab et al. (1992b) |
| Christensen et al. (1996) | Merchen and Satter (1983) | Seymour et al. (1992) |
| Cunningham et al. (1993) | Moller (1985) | Song and Kennelly (1989) |
| Cunningham et al. (1994) | Murphy et al. (1987) | Stensig and Robinson (1997) |
| Cunningham et al. (1996) | Narasimhalu et al. (1989) | Stern et al. (1983) |
| Doreau et al. (1991) | Ohajuruka et al. (1991) | Stern et al. (1985) |
| Erasmus et al. (1992) | Oldham et al. (1979) | Stokes et al. (1991b) |
| Erasmus et al. (1994b) | Oliveira et al. (1995) | Tamminga et al. (1979) |
| Espindola et al. (1997) | O'Mara et al. (1997b) | Teller et al. (1992) |
| Feng et al. (1993) | Overton et al. (1995) | Tice et al. (1993) |
| Herrera-Saldana et al. (1990) | Palmquist et al. (1993) | van Vuuren et al. (1992) |
| Holden et al. (1994a) | Pantoja et al. (1995) | Waltz et al. (1989) |
| Joy et al. (1997) | Pantoja et al. (1994) | Weisbjerg et al. (1992) |
| Kalscheur et al. (1997a) | Pena et al. (1986) | Windschitl and Stern (1988) |
| Kalscheur et al. (1997b) | Pires et al. (1997) | Yang et al. (1997) |
| Khorasani et al. (1996a) | Poore et al. (1993) | Yoon and Stern (1996) |
| King et al. (1990) | Prange et al. (1984) | Zerbini et al. (1988) |
| Klusmeyer et al. (1991a) | Putnam et al. (1997) | Zhu et al. (1997) |

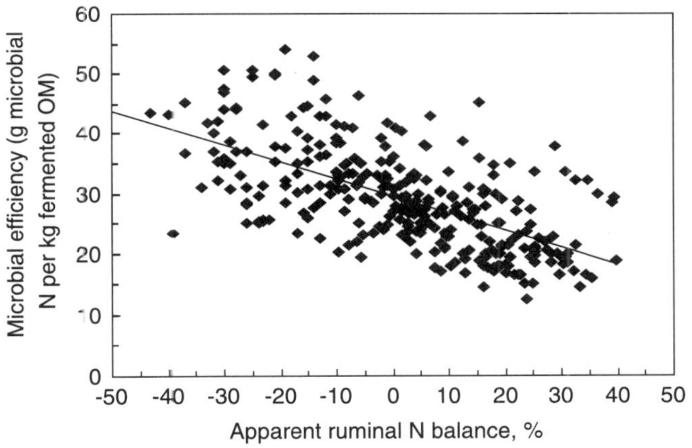


FIGURE 5-4 Relationship between measured efficiency of microbial protein synthesis (g microbial N/kg rumen fermented OM) and apparent ruminal N balance (microbial efficiency = 29.74 − 0.30 apparent ruminal N digestibility percent, $r^2 = 0.41$, $P < 0.001$, Sy = 6.49, n = 306).

The *Nutrient Requirements of Dairy Cattle* (National Research Council, 1989) report assumed a net recycling of 15 percent of dietary N intake or an apparent ruminal N balance of −15 percent. The average apparent ruminal N balance in the literature data set was plus 1.0 percent suggesting that on average net recycling of N to the rumen was zero. If under practical circumstances, ruminal N balance ranges from +20 to −20 percent, efficiency of microbial protein synthesis would vary from 24 to 36 g N/kg of OM fermented in the rumen and would have a major impact on estimated microbial protein production.

The implication is that as availability of N increases in relation to fermented OM, efficiency of microbial protein synthesis decreases. If ruminal N availability is relatively high compared to fermented OM, then output of microbial N per unit of fermented OM decreases, indicating that microbial utilization of N and energy becomes uncoupled and energy utilization for microbial protein synthesis becomes less efficient because the excess N is not used by the rumen microbes (Clark et al., 1992). Systems for predicting microbial N production as fixed linear functions are likely to over predict microbial protein production, particularly at high intakes of ruminally fermented OM. This would be true regardless of whether microbial N was predicted directly from ruminally fermented OM or indirectly using total tract digestible OM (TTDOM) intake or energy intake as an indicator of ruminally fermented OM.

The 1989 *Nutrient Requirements of Dairy Cattle* (National Research Council, 1989) report assumed an efficiency of use of apparent ruminally degraded N (RDP) of 0.9. If N recycling is set to zero, then net RDP required would be 1.11 × microbial N. The mean RDP to microbial N ratio (RDP:MN) in the data set was 1.18 or about 1.2. Although deficits in RDP for microbial N synthesis can be made up through N recycling, the impact of low RDP availability on rumen fermentation is not well understood nor could it be defined using the current literature data set. Therefore, the mean RDP to microbial N ratio of 1.18 was used to define RDP requirements assuming an apparent ruminal N balance of zero.

Ruminally fermented OM is not practical to use as a direct index of available energy for microbial growth as there are not adequate means by which rumen fermentability of an individual feedstuff or diet can be predicted. Previously cited techniques for predicting TDN offered a more practical indirect indicator of ruminally fermented OM. This is similar to the use of $NE_L$ intake in *Nutrient Requirements of Dairy Cattle* (National Research Council, 1989) publication. In a summary of experiments with dairy cows fed diets containing as much as 7 percent of added dietary fat, rumen fermentability of the diet was reduced by an amount equivalent to the amount of fat added to the diet and total microbial N production was unaffected (Erdman, 1995). Because the increase in efficiency of microbial protein synthesis was due to a reduction in fermented OM and not an increase in microbial N synthesis, TTDOM was used as an indirect indicator of fermentable energy. This can be calculated by adjusting the contribution of fat to TDN by a factor of 1.25 where: TTDOM = TDN − [(EE − 1) × 1.25]. The factor of 1.25 corresponds to the increase in energy content of absorbed ether extract (EE) versus other dietary components and EE is adjusted downward to account for the 1 percent dietary EE of non-fatty acid origin.

To correct for differences in microbial efficiency due to availability of RDN in relation to microbial N, the microbial efficiency values were adjusted in the literature data set using the equation (g microbial N/kg of TTDOM = 32.78 − 8.29 RDN:MN, $r^2 = 0.35$, $P < 0.001$, Sy = 4.8, n = 270). The microbial N yields adjusted to a common RDN:MN availability of 1.2 were then regressed against TTDOM. The results are shown in Figure 5-5.

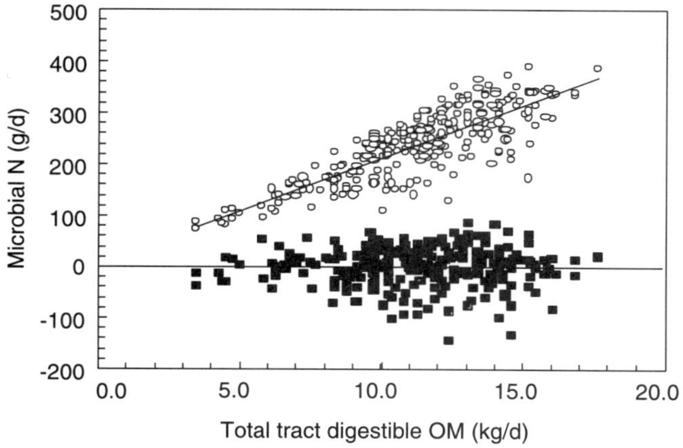


FIGURE 5-5 Plot of adjusted (open circles) and residuals (squares) for measured microbial N (g/d) versus measured total tract digestible OM (kg/d). (Microbial N = 21.03 total tract digestible OM. $r^2 = 0.69$, $P < 0.001$, Sy = 38.1, n = 266).

Microbial N flow corrected to 1.2 RDN:MN was related linearly to TTDOM at all levels of TTDOM intakes. This was also true for the relationship with both $NE_L$ and TDN intake. Calculated intercepts were not different from zero and regression coefficients using zero intercepts were 21.03, 20.32, and 8.21 g microbial N per kilogram TTDOM, per kilogram TDN, and per Mcal $NE_L$, respectively. Each equation had a standard error of prediction of 38 g. If coefficients were converted to a microbial CP basis (N × 6.25), corresponding coefficients would be 131, 127, and 51 g respectively. The coefficient (127) for TDN is identical to the adapted Burrough's value (130.5) and the value (130) used in Level I of the *Nutrient Requirements of Beef Cattle* report (National Research Council, 1996) suggesting that a common value (130) could be used for both growing animals and lactating dairy cows. In this volume, 130 g of microbial CP/kg discounted TDN is used to estimate microbial protein synthesis. Because there is no intercept in these equations, the microbial protein and net absorbed protein values can be assigned to individual feeds, which was not possible in the *Nutrient Requirements of Dairy Cattle* (National Research Council, 1989) report.

In summary, it is assumed that the yield of MCP is 130 g/kg of TDN (discounted) intake and that the requirement for RDP is 1.18 × MCP yield. Therefore, yield of MCP is calculated as 0.130 × TDN (discounted TDN, see Chapter 2) when RDP intake exceeds 1.18 × MCP yield. When RDP intake is less than 1.18 × TDN-predicted MCP, then MCP yield is calculated as 0.85 of RDP intake (1.00/1.18 = 0.85).

### *Predicting Passage of Rumen Undegradable Feed Protein*

The values for RUP reported in the previous edition of *Nutrient Requirements of Dairy Cattle* (National Research Council, 1989) were based on in vivo and in situ estimates from cattle and sheep and in many cases represented few observations. Subsequent to the *Nutrient Requirements of Dairy Cattle* (National Research Council, 1989) publication, a wealth of data has been published that have provided estimates of RUP concentrations in feedstuffs. Approaches have included in vivo, in situ, and in vitro (enzymatic, inhibitor, nitrogen solubility and protein fractionation, continuous culture fermentation, gel electrophoresis, and near-infrared reflectance spectroscopy) techniques (Hoffman et al., 1999; Michalet-Doreau and Ould-Bah, 1992; Nocek, 1988; Stern et al., 1997). Although often used as the standard by which other methods are evaluated, the in vivo approach requires the use of cannulated animals and, therefore, is subject to errors associated with cannula placement and the use of microbial and digesta flow markers.

The in situ procedure has emerged as the most widely used approach for estimating RUP (Stern et al., 1997) and is used in this edition. The procedure has been modified and adopted in several countries (Lindberg, 1985; Michalet-Doreau and Ould-Bah, 1992; Nocek, 1988; Stern et al., 1997; Vanzant et al., 1998). Adherence to guidelines for standardizing factors known to affect the results (Michalet-Doreau and Ould-Bah, 1992; Nocek, 1988; Stern et al., 1997) have increased considerably the reproducibility of the measurements within and among laboratories.

As described in the section "Kinetics of Ruminal Protein Degradation", the in situ procedure can be used to identify and quantify at least three N fractions which commonly are referred to as the A, B, and C fractions, and the rate of degradation (Kd) of fraction B. Fraction A includes NPN, rapidly solubilized protein, and protein in particles of smaller size than the porosity of the Dacron polyester or nylon bags into which the feedstuff is placed during incubation in the rumen. The different forms of N in fraction A cannot be separated by using the in situ procedure, nor can the rate be determined at which fraction A is degraded. Fraction C is estimated by a defined end-point of degradation, which corresponds to the lowest percent residual beyond which no further ruminal degradation occurs (Nocek and English, 1986). Different approaches have been described to combine estimates of the Kd of fraction B with rates of passage (Kp) from the rumen to estimate RUP (see Michalet-Doreau and Ould-Bah, 1992; Stern et al., 1997; and Bach et al., 1998, for review). The portion of fraction B determined not to be degraded, plus fraction C, is assumed to be RUP. Important assumptions with the in situ method are that "disappearance" from the bag is synonymous with degradation and that any N that has disappeared from the bag, including N associated with rapidly degradable proteins that are likely to be hydrolyzed as peptides (Broderick and Wallace, 1988), has been degraded and can be used by ruminal microorganisms.

In situ data from 190 cattle experiments were reviewed. The experiments involved 1326 individual feedstuff observations. Most of the publications were published between 1988 and 1998. Experiments involving sheep were not used because rumen degradation kinetics have been shown to differ between sheep and cows (Sebek and Everts, 1999; Siddons and Paradine, 1983; Prigge et al., 1984; Uden and Van Soest, 1984). Rarely were all three fractions reported, and sometimes Kd was not reported. In cases of incomplete information, the data were discarded unless enough information was provided to solve for the missing parameter by using either of the two equations, RDP = A + B[Kd/(Kd + Kp)] or RUP = B[Kp/(Kp + Kd)] + C. For observations in which no C fraction was reported, but the sum of the A and B fractions was less than 100, the residual was considered to be the C fraction. In the majority of observations where the protein fractions and Kd were estimated by using the model of Ørskov and McDonald (1979), or the linear approach of Mathers and Miller (1981), the sum of the A and B fractions equaled 100 (i.e., B and C were "lumped" together and Kd was for the "B + C" fractions). In general, those data were considered acceptable if a small to negligible C fraction could be expected (e.g., most energy feeds, unprocessed oil-seeds, or unprocessed oil-seed meals). However, for forages or for feedstuffs that were heat processed, or feedstuffs where a moderate to large C fraction could be expected (e.g., blood meal, corn gluten meal), if the sum of the A and B fractions equaled 100, then those data were not used. In situations in which an assumed value for Kp was needed to calculate RDP, RUP, or a missing N fraction, an assumed rate of 5 %/h was used. If needed and not reported, RDP was calculated as 100–RUP and RUP was calculated as 100 − RDP. Some authors included a lag term for model-fitting procedures. However, lag was not considered for purposes of solving for missing information.

Of the total 1326 feedstuff observations, 801 observations from 170 experiments (Table 5-5) were considered acceptable for inclusion into the feed library (Tables 15-2a,b). Most of the rejected data were of feedstuffs that were either experimental in nature or uncommon to North America. Other reasons for not accepting data included clear deviations from recommended procedures, reported estimates of protein fractions that exceeded 100% of CP, or no reported C fraction when one would be expected.

A number of diet-related factors such as ruminal pH, frequency of feeding, particle size, and Kp can affect the estimates of Kd (see reviews by Lindberg, 1985; Michalet-Doreau and Ould-Bah, 1992; Nocek, 1988; Vanzant et al., 1998). However, sufficient data were not available to allow for more than one set of Kd values to be summarized for those factors. The RDP or RUP fraction of CP can be calculated for each feedstuff by the two equations:

$$RDP = A + B[Kd/(Kd + Kp)] \qquad (5\text{-}1)$$

where:

RDP = RDP of the feedstuff, percentage of CP
A = Fraction A, percentage of CP
B = Fraction B, percentage of CP
Kd = rate of degradation of the B fraction, %/h
Kp = rate of passage from the rumen, %/h

$$RUP = B[Kp/(Kd + Kp)] + C \qquad (5\text{-}2)$$

where:

RUP = RUP of the feedstuff, percentage of CP
B = Fraction B, percentage of CP
Kd = rate of degradation of the B fraction, %/h
Kp = rate of passage from the rumen, %/h
C = Fraction C, percentage of CP

The sum of RDP plus RUP equals 100%.

TABLE 5-5 Studies Reporting In Situ Determined Estimates of N Fractions and Rates of Protein Degradations That Were Used in Preparing This Edition

| | | |
|---|---|---|
| Akayezu et al. (1997) | Herrera-Saldana et al. (1990) | Robinson et al. (1991a) |
| Aldrich et al. (1996) | Hoffman et al. (1993) | Robinson et al. (1991b) |
| Alexandrov (1998) | Hongerholt and Muller (1998) | Robinson and Kennelly (1988a) |
| Antoniewicz et al. (1995) | Hristov (1998) | Robinson and Kennelly (1988b) |
| Arieli and Adin (1994) | Hristov and Sandev (1998) | Robinson and McNiven (1993) |
| Arieli et al. (1989) | Ibrahim et al. (1995) | Robinson and McNiven (1994) |
| Arieli et al. (1995) | Janicki and Stallings (1988) | Robinson and McQueen (1994) |
| Armentano et al. (1997) | Jones-Endsley et al. (1997) | Romagnolo et al. (1994) |
| Armentano et al. (1993) | Keady and Steen (1996) | Rooke et al. (1985) |
| Armentano et al. (1983) | Keady et al. (1994) | Schroeder et al. (1996) |
| Armentano et al. (1986) | Kenelly et al. (1988) | Seymour and Polan (1986) |
| Balde et al. (1993) | Khalili et al. (1994) | Sicilano-Jones, J. L., Personal communication. |
| Barney, N. C., Personal communication. | Khalili et al. (1992) | Sievert and Shaver (1993) |
| Batajoo and Shaver (1998) | Khorasani et al. (1996a) | Singh et al. (1995) |
| Beauchemin et al. (1997) | Khorasani et al. (1994a, b) | Song and Kennelly (1989) |
| Beckers et al. (1995) | Khorasani et al. (1992) | Stallings et al. (1991) |
| Beever et al. (1986) | Khorasani et al. (1993) | Stanford et al. (1996) |
| Ben Salem et al. (1993) | Kibelolaud et al. (1993) | Steg et al. (1994) |
| Berzaghi et al. (1997) | Kirkpatrick and Kennelly (1987) | Stutts et al. (1988) |
| Bohnert et al. (1998) | Klover et al. (1998) | Subuh et al. (1994) |
| Boila and Ingalls (1992) | Kowalski et al. (1997) | Susmel et al. (1993) |
| Boila and Ingalls (1994) | Lehman et al. (1995) | Susmel et al. (1991) |
| Brown and Pate (1997) | Lu et al. (1988) | Susmel et al. (1990) |
| Calsamiglia et al. (1995b) | Lykos and Varga (1995) | Tamminga et al. (1991) |
| Carey et al. (1993) | Maiga et al. (1997) | Valentine and Bartsch (1988) |
| Caton et al. (1994) | Makoni et al. (1991) | van der Aar et al. (1984) |
| Cecava, M. J., Personal communication. | Manyuchi et al. (1992) | van der Koelan et al. (1992) |
| Coblentz et al. (1999) | Marshall et al. (1993) | Vanhatalo et al. (1995) |
| Coblentz et al. (1997) | McKinnon et al. (1995) | van Vuuren et al. (1989) |
| Coblentz et al. (1998) | McNiven et al. (1994) | van Vuuren et al. (1992) |
| Cody et al. (1990) | Michalet-Doreau and Cerneau (1991) | van Vuuren et al. (1991) |
| Cozzi et al. (1995) | Michalet-Doreau and Nozière (1998) | van Vuuren et al. (1993) |
| Cozzi et al. (1993) | Michalet-Doreau and Ould-Bah (1992) | Vanzant et al. (1996) |
| Cozzi and Polan (1994) | Mir et al. (1993) | Varvikko and Vanhatalo (1992) |
| Cushnahan et al. (1995) | Mir et al. (1992) | Vasquez-Anon et al. (1993) |
| Dawson and Mayne (1997) | Mupeta et al. (1997) | Vieira et al. (1997) |
| Dawson and Mayne (1998) | Murphy and Kennelly (1987) | Vik-Mo (1989) |
| Deacon et al. (1988) | Murphy et al. (1993) | von Keyserlingk and Mathison (1993) |
| Deacon et al. (1988) | Mustafa et al. (1996) | von Keyserlingk and Mathison (1989) |
| Denham et al. (1989) | Mustafa et al. (1997) | von Keyserlingk et al. (1996) |
| DePeters and Bath (1986) | Napoli and Santini (1989) | Walhain et al. (1992) |
| DeVisser et al. (1998) | Negi et al. (1988) | Waltz and Stern (1989) |
| England et al. (1997) | Nocek et al. (1979) | Waltz et al. (1989) |
| Erasmus (1993) | Nocek and Grant (1987) | Wanderly et al. (1999) |
| Erdman et al. (1986) | Olson et al. (1994) | Wang et al. (1997) |
| Erdman and Vandersall (1983) | O'Mara et al. (1997a, b) | Wattiaux et al. (1994) |
| Erdman et al. (1987) | O'Mara et al. (1998) | Wen-Shyg et al. (1995) |
| Erickson et al. (1986) | Petit et al. (1994) | Windschitl and Stern (1988) |
| Faldet et al. (1991) | Petit and Tremblay (1992) | Xu et al. (1996) |
| Ganesh and Grieve (1990) | Peyraud et al. (1997) | Yan et al. (1998) |
| Givens et al. (1997) | Piepenbrink and Schingoethe (1998) | Yang et al. (1997) |
| Goelema et al. (1998) | Pires et al. (1997) | Yang et al. (1996) |
| Gordon and Peoples (1986) | Polan et al. (1997) | Yang et al. (1999) |
| Grings et al. (1991) | Polan et al. (1998) | Yong-Gang et al. (1994) |
| Grings et al. (1992a) | Powers et al. (1995) | Yoon et al. (1996) |
| Grings et al. (1992b) | Prakash et al. (1996) | Zerbini and Polan (1985) |
| Ha and Kennelly (1984) | Rioux et al. (1995) | |

The use of the equations presented above requires for each feedstuff an estimate of the rate of passage ($K_p$) from the rumen. For the purpose of developing equations that would predict rates of passage, 275 experiments were reviewed in which estimates of $K_p$ were reported for a variety of feedstuffs. Three equations were developed and have been adopted for use in this publication:

Equation for estimating $K_p$ of wet forages (i.e., silages and fresh forages)

$$K_p = 3.054 + 0.614X_1$$

where:

$K_p$ = rate of passage from the rumen, %/h
$X_1$ = DMI, percentage of BW

Equation for estimating $K_p$ of dry forages

$$K_p = 3.362 + 0.479X_1 - 0.007X_2 - 0.017X_3$$

where:

$K_p$ = rate of passage from the rumen, %/h
$X_1$ = DMI, percentage of BW
$X_2$ = concentrate, percentage of diet DM
$X_3$ = NDF of feedstuff, percentage of DM

Equation for estimating Kp of concentrates

$$K_p = 2.904 + 1.375X_1 - 0.020X_2$$

where:

$K_p$ = rate of passage from the rumen, %/h
$X_1$ = DMI, percentage of BW
$X_2$ = concentrate, percentage of diet DM

The equations were derived from experiments in which rare earth elements were used as $K_p$ markers. Studies involving Cr-mordanted feeds and Cr-mordanted NDF were not used to estimate $K_p$ of feeds. No significant independent variables could be identified for predicting $K_p$ of concentrates when the data set included these studies. The subcommittee recognized that intrinsic properties of feedstuffs, such as particle size and density, functional specific gravity, and processing of grains are not considered by the equations. Those factors, in addition to others (e.g., ruminal pH, feeding frequency, and use of ionophores) (see reviews by Owens and Goetsch, 1986 and Firkins et al., 1998), could not be considered because data are too sparse to make adjustments for those factors. Nonetheless, data from which the equations were developed for estimating $K_p$ are diverse with respect to DMI (2.7 to 26.8 kg/d), body weight (120 to 745 kg), DMI as percentage of body weight (0.8 to 4.4%), concentrate in dietary DM (0 to 85%), and represent estimates of $K_p$ obtained in growing, lactating, and nonlactating cattle.

Standardized methods have been proposed (AFRC, 1992; Lindberg, 1985; Madsen et al., 1995; Michalet-Doreau and Ould-Bah, 1992; Nocek, 1988; Ørskov, 1982; Vanzant et al., 1998; Wilkerson et al., 1995) for the in situ procedure of estimating RUP of feedstuffs. Those reviews agree generally about most procedural aspects, but the committee deemed it necessary to augment the recommendations in those reviews to foster a more complete reporting of data such that future summaries possibly may account for factors (e.g., ruminal pH, DMI) that may affect estimates of Kd. The recommendations by the committee are shown in Table 5-6.

The committee encourages the development and acceptance of an alternative method for quantifying N fractions and Kd that can be adopted by commercial feed testing laboratories for estimating RUP of feedstuffs. Chemical approaches are the most attractive for quantifying N fractions in feedstuffs because those procedures can be performed under routine laboratory conditions. The most sophisticated approach described to date is the use of the detergent system developed by Goering and Van Soest (1970) for analysis of carbohydrates in conjunction with extraction with borate phosphate buffer (Krisnamoorthy et al., 1982; Fox et al., 1990; Chalupa et al., 1991; Sniffen et al., 1992). As discussed previously, this method partitions CP into five fractions (A, B1, B2, B3, and C) according to rates of ruminal degradation and is the method that is used in the CNCPS (Sniffen et al., 1992). Protein degradability is calculated on the basis of pool size and rates of degradation of protein fractions in combination with ruminal passage rate.

### *Digestibility of Rumen Undegradable Feed Protein*

The previous edition of *Nutrient Requirements of Dairy Cattle* (National Research Council, 1989) recognized that intestinal digestion of feed proteins may differ. However, because of the lack of sufficient data at the time, a constant digestibility value of 80 percent was used for RUP of all feedstuffs. This value was selected because it approximated the average calculated true absorption of both nonammonia-N and RUP as measured in vivo (see Tables 13 and 14 in *Nutrient Requirements of Dairy Cattle* 1989 report). The current edition of *Nutrient Requirements of Beef Cattle* (National Research Council, 1996) also assumes that all RUP is 80 percent digestible.

Other feeding standards have attempted to account for differences in RUP digestibility among feedstuffs. However, the approaches have differed. For example, it is assumed in the UK Metabolizable Protein System (Webster, 1987) that acid detergent insoluble nitrogen (ADIN) is both undegradable in the rumen and indigestible in the small intestine. The equation of Webster et al. (1984) was adopted in that publication to predict digestible RUP from ADIN values [g/kg DM = 0.90 (RUP N-ADIN)/RUP N]. However, more recent data raise concerns about the appropriateness of using ADIN to predict RUP digestibility. Although a good relationship between ADIN and N indigestibility has been demonstrated for most forages (Goer-

TABLE 5-6 Recommended Procedures and Reporting Details for a Standardized In Situ Procedure for Measuring Ruminal Degradability of Protein in Dairy Cattle[a]

| Item | Recommendation |
|---|---|
| *Diet* | |
| Type | Similar to that of desired application. Report ingredient and chemical composition (minimum of DM, CP, NDF, and ash) |
| Feeding level | Similar to that of desired application; report DMI and ruminal pH |
| Feeding frequency | 2 times/d if not fed for *ad libitum* DMI |
| *Evaluated feedstuff* | |
| Chemical composition | Report (minimum) DM, CP, NDF, and ash |
| Physical characteristics | Report specifics about processing of feedstuffs (e.g., steam-flaked, 0.39 kg/L; heated, 150 °C, 3 h) |
| Sample processing | 2-mm screen size (Wiley mill) |
| *Bag* | |
| Material | Polyester |
| Pore size | 40 to 60 μ |
| *Incubation procedure* | |
| Number of animals | 2; report BW |
| Number of days | 2 |
| Number of replications | 1 |
| Presoaking | Recommended |
| Ruminal position | Ventral rumen |
| Insertion/removal | Remove simultaneously |
| Incubation times, h | 0, 2, 4, 8, 16, 24, and 48 (include 72 for forages). Report time zero washout so a lag time can be calculated. |
| Rinsing | Machine (5 times at 1 min/rinse) |
| Standard substrate | Recommended |
| *Microbial correction* | Required |
| *Mathematic model* | Non-linear |

[a]Adapted and modified from AFRC, 1992; Lindberg, 1985; Madsen et al., 1995; Michalet-Doreau and Ould-Bah, 1992; Nocek, 1988; Ørskov, 1982; Vanzant et al., 1998; Wilkerson et al., 1995.

ing et al., 1972; Yu and Thomas, 1976) and other feeds that were not heat processed (Waters et al., 1992), others have reported that ADIN is partially digestible and that a poor relationship exists between ADIN and N digestibility in nonforage plant protein sources that have been subjected to heat treatment (e.g., Nakamura et al., 1994a; Rogers et al., 1986; Cleale et al., 1987; Weiss et al., 1989; Harty et al., 1998; Waters et al., 1992). In each of the latter studies, the evaluated feedstuffs were distiller's products and other grain-byproducts that had been subjected to sufficient heat and moisture to induce the Maillard reactions and thus have "added" ADIN. These data indicate that much of the ADIN from these products is digestible but it is not clear whether this involves ruminal digestion, postruminal digestion, or both. Nakamura et al. (1994b) confirmed that significant amounts of ADIN in heat-damaged corn gluten meal and distillers grains were digestible but that the absorbed N from the heat-damaged protein was not used for growth by lambs and cattle. Waters et al. (1992) also confirmed the findings of Van Soest et al. (1987) that high tannin feeds bind protein in the gut which appears as ADIN in feces. The result was a high negative mean value (−89 percent) for apparent digestibility of ADIN in digestibility trials with sheep in which diets contained high tannin feeds. In contrast, diets that contained distillers products resulted in high positive values (62 percent) for ADIN digestibility whereas diets consisting only of "conventional" feeds resulted in a mean digestibility value for ADIN of 2 percent (Waters et al., 1992). Observations such as these indicate that ADIN is probably a useful indicator of nonusable N but that it may not be useful for estimating digestibility of RUP. In the French PDI System (Jarrige, 1989), variable digestibility values for RUP (0.25 to 0.95) are assigned to feedstuffs. Digestibility values were calculated from results of digestibility experiments with sheep using the assumption that the between-feed differences in fecal N excretion per unit of DMI results from indigestible dietary protein.

Other methods for estimating the intestinal digestibility of RUP include in vivo procedures, nonruminant animal bioassay, the in situ mobile nylon bag technique, and in vitro techniques (e.g., lysine availability test and enzymatic methods) (Stern et al., 1997). Although used as the standard by which other methods are evaluated, the in vivo approach requires the use of cannulated animals and is subject to inherent animal variation and errors associated with cannula placement and the use of microbial and digesta flow markers. The most widely used approach for estimating the true intestinal digestibility of the RUP fraction of feedstuffs is the mobile bag technique. Although requiring the need for ruminally and duodenally cannulated animals, the technique is relatively easy and it provides a more direct and physiologic approach than the use of ADIN. Using this method, small amounts of washed, ruminally undegraded feed residues are placed in bags. The bags are then usually preincubated in a pepsin/HCl solution for 1 to 3 h, inserted into the duodenum of cannulated ruminants, and then recovered either from an ileal cannula or (more typically because of convenience) from the feces. A comparison of ileal and fecal recovery of mobile bags provides similar estimates of RUP digestibility (Beckers et al., 1996; Boila and Ingalls, 1994, 1995; Hvelplund, 1985; Jarosz et al., 1994; Moshtaghi Nia and Ingalls, 1995; Todorov and Griginov, 1991; Vanhatalo and Ketoja, 1995). Recovered bags are washed thoroughly to remove endogenous and other contaminating protein and analyzed for N or AA content. Therefore, estimates of RUP digestibility obtained using this technique are considered to be estimates of true rather than apparent digestibility. Factors that can potentially affect the accuracy of the estimates of intestinal digestibility obtained using the mobile bag technique have been reviewed (Beckers et al., 1996; Stern et al., 1997) and a standardized procedure for its use has been recommended (Madsen et al., 1995). Studies have indicated good correlation between results from fecal collection of bags and in vivo intestinal CP digestion (Hvelplund, 1985; Todorov and Griginov, 1991).

Calsamiglia and Stern (1995) developed a three-step in vitro procedure that provides an alternative to the use of intestinally cannulated ruminants for estimating intestinal digestibility of the RUP fraction of feed proteins. The procedure consists of: (1) incubating ruminally undegraded feed residues for 1 h in 0.1N HCl solution containing 1 g/L of pepsin, (2) neutralizing the mixture with 1N NaOH and a pH 7.8 phosphate buffer containing pancreatin followed by a 24-h incubation, and (3) precipitation of undigested proteins with a 100 percent (wt/vol) trichloracetic acid solution. Pepsin-pancreatin digestion of protein is calculated as TCA-soluble N divided by the amount of N in the sample (Dacron bag residue) used in the assay. The authors reported an excellent correlation ($r = 0.91$) with in vivo estimates of intestinal CP digestion when using ruminally undegraded feed residues from 16-h ruminal incubations.

To arrive at estimates of RUP digestibility for this publication, 54 studies were summarized (Table 5-7). The mobile bag technique with recovery of the bags from the feces was used in 48 studies and the in vitro procedure of Calsamiglia and Stern (1995) was used in 6 studies. Porosity of bag material used in the mobile bag technique studies ranged from 9 to 53 μm. Comparative data within studies in which the effect of bag pore size on protein digestibility was measured indicated that digestibility tended to increase slightly with increasing pore size. Beckers et al. (1996) obtained digestibility values of 87 and 92 percent, 72 and 75 percent, and 64 and 69 percent for ruminal residues of soybean meal, wheat bran, and meat and bone meal when pore size was 10 and 43 μm, respectively. Hvelplund (1985) obtained values of 95 and 97 percent, 87 and 87 percent, and 74 and 75 percent for residues of soybean meal, coconut cakes, and rapeseed meal when pore size was 9 and 22 μm. Porosities of 40 to 53 μm were used in all but twelve studies identified for this data set. Mobile bags containing the ruminal residues were preincubated in a pepsin/HCl solution before placement in the duodenum in 75 percent of the studies. Studies not employing pepsin/HCl preincubation were retained in the data set because comparative data in studies that have evaluated the importance of pepsin/HCl preincubation indicate that it is not a necessary step when the mobile bag technique includes preincubation of feeds in the rumen (Vanhatalo et al., 1995; Voigt et al., 1985). For feeds in which data were limited or did not exist, the values reported by Jarrige (1989) in Table 13.3 of *Ruminant Nutrition: Recommended Allowances and Feed Tables* were used. The mean values used in this revision (Tables 15-2a,b) are rounded to the nearest 5 percentage units to emphasize the lack of precision involved in arriving at mean values.

### *Predicting Passage of Endogenous Protein*

Predicted passage of protein to the small intestine in the previous *Nutrient Requirements of Dairy Cattle* publication (National Research Council, 1989) was assumed to originate entirely from ruminally synthesized microbial protein and RUP. However, research indicates that endogenous protein N also contributes to N passage to the duodenum and maybe should be considered in models designed to predict passage of protein to the small intestine. Sources of endogenous protein that may contribute to duodenal protein include: (1) mucoproteins in saliva, (2) epithelial cells from the respiratory tract, (3) cellular debris from the sloughing and abrasion of the epithelial tissue of the mouth, esophagus, and the reticulo-rumen, (4) cellular debris from the sloughing and abrasion of the epithelial tissue of the omasum and abomasum, and (5) enzyme secretions into the abomasum. Significant amounts of the first three sources of endogenous protein probably are degraded by ruminal microorganisms, and therefore do not contribute in their entirety to protein passage to the small intestine.

Attempts to measure passage of endogenous protein N to the small intestine of ruminants are limited because of the difficulty of being able to distinguish endogenous N from microbial N and feed N in duodenal digesta. Several different approaches have been used. One approach has been to measure the flow of nonammonia-N (NAN) through the rumen and abomasum when cows and steers were nourished totally on volatile fatty acids infused into the rumen. Using this approach, Ørskov et al. (1986) obtained mean flows of NAN from the rumen of two nonlactating, pregnant Holstein cows (650 and 700 kg) of 8.3 g/d or 51 mg/kg $BW^{0.75}$; for two steers (307 and 405 kg), the flows were 5.1 g/d or 58.2 mg/kg $BW^{0.75}$. Ørskov et al.

TABLE 5-7 Published Studies That Were Summarized for the Purpose of Arriving at Estimates of Intestinal Digestibility of the RUP Fraction of Feedstuffs

| | | |
|---|---|---|
| Antoniewicz et al. (1992) | Hvelplund et al. (1994) | Prestløkken (1999) |
| Arieli et al. (1989) | Hvelplund et al. (1991) | Rae and Smithard (1985) |
| Beckers et al. (1996) | Jarosz et al. (1994) | Rooke (1985) |
| Boila and Ingalls (1994) | Kendall et al. (1991) | Steg et al. (1994) |
| Boila and Ingalls (1995) | Kibelolaud et al. (1993) | Todorov and Girginov (1991) |
| Calsamiglia and Stern (1995) | Kopecný et al. (1998) | Vanhatalo et al. (1995) |
| Calsamiglia et al. (1995a) | Liu et al. (1994) | Vanhatalo and Ketoja (1995) |
| Cros et al. (1992a) | Maiga et al. (1996) | Vanhatalo and Varvikko (1995) |
| Cros et al. (1992b) | Masoero et al. (1994) | Vanhatalo et al. (1996) |
| Dakowski et al. (1996) | Mhgeni et al. (1994) | van Straalen and Huisman (1991) |
| Deacon et al. (1988) | Moshtaghi Nia and Ingalls (1992) | van Straalen et al. (1993) |
| de Boer et al. (1987) | Moshtaghi Nia and Ingalls (1995) | van Straalen et al. (1997) |
| Erasmus et al. (1994a) | Mupeta et al. (1997) | Varvikko and Vanhatalo (1992) |
| Frydrych (1992) | Mustafa et al. (1998) | Volden and Harstad (1995) |
| Goelema et al. (1998) | O'Mara et al. (1997a) | von Keyserlingk et al. (1998) |
| Hindle et al. (1995) | Palmquist et al. (1993) | Walhain et al. (1992) |
| Howie et al. (1996) | Pereira et al. (1998) | Wang et al. (1999) |
| Hvelplund (1985) | Piepenbrink and Schingoethe (1998) | Weisbjerg et al. (1996) |

(1986) used the same approach with growing cattle and lambs but measured flows of NAN through both the rumen and abomasum. In this experiment with four steers (240 to 315 kg), they reported flows of total N and NAN through the rumen of 9.9 and 5.8 g/d (145 and 85 mg/kg $BW^{0.75}$) and flows through the abomasum of 17.0 and 13.4 g/d (248 and 195 mg/kg $BW^{0.75}$). In lambs (40 to 50 kg), respective flows of N and NAN from the rumen and abomasum were 103 and 76 and 244 and 181 mg/kg $BW^{0.75}$. In both steers and lambs, the contribution of the omasum and abomasum to the total endogenous N leaving the abomasum was greater than the contributions from the other sources.

A more physiologic approach for obtaining estimates of passage of endogenous N to the small intestine of cattle has been to measure flows of N fractions when diets considered free of rumen digestible protein are fed. In this case, flows of endogenous N are estimated as the difference between the sum of N intake and measured flows to the duodenum of microbial N and flows of total NAN. Hannah et al. (1991) and Lintzenich et al. (1995) fed dormant bluestem-range hay (2.3 and 2.8 percent CP, respectively) as the sole source of dietary energy and protein to Holstein steers (370 to 424 kg). Ad libitum intake of DM was 0.7 to 0.8 percent of BW (about 3.1 kg/d in both studies). Flows of endogenous N to the small intestine were calculated to be 278 (Hannah et al., 1991) and 279 mg/kg $BW^{0.75}$ (Lintzenich et al., 1995). Hart and Leibholz (1990) fed variable amounts of alkali-treated wheat straw (1.7 to 4.1 kg/d) to 300 kg steers fitted with ruminal and abomasal (distal pyloric region) cannulas. The hay was demonstrated to be free of rumen digestible protein. The average flow of endogenous N to the abomasum was 325 mg/kg $BW^{0.75}$. The flow of endogenous N from the rumen to the omasum increased with increasing DMI, averaging 2.2 g/kg DMI (87 mg/kg $BW^{0.75}$), whereas the contribution of the omasum to flow of endogenous N to the abomasum appeared unaffected by DMI, averaging 17.2 g N/d.

Brandt et al. (1980) used an alternative approach that allowed for the provision of N for ruminal microorganisms. Two lactating cows fitted with ruminal and duodenal cannulas were fed twelve daily meals of (kg/d) 4.86 cellulose, 0.48 straw, and 3.0 concentrate (corn starch, sugar, oil, and minerals). The basal diet was supplemented with constant ruminal infusions of $^{15}N$-enriched urea. From measured $^{15}N$ surpluses in duodenal NAN, microbial N, and milk N they determined that 3.6 g of endogenous protein N passed to the duodenum of dairy cows for each kilogram of OM that passes to the small intestine. Assuming that dietary DM approximates 90 to 93 percent OM and that 60 to 65 percent of OM intake passes to the small intestine of dairy cows (Clark et al., 1992), then approximately 2.1 g of endogenous N passes to the small intestine for each kilogram of DM consumed ($3.6 \text{ g} \times 0.915 \times 0.625 = 2.1 \text{ g}$). The authors concluded that with normal diets, endogenous protein N may constitute 9 to 12 percent of NAN passing to the small intestine.

Vérité and Peyraud (1989) reported a regression equation that was developed to determine the contributions of microbial N, feed N, and endogenous N to passage of NAN to the small intestine. It was assumed in the regression model that flow of endogenous N to the small intestine is proportional to the intake of nondigestible OM (OM not digested in the entire digestive tract). Using a data set involving 405 measurements of NAN passage in sheep, growing cattle and cows, the resulting equation indicated that flow of endogenous N to the small intestine is equal to 5.3 g/kg of nondigestible OM intake, or approximately 1.7 g/kg DMI.

In summary, it is apparent that significant amounts of endogenous N may pass to the small intestine. The quantity that passes to the duodenum in an animal of a given BW appears to be correlated closely to intake of indigestible OM. However, because OM digested in the rumen is not calculated in the model, for purpose of simplicity it was decided to predict passage of endogenous N to the duodenum from DMI. The equation selected for use in this publication is: endogenous N (g/d) = 1.9 × DMI (kg/d). The value of 1.9 is less than the value of 2.1 reported by Brandt et al. (1980) and was selected for use in this model because it yields a mean bias closest to zero for predicting non-ammonia-non-microbial N in the model (see next section). The value of 1.9 also provides estimates of endogenous N that are consistent with the above cited data. For example, using a cow weighing 600 kg and consuming 25 kg of dry matter, the predicted flow of endogenous N is 47.5 g/d, or 392 mg/kg $BW^{0.75}$. The value of 392 mg/kg $BW^{0.75}$ is 58 percent higher than the measured flow of 248 mg/kg $BW^{.75}$ in steers maintained by intragastric infusion and consuming no feed (Ørskov et al., 1986).

*Evaluation of Model for Predicting Flows of N Fractions*

The described approaches to predicting passage of MCP, RUP, and ECP to the small intestine were validated using 99 published studies that reported flows of N fractions [non-ammonia N (NAN), microbial N (MN), and non-ammonia-non-microbial N (NANMN)] to the small intestine (Table 5-8). Selected studies were limited to those in which duodenal N flow was partitioned into NAN, MN, and NANMN; data were not used if it was not explicitly clear that ammonia-N was measured and subtracted from total N for reporting flows of NAN. Of the 99 selected studies, 27 used growing cattle (106 treatment means) and 72 used lactating and non-lactating dairy cows (284 treatment means). The animals (155 to 785 kg BW) were fed a diversity of diets (e.g., 0 to 90% concentrate, mean = 50%; 8.0 to 24.8% CP, mean = 16.2%; and 7.2 to 12.8% RDP, mean 10.9%) at variable intakes of DM (0.95 to 4.40% of BW; mean = 2.86%). Although independently selected by a blind collaborator, 56 of the 72 studies involving cows in the 99-study data base used for evaluation were used for developing the equation for predicting passage of MCP. None of the growing cattle studies were used in developing the equation for predicting passage of MCP.

Figures 5-6, 5-7, and 5-8 are plots of predicted vs. measured flows and of residuals (predicted-measured) vs. measured flows for MN, NANMN (ruminally undegraded feed N + endogenous N), and NAN for cows. The plots for growing cattle showed the same tendencies as those for the cows so only the plots for cows are presented. On average, for all variables and for both growing cattle and cows, discrepancies were small between predicted and measured flows. Mean biases of prediction for MN, NANMN, and NAN for growing cattle and cows were (g/d) −0.75, +0.44, −1.9 and +0.52, −0.12, +0.14, respectively. Mean biases of prediction for MN, NANMN, and NAN for the combined data set were (g/d) +0.18, −0.01, and −0.37. In 57 percent of the cases for growing cattle and 28 percent of the cases for cows (36 percent of the total cases), passage of microbial CP was restricted by the availability of RDP and therefore, predicted by RDP intake (0.85 × RDP intake).

The degree of the negative slope-bias that is evident in the residual plots are of concern. However, some negative slope-bias was expected because of errors in measurement. A negative slope-bias was expected for NAN (Figure 5-8) because of errors associated with quantifying passage of digesta to the small intestine. Because measurements of digesta passage require the use of markers, flows can be under- or over-estimated to varying degrees. A greater negative slope-bias was expected for MN (Figure 5-6) and NANMN (Figure 5-7) because errors in measurement include errors in quantifying passage as well as estimating the content of MN in NAN. Primarily because of the error associated with the use of markers for estimating MN in NAN, estimates may be lower or higher than actual. To help determine if the negative slope-biases were attributable to the data used for evaluation, the model, or both, the residuals were regressed on some variables that were reported in most of the studies and considered to possibly influence the prediction accuracy of the model. These variables included BW, DMI (percent of BW and kg/d), concentrate intake (percent of DMI), diet CP (percent of DM), and CP intake. None of these factors contributed appreciably to the negative slope biases. Therefore, it was concluded that errors in the structure of the model are probably major contributors to the negative slope biases. The series of equations used for predicting flows of N fractions includes some nonlinear equations. Therefore, because of its nonlinear nature, the model is sensitive to generating bias predictions because of errors in model input (i.e., errors in measuring the independent variables).

*Predicting Passage of Metabolizable Protein*

Microbial CP as provided by bacteria and protozoa is considered to contain 80 percent true protein; the remaining 20 percent of MCP is considered to be provided by nucleic acids (National Research Council, 1989). The true protein of MCP is assumed to be 80 percent digestible (National Research Council, 1989). Consequently, the conversion of MCP to MP is assumed to be 64 percent. Ruminally undegraded feed CP is assumed to be 100 percent true protein (National Research Council, 1989). As dis-

TABLE 5-8 Studies Used to Evaluate the Model Equations for Predicting Flows of MCP, RUP plus ECP, and NAN Flows to the Small Intestine

| | | |
|---|---|---|
| Aldrich et al. (1995) | Klusmeyer et al. (1990) | Robinson et al. (1985) |
| Aldrich et al. (1993a) | Köster et al. (1997) | Rode et al. (1985) |
| Aldrich et al. (1993b) | Kung et al. (1983) | Rooke et al. (1985) |
| Armentano et al. (1986) | Lardy et al. (1993) | Santos et al. (1984) |
| Beauchemin et al. (1999) | Lu et al. (1988) | Sarwar et al. (1991) |
| Bernard et al. (1988) | Lykos et al. (1997) | Schwab et al. (1992a) |
| Bohnert et al. (1999) | Lynch et al. (1991) | Schwab et al. (1992b) |
| Cameron et al. (1991) | Mabjeesh et al. (1996) | Song and Kennelly (1989) |
| Cecava et al. (1993) | Mansfield and Stern (1994) | Stern et al. (1983) |
| Cecava and Parker (1993) | McCarthy et al. (1989) | Stern et al. (1985) |
| Christensen et al. (1993a, b) | Merchen and Satter (1983) | Stokes et al. (1991b) |
| Christensen et al. (1996) | Milton et al. (1997) | Tesfa (1993) |
| Crocker et al. (1998) | Murphy et al. (1993) | Tice et al. (1993) |
| Cunningham et al. (1993) | Murphy et al. (1994) | van Vuuren et al. (1992) |
| Cunningham et al. (1994) | Narasimhalu et al. (1989) | van Vuuren et al. (1993) |
| Cunningham et al. (1996) | Ohajuruka et al. (1991) | Volden (1999) |
| Elizalde et al. (1999) | Oliveira et al. (1995) | Waltz et al. (1989) |
| Erasmus et al. (1992) | O'Mara et al. (1998) | Wessels et al. (1996) |
| Erasmus et al. (1994b) | O'Mara et al. (1997b) | Yang et al. (1997) |
| Espindola et al. (1997) | Overton et al. (1995) | Yang et al. (1999) |
| Feng et al. (1993) | Pantoja et al. (1995) | Yoon and Stern (1996) |
| Glenn et al. (1989) | Pantoja et al. (1994) | Younker et al. (1998) |
| Goetsch et al. (1987) | Pena et al. (1986) | Zerbini et al. (1988) |
| Holden et al. (1994a) | Peyraud et al. (1997) | Zhu et al. (1997) |
| Holden et al. (1994b) | Pires et al. (1997) | Zinn (1988) |
| Johnson et al. (1998) | Poore et al. (1993) | Zinn (1993a) |
| Joy et al. (1997) | Prange et al. (1984) | Zinn (1993b) |
| Kalscheur et al. (1997a) | Putnam et al. (1997) | Zinn (1995) |
| Kalscheur et al. (1997b) | Rangngang et al. (1997) | Zinn et al. (1995) |
| Keery et al. (1993) | Rinne et al. (1997) | Zinn and Plascencia (1993) |
| Khorasani et al. (1996b) | Robinson (1997) | Zinn et al. (1994) |
| Klusmeyer et al. (1991a) | Robinson and Sniffen (1985) | Zinn and Shen (1998) |
| Klusmeyer et al. (1991b) | Robinson et al. (1994) | Zinn et al. (1996) |

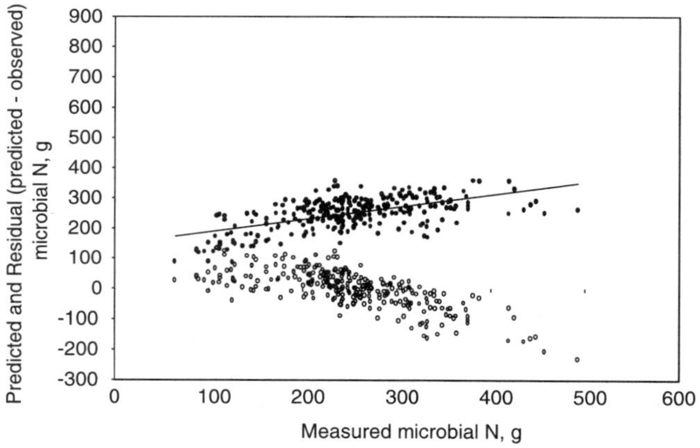


FIGURE 5-6 Plot of predicted vs. measured (filled circles) and residuals (predicted-measured; open circles) vs. measured flows of microbial N to the small intestine of dairy cows ($y = 0.4109x + 146.5$; $r^2 = 0.35$; mean bias $= + 0.52$; RMSPE $= 63.1$; $n = 284$).

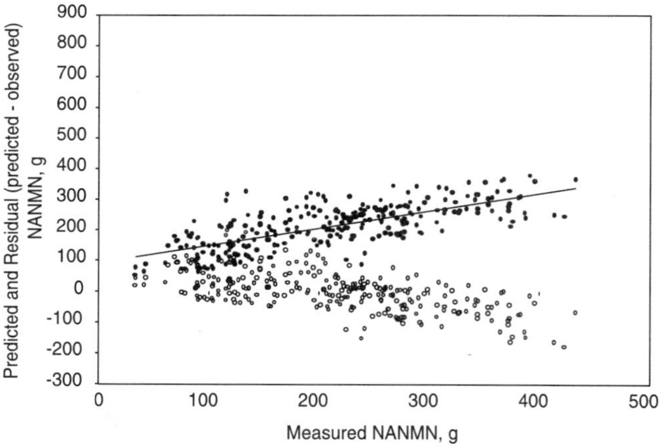


FIGURE 5-7 Plot of predicted vs. measured (filled circles) and residuals (predicted-measured; open circles) vs. measured flows of NANMN (rumen undegradable N plus endogenous N) to the small intestine of dairy cows ($y = 0.5701x + 91.193$; $r^2 = 0.51$; mean bias $= -0.12$; RMSPE $= 63.1$; $n = 275$).

cussed previously, estimates of intestinal digestibility have been assigned to the RUP fraction of each feedstuff; assigned values vary from 50 to 100 percent. Therefore, the contribution of RUP to MP is variable and dependent on feed type. Published data on the content and digestibility of true protein in ECP is extremely limited. Ørskov et al. (1986) reported that NAN constituted 79 percent of total N in ruminal fluids and 74 percent of total N in abomasal fluids collected from 40-50 kg lambs nourished by N-free ruminal infusions of volatile fatty acids. Using a

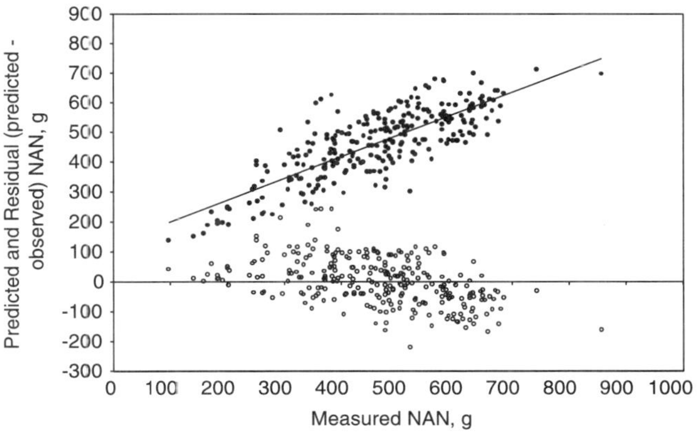


FIGURE 5-8 Plot of predicted vs. measured (filled circles) and residuals (predicted-measured; open circles) vs. measured flows of NAN (microbial N + rumen undegradable N + endogenous N) to the small intestine of dairy cows ($y = 0.7251x + 127.1$; $r^2 = 0.54$; mean bias = +0.14; RMSPE = 78.3; n = 275).

similar approach, Guilloteau (1986) found that 30 percent of abomasal endogenous N was AA-N. Based on these two experiments, the true protein content of ECP passing to the duodenum is assumed to be 50 percent. The true protein of ECP is assumed to be 80 percent digestible; consequently, the conversion of ECP to MP is assumed to be 40 percent.

## METABOLIZABLE PROTEIN REQUIREMENTS

Previous National Research Council (1985, 1989) requirements for MP were based on the factorial method. The same approach is used in this edition. The protein requirement includes that needed for maintenance and production. The maintenance requirement consists of urinary endogenous N, scurf N (skin, skin secretions, and hair), and metabolic fecal N. The requirement for production includes the protein needed for the conceptus, growth, and lactation.

### *MP Requirements for Maintenance*

Swanson (1977) derived the equation used to estimate the endogenous urinary protein requirement. The equation of Swanson ($UPN = 2.75 \times BW^{0.50}$) was in net protein units and was used as such in the previous *Nutrient Requirements of Dairy Cattle* publication (National Research Council, 1989). The protein system used in this version is based on MP. Assuming an efficiency of converting MP to net protein of 0.67 (National Research Council, 1989), the endogenous urinary protein requirement in MP units is $4.1 \times BW^{0.50}$.

The original equation of Swanson (1977) for predicting protein requirements for scurf protein also was in units of net protein ($SPN = 0.2\ BW^{0.60}$) and used in the previous *Nutrient Requirements of Dairy Cattle* publication (National Research Council, 1989). Assuming an efficiency of converting MP to net protein of 0.67 (National Research Council, 1989), the scurf protein requirement in MP units is $0.3 \times BW^{0.60}$.

In the last edition (National Research Council, 1989), metabolic fecal protein (MFP) was calculated using an equation based on intake of indigestible DM (IDM) (i.e., MFP, g/d = 90 × IDM, kg/d). Because of the errors associated with estimating the indigestibility of diets, the committee chose to calculate MFP directly from DM intake (DMI). Estimates of MFP have been made by two methods (Swanson, 1982). The first is by feeding diets of differing content of CP and regressing intake of digestible CP on intake of CP. The intercept is estimated MFP. Using this approach, Waldo and Glenn (1984) obtained a proportional intercept of 0.029 on the lactating dairy cow data of Conrad et al. (1960). Also using lactating cows, Boekholt (1976) obtained a proportional intercept of 0.033. Using sheep and cattle fed forage diets, Holter and Reid (1959) obtained an intercept of 0.034. The other approach for estimating MFP is to measure fecal N output when animals are fed low CP diets and subtract from fecal N an estimate of undigested feed N. Using this approach, Swanson (1977) estimated metabolic fecal N for ruminating cattle fed 70 natural and semi-synthetic low protein diets. By subtracting 10 percent of feed N from fecal N, Swanson (1977) obtained a mean estimate of metabolic fecal N of 4.7 g /kg DMI (29.4 g CP/kg of DMI). Based on the above data, the committee chose to calculate MFP (g/d) as: MFP = 30 × DMI (kg).

Metabolic fecal protein consists of bacteria and bacterial debris synthesized in the cecum and large intestine, keratinized cells, and a host of other compounds (Swanson, 1982). Using different solvents and centrifugation techniques, Mason (1979) reported that about 30 percent of the nonfeed portion of fecal N was soluble and about 70 percent was bacterial and endogenous debris. Quantitative data on the contribution of undigested bacterial CP synthesized in the rumen to metabolic fecal N are limited. In a series of experiments using cannulated lambs, Mason and White (1971) observed no degradation in the small intestine of the 2,6-diaminopimelic acid (DAPA)-containing fraction of bacterial cell-wall material. Based on differences in the quantities of DAPA passing through the terminal ileum and passing out of the rectum, the authors reported an 80 percent loss (apparent) of DAPA when the lambs were fed concentrate diets and a 30 percent loss when forage diets were fed. The true losses of the DAPA-containing material that originated in the rumen would be higher than the reported values to the extent that hindgut synthesis of bacterial CP occurred, an event that is influenced by the availability of energy in the hindgut (Mason et al., 1981). Measurements of the amount of undigested ruminal bacterial CP that appears in the feces of dairy cattle fed a variety of diets are needed. Although uncertain of the amount of undigested ruminal bacterial CP that appears in the feces of dairy cattle, the subcommittee chose to assume that 50 percent of model estimated, intestinally indigestible MCP appears in the feces and that the other 50 percent is digested in the hindgut. Therefore, the equation for predicting the MP requirements for MFP (g/d) is: MP $= [(\text{DMI (kg)} \times 30) - 0.50((\text{bacterial MP}/0.80)\text{-bacterial MP})]$.

In this edition, endogenous crude protein secretions are considered to contribute to MP supply. In view of the lack of published data, the efficiency of use of the absorbed MP for endogenous MP is assumed to be 0.67. Therefore the equation to calculate the MP requirement for endogenous MP is: endogenous MP/0.67.

In summary, the overall equation for predicting the MP requirement for maintenance (g/d) is: MP $= 4.1 \times BW^{0.50}$ (kg) $+ 0.3 \times BW^{0.60}$ (kg) $+ [(\text{DMI (kg)} \times 30) - 0.50((\text{bacterial MP}/0.8)\text{-bacteria MP})] +$ endogenous MP/0.67.

*Protein Requirements for Pregnancy*

Dry cows require nutrients for maintenance, growth of the conceptus, and perhaps growth of the dam. Estimating nutrient requirements for pregnancy by the factorial method requires knowledge of the rates of nutrient accretion in conceptus tissues (fetus, placenta, fetal fluids, and uterus) and the efficiency with which dietary nutrients are utilized for growth of the conceptus. Data are limited for dairy cattle.

This document differs from the last edition (National Research Council, 1989) for estimates of protein requirements for gestation during the last two months of pregnancy. Current estimates are from Bell et al. (1995). Other estimates are available, but they were obtained from beef cattle, dairy breeds other than Holsteins, or from research conducted more than 25 years ago. However, estimates from Bell et al. (1995) do not vary greatly from previous estimates and thus support the requirements published in the 1989 National Research Council report. Bell et al. (1995) measured rates of growth and conceptus chemical composition in multiparous Holstein cows that were serially slaughtered from 190 to 270 d of pregnancy. A quadratic regression equation best described protein accretion in the gravid uterus.

Estimates were derived from cows with a mean BW of 714 kg that carried a single fetus. Estimates of protein requirements to support pregnancy are solely a function of day of gestation and calf BW. The requirement for metabolizable protein to meet the demands of pregnancy (MPPreg) was derived from the equation of Bell et al. (1995), which includes conceptus weight, calf birth weight and days of gestation as variables. The efficiency with which MP is used for pregnancy (EffMPPreg) is assumed to be 0.33. Because the experiments conducted by Bell included only animals more than 190 days pregnant and because the requirements for pregnancy are small before this time, pregnancy requirements are calculated only for animals more than 190 days pregnant. If the animal is between 190 and 279 days pregnant, the equation to compute the weight of the conceptus (CW) is:

$$CW = (18 + ((\text{DaysPreg} - 190) \times 0.665)) \times (\text{CBW}/45)$$

Where DaysPreg = days pregnant and CBW = calf birth weight.

The average daily gain due to pregnancy (ADGPreg) is: ADGPreg $= 665 \times (\text{CBW}/45)$.

The MPPreg is MPPreg $= (((0.69 \times \text{DaysPreg}) - 69.2) \times (\text{CBW}/45))/\text{EffMPPreg}$.

In the model, animals more than 279 days pregnant have the same requirements as animals that are 279 days pregnant.

*Protein Requirement for Lactation*

Protein required for lactation is based on the amount of protein secreted in milk. The equation for calculating protein in milk (kg/d) is (YProtn) = milk production, kg/d × (milk true protein / 100). The efficiency of use of MP for lactation is assumed to be 0.67. Use of this efficiency value in this edition's model resulted in MP balances of zero or less for 61 of the 206 diet treatments reported in the studies presented in Table 5-2. In all cases, cows were in early to mid lactation and averaged 30.9 kg/d of milk (range = 18.8 to 44.0). Crude protein, RDP, and RUP in diet DM averaged 16.1 percent (range = 13.8 to 20.8), 10.9 percent (range = 7.8 to 14.7), and 5.2 percent (range = 2.8 to 8.9). The equation to calculate MP requirement for lactation (MPLact) is (g/d) MPLact $= (\text{YProtn}/0.67) \times 1000$.

*Protein Requirements for Growth*

The protein requirements for heifers and steers are from the *Nutrient Requirements of Beef Cattle* (National Research Council, 1996) (see growth section Chapter 11). The net protein requirement (NP, g/d) for growth is calculated using retained energy (RE), average daily weight gain (WG), and equivalent shrunk BW (EQSBW). The following equations are needed: if WG = 0 then NPg = 0 otherwise NPg $= \text{WG} \times (268-(29.4 \times (\text{RE} / \text{ADG})))$. If (EQSBW < or = 478 kg) then efficiency of use of MP for growth (EffMP_NPg) $= (83.4-(0.114 \times \text{EQSBW}))$ /

100 otherwise EffMP_NPg = 0.28908. Metabolizable protein for growth in g/d (MPGrowth) = NPg / EffMP_NPg.

## AMINO ACIDS

Absorbed AA provided by ruminally synthesized MCP, RUP, and ECP are essential as the building blocks for the synthesis of tissue and milk proteins. Although to a lesser extent, absorbed AA are required also as precursors for the synthesis of other body metabolites. Amino acids other than leucine also serve as precursors for gluconeogenesis and all can be converted to fatty acids or serve as immediate sources of metabolic energy when oxidized to $CO_2$. The metabolic fate of AA in ruminants has been reviewed (Lobley, 1992).

Amino acids in plant and animal proteins and those produced industrially in pure form for the feed industry by fermentative technology (lysine, threonine, and tryptophan) are of the L-form. In contrast, methionine produced by chemical synthesis is a DL-racemic mixture. Small amounts of D-AA exist in bacterial cell walls and in free form in a number of plants. Biologic use of absorbed D-AA requires conversion to the L-isomer, the efficiency of which is both AA and species dependent (Baker, 1994). The conversion of D-methionine to L-methionine has been of some concern in cattle nutrition because of the commercial availability of various types of ruminally protected DL-methionine. Titgemeyer and Merchen (1990a) noted a tendency for lower N retention when steers were infused abomasally with DL-methionine than with L-methionine. However, Campbell et al. (1996) concluded that D-methionine was used as effectively as L-methionine for N retention of growing cattle. Doyle (1981) and Reis et al. (1989) concluded that D-methionine was used as efficiently as L-methionine for wool growth.

### *Essential vs. Nonessential Amino Acids*

Of the twenty primary AA that occur in proteins, ten are usually classified as being "essential" (or indispensable). These include arginine (Arg), histidine (His), isoleucine (Ile), leucine (Leu), lysine (Lys), methionine (Met), phenylalanine (Phe), threonine (Thr), tryptophan (Trp), and valine (Val). Amino acids termed essential either cannot be synthesized by animal tissues or if they can (Arg and His), not at rates sufficient to meet requirements, particularly during the early stages of growth or for high levels of production. It is understood that when EAA are absorbed in the profile as required by the animal, the requirements for total EAA is reduced and their efficiency of use for protein synthesis is maximized (Heger and Frydrych, 1989) Amino acids classified as "nonessential" (or dispensable) are those which are readily synthesized from metabolites of intermediary metabolism and amino groups from surplus AA. Unlike the EAA, there remains little evidence that the profile of absorbed nonessential AA (NEAA) is important for efficiency of use of absorbed AA for protein synthesis. If one or more of the NEAA are in short supply relative to metabolic need, most of the evidence indicates they can be synthesized in adequate amounts from one another or from one or more of the EAA that are absorbed in excess of need.

The classification of AA as being essential or nonessential originates from research with nonruminant animals. Research with dairy cattle is extremely limited. However, the early isotopic tracer studies of Black et al. (1957) and Downes (1961), using dairy cattle and sheep, indicated that the classification is similar to that of non-ruminants. Other studies in a more indirect way support that conclusion. For example, it was demonstrated that postruminal administration of mixtures of NEAA did not substitute for mixtures of EAA in supporting N retention of postweaned calves (Schwab et al., 1982) or milk protein production in lactating cows (Oldham et al., 1979; Schwab et al., 1976). Using the total intragastric nutrition technique, Fraser et al. (1991) observed that exclusion of NEAA from a supplemental mixture of EAA and NEAA decreased urinary N excretion without affecting productive N (milk N + retained N). Schwab et al. (1976) observed that increases in milk protein yields were generally of the same magnitude as for casein when only the 10 standard EAA were infused into the abomasum. Collectively, these observations indicate that when AA supplies approach requirements for total absorbable AA, requirements for total NEAA are met before the requirements for the most limiting of the EAA and that individual NEAA absorbed in amounts less than required for metabolic need can be synthesized in adequate amounts such that animal performance is not affected. These observations are consistent with those observed in *Nutrient Requirements of Swine* (National Research Council, 1998) and *Nutrient Requirements of Poultry* (National Research Council, 1994).

Although there is no evidence that NEAA as a group of AA become more limiting than EAA when dairy cattle are fed conventional diets, research is too limited to rule out the potential importance of selected NEAA to dairy cattle nutrition and production. For example, it is well-documented in nonruminants such as swine and poultry that the EAA, Met and Phe, are precursors to the synthesis of the NEAA, cysteine and tyrosine, respectively. Research indicates also that cysteine and its oxidation product cystine can satisfy approximately 50 percent of the need for total sulfur AA and that tyrosine can satisfy approximately 50 percent of the need for tyrosine + Phe (National Research Council, 1998; National Research Council, 1994). However, there are no reports involving dairy cattle as to the extent that cysteine/cystine and tyrosine can spare Met and

Phe in MP for maintenance and productive functions. Such information is ultimately needed to balance diets for AA and to know when cysteine/cystine or tyrosine in RUP can substitute for Met and Phe. A single study by Ahmed and Bergen (1983) indicated that as much as 58 percent of the total sulfur AA requirement of growing cattle can be met by cysteine and cystine. There are no reports that provide an example of the Met-sparing effect of cysteine/cystine in lactating dairy cows. Pruekvimolphan et al. (1997) concluded from an experiment with lactating dairy cows fed a Met-deficient diet that cystine in feather meal probably cannot substitute for Met in MP.

The percentage contributions of cysteine/cystine to total sulfur AA and of tyrosine to tyrosine + Phe of ruminal microorganisms and of feedstuffs are presented in Table 5-9. If cysteine/cystine can satisfy approximately 50 percent of the sulfur AA requirements and tyrosine can satisfy approximately 50 percent of the tyrosine + Phe requirements of dairy cattle, then it would appear there may often be an obligatory use of Met and Phe for cysteine and tyrosine synthesis. In cases where this exists, feedstuffs with higher concentrations of cysteine/cystine and tyrosine in RUP would be important in reducing the need for Met and Phe in MP. An eventual understanding of the extent that cysteine/cystine can contribute to the requirements of total sulfur AA in MP is particularly important as Met has been identified as one of the most limiting EAA for growth and milk protein production. An apparent example of the Phe-sparing effect of tyrosine was provided by Rae and Ingalls (1984) who reported increased milk yields with supplemental tyrosine when cows were fed large amounts (17 percent of DM) of formaldehyde-treated canola meal. Substantial amounts of tyrosine have been shown to be destroyed or rendered unavailable by formaldehyde treatment (Rae et al., 1983; Sidhu and Ashes, 1977). The milk yield response of cows in the study by Rae and Ingalls (1984) may have resulted because of decreased bioavailability of tyrosine and an increased requirement for Phe to synthesize tyrosine.

Two NEAA that have received limited attention in regards to their importance to milk production in dairy cows are proline and glutamine. Bruckental et al. (1991) reported increased content and yield of fat in milk when proline was infused into the duodenum of early and midlac-

TABLE 5-9 Mean Percentage Contributions of Cysteine (and its oxidation product cystine) to Total Sulfur Amino Acids (methionine + cysteine + cystine) and of Tyrosine to Tyrosine + Phenylalanine in Ruminal Microbes and Feedstuffs

| | Cysteine | Tyrosine |
|---|---|---|
| *Ruminal microbes*[a] | | |
| Bacteria | 36 | 47 |
| Protozoa | 40 | 46 |
| *Forages*[b] | | |
| Alfalfa hay | 48 | 41 |
| Alfalfa silage | 37 | 39 |
| Corn silage | 47 | 35 |
| Grass hay | 47 | 39 |
| Grass pasture | | |
| Grass silage | 39 | — |
| Oat silage | 28 | — |
| Rye silage | 36 | — |
| Sorghum silage | 33 | — |
| Wheat silage | 34 | — |
| *Grains and energy feeds*[b] | | |
| Barley | 57 | 38 |
| Corn | 50 | 44 |
| Corn gluten feed | 57 | 45 |
| Cottonseed | 51 | — |
| Oats | 63 | 40 |
| Sorghum | 51 | 42 |
| Triticale | 58 | 38 |
| Wheat | 58 | 39 |
| *Fibrous byproduct feeds*[b] | | |
| Beet pulp | 47 | 57 |
| Citrus pulp | 57 | 38 |
| Cottonseed hulls | 47 | — |
| Rice bran | 52 | 42 |
| Soybean hulls | 60 | — |
| Wheat bran | 57 | 42 |
| *Plant proteins*[b] | | |
| Brewer's grains, dry | 52 | 40 |
| Brewer's grains, wet | 50 | — |
| Canola meal | 58 | 44 |
| Corn distillers grain w/sol. | 51 | 38 |
| Corn gluten meal | 43 | 46 |
| Cottonseed meal | 51 | 36 |
| Fava beans | 61 | 46 |
| Linseed meal | 50 | — |
| Lupin | 65 | 53 |
| Peas, field | 60 | 42 |
| Peanut meal | 54 | 45 |
| Rapeseed meal | 55 | 44 |
| Safflower meal | 53 | 42 |
| Soybean meal | 51 | 43 |
| Sunflower meal | 44 | 37 |
| *Animal proteins*[b] | | |
| Blood meal | 52 | 31 |
| Feather meal | 87 | 38 |
| Fish meal, menhaden | 24 | 45 |
| Fish meal, anchovy | 24 | 45 |
| Meat meal | 44 | 39 |
| Meat and bone meal | 42 | 40 |
| Skim milk powder | 24 | 51 |
| Whey, wet | 59 | 41 |

[a]Values were calculated from mean AA concentrations as reported by Martin et al. (1996) and Storm and Ørskov (1983).

[b]Contributions of cysteine to total sulfur AA were calculated from AA concentrations presented in Tables 15-2a,b. Contributions of tyrosine to tyrosine + phenylalanine were calculated largely from AA concentrations presented in the Degussa book (Fickler et al., 1996); the remaining values were calculated from data presented in *Nutrient Requirements of Swine* (National Research Council, 1998).

tation cows. Proline infusion increased content and yield of protein in milk during midlactation but not in early lactation. In the same study, it was observed that proline infusion reduced mammary gland uptake of Arg by 40 to 50 percent. Glutamine has been hypothesized to be one of the first-limiting AA for milk protein synthesis in cows during early lactation (Meijer et al., 1993, 1995). The reasons for glutamine being suggested to be deficient were low concentrations of free glutamine in plasma of cows during early lactation and increased metabolic requirements during periods of energy deficiency. However, there are no reported studies in which intestinal supplies of glutamine were increased in cows during early lactation and lactational responses measured. Increasing duodenal supplies during late lactation did not increase content or yield of protein in milk (Meijer and van der Koelen, 1994). Proline and glutamine (including its intermediate precursor glutamic acid) are similar in that: (1) concentrations of both are considerably higher in milk casein (11.6 and 22.3 percent, respectively) than in the true protein fraction of either ruminal bacteria (3.5 and 12.6 percent, respectively) or of most feedstuffs (Fickler et al., 1996; Storm and Ørskov, 1983), (2) extraction by the lactating mammary gland is considerably less than the quantities secreted in milk protein (Clark, 1975; Clark et al., 1978; Illg et al., 1987), and (3) both can be synthesized in the mammary gland from Arg, an EAA, and ornithine (Clark et al., 1975; Mepham and Linzell, 1967; Mezl and Knox, 1977). Glutamine has received widespread attention in humans because of its numerous physiologic roles and its increased requirements during stress and illness. The additional quantities of glutamine required for stress and mild illness can be met by adaptive mechanisms for biosynthesis and utilization (Neu et al., 1996). However, during serious or long illness, glutamine producing tissues are unable to meet increased needs and thus, glutamine becomes conditionally essential (Young and El-Khoury, 1995). Currently, there are no reports of glutamine becoming a conditionally EAA for dairy cattle. However, such might be expected, particularly in young calves and early postpartum cows, when nutritional status is compromised for extended periods of time because of disease and metabolic disorders.

*Limiting Essential Amino Acids*

As noted in the previous section, research indicates that the dairy animal's requirement for total NEAA for growth and milk protein production are met before the requirement for at least the most limiting of the EAA. If this is true, then it follows that the efficiency of use of MP for protein synthesis will be determined by how well the profile of EAA in MP matches the profile required by the animal and by the amount of total EAA in MP. This logic has led to an interest in identifying the EAA that are most limiting when dairy cattle are fed diets that differ in ingredient composition. Knowledge of how the sequence of AA limitation is influenced by diet composition is useful for selecting feed protein supplements that will improve the profile of AA in MP. Also, knowledge of the first limiting EAA when a diet of known composition is fed is requisite information for initial studies to determine AA requirements.

Lysine and Met have been identified most frequently as first-limiting EAA in MP of dairy cattle. The most direct evidence of their limitation has been observed by infusing individual AA or combinations of EAA into the abomasum or duodenum and measuring effects on N retention and milk protein production. Feeding ruminally inert supplements of ruminally protected Met (RPMet) and ruminally protected Lys (RPLys) and measuring effects on weight gains of growing cattle and milk protein production of lactating cows have confirmed and extended the results of infusion studies. Use of the reflex closure of the reticular groove also has provided a means of delivering AA to the small intestine of weaned calves (Abe et al., 1997, 1998).

Use of the above approaches indicate that the sequence of Lys and Met limitation is determined by their relative concentrations in RUP. For example, Lys was identified as first limiting for young post-weaned calves (Abe et al., 1997), growing cattle (Abe et al., 1997; Burris et al., 1976; Hill et al., 1980), and lactating cows (King et al., 1991; Polan et al., 1991; Schwab et al., 1992a) when corn and feeds of corn origin provided most or all of dietary RUP. In contrast, Met was identified as first-limiting for young post-weaned calves (Donahue et al., 1985; Schwab et al., 1982), growing cattle (Hopkins et al., 1999; Klemesrud and Klopfenstein, 1994; Lusby, 1994; Robert et al., 1999) and lactating cows (e.g., Armentano et al., 1997; Rulquin and Delaby, 1997; Robert et al., 1994; Schingoethe et al., 1988) when smaller amounts of corn were fed, when high forage diets were fed, or when most of the supplemental RUP was provided by soybean products, animal-derived proteins, or a combination of the two. Relative to concentrations in ruminal bacteria, feeds of corn origin are low in Lys and similar in Met whereas soybean products and most animal-derived proteins are similar in Lys and low in Met (Table 5-10). Lysine and Met were identified as co-limiting when lactating cows were fed diets without (Schwab et al., 1976) or with minimal protein supplementation (Rulquin, 1987).

That Lys and Met are often the first two limiting EAA for both growth and milk protein production may be expected. First, Met was identified as first limiting (Richardson and Hatfield, 1978; Titgemeyer and Merchen, 1990b) and Lys was identified as second limiting (Richardson and Hatfield, 1978) in MCP for N retention of growing cattle. Second, most feedstuffs have lower amounts of Lys and Met, particularly of Lys, in total EAA than in MCP (Table 5-10). And last, contributions of Lys and Met to total EAA in body lean tissue and milk are similar (Table 5-10).

TABLE 5-10 A Comparison of the EAA Profiles of Body Tissue and Milk With That of Ruminal Bacteria and Protozoa and Common Feeds

| Item | Arg | His | Ile | Leu | Lys | Met | Phe | Thr | Trp | Val | EAA |
|---|---|---|---|---|---|---|---|---|---|---|---|
| | (% of total EAA) | | | | | | | | | | (%CP) |
| *Animal products* | | | | | | | | | | | |
| Lean tissue[a] | 16.8 | 6.3 | 7.1 | 17.0 | 16.3 | 5.1 | 8.9 | 9.9 | 2.5 | 10.1 | — |
| Milk[b] | 7.2 | 5.5 | 11.4 | 19.5 | 16.0 | 5.5 | 10.0 | 8.9 | 3.0 | 13.0 | — |
| *Rumen microbes* | | | | | | | | | | | |
| Bacteria[c] | 10.2 | 4.0 | 11.5 | 16.3 | 15.8 | 5.2 | 10.2 | 11.7 | 2.7 | 12.5 | — |
| Bacteria[d] | 10.6 | 4.3 | 11.6 | 15.5 | 17.3 | 4.9 | 10.0 | 11.0 | 2.6 | 12.2 | — |
| Protozoa[e] | 9.3 | 3.6 | 12.7 | 15.8 | 20.6 | 4.2 | 10.7 | 10.5 | 2.8 | 9.7 | — |
| *Forages*[f,g] | | | | | | | | | | | |
| Legume (alfalfa) hay | 12.5 | 4.7 | 10.3 | 17.9 | 12.4 | 3.8 | 11.6 | 10.6 | 3.6 | 12.7 | 41.2 |
| Legume (alfalfa) silage | 10.9 | 4.7 | 11.1 | 17.9 | 12.1 | 3.8 | 11.7 | 10.7 | 2.7 | 14.1 | 35.6 |
| Corn silage, normal | 6.2 | 5.7 | 10.6 | 27.2 | 7.9 | 4.8 | 12.1 | 10.1 | 1.4 | 14.1 | 31.6 |
| Grass hay | 11.7 | 4.9 | 10.0 | 18.8 | 10.5 | 3.9 | 11.8 | 10.9 | 3.7 | 13.6 | 33.1 |
| Grass silage | 9.4 | 5.1 | 10.9 | 18.8 | 10.1 | 3.7 | 13.4 | 10.2 | 3.3 | 15.0 | 32.6 |
| *Grains*[f] | | | | | | | | | | | |
| Barley | 13.4 | 6.1 | 9.2 | 18.5 | 9.6 | 4.5 | 13.5 | 9.1 | 3.1 | 13.0 | 37.7 |
| Corn, grain, cracked | 11.5 | 7.8 | 8.2 | 27.9 | 7.1 | 5.3 | 11.5 | 8.8 | 1.8 | 10.0 | 40.1 |
| Corn gluten feed | 10.9 | 8.3 | 8.8 | 25.4 | 7.7 | 4.5 | 10.4 | 9.8 | 1.6 | 12.6 | 35.4 |
| Oats | 16.6 | 5.9 | 9.1 | 17.7 | 10.1 | 4.2 | 12.5 | 8.4 | 2.9 | 12.6 | 41.2 |
| Sorghum | 9.4 | 5.7 | 9.3 | 31.9 | 5.4 | 4.2 | 12.3 | 7.8 | 2.5 | 11.6 | 42.8 |
| Wheat | 13.6 | 7.1 | 9.6 | 19.3 | 8.1 | 4.6 | 13.3 | 8.4 | 3.5 | 12.3 | 34.4 |
| *Plant proteins*[f] | | | | | | | | | | | |
| Brewers grains, dry | 14.7 | 5.1 | 9.8 | 20.0 | 10.4 | 4.3 | 11.7 | 9.1 | 2.5 | 12.1 | 39.2 |
| Canola meal | 16.5 | 6.6 | 9.0 | 15.9 | 13.2 | 4.4 | 9.5 | 10.4 | 3.4 | 11.1 | 42.6 |
| Corn DDG w/sol. | 10.7 | 6.6 | 9.8 | 25.4 | 5.9 | 4.8 | 12.9 | 9.1 | 2.3 | 12.4 | 37.8 |
| Corn gluten meal | 7.1 | 4.7 | 9.1 | 37.2 | 3.7 | 5.2 | 14.1 | 7.5 | 1.2 | 10.3 | 45.2 |
| Cottonseed meal | 26.0 | 6.6 | 7.3 | 13.8 | 9.7 | 3.7 | 12.5 | 7.6 | 2.8 | 10.0 | 42.6 |
| Linseed meal | 20.9 | 4.8 | 11.0 | 14.5 | 8.7 | 4.2 | 11.1 | 8.9 | 3.7 | 12.3 | 42.2 |
| Peanut meal | 27.6 | 6.0 | 8.1 | 15.9 | 8.3 | 2.9 | 12.1 | 6.7 | 2.4 | 9.8 | 40.1 |
| Safflower meal | 22.4 | 6.5 | 7.3 | 16.7 | 8.1 | 3.7 | 11.7 | 7.1 | 3.6 | 12.9 | 39.0 |
| Soybean meal | 16.2 | 6.1 | 10.1 | 17.2 | 13.9 | 3.2 | 11.6 | 8.7 | 2.8 | 10.2 | 45.3 |
| Sunflower meal | 20.8 | 6.2 | 9.9 | 15.2 | 8.0 | 5.6 | 11.0 | 8.7 | 2.9 | 11.7 | 42.2 |
| *Animal proteins*[f] | | | | | | | | | | | |
| Blood meal, ring dried | 7.8 | 11.3 | 2.2 | 22.7 | 15.9 | 2.1 | 12.1 | 7.7 | 2.8 | 15.4 | 56.4 |
| Feather meal | 16.2 | 2.7 | 11.4 | 19.9 | 6.0 | 1.8 | 11.6 | 11.1 | 1.7 | 17.6 | 42.7 |
| Fish meal, menhaden | 13.1 | 6.4 | 9.2 | 16.2 | 17.2 | 6.3 | 9.0 | 9.4 | 2.4 | 10.8 | 44.5 |
| Meat and bone meal | 19.5 | 5.3 | 7.7 | 17.2 | 14.5 | 3.9 | 9.4 | 9.1 | 1.6 | 11.8 | 35.7 |
| Whey, dry | 5.0 | 4.5 | 12.1 | 21.2 | 17.6 | 3.3 | 7.0 | 14.1 | 3.5 | 11.7 | 42.2 |

[a]From Ainslie et al. (1993); average values of empty, whole body carcasses as reported in 3 studies.
[b]Each value is an average of 3 observations from Jacobson et al. (1970), McCance and Widdowson (1978), and Waghorn and Baldwin (1984).
[c]From Clark et al. (1992); average values from 61 dietary treatments.
[d]From Storm and Ørskov (1983); average values from 62 literature reports.
[e]From Storm and Ørskov (1983); average values from 15 literature reports.
[f]Calculated from values presented in this edition of *Nutrient Requirements of Dairy Cattle* feed table.
[g]Legume and grass hays and silages are mid-maturity.

Responses of growing cattle to improved supplies of Lys and Met in MP include variable increases in BW gains and feed efficiency (Hopkins et al., 1999; Robert et al., 1999; Veira et al., 1991) and variable decreases in urinary N excretion (Abe et al., 1997, 1998; Campbell et al., 1996, 1997; Donahue et al., 1985; Schwab et al., 1982). Production responses of lactating dairy cows to increased supplies of Lys and Met in MP include variable increases in content and yield of protein in milk, milk yield, and feed intake. The nature of production responses of lactating cows to increased postruminal supplies of Lys and Met have been reviewed (Rulquin and Vérité, 1993; Schwab 1995b, 1996a; Garthwaite et al., 1998). Collectively, these reviews and other more recent studies (Piepenbrink et al., 1999; Nocek et al., 1999; Sniffen et al., 1999a,b; Freeden et al., 1999; Rode et al., 1999; Wu et al., 1999; Nichols et al., 1998; Rulquin and Delaby, 1997) indicate: (1) that content of protein in milk is more responsive than milk yield to supplemental Lys and Met, particularly in post-peak lactation cows, (2) that increases in milk protein percentage are independent of milk yield, (3) that casein is the most influenced milk protein fraction, (4) that increases in milk protein production to increased supplies of either Lys or Met in MP are the most predictable when the resulting predicted supply of the other AA in MP is near or at estimated requirements (Rulquin et al., 1993; Schwab, 1996a; Sloan et al., 1998), (5) that milk yield responses to Lys and Met are more common in cows during early lactation than in mid or late lactation cows, and (6) production responses to increased supplies of Lys and Met in MP typically are greater when CP in diet DM approximates normal levels (14 to 18 percent) than when it is lower or higher. That milk protein percentage is more sensitive than milk yield to improved concentrations of Lys and Met in MP of post-peak lactation cows was demonstrated by Chapoutot et al. (1992). The authors used a multiple switch-back experiment to determine individual responses of 40 post-peak lactation cows to ruminally protected Lys and Met. The RPAA blend was fed in amounts to provide 23 g/d of digestible Lys and 7 g/d of digestible Met. They observed that 37 cows responded with greater content of milk protein, 31 responded with greater protein yield, and 16 responded with more milk.

In addition to the effects on milk protein production, there are reports also of increased percentages of fat in milk with increased amounts of Met or Met plus Lys in MP. These increases in milk fat have been observed in postruminal infusion studies (Socha et al., 1994b) and when Met (Brunschwig and Augeard, 1994; Brunschwig et al., 1995; Yang et al., 1986) or Met and Lys (Bremmer et al., 1997; Canale et al., 1990; Rogers et al., 1987; Xu et al., 1998) were supplied in ruminally protected forms. The increases in milk fat generally have been observed in association with increases in milk protein but increases also have been observed without increases in milk protein (Varvikko et al., 1999). Increases in percentages of fat in milk with improved Met and Lys nutrition also have not been predictable. For example, the infusion of graded amounts of Met (0, 3.5, 7.0, 10.5, and 16.0 g/d) into the duodenum of post-peak lactation cows fed a corn-based diet supplemented with soybean products and blood meal increased percentages in milk of both fat (3.73, 3.86, 3.78, 3.91, and 4.15) and true protein (3.00, 3.07, 3.09, 3.13, and 3.15) (Socha et al., 1994b). However, when the same cows fed the same feedstuffs were infused with similar amounts of Met during peak lactation (Socha et al., 1994c) or mid lactation (Socha et al., 1994a), percentages of fat in milk did not change but protein in milk increased.

It is not clear why increased amounts of Met and Lys in MP may sometimes increase fat content of milk. One reason may involve a possible effect of Met on de novo synthesis of short- and medium-chain fatty acids in the mammary gland. This was suggested by Pisulewski et al. (1996) who demonstrated that the infusion of Met into the duodenum of early lactation cows increased proportions of short- and medium-chain fatty acids and decreased proportions of long-chain fatty acids in milk fat. Christensen et al. (1994) reported a similar trend in the fatty acid composition of milk when lactating cows were fed ruminally protected Met and Lys. However, others did not observe an effect of increased postruminal supplies of Met on fatty acid composition of milk (Casper et al., 1987; Chow et al., 1990; Karunanandaa et al., 1994; Kowalski et al., 1999; Rulquin and Delaby, 1997; Varvikko et al., 1999). Another reason may relate to the role of AA in the intestinal and hepatic synthesis of chylomicrons and very low density lipoproteins (VLDL). Required substrates for the synthesis of chylomicrons and VLDL, in addition to the presence of the long-chain fatty acids that stimulate their formation, include apolipoproteins and phospholipids (Bauchart et al., 1996). The synthesis of apolipoproteins requires AA. The synthesis of phosphatidylcholine (lecithin), the most abundant phospholipid, requires choline. It has been demonstrated that a portion of the dairy cows' requirement for Met is as a methyl donor for choline synthesis (Sharma and Erdman, 1988) and that in some studies (Sharma and Erdman,1988,1989; Erdman, 1994), but not in others (Erdman and Sharma, 1991; Grummer et al., 1987), choline can be a limiting nutrient for milk fat synthesis. That Met and Lys may sometimes be limiting for the synthesis of chylomicrons or VLDL such that the availability of long-chain fatty acids for milk fat synthesis is reduced has not been demonstrated. However, there is limited evidence that formation or secretion of these lipoproteins can be enhanced with improved Met and Lys nutrition (Auboiron et al., 1995; Durand et al., 1992). Decreases in plasma nonesterified fatty acids concentrations in preruminant calves (Auboiron et al., 1995; Chilliard et al., 1994) and lactating cows (Pisulewski et al., 1996; Rulquin and Delaby, 1997) with increased amounts of Met in MP have been reported. However, decreases in plasma nonesterified fatty acids concentrations are generally considered to reflect reduced mobilization of fatty acids from body reserves rather than increased utilization.

Attempts to identify EAA that may become limiting after Lys and Met in dairy cattle are limited. Using the total intragastric nutrition technique, Fraser et al. (1991) concluded that His was limiting after Met and Lys for lactating cows when casein was the infused protein. Similar conclusions could not be drawn from the abomasal infusion experiments of Schwab et al. (1976) and Rulquin (1987) when lactating cows were fed diets of conventional ingredients. Rulquin (1987) concluded that Thr was not limiting after Lys and Met. Schwab et al. (1976) concluded from five infusion experiments that the sequence of limiting EAA after Lys and Met for lactating cows will be determined by the ingredient composition of the diet. Amino acid extraction efficiencies, transfer efficiencies, and ratios of uptake to output have been used in many studies to evaluate the order of limiting AA. Nichols et al. (1998) and Piepenbrink et al. (1999) concluded that AA extraction efficiency is the most accurate of the three methods for estimating the sequence of AA limitation because no errors from estimates of blood flow are involved. Use of this method identified Phe and Ile as most frequently limiting after Lys and Met (Nichols et al., 1998; Piepenbrink et al.,

1998; Liu et al., 2000) when corn-based diets are supplemented with common protein supplements such as soybean meal, corn distillers dried grains, canola meal, or a mixture of canola meal, corn gluten meal, blood meal, and fish meal.

Although research is limited, there is little direct evidence to indicate that other EAA might be more limiting than either Lys or Met. Two exceptions may be Arg and His. Abomasal infusion of Arg (13.7 g/d) increased N retention of 159-kg Holstein steers fed direct-cut vegetative wheat silage (12.3 percent CP) as the sole feed. In contrast, abomasal (178 g/d) and intravenous (112 g/d) infusions of Arg did not affect milk production or milk composition when post-peak lactating Holstein cows (544 kg) were fed a 15.3 percent CP diet of alfalfa-grass silage, corn silage, corn, and soybean meal (Vicini et al., 1988). Vanhatalo et al. (1999) concluded that His was the first-limiting EAA when post-peak lactating Finnish Aryshire cows were fed a grass silage-based diet without feeds of corn origin and without protein supplementation. The diet contained 56 percent grass silage ensiled with an acid-based additive, 18 percent barley, 18 percent oats, 6.7 percent beet pulp, and 1.3 percent minerals and vitamins. The abomasal infusion of 6.5 g/d His increased yields of milk (23.6 vs. 22.9 kg/d) and milk protein (721 vs. 695 g/d) but not milk protein content. The infusions of either 6.0 g/d of Met or 19.0 g/d of Lys or both in combination with 6.5 g/d of His did not further increase milk protein production. Factors that probably contributed to His being first limiting in the study by Vanhatalo et al. (1999) are: (1) the low content of RUP in dietary DM, (2) the low content of His in microbial protein as compared to feed proteins (Table 5-10), and (3) the low content of His in barley and oats as compared to corn (Table 5-10). Mackle et al. (1999) found no response in milk yield or milk composition when Holstein cows in early lactation fed a 16.2 percent CP diet (based on alfalfa hay, corn, and soybean products) were abomasally infused with branched-chain AA (55.5, 39.0, and 55.5 g/d of Leu, Ile, and Val, respectively). Hopkins et al. (1994) provided daily intraperitoneal infusions of branched-chain AA plus Arg (46.1, 31.4, 38.3, and 25.0 g/d of Leu, Ile, Val, and Arg, respectively) over a 2-h period each day to Holstein cows in early lactation fed 13.6 percent CP diets that contained 15.0 or 22.4 percent ADF, respectively. The infusion of AA did not increase the content or yield of protein in milk but it did appear to attenuate the decreases in content and yield of fat in milk, when cows were fed the low fiber diet. Analysis of milk fat for fatty acids indicated that the infused AA may have increased *de novo* synthesis of $C_4$ to $C_{16}$ fatty acids, particularly the $C_{16}$ fatty acids. It is well-documented that Arg and the branched-chain AA are taken up by the mammary gland well in excess of their direct output in milk protein (Clark et al., 1978; Nichols et al., 1998; Piepenbrink et al., 1999) and that they can be converted to NEAA or utilized as energy sources in the mammary gland (Mepham, 1982; Wohlt et al., 1977).

### *Predicting Passage to the Small Intestine*

As reviewed in the previous section, the efficiency of use of MP by dairy cattle is influenced by its content of EAA. To advance AA nutrition research (e.g., to define the ideal content of EAA in MP) and to implement the results of such research (e.g., to select protein and AA supplements to optimize the balance of EAA in MP) models are needed that predict accurately the EAA composition of duodenal protein. In recognition of this need, it was the goal of the subcommittee to extend the use of the MP system developed for this revision of *Nutrient Requirements of Dairy Cattle* to one that would predict directly the EAA composition of duodenal protein. The EAA content of MP and flow to the duodenum of the individual digestible EAA could be calculated from knowledge of: (1) the predicted EAA composition of duodenal protein; (2) the predicted contribution of each protein fraction (microbial protein, the RUP fraction of each feedstuff, and endogenous protein) to the total flow of each EAA; (3) the digestibility coefficients assigned to microbial protein, the RUP fraction of each feedstuff, and endogenous protein; and (4) the predicted flows of MP.

The subcommittee considered both factorial and multivariate regression approaches. Prediction models based on the factorial method require the assignment of AA values to model-predicted supplies of ruminally synthesized microbial protein, ruminally undegraded feed proteins, and if predicted, endogenous protein. The challenge associated with such an approach is to have the predicted flows of protein fractions and their assigned AA values be accurate. Indeed, it can be assumed that there are errors in predicting flows of protein fractions as well as in assigning AA values to each fraction. To the extent that this occurs, then at each step in the factorial process, errors of prediction are aggregated, and depending on the number of steps involved, the aggregated error can be quite large. The net result of such errors are biases of prediction of mean values.

Two examples of published factorial approaches for predicting AA passage to the small intestine are the AA submodel of the Cornell Net Carbohydrate and Protein System (CNCPS) (O'Connor et al., 1993) and the AA submodel developed by Rulquin et al. (1998). The CNCPS AA submodel, adopted in conjunction with the CNCPS model for Level II of the *Nutrient Requirements of Beef Cattle* (National Research Council, 1996) model, was developed to predict directly the absolute flows of each of the EAA. The AA submodel of Rulquin et al. (1998), which uses the PDI system (INRA, 1989) to predict flows of protein fractions, was developed to predict directly the content of AA in duodenal protein and not the absolute flows of the individual AA. This approach provided for a true integration of the AA submodel with the protein model. The *Nutrient Requirements of Beef Cattle* (National Research Council, 1996) and Rulquin et al. (1998) models differ in the AA values assigned to microbial protein and RUP. In the *Nutrient Requirements of Beef Cattle* (National Research Council, 1996) model, predicted flows of microbial protein are partitioned into cell wall and non-cell wall fractions and estimated EAA compositions of each (O'Connor et al., 1993) are assigned. The EAA values assigned to the predicted digestible RUP fractions of feedstuffs are those of the insoluble protein fraction of feedstuffs and not of total CP (O'Connor et al., 1993). In the model of Rulquin et al. (1998), the average AA composition of liquid-associated bacteria from 66 publications are assigned to microbial protein. The AA profile of the RUP fraction of feedstuffs is assumed to be the same as in the original feedstuff. The two submodels also differ in that endogenous protein is considered in the model of Rulquin et al. (1998) but not in the *Nutrient Requirements of Beef Cattle* (National Research Council, 1996) model.

Both models were tested against published AA flow data and reasonable results were obtained. However, in both cases, the evaluation studies indicated biases of prediction for individual AA. Based on slopes of regression lines that related observed flows obtained from 200 diets (as reported in 12 lactating cow studies and 9 nonlactating cow studies) to predicted flows, O'Connor et al. (1993) observed that the CNCPS model over-predicted flows of Thr and Leu and under-predicted flows of Arg. Rulquin et al. (1998) tested their model against abomasal and duodenal digesta AA compositions measured in 133 dairy cow diets and 49 growing cattle diets. Mean percentage differences between predicted and measured concentrations (g/100 g AA) were: Arg (−5.6%), His (+0.9%), Ile (−1.5%), Leu (−5.8%), Lys (−4.7%), Met (+12.3%), Thr (−0.2%), Phe (+0.4%), and Val (+0.8%). As a result of these biases, the authors adjusted the initial model by covariance (i.e., regression) analysis. This improved the accuracy of prediction. In summary, if the two described models were perfect both in structure (i.e., all of the contributing variables were included) and parameters (i.e., assigned constants were correct), and measured profiles of AA in duodenal digesta protein used for evaluation were without systematic errors, then a comparison of predicted values with measured values would have revealed no biases of prediction of mean values.

In contrast to the described factorial models in which both the structure and the parameters were determined on theoretic grounds, the multivariate regression or semi-factorial approach allows for some of the parameters to be determined by regression. This allows the model (i.e., equations) to adapt to the measured data, and allows for at least partial correction of the errors of the mechanistically determined variables. The result is that semi-mechanistic models generally are better at predicting (forecasting) than full mechanistic models when forecasting is within the inference range of the model. Because of the potential for increased accuracy of prediction, and because the approach eliminated the need to assign AA values to ruminally synthesized microbial protein and endogenous protein (AA values had to be assigned only to feedstuffs), the semi-mechanistic method was the method of choice by the subcommittee for predicting the content of EAA in total EAA of duodenal protein. This approach required the development of an equation for each of the EAA and one for predicting flows of total EAA.

The approach used for developing the AA submodel was as follows. A data set of observed abomasal and duodenal AA flows was compiled from 57 published studies involving 199 treatment means (Table 5-11). The data set included 155 treatment means from cows (lactating and dry) and 44 treatment means from growing cattle (dairy and beef). Only one experiment reported flows of Trp; thus, no equation could be developed for predicting the content of Trp in total EAA of duodenal protein. For data to be included in the final data set, the following requirements had to be met: (1) DMI was reported or could be calculated from the information given, (2) ingredient composition of diets was reported, (3) feedstuffs used in the experiments were represented in the feed library of the model for N fractions, $K_d$, and AA composition, and (4) flows (g/d) to the duodenum of Arg, His, Ile, Leu, Lys, Met, Phe, Thr, and Val were reported. An exception was made in regard to requirement # 3 in that N fractions and $K_d$ for barley straw were used for oat straw, but the AA composition of oat straw was used. The first three requirements were necessary because the information is model-required data. For experiments that employed a factorial arrangement of treatments and reported main effect means only, data were used only if one of the main effects was not related to diet (e.g., for an experiment with main effects of protein source and feeding frequency, data for the main effect of protein source was used). Body weights of animals had to be estimated for 15 of the 57 published studies; in all cases, these 15 studies involved cows. Body weights were estimated from reported information on breed, stage of lactation, and BW reported by the same authors in other papers.

The 199 treatment means for duodenal flows of each EAA in the final data set represented 199 unique and diverse diets fed to cattle ranging in BW from 191 to 717 kg. Intake of DM ranged from 3.6 to 26.7 kg/d. Feedstuffs, their frequency of use, and the means and ranges of their contribution to diet DM are summarized in Table 5-12. Diets varied in percent concentrate (0 to 86%, mean = 46%), dietary CP (8.5 to 29.6%, mean = 16.2%), dietary RDP (4.6 to 18.2, mean = 10.7%), and dietary RUP (2.2 to 11.9%, mean = 5.5%). The descriptive statistics of the

TABLE 5-11 Experiments Used to Develop Equations for Predicting Amino Acid Passage to the Small Intestine

| | | |
|---|---|---|
| Aldrich et al. (1995) | Klusmeyer et al. (1991b) | Robinson (1997) |
| Aldrich et al. (1993a) | Klusmeyer et al. (1990) | Robinson et al. (1991a) |
| Aldrich et al. (1993b) | Lardy et al. (1993) | Robinson et al. (1994) |
| Armentano et al. (1986) | Lynch et al. (1991) | Santos et al. (1984) |
| Bernard et al. (1988) | Mabjeesh et al. (1996) | Schwab et al. (1992a) |
| Bohnert et al. (1999) | Mansfield and Stern (1994) | Schwab et al. (1992b) |
| Cameron et al. (1991) | McCarthy et al. (1989) | Stern et al. (1983) |
| Cecava et al. (1993) | McNiven et al. (1995) | Stern et al. (1985) |
| Cecava and Parker (1993) | Merchen and Satter (1983) | Titgemeyer et al. (1988) |
| Christensen et al. (1993a, b) | Murphy et al. (1993) | van Vuuren et al. (1992) |
| Christensen et al. (1996) | Narasimhalu et al. (1989) | van Vuuren et al. (1993) |
| Cunningham et al. (1993) | O'Mara et al. (1998) | Volden (1999) |
| Cunningham et al. (1994) | O'Mara et al. (1997b) | Waltz et al. (1989) |
| Cunningham et al. (1996) | Overton et al. (1995) | Wessels et al. (1996) |
| Erasmus et al. (1992) | Palmquist et al. (1993) | Zerbini et al. (1988) |
| Erasmus et al. (1994b) | Pena et al. (1986) | Zinn (1988) |
| Holden et al. (1994b) | Pisulewski et al. (1996) | Zinn (1993b) |
| Keery et al. (1993) | Prange et al. (1984) | Zinn and Shen (1998) |
| Klusmeyer et al. (1991a) | Putnam et al. (1997) | |

TABLE 5-12 Feedstuffs and the Extent of Their Use in the 199 Diets in the Data Set Used to Develop Equations to Predict the Content of Individual EAA in Total EAA of Duodenal Protein

| Feedstuff | N[a] | Contribution to dietary DM (%) | | Feedstuff | N[a] | Contributions to dietary DM (%) | |
|---|---|---|---|---|---|---|---|
| | | Mean | Range | | | Mean | Range |
| *Forages* | | | | *Protein supplements* | | | |
| Corn silage | 108 | 35 | 8–80 | Alfalfa meal | 5 | 9 | 5–10 |
| Grass, fresh | 10 | 87 | 56–100 | Blood meal | 22 | 4 | 0.6–10 |
| Grass, hay | 26 | 21 | 5–100 | Brewers grains, dry | 2 | 34 | 25–44 |
| Grass, silage | 17 | 58 | 38–100 | Brewers grains, wet | 1 | 32 | — |
| Grass-legume, silage | 18 | 19 | 11–26 | Canola meal | 10 | 12 | 4–20 |
| Legume, fresh | 5 | 86 | 65–100 | Casein | 4 | 3 | 2–4 |
| Legume, hay | 61 | 17 | 5–65 | Corn distillers grains | 14 | 8 | 4–28 |
| Legume, silage | 37 | 33 | 8–65 | Corn gluten meal | 17 | 6 | 1–19 |
| Oat, silage | 10 | 18 | 9–30 | Feather meal | 6 | 4 | 0.3–10 |
| Oat, straw | 13 | 6 | 3–95 | Feather meal with viscera | 3 | 4 | 2–6 |
| Sorghum, sudan hay | 7 | 11 | 10–12 | Fish meal, anchovy | 1 | 5 | — |
| Sorghum, sudan, silage | 6 | 68 | 66–70 | Fish meal, menhaden | 23 | 5 | 2–13 |
| Wheat, silage | 8 | 33 | 23–45 | Meat meal | 5 | 2 | 0.3–9 |
| Wheat, straw | 1 | 25 | — | Rapeseed meal | 7 | 6 | 1–19 |
| *Energy feeds* | | | | Soybean meal, expeller | 6 | 8 | 4–15 |
| Barley, grain | 24 | 26 | 4–46 | Soybean meal, heated | 3 | 11 | 5–15 |
| Barley, grain, heated | 1 | 46 | | Soybean meal, nonenz browned | 2 | 17 | 16–17 |
| Barley, grain, steam-rolled | 12 | 36 | 12–50 | Soybean meal, solvent | 78 | 9 | 0.3–20 |
| Corn, grain | 119 | 24 | 1–49 | Sunflower meal | 2 | 12 | 10–13 |
| Corn, grain and cob | 6 | 40 | 37–42 | Urea | 66 | 0.5 | 0.1–2.0 |
| Corn, grain, high moisture | 19 | 25 | 2–32 | *Energy and protein feeds* | | | |
| Corn, grain, steam-flaked | 7 | 51 | 16–65 | Cottonseed, whole, extruded | 1 | 42 | — |
| Corn, hominy | 1 | 22 | — | Cottonseed, whole, heated | 1 | 43 | — |
| Corn, starch | 19 | 5 | 0.3–17 | Cottonseed, whole, raw | 1 | 41 | — |
| Fat | 33 | 3 | 0.2–6 | Soybean seed, raw | 5 | 12 | 6–20 |
| Molasses | 75 | 4 | 0.5–13 | Soybean seed, roasted | 5 | 17 | 16–19 |
| Oats, grain | 5 | 21 | 17–25 | *Byproduct feeds* | | | |
| Sorghum, grain | 1 | 10 | — | Beet pulp | 7 | 18 | 9–36 |
| Sugar/dextrose | 2 | 3 | — | Corn gluten feed | 9 | 14 | 6–32 |
| Wheat, grain | 5 | 23 | 5–29 | Soy hulls | 21 | 15 | 0.3–36 |
| Wheat, grain, steam. flaked | 2 | 51 | 50–52 | Tapioca | 4 | 7 | 2–20 |
| | | | | Wheat middlings | 16 | 8 | 0.2–34 |

[a]Number of diets in which the feedstuff was an ingredient.

animal, diet, and EAA flow data used in the development of the equations are presented in Table 5-13. All of the required animal and diet data for the 199 diets were entered into this edition's model for predicted intakes of RUP and RDP and for predicted duodenal flows of MCP, RUP, and endogenous CP. The CP content of feedstuffs was obtained from the experiment if reported; otherwise, model default values (±1.0 SD) were used.

The following approach was used to identify the independent variables and a model structure that would most accurately predict the content of each EAA (except Trp) in total EAA of duodenal protein and flows of individual EAA to the small intestine. The first step involved calculating the content of each EAA in total EAA of the RUP fraction of each diet in the data set. The three equations used for this purpose are presented; Lys is used as the example EAA.

$$RUPLys = \Sigma_f (DMI_f \times CP_f \times RUP_f \times Lys_f \times 0.001) \quad (5\text{-}3)$$

where:
RUPLys = amount of Lys supplied by total diet RUP, g
$DMI_f$ = intake of DM of each feedstuff contributing RUP, kg
$CP_f$ = crude protein content of each feedstuff contributing RUP, g/100 g DM
$RUP_f$ = ruminally undegraded protein content of each feedstuff contributing RUP, g/100 g CP
$Lys_f$ = lysine content of each feedstuff contributing RUP, g/100 g CP

$$RUPEAA = RUPArg + RUPHis + RUPIle + RUPLeu + RUPLys + RUPMet + RUPPhe + RUPThr + RUPTrp + RUPVal \quad (5\text{-}4)$$

where:
RUPEAA = amount of essential AA supplied by RUP, g

$$RUPLysPctRUPEAA = 100 \times (RUPLys/RUPEAA) \quad (5\text{-}5)$$

where:
RUPLysPctRUPEAA = Lys as percentage of essential AA in RUP, each g/100 g essential AA.

The content of each EAA in total EAA of the RUP fraction of each diet was estimated in recognition of the belief that the resulting values would be significant predictors of the contributions that each EAA makes to total EAA in duodenal protein. Multivariate analysis of measurements of AA passage to the small intestine indicated that the concentrations of individual AA in RUP and the proportional contribution of RUP to total protein passing to the duodenum explained most of the variation in AA profiles of duodenal protein (Rulquin and Vérité, 1993). Dietary RUP and the percentage contributions of Lys and Met to total EAA in diet RUP also emerged as significant independent variables in regression equations developed for predicting concentrations of Lys and Met in total EAA of duodenal protein of lactating dairy cows (Schwab, 1996b; Socha, 1994).

The second step involved the identification of significant independent variables to develop equations to predict percentages of each EAA (excluding Trp) and total EAA in duodenal protein. Variables that were evaluated as potential significant predictors of the content of each EAA in total EAA (e.g., g/100 g total EAA) of duodenal protein were: "Trial," dietary CP and predicted dietary RUP as

TABLE 5-13 Descriptive Statistics of the Data Used for Developing Equations for Predicting Content of Individual EAA in Total EAA of Duodenal Protein and for Predicting Flows of Total EAA to the Small Intestine

| Item | Mean | Median | Minimum | Maximum | SD |
|---|---|---|---|---|---|
| Animal characteristics | | | | | |
| DMI, kg/d | 15.5 | 16.4 | 3.6 | 26.7 | 6.4 |
| BW, kg | 515.2 | 568.0 | 191.0 | 717.0 | 128.0 |
| DMI, %BW | 2.9 | 2.9 | 1.3 | 4.4 | 0.8 |
| Diet characteristics, %DM | | | | | |
| CP | 16.2 | 16.5 | 8.5 | 29.6 | 2.7 |
| RUP[a] | 5.5 | 5.3 | 2.2 | 11.9 | 1.6 |
| Concentrate | 46.3 | 50.0 | 0.0 | 85.7 | 18.0 |
| AA in duodenal protein, %EAA | | | | | |
| Arg | 10.4 | 10.3 | 7.1 | 16.1 | 1.2 |
| His | 5.0 | 4.9 | 3.1 | 9.2 | 0.8 |
| Ile | 10.8 | 10.9 | 6.4 | 14.5 | 1.4 |
| Leu | 20.2 | 20.4 | 9.6 | 28.5 | 2.5 |
| Lys | 14.4 | 14.7 | 9.7 | 18.0 | 1.4 |
| Met | 4.3 | 4.1 | 2.2 | 7.1 | 0.9 |
| Phe | 11.3 | 11.2 | 9.8 | 15.1 | 0.7 |
| Thr | 11.1 | 11.1 | 8.9 | 13.8 | 0.8 |
| Val | 12.5 | 12.6 | 9.0 | 15.7 | 1.2 |
| EAA flow to duodenum, g/d | 894.1 | 938.5 | 169.2 | 1970.0 | 463.7 |

[a]Predicted by the model.

percentages of dietary DM, the percentage of each EAA in dietary RUP (e.g., RUPLys, g/100 g RUP), the percentage of each EAA in total EAA of dietary RUP (e.g., RUPLysPctRUPEAA, g/100 g), and the percentage of predicted RUP in predicted flows of total duodenal protein (predicted MCP + predicted RUP + predicted endogenous protein). The potential independent variables considered for predicting flows of total EAA to the duodenum were: "Trial," dietary CP and predicted dietary RUP as percentages of diet DM, the percentage of total EAA in dietary RUP, RUPEAA intake (g/d), predicted flows of endogenous protein (g/d), and model predicted MCP (g/d). Trial was included in all models as a class variable to account for variation caused by independent variables or factors that are not continuous (e.g., feeding frequency, sampling methods, microbial markers used, etc.) and for which their inclusion risks overparameterization of the model. Significant independent variables were identified by using the backward elimination procedure of multiple regression. Briefly, independent variables, their squared terms (except for "Trial"), and all possible two-way interactions (excluding interactions with "Trial") were entered into the model. The following algorithm was used to reduce the model to significant ($P < 0.05$) independent variables. First, non-significant ($P > 0.05$) interactions were removed sequentially from the model. Second, non-significant main effects were removed from the model if no interactions or squared term of the main effect was significant. Third, if variance inflation factors (VIF) were all less than 100 then the model was accepted. If a term had a VIF greater than 100, it was removed. If more than one had a VIF greater than 100, the term with the largest $P$ value was removed. In that case, all steps were repeated until an accepted model was obtained at the third step. When an apparently acceptable model was generated, the Difference in Fits Statistic (DFFITS) was used as the basis for omitting outliers; absolute values of DFFITS $\geq 2$ were omitted (Bowerman and O'Connell, 1990). The variables that emerged as significant predictors of the content of individual EAA in total EAA of duodenal protein were Trial, each EAA as a percentage of EAA in RUP, and RUP as a percentage of total duodenal protein.

The third step involved the use of PROC MIXED of SAS (a random effects model) to develop the final equations. This was done to yield more accurate parameter estimates and to increase the utility of the prediction equations for purpose of field application (i.e., Trial effects would be unknown). In brief, two random coefficient models for each EAA and for total EAA were fitted for the prediction equations generated by using PROC GLM. The first random coefficient model utilized unstructured covariance to test whether the intercept and slope within trials were significantly ($P < 0.05$) correlated, which was not the case for any of the equations. The second random coefficients model, which models a different variance component for each random effect (the default structure), then was used to generate the final prediction equations.

Arginine

$$Y = 7.31 + 0.251X_1 \text{ (RMSE} = 0.278)$$

where:
$Y$ = Arg, % of EAA in duodenal protein
$X_1$ = Arg, % of EAA in RUP

Histidine

$$Y = 2.07 + 0.393X_1 + 0.0122X_2 \text{ (RMSE} = 0.156)$$

where:
$Y$ = His, % of EAA in duodenal protein
$X_1$ = His, % of EAA in RUP
$X_2$ = RUP, % of duodenal protein (MCP + RUP + endogenous CP)

Isoleucine

$$Y = 7.59 + 0.391X_1 - 0.0123X_2 \text{ (RMSE} = 0.174)$$

where:
$Y$ = Ile, % of EAA in duodenal protein
$X_1$ = Ile, % of EAA in RUP
$X_2$ = RUP, % of duodenal protein (MCP + RUP + endogenous CP)

Leucine

$$Y = 8.53 + 0.410X_1 + 0.0746X_2 \text{ (RMSE} = 0.541)$$

where:
$Y$ = Leu, % of EAA in duodenal protein
$X_1$ = Leu, % of EAA in RUP
$X_2$ = RUP, % of duodenal protein (MCP + RUP + endogenous CP)

Lysine

$$Y = 13.66 + 0.3276X_1 - 0.07497X_2 \text{ (RMSE} = 0.400)$$

where:
$Y$ = Lys, % of EAA in duodenal protein
$X_1$ = Lys, % of EAA in RUP
$X_2$ = RUP, % of duodenal protein (MCP + RUP + endogenous CP)

Methionine

$$Y = 2.90 + 0.391X_1 - 0.00742X_2 \text{ (RMSE} = 0.168)$$

where:
$Y$ = Met, % of EAA in duodenal protein
$X_1$ = Met, % of EAA in RUP
$X_2$ = RUP, % of duodenal protein (MCP + RUP + endogenous CP)

Phenylalanine

$$Y = 7.32 - 0.244X_1 + 0.0290X_2 \text{ (RMSE} = 0.194)$$

where:

$Y$ = Phe, % of EAA in duodenal protein
$X_1$ = Phe, % of EAA in RUP
$X_2$ = RUP, % of duodenal protein (MCP + RUP + endogenous CP)

Threonine

$$Y = 7.55 + 0.450X_1 - 0.0212X_2 \text{ (RMSE} = 0.167)$$

where:

$Y$ = Thr, % of EAA in duodenal protein
$X_1$ = Thr, % of EAA in RUP
$X_2$ = RUP, % of duodenal protein (MCP + RUP + endogenous CP)

Valine

$$Y = 8.68 + 0.314X_1 \text{ (RMSE} = 0.216)$$

where:

$Y$ = Val, % of EAA in duodenal protein
$X_1$ = Val, % of EAA in RUP

Total essential amino acids

$$Y = 30.9 + 0.863X_1 + 0.433X_2 \text{ (RMSE} = 58.8)$$

where:

$Y$ = EAA in duodenal protein, g
$X_1$ = EAA supplied by RUP, g
$X_2$ = MCP, g

The model predicts flows (g/d) of individual EAA to the small intestine by multiplying predicted concentrations of each EAA in duodenal total EAA by predicted flows of total EAA. Plots of predicted vs. measured values and of residuals (predicted − measured) vs. measured values for Lys, Met, and total EAA are presented in Figures 5-9 through 5-11.

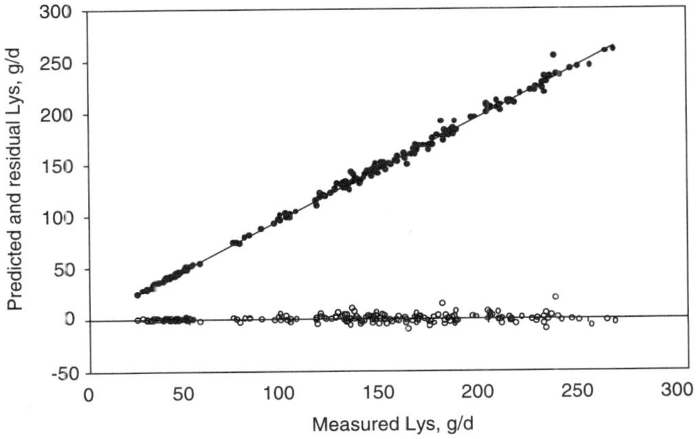


FIGURE 5-9 Plot of predicted vs. measured (filled circles) and residuals (predicted − measured; open circles) vs. measured (Lys, g/d) (from predicted Lys, percent of EAA and predicted EAA, g/d) (mean bias = $2.4 \times 10^{-2}$; RMSPE = 3.5; n = 186).

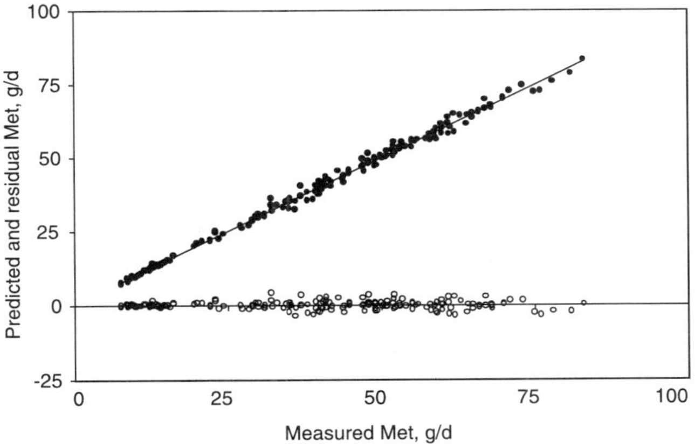


FIGURE 5-10 Plot of predicted vs. measured (filled circles) and residuals (predicted − measured; open circles) vs. measured Met, g/d (from predicted Met, percent of EAA and predicted EAA, g/d) (mean bias = $2.2 \times 10^{-3}$; RMSPE = 1.3; n = 182).

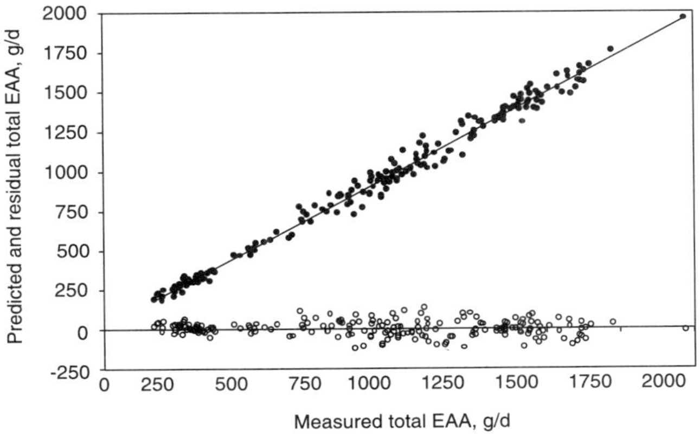


FIGURE 5-11 Plot of predicted vs. measured (filled circles) and residuals (predicted − measured; open circles) vs. measured flow of total EAA (mean bias = $3.06 \times 10^{-5}$; RMSPE = 47.8; n = 196).

The subcommittee also evaluated the use of a semi-mechanistic approach to predict directly the "flows" of individual EAA to the duodenum. Using the same data base, the theoretically based model structure for each EAA was $Y = \beta_0 + \beta_1X_1 + \beta_2X_2$ where: Y = flow to duodenum(g), $\beta_0$ = parameter estimate for contribution of endogenous protein (g), $\beta_1$ = parameter estimate of the fractional contribution of RUP to flows from RUP, $X_1$ = model predicted flow of the EAA (g), $\beta_2$ = parameter estimate of the fractional content of the EAA in MCP, and $X_2$ = model predicted flow of MCP (g). The parameter estimates that resulted appeared reasonable, indicating that the model does an adequate job of predicting flows of MCP and RUP and that the content of EAA in MCP is similar to mean values reported in the literature (e.g., Clark et al., 1992). A comparison of the root mean square prediction errors (RMSPE) obtained from two sets of residual plots ("g/d" and "% of total EAA") for each of the two approaches is presented in Table 5-14.

The residual plots indicated that the equations that predict percentages directly predict more accurately both the "percentages" of individual EAA in duodenal total EAA and "flows" (g/d) of individual EAA. The lower RMSPE for predicting "percentages" and "flows" when percentages are predicted directly (and flows are calculated) result partially because errors of prediction are "condensed" into two variables (i.e., the prediction of the percentage and prediction of total EAA, from which the product yields prediction of flow). In contrast, prediction errors of all nine EAA are aggregated into total EAA and subsequently into the calculation of percentages for the more theoretically based model. Thus, the equations that predict directly the percentages of each EAA in total EAA of duodenal protein were accepted for use in this publication.

Knowledge of predicted flows of digestible EAA and the EAA content of MP is more important than knowing the predicted flows of total EAA and the EAA content of total duodenal protein. This is because the AA in undigested protein are not absorbed and do not contribute to meeting the AA requirements of the animal. The EAA composition of MP will generally be different from that of total duodenal protein. This is because of differences among feedstuffs in both the digestibility and the EAA composition of their RUP fractions, differences in the proportional contributions that microbial protein and RUP make to total EAA passage, and mean differences in the digestibility of microbial protein and total dietary RUP. Because undigested AA do not contribute to meeting the AA requirements of the animal, and because the AA composition of MP is likely to differ from the AA composition of total duodenal protein, it is desirable also to express EAA requirements in terms of digestible (i.e., metabolizable) requirements rather than on the basis of total flows. In recognition of the need for research aimed at defining AA requirements and the need for models designed to predict as accurately as possible passage of digestible EAA to the small intestine, the model was extended to predict flows of digestible EAA and the EAA composition of MP. The following 9 equations are used; again, Lys is used as the example EAA.

$$\text{RUPLys} = \Sigma_f\,(\text{DMI}_f \times \text{CP}_f \times \text{RUP}_f \times \text{Lys}_f \times 0.01) \tag{5-6}$$

where:

RUPLys = amount of Lys supplied by total diet RUP, g

$\text{DMI}_f$ = intake of DM of each feedstuff contributing RUP, kg

$\text{CP}_f$ = crude protein content of each feedstuff contributing RUP, g/100 g DM

$\text{RUP}_f$ = ruminally undegraded protein content of each feedstuff contributing RUP, g/100 g CP

$\text{Lys}_f$ = lysine content of each feedstuff contributing RUP, g/100 g CP

The preceeding equation is used to calculate for each feedstuff, and subsequently the diet, the amount of Lys supplied by RUP. Equation 5-6 is extended in the following manner to calculate the amount of digestible Lys supplied by RUP, which weights feedstuffs appropriately for differences of digestibility of RUP and concentration of Lys among feeds.

$$\text{dRUPLys} = \Sigma_f\,(\text{DMI}_f \times \text{CP}_f \times \text{RUP}_f \times \text{RUPdigestibility}_f \times \text{Lys}_f \times 0.001) \tag{5-7}$$

where:

dRUPLys = amount of digestible Lys supplied by total diet RUP, g

$\text{DMI}_f$ = intake of DM of each feedstuff contributing RUP, kg

$\text{CP}_f$ = crude protein content of each feedstuff contributing RUP, g/100 g DM

$\text{RUP}_f$ = ruminally undegraded protein content of each feedstuff contributing RUP, g/100 g CP

TABLE 5-14 Comparison of Root Mean Square Prediction Errors (RMSPE) Obtained from Plots of Residuals (predicted-measured vs. measured) for Equations That Predicted Directly the Flow of Each EAA With Those Accepted for Use in the Model That Predict Directly the Percentage of Each EAA in Total EAA of Duodenal Protein

| | Flow | | Percentage | |
|---|---|---|---|---|
| Amino acid | RMSPE from plots for % | RMSPE from plots for g/d[a] | RMSPE from plots for % | RMSPE from plots for g/d[b] |
| Arg | 0.46 | 6.1 | 0.24 | 2.8 |
| His | 0.26 | 3.0 | 0.13 | 1.3 |
| Ile | 0.34 | 4.4 | 0.14 | 1.3 |
| Leu | 0.51 | 9.4 | 0.45 | 4.8 |
| Lys | 0.45 | 7.0 | 0.33 | 3.5 |
| Met | 0.22 | 2.7 | 0.14 | 1.3 |
| Phe | 0.28 | 5.9 | 0.16 | 1.5 |
| Thr | 0.25 | 5.6 | 0.14 | 1.5 |
| Val | 0.22 | 5.4 | 0.17 | 1.7 |
| Total EAA | | 40.6 | | 47.8 |

[a] Percentages of each EAA in duodenal total EAA were calculated from predicted flows of individual EAA.
[b] Flows of each EAA to the duodenum were calculated from predicted flows of total EAA and predicted percentages of each EAA in duodenal total EAA.

$RUPdigestibility_f$ = digestibility coefficient of ruminally undegraded protein for each feedstuff contributing RUP, g/100 g RUP
$Lys_f$ = lysine content of each feedstuff contributing RUP, g/100 g CP

The preceeding two equations then are combined to yield the calculation of digestible RUPLys as a percentage of total RUPLys for the diet.

$$\text{PctdRUPLys} = 100 \times (\text{dRUPLys}/\text{RUPLys}) \quad (5\text{-}8)$$

where:
PctdRUPLys = digestibility coefficient for Lys supplied by RUP, g/100 g
dRUPLys = amount of digestible Lys supplied by total diet RUP, g
RUPLys = amount of Lys supplied by total diet RUP, g

In order to calculate the supply of total digestible Lys, two "pools" must be considered. The first pool is the amount supplied by RUP. The equation for predicting total EAA has associated with it a coefficient of 0.863 for RUPEAA, which indicates that the total EAA supplied by RUP (thus, individual AA supplied by RUP) is "discounted" by 13.8 percent (i.e, 100 − 86.3). Theoretically, the total flow (g/d) of Lys from RUP can be calculated.

$$\text{TotalRUPLysFlow} = 0.863 \times \text{RUPLys} \quad (5\text{-}9)$$

where:
TotalRUPLysFlow = adjusted total supply of Lys from RUP, g
RUPLys = amount of Lys supplied by total diet RUP, g

The second "pool" is the amount of Lys supplied from MCP and endogenous CP, and is calculated by difference from total Lys flow and the supply of Lys from RUP as calculated in Equation 5-9.

$$\text{TotalMCPEndoLysFlow} = \text{LysFlow} - \text{TotalRUPLysFlow} \quad (5\text{-}10)$$

where:
TotalMCPEndoLysFlow = supply of Lys from MCP and endogenous CP, g
LysFlow = total amount of Lys in duodenal protein, g
TotalRUPLysFlow = adjusted total supply of Lys from RUP, g

The amount of digestible Lys supplied by each of the two pools and total digestible Lys is calculated as follows:

$$\text{dTotalRUPLys} = \text{TotalRUPLysFlow} \times \text{PctdRUPLys} \times 0.01 \quad (5\text{-}11)$$

where:

dTotalRUPLys = supply of digestible Lys from RUP, g
TotalRUPLysFlow = adjusted total supply of Lys from RUP, g
PctdRUPLys = digestibility coefficient for Lys supplied from RUP (i.e., Equation 5-8), g/100g

$$\text{dTotalMCPEndoLys} = 0.80 \times \text{TotalMCPEndoLysFlow} \quad (5\text{-}12)$$

where:

dTotalMCPEndoLysFlow = supply of Lys from MCP and endogenous CP, g

$$\text{TotalDigestibleLys} = \text{Equation 5-11} + \text{Equation 5-12} \quad (5\text{-}13)$$

The final step is to calculate digestible Lys as percentage of MP.

$$\text{dLysPctMP} = 100 \times (\text{TotalDigestibleLys}/(\text{MPBact} + \text{MPFeed} + \text{MPEndo})) \quad (5\text{-}14)$$

where:
dLysPctMP = digestible Lys as percentage of MP, %
TotalDigestibleLys = total amount of digestible Lys (i.e., Equation 5-13), g
MPBact = model predicted MP from MCP, g
MPFeed = model predicted MP from RUP, g
MPEndo = model predicted MP from endogenous CP, g

### *Requirements for Lysine and Methionine in Metabolizable Protein for Lactating Cows*

The AA requirements of dairy cattle are not known with much certainty. Attempts have been made to quantify AA requirements of cattle using the factorial approach (Oldham, 1981; O'Connor et al., 1993). The factorial method is a mathematic approach of calculating requirements from a segmentation of the requirements into individual and independent components, and from knowledge of pool sizes and the rates by which nutrients move through digestive and metabolic pools. More specifically, calculating requirements for absorbed AA using this approach requires at a minimum a knowledge of: (1) net protein requirements for maintenance, growth, pregnancy, and lactation, (2) AA composition of products, and (3) efficiencies of use of absorbed AA for maintenance and product formation. The Cornell Net Carbohydrate and Protein System for evaluating cattle diets and the associated AA submodel (O'Connor et al., 1993) is the most tested of the AA factorial models published to date in the United States. It was the opinion of the subcommittee, however, that current knowledge is too limited, both for model construction and model evaluation, to put forth a model that quantifies AA requirements for dairy cattle. Indeed, there have been few direct attempts to quantify AA requirements of dairy cattle (Campbell et al., 1997; Fenderson and Bergen, 1975; Titgemeyer et al., 1988; Williams and Smith, 1974). This is due largely to the technical difficulties involved in providing graded amounts of a limiting AA to sites of absorption in ruminants at various production levels, while simultaneously measuring AA flows to the small intestine and weight gains or milk production.

An alternate and more direct approach to defining AA requirements is to use the dose-response approach to estimate required AA concentrations in MP for maximal use of MP for protein synthesis. Thus far, the most progress has been made for Lys and Met in lactating cows. Two dose-response approaches have been used. The first is the "direct" dose-response approach, whereby postruminal supplies of Lys (Rulquin et al., 1990; Schwab et al., 1992b) or Met (Pisulewski et al., 1996; Socha et al., 1994a,b,c) were increased in graded fashion via intestinal infusion and production responses and AA flows to the small intestine were measured. A constant amount of supplemental Met was provided in each of the Lys experiments and a constant amount of supplemental Lys was provided in each of the Met experiments to reduce the possibility that they would limit responses. This approach indicated that for cows fed corn-based diets, Lys must contribute about 7.0 percent and Met about 2.5 percent of total AA in duodenal digesta for maximum content and yield of protein in milk.

The second method for estimating the optimum amounts of Lys and Met in MP for lactating cows is an "indirect" dose-response approach. This approach was used by Rulquin et al. (1993) and involved five steps: (1) predicting concentrations of digestible Lys and Met in protein truly digested in the small intestine (PDI) for control and treatment groups in experiments in which postruminal supplies of Lys, Met, or both were increased (either by intestinal infusion or by feeding in ruminally protected form) and production responses were measured, (2) identifying "fixed" concentrations of Lys and Met in PDI that were intermediate to the lowest and highest values in the greatest number of Lys experiments and Met experiments, respectively, (3) calculating by linear regression a "reference production value" for each production parameter in each Lys experiment that corresponded to the "fixed" level of Lys in PDI and in each Met experiment that corresponded to the "fixed" level of Met in PDI, (4) calculating "production responses" (plus and minus values) for control and treatment groups relative to the "reference production values," and (5) regressing the production responses on the predicted concentrations of Lys and Met in PDI. Experiments involving ruminally protected Lys or Met were limited to those in which data on ruminal stability and postruminal release of Lys and Met had been obtained in the author's laboratory.

Using the described approach, Rulquin et al. (1993) obtained curvilinear (monomolecular) dose-response relationships for content and yield of milk protein to increasing concentrations of Lys in PDI. The authors reported that concentrations of Met in PDI had no apparent effect on milk protein responses to Lys in PDI. In contrast, concentrations of Lys lower than 6.5 percent of PDI limited responses to increases in Met. Thus, curvilinear dose-response relationships for content and yield of milk protein to increasing concentrations of Met in PDI were obtained from the data for Lys concentrations greater than 6.5 percent of PDI. Assuming that Lys and Met requirements were met when protein yield responses were slightly below the maximum attainable values (as determined from the derived exponential equations), the authors concluded that the requirements for Lys and Met in PDI are the amounts that would result in the production of 16 g less milk protein (i.e., 0.5 kg milk containing 3.2 percent true protein) than the maximum attainable values. Using the derived equations, the calculated requirements for Lys and Met in PDI were 7.3 percent and 2.5 percent, respectively.

The "indirect" dose-response approach described by Rulquin et al. (1993) was used in this revision to determine the requirements for Lys and Met in MP for lactating cows. A unique and practical feature of this approach is that the requirement values are estimated using the same model as that used to estimate the contributions of feedstuffs to AA passage to the small intestine. Experiments were identified in which Lys (18 experiments; 63 treatments) or Met (27 experiments; 87 treatments) was infused continuously into the abomasum or duodenum or fed in ruminally protected form (Table 5-15). Experiments were not considered if diet or feed intake information was insufficient for model input, or if Lys and Met were supplemented together and there was no corresponding control where one of the two AA was supplemented at the same concentration. Of the 36 different experiments that were identified (9 experiments involved the administration of one or more quantities of both Lys and Met), 24 were Latin squares and of these 18 were infusion experiments. Experiments in which ruminally protected products were fed were restricted to those that had data for viability reported in peer-reviewed literature and estimates of ruminal escape were 80 percent or higher. Experiments involving rumina-

TABLE 5-15 Studies Used to Determine the Dose-Response Relationships for Lysine and Methionine in Metabolizable Protein

| | |
|---|---|
| Armentano et al. (1997) | Rogers et al. (1987) |
| Casper et al. (1987) | Rulquin and Delaby (1997) |
| Casper and Schingoethe (1988) | Rulquin and Delaby (1994) |
| Guinard and Rulquin (1994) | Rulquin et al. (1994) |
| Illg et al. (1987) | Schingoethe et al. (1988) |
| King et al. (1991) | Schwab et al. (1976) |
| Munneke et al. (1991) | Schwab et al. (1992a) |
| Papas et al. (1984a) | Schwab et al. (1992b) |
| Papas et al. (1984b) | Socha (1994) |
| Piepenbrink et al. (1999) | Socha et al. (1994a) |
| Pisulewski et al. (1996) | Socha et al. (1994b) |
| Polan et al. (1991) | Yang et al. (1986) |

lly protected products with published estimates of ruminal escape less than 80 percent were not used because of the concern that ruminally released Met may affect ruminal fermentation and AA passage to the small intestine. All experiments utilized Holstein cows. All but 2 experiments involved early and mid lactation cows. Ten experiments involved both multiparous and primiparous cows and 26 experiments involved only multiparous cows. Cows produced an average of 31.5 kg milk in the Lys experiments (range = 20.7 to 46.3 kg) and an average of 33.7 kg milk in the Met experiments (range = 20.9 to 43.1 kg).

To calculate concentrations of Lys and Met in MP, all cow and diet data were entered into the model. Published nutrient composition of the individual ingredients was used when available; otherwise, model default values were used. When nutrient composition of ingredients was not published but nutrient composition of the total diet was included, nutrient composition of individual ingredients (usually only the forages) was changed so that the composition of the diet was the same as the published composition. In all cases, model default values were used for the AA composition of feeds. Contributions of supplemental Lys and Met to predicted flows of digestible Lys and Met originating from the basal diet were estimated as follows: (1) the intestinal availability of infused Lys and Met was considered to be 100 percent, (2) ruminally protected sources of Lys and Met containing polymers in the surface coating (see next section, "Ruminally Protected Amino Acids") were considered to have a ruminal escape of 90 percent and an intestinal digestibility coefficient of 90 percent (Rogers et al., 1987; Schwab, 1995a) so 81 percent (0.90 × 0.90) of the fed amounts of Lys and Met was considered digestible, and (3) the ruminally protected Met product, Ketionin (Rumen Kjemi; Oslo, Norway), was considered to have a ruminal escape of 80 percent and an intestinal digestibility of 75 percent (Schwab, 1995a; Yang et al., 1986) so 60 percent of the fed amounts of Met was considered digestible.

Predicted concentrations of Lys in MP varied between 4.33 percent and 9.83 percent and for Met between 1.70 percent and 3.36 percent. The "fixed" concentration of Lys in MP that was selected (6.67 percent) to calculate the required "reference production values" was intermediate to the lowest and highest concentrations in 16 of the 18 Lys experiments. This eliminated the experiments of Polan et al. (1991) (6 treatments with predicted concentrations of Lys in MP between 4.32 percent and 5.87 percent) and Rogers et al. (1987) (4 treatments with predicted concentrations of Lys in MP between 6.76 and 7.55 percent). The "fixed" concentration of Met in MP (2.06 percent) that was selected was intermediate to the lowest and highest concentrations in all of the 27 Met experiments. The "reference production values" for each experiment and the "production responses" (plus and minus values) for each production parameter for each treatment were calculated as described above. The final database contained 53 observations for Lys and 87 observations for Met.

As observed by Rulquin et al. (1993), changes in milk yield, milk fat content, and milk fat yield to changes in concentrations of Lys and Met in MP were small and inconsistent. These observations were expected (see section, "Limiting Essential Amino Acids"). Therefore, no attempt was made to use these production measurements as response criteria for establishing requirements for Lys and Met in MP.

Four statistical models were used to describe the relationships between increasing concentrations of Lys and Met in MP and milk protein content and yield responses. These were: (1) a straightforward quadratic model (SAS, GLM procedure), (2) a negative exponential curve model (SAS, NLIN procedure), (3) a segmented quadratic model with a plateau (SAS, NLIN procedure), and (4) a rectilinear model (referred to in the literature as a linear abrupt threshold and plateau model, essentially consisting of a straight line followed by a plateau) (SAS, NLIN procedure). Analyses involving all models indicated that low concentrations of Met in MP limited responses to increasing concentrations of Lys in MP and that low concentrations of Lys in MP limited responses to increasing concentrations of Met in MP. The final regression analysis for Lys was limited to data where Met was 1.95 percent or more of MP (n = 41 of 53) and for Met it was limited to data where Lys was 6.50 percent or more of MP (n = 48 of 87). Using these restricted databases, the rectilinear model was either equal to or superior to the other models for describing protein content and protein yield responses to increasing amounts of both Lys and Met in MP. Based on these findings, the rectilinear model was accepted as the final model. An advantage of the rectilinear model is that the breakpoint in the nutrient dose-response line provides an objective, mathematically determined estimate of nutrient requirements. However, a requirement predicted by this type of break-point analysis is usually lower than that predicted by a curvilinear model because of the implicit smoothness constraint of curvilinear models. The appropriateness of different models for defining AA requirements have been discussed (Baker, 1986; Fuller and Garthwaite, 1993; Owens and Pettigrew, 1989).

The plots of predicted concentrations of Lys and Met in MP and the corresponding responses for milk protein content for all data are presented in Figure 5-12; the equivalent plots for milk protein yield are in Figure 5-13. The rectilinear dose-response relationships for the restricted databases are in the same figures. There are several noteworthy observations. First, the breakpoint estimates for the required concentrations of Lys and Met in MP for maximal yield of milk protein (7.08 percent and 2.35 percent, respectively; Figure 5-13) are similar to those

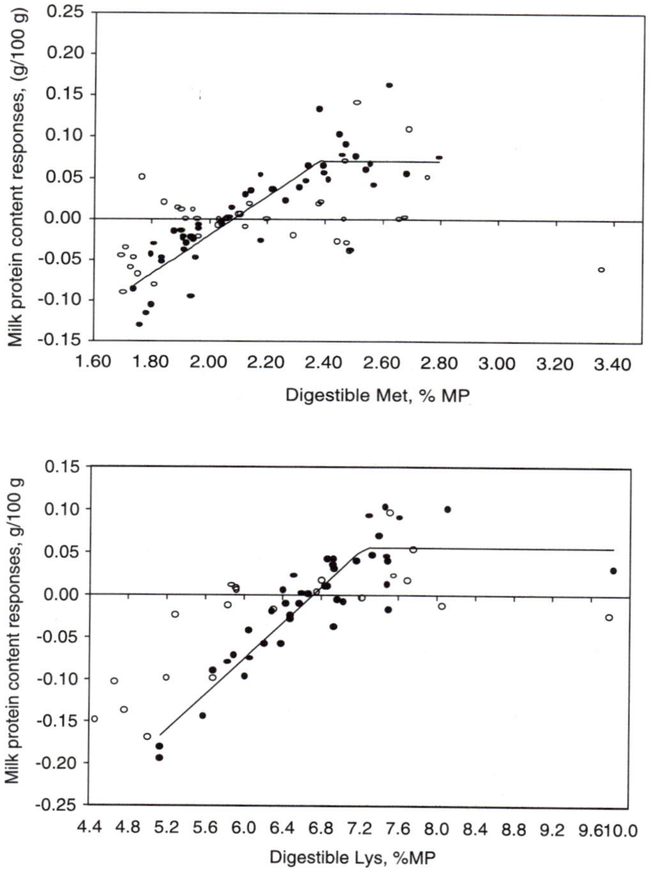


FIGURE 5-12 Milk protein content responses as a function of digestible Lys and Met concentrations in MP. Regression analysis for Lys was limited to data where Met was 1.95 percent or more of MP (filled circles) [$y = -0.712 + 0.106x$ for the linear part of the model and $y = -0.712 + 0.106 \times 7.24$ for the plateau (SE = 0.12 for x value of breakpoint); $r^2 = 0.85$; SE = 0.029; n = 41]. Regression analysis for Met was limited to data where Lys was 6.50 percent or more of MP (filled circles) [$y = -0.496 + 0.238x$ for the linear part of the model and $y = -0.496 + 0.238 \times 2.38$ for the plateau (SE = 0.07 for x value of breakpoint); $r^2 = 0.76$; SE = 0.033; n = 48]. The "trial" effect was not significant and therefore, not included in the model.

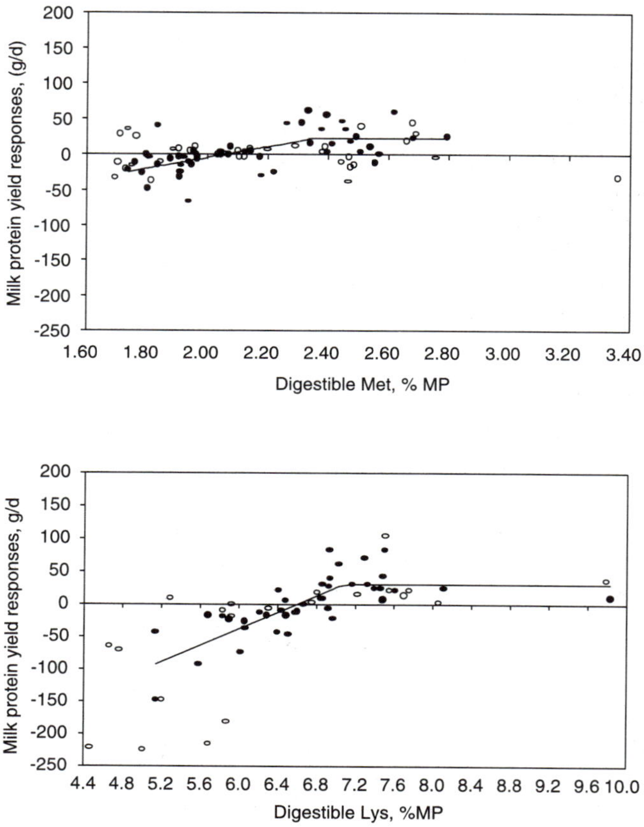


FIGURE 5-13 Milk protein yield responses as a function of digestible Lys and Met concentrations in MP. Regression analysis for Lys was limited to data where Met was 1.95 percent or more of MP (filled circles) [$y = -419.6 + 63.62x$ for the linear part of the model and $y = -419.6 + 63.62 \times 7.08$ for the plateau (SE = 0.18 for x value of breakpoint); $r^2 = 0.62$; SE = 27.9; n = 41]. Regression analysis for Met was limited to data where Lys was 6.50 percent or more of MP (filled circles) [$y = -159.1 + 77.30x$ for the linear part of the model and $y = -159.1 + 77.30 \times 2.35$ for the plateau (SE = 0.13 for x value of breakpoint); $r^2 = 0.40$; SE = 21.8; n = 48]. The "trial" effect was not significant and therefore, not included in the model.

required for maximal content of milk protein (7.24 percent and 2.38 percent; Figure 5-12). For both AA, the nutrient-response relationships were determined more accurately for protein content than for protein yield

Based on these results, it is concluded that optimal use of MP for the combined functions of maintenance and milk protein production requires concentrations of Lys and Met in MP (as determined by this edition's model) that approximate 7.2 percent and 2.4 percent, respectively. Second, the resultant requirement values are strikingly similar to the values of 7.3 percent and 2.5 percent proposed by Rulquin et al. (1993). As noted previously, the requirements proposed by Rulquin et al. (1993) were calculated to be somewhat less than required for maximum response as determined using an exponential representation of milk protein yield responses. Third, the observed optimum concentrations of Lys and Met in MP for the combined functions of maintenance and milk protein production (7.3 percent and 2.4 percent) are within their reported concentrations in milk protein (7.1 to 8.2 percent and 2.4 to 2.7 percent, respectively) (Rulquin et al., 1993; Waghorn and Baldwin, 1984). This observation may be considered as providing evidence of the reasonableness of the observed requirements. And last, an examination of Figures 16-4 and 16-5 indicates that implementation of diet formulation strategies that increase Lys and Met in MP to concentrations that approach or meet the requirement levels can result in more actual milk than MP allowable milk. Indeed, achieving the optimum concentrations of the most limiting AA in MP is the first step in balancing diets for AA. The subcommittee encourages more research aimed at determining the ideal profile of EAA in MP of growing cattle and lactating cows. The results of such efforts are needed to combine protein supplements and ruminally protected AA in ways to meet AA requirements of dairy cattle with minimal MP, and thus, minimal RUP.

### *Ruminally Protected Amino Acids*

As discussed, Lys and Met are two of the most limiting AA for protein synthesis in dairy cattle fed corn-based diets. A challenge in diet formulation, particularly for animals requiring higher RUP diets, is to achieve the desired concentrations of both Lys and Met in MP by relying solely on feed protein supplements. Supplements of crystalline Lys and Met have not been considered efficacious because of rapid deamination in the rumen (Chalupa, 1976; Onodera, 1993). Thus, a considerable effort has been made to develop technologies for supplying Met and Lys in forms that would allow them to escape ruminal degradation without compromising substantially their digestibility in the small intestine. The physical-chemical properties of Lys are such that application of most technologies are currently limited to Met.

The methods that have been evaluated for protecting free AA from ruminal degradation have been reviewed (Loerch and Oke, 1989; Schwab, 1995a). Technologically, the approaches in current use fall into one of three categories: (1) surface coating with a fatty acid/pH-sensitive polymer mixture, (2) surface coating or matrices involving fat or saturated fatty acids and minerals, and (3) liquid sources of Met hydroxy analog (DL-2-hydroxy-4-methylthiobutanoic acid; HMB).

Technology # 1 provides for a postruminal delivery system that is independent of digestive enzyme function and dependent on the differences in pH between the rumen and abomasum. The resulting ruminally inert products have an apparent high coefficient of rumen protection (Mbanzamihigo et al., 1997; Robert and Williams, 1997; Schwab, 1995a) and possess high intestinal release coefficients of the coated AA (Robert and Williams, 1997). This technology appears to be the most effective in increasing Met in MP as evidenced by the largest increases in blood Met concentrations (Blum et al., 1999; Robert et al., 1997).

Several variations of technology # 2 have been evaluated (Loerch and Oke, 1989; Schwab, 1995a). The physical-chemical properties of Lys are such that this technology has generally been limited to Met. The technology relies in identifying a combination of process and materials that provides a coating or matrix that gives a reasonable degree of protection against ruminal degradation, provided by the relatively inert characteristics of saturated fat in the rumen, while providing also for a reasonable degree of intestinal release. The apparent bioavailability of Met (ruminal escape × intestinal release) from RPMet products using this approach is less than RPMet products utilizing technology # 1 (Bach and Stern, 2000; Berthiaume et al., 2000; Blum et al., 1999; Mbanzamihigo et al., 1997; Overton et al., 1996).

Technology # 3 (i.e., liquid HMB) is currently being evaluated as an alternative to coated or encapsulated forms of Met. The Ca salt of HMB, commonly known as Met hydroxy analog, has been studied extensively as a supplement for increasing milk and milk fat production (Loerch and Oke, 1989). The Ca salt of HMB is no longer manufactured but liquid HMB is available and is used in the poultry and swine industry as a substitute for Met. It is well documented in nonruminants that following absorption, HMB is first converted to the α-keto analog of Met and then transaminated to L-Met (Baker, 1994). The combined efficiencies of absorption and conversion rates to Met in nonruminants is still being questioned. Baker (1994) summarized the efficiency estimates for dietary HMB and concluded that appropriate "Met bioavailability" values (molar basis) for rats, chickens, and pigs were 70, 80, and 100 percent, respectively. Comparable "Met bioavailability" data (ruminal escape × intestinal absorption × conversion to Met) is not available for ruminants. However, studies indicate that HMB is more resistant to ruminal degradation than free Met (Belasco, 1972, 1980; Patterson and Kung, 1988), that it can be absorbed across the ruminal and omasal epithelium (McCollum et al., 2000), and that ruminants possess the enzymes involved in the conversion of HMB to Met (Belasco, 1972, 1980; Papas et al., 1994). The study of Koenig et al. (1999) is the only reported attempt to quantify ruminal escape and intestinal absorption of liquid HMB in dairy cattle. In this study, a 90-g pulse-dose of HMB was given to lactating dairy cows fed a diet containing 30 g/d HMB. Based on fractional rate constants for ruminal and duodenal disappearance of HMB and passage of liquid, the workers reported that 50 percent of the HMB escaped ruminal degradation. However, the extent to which dietary HMB substitutes for absorbed Met for protein synthesis remains questionable because of observed minimal effects on blood Met concentrations (Johnson et al., 1999; Robert et al., 1997) and milk protein concentrations (Johnson et al., 1999; Rode et al., 1998).

## REFERENCES

Abe, M., T. Iriki, M. Funaba, and S. Onda. 1998. Limiting amino acids for a corn and soybean meal diet in weaned calves less than three months of age. J. Anim. Sci. 76:628–636.

Abe, M., T. Iriki, and M. Funaba. 1997. Lysine deficiency in postweaned calves fed corn and corn gluten meal diets. J. Anim. Sci. 75:1974–1982.

Agricultural and Food Research Council (AFRC). 1984. The Nutrient Requirements of Ruminant Livestock. Supplement No. 1. Commonwealth Agricultural Bureaux, Slough, England.

Agricultural and Food Research Council (AFRC). 1992. Nutritive requirements of ruminant animals: Protein. Nutr. Abstr. Rev. (Ser. B) 62:787–835.

Aharoni, Y., A. Arieli, and H. Tagari. 1993. Lactational response of dairy cows to change of degradability of dietary protein and organic matter. J. Dairy Sci. 76:3514–3522.

Ahmed, B. M., and W. G. Bergen. 1983. Metionine-cyst(e)ine relationship in steers. J. Anim. Sci. 57(Suppl.1):110. (Abstr.)

Ainslie, S. J., D. G. Fox, T. C. Perry, D. J. Ketchen, and M. C. Barry. 1993. Predicting amino acid adequacy of diets fed to Holstein steers. J. Anim. Sci. 71:1312–1319.

Aitchison, T. E., D. R. Mertens, A. D. McGilliard, and N. L. Jacobson. 1976. Effect of nitrogen solubility on nitrogen utilization in lactating dairy cattle. J. Dairy Sci. 59:2056–2062.

Akayezu, J. M., W. P. Hansen, D. E. Otterby, B. A. Crooker, and G. D. Marx. 1997. Yield response of lactating Holstein dairy cows to dietary fish meal or meat and bone meal. J. Dairy Sci. 80:2950–2963.

Aldrich, J. M., L. A. Holden, L. D. Muller, and G. A. Varga. 1996. Rumen availabilities of nonstructural carbohydrate and protein estimated from in situ incubation of ingredients versus diets. Anim. Feed Sci. Technol. 63:257–271.

Aldrich, C. G. N. R. Merchen, D. R. Nelson, and J. A. Barmore. 1995. The effects of roasting temperature applied to whole soybeans on site of digestion by steers: II. Protein and amino acid digestion. J. Anim. Sci. 73:2131–2140.

Aldrich, J. M., L. D. Muller, and G. A. Varga. 1993a. Effect of somatatropin administration and duodenal infusion of methionine and lysine on lactational performance and nutrient flow to the small intestine. Br. J. Nutr. 69:49–58.

Aldrich, J. M., L. D. Muller, G. A. Varga, and L. C. Griel, Jr. 1993b. Nonstructural carbohydrate and protein effects on rumen fermentation, nutrient flow, and performance of dairy cows. J. Dairy Sci. 76:1091–1105.

Alexandrov, A. N. 1998. Effect of ruminal exposure and subsequent microbial contamination on dry matter and protein degradability of various feedstuffs. Anim. Feed Sci. Technol. 71:99–107.

Anderson, G. W., and B. A. Barton. 1988. Reproductive efficiency: potential nutrition-management interactions. Page 107 *in* Proc. Winter Dairy Management Schools. Cornell University, Ithaca, NY.

Annexstad, R. J., M. D. Stern, D. E. Otterby, J. G. Linn, and W. P. Hansen. 1987. Extruded soybeans and corn gluten meal as supplemental protein sources for lactating dairy cattle. J. Dairy Sci. 70:814–822.

Annison, E. F. 1956. Nitrogen metabolism in the sheep. Protein digestion in the rumen. Biochem. J. 64:705–714.

Antoniewicz, A. M., J. Kowalczyk, J. Kanski, Z. Gorska-Matusiak, and M. Nalepka. 1995. Rumen degradability of crude protein of dried grass and lucerne forage measured by in sacco incubation and predicted by near infrared spectroscopy. Anim. Feed Sci. Technol. 54:203–216.

Antoniewicz, A. M., A. M. van Vuuren, C. J. van der Koelen, and I. Kosmala. 1992. Intestinal digestibility of rumen undegraded protein of formaldehyde-treated feedstuffs measured by mobile bag and in vitro technique. Anim. Feed Sci. Technol. 39:111–124.

Argyle, J. L., and R. L. Baldwin. 1989. Effects of amino acids and peptides on rumen microbial growth yields. J. Dairy Sci. 72:2017–2027.

Arieli, A., and G. Adin. 1994. Effect of wheat silage maturity on digestion and milk yield in dairy cows. J. Dairy Sci. 77:237–243.

Arieli, A., I. Bruckental, O. Kedar, and D. Sklan. 1995. In sacco disappearance of starch nitrogen and fat in processed grains. Anim. Feed Sci. Technol. 51:287–295.

Arieli, A., S. Mabjeesh, H. Tagari, I. Bruckental, and S. Zamwell. 1993. Evaluation of protein flow to the duodenum in dairy cattle by in sacco method. Livest. Prod. Sci. 35: 283–292.

Arieli, A., A. Ben-Moshe, S. Zamwel, and H. Tagari. 1989. In situ evaluation of the ruminal and intestinal digestibility of heat-treated whole cottonseeds. J. Dairy Sci. 72:1228–1233.

Armentano, L. E., S. J. Bertics, and G. A. Ducharme. 1997. Response of lactating cows to methionine or methionine plus lysine added to high protein diets based on alfalfa and heated soybeans. J. Dairy Sci., 80:1194–1199.

Armentano, L. E., S. J. Bertics, and J. Riesterer. 1993. Lack of response to addition of degradable protein to a low protein diet fed to midlactation dairy cows. J. Dairy Sci. 76:3755–3762.

Armentano, L. E., T. A. Herrington, C. E. Polan, A. J. Moe, J. H. Herbein, and P. Umstadt. 1986. Ruminal degradation of dried brewers grains, wet brewers grains, and soybean meal. J. Dairy Sci. 69:2124–2133.

Armentano, L. E., T. A. Herrington, and C. E. Polan. 1983. Ruminal degradation of dried brewers grains, wet brewers grains, and soybean meal in situ and in vitro. J. Dairy Sci. 66(Suppl. 1):171(Abstr.).

Armstead, I. P., and J. R Ling. 1993. Variations in the uptake and metabolism of peptides and amino acids by mixed ruminal bacteria in vitro. Appl. Environ. Microbiol 59:3360–3366.

Atwal, A. S., S. Mahadevan, M. S. Wolynetz, and Y. Yu. 1995. Increased milk production of cows in early lactation fed chemically treated soybean meal. J. Dairy Sc. 78:595–603.

Auboiron, S., D. Durand, J. C. Robert, M. J. Chapman, and D. Bauchart. 1995. Effect of dietary fat and L-methionine on the hepatic metabolism of very-low density lipoproteins in the preruminant calf, *Bos* spp. Reprod. Nutr. Dev. 35:167–168.

Bach, A., and M. D. Stern. 2000. Measuring resistance to ruminal degradation and bioavailability of ruminally protected methionine. Anim. Feed Sci. Technol. 84:23–32.

Bach, A., M. D. Stern, N. R. Merchen, and J. K. Drackley. 1998. Evaluation of selected mathematical approaches to the kinetics of protein degradation in situ. J. Anim. Sci. 76:2885–2893.

Baker, D. H. 1986. Problems and pitfalls in animal experiments designed to establish dietary requirements for essential nutrients. J. Nutr. 116:2339–2349.

Baker, D. H. 1994. Utilization of precursors for L-amino acids. Page 37–47 in Amino Acids in Farm Animal Nutrition. J.P.F. D'Mello, ed. Cab International.

Baker, L. D., J. D. Ferguson, and W. Chalupa. 1995. Responses in urea and true protein of milk to different protein feeding schemes for dairy cows. J. Dairy Sci. 78:2424–2434.

Balde, A. T., J. H. Vandersall, R. A. Erdman, J. B. Reeves, III, and B. P. Glenn. 1993. Effect of stage of maturity of alfalfa and orchardgrass on in situ dry matter and crude protein degradability and amino acid composition. Anim. Feed Sci. Technol. 44:29–43.

Barney, N. C. Personal communication.

Barney, D. J., D. G. Grieve, G. K. Macleod, and L. G. Young. 1981. Response of cows to dietary crude protein during midlactation. J. Dairy Sci. 64:655–661.

Barton, B. A. 1996a. Effects of dietary crude protein, breed, parity, and health status on the fertility of dairy cows. J. Dairy Sci. 70:2225–2236.

Barton, B. A. 1996b. Determining if reproduction is affected by a nutrient imbalance. Pages 17–32 *in* Proc. Tri-State Dairy Nutrition Conf.

Batajoo, K. K., and R. D. Shaver. 1998. In situ dry matter, crude protein, and starch degradabilities of selected grains and by-products. Anim. Feed Sci. Technol. 71:165–176.

Bauchart, D. 1993. Lipid absorption and transport in ruminants. J. Dairy Sci. 76:3864–3881.

Bauchart, D., D. Gruffat, and D. Durand. 1996. Lipid absorption and hepatic metabolism in ruminants. Proc. Nutr. Soc. 55:39–47.

Beam, S. W., and W. R. Butler. 1997. Energy balance and ovarian follicle development prior to the first ovulation postpartum in dairy cows receiving three levels of dietary fat. Biol. Repro. 56:133–142.

Beauchemin, K. A., W. Z. Yang, and L. M. Rode. 1999. Effects of grain source and enzyme additive on site and extent of nutrient digestion in dairy cows. J. Dairy Sci. 82:378–390.

Beauchemin, K. A., L. M. Rode, and M. V. Eliason. 1997. Chewing activities and milk production of dairy cows fed alfalfa as hay, silage, or dried cubes of hay or silage. J. Dairy Sci. 80:324–333.

Beckers, Y., A. Théwis, and B. Madoux. 1996. Intestinal digestibility of rumen undegraded N of concentrates measured by the mobile nylon bag technique. Anim. Feed Sci. Technol. 61:305–323.

Beckers, Y., A. Théwis, B. Madoux, and E. François. 1995 Studies on the in situ nitrogen degradability corrected for bacterial contamination of concentrate feeds in steers. J. Anim. Sci. 73:220–227.

Beever, D. E., H. R. Losada, D. L. Gale, M. C. Spooner, and M. S. Dhanoa. 1987. The use of monensin or formaldehyde to control the digestion of nitrogenous constituents of perennial ryegrass (*Lolium perenne* cv. Melle) and white clover (*Trifolium repens* cv. Blanca) in the rumen of cattle. Br. J. Nutr. 57:57–67.

Beever, D. E., M. S. Dhanoa, H. R. Losada, R. T. Evans, S. B. Cammell, and J. France. 1986. Br. J. Nutr. 56:439–454.

Beever, D. E., D. J. Thomson, and S. B. Cammell. 1976. The digestion of frozen and dried grass by sheep. J. Agric. Sci., Camb. 86:443–452.

Belasco, I. J. 1972. Stability of methionine hydroxy analog in rumen fluid and its conversion in vitro to methionine by calf liver and kidney. J. Dairy Sci. 55:353–357.

Belasco, I. J. 1980. Fate of carbon-14 labeled methionine hydroxy analog and methionine in the lactating dairy cow. J. Dairy Sci. 63:775–784.

Bell, A. W., R. Sleptis, and R. A. Ehrhardt. 1995. Growth and accretion of energy and protein in the gravid uterus during late pregnancy in Holstein cows. J. Dairy Sci. 78:1954–1961.

Benchaar, C., C. Bayourthe, R. Moncoulon, and M. Vernay. 1991. Ruminal digestion and intestinal absorption of lupine proteins extruded in the lactating cow. Reprod. Nutr. Dev. 316:655–665.

Benchaar, C., M. Vernay, C. Bayourthe, and R. Moncoulon. 1994a. Effects of extrusion of whole horse beans on protein digestion and amino acid absorption in dairy cows. J. Dairy Sci. 77:1360–1371.

Benchaar, C., R. Moncoulon, C. Bayourthe, and M. Vernay. 1994b. Effects of a supply of raw or extruded white lupin seeds on protein digestion and amino acid absorption in dairy cows. J. Anim. Sci. 72:492–501.

Bendall, J. R. 1964. Meat proteins. Page 225 in Symposium on Foods: Proteins and Their Reactions. H. W. Schultz (ed.). AVI Publication Co., Inc., Westport, CT.

Ben Salem, H., R. Krzeminski, A. Ferlay, and M. Doreau. 1993. Effect of lipid supply on in vivo digestion in cows: comparison of hay and corn silage diets. Can. J. Anim. Sci. 73:547–557.

Bernard, J. K., H. E. Amos, M. A. Froetschel, and J. J. Evans. 1988. Influence of supplemental energy and protein on protein synthesis and crude protein reaching the abomasum. J. Dairy Sci. 71:2658–2669.

Berthiaume, R., H. Lapierre, M. Stevenson, N. Cote, and B. W. McBride. 2000. Comparison of the in situ and in vivo intestinal disappearance of ruminally protected methionine. J. Dairy Sci. 83:(In press).

Bertrand, J. A., F. E. Pardue, and T. C. Jenkins. 1998. Effect of ruminally protected amino acids on milk yield and composition of Jersey cows fed whole cottonseed. J. Dairy Sci. 81:2215–2220.

Berzaghi, P., G. Cozzi, and I. Andrighetto. 1997. The use of near infrared analysis for in situ studies. J. Dairy Sci. 80:3263–3270.

Black, A. L., M. Kleiber, A. H. Smith, and D. N. Stewart. 1957. Acetate as a precursor of amino acids of casein in the intact dairy cow. Biochem. Biophys. Acta. 23:54.

Blauwiekel, R., and R. L. Kincaid. 1986. Effect of crude protein and solubility on performance and blood constituents of dairy cows. J. Dairy Sci. 69:2091–2098.

Blauwiekel, R., S. Xu, J. H. Harrison, K. A. Loney, R. E. Riley, and M. C. Calhoun. 1997. Effect of whole cottonseed, gossypol, and ruminally protected lysine supplementation on milk yield and composition. J. Dairy Sci. 80:1358–1365.

Blauwiekel, R., W. H. Hoover, S. D. Slider, and T. K. Miller. 1990. Effects of fish meal protein supplementation on milk yield and composition and blood constituents of dairy cows. J. Dairy Sci. 73:3217–3221.

Blethen, D. B., J. E. Wohlt, D. K. Jasaitis, and J. L. Evans. 1990. Feed protein fractions: relationship to nitrogen solubility and degradability. J. Dairy Sci. 73:1544–1551.

Blum, J. W., R. M. Bruckmaier, and F. Jans. 1999. Rumen-protected methionine fed to dairy cows: bioavailability and effects on plasma amino acid pattern and plasma metabolite and insulin concentrations. J. Dairy Sci. 82:1991–1998.

Boehme, W. R. 1982. Protein products of the rendering industry. Page 173 *in* CRC Handbook of Processing and Utilization in Agriculture. Vol 1. Animal Products. I. A. Wolff (ed.). CRC Press, Inc., Boca Raton, FL.

Boekholt, H. A. 1976. Nitrogen metabolism of the lactating cow and the role of gluconeogenesis from amino acids. Meded. Landbouwhogesch. Wageningen 76:10.

Bohnert, D. W., B. T. Larson, M. L. Bauer, A. F. Branco, K. R. McLeod, D. L. Harmon, and G. E. Mitchell, Jr. 1999. Nutritional evaluation of poultry by-product meal as a protein source for ruminants: Small intestinal amino acid flow and disappearance in steers. J. Anim. Sci. 77:1000–1007.

Bohnert, D. W., B. T. Larson, M. L. Bauer, A. F. Branco, K. R. McLeod, D. L. Harmon, and G. E. Mitchell, Jr. 1998. Nutritional evaluation of poultry by-product meal as a protein source fro ruminants: effects on performance and nutrient flow and disappearance in steers. J. Anim. Sci. 76:2474–2484.

Boila, R.J., and J. R. Ingalls. 1995. Prediction of rumen undegradable amino acids that are digested post-ruminally. Can. J. Anim. Sci. 75: 583–592.

Boila, R. J., and J. R. Ingalls. 1994. The post-ruminal digestion of dry matter, nitrogen and amino acids in wheat-based distillers dried grains and canola meal. Anim. Feed. Sci. Technol. 49:173–188.

Boila, R. J., and J. R. Ingalls. 1992. In situ rumen digestion and escape of dry matter, nitrogen and amino acids in canola meal. Can. J. Anim. Sci. 72:891–901.

Bowerman, B. L., and R. T. O'Connell. 1990. Linear statistical models: An applied approach. 2nd ed. PWS-Kent Publishing Co., Boston, MA.

Bowman, J. M., D. G. Grieve, J. G. Buchanan-Smith, and G. K. Macleod. 1988. Response of dairy cows in early lactation to sodium hydroxide-treated soybean meal. J. Dairy Sci. 71:982–989.

Brandt, M., K. Rohr, and P. Lezien. 1980. Bestimmung des endogenen Protein-N im Duodenalchymus von Milchkhen mit Hilfe von $^{15}$N. J. Anim. Physiol. Anim. Nutr. 44:26.

Bremmer, D. R., T. R. Overton, and J. H Clark. 1997. Production and composition of milk from Jersey cows administered bovine somatotropin and fed ruminally protected amino acids. J. Dairy Sci. 80:1374–1380.

Broderick, G. A. 1992. Relative value of fish meal versus solvent soybean meal for lactating dairy cows fed alfalfa silage as sole forage. J. Dairy Sci. 75:174–183.

Broderick, G. A. 1998. Can cell-free enzymes replace rumen microorganisms to model energy and protein supply? Pages 99-114 in In vitro Techniques for Measuring Nutrient Supply to Ruminants. E. R. Deaville, E. Owens, A. T. Adesogan, C. Rymer, J. A. Huntington, and T. L. J. Lawrence (eds.) Occasional Publication No. 22, British Society of Animal Sciences, Edinburgh.

Broderick, G. A., R. J. Wallace, and E. R. Ørskov. 1991. Control of rate and extent of protein degradation. Pages 541–592 in Physiological Aspects of Digestion and Metabolism in Ruminants. T. Tsuda, Y. Sasaki, and R. Kawashima (eds.) Academic Press, Orlando, FL.

Broderick, G. A., and R. J. Wallace. 1988. Effects of dietary nitrogen source on concentrations of ammonia, free amino acids and fluorescamine-reactive peptides in the sheep rumen. J. Anim. Sci., 66: 2233–2238.

Broderick, G. A., D. B. Ricker, and L. S. Driver. 1990. Expeller soybean meal and corn by-products versus solvent soybean meal for lactating dairy cows fed alfalfa silage as sole forage. J. Dairy Sci. 73:453–462.

Brown, W. F., and F. M. Pate. 1997. Cottonseed meal or feather meal supplementation of ammoniated tropical grass hay for yearling cattle. J. Anim. Sci. 75:1666–1673.

Bruckental, I., D. Dori, M. Kaim, H. Lehrer, and Y. Folman. 1989. Effects of source and level of protein on milk yield and reproductive performance of high-producing primiparous and multiparous dairy cows. Anim. Prod. 48:319–329.

Bruckental, I., I. Ascarelli, B. Yosif, and E. Alumot. 1991. Effect of duodenal proline infusion on milk production and composition in dairy cows. Anim. Prod. 53:299–303.

Brunschwig, P., and P. Augeard. 1994. Acide aminé protégé: effet sur la production et la composition du lait des vaches sur régime ensilage de maïs. Journées de Recherches sur l'alimentation et la nutrition des Herbivores 16-17 INRA Theix.

Brunschwig, P., P. Augeard, B. K. Sloan, and K. Tanan. 1995. Feeding of protected methionine from 10d pre-calving and at the beginning of lactation to dairy cows fed a maize silage based ration. Recontres Recherches Ruminants 2:249.

Burris, W. R., J. A. Boling, N. W. Bradley, and A. W. Young. 1976. Abomasal lysine infusion in steers fed a urea supplemented diet. J. Anim. Sci. 42:699–705.

Burroughs, W.A., A.H. Trenkle, and R.L. Vetter. 1974. A system of protein evaluation for cattle and sheep involving metabolizable protein (amino acids) and urea fermentation potential of feedstuffs. Vet Med. Small Anim. Clin. 69:713–722.

Butler, W. R. 1998. Review: Effect of protein nutrition on ovarian and uterine physiology in dairy cattle. J. Dairy Sci. 81:2533–2539.

Butler, W. R., J. J. Calaman, and S. W. Beam. 1995. Plasma and milk urea nitrogen in relation to pregnancy rate in lactating dairy cattle. J. Anim. Sci. 74:858–865.

Calsamiglia, S., and M. D. Stern. 1995. A three-step in vitro procedure for estimating intestinal digestion of protein in ruminants. J. Anim. Sci. 73:1459–1465.

Calsamiglia, S., G. Caja, M. D. Stern, and B. A. Crooker. 1995a. Effects of ruminal versus duodenal dosing of fish meal on ruminal fermentation and milk composition. J. Dairy Sci. 78:1999–2007.

Calsamiglia, S., M. D. Stern, and J. L. Firkins. 1995b. Effects of protein source on nitrogen metabolism in continuous culture and intestinal digestion in vitro. J. Anim. Sci. 73:1819–1827.

Cameron, M. R., T. H. Klusmeyer, G. L. Lynch, J. H. Clark, and D. R, Nelson. 1991. Effects of urea and starch on rumen fermentation, nutrient passage to the duodenum, and performance of cows. J. Dairy Sci. 74:1321–1336.

Campbell, C. G., E. C. Titgemeyer, and G. St-Jean. 1997. Sulfur amino acid utilization by growing steers. J. Anim. Sci. 75:230–238.

Campbell, C. G., E. C. Titgemeyer, and G. St-Jean. 1996. Efficiency of D- vs L-methionine utilization by growing steers. J. Anim. Sci. 74:2482–2487.

Canale, C. J., L. D. Muller, H. A. McCahon, T. J. Whitsel, G. A. Varga, and M. J. Lormore. 1990. Dietary fat and ruminally protected amino acids for high producing dairy cows. J. Dairy Sci. 73:135–141.

Canfield, R. W., C. J. Sniffen, and W. R. Butler. 1990. Effects of excess degradable protein on postpartum reproduction and energy balance in dairy cattle. J. Dairy Sci. 73:2342–2349.

Carey, D. A., J. S. Caton, and M. Biondini. 1993. Influence of energy source on forage intake, digestibility, in situ forage degradation, and ruminal fermentation in beef steers fed medium-quality brome hay. J. Anim. Sci. 71:2260–2269.

Carroll, D. J., B. A. Barton, G. W. Anderson, and R. D. Smith. 1988. Influence of protein intake and feeding strategy on reproductive performance of dairy cows. J. Dairy Sci. 71:3470–3481.

Carroll, D. J., G. W. Anderson, and B. A. Barton. 1987. The influence of level of crude protein on the reproductive performance of the early lactation cow. J. Dairy Sci. 70 (Suppl. 1):207. (Abstr.)

Casper, D. P., and D. J. Schingoethe. 1988. Protected methionine supplementation to a barley-based diet for cows during early lactation. J. Dairy Sci. 71:164–172.

Casper, D. P., D. J. Schingoethe, and W. A. Eisenbeisz. 1990. Response of early lactation dairy cows fed diets varying in source of nonstructural carbohydrate and crude protein. J. Dairy Sci. 73:1039–1050.

Casper, D.P., H. A. Maiga, M. J. Brouk, and D. J. Schingoethe. 1999. Synchronization of carbohydrate and protein sources on fermentation and passage rates in dairy cows. J. Dairy Sci. 82:1779–1790.

Casper, D. P., D. J. Schingoethe, C.-M. J. Yang, and C. R. Mueller. 1987. Protected methionine supplementation with extruded blend of soybeans and soybean meal for dairy cows. J. Dairy Sci. 70:321–330.

Caton, J. S., V. I. Burke, V. L. Anderson, L. A. Burgwald, P. L. Norton, and K. C. Olson. 1994. Influence of crambe meal as a protein source on intake, site of digestion, ruminal fermentation, and microbial efficiency in beef steers fed grass hay. J. Anim. Sci. 72:3238–3245.

Cecava, M. J. Personal communication.

Cecava, M. J., and J. E. Parker. 1993. Intestinal supply of amino acids in steers fed ruminally degradable and undegradable crude protein sources alone and in combination. J. Anim. Sci. 71:1596–1605.

Cecava, M. J., D. L. Hancock, and J. E. Parker. 1993. Effects of zinc-treated soybean meal on ruminal fermentation and intestinal amino acid flows in steers fed corn silage-based diets. J. Anim. Sci. 71:3423–3431.

Cecava, M. J., N. R. Merchen, L. L. Berger, R. I. Mackie, and G. C. Fahey, Jr. 1991. Effects of dietary energy level and protein source on nutrient digestion and ruminal nitrogen metabolism in sheep. J. Anim. Sci. 69:2230–2243.

Chalupa, W. 1976. Degradation of amino acids by mixed rumen microbial population. J. Anim. Sci. 43:829–834.

Chalupa, W., and J. E. Chandler. 1975. Methionine and lysine nutrition of growing cattle. J. Anim. Sci. 394. (Abstr.)

Chalupa, W., C. J. Sniffen, D. G. Fox and P. J. Van Soest. 1991. Model generated protein degradation nutritional information. Proc. Cornell Nutr. Conf., p. 44, Ithaca, NY.

Chan, S. C., J. T. Huber, C. B. Theurer, Z. Wu, K. H. Chen, and J. M. Simas. 1997. Effects of supplemental fat and protein source on ruminal fermentation and nutrient flow to the duodenum in dairy cows. J. Dairy Sci. 80:152–159.

Chapoutot, P., P. Schmidely, D. Sauvant, J. C. Robert, and B. Sloan. 1992. Influence of a ruminally protected blend of methionine and lysine (ML) on the dairy cow nutrition and production. J. Dairy Sci. 75(Suppl. 1):199. (Abstr.)

Chen, G., and J. B. Russell. 1988. Fermentation of peptides and amino acids by a monensin-sensitive ruminal peptostreptococcus. Appl. Environ. Microbiol. 54:2742–2749.

Chen, G., and J. B. Russell. 1989. More monensin-sensitive, ammonia-producing bacteria from the rumen. Appl. Environ. Microbiol. 55:1052–1057.

Chen, G., C. J. Sniffen, and J. B. Russell. 1987. Concentration and estimated flow of peptides from the rumen of dairy cattle: Effects of protein solubility and feeding frequency. J. Dairy Sci. 70:983–992.

Chen, K. H., J. T. Huber, C. B. Theurer, D. V. Armstrong, R. C. Wanderley, J. M. Simas, S. C. Chan, and J. L. Sullivan. 1993. Effect of protein quality and evaporative cooling on lactational performance of Holstein cows in hot weather. J. Dairy Sci. 76:819–825.

Cherney, D. J. R., J. J. Volenec, and J. H. Cherney. 1992. Protein solubility and degradation in vitro as influenced by buffer and maturity of alfalfa. Anim. Feed Sci. Technol. 37:9–20.

Chikunya, S., C. J. Newbold, L. Rode, X. B. Chen, and R. J. Wallace. 1996. The influence of non protein nitrogen, preformed amino acids and protein on microbial activity in the rumen of sheep receiving diets containing rapidly and slowly degraded fiber sources. Anim. Feed Sci. Technol. 63:333–340.

Chilliard, Y., C. Audigier, D. Durand, S. Auboiron, and D. Bauchart. 1994. Effects of portal infusions of methionine on plasma concentrations and estimated hepatic balances in underfed preruminant calves. Ann. Zootech. 43:299.

Chow, J. M., E. J. DePeters, and R. L. Baldwin. 1990. Effect of rumen-protected methionine and lysine on casein in milk when diets high in fat or concentrate are fed. J. Dairy Sci. 73:1051–1061.

Christensen, R. A., T. R. Overton, J. H. Clark, J. K. Drackley, D. R. Nelson, and S. A. Blum. 1996. Effects of dietary fat with or without nicotinic acid on nutrient flow to the duodenum of dairy cows. J. Dairy Sci. 79:1410–1424.

Christensen, R. A., M. R. Cameron, J. H. Clark, J. K. Drackley, J. M. Lynch, and D. M. Barbano. 1994. Effects of amount of protein and ruminally protected amino acids in the diet of dairy cows fed supplemental fat. J. Dairy Sci. 77:1618–1629.

Christensen, R. A., G. L. Lynch, J. H. Clark, and Y. Yu. 1993a. Influence of amount and degradability of protein on production of milk and milk components by lactating Holstein cows. J. Dairy Sci. 76:3490–3496.

Christensen, R. A., M. R. Cameron, T. H. Klusmeyer, J. P. Elliott, J. H. Clark D. R. Nelson, and Y. Yu. 1993b. Influence of amount and degradability of dietary protein on nitrogen utilization by dairy cows. J. Dairy Sci. 76:3497–3513.

Clark, J. H. 1975. Lactational responses to postruminal administration of protein and amino acids. J. Dairy Sci. 58:1178–1197.

Clark, J. H., H. R. Spires, and C. L Davis. 1978. Uptake and metabolism of nitrogenous components by the lactating mammary gland. Fed. Proc. 37:1233–1238.

Clark, J. H., R. G. Derrig, C. L. Davis, and H. R. Spires. 1975. Metabolism of arginine and ornithine in the cow and rabbit mammary tissue. J. Dairy Sci. 58:1808–1813.

Clark, J. H., T. H. Klusmeyer, and M. R. Cameron. 1992. Microbial protein synthesis and flows of nitrogen fractions to the duodenum of dairy cows. J. Dairy Sci. 75:2304–2323.

Cleale, R. M., IV, T. J. Klopfenstein, R. A. Britton, L. D. Satterlee, and S. R. Lowry. 1987. Induced non-enzymatic browning of soybean meal. III. Digestibility and efficiency of protein utilization by ruminants of soybean meal treated with xylose or glucose. J. Anim. Sci. 65:1327–1335.

Coblentz, W. K., I.E.O. Abdelgadir, R. C. Cochran, J. O. Fritz, W. H. Fick, K. C. Olson, and J. E. Turner. 1999. Degradability of forage proteins by in situ and in vitro enzymatic methods. J. Dairy Sci. 82:343–354.

Coblentz, W. K., J. O. Fritz, W. H. Fick, R. C. Cochran, and J. E. Shirley. 1998. In situ dry matter, nitrogen, and fiber degradation of alfalfa, red clover, and Eastern gamagrass at four maturities. J. Dairy Sci. 81:150–161.

Coblentz, W. K., J. O. Fritz, R. C. Cochran, W. L. Rooney, and K. K. Bolsen. 1997. Protein degradation in response to spontaneous heating in alfalfa hay by in situ and ficin methods. J. Dairy Sci. 80:700–713.

Cody, R. F., J. J. Murphy, and D. J. Morgan. 1990. Effect of supplementary crude protein level and degradability in grass silage-based diets on performance of dairy cows, and digestibility and abomasal nitrogen flow in sheep. Anim. Prod. 51:235–244.

Coleman, G. S. 1985. Possible causes of the high death rate of ciliate protozoa in the rumen. J. Agric. Sci., Camb. 105:39–43.

Conrad, H. R., J. W. Hibbs, and A. D. Pratt. 1960. Nitrogen metabolism in dairy cattle. I. Efficiency of nitrogen utilization by lactating cows fed various forges. Ohio Agric. Exp. Stn. Res. Bull. No. 861. Wooster, Ohio State University.

Cooper, P. B., and J. R. Ling. 1985. The uptake of peptides and amino acids by rumen bacteria. Proc. Nutr. Soc. 44:144A.

Cotta, M. A., and R. B. Hespell. 1984. Protein and amino acid metabolism of rumen bacteria. Pages 122–136 *in* Control of Digestion and Metabolism in Ruminants. L. P. Milligan, W. L. Grovum, and A. Dobson (ed.). Prentice-Hall Englewood Cliffs, NJ.

Cotta, M. A., and J. B. Russell. 1982. Effect of peptides and amino acids on efficiency of rumen bacterial protein synthesis in continuous culture. J. Dairy Sci. 65:226–234.

Cozzi, G., and C. E. Polan. 1994. Corn gluten meal or dried brewers grains as partial replacement for soybean meal in the diet of Holstein cows. J. Dairy Sci. 77:825–834.

Cozzi, G., I. Andrighetto, P. Berzaghi, and C. E. Polan. 1995. In situ ruminal disappearance of essential amino acids in protein feedstuffs. J. Dairy Sci. 78:161–171.

Cozzi, G., G. Bittante, and C. E. Polan. 1993. Comparison of fibrous materials as modifiers of in situ ruminal degradation of corn gluten meal. J. Dairy Sci. 76:1106–1113.

Crawford, R. J., W. H. Hoover, C. J. Sniffen, and B. A. Crooker. 1978. Degradation of feedstuff nitrogen in the rumen *vs* nitrogen solubility in three solvents. J. Anim. Sci. 46:1768–1775.

Crawley, D. D., and L. H. Kilmer. 1995. Effects of level and source of rumen degradable protein fed prepartum on postpartum performance of dairy cows. J. Dairy Sci. 78 (Suppl. 1):266. (Abstr.)

Crish, E. M., J. E. Wohlt, and J. L. Evans. 1986. Insoluble nitrogen for milk production in Holstein cows via increases in voluntary intake and nitrogen utilization. J. Dairy Sci. 69:1576–1586.

Crocker, L. M., E. J. DePeters, J. G. Fadel, H. Perez-Monti, S. J. Taylor, J. A. Wyckoff, and R. A. Zinn. 1998. Influence of processed corn grain in diets of dairy cows on digestion of nutrients and milk composition. J. Dairy Sci. 81:2394–2407.

Crooker, B. A., C. J. Sniffen, W. H. Hoover, and L. L. Johnson. 1978. Solvents for soluble nitrogen measurements in feedstuffs. J. Dairy Sci. 61:437–447.

Cros, P., M. Vernay, C. Bayourthe, and R. Moncoulon. 1992a. Influence of extrusion on ruminal and intestinal disappearance of amino acids in whole horsebean. Can. J. Anim. Sci. 72: 359–366.

Cros, P., R. Moncoulon, C. Bayourthe, and M. Vernay. 1992b. Effect of extrusion on ruminal and intestinal disappearance of amino acids in white lupin seed. Can. J. Anim. Sci. 72: 89–96.

Cruz Soto, R., S. A. Muhammad, C. J. Newbold., C. S. Stewart, and R. J. Wallace. 1994. Influence of peptides, amino acids and urea on microbial activity in the rumen of sheep receiving grass hay and on the growth of rumen bacteria in vitro. Anim. Feed. Sci. Technol. 49:151–161.

Cunningham, K. D., M. J. Cecava, and T. R. Johnson. 1993. Nutrient digestion, nitrogen, and amino acid flows in lactating cows fed soybean hulls in place of forage or concentrate. J. Dairy Sci. 76:3523–3535.

Cunningham, K. D., M. J. Cecava, and T. R. Johnson. 1994. Flows of nitrogen and amino acids in dairy cows fed diets containing supplemental feather meal and blood meal. J. Dairy Sci. 77:3666–3675.

Cunningham, K. D., M. J. Cecava, T. R. Johnson, and P. A. Ludden. 1996. Influence of source and amount of dietary protein on milk yield by cows in early lactation. J. Dairy Sci. 79:620–630.

Cushnahan, A., C. S. Mayne, and E. F. Unsworth. 1995. Effects of ensilage of grass on performance and nutrient utilization by dairy cattle 2. Nutrient metabolism and rumen fermentation. Anim. Feed Sci. Technol. 60:347–359.

Dakowski, P., M. R. Weisbjerg, and T. Hvelplund. 1996. The effect of temperature during processing of rape seed meal on amino acid degradation in the rumen and digestion in the intestine. Anim. Feed. Sci. Technol. 58: 213–226.

Dale, N. 1996. Variation in feed ingredient quality: oilseed meals. Anim. Feed Sci. Technol. 59:129–135.

Dawson, L.E.R., and C. S. Mayne. 1998. The effect of silage fermentation characteristics on dry matter intake of steers. Anim. Sci. 66:105–113.

Dawson, L.E.R., and C. S. Mayne. 1997. The effect of infusion of putrescine and gamma amino butyric acid on the intake of steers offered grass silage containing three levels of lactic acid. Anim. Feed Sci. Technol. 66:15–29.

de Boer, G., J. J. Murphy, and J. J. Kennelly. 1987. Mobile nylon bag for estimating intestinal availability of rumen undegradable protein. J. Dairy Sci. 70:977–982.

De Gracia, M., F. G. Owen, and S. R. Lowry. 1989. Corn gluten meal and blood meal mixture for dairy cows in midlactation. J. Dairy Sci. 72:3064–3069.

Deacon, M. A., G. deBoer, and J. J. Kennelly. 1988. Influence of Jet-Sploding and extrusion on ruminal and intestinal disappearance of canola soybeans. J. Dairy Sci. 71:745–753.

Denham, S. C., G. A. Morantes, D. B. Bates, and J. E. Moore. 1989. Comparison of two models used to estimate in situ nitrogen disappearance. J. Dairy Sci. 72:708–714.

DePeters, E. J., and D. L. Bath. 1986. Canola meal versus cottonseed meal as the protein supplement in dairy diets. J. Dairy Sci. 69:148–154.

DeVisser, H., A. Klop, C. J. van der Koelen, and A. M. van Vuuren. 1998. Starch supplementation of grass harvested at two stages of maturity prior to ensiling: intake, digestion, and degradability by dairy cows. J. Dairy Sci. 81:2221–2227.

Dewhurst, R. J., D. R. Davies, and R. J. Merry. 2000. Microbial protein supply from the rumen. Anim. Feed Sci. Technol. 85:1–21.

Dhiman, T. R., and L. D. Satter. 1993. Protein as the first-limiting nutrient for lactating dairy cows fed high proportions of good quality alfalfa silage. J. Dairy Sci. 76:1960–1971.

Dijkstra, J. 1994. Simulation of the dynamics of protozoa in the rumen. Br. J. Nutr. 72:679–699.

Donahue, P. B., C. G., J. D. Quigley, III, and W. E. Hylton. 1985. Methionine deficiency in early weaned dairy calves fed pelleted rations based on corn and alfalfa or corn and soybean proteins. J. Dairy Sci. 68:681–693.

Doreau, M., F. Legay, and D. Bauchart. 1991. Effect of source and level of supplemental fat on total and ruminal organic matter and nitrogen digestion in dairy cows. J. Dairy Sci. 74:2233–2242.

Downes, A. M. 1961. On the amino acids essential for the tissues of the sheep. Aust. J. Biol. Sci. 14:254.

Doyle, P. T. 1981. Sulfur and methionine metabolism in sheep. V. Utilization of methionine isomers. Aust. J. Biol. Sci. 34:47–59.

Durrand, D., Y. Chilliard, and D. Bauchart. 1992. Effects of lysine and methionine on in vivo hepatic secretion of VLDL in the high yielding dairy cow. J. Dairy Sci. 75 (Suppl. 1):279 (Abstr.).

Elizalde, J. C., N. R. Merchen, and D. B. Faulkner. 1999. Supplemental cracked corn for steers fed fresh alfalfa: II. Protein and amino acid digestion. J. Anim. Sci. 77:467–475.

Elrod, C. C., and W. R. Butler. 1993. Reduction of fertility and alteration of uterine pH in heifers fed excess ruminally degradable protein. J. Anim. Sci. 71:694–701.

England, M. L., G. A. Broderick, R. D. Shaver, and D. K. Combs. 1997. Comparison of in situ and in vitro techniques for measuring ruminal degradation of animal by-product proteins. J. Dairy Sci. 80:2925–2931.

Erasmus, L. J. 1993. Ruminal degradation of protein of various feedstuffs and its affect on post ruminal amino acid flow in high producing dairy cows. Ph. D. Diss. Univ. Pretoria, South Africa.

Erasmus, L. J., P. M. Botha, and H. H. Meissner. 1994a. Effect of protein source on ruminal fermentation and passage of amino acids to the small intestine of lactating cows. J. Dairy Sci. 77:3655–3665.

Erasmus, L. J., P. M. Botha, C. W. Cruywagen, and H. H. Meissner. 1994b. Amino acid profile and intestinal digestibility in dairy cows of rumen-undegradable protein from various feed stuffs. J. Dairy Sci. 77:541–551.

Erasmus, L. J., P. M. Botha, and A. Kistner. 1992. Effect of yeast culture supplement on production, rumen fermentation, and duodenal nitrogen flow in dairy cows. J. Dairy Sci. 75:3056–3065.

Erdman, R. A. 1994. Production responses in field study herds fed rumen protected choline. J. Dairy Sci. 77(Suppl. 1):186. (Abstr.)

Erdman, R. A. 1995. Factors affecting microbial protein flow in dairy cows. Four-State Dairy Nutrition and Management Conference. LaCrosse, Wisconsin.

Erdman, R. A., and B. K. Sharma. 1991. Effect of dietary rumen-protected choline in lactating dairy cows. J. Dairy Sci. 74:1641–1647.

Erdman, R. A., and J. H. Vandersall. 1983. Effect of rumen protein degradability on milk yield of dairy cows in early lactation. J. Dairy Sci. 66:1873–1880.

Erdman, R. A., J. H. Vandersall, E. Russek-Cohen, and G. Switalski. 1987. Simultaneous measures of rates of ruminal digestion and passage of feeds for prediction of ruminal nitrogen and dry matter digestion in lactating dairy cows. J. Anim. Sci. 64:565–577.

Erdman, R. A., G. H. Proctor, and J. H. Vandersall. 1986. Effect of rumen ammonia concentration on in situ rate and extent of digestion of feedstuffs. J. Dairy Sci. 69:2312–2320.

Erickson, P. S., M. R. Murphy, and C. L. Davis. 1986. Malt sprouts as a source of supplemental protein for ruminants. J. Dairy Sci. 69:2959–2962.

Espindola, M. S., E. J. DePeters, J. G. Fadel, R. A. Zinn, and H. Perez-Monti. 1997. Effects on nutrient digestion of wheat processing and method of tallow addition to the diets of lactating dairy cows. J. Dairy Sci. 80:1160–1171.

Fairbairn, R., I. Alli, and B. E. Baker. 1988. Proteolysis associated with the ensiling of chopped alfalfa. J. Dairy Sci. 71:152–158.

Faldet, M. A., V. L. Voss, G. A. Broderick, and L. D. Satter. 1991. Chemical, in vitro, and in situ evaluation of heat treated soybean proteins. J. Dairy Sci. 74:2548–2554.

Fenderson, C. L., and W. G. Bergen. 1975. An assessment of essential amino acid requirements of growing steers. J. Anim. Sci. 41:1759–1766.

Feng, P., W. H. Hoover, T. K. Miller, and R. Blauwiekel. 1993. Interactions of fiber and nonstructural carbohydrates on lactation and ruminal function. J. Dairy Sci. 76:1324–1333.

Ferguson, J. D., and W. Chalupa. 1989. Impact of protein nutrition on reproduction in dairy cows. J. Dairy Sci. 72:746–766.

Ferguson, J. D., T. Blanchard, D. T. Galligan, D. C. Hoshall, and W. Chalupa. 1988. Infertility in dairy cattle fed a high percentage of protein degradable in the rumen. J. Am. Vet. Assoc. 192:659–662.

Ferguson, K. A. 1975. The protection of dietary proteins and amino acids against microbial fermentation in the rumen. Pages 448–464 *in* Digestion and Metabolism in the Ruminant. I. W. McDonald and A. C. I. Warner (eds.). University of New England Publishing Unit, Armidale, NSW, Australia.

Ffoulkes, D., and R. A. Leng. 1988. Dynamics of protozoa in the rumen of cattle. Br. J. Nutr. 59:429–436.

Fickler, J., J. Fontaine, and W. Heimbeck. 1996. The Amino Acid Composition of Feedstuffs, Degussa Corporation, Ridgefield Park, NJ.

Firkins, J. L., M. S. Allen, B. S. Oldick, and N. R. St-Pierre. 1998. Modeling ruminal digestibility of carbohydrates and microbial protein flow to the duodenum. J. Dairy Sci. 81:3350–3369.

Fox, D. G., C. J. Sniffen, J. D. O'Conner, J. B. Russell, and P. J. Van Soest. 1990. The search: agriculture. Cornell Univ. Agric. Exp. Sta. No. 34., Ithaca.

Fraser, D. L., E. R. Ørskov, F. G. Whitelaw, and M. F. Franklin. 1991. Limiting amino acids in dairy cows given casein as the sole source of protein. Livestock Prod. Sci., 28:235–252.

Freeden, A. H., W. Chalupa, W. E. Julien, C. J. Sniffen, H. Sato, T. Fujieda, T. Ueda, and H. Suzuki, 1999. Effects of rumen-protected LYS and MET to periparturient cows on their productivity during 24 weeks post-partum. J. Dairy Sci. 82(Suppl. 1):121. (Abstr.)

Frydrych, Z. 1992. Intestinal digestibility of rumen undegraded protein of various feeds as estimated by the mobile bag technique. Anim. Feed Sci. Technol. 37:161–172.
Fuller, M. F., and P. Garthwaite. 1993. The form of response of body protein accretion to dietary amino acid supply. J. Nutr. 123:957–963.
Ganesh, D., and D. G. Grieve. 1990. Effect of roasting raw soybeans at three temperatures on in situ dry matter and nitrogen disappearance in dairy cows. J. Dairy Sci. 73:3222–3230.
Garcia, A. D., W. G. Olson, D. E. Otterby, J. G. Linn, and W. P. Hansen. 1989. Effects of temperature, moisture, and aeration on fermentation of alfalfa silage. J. Dairy Sci. 72:93–103.
Garcia-Bojalil, C. M., C. R. Staples, C. A. Risco, J. D. Savio, and W. W. Thatcher. 1998b. Protein degradability and calcium salts of long-chain fatty acids in the diets of lactating dairy cows: reproductive responses. J. Dairy Sci. 81:1385–1395.
Garcia-Bojalil, C. M., C. R. Staples, C. A. Risco, J. D. Savio, and W. W. Thatcher. 1998a. Protein degradability and calcium salts of long-chain fatty acids in the diets of lactating dairy cows: productive responses. J. Dairy Sci. 81:1374–1384.
Garthwaite, B. D., C. G. Schwab, and B. K. Sloan. 1998. Amino acid nutrition of the transition and early lactation cow. Proc. Cornell Nutr. Conf. pp. 38–50, Ithaca, NY.
Givens, D. I., E. R. Deaville, and A. R. Moss. 1997. The effect of fertilizer nitrogen on the solubility and rumen degradability of dry matter and nitrogen in wheat grain. Anim. Feed Sci. Technol. 66:247–256.
Glenn, B. P., G. A. Varga, G. B. Huntington, and D. R. Waldo. 1989. Duodenal nutrient flow and digestibility in Holstein steers fed formaldehyde- and formic acid-treated alfalfa or orchardgrass silage at two intakes. J. Anim. Sci. 67:513–528.
Goelema, J. O., A. Smits, L. M. Vaessen, and A. Wemmers. 1999. Effects of pressure toasting, expander treatment and pelleting on in vitro and in situ parameters of protein and starch in a mixture of broken peas, lupins and faba beans. Anim. Feed Sci. Technol. 78:109–126.
Goelema, J. O., M. A. M. Spreeuwenberg, G. Hof, A. F. B. van der Poel, and S. Tamminga. 1998. Effect of pressure toasting on the rumen degradability and intestinal digestibility of whole and broken peas, lupins and faba beans and a mixture of these feedstuffs. Anim. Feed Sci. Technol. 76:35–50.
Goering, H. K., and P. J. Van Soest. 1970. Forage fiber analysis. (Apparatus, reagents, procedures and some applications). Agric. Handbook No. 379.
Goering, H. K., C. H. Gordon, R. W. Hemken, D. R. Waldo, P. J. van Soest, and L. W. Smith. 1972. Analytical estimates of nitrogen digestibility in heat damaged forages. J. Dairy Sci. 55:1275–1280.
Goetsch, A. L., F. N. Owens, M. A. Funk, and B. E. Doran. 1987. Effects of whole or ground corn with different forms of hay in 85 percent concentrate diets on digestion and passage rate in beef heifers. Anim. Feed Sci. Technol. 18:151–164.
Gordon, F. J., and A. C. Peoples. 1986. The utilization of wilted and unwilted silages by lactating cows and the influence of changes in the protein and energy concentration of the supplement offered. Anim. Prod. 43:355–366.
Grant, R. J., and S. G. Haddad. 1998. Effect of a mixture of feather and blood meals on lactational performance of dairy cows. J. Dairy Sci. 81:1358–1363
Grings, E. E., R. E. Roffler, and D. P. Deitelhoff. 1992a. Evaluation of corn and barley as energy sources for cows in early lactation fed alfalfa-based diets. J. Dairy Sci. 75:193–200.
Grings, E. E., R. E. Roffler, and D. P. Deitelhoff. 1992b. Responses of dairy cows to additions of distillers dried grains with solubles in alfalfa-based diets. J. Dairy Sci. 75:1946–1953.
Grings, E. E., R. E. Roffler, and D. P. Deitelhoff. 1991. Response of dairy cows in early lactation to additions of cottonseed meal in alfalfa-based diets. J. Dairy Sci. 74:2580–2587.
Griswold, K. E., W. H. Hoover, T. K. Miller, and W. V. Thayne. 1996. Effect of form of nitrogen on growth of ruminal microbes in continuous culture. J. Anim. Sci. 74:483–491.
Grum, D. E., W. L. Shockey, and W. P. Weiss. 1991. Electrophoretic examination of alfalfa silage proteins. J. Dairy Sci. 74:146–154.
Grummer, R. C. 1991. Effect of feed on the composition of milk fat. J. Dairy Sci. 74:3244–3257.
Grummer, R. R., K. Slark, S. J. Bertics, M. L. Luck, and J. A. Barmore. 1996. Soybeans versus animal sources of rumen-undegradable protein and fat for early lactation dairy cows. J. Dairy Sci. 79:1809–1816.
Grummer, R. R., L. E. Armentano, and M. S. Marcus. 1987. Lactation response to short-term abomasal infusion of choline, inositol, and soy lecithin. J. Dairy Sci. 70:2518–2524.
Guilloteau, P. 1986. Digestion des proteines chez le jeune ruminant. These de doctorates-sciences, specialite sciences naturelles. Universite de Paris VI. 246 p.
Guinard, J., and H. Rulquin. 1994. Effects of graded amounts of duodenal infusions of lysine on the mammary uptake of major milk precursors in dairy cows. J. Dairy Sci. 77:3565–3576.
Ha, J. K., and J. J. Kennelly. 1984. Effect of protein on nutrient digestion and milk production by Holstein cows. J. Dairy Sci. 67:2302–2307.
Hadwell, D. L., and J. L. Sommerfeldt. 1988. Chickpeas as a protein and energy supplement for high producing dairy cows. J. Dairy Sci. 71:762–772.
Hannah, S. M., R. C. Cochran, E. S. Vanzant, and D. L. Harmon. 1991. Influence of protein supplementation on site and extent of digestion, forage intake, and nutrient flow characteristics in steers consuming dormant bluestem-range forage. J. Anim. Sci. 69:2624–2633.
Harris, B. Jr., D. E. Dorminey, W. A. Smith, H. H. Van Horn, and C. J. Wilcox. 1992. Effects of feather meal at two protein concentrations and yeast culture on production parameters in lactating dairy cows. J. Dairy Sci. 75:3524–3530.
Hart, F. J., and J. Leibholz. 1990. A note on the flow of endogenous protein to the omasum and abomasum of steers. Anim. Prod. 51:217–219.
Harty, S. R., J-M. Akayezu, J. G. Linn, and J. M. Cassady. 1998. Nutrient composition of distillers grains with added solubles. J. Dairy Sci. 81:1201. (Abst.)
Heger, J., and Z. Frydrych. 1989. Efficiency of utilization of amino acids. Pages 31–56 *in* Absorption and Utilization of Amino Acids, Vol. 1. M. Friedman, ed. CRC Press, Inc., Boca Raton, FL.
Henderson, S. J., H. E. Amos, and J. J. Evans. 1985. Influence of dietary protein concentration and degradability on milk production, composition, and ruminal protein metabolism. J. Dairy Sci. 68:2227–2237.
Henning, P. H., D. G. Steyn, and H. H. Meissner. 1993. Effect of synchronization of energy and nitrogen supply on ruminal characteristics and microbial growth. J. Anim. Sci. 71:2516–2528.
Henson, J. E., D. J. Schingoethe, and H. A. Maiga. 1997. Lactational evaluation of protein supplements of varying ruminal degradabilities. J. Dairy Sci. 80:385–392.
Herrera-Saldana, R., R. Gomez-Alarcaon, M. Tobrabi, and T. Huber. 1990. Influence of synchronizing protein and starch degradation in the rumen on nutrient utilization and microbial protein synthesis. J. Dairy Sci. 73:142–148.
Higginbotham, G. E., M. Torabi, and J. T. Huber. 1989. Influence of dietary protein concentration and degradability on performance of lactating cows during hot environmental temperatures. J. Dairy Sci. 72:2554–2564.
Hill, G. M., J. A. Boling, and N. W. Bradley. 1980. Postruminal lysine and methionine infusion in steers fed a urea-supplemented diet adequate in sulfur. J. Dairy Sci. 63:1242–1247.
Hindle, V. A., A. Steg, A. M. van Vuuren, and J. Vroons-de Bruin. 1995. Rumen degradation and post-ruminal digestion of palm kernel by-products in dairy cows. Anim. Feed Sci. Technol. 51:103–121.

Hino, T., and J. B. Russell. 1987. Relative contributions of ruminal bacteria and protozoa to the degradation of protein *in vitro*. J. Anim. Sci. 64:261–270.

Hoffman, P. C., and L. E. Armentano. 1988. Comparison of brewers wet and dried grains and soybean meal as supplements for dairy cattle. Nutr. Reports Int'l 38:655–663.

Hoffman, P. C., N. M. Brehm, L. M. Bauman, J. B. Peters, and D. J. Undersander. 1999. Prediction of laboratory and in situ protein fractions in legume and grass silages using near-infrared reflectance spectroscopy. J. Dairy Sci. 82:764–770.

Hoffman, P. C., S. J. Sievert, R. D. Shaver, D. A. Welch, and D. K. Combs. 1993. In situ dry matter, protein, and fiber degradation of perennial forages. J. Dairy Sci. 76:2632–2643.

Hoffman, P. C., R. R. Grummer, R. D. Shaver, G. A. Broderick, and T. R. Drendel. 1991. Feeding supplemental fat and undegraded intake protein to early lactation dairy cows. J. Dairy Sci. 74:3468–3474.

Holden, L. A., B. P. Glenn, R. A. Erdman, and W. E. Potts. 1994a. Effects of alfalfa and orchardgrass on digestion by dairy cows. J. Dairy Sci. 77:2580–2594.

Holden, L. A., L. D. Muller, G. A. Varga, and P. J. Hillard. 1994b. Ruminal digestion and duodenal nutrient flows in dairy cows consuming grass as pasture, hay, or silage. J. Dairy Sci. 77:3034–3042.

Holter, J. A., and J. T. Reid. 1959. Relationship between the concentrations of crude protein and apparently digestible protein in forages. J. Anim. Sci. 18:1339–1349.

Holter, J. B., H. H. Hayes, W. E. Urban Jr., S. Ramsey, and H. Rideout. 1992. Response of Holstein cows to corn gluten meal used to increase undegradable protein in early or later lactation. J. Dairy Sci. 75:1495–1506.

Hongerholt, D. D., and L. D. Muller. 1998. Supplementation of rumen undegradable protein to the diets of early lactation Holstein cows on grass pasture. J. Dairy Sci. 81:2204–2214.

Hoover, W. H., and S. R. Stokes. 1991. Balancing carbohydrates and protein for optimum rumen microbial yield. J. Dairy Sci. 74:3630–3644.

Hopkins, B. A., A. H. Rakes, T. E. Daniel, C. A. Zimmerman, and W. J. Croom, Jr. 1994. Effects of intraperitoneal L-leucine, L-isoleucine, L-valine, and L-arginine on milk fat depression in early lactation cows. J. Dairy Sci. 77:1084–1092.

Hopkins, D. I., W. E. Kunkle, A. C. Hammond, D. B. Bates, and B. A. Reiling. 1999. Effects of bypass methionine on the performance of growing cattle fed bermudagrass hay supplemented with molasses-based supplements. J. Anim. Sci. 71(Suppl.1):202. (Abstr.)

Howard, H. J., E. P. Aalseth, G. D. Adams, L. J. Bush, R. W. McNew, and L. J. Dawson. 1987. Influence of dietary protein on reproductive performance of dairy cows. J. Dairy Sci. 70:1563–1571.

Howie, S. A., S. Calsamiglia, and M. D. Stern. 1996. Variation in ruminal degredation and intestinal digestion of animal byproduct proteins. Anim. Feed. Sci. Technol. 63:1–7.

Hristov, A. 1998. Nitrogen fractions and in sacco dry matter and crude protein degradability of fresh and frozen alfalfa. Anim. Feed Sci. Technol. 71:351–355.

Hristov, A. N., and S. G. Sandev. 1998. Proteolysis and rumen degradability of protein in alfalfa preserved as silage, wilted silage, or hay. Anim. Feed Sci. Technol. 72:175–181.

Hristov, A. N., and G. A. Broderick. 1996. Synthesis of microbial protein in ruminally cannulated cows fed alfalfa silage, alfalfa hay, or corn silage. J. Dairy Sci. 79:1627–1637.

Hristov, A. N., T. A. McAllister, and K. J. Cheng. 1997. Effect of carbohydrate level and ammonia availability on utilization of alpha amino nitrogen by mixed ruminal microorganisms in vitro. Proc. Western Section, Amer. Soc. Anim. Sci. 48:186–189.

Hughes, A. D. 1970. The non-protein nitrogen composition of grass silages. II. The changes occurring during the storage of silage. J. Agr. Sci. 75:421–431.

Hurrell, R. F., and R. A. Finot. 1985. Effect of food processing on protein digestibility and amino acid availability. Pages 233–258 *in* Digestiblity and Amino Acid Availability in Cereals and Oilseeds. J. W. Finely and D.T. Hopkins (eds.). American Association of Cereal Chemists, St. Paul, MN.

Hussein, H. S., R. M. Jordan, and M. D. Stern. 1991. Ruminal protein metabolism and intestinal amino acid utilization as affected by dietary protein and carbohydrate sources in sheep. J. Anim. Sci. 69:2143–2151.

Huyler, M. T., R. L. Kincaid, and D. F. Dostal. 1999. Metabolic and yield responses of multiparous Holstein cows to prepartum rumen-undegradable protein. J. Dairy Sci. 82:527–536.

Hvelplund, T. 1985. Digestibility of rumen microbial protein and undegraded dietary protein estimated in the small intestine of sheep and by in sacco procedure. Acta. Agric. Scand. Suppl. 25:132–144.

Hvelplund, T., M. R. Weisbjerg, and L. S. Anderson. 1991. Estimation of the true digestibility of rumen undegraded dietary protein in the small intestine of ruminants by the mobile bag technique. Acta. Agric. Scand. Sect. A, Anim. Sci. 42:34–39.

Hvelplund, T., F. D. DeB Hovell, E. R. Ørskov, and D. J. Kyle. 1994. True intestinal digestibility of protein estimated with sheep on intragastric infusion and with the mobile bag technique. Proc. Soc. Nutr. Physiol. 3:64.

Ibrahim, M.N.M., S. Tamminga, and G. Zemmelink. 1995. Degradation of tropical roughages and concentrate feeds in the rumen. Anim. Feed Sci. Technol. 54:81–92.

Illg, D. J., J. L. Sommerfeldt, and D. J. Schingoethe. 1987. Lactational and systemic responses to the supplementation of protected methionine in soybean meal diets. J. Dairy Sci. 70:620–629.

Institute National de la Recherche Agronomique. 1989. Ruminant Nutrition: Recommended Allowances and Feed Tables. R. Jarrige, ed. John Libbey Eurotext, Paris.

Jacobson, D. R., H. H. Van Horn, and C. J. Sniffen. 1970. Lactating ruminants. Fed. Proc. 29:39–40.

Janicki, F. J., and C. C. Stallings. 1988. Degradation of crude protein in forages determined by in vitro and in situ procedures. J. Dairy Sci. 71:2440–2448.

Jaquette, R. D., A. H. Rakes, and W. J. Croom, Jr. 1986. Effects of dietary protein on milk, rumen, and blood parameters in dairy cattle fed low fiber diets. J. Dairy Sci. 69:1026–1034.

Jaquette, R. D., A. H. Rakes, and W. J. Croom, Jr. 1987. Effect of amount and source of dietary nitrogen on milk fat depression in early lactation dairy cows. J. Dairy Sci. 70:1202–1210.

Jarosz, L., T. Hvelplund, M. R. Weisbjerg, and B. B. Jensen. 1994. True digestibility of protein in the small intestine and the hind gut of cows measured with the mobile bag technique using $^{15}$N-labelled roughage. Acta Agric. Scand., Sect. A, Anim. Asci. 44:146–151.

Jarrige, R. 1989. Ruminant Nutrition: Recommended Allowances and Feed Tables. Institut National de la Recherche Agronomique, Libbey, Eurotext, Paris, France.

Johnson H. E., N. L. Whitehouse, B. D. Garthwaite, M. S. Piepenbrink, and C. G. Schwab. 1999. Supplementation of corn and barley-based diets of late gestation and early lactation cows with liquid methionine hydroxy analog (HMB). J. Dairy Sci. 82(Suppl. 1):65. (Abstr.)

Johnson, L. M., J. H. Harrison, and R. E. Riley. 1998. Estimation of the flow of microbial nitrogen to the duodenum using urinary uric acid or allantoin. J. Dairy Sci. 81:2408–2420.

Jones, D. F., W. H. Hoover, and T. K. Miller Webster. 1998. Effects of concentrations of peptides on microbial metabolism in continuous culture. J. Anim. Sci. 76:611–616.

Jones-Endsley, J. M., M. J. Cecava, and T. R. Johnson. 1997. Effects of dietary supplementation on nutrient digestion and the milk yield of intensively grazed lactating dairy cows. J. Dairy Sci. 80:3283–3292.

Jordan, E. R., and L. V. Swanson. 1979. Effect of crude protein on reproductive efficiency, serum total protein, and albumin in the high producing dairy cow. J. Dairy Sci. 62:58–63.

Jordan, E. R., T. E. Chapman, D. W. Holtan, and L. V. Swanson. 1983. Relationship of dietary crude protein to composition of uterine secretions and blood in high-producing dairy cows. J. Dairy Sci. 66:1854–1862.

Jouany, J. P. 1996. Effect of rumen protozoa on nitrogen utilization by ruminants. J. Nutr. 126:1335S–1346S.

Jouany, J. P., and K. Ushida. 1999. The role of protozoa in feed digestion. Review. AJAS 12:113–128.

Joy, M. T., E. J. DePeters, J. G. Fadel, and R. A. Zinn. 1997. Effects of corn processing on the site and extent of digestion in lactating cows. J. Dairy Sci. 80:2087–2097.

Kaim, M., H. Neumark, Y. Folman, and W. Kaufmann. 1987. The effect of two concentrations of dietary protein and of formaldehyde-treated soya-bean meal on the performance of high-yielding dairy cows. Anim. Prod. 4:333–345.

Kaim, M., Y. Folman, H. Neumark, and W. Kaufmann. 1983. The effect of protein intake and lactation number on post-partum body weight loss and reproductive performance of dairy cows. Anim. Prod. 37:229–235.

Kalscheur, K. F., B. B. Teter, L. S. Piperova, and R. A. Erdman. 1997a. Effect of dietary forage concentration and buffer addition on duodenal flow of *Trans*-$C_{18:1}$ fatty acids and milk fat production in dairy cows. J. Dairy Sci. 80:2104–2114.

Kalscheur, K. F., B. B. Teter, L. S. Piperova, and R. A. Erdman. 1997b. Effect of fat source on duodenal flow of *Trans*-$C_{18:1}$ fatty acids and milk fat production in dairy cows. J. Dairy Sci. 80:2115–2126.

Kalscheur, K. F., J. H. Vandersall, R. A. Erdman, R. A. Kohn, and E. Russek-Cohen. 1999a. Effects of dietary crude protein concentration and degradability on milk production responses of early, mid, and late lactation dairy cows. J. Dairy Sci. 82:545–554.

Kalscheur, K. F., R. A. Kohn, and B. P. Glenn. 1999b. Effect of increasing ruminally degraded protein on lactation performance of dairy cows. J. Dairy Sci. 82 (Suppl. 1):95. (Abstr.)

Karunanandaa, K., L. E. Goodling, G. A. Varga, L. D. Muller, W. W. McNeill, T. W. Casssidy, and T. Lykos. 1994. Supplemental dietary fat and ruminally protected amino acids for lactating Jersey cows. J. Dairy Sci. 77:3417–3425.

Kaufmann, W., and Lüpping, W. 1982. Protected proteins and protected amino acids for ruminants. In: Protein Contribution of Feedstuffs for Ruminants: Application to feed formulation (E.L Miller,., I.H. Pike, and A.J.H. Van Es, eds.) pp. 36–75. Butterworth Scientific, London, England.

Keady, T.W.J., and R.W.J. Steen. 1996. Effects of applying a bacterial inoculant to silage immediately before feeding on silage intake, digestibility, degradability and rumen volatile fatty acid concentrations in growing beef cattle. Grass Forage Sci. 51:155–162.

Keady, T.W.J., R.W.J. Steen, D. J. Kilpatrick, and C. S. Mayne. 1994. Effects of inoculant treatment on silage fermentation, digestibility and intake by growing cattle. Grass Forage Sci. 49:284–294.

Keery, C. M., H. E. Amos, and M. A. Froetschel. 1993. Effects of supplemental protein source on intraruminal fermentation, protein degradation, and amino acid absorption. J. Dairy Sci. 76:514–524.

Kendall, E. M., J R. Ingalls, and R. J. Boila. 1991. Variability in the rumen degradability and postruminal digestion of the dry matter, nitrogen and amino acids of canola meal. Can. J. Anim. Sci. 71:739–754.

Kenelly, J. J., D. L. Dalton, and J. K. Ha. 1988. Digestion and utilization of high moisture barley by lactating dairy cows. J. Dairy Sci. 71:1259–1266.

Kerry, C. M., and H. E. Amos. 1993. Effects of source and level of undegraded intake protein on nutrient use and performance of early lactation cows. J. Dairy Sci. 76:499–513.

Khalili, H., P. O Osuji, N. N. Umunna, and S. Crosse. 1994. The effects of forage type (maize-lablab or oat-vetch) and level of supplementation (wheat middlings) on food intake, diet apparent digestibility, purine excretion and milk production of crossbred (*Bos taurus* × *Bos indicus*) cows. Anim. Prod. 58:321–382.

Khalili, H., T. Varvikko, and S. Crosse. 1992. The effects of forage type and level of concentrate supplementation on food intake, diet digestibility and milk production of crossbred cows (*Bos taurus* × *Bos indicus*). Anim. Prod. 54:183–189.

Khorasani, G. R., E. K. Okine, and J. J. Kennelly. 1996a. Forage source alters nutrient supply to the intestine without influencing milk yield. J. Dairy Sci. 79:862–872.

Khorasani, G. R., G. De Boer, and J. J. Kennelly. 1996b. Response of early lactation cows to ruminally undegradable protein in the diet. J. Dairy Sci. 79:446–453.

Khorasani, G. R., G. deBoer, B. Robinson, and J. J. Kennelly. 1994a. Influence of dietary protein and starch on production and metabolic responses of dairy cows. J. Dairy Sci. 77:813–824.

Khorasani, G. R., P. H. Robinson, and J. J. Kennelly. 1994b. Evaluation of solvent and expeller linseed meals as protein sources for dairy cattle. Can. J. Anim. Sci. 74:479–485.

Khorasani, G. R., P. H. Robinson, and J. J. Kennelly. 1993. Effects of canola meal treated with acetic acid on ruminal degradation and intestinal digestibility in lactating dairy cows. J. Dairy Sci. 76:1607–1616.

Khorasani, G. R., G. deBoer, P. H. Robinson, and J. J. Kennelly. 1992. Effect of canola fat on ruminal and total tract digestion, plasma hormones, and metabolites in lactating cows. J. Dairy Sci. 75:492–501.

Kibelolaud, A. R., M. Vernay, C. Bayourthe, and R. Moncoulon. 1993. Effect of extruding on ruminal disappearance and lower gastrointestinal tract digestion of white lupin seeds. Can. J. Anim. Sci. 73: 571–579.

Kim, Y. K., D. J. Schingoethe, D. P. Casper, and F. C. Ludens. 1991. Lactational response of dairy cows to increased dietary crude protein with added fat. J. Dairy Sci. 74:3891–3899.

King, K. J., J. T. Huber, M. Sadik, W. G. Bergen, A. L. Grant, and V. L. King. 1990. Influence of dietary protein sources on the amino acid profiles available for digestion and metabolism in lactating cows. J. Dairy Sci. 73:3208–3216.

King, K. J., W. G. Bergen, C. J. Sniffen, A. L. Grant, D. B. Grieve, V. L. King, and N. K. Ames. 1991. An assessment of absorbable lysine requirements in lactating cows. J. Dairy Sci. 74:2530–2539.

Kirkpatrick, B. K., and J. J. Kennelly. 1987. In situ degradability of protein and dry matter from single protein sources and from a total diet. J. Anim. Sci. 65:567–576.

Klemesrud, M. J., and T. J. Klopfenstein. 1994. Addition of ruminal escape methionine and lysine to meat and bone meal. J. Dairy Sci. 77(Suppl. 1):94. (Abstr.)

Klover, E., L. D. Muller, G. A. Varga, and T. J. Cassidy. 1998. Synchronization of ruminal degradation of supplemental carbohydrate with pasture nitrogen in lactating dairy cows. J. Dairy Sci. 81:2017–2028.

Klusmeyer, T. H., G. L. Lynch, J. H. Clark, and D. R. Nelson. 1991a. Effects of calcium salts of fatty acids and protein source on ruminal fermentation and nutrient flow to duodenum of cows. J. Dairy Sci. 74:2206–2219.

Klusmeyer, T. H., G. L. Lynch, J. H. Clark, and D. R. Nelson. 1991b. Effects of calcium salts of fatty acids and proportion of forage in diet on ruminal fermentation and nutrient flow to duodenum of cows. J. Dairy Sci. 74:2220–2232.

Klusmeyer, T. H., R. D. McCarthy, Jr., J. H. Clark, and D. R. Nelson. 1990. Effects of source and amount of protein on ruminal fermentation and passage of nutrients to the small intestine of lactating cows. J. Dairy Sci. 73:3526–3537.

Koenig, K. M., L. M. Rode, C. D. Knight, and P. R. McCullough. 1999. Ruminal escape, gastrointestinal absorption, and response of serum methionine to supplementation of liquid methionine hydroxy analog in dairy cows. J. Dairy Sci. 82:355–361.

Komaragiri, M. V. S., and R. A. Erdman. 1997. Factors affecting body tissue mobilization in early lactation dairy cows. 1. Effect of dietary protein on mobilization of body fat and protein. J. Dairy Sci. 80:929–937.

Kopecný, J., and R. J. Wallace. 1982. Cellular location and some properties of proteolytic enzymes of rumen bacteria. Appl. Environ. Microbiol. 43:1026–1033.

Kopecný, J., O. Tománková, and P. Homolka. 1998. Comparison of protein digestibility of rumen undegraded protein estimated by an enzymatic and mobile bag method: feeds for ruminants and anaerobic fungus. Anim. Feed Sci. Technol. 71:109–116.

Köster, H. H., R. C. Cochran, E. C. Titgemeyer, E. S. Vanzant, T. G. Nagaraja, K. K. Kreikemeier, and G. St. Jean. 1997. Effect of increasing proportion of supplemental nitrogen from urea on intake and utilization of low-quality, tallgrass-prairie forage by beef steers. J. Anim. Sci. 75:1393–1399.

Kowalski, Z. M., P. M. Pisulewski, and M. Spanghero. 1999. Effects of calcium soaps of rapeseed fatty acids and protected methionine on milk yield and composition in dairy cows. J. Dairy Res. 66:475–487.

Kowalski, Z. M., A. Marszaek, and C. R. Mills. 1997. The use of Ca salts of rape seed fatty acids to protect protein against degradation in the rumen. Anim. Feed Sci. Technol. 65:265–274.

Krishnamoorthy, U., T. V. Muscato, C. J. Sniffen, and P. J. Van Soest. 1982. Nitrogen fractions in selected feedstuffs. J. Dairy Sci., 65: 217–225.

Kung, L., JR., J. T. Huber, and L. D. Satter. 1983. Influence of nonprotein nitrogen and protein of low rumen degradability on nitrogen flow and utilization in lactating dairy cows. J. Dairy Sci. 66:1863–1872.

Lardy, G. P., G. E. Catlett, M. S. Kerley, and J. A. Paterson. 1993. Determination of the ruminal excape value and duodenal amino acid flow of rapeseed meal. J. Anim. Sci. 71:3096–3104.

Laycock, K. A., and E. L. Miller. 1981. Nitrogen solubility and protein degradability of commercially and laboratory prepared rapeseed and soya-bean meals. Proc. Nutr. Soc. 40:103A.

Lees, J. A., J. D. Oldham, W. Haresign, and P. C. Garnsworthy. 1990. The effects of patterns of rumen fermentation on the response by dairy cows to dietary protein concentration. Brit. J. Nutr. 63:177–186.

Lehman, K. B., E. K. Okine, G. W. Mathison, and J. Helm. 1995. In situ degradabilities of barley grain cultivars. Can. J. Anim. Sci. 75:485–487.

Leng, R. A., and J. V. Nolan. 1984. Nitrogen metabolism in the rumen. J. Dairy Sci. 67:1072–1089.

Leng, R. A., D. Dellow, and G. Waghorn. 1986. Dynamics of large ciliate protozoa in the rumen of cattle fed on diets of freshly cut grass. Br. J. Nutr. 56:455–462.

Leonard, M., and E. Block. 1988. Effect of ration protein content and solubility on milk production of primiparous Holstein heifers. J. Dairy Sci. 71:2709–2722.

Licitra, G., T. M. Hernandez, and P. J. Van Soest. 1996. Standardization of procedures for nitrogen fractionation of ruminant feeds. Anim. Feed Sci. Technol. 57:347–358.

Lindberg, J. E. 1985. Estimation of rumen degradability of feed protein with the in sacco technique and various in vitro methods: A review. Acta Agric. Scand. Suppl. 25:64–97.

Ling, J. R., and I. P Armstead. 1995. The in vitro uptake and metabolism of peptides and amino acids by five species of rumen bacteria. J. Appl. Bacteriol. 78:116–124.

Lintzenich, B. A., E. S. Vanzant, R. C. Cochran, J. L. Beaty, R. T. Brandt, Jr., and G. St. Jean. 1995. Influence of processing supplemental alfalfa on intake and digestion of dormant bluestem-range forage by steers. J. Anim. Sci. 73:1187–1195.

Liu, C., D. J. Schingoethe, and G. A. Stegeman. 2000. Corn distillers grains verus a blend of protein supplements with or without ruminally protected amino acids for lactating cows. J. Dairy Sci. 83:(In press).

Liu, Y., L., A. Steg, and V. A. Hindle. 1994. Rumen degradation and intestinal digestion of crambe and other oilseed by-products in dairy cows. Anim. Feed Sci. Technol. 45:397–409.

Lobley, G. E. 1992. Control of the metabolic fate of amino acids in ruminants: A review. J. Anim. Sci. 70:3264–3275.

Loerch, S. G., and B. O. Oke. 1989. Rumen protected amino acids in ruminant nutrition. *In* Absorption and Utilization of Amino Acids. Vol. III (M. Friedman, ed.) pp. 187–200. CRC Press. Boca Raton, FL.

Lu, C. D., N. A. Jorgensen, and L. D. Satter. 1988. Site and extent of nutrient digestion in lactating dairy cows fed alfalfa protein concentrate or soybean meal. J. Dairy Sci. 71:697–704.

Lundquist, R. G., D. E. Otterby, and J. G. Linn. 1986. Influence of formaldehyde-treated soybean meal on milk production. J. Dairy Sci. 69:1337–1345.

Lusby, K. S. 1994. Performance of beef calves supplemented with protein or energy with or without Smartamine-M. Pages 173–178 *in* 1994 Oklahoma State University Animal Science Research Report.

Lykos, T., and G. A. Varga. 1995. Effects of processing method on degradation characteristics of protein and carbohydrate sources in situ. J. Dairy Sci. 78:1789–1801.

Lykos, T, G. A. Varga, and D. Casper. 1997. Varying degradation rates of total nonstructrual carbohydrates: Effects on ruminal fermentation, blood metabolites, and milk production and composition in high producing Holstein cows. J. Dairy Sci. 80:3341–3355.

Lynch, G. L., T. H. Klusmeyer, M. R. Cameron, J. H. Clark, and D. R. Nelson. 1991. Effects of somatatropin and duodenal infusion of amino acids on nutrient passage to duodenum and performance of dairy cows. J. Dairy Sci. 74:3117–3127.

Mabjeesh, S. J., A. Ariele, I. Bruckental, S. Zamwell, and H. Tagari. 1996. Effect of type of protein supplementation on duodenal amino acid flow and absorption in lactating dairy cows. J. Dairy Sci. 79:1792–1801.

Mabjeesh, S. J., A. Arieli, I. Bruckental, S. Zamwell, and H. Tagari. 1997. Effect of ruminal degradability of crude protein and nonstructural carbohydrates on the efficiency of bacterial crude protein synthesis and amino acid flow to the abomasum of dairy cows. J. Dairy Sci. 80:2939–2949.

Mackle, T. R., Dwyer, D. A., and D. E. Bauman. 1999. Effects of branched-chain amino acids and sodium caseinate on milk protein concentration and yield from dairy cows. J. Dairy Sci. 82:161–171.

Macleod, G. K., and L. W. Cahill. 1987. Canola meal as a protein supplement in corn based dairy rations. Guelph Dairy Research Report; June pp. 100–108.

Madsen, J. 1986. Influence of feeding level on digestion and protein passage to the duodenum in cows fed high concentrate diets. Acta Agric. Scand. 36:275–285.

Madsen, J., and T. Hvelplund. 1990. Protein degradation in the rumen. Pages 103–124 *in* A Study of the Quantitative Nitrogen Metabolism in the Gastro-intestinal Tract, and the Resultant New Protein Evaluation System for Ruminants. The AAT-BPV System. T. Hvelplund and J. Madsen, eds. Institute of Animal Science, The Royal Veterinary and Agricultural University, Copenhagen.

Madsen, J., T. Hvelplund, M. R. Weisbjerg, J. Bertilsson, I. Olsson, R. Spörndly, O. M. Harstad, H. Volden, M. Tuori, T. Varvikko, P. Huntanen, and B. L. Olafsson. 1995. The AAT/PBV protein evaluation system for ruminants. A revision. The Norwegian J. Agric. Sci., Suppl. No. 19:1–37 (ISSN 0802-1600).

Maeng, W. J., and R. L. Baldwin. 1976. Factors influencing rumen microbial growth rates and yields: Effects of urea and amino acids over time. J. Dairy Sci. 72:2002–2016.

Maeng, W. J., H. Park, and H. J. Kim. 1997. The role of carbohydrate supplementation in microbial protein synthesis in the rumen. *In* Rumen Microbes and Digestive Physiology in Ruminants (Onodera et al, eds.), pp. 107–119. Japan Sci. Soc. Press, Tokyo/S. Karger, Basel.

Mahadevan, S., J. D. Erfle, and F. D. Sauer. 1980. Degradation of soluble and insoluble proteins by *Bacteroides amylophilus* protease and by rumen microorganisms. J. Anim. Sci. 50:723–728.

Maiga, H. A., D. J. Schingoethe, and J. Ellison Henson. 1997. Ruminal degradation, amino acid composition, and intestinal digestibility of the residual components of five protein supplements. J. Dairy Sci. 79:1647–1653.

Maiga, H. A., D. J. Schingoethe, and J. E. Henson. 1996. Ruminal degradation, amino acid composition, and intestinal digestibility of the residual components of five protein supplements. J. Dairy Sci. 79: 1647–1653.

Makoni, N. F., J. A. Shelford, and L. J. Fisher. 1991. The rate and extent of silage nitrogen degradation in the rumen as influenced by wilting and duration of regrowth. Can. J. Anim. Sci. 71:245–248.

Mangan, J. L. 1972. Quantitative studies on nitrogen metabolism in the bovine rumen. The rate of proteolysis of casein and ovalbumin and the release and metabolism of free amino acids. Br. J. Nutr. 27:261–283.

Mansfield, H. R., and M. D. Stern. 1994. Effects of soybean hulls and lignosulfonate-treated soybean meal on ruminal fermentation in lactating dairy cows. J. Dairy Sci. 77:1070–1083.

Manson, F. J., and J. D. Leaver. 1988. The influence of dietary protein intake and of hoof trimming on lameness in dairy cattle. Anim. Prod. 47:191–199.

Mantysaari, P. E., C. J. Sniffen, T. V. Muscato, J. M. Lynch, and D. M. Barbano. 1989. Performance of cows in early lactation fed isonitrogenous diets containing soybean meal or animal by-product meals. J. Dairy Sci. 72:2958–2967.

Manyuchi, B., T. Smith, and S. Mikayiri. 1992. The use of poultry litter in ruminant diets 1. Poultry litter and cotton seed meal as supplements for weaner steers grazing natural pasture during the dry season or sheep fed natural pasture hay in pens. Zimbabwe J. Agric. Res. 30:91–103.

Marshall, S. A., C. P. Campbell, and J. G. Buchanan-Smith. 1993. Proteolysis and rumen degradability of alfalfa silages preserved with a microbial inoculant, spent-sulphite liquor, formic acid, or formaldehyde. Can J. Anim. Sci. 73:559–570.

Martin. C., L. Bernard, and B. Michalet-Doreau. 1996. Influence of sampling time and diet on amino acid composition of protozoal and bacterial fractions from bovine ruminal contents. J. Anim. Sci. 74:1157–1163.

Masoero, F., L. Fiorentini, F. Rossi, and A. Piva. 1994. Determination of nitrogen intestinal digestibility in ruminants. Anim. Feed Sci. Technol. 48: 253–263.

Mason, V. C. 1979. The quantitative importance of bacterial residues in the non-dietary faecal nitrogen of sheep. 2. Estimates of bacterial nitrogen in faecal material from 47 digestibility trials. Z. Tierphysiol., Tierernährg. U. Futtermittelkde. 41:131–139.

Mason, V. C., and F. White. 1971. The digestion of bacterial mucopeptide constituents in the sheep. 1. The metabolism of 2,6-diaminopimelic acid. J. Agric. Sci., Camb. 77:91–98.

Mason, V. C., P. Kessank, J. C. Onontwu, and M. P. Narang. 1981. Z. Tierphysiol., Tierernährg. U. Futtermittelkde. 45:174–184.

Mathers, J.C., and E. L. Miller. 1981. Quantitative studies of food protein degradation and the energetic efficiency of microbial protein synthesis in the rumen of sheep given chopped lucerne and rolled barley. Br. J. Nutr. 45:587–604.

Mbanzamihigo, L., E. Vandycke, and D. I. Demeyer. 1997. Degradation of methionine by rumen contents in vitro and efficiency of its protection. Anim. Feed Sci. Tech. 67:339–347.

McCance, R. A., and E. Widdowson. 1978. *In*: The Composition of Foods, 4th ed. D.A.T. Southgate and A.A. Paul, eds. HMSO, London, Engl.

McCarthy, R. D. Jr., T. H. Klusmeyer, J. L. Vicini, J. H. Clark, and D. R. Nelson. 1989. Effects of source of protein and carbohydrate on ruminal fermentation and passage of nutrients to the small intestine of lactating cows. J. Dairy Sci. 72:2002–2016.

McCollum, M. Q., M. Vázquez-Añón, J. J. Dibner, and K. E. Webb, Jr. 2000. Absorption of 2-hydroxy-4-(methylthio)butanoic acid by isolated sheep ruminal and omasal epithelia. J. Anim. Sci. 78:1078–1083.

McCormick, M. E., D. D. French, T. F. Brown, G. J. Cuomo, A. M. Chapa, J. M. Fernandez, J. F. Beatty, and D. C. Blouini. 1999. Crude protein and rumen undegradable protein effects on reproduction and lactation performance of Holstein cows. J. Dairy Sci. 82:2697–2708.

McGuffey, R. K., H. B. Green, and R. P. Basson. 1990. Lactation response of dairy cows receiving bovine somatotropin and fed rations varying in crude protein and undegradable intake protein. J. Dairy Sci. 73:2437–2443.

McKinnon, J. J., A. F. Mustafa, and R.D.H. Cohen. 1995. Nutritional evaluation and processing of canola hulls for ruminants. Can. J. Anim. Sci. 75:231–237.

McNiven, M. A., M. R. Weisbjerg, and T. Hvelplund. 1995. Influence of roasting or sodium hydroxide treatment of barley on digestion in lactating cows. J. Dairy Sci. 78:1106–1115.

McNiven, M. A., R.M.G. Hamilton, P. H. Robinson, and J. W. deLeeuw. 1994. Effect of flame roasting on the nutritional quality of common cereal grains for non-ruminants and ruminants. Anim. Feed Sci. Technol. 47:31–40.

Meijer, G. A. L., and C. J. van der Koelen. 1994. Duodenal infusion of glutamine does not affect protein synthesis in late lactation dairy cows. J. Dairy Sci. 77(Suppl. 1):242. (Abstr.)

Meijer, G. A. L., J. van der Meulen, and A. M. van Vuuren. 1993. Glutamine is a potentially limiting amino acid for milk production in dairy cows: A hypothesis. Metabolism 42: 358–364.

Meijer, G. A. L., J. van der Meulen, J. G. M. Bakker, C. J. van der Koelen and A. M. van Vuuren. 1995. Free amino acids in plasma and muscle of high yielding dairy cows in early lactation. J. Dairy Sci. 78:1131–1141.

Mepham, T. B. 1971. Amino acid utilization by the lactating mammary gland. Page 297 *in* Lactation. (I. R. Falconer, ed.) Butterworths, London.

Mepham, T. B. 1982. Amino acid utilization by lactating mammary gland. J. Dairy Sci. 65:287–298.

Mepham, T. B., and J. L. Linzell. 1967. Urea formation by the lactating goat mammary gland. Nature 214:507–518.

Merchen, N. R., and L. D. Satter. 1983. Changes in nitrogenous compounds and sites of digestion of alfalfa harvested at different moisture contents. J. Dairy Sci. 66:789–801.

Messman, M. A., W. P. Weiss, and M. E. Koch. 1994. Changes in total and individual proteins during drying, ensiling, and ruminal fermentation of forages. J. Dairy Sci. 77:492–500.

Mezl, V. A., and W. E. Knox. 1977. Metabolism of arginine in lactating rat mammary gland. Biochem. J. 164:105–113.

Mhgeni, D. M., T. Hvelplund, and M. R. Weisbjerg. 1994. Intestinal digestibility of rumen undegraded dietary protein from tropical roughages estimated by the mobile bag technique. Acta Agric. Scand., Sect. A, Anim. Sci. 44:230–235.

Michalet-Doreau, B., and P. Cerneau. 1991. Influence of foodstuff particle size on in situ degradation of nitrogen in the rumen. Anim. Feed Sci. Technol. 35:69–81.

Michalet-Doreau, B., and P. Nozière. 1998. Validation of in situ nitrogen degradation measurements: comparative proteolytic activity of solid-adherent microorganisms isolated from rumen content and nylon bags containing various feeds. Anim. Feed Sci. Technol. 70:41–47.

Michalet-Doreau, B., and M. Y. Ould-Bah. 1992. *In vitro* and *in sacco* methods for the estimation of dietary nitrogen degradability in the rumen: a review. Anim. Feed Sci. and Technol. 40:57–86.

Milton, C. T., R. T. Brandt, Jr., and E. C. Titgemeyer. 1997. Urea in dry-rolled corn diets: Finishing steer performance, nutrient digestion, and microbial protein production. J. Anim. Sci. 75:1415–1424.

Mir, P. S., Z, Mir, and L. Townley-Smith. 1993. Comparison of the nutrient content and in situ degradability of fenugreek (*Trigonella foenum-graecum*) and alfalfa hays. Can J. Anim. Sci. 73:993–996.

Mir, Z., P. S. Mir, S. Bittman, and L. J. Fisher. 1992. Ruminal degradation characteristics of corn and corn-sunflower intercropped silages prepared at two stages of maturity. Can. J. Anim. Sci. 72:881–889.

Moller, P. D. 1985. Results of grass silage based rations on the nitrogen absorption in the gastro-intestinal tract of dairy cows applied in the Nordic protein evaluation system. Acta Agric. Scand. Suppl. 25:49–63.

Moshtaghi Nia, S. A., and J. R. Ingalls. 1992. Effect of heating on canola meal protein degradation in the rumen and digestion in the lower gastrointestinal tract of steers. Can. J. Anim. Sci. 72: 83–88.

Moshtaghi Nia, S. A., and J. R. Ingalls. 1995. Evaluation of moist heat treatment of canola meal on digestion in the rumen, small intestine, large intestine, and total digestive tract of steers. Can. J. Anim. Sci. 75: 279–283.

Munneke, R. L., D. J. Schingoethe, and D. P. Casper. 1991. Lactational evaluation of ruminally protected methionine in diets containing extruded soybeans and urea. J. Dairy Sci. 74:227–233.

Mupeta, B., M. R. Weisbjerg, T. Hvelplund, and J. Madsen. 1997. Digestibility of amino acids in protein rich tropical feeds for ruminants estimated with the mobile bag technique. Anim. Feed Sci. Technol. 69: 271–280.

Murphy, J. J., and J. J. Kennelly. 1987. Effect of protein concentration and protein source on the degradability of dry matter and protein in situ. J. Dairy Sci. 70:1841–1849.

Murphy, T. A., S. C. Loerch, and B. A. Dehority. 1994. The influence of restricted feeding on site and extent of digestion and flow of nitrogenous compounds to the duodenum in steers. J. Anim. Sci. 72:2487–2496.

Murphy, M., H. Khalili, and P. Huhtanen. 1993. The substitution of barley by other carbohydrates in grass silage based diets to dairy cows. Anim. Feed Sci. Technol. 41:279–296.

Murphy, M., P. Uden, D. L. Palmquist, and H.Wiktorsson. 1987. Rumen and total diet digestibilities in lactating cows fed diets containing full-fat rapeseed. J. Dairy Sci. 70:1572–1582.

Mustafa, A. F., D. A. Christensen, and J. J. McKinnon. 1998. Effects of moist heat treatment on crude protein composition and degradability of field peas. Can. J. Anim. Sci. 78:453–456.

Mustafa, A. F., J. J. McKinnon, P. A. Thacker, and D. A. Christensen. 1997. Effect of borage meal on nutrient digestibility and performance of ruminants and pigs. Anim. Feed Sci. Technol. 64:273–285.

Mustafa, A. F., D. A. Christensen, and J. J. McKinnon. 1996. Chemical characterization and nutrient availability of high and low fiber canola meal. Can. J. Anim. Sci. 76:579–586.

Nakamura, T., T. J. Klopfenstein, and R. A. Britton. 1994a. Evaluation of acid detergent insoluble nitrogen as an indicator of protein quality in nonforage proteins. J. Anim. Sci. 72:1043–1048.

Nakamura, T., T. J. Klopfenstein, D. J. Gibb, and R. A. Britton. 1994b. Growth efficiency and digestibility of heated proteins fed to growing ruminants. J. Anim. Sci. 72:774–782.

Nakamura, T., T. J. Klopfenstein, F. G. Owen, R. A. Britton, R. J. Grant, and T. S. Winowiski. 1992. Nonenzymatically browned soybean meal for lactating dairy cows. J. Dairy Sci. 75:3519–3523.

Napoli, G. M., and F. J. Santini. 1989. The effect of a protein energy supplement on pasture protein and fibre digestion in the rumen of grazing steers. Anim. Feed Sci. Technol. 25:39–53.

Narasimhalu, P., E. Teller, M. Vanbelle, M. Foulon, and F. Dasnoy. 1989. Apparent digestibility of nitrogen in rumen and whole tract of Friesan cattle fed direct-cut and wilted grass silages. J. Dairy Sci. 72:2055–2061.

National Research Council. 1985. Ruminant Nitrogen Usage. Washington D.C.: National Academy Press.

National Research Council. 1989. Nutrient Requirements of Dairy Cattle, 6th rev. ed. Washington, D.C.: National Academy Press.

National Research Council. 1994. Nutrient Requirements of Poultry, 9th rev. ed. Washington, D.C.: National Academy Press.

National Research Council. 1996. Nutrient Requirements of Beef Cattle, 7th rev. ed. Washington, D.C.: National Academy Press.

National Research Council. 1998. Nutrient Requirements of Swine, 10th rev. ed. Washington, D.C.: National Academy Press. 189 pp.

Negi, S. S., B. Singh, and H.P.S. Makkar. 1988. Rumen degradability of nitrogen in typical cultivated grasses and leguminous fodders. Anim. Feed Sci. Technol. 22:79–89.

Neu, J., V. Shenoy, and R. Chakrabarti. 1996. Glutamine nutrition and metabolism: Where do we go from here? FASEB J. 10:829–837.

Newbold, J. R., and S. R. Rust. 1992. Effect of asynchronous nitrogen and energy supply on growth of ruminal bacteria in batch culture. J. Anim. Sci. 70:538–546.

Nichols, J. R., D. J. Schingoethe, H. A. Maiga, M. J. Brouk, and M. S. Piepenbrink. 1998. Evaluation of corn distillers grains and ruminally protected lysine and methionine for lactating dairy cows. J. Dairy Sci. 81:482–491.

Nocek, J. E. 1988. *In situ* and other methods to estimate ruminal protein and energy digestibility: a review. J. Dairy Sci. 71:2051–2069.

Nocek, J. E., and A. L. Grant. 1987. Characterization of in situ nitrogen and fiber digestion and bacterial nitrogen contamination of haycrop forages preserved at different dry matter percentages. J. Anim. Sci. 64:552–564.

Nocek, J. E., and J. E. English. 1986. *In situ* degradation kinetics: evaluation of rate determinationprocedure. J. Dairy Sci., 69:77–87.

Nocek, J. E., G. D. Young, W. Chalupa, C. J. Sniffen, W. E. Julien, T. Ueda, T. Fujieda, I. Shinzato, H. Sato, and H. Suzuki. 1999. The effect of rumen-protected lysine on production performance of lactating dairy cows. J. Dairy Sci. 82(Suppl. 1):94. (Abstr.)

Nocek, J. E., K. A. Cummins, and C. E. Polan. 1979. Ruminal disappearance of crude protein and dry matter in feeds and combined effects in formulated diets. J. Dairy Sci. 62:1587–1598.

Noel, R. J. 2000. Official feed terms. Pages 187–200 In Association of American Feed Control Officials, Official Publication 2000.

Nolan, J. V. 1975. Quantitative models of nitrogen metabolism in sheep. In: Digestion and Metabolism in the Ruminant (McDonald, I. W. and A.C. I. Warner, eds.), pp 416–431. University of New England Publishing Unit, Armidale, Australia.

Nolan, J. V. 1993. Nitrogen kinetics. Pages 123–163 *in* Quantitative Aspects of Ruminant Digestion and Metabolism. J. M. Forbes and J. France (eds.). CAB International Wallingford, UK.

Nugent, J. H. A., and J. L. Mangan. 1978. Rumen proteolysis of fraction I leaf protein, casein, and bovine serum albumin. Proc. Nutr. Soc. 37:48A.

Nugent, J. H. A., and J. L. Mangan. 1981. Characteristics of the rumen proteolysis of Fraction 1 (18S) leaf protein from lucerne (*Medicago sativa L.*). Br. J. Nutr. 46:39–58.

Nugent, J. H. A., W. T. Jones, D. J. Jordan, and J. L. Mangan. 1983. Rates of proteolysis in the rumen of the soluble proteins casein, Fraction 1 (18S) leaf protein, bovine serum albumin, and bovine submaxillary mucoprotein. Br. J. Nutr. 50:357–368.

O'Connor, J. D., C. J. Sniffen, D. G. Fox, and W. Chalupa. 1993. A net carbohydrate and protein system for evaluating cattle diets: IV. Predicting amino acid adequacy. J. Anim. Sci. 71: 1298–1311.

O'Mara, F. P., G. K. Stakelum, P. Dillon, J. J. Murphy, and M. Rath. 1997a. Rumen fermentation and nutrient flows for cows fed grass and grass supplemented with molassed beet pulp pellets. J. Dairy Sci. 80:2466–2474.

O'Mara, F. P., J. J. Murphy, and M. Rath. 1997b. The amino acid composition of protein feedstuffs before and after ruminal incubation and after subsequent passage through the intestines of dairy cows. J. Anim. Sci. 75:1941–1949.

O'Mara, F. P., J. J. Murphy, and M. Rath. 1998. Effect of amount of dietary supplement and source of protein on milk production, ruminal fermentation, and nutrient flows in dairy cows. J. Dairy Sci. 81:2430–2439.

Ohajuruka, O. A., Z. Wu, and D. L. Plamquist. 1991. Ruminal metabolism, fiber, and protein digestion by lactating cows fed calcium soap or animal-vegetable fat. J. Dairy Sci. 74:2601–2609.

Oldham, J. D. 1981. Amino acid requirements for lactation in high-yielding dairy cows. In Recent Developments in Ruminant Nutrition. W. Haresign and D. J. A. Cole (eds.), pp 49–81. Butterworths, London.

Oldham, J. D., J. D. Sutton, and A. B. McAllan. 1979. Protein digestion and utilization by dairy cows. Ann. Rech. Vet. 10:290–293.

Oldick, B. S., and J. L. Firkins. 1996. Imbalanced, inadequate diets effect reproduction performance, bottom line. Feedstuffs. 51:12–14,25.

Oliveira, J. S., J. T. Huber, J. M. Simas, C. B. Theurer, and R. S. Swingle. 1995. Effect of sorghum grain processing on site and extent of digestion of starch in lactating dairy cows. J. Dairy Sci. 78:1318–1327.

Olson, K. C., J. S. Caton, D. R. Kirby, and P. L. Norton. 1994. Influence of yeast culture supplementation and advancing season on steers grazing mixed-grass prairie in the Northern Great Plains: I. Dietary composition, intake, and in situ nutrient disappearance. J. Anim. Sci. 72:2149–2157.

Onodera, R. 1993 Methionine and lysine metabolism in the rumen and the possible effects of their metabolites on the nutrition and physiology of ruminants. Amino Acids 5:217–232.

Opstvedt, J., R. Miller, R. W. Hardy, and J. Spinelli. 1984. Heat-induced changes in sulfhydryl groups and disulfide bonds in fish protein and their effect on protein and amino acid digestibility in rainbow trout (*Salmo gaifdneri*). J. Agric. Food Chem. 32:929–935.

Ørskov, E. R. 1982. Protein Nutrition in Ruminants. Academic Press Inc., San Diego, CA.

Ørskov, E. R., and I. McDonald. 1979. The estimate of protein degradability in the rumen from incubation measurements weighted according to rate of passage. J. Agric. Sci. (Camb.) 92:499–503.

Ørskov, E. R., N. A. MacLeod, and D. J. Kyle. 1986. Flow of nitrogen from the rumen and abomasum in cattle and sheep given protein-free nutrients by intragastric infusion. Br. J. Nutr. 56:241–248.

Orten, J. M., and O. W. Neuhaus. 1975. Human Biochemistry. Ninth Edition. C. V. Mosby Company, Saint Louis, MO.

Overton, T. R., D. W. LaCount, T. M. Cicela, and J. H. Clark. 1996. Evaluation of a ruminally protected methionine product for lactating dairy cows. J. Dairy Sci. 79:631–638.

Overton, T. R., M. R. Cameron, J. P. Elliott, J. H. Clark, and D. R. Nelson. 1995. Ruminal fermentation and passage of nutrients to the duodenum of lactating cows fed mixtures of corn and barley. J. Dairy Sci. 78:1981–1998.

Owen, F. G., and L. L. Larson. 1991. Corn distillers dried grains versus soybean meal in lactation diets. J. Dairy Sci. 74:972–979.

Owens, F. N., and A. L. Goetsch. 1986. Digesta passage and microbial protein synthesis. Pages 196–226 *in* Control of Digestion and Metabolism in Ruminants. L. P. Milligan, W. L. Grovum, and A. Dobson, ed. Prentice-Hall, Englewood Cliffs, NJ.

Owens, F. N., and J. E. Pettigrew. 1989. Subdividing amino acid requirements into portions for maintenance and growth. In Absorption and Utilization of Amino Acids. Vol. I (M. Friedman, ed.) pp. 15–30. CRC Press, Boca Raton, FL.

Palmquist, D. L., M. R. Weisbjerg, and T. Hvelplund. 1993. Ruminal, intestinal, and total digestibilities of nutrients in cows fed diets high in fat and undegradable protein. J. Dairy Sci. 76:1353–1364.

Palmquist, D. L., and W. P. Weiss. 1994. Blood and hydrolyzed feather meals as sources of undegradable protein in high fat diets for cows in early lactation J. Dairy Sci. 77:1630–1643.

Palmquist, D. L., M. R. Weisbjerg, and T. Hvelplund. 1993. Ruminal, intestinal, and total digestibilities of nutrients in cows fed diets high in fat and undegradable protein. J. Dairy Sci. 76:1353–1364.

Pantoja, J., J. L Firkins, and M. L. Eastridge. 1995. Site of digestion and milk production by cows fed fats differing in saturation, esterification, and chain length. J. Dairy Sci. 78:2247–2258.

Pantoja, J., J. L. Firkins, M. L. Eastridge, and B. L. Hull. 1994. Effects of fat saturation and source of fiber on site of nutrient digestion and milk production by lactating dairy cows. J. Dairy Sci. 77:2341–2356.

Papas, A. M., C. J. Sniffen, and T. V. Muscato. 1984a. Effectiveness of rumen protected methionine for delivering methionine postruminally in dairy cows. J. Dairy Sci. 67:545–552.

Papas, A. M., J. L. Vicini, J. H. Clark, and S. Peirce-Sandner. 1984b. Effects of rumen-protected methionine on plasma free amino acids and production by dairy cows. J. Nutr. 114:2221–2227.

Papas, A., G. A .B. Hall, E. E. Hatfield, and F. N. Owens. 1974. Response of lambs to oral or abomasal supplementation of methionine hydroxy analog or methionine. J. Nutr. 104:653–659.

Paster, B. J., J. B. Russell, C. M. J., Yang J. M. Chow, C. R. Woese, and R. Tanner. 1993. Phylogeny of the ammonia-producing ruminal bacteria *Peptostreptococcus anaerobius, Clostridium sticklandii*, and *Clostridium aminophilum* sp. nov. Int. J. System. Bacteriol. 43:107–110.

Patterson, J. A., and L. Kung, Jr. 1988. Metabolism of DL-methionine and methionine analogs by rumen microorganisms. J. Dairy Sci. 71:3292–3301.

Pena, F., H. Tagari, and L. D. Satter. 1986. The effect of heat treatment of whole cottonseed on site and extent of protein digestion in dairy cows. J. Anim. Sci. 62:1423–1433.

Pereira, J. C., M. D. Carro, J. González, M. R. Alvir, and C. A. Rodríguez. 1998. Rumen degradability and intestinal digestibility of brewers grains as affected by origin and heat treatment and of barley rootlets. Anim. Feed Sci. Technol. 74:107–121.

Petit, H. V., and G. F. Tremblay. 1992. In situ degradability of fresh grass and grass conserved under different harvesting methods. J. Dairy Sci. 75:774–781.

Petit, H. V., P. Savoie, D. Tremblay, G. T. Dos Santos, and G. Butler. 1994. Intake, digestibility, and ruminal degradability of shredded hay. J. Dairy Sci. 77:3043–3050.

Peyraud, J. L., L. Astigarraga, and P. Faverdin. 1997. Digestion of fresh perennial ryegrass fertilized at two levels of nitrogen by lactating dairy cows. Anim. Feed Sci. Technol. 64:155–171.

Piepenbrink, M. S., and D. J. Schingoethe. 1998. Ruminal degradation, amino acid composition, and estimated intestinal digestibilities of four protein supplements. J. Dairy Sci. 81:454–461.

Piepenbrink, M. S., C. G. Schwab, B. K. Sloan, and N. L.Whitehouse. 1999. Importance of dietary concentrations of absorbable lysine on maximizing milk protein production of mid-lactation cows. J. Dairy Sci. 82(Suppl. 1):93. (Abstr.)

Piepenbrink, M. S., D. J. Schingoethe, M. J. Brouk, and G. A. Stegeman. 1998. Systems to evaluate the protein quality of diets fed to lactating cows. J. Dairy Sci. 81:1046–1061.

Pires, A. V., M. L. Eastridge, J. L. Firkins, and Y. C. Lin. 1997. Effects of heat treatment and physical processing of cottonseed on nutrient digestibility and production performance by lactating cows. J. Dairy Sci. 80:1685–1694.

Pisulewski, P. M., H. Rulquin, J. L. Peyraud, and R. Verite. 1996. Lactational and systemic responses of dairy cows to postruminal infusions of increasing amounts of methionine. J. Dairy Sci. 79:1781–1791.

Polan, C. E., D. E. Stieve, and J. L. Garrett. 1998. Protein preservation and ruminal degradation of ensiled forage treated with heat, formic acid, ammonia, or microbial inoculant. J. Dairy Sci. 81:765–776.

Polan, C. E., G. Cozzi, P. Berzaghi, and I. Andrighetto. 1997. A blend of animal and cereal protein or fish meal as partial replacement for soybean meal in the diets of lactating Holstein cows. J. Dairy Sci. 80:160–166.

Polan, C. E., K. A. Cummins, C. J. Sniffen, T. V. Muscato, J. L. Vicini, B.A. Crooker, J. H. Clark, D. G. Johnson, D. E. Otterby, B. Guillaume, L. D. Muller, G. A. Varga, R. A. Murray, and S. B. Peirce-Sandner. 1991. Responses of dairy cows to supplemental rumen-protected forms of methionine and lysine. J. Dairy Sci. 74:2997–3013.

Polan, C. E., T. A. Herrington, W. A. Wark, and L. E. Armentano. 1985. Milk production response to diets supplemented with dried brewers grains, wet brewers grains, or soybean meal. J. Dairy Sci. 68:2016–2026.

Poore, M. H., J. A. Moore, T. P. Eck, R. S. Swingle, and C. B. Theurer. 1993. Effect of fiber source and ruminal starch degradability on site and extent of digestion in dairy cows. J. Dairy Sci. 76:2244–2253.

Powers, W. J., H. H. Van Horn, B. Harris, Jr., and C. J. Wilcox. 1995. Effects of variable sources of distillers dried grains plus solubles on milk yield and composition. J. Dairy Sci. 78:388–396.

Prakash, P., D. V. Reddy, R. Ramachandra Reddy, and N. Krishna. 1996. The catalytic effect of supplementation of protein meals on utilization of rice straw-poultry droppings-rice bran diet in buffaloes. Anim. Feed Sci. Technol. 63:229–245.

Prange, R. W., M. D. Stern, N. A. Jorgensen, and L. D. Satter. 1984. Site and extent of protein digestion in lactating cows fed alfalfa silage or baled alfalfa hay. J. Dairy Sci. 67:2308–2314.

Prestløkken, E. 1999. In situ ruminal degradation and intestinal digestibility of dry matter and protein in expanded feedstuffs. Anim. Feed Sci. Technol. 71:1–23.

Prigge, E. C., M. J. Baker, and G. A. Varga. 1984. Comparative digestion, rumen fermentation and kinetics of forage diets by steers and wethers. J. Anim. Sci. 59:237–245.

Prins, R. A., J. C. Van Gestel, and G. H. M. Counotte. 1979. Degradation of amino acids and peptides by mixed rumen microorganisms. Z. Tierphysiol. Tierernahr. Futtermittelk. 42:333–339.

Pruekvimolphan S., R. R. Grummer, and S. J. Bertics. 1997. Effects of feather meal on lactation performance of dairy cows fed methionine deficient diets. J. Dairy Sci. 80(Suppl. 1):248. (Abstr.)

Punia, B. S., J. Leibholz, and G. J. Faichney. 1992. Rate of production of protozoa in the rumen and flow of protozoal nitrogen to the duodenum in sheep and cattle given a pelleted diet of lucerne hay and barley. J. Agric. Sci., Camb. 118:229–236.

Putnam, D. E., C. G. Schwab, M. T. Socha, N. L. Whitehouse, N. A. Kierstead, and B. D. Garthwaite. 1997. Effect of yeast culture in the diets of early lactation dairy cows on ruminal fermentation and passage of nitrogen fractions and amino acids to the small intestine. J. Dairy Sci. 80:374–384.

Rae, R. C., and J. R. Ingalls. 1984. Lactational response of dairy cows to oral administration of L-tyrosine. J. Dairy Sci. 67:1430–1438.

Rae, R. C., and R. R. Smithard. 1985. Estimation of true nitrogen digestibility in cattle by a modified nylon bag technique. Proc. Nutr. Soc. 44:116A.

Rae, R. C., J. R. Ingalls, and J. A. McKirdy. 1983. Effect of dietary crude protein level and formaldehyde treated canola meal on milk production and nitrogen utilization during early lactation. Can. J. Anim. Sci. 63:905–915.

Ragland-Gray, K. K., H. E. Amos, M. A. McCann, C. C. Williams, J. L. Sartin, C. R. Barb, and F. M. Kautz. 1997. Nitrogen metabolism and hormonal responses of steers fed wheat silage and infused with amino acids or casein. J. Anim. Sci. 75:3038–3045.

Rangngang, M. B., M. L. Nelson, and S. M. Parish. 1997. Ruminal undegradability of blood meal and effects of blood meal on ruminal and postruminal digestion in steers consuming vegetative orchardgrass hay. J. Anim. Sci. 75:2788–2795.

Reis, P. J., D. A. Tunks, and L. F. Sharry. 1989. Incorporation of abomasal and intravenous doses of [$^{35}$S] cysteine and [$^{35}$S] methionine into wool. J. Agric. Sci. 112:313–319.

Richardson, C. R., and E. E. Hatfield. 1978. The limiting amino acid in growing cattle. J. Anim. Sci. 46:740–745.

Rinne, M., S. Jaakkola, and P. Huhtanen. 1997. Grass maturity effects on cattle fed silage-based diets. 1. Organic matter digestion, rumen fermentation and nitrogen utilization. Anim. Feed Sci. Technol. 67:1–17.

Rioux, R., G. T. Dos Santos, H. V. Petit, and J. G. Proulx. 1995. Effect of cultivars on in vitro and ruminal degradation of the nitrogen fraction in birdsfoot trefoil silages. J. Dairy Sci. 78:1766–1773.

Robert, J. C., and P. E. V. Williams. 1997. Influence of forage type on the intestinal availability of methionine from a rumen protected form. J. Dairy Sci. 80(Suppl. 1):248. (Abstr.)

Robert, J. C., B. K. Sloan, and S. Bourdeau. 1994. The effects of supplementation of corn silage plus soybean meal diets with rumen protected methionine on the lactational performance of dairy cows in early lactation. J. Dairy Sci. 77(Suppl. 1):92. (Abstr.)

Robert, J. C., B. K. Sloan, N. Jouan, and J. Math. 1999. Influence of supplementation with protected methionine on the growth of heifers. J. Dairy Sci. 82(Suppl. 1):91. (Abstr.)

Robert, J. C., P. E. V. Williams, and B. Bouza. 1997. Influence of source of methionine and protection technology on the postruminal delivery and supply to the blood of dairy cows of an oral supply of methionine. J. Dairy Sci. 80(Suppl. 1):248. (Abstr.)

Robinson, P. H. 1997. Modifying duodenal flow of amino acids by manipulation of dietary protein sources. Can. J. Anim. Sci. 77:241–251.

Robinson, P. H., and J. J. Kennelly. 1988a. Ammonia or sulphur dioxide treatment of high-moisture barley on in situ rumen degradability and in situ whole-tract digestibility. Can. J. Anim. Sci. 68:779–786.

Robinson, P. H., and J. J. Kennelly. 1988b. Influence of intake of rumen undegradable protein on milk production of late lactation Holstein cows. J. Dairy Sci. 71:2135–2142.

Robinson, P. H., and J. J. Kennelly. 1988b. Influence of ammoniation of high moisture barley on its in situ rumen degradation and influence on rumen fermentation in dairy cows. Can. J. Anim. Sci. 68:839–851.

Robinson, P. H., and M. A. McNiven. 1994. Influence of flame roasting and feeding frequency of barley on performance of dairy cows. J. Dairy Sci. 77:3631–3643.

Robinson, P. H., and M. A. McNiven. 1993. Nutritive value of raw and roasted sweet white lupins (*Lupinus albus*) for lactating dairy cows. Anim. Feed Sci. Technol. 43:275–290.

Robinson, P. H., and R. E. McQueen. 1994. Influence of supplemental protein source and feeding frequency on rumen fermentation and performance in dairy cows. J. Dairy Sci. 77:1340–1353.

Robinson, P. H., and C. J. Sniffen. 1985. Forestomach and whole tract digestibility for lactating cows as influenced by feeding frequency. J. Dairy Sci. 68:857–867.

Robinson, P. H., M. Gill, and J. J. Kennelly. 1997. Influence of time of feeding a protein meal on ruminal fermentation and forestomach digestion in diary cows. J. Dairy Sci. 80:1366–1373.

Robinson, P. H., G. R. Khorasani, and J. J. Kennelly. 1994. Forestomach and whole tract digestion in lactating dairy cows fed canola meal treated with variable levels of acetic acid. J. Dairy Sci. 77:552–559.

Robinson, P. H., G. de Boer, and J. J. Kennelly. 1991a. Influence of source of rumen-degraded nitrogen and whole tract digestion, plasma hormone and metabolite concentrations as well as milk yield and composition in dairy cows. Can. J. Anim. Sci. 71:417–428.

Robinson, P. H., G. de Boer, and J. J. Kennelly. 1991b. Effect of bovine somatatropin and protein on rumen fermentation and forestomach and whole tract digestion in dairy cows. J. Dairy Sci. 74:3505–3517.

Robinson, P. H., R. E. McQueen, and P. L. Burgess. 1991c. Influence of rumen undegradable protein levels on feed intake and milk production of dairy cows. J. Dairy Sci. 74:1623–1631.

Robinson, P. H., C. J. Sniffen, and P. J. Van Soest. 1985. Influence of level of feed intake on digestion and bacterial yield in the forestomachs of dairy cattle. Can. J. Anim. Sci. 65:437–444.

Rode, L. M., and L. D. Satter. 1988. Effect of amount and length of alfalfa hay in diets containing barley or corn on site of digestion and rumen microbial protein synthesis in dairy cows. Can J. Anim. Sci. 68:445–454.

Rode, L. M., C. D. Knight, K. A. Andrews, and K. M. Koenig. 1998. Effects of pre- and post-partum Alimet® supplementation on milk production of dairy cows. J. Dairy Sci. 81(Suppl. 1):294. (Abstr.)

Rode, L. M., D. C. Weakley, and L. D. Satter. 1985. Effect of forage amount and particle size in diets of lactating dairy cows on site of digestion and microbial protein synthesis. Can. J. Anim. Sci. 65:101–111.

Rode, L., T. Fujieda, H. Sato, H. Suzuki, W. E. Julien, W. V. Chalupa, and C. J. Sniffen 1999. Rumen-protected amino (RPAA) acid supplementation pre- and postpartum in commercial herds. J. Dairy Sci. 82(Suppl. 1):121 (Abstr.)

Rodwell, V. W. 1985. Proteins. *In:* D. W. Martin, Jr., P. A. Mayes, V. W. Rodwell, and D. K. Granner (Ed.) Harper's Review of Biochemistry, Twentieth Edition. pp. 32–40. Lange Medical Publications, Los Altos, CA.

Roe, M. B., C. J. Sniffen, and L. E. Chase. 1990. Techniques for measuring protein fractions in feedstuffs. Proc. Cornell Nutr. Conf., p. 81–88, Ithaca, NY.

Roffler, R. E., J. E Wray, and L. D. Satter. 1986. Production responses in early lactation to additions of soybean meal to diets containing predominantly corn silage. J. Dairy Sci. 69:1055–1062.

Rogers, J. A., H. R. Conrad, B. A. Dehority, and J. A. Grubb. 1986. Microbial numbers, rumen fermentation, and nitrogen utilization of steers fed wet or dried brewers grains. J. Dairy Sci. 69:745–753.

Rogers, J A., U. Krishnamoorthy, and C. J. Sniffen. 1987. Plasma amino acids and milk protein production by cows fed rumen-protected methionine and lysine. J. Dairy Sci. 70:789–798.

Romagnolo, D., C. E. Polan, and W. E. Barbeau. 1994. Electrophoretic analysis of ruminal degradability of corn proteins. J. Dairy Sci. 77:1093–1099.

Rooke, J. A. 1985. The nutritive values of feed proteins and feed protein residues resistant to degradation by rumen microorganisms. J. Sci. Food Agric. 36:629–637.

Rooke, J A., H. A. Greife, and D. G. Armstrong. 1985. The digestion by cattle of silage-containing diets fed at two dry matter intakes. Br. J. Nutr. 53:691–708.

Roseler, D. K., J. D. Ferguson, C. J. Sniffen, and J. Herrema. 1993. Dietary protein degradability effects on plasma and milk urea nitrogen and milk nonprotein nitrogen in Holstein cows. J. Dairy Sci. 76:525–534.

Rulquin, H. 1987. Determination de certains acides amines limitants chez la vache laitiere par la methode administrations post-ruminales. Reprod. Nutr. Develop. 27(1B):299–300.

Rulquin, H., and L. Delaby. 1994. Lactational responses of dairy cows to graded amounts of rumen-protected methionine. J. Dairy Sci. 77(Suppl. 1):91 (Abstr.)

Rulquin, H., and L. Delaby. 1997. Effects of the energy balance of dairy cows on lactational responses to rumen-protected methionine. J. Dairy Sci. 80:2513–2522.

Rulquin. H., and R. Vérité. 1993. Amino acid nutrition of dairy cows: production effects and animal requirements. Pages 55–77 *in* Recent Advances in Animal Nutrition. P. C. Garnsworthy and D. J. A. Cole, eds. Nottingham University Press.

Rulquin, H., J. Guinard, and R. Vérité. 1998. Variation of amino acid content in the small intestine digesta of cattle: Development of a prediction model. Livestock Prod. Sci. 53:1–13.

Rulquin, H., C. Hurtaud, and L. Delaby. 1994. Effects of dietary protein level on lactational responses of dairy cows to rumen-protected methionine and lysine. Ann. Zootech. 43:245.

Rulquin, H., L. Le Henaff, and R. Vérité. 1990. Effects on milk protein yield of graded levels of lysine infused into the duodenum of dairy cows fed diets with two levels of protein. Reprod. Nutr. Dev. 30(Suppl. 2):238 (Abstr.).

Rulquin, H., P. M. Pisulewski, R. Vérité, and J. Guinard. 1993. Milk production and composition as a function of postruminal lysine and methionine supply: a nutrient-response approach. Livest. Prod. Sci., 37:69–90.

Rulquin, H., R. Vérité, J. Guinard, and P. M. Pisulewski. 1995. Dairy cows requirements for amino acids. Pages 143–160 *in* Animal Science Research and Development: Moving Toward a New Century. M. Ivan, ed., ISBN 0-662-23589-4, Centre for Food and Animal Research, Ottawa, Canada.

Russell, J. B., and C. J. Sniffen. 1984. Effect of carbon-4 and carbon-5 volatile fatty acids on growth of mixed rumen bacteria in vitro. J. Dairy Sci. 67:987–994.

Russell, J. B., C. J. Sniffen, and P. J. Van Soest. 1983. Effect of carbohydrate limitation on degradation and utilization of casein by mixed rumen bacteria. J. Dairy Sci. 66:763–775.

Russell, J. B., H. J. Strobel, and G. Chen. 1988. Enrichment and isolation of a ruminal bacterium with a very high specific activity of ammonia production. Appl. Environ. Microbiol. 54: 872–877.

Russell, J. B., J. D. O'Connor, D. G. Fox, P. J. Van Soest, and C. J. Sniffen. 1992. A net carbohydrate and protein system for evaluating cattle diets: I. Ruminal fermentation. J. Anim. Sci. 70:3551–3561.

Salter, D. N., K. Daneshaver, and R. H. Smith. 1979. The origin of nitrogen incorporated into compounds in the rumen bacteria of steers given protein- and urea-containing diets. Br. J. Nutr. 41:197–209.

Santos, F. A. P., J. E. P. Santos, C. B. Theurer, and J. T. Huber. 1998a. Effects of rumen-undegradable protein on dairy cow performance: A 12-year literature review. J. Dairy Sci. 81:3182–3213.

Santos, F. A. P., J. T. Huber, C. B. Theurer, R. S. Swingle, J. M. Simas, K. H. Chen, and P. Yu. 1998b. Milk yield and composition of lactating cows fed steam-flaked sorghum and graded concentrations of ruminally degradable protein. J. Dairy Sci. 81:215–220.

Santos, K. A., M. D. Stern, and L. D. Satter. 1984. Protein degradation in the rumen and amino acid absorption in the small intestine of lactating dairy cattle fed various protein sources. J. Anim. Sci. 58:244–255.

Sarwar, M., J. L. Firkins, and M. L. Eastridge. 1991. Effect of replacing neutral detergent fiber of forage with soyhulls and corn gluten feed for dairy heifers. J. Dairy Sci. 74:1006–1017.

Satter, L. D. 1986. Protein supply from undegraded dietary protein. J. Dairy Sci. 69:2734–2749.

Sauvant D., and J. van Milgen. 1995. Dynamic aspects of carbohydrate and protein breakdown and the associated microbial matter synthesis. *In* Ruminant Physiology: Digestion, Metabolism, Growth and Reproduction: Proceedings of the Eighth International Symposium on Ruminant Physiology. Ferdinand Enke Verlag, Stuttgart, Germany.

Schingoethe, D. J., D. P. Casper, C. Yang, D. J. Illg, J. L. Sommerfeldt, and C. R. Mueller. 1988. Lactational response to soybean meal, heated soybean meal, and extruded soybeans with ruminally protected methionine. J. Dairy Sci. 71:173–180.

Schroeder, G. E., L. J. Erasmus, and H. H. Meissner. 1996. Chemical and protein quality parameters of heat processed sunflower oilcake for dairy cattle. Anim. Feed Sci. Technol. 58:249–265.

Schwab, C. G. 1995a. Protected proteins and amino acids for ruminants. Pages 115–141 *in* R.J. Wallace and A. Chesson, eds. Biotechnology in Animal Feeds and Animal Feeding. V.C.H. Press, Weinheim, Germany.

Schwab, C. G. 1995b. Rumen-protected amino acids—their role in nutrition of high-producing ruminants. Pages 161–175 *in* M. Ivan, ed., Animal Science Research and Development: Moving Toward a New Century. ISBN 0-662-23589-4, Centre for Food and Animal Research, Ottawa, Canada.

Schwab, C. G. 1996a. Amino acid nutrition of the dairy cow: Current status. Proc. Cornell Nutr. Conf., p. 184–198, Ithaca, NY.

Schwab, C. G. 1996b. Rumen-protected amino acids for dairy cattle: Progress towards determining lysine and methionine requirements. Anim. Feed Sci. Technol. 59:87–101.

Schwab, C. G., C. K. Bozak, N. L. Whitehouse, and M.M.A. Mesbah. 1992a. Amino acid limitation and flow to the duodenum at four stages of lactation. I. Sequence of lysine and methionine limitation. J. Dairy Sci. 75:3486–3502.

Schwab, C. G., C. K. Bozak, N. L. Whitehouse, and V. M. Olson. 1992b. Amino acid limitation and flow to duodenum at four stages of lactation. 2. Extent of lysine limitation. J. Dairy Sci. 75:3503–3518.

Schwab, C. G., L. D. Satter, and A. B. Clay. 1976. Response of lactating dairy cows to abomasal infusion of amino acids. J. Dairy Sci. 59:1254–1270.

Schwab, C. G., S. J. Muise, W. E. Hylton, and J. J. Moore, III. 1982. Response to abomasal infusion of methionine of weaned dairy calves fed a complete pelleted starter ration based on by-product feeds. J. Dairy Sci. 65:1950–1961.

Scollan, N. D., H. J. Kim, W. J. Maeng, H. Park, M. A. Neville, R.T. Evans, and A. B. McAllan. 1996. The effect of cereal carbohydrate supplementation on nutrient flow to the duodenum and microbial protein synthesis in steers fed grass silage. *In* Proceedings of the XI the International Silage Conference (Jones, D. I. H. et al., eds.) pp. 228–229.

Sebek, L. B., and H. Everts. 1999. *In situ* degradation of dry matter and crude protein in ewes and dairy cows. Anim. Sci. 68:801–808.

Seymour, W. M., and C. E. Polan. 1986. Dietary energy regulation during gestation on subsequent lactational response to soybean meal or dried brewers grains. J. Dairy Sci. 69:2837–2845.

Seymour, W. M., C. E. Polan, and J. H. Herbein. 1992. In vivo degradation of protein in diets formulated for two degradabilities. J. Dairy Sci. 75:2447–2453.

Shabi, Z., A. Arieli, I. Bruckental, Y. Aharoni, S. Zamwel, A. Bor, and H. Tagari. 1998. Effect of the synchronization of the degradation of dietary crude protein and organic matter and feeding frequency on ruminal fermentation and flow of digesta in the abomasum of dairy cows. J. Dairy Sci. 81:1991–2000.

Sharma, B. K., and R. A. Erdman. 1988. Abomasal infusion of choline and methionine with or without 2-amino-2-methyl-1-propanol for lactating dairy cows. J. Dairy Sci. 71:2406–2411.

Sharma, B. K., and R. A. Erdman. 1989. Effects of dietary and abomasally infused choline on milk production responses of lactating dairy cows. J. Nutr. 119:248–254.

Sicilano-Jones, J. L. Personal communication.

Siddons, R. C., and J. Paradine. 1983. Protein degradation in the rumen of sheep and cattle. J. Sci. Food and Agric. 34:701–708.

Sidhu, G. S., and J. R. Ashes. 1977. Amino acid availability from protected protein—a critical factor for response in milk production. Proc. Nutr. Soc. Aust. 2:81. (Abstr.)

Sievert, S. J., and R. D. Shaver. 1993. Effect of nonfiber carbohydrate level and *Aspergillus oryzae* fermentation extract on intake, digestion, and milk production in lactating dairy cows. J. Anim. Sci. 71:1032–1040.

Sinclair, L. A., P. C. Garnsworthy, J. R. Newbold, and P. J. Buttery. 1993. Effect of synchronizing the rate of dietary energy and nitrogen release on rumen fermentation and microbial protein synthesis in sheep. J. Agric. Sci. Camb. 120:251–263.

Sinclair, L. A., P. C. Garnsworthy, J. R. Newbold, and P. J. Buttery. 1995. Effects of synchronizing the rate of dietary energy and nitrogen release in diets with similar carbohydrate composition on rumen fermentation and microbial protein synthesis in sheep. J. Agric. Sci. 124:463–472.

Singh, C. K., P. H. Robinson, and M. A. McNiven. 1995. Evaluation of raw and roasted lupin seeds as protein supplements for lactating cows. Anim. Feed Sci. Technol. 52:63–76.

Sloan, B. K., B. D. Garthwaite, and C. G. Schwab. 1998. Practical formulation of dairy cow diets for digestible amino acids to improve nitrogen efficiency and the bottom line. Proc. Cornell Nutr. Conf., p. 51–64, Ithaca, NY.

Sloan, B. K., P. Rowlinson, and D. G. Armstrong. 1988. The influence of a formulated excess of rumen degradable protein or undegradable protein on milk production in dairy cows in early lactation. Anim. Prod. 46:13–22.

Sniffen, C. J. 1974. Nitrogen utilization as related to solubility of NPN and protein in feeds. Proc. Cornell Nutr. Conf., p. 12–18, Ithaca, NY.

Sniffen, C. J., J. D. O'Connor, P. J. Van Soest, D. G. Fox, and J. B. Russell. 1992. A net carbohydrate and protein system for evaluating cattle diets: II. carbohydrate and protein availability. J. Anim. Sci., 70:3562–3577.

Sniffen, C. J., C. S. Ballard, D. S. Tsang, W. Chalupa, W. E. Julien, B. Perkins, T. Fujieda, T. Ueda, and H. Suzuki. 1999a. Effect of rumen-protected amino acids (RPAA) on performance of lactating Holstein cows. J. Dairy Sci. 82(Suppl. 1):94. (Abstr.)

Sniffen, C. J., D. S. Tsang, C. S. Ballard, W. Chalupa, W. E. Julien, T. Fujieda, T. Ueda, H. Sato, and H. Suzuki. 1999b. Effect of rumen-protected lysine and methionine supplementation with different sources of metabolizable protein on milk production of high producing dairy cows. J. Dairy Sci. 82(Suppl. 1):94. (Abstr.)

Socha, M. T. 1994. Determining the methionine requirements of lactating dairy cows. Thesis. Ph. D. dissertation University of New Hampshire. 174 p.

Socha, M. T., C. G. Schwab, D. E. Putnam, N. A. Kierstead, N. L. Whitehouse, B. D. Garthwaite, and G. A. Ducharme. 1994a. Determining methionine requirements of dairy cows during midlactation by postruminally infusing incremental amounts of methionine. J. Dairy Sci. 77(Suppl. 1):93. (Abstr.)

Socha, M. T., C. G. Schwab, D. E. Putnam, N. A. Kierstead, N. L. Whitehouse, B. D. Garthwaite, and G. A. Ducharme. 1994c. Determining methionine requirements of dairy cows during peak lactation by postruminally infusing incremental amounts of methionine. J. Dairy Sci. 77(Suppl. 1):92. (Abstr.)

Socha, M. T., C. G. Schwab, D. E. Putnam, N. L. Whitehouse, N. A. Kierstead, B. D. Garthwaite, and G. A. Ducharme. 1994b. Determining methionine requirements of dairy cows during early lactation by postruminally infusing incremental amounts of methionine. J. Dairy Sci. 77(Suppl. 1):65. (Abstr.)

Song, M. K., and J. J. Kennelly. 1989. Effect of ammoniated barley silage on ruminal fermentation, nitrogen supply to the small intestine, ruminal and whole tract digestion, and milk production of Holstein cows. J. Dairy Sci. 72:2981–2990.

Spain, J. N., C. E. Polan, and B. A. Watkins. 1995. Evaluating effects of fish meal on milk fat yield of dairy cows. J. Dairy Sci. 78:1142–1153.

Spicer, L. A., C. B. Theurer, J. Sowe, and T. H. Noon. 1986. Ruminal and postruminal utilization of nitrogen and starch from sorghum grain, corn, and barley based diets by beef steers. J. Anim Sci. 65:521–529.

Stallings, C. C., Y. M. Acosta, and C. E. Polan. 1991. Predicting diet protein degradability from individual ingredient estimations in diets containing barley silages. J. Dairy Sci. 74:3486–3491.

Staples, C. R., W. W. Thatcher, and J. H. Clark. 1990. Relationship between ovarian activity and energy status during the early postpartum period of high producing dairy cows. J. Dairy Sci. 73:938–947.

Stanford, K., T. A. McAllister, B. M. Lees, Z. J. Xu, and K. J. Cheng. 1996. Comparison of sweet white lupin seed, canola meal and soybean meal as protein supplements for lambs. Can. J. Anim. Sci. 76:215–219.

Steg, A., W. M. van Straalen, V. A. Hindle, W. A. Wesink, F. M. H. Dooper, and R. L. M. Schils. 1994. Rumen degradation and intestinal digestion of grass and clover at two maturity levels during the season in dairy cows. Grass Forage Sci. 49:378–390.

Stensig, T., and P. H. Robinson. 1997. Digestion and passage kinetics of forage fiber in dairy cows as affected by fiber-free concentrate in the diet. J. Dairy Sci. 80:1339–1352.

Stern, M. D., A. Bach, and S. Calsamiglia. 1997. Alternative techniques for measuring nutrient digestion in ruminants. J. Anim Sci. 75:2256–2276.

Stern, M. D., and L. D. Satter. 1984. Evaluation of nitrogen solubility and the dacron bag technique as methods for estimating protein degradation in the rumen. J. Anim. Sci. 58:714–724.

Stern, M. D., G. A. Varga, J. H. Clark, J. L. Firkins, J. T. Huber, and D. L. Palmquist 1994. Evaluation of chemical and physical properties of feeds that affect protein metabolism in the rumen. J. Dairy Sci. 77:2762–2786.

Stern, M. D., K. A. Santos, and L. D. Satter. 1985. Protein degradation in rumen and amino acid absorption in small intestine of lactating cattle fed heat-treated whole soybeans. J. Dairy Sci. 68:45–56.

Stern, M. D., L. M. Rode, R. W. Prange, R. H. Stauffacher, and L. D. Satter. 1983. Ruminal protein degradation of corn gluten meal in lactating dairy cattle fitted with duodenal T-type cannulae. J. Anim. Sci. 56:194–205.

Stern, M. D., W. H. Hoover, C. J. Sniffen, B. A. Crooker, and P. H. Knowlton. 1978. Effects of nonstructural carbohydrate, urea and soluble protein level on microbial protein synthesis in continuous culture of rumen contents. J. Anim. Sci. 47:944–951.

Stokes, S. R., W. H. Hoover, T. K. Miller, and R. P. Manski. 1991a. Impact of carbohydrate and protein levels on bacterial metabolism in continuous culture. J. Dairy Sci. 74:860–870.

Stokes, S. R., W. H. Hoover, T. K. Miller, and R. Blauweikel. 1991b. Ruminal digestion and microbial utilization of diets varying in type of carbohydrates and protein. J. Dairy Sci. 74:871–881.

Storm, E., and E. R. Ørskov. 1983. The nutritive value of rumen microorganisms in ruminants. 1. Large scale isolation and chemical composition of rumen micro-organisms. Br. J. Nutr. 50:463–470.

Stutts, J. A., W. A. Nipper, R. W. Adkinson, J. E. Chandler, and A. S. Achacoso. 1988. Protein solubility, in vitro ammonia concentration, and in situ disappearance of extruded whole cottonseed and other protein sources. J. Dairy Sci. 71:3323–3333.

Subuh, A.M.H., T. G. Rowan, and T.L.J. Lawrence. 1994. Effect of heat or formaldehyde treatment and differences in basal diet on the rumen degradability of protein in soyabean meal and in rapeseed meals of different glucosinolate content. Anim. Feed Sci. Technol. 49:297–310.

Susmel, P., C. R. Mills, M. Colitti, and B. Stefanon. 1993. In vitro solubility and degradability of nitrogen in concentrate ruminant feeds. Anim. Feed Sci. Technol. 42:1–13.

Susmel, P., M. Spanghero, B. Stefanon, C. R. Mills, and C. Cargnelutti. 1991. Effect of NDF concentration and physical form of fescue hay on rumen degradability, intake, and rumen turn-over of cows. Anim. Prod. 53:305–313.

Susmel, P., B. Stefanon, C. R. Mills, and M. Spanghero. 1990. Rumen degradability of organic matter, nitrogen and fibre fractions in forages. Anim. Prod. 51:515–526.

Swanson, E. W. 1977. Factors for computing requirements of protein for maintenance of cattle. J. Dairy Sci. 60:1583–1593.

Swanson, E.W. 1982. Estimation of metabolic protein requirements to cover unavoidable losses of endogenous nitrogen in maintenance of cattle. Pp. 183–197 in Protein Requirement for Cattle: Symposium. F.N. Owens, ed. MP-109, Oklahoma State University, Stillwater.

Tamminga, S., R. Ketelaar, and A. M. van Vuuren. 1991. Degradation of nitrogenous compounds in conserved forages in the rumen of dairy cows. Grass Forage Sci. 46:427–435.

Tamminga, S., van der Koelen, C. J., and van Vuuren, A. M. 1979. Effect of the level of feed intake on nitrogen entering the small intestine of dairy cows. Livestock Prod. Sci. 6:255–262.

Teller, E., M. Vanbelle, M. Foulon, G. Collignon, and B. Matatu. 1992. Nitrogen metabolism in rumen and whole digestive tract of lactating dairy cows fed grass silage. J. Dairy Sci. 75:1296–1304.

Tesfa, A. T. 1993. Effects of rape-seed oil supplementation on digestion, microbial protein synthesis and duodenal microbial amino acid composition in ruminants. Anim. Feed Sci. Technol. 41:313–328.

Tice, E. M., M. L. Eastridge, and J. L. Firkins. 1993. Raw soybeans and roasted soybeans of different particle sizes. 1. Digestibility and utilization by lactating cows. J. Dairy Sci. 76:224–235.

Titgemeyer, E. C., and N. R. Merchen. 1990a. Sulfur-containing amino acid requirements of rapidly growing steers. J. Anim. Sci. 68:2075–2083.

Titgemeyer, E. C., and N. R. Merchen. 1990b. The effect of abomasal methionine supplementation on nitrogen retention of growing steers postruminally infused with casein or nonsulfur-containing amino acids. J. Anim. Sci. 68:750–757.

Titgemeyer, E. C., N. R. Merchen, and L. L. Berger. 1989. Evaluation of soybean meal, corn gluten meal, blood meal and fish meal as sources of nitrogen and amino acids disappearing from the small intestine of steers. J. Anim. Sci., 67:262–275.

Titgemeyer, E. C., N. R. Merchen, L. L. Berger, and L. E. Deetz. 1988. Estimates of lysine and methionine requirements of growing steers fed corn silage-based or corn-based diets. J. Dairy Sci. 71:421–434.

Todorov, N. A., and D. G. Griginov. 1991. Comparison of the infusion method, mobile bag technique and in vitro method for determination of the true protein digestibility in small intestine of cattle. 6th Int. Symp. Protein Metabolism and Nutrition Herning, Denmark, p. 80–82.

Uden, P., and P. J. Van Soest. 1984. Investigations of the *in situ* bag technique and a comparison of the fermentation in heifers, sheep, ponies and rabbits. J. Anim. Sci. 58:213–221.

Van Barneveld, R. J., E. S. Batterham, and B. W. Norton. 1994a. The effects of heat on amino acids for growing pigs. 1. A comparison of ileal and faecal digestibilities of amino acids in raw and heat-treated field peas (Pisum sativum cultivar Dundale). Br. J. Nutr. 72:243–256.

Van Barneveld, R. J., E. S. Batterham, and B. W. Norton. 1994b. The effects of heat on amino acids for growing pigs. 2. Utilization of ileal-digestible lysine from heat-treated field peas (Pisum sativum cultivar Dundale). Br. J. Nutr. 72:221–241.

Van Barneveld, R. J., E. S. Batterham, and B. W. Norton. 1994c. The effects of heat on amino acids for growing pigs. 3. The availability of lysine from heat-treated field peas (Pisum sativum cultivar Dundale) determined using the slope-ratio assay.. Br. J. Nutr. 72:257–275.

van der Aar, P. J., L. L. Berger, G. C. Fahey, Jr., and N. R. Merchen. 1984. Effects of alcohol treatment of soybean meal on ruminal escape of soybean meal protein. J. Anim. Sci. 59:483–489.

van der Koelan, C. J., P. W. Goedhart, A. M. van Vuuren, and G. Savoini. 1992. Sources of variation of the in situ nylon bag technique. Anim. Feed Sci. Technol. 38:35–42.

Van Gylswyk, N. O. 1990. Enumeration and presumptive identification of some functional groups of bacteria in the rumen of dairy cows fed silage-based diets. FEMS Microbiol. Ecol. 73:243–254.

Van Kessel, J. S., and J. B. Russell. 1997. The endogenous polysaccharide utilization rate of mixed ruminal bacteria and the effect of energy starvation on ruminal fermentation rates. J. Dairy Sci. 80:2442–2448.

Van Soest, P. J. 1994. Nutritional Ecology of The Ruminant. Second Edition. Cornell University Press, Ithaca, NY.

Van Soest, P. J., N. L. Conklin, and P. J. Horvath. 1987. Tannins in foods and feeds. Proc. Cornell Nutr. Conf. For Feed Manufactures, Ithaca, NY, Cornell University, Syracuse, NY, p. 115–122.

van Straalen, W. M., and G. Huisman. 1991. The digestibility of bypass crude protein from grass silage in the intestine of dairy cows measured by the mobile nylon bag technique. 6th Int. Symp. Protein Metabolism and Nutrition Herning, Denmark, p. 83–85.

van Straalen, W. M., F. M. H. Dooper, A. M. Antoniewicz, I. Kosmala, and A. M. van Vuuren. 1993. Intestinal digestibility in dairy cows of protein from grass and clover measured with mobile nylon bag and other methods. J. Dairy Sci. 76:2970–2981.

van Straalen, W. M., J. J. Odinga, and W. Mostert. 1997. Digestion of feed amino acids in the rumen and small intestine of dairy cows measured with nylon-bag techniques. Br. J. Nutr. 77:83–97.

van Vuuren, A. M., C. J. van der Koelen, and J. Vroons-de Bruin. 1993. Ryegrass versus corn starch or beet pulp fiber diet effects on digestion and intestinal amino acids in dairy cows. J. Dairy Sci. 76:2692–2700.

van Vuuren, A. M., F. Krol-Kramer, R. A. van der Lee, and H. Corbijn. 1992. Protein digestion and intestinal amino acids in dairy cows fed fresh *Lolium perenne* with different nitrogen contents. J. Dairy Sci. 75:2215–2225.

van Vuuren, A. M., S. Tamminga, and R. S. Ketelaar. 1991. In sacco degradation of organic matter and crude protein of fresh grass (*Lolium perenne*) in the rumen of grazing cows. J. Agric. Sci. (Camb.) 116:429–436.

van Vuuren, A. M., K. Bergsma, F. Krol-Kramer, and J.A.C. van Beers. 1989. Effects of addition of cell wall degrading enzymes on the chemical composition and the in sacco degradation of grass silage. Grass Forage Sci. 44:223–230.

Valentine, S. C., and B. D. Bartsch. 1988. Degradation of dry matter, crude protein, fat, crude fibre and nitrogen-free-extract in milled barley and lupin grains incubated in nylon bags in the rumen of dairy cows. J. Agric. Sci. (Camb.) 110:395–398.

Vanhatalo, A., and E. Ketoja. 1995. The role of the large intestine in post-ruminal digestion of feeds as measured by the mobile-bag method in cattle. Br. J. Nutr. 73:491–505.

Vanhatalo, A., and T. Varvikko. 1995. Effect of rumen degradation on intestinal digestion of nitrogen of $^{15}$N-labelled rapeseed meal and straw measured by the mobile-bag method in cows. J. Agric. Sci. (Camb.). 125:253–261.

Vanhatalo, A., I. Aronen, and T. Varvikko. 1995. Intestinal nitrogen digestibility of heat-moisture treated rapeseed meals as assessed by the mobile-bag method in cows. Anim. Feed Sci. Technol. 55:139–152.

Vanhatalo, A., P. Dakowski, and P. Huhtanen. 1996. Effects of stage of growth and duration of rumen incubation time on intestinal digestibility of rumen-undegradable nitrogen of grass by mobile-bag method in cows. Acta Agric. Scand., Sect. A, Anim. Sci. 46:1–10.

Vanhatalo, A., P. Huhtanen, V. Toivonen, and T. Varvikko. 1999. Response of dairy cows fed grass silage diets to abomasal infusions of histidine alone or in combinations with methionine and lysine. J. Dairy Sci. 82:2674–2685.

Vanzant, E. S., R. C. Cochran, and E. C. Titgemeyer. 1998. Standardization of in situ techniques for ruminant feedstuff evaluation. J. Anim. Sci. 76:2717–2729.

Vanzant, E. S., R. C. Cochran, E. E. Titgemeyer, S. D. Stafford, K. C. Olson, D. E. Johnson, and G. St. Jean. 1996. In vivo and in situ measurements of forage protein degradation in beef cattle. J. Anim. Sci. 74:2773–2784.

Varvikko, T., A. Vanhatalo, T. Jalava, and P. Huhtanen. 1999. Lactation and metabolic responses to graded abomasal doses of methionine and lysine in cows fed grass silage diets. J. Dairy Sci. 82:2659–2673.

Varvikko, T., and A. Vanhatalo. 1992. Effect of supplementary energy and protein feeding on the true digestion of grass-silage organic matter, cell walls and nitrogen estimated by the combined synthetic-fiber-bag method in cows. Can. J. Anim. Sci. 72:671–678.

Vasquez-Anon, M., A. J. Heinrichs, J. M. Aldrich, and G. A. Varga. 1993. Effect of postweaning age on rate of protein disappearance in calves weaned at 5 weeks of age. J. Dairy Sci. 76:2749–2757.

Veira, D. M., J. R. Seoane, and J. G. Proulx. 1991. Utilization of grass silage by growing cattle: Effect of a supplement containing ruminally protected amino acids. J. Anim. Sci. 69:4703–4709.

Vérité, R., and J. L. Peyraud. 1989. Protein: the PDI system. In : Jarrige, R. (Ed.): Ruminant Nutrition: Recommended Allowances and Feed Tables. INRA. John Libbey, Paris. pp. 33–48.

Vicini, J. L., J. H. Clark, W. L. Hurley, and J. M. Bahr. 1988. Effects of abomasal or intravenous administration of arginine on milk production, milk composition, and concentrations of somatotropin and insulin in plasma of dairy cows. J. Dairy Sci. 71:658–665.

Vieira, R.A.M., J. Pereira, P.A.M. Malafaia, and A. C. de Queiroz. 1997. The influence of elephant-grass (*Pennisetum purpureum* Schum., Mineiro variety) growth on the nutrient kinetics in the rumen. Anim. Feed Sci. Technol. 67:151–161.

Vik-Mo, L. 1989. Degradability of forages in sacco. 2. Silages of grasses and red clover at two cutting times, with formic acid and without additive. Acta Agric. Scand. 39:53–64.

Virtanen, A. I. 1966. Milk production of cows on protein-free feed. Science. 153:1603–1614.

Voigt, J., B. Piatkowski, H. Englemann, and E. Rudolph. 1985. Measurement of the postruminal digestibility of crude protein by the bag technique in cows. Arch. Tierernaehr. 8:555–562.

Volden, H. 1999. Effects of level of feeding and ruminally undegraded protein on ruminal bacterial protein synthesis, escape of dietary protein, intestinal amino acid profile, and performance of dairy cows. J. Anim. Sci. 77:1905–1918.

Volden, H., and O. M. Harstad. 1995. Effect of rumen incubation on the true digestibility of feed protein in the digestive tract determined by nylon bag techniques. Acta Agric. Scand., Sect. A, Anim. Sci. 45:106–115.

von Keyserlingk, G.E.M., and G. W. Mathison. 1993. The effect of ruminal escape protein and ambient temperature on the efficiency of utilization of metabolizable energy by lambs. J. Anim. Sci. 71:2206–2217.

von Keyserlingk, M.A.G., and G. W. Mathison. 1989. Use of the in situ technique and passage rate constants in predicting voluntary intake and apparent digestibility of forages by steers. Can. J. Anim. Sci. 69:973–987.

von Keyserlingk, M. A. G., J. A. Shelford, R. Purchala, M. L. Swift, and L. J. Fisher. 1998. In situ disappearance of amino acids from the grass silages in the rumen and intestine of cattle. J. Dairy Sci. 81:140–149.

von Keyserlingk, M. A. G., M. L. Swift, R. Puchala, and J. A. Shelford. 1996. Degradability characteristics of dry matter and crude protein of forages in ruminants. Anim. Feed Sci. Technol. 57:291–311.

Voss, V. L., D. Stehr, L. D. Satter, and G. A. Broderick. 1988. Feeding lactating dairy cows proteins resistant to ruminal degradation. J. Dairy Sci. 71:2428–2439.

Waghorn, G. C., and R. L. Baldwin. 1984. Model of metabolite flux within mammary gland of the lactating cow. J. Dairy Sci. 67:531–544.

Wagner, D. G., and J. K. Loosli. 1967. Studies on the energy requirements of high- producing dairy cows. Cornell Exp. Agric. Stn. Mem. No. 400. Ithaca, N.Y., Cornell University Press.

Waldo, D. R., and B. P. Glenn. 1984. Comparison of new protein systems for lactating dairy cows. J. Dairy Sci. 67:1115–1133.

Walhain, P., M. Foucart, and A. Théwis. 1992. Influence of extrusion on ruminal and intestinal disappearance in sacco of pea (*Psium sativum*) proteins and starch. Anim. Feed Sci. Technol. 38:43–55.

Wallace, R. J. 1983. Hydrolysis of $^{14}$C-labelled proteins by rumen microorganisms and by proteolytic enzymes prepared from rumen bacteria. Br. J. Nutr. 50:345–355.

Wallace, R. J. 1985. Adsorption of soluble proteins to rumen bacteria and the role of adsorption in proteolysis. Br. J. Nutr. 53:399–408.

Wallace, R. J. 1994. Amino acid and protein synthesis, turnover, and breakdown by rumen microorganisms. In: Principles of Protein Metabolism in Ruminants (Asplund, J. M., ed.), pp 71–111, CRC Press, Boca Raton, Florida.

Wallace, R. J. 1996. Ruminal microbial metabolism of peptides and amino acids. J. Nutr. 126:1326S–1334S.

Wallace, R. J. 1997. Peptide metabolism and its efficiency in ruminant production. In Rumen Microbes and Digestive Physiology in Ruminants (Onodera, R. et al., eds.), pp 95–105. Japan Sci. Soc. Press, Tokyo/S Karger, Basel.

Wallace, R. J., and C. A. Munro. 1986. Influence of the rumen anaerobic fungus *Neocallimastix frontalis* on the proteolytic activity of a defined mixture of rumen bacteria growing on a solid substrate. Lett. Appl. Microbiol. 3:23–26.

Wallace, R. J., and K. N. Joblin. 1985. Proteolytic activity of a rumen anaerobic fungus. Fed. Eur. Microbiol. Soc. Microbial. Lett. 29:19.

Wallace, R. J., C, Atasoglu, and C. J. Newbold. 1999. Role of peptides in rumen microbial metabolism. Review. AJAS 12:139–147.

Waltz, D. M., and M. D. Stern. 1989. Evaluation of various methods for protecting soya-bean protein from degradation by rumen bacteria. Anim. Feed Sci. Technol. 25:111–122.

Waltz, D. M., M. D. Stern, and D. J. Illg. 1989. Effect of ruminal protein degradation of blood meal and feather meal on the intestinal amino acid supply to lactating cows. J. Dairy Sci. 72:1509–1518.

Wanderly, R. C., G. A. Alhadhrami, M. Pessarkli, J. L. Aquino-Ramos, and J. T. Huber. 1999. An assessment of the microbial colonization of forage in the rumen of dairy cows and camels. Anim. Feed Sci. Technol. 76:207–218.

Wang, Y., T. A. McAllister, M. D. Pickard, Z. Xu, L. M. Rode, and K. -J. Cheng. 1999. Effect of micronizing full fat canola seed on amino acid disappearance in the gastrointestinal tract of dairy cows. J. Dairy Sci. 82:537–544.

Wang, Y., T. A. McAllister, D. R. Zobell, M. D. Pickard, L. M. Rode, S. Mir, and K. J. Cheng. 1997. The effect of micronization of full-fat canola seed on digestion in the rumen and total tract of dairy cows. Can. J. Anim. Sci. 77:431–440.

Waters, C. J., M. A. Kitcherside, and A. J. F. Webster. 1992. Problems associated with estimating the digestibility of undegraded dietary nitrogen from acid-detergent insoluble nitrogen. Anim. Feed Sci. Technol. 39:279–291.

Wattiaux, M. A., D. K. Combs, and R. D. Shaver. 1994. Lactational responses to ruminally undegradable protein by dairy cows fed diets based on alfalfa silage. J. Dairy Sci. 77:1604–1617.

Webb, K. E., J. C. Matthews, and D. B. DiRienzo. 1992. Peptide absorption: A review of current concepts and future perspectives. J. Anim. Sci. 70:3248–3257.

Webster, A. J. F. 1987. Metabolizable protein- the U.K. approach. *In*: G. Alderman and R. Jarrige (eds.), Feed Evaluation and Protein Requirement System for Ruminants. Commission of European Communities, EUR 10657 EN, Luxembourg, p. 47–54.

Webster, A. J. F., M. A. Kitcherside, J. R. Keirby, and P. A. Hall. 1984. Evaluation of protein feeds for dairy cows. Anim. Prod. 8:548.

Weigel, D. J., J. P. Elliott, and J. H. Clark. 1997. Effects of amount and ruminal degradability of protein on nutrient digestibility and production by cows fed tallow. J. Dairy Sci. 80:1150–1159.

Weisbjerg, M. R., C. F., Boersting, and T. Hvelplund. 1992. The influence of tallow on rumen metabolism, microbial biomass synthesis and fatty acid composition of bacteria and protozoa. Acta Agric. Scand. 42:138–147.

Weisbjerg, M. R , T. Hvelplund, S. Hellberg, S. Olsson, and S. Sanne. 1996. Effective rumen degradability and intestinal digestibility of individual amino acids in different concentrates determined in situ. Anim. Feed Sci. Technol. 62:179–188.

Weiss, W. P., D. O. Erickson, G. M. Erickson, and G. R. Fisher. 1989. Barley distillers grains as a protein supplement for dairy cows. J. Dairy Sci. 72:980–987.

Wen-Shyg, P. C. C. Kuen-Jaw, K. Kwen-Sheng, H. Jenn-Chung, and Y. Bi. 1995. Studies on the protein degradabilities of feedstuffs in Taiwan. Anim. Feed Sci. Technol. 55:215–226.

Wessels, R. H., E. C. Titgemeyer, C. K. Armendariz, and G. St. Jean. 1996. Lasalocid effects on ruminal degradation of protein and postruminal supply of amino acids in Holstein steers. J. Dairy Sci. 79:1802–1808.

Wheeler, J. G., H. E. Amos, M. A. Froetschel, J. C. Coomer, T. Maddox, and J. M. Fernandez. 1995. Responses of early lactation cows fed winter and summer annual forages and undegradable intake protein. J. Dairy Sci. 78:2767–2781.

Wilkerson, V. A., T. J. Klopfenstein, and W. W. Stroup. 1995. A collaborative study of in situ forage protein degradation. J. Anim. Sci. 73:583–588.

Williams, A. P., and R. H. Smith. 1974. Concentrations of amino acids and urea in the plasma of the ruminating calf and estimation of the amino acid requirements. Br. J. Nutr. 32:421–433.

Windschitl, P. M. 1991. Lactational performance of high producing dairy cows fed diets containing salmon meal and urea. J. Dairy Sci. 74:3475–3485.

Windschitl, P. M., and M. D. Stern. 1988. Evaluation of calcium lignosulfonate-treated soybean meal as a source of rumen protected protein for dairy cattle. J. Dairy Sci. 71:3310–3322.

Wohlt, J. E., J. H. Clark, R. G. Derrig, and C. L. Davis. 1977. Valine, leucine, and isoleucine metabolism by lactating bovine mammary tissue. J. Dairy Sci. 60:1875–1882.

Wohlt, J. E., S. L. Chmiel, P. K. Zajac, L. Backer, D. B. Blethen, and J. L. Evans. 1991. Dry matter intake, milk yield and composition, and nitrogen use in Holstein cows fed soybean, fish, or corn gluten meals. J. Dairy Sci. 74:1609–1622.

Wright, T. C. 1996. Effects of rumen-undegradable protein and feed intake on milk protein production in dairy cows. Thesis. University of Guelph. 92 p.

Wu, Z., and L. D. Satter. 2000. Milk production during the complete lactation of dairy cows fed diets containing different amounts of protein. J. Dairy Sci. 83:1042–1051.

Wu, Z., C. Le Guilloux, and L. D. Satter. 1999. Supplementing rumen protected methionine to lactating cows fed different amounts of protein. J. Dairy Sci. 82(Suppl. 1):65. (Abstr.)

Wu, Z., R. J. Fisher, C. E. Polan, and C. G. Schwab. 1997. Lactational performance of cows fed low or high ruminally undegradable protein prepartum and supplemental methionine and lysine postpartum. J. Dairy Sci., 80:722–729.

Xu, S., J. H. Harrison, and R. E. Riley. 1996. Characteristics of nitrogen fractions and amino acids of feedstuffs common to the Pacific Northwest. Professional Anim. Scientist 12:223–237.

Xu, S., J. H. Harrison, W. Chalupa, C. Sniffen, W. Julien, H. Sato, T. Fujieda, H. Watanabe, T. Ueda, and H. Suzuki. 1998. The effect of ruminal bypass lysine and methionine on milk yield and composition of lactating cows. J. Dairy Sci. 81:1062–1077.

Yan, T., D. C. Patterson, F. J. Gordon, and D. J. Kilpatrick. 1998. Effects of bacterial inoculation of unwilted and wilted grass silages 1. Rumen microbial activity, silage nutrient degradability and digestibility. J. Agric. Sci. (Camb.) 131:103–112.

Yang, W. Z, K. A. Beauchemin, and L. M. Rode. 1999. Effects of an enzyme feed additive on extent of digestion and milk production of lactating dairy cows. J. Dairy Sci. 82:391–403.

Yang, W. Z., K. A. Beauchemin, K. M. Koenig, and L. M. Rode. 1997. Comparison of hull-less barley, barley, or corn for lactating cows: Effects on extent of digestion and milk production. J. Dairy Sci. 80:2475–2486.

Yang, W. Z., K. A. Beauchemin, and L. M. Rode. 1996. Ruminal digestion kinetics of temper-rolled hulless barley. Can. J. Anim. Sci. 76:629–632.

Yang, C.-M.J., D. J. Schingoethe, and D. P. Casper. 1986. Protected methionine and heat-treated soybean meal for high producing dairy cows. J. Dairy Sci. 69:2348–2357.

Yong-Gang, L., A. Steg, and V. A. Hindle. 1994. Rumen degradation and intestinal digestion of crambe and other oilseed by-products in dairy cows. Anim. Feed Sci. Technol. 45:397–409.

Yoon, I. K., and M. D. Stern. 1996. Effects of *Saccharomyces cerevisiae* and *Aspergillus oryzae* cultures on ruminal fermentation in dairy cows. J. Dairy Sci. 79:411–417.

Yoon, I. K., K. J. Lindquist, D. D. Hongerholt, M. D. Stern, B. A. Crooker, and K. D. Short. 1996. Variation in menhaden fish meal characteristics and their effects on ruminal protein degradation as assessed by various techniques. Anim. Feed Sci. Technol. 60:13–27.

Young, V. R., and A. E. El-Khoury. 1995. The notion of the nutritional essentiality of amino acids revisited with a note of the indispensable amino acid requirements in adults. *In* Amino Acid Metabolism and Therapy in Health and Nutritional Disease (L. Cynober, ed), pp. 191–233, CRC Press, Boca Raton, FL, USA.

Younker, R. S., S. D. Winland, J. L. Firkins, and B. L. Hull. 1998. Effects of replacing forage fiber or nonfiber carbohydrates with dried brewers grains. J. Dairy Sci. 81:2645–2656.

Yu, Y., and J. W. Thomas. 1976. Estimation of the extent of heat damage in alfalfa haylage by laboratory measurement. J. Anim. Sci. 42:766–774.

Zerbini, E., and C. E. Polan. 1985. Protein sources evaluated for ruminating Holstein calves. J. Dairy Sci. 68:1416–142

Zerbini, E., C. E. Polan, and J. H. Herbein. 1988. Effect of dietary soybean meal and fish meal on protein digesta flow in Holstein cows during early and midlactation. J. Dairy Sci. 71:1248–1258.

Zhu, J. S., S. R. Stokes, and M. R. Murphy. 1997. Substitution of neutral detergent fiber from forage with neutral detergent fiber from by-products in the diets of lactating cows. J. Dairy Sci. 80:2901–2906.

Zimmerman, C. A., A. H. Rakes, R. D. Jaquette, B. A. Hopkins, and W. J. Croom, Jr. 1991. Effects of protein level and forage source on milk production and composition in early lactation dairy cows. J. Dairy Sci. 74:980–990.

Zimmerman, C. A., A. H. Rakes, T. E. Daniel, and B. A. Hopkins. 1992. Effect of total and rumen undegradable protein on the performance of cows fed low fiber diets. J. Dairy Sci. 75:1954–1964.

Zinn, R. A. 1993a. Characteristics of ruminal and total tract digestion of canola meal and soybean meal in a high-energy diet for feedlot cattle. J. Anim. Sci. 71:796–801.

Zinn, R. A. 1993b. Influence of processing on the comparative feeding value of barley for feedlot cattle. J. Anim. Sci. 71:3–10.

Zinn, R. A. 1995. Characteristics of digestion of linted and lint-free cottonseed in diets for feedlot cattle. J. Anim. Sci. 73:1246–1250.

Zinn, R. A., 1988. Crude protein and amino acid requirements of growing-finishing Holstein steers gaining 1.43 kilograms per day. J. Anim. Sci. 66:1755–1763.

Zinn, R. A., A. Plascencia, and R. Barajas. 1994. Interaction of forage level and monensin in diets for feedlot cattle on growth performance and digestive function. J. Anim. Sci. 72:2209–2215.

Zinn, R. A., and A. Plascencia. 1993. Interaction of whole cottonseed and supplemental fat on digestive function in cattle. J. Anim. Sci. 71:11–17.

Zinn, R. A., and Y. Shen. 1998. An evaluation of ruminally degradable intake protein and metabolizable amino acid requirements of feedlot calves. J. Anim. Sci. 76:1280–1289.

Zinn, R. A., C. F. Adam, and M. S. Tamayo. 1995. Interaction of feed intake level on comparative ruminal and total tract digestion of dry-rolled and steam-flaked corn. J. Anim. Sci. 73:1239–1245.

Zinn, R. A., Y. Shen, C. F. Adam, M. Tamayo, and J. Rosalez. 1996. Influence of dietary magnesium level on metabolic and growth-performance responses of feedlot cattle to laidlomycin propionate. J. Anim. Sci. 74:1462–1469.

# 6 Minerals

A number of inorganic elements are essential for normal growth and reproduction of animals. Those required in gram quantities are referred to as macrominerals and this group includes calcium, phosphorus, sodium, chlorine, potassium, magnesium, and sulfur. The macrominerals are important structural components of bone and other tissues and serve as important constituents of body fluids. They play vital roles in the maintenance of acid-base balance, osmotic pressure, membrane electric potential and nervous transmission. Those elements required in milligram or microgram amounts are referred to as the trace minerals. This group includes cobalt, copper, iodine, iron, manganese, molybdenum, selenium, zinc, and perhaps chromium and fluorine. Other elements have been suggested to be essential based on studies in other species but these are generally not considered to ever be of practical importance in dairy cattle. The trace minerals are present in body tissues in very low concentrations and often serve as components of metalloenzymes and enzyme cofactors, or as components of hormones of the endocrine system. A factorial approach was used to describe the requirements for both the macro- and trace minerals whenever such an approach could be supported by research data.

Maintenance requirements as described in this model will include the endogenous fecal losses and insensible urinary losses. Though technically not correct, it will also include losses incurred through sweat. The lactation requirement will be defined as the concentration of the mineral in milk multiplied by the 4 percent FCM milk yield. The pregnancy requirement is defined as the amount of mineral retained within the reproductive tract (fetus, uterine contents, and uterus) at each day of gestation. For most minerals, the requirement of the animal pregnant for <190 days is small and not considered in the model. The growth requirement is expressed as the amount of mineral retained/kg body weight gained and entered into the model as expected average daily gain (ADG).

The sum of the maintenance, lactation, pregnancy, and growth requirements is the true requirement of the tissues for the mineral, and is referred to as the "requirement for absorbed mineral." The diet must supply this amount to the tissues. Not all the mineral in a diet is available for absorption. Where data permitted, the availability of minerals from forages, concentrates, and inorganic sources was assigned an absorption coefficient. The model evaluates the absorbable mineral content of a diet by determining the available mineral provided by each constituent of the diet and comparing the sum of the amount of mineral available from the diet with the requirement of the animal for absorbed mineral.

For all minerals considered essential, detrimental effects on animal performance can be demonstrated from feeding excessive amounts. Generally, the dietary amount required for optimal performance is well below amounts found to be detrimental to performance. However, toxicity from several of the essential minerals, including fluorine, selenium, molybdenum, and copper are unfortunately problems that can occur under practical feeding conditions. The National Research Council (1980) described signs of toxicosis and the dietary concentrations of minerals that are considered excessive. Certain elements such as lead, cadmium, and mercury are discussed because they should always be considered toxic and are of practical concern because toxicosis from these elements unfortunately occasionally occurs.

Concentrations of mineral elements in both concentrate and forage feedstuffs vary greatly (Adams, 1975; Coppock and Fettman, 1977; Kertz, 1998). Reliable or typical analyses of concentrations of some mineral elements (e.g., chloride and various micromineral elements) in many feedstuffs are unavailable (Henry, 1995c). Also, concentrations among samples of the same feed type may be quite variable depending upon such factors as fertilization and manure application rates, soil type, and plant species (Butler and Jones, 1973). Concentrations in byproducts or coproducts also are variable and influenced by the method of processing to produce the feedstuff. Therefore, laboratory analyses of feeds for macro- and micromineral element content is critically important for precise and accurate diet formulation to meet requirements at least cost. Laboratory analyses using wet chemistry methods is critical for accurate determination. Near infrared reflectance spectroscopy (NIRS) is not reliable (Shenk and Westerhaus, 1994).

Estimates of mean concentrations and of variation (standard deviations) in mineral element content of many commonly used feedstuffs are given in Table 15-1 of this publication. Compositions of inorganic mineral sources commonly used in diet supplementation are presented in Table 15-3.

## MACROMINERALS

### *Calcium*

#### FUNCTIONS

Extracellular calcium is essential for formation of skeletal tissues, transmission of nervous tissue impulses, excitation of skeletal and cardiac muscle contraction, blood clotting, and as a component of milk. Intracellular calcium, while 1/10,000 of the concentration of extracellular calcium, is involved in the activity of a wide array of enzymes and serves as an important second messenger conveying information from the surface of the cell to the interior of the cell.

About 98 percent of the calcium in the body is located within the skeleton where calcium, along with phosphate anion, serves to provide structural strength and hardness to bone. The other 2 percent of the calcium in the body is found primarily in the extracellular fluids of the body. Normally the concentration of calcium in blood plasma is 2.2 to 2.5 mM (9 to 10 mg/dl, or 4.4 to 5 mEq/L) in the adult cow, with slightly higher values in calves. Between 40 and 45 percent of total calcium in plasma is bound to plasma proteins, primarily albumin, and another 5 percent is bound to organic components of the blood such as citrate or inorganic elements. From 45 to 50 percent of total calcium in plasma exists in the ionized, soluble form; the amount being closer to 50 percent at low blood pH and closer to 45 percent when blood pH is elevated. The ionized calcium concentration of the plasma must be maintained at a relatively constant value of 1 to 1.25 mM to ensure normal nerve membrane and muscle end plate electric potential and conductivity, which has forced vertebrates to evolve an elaborate system to maintain calcium homeostasis. This system attempts to maintain a constant concentration of extracellular calcium concentration by increasing calcium entry into the extracellular fluids whenever there is a loss of calcium from the extracellular compartment. When the loss of calcium exceeds entry, hypocalcemia can occur and this results in loss of nerve and muscle function, which can in some instances lead to recumbency and the clinical condition referred to as milk fever. During vitamin D intoxication, calcium enters the extracellular compartment faster than it leaves resulting in hypercalcemia, which can lead to soft tissue deposition of calcium.

#### CALCIUM HOMEOSTASIS

Calcium leaves the extracellular fluids during bone formation, in digestive secretions, sweat, and urine. An especially large loss of calcium to milk occurs during lactation in the cow. Calcium lost via these routes can be replaced from dietary calcium, from resorption of calcium stored in bone, or by resorbing a larger portion of the calcium filtered across the renal glomerulus, i.e., reducing urinary calcium loss. Whenever the loss of calcium from the extracellular fluids exceeds the amount of calcium entering the extracellular fluids there is a decrease in the concentration of calcium in plasma. The parathyroid glands monitor the concentration of calcium in carotid arterial blood and secrete parathyroid hormone when they sense a decrease in blood calcium. Parathyroid hormone immediately increases renal reabsorption mechanisms for calcium to reduce the loss of urinary calcium, and will stimulate processes to enhance intestinal absorption of calcium and resorption of calcium from bone.

Ultimately dietary calcium must enter the extracellular fluids to permit optimal performance of the animal. Calcium absorption can occur by passive transport between epithelial cells across any portion of the digestive tract whenever ionized calcium in the digestive fluids directly over the mucosa exceeds 6 mM (Bronner, 1987). These concentrations are reached when calves are fed all milk diets and when cows are given oral calcium drenches for prevention of hypocalcemia (Goff and Horst, 1993). In nonruminant species, studies suggest that as much as 50 percent of dietary calcium absorption can be passive (Nellans, 1988). It is unknown how much passive absorption of calcium occurs from the diets typically fed to dairy cattle but the diluting effect of the rumen would likely reduce the degree to which passive calcium absorption would occur. Active transport of calcium appears to be the major route for calcium absorption in mature ruminants and this process is controlled by 1,25-dihydroxyvitamin D, the hormone derived from vitamin D. By carefully regulating the amount of 1,25-dihydroxyvitamin D produced, the amount of dietary calcium absorbed can be adjusted to maintain a constant concentration of extracellular calcium (DeLuca, 1979; Bronner, 1987; Wasserman, 1981).

When dietary calcium is insufficient to meet the requirements of the animal, calcium will be withdrawn from bone to maintain a normal concentration of extracellular calcium. If dietary calcium is severely deficient for a prolonged period the animal will develop severe osteoporosis to the point of developing fractures—still, because the desire to maintain a normal concentration of extracellular calcium is so strong, plasma calcium will only be slightly lower than normal. A sudden large increase in loss of calcium from the extracellular pool can result in acute hypocalcemia before the calcium homeostatic mechanisms can act. This is discussed further in the section on milk fever (Chapter 9).

### REQUIREMENT FOR ABSORBED CALCIUM

The amount of calcium that must enter the extracellular compartment for maintenance, growth, pregnancy, and lactation is fairly well known and essentially the same equations were used to predict these amounts as were used in the 1989 National Research Council publication *Nutrients Requirements of Dairy Cattle*.

*Maintenance* For maintenance of nonlactating cattle, the absorbed calcium required is 0.0154 g/kg body weight (Visek et al., 1953; Hansard et al., 1957). For lactating animals the maintenance requirement is increased to 0.031 g/kg live BW (Martz et al., 1990). The increase in lactating cows reflects the impact increased dry matter intake (DMI) has on intestinal secretion of calcium during digestion.

*Growth* Growth of cattle requires more calcium when animals are young and actively accruing bone and less as they reach mature skeletal size. The Agricultural and Food Research Council (1991) developed an allometric equation to describe the calcium requirement of growing calves which will be adopted in this model. The requirement for absorbed calcium/kg average daily gain is:

$$\text{Ca (g/day)} = (9.83 \times (MW^{0.22}) \times (BW^{-0.22})) \times WG$$

where MW = expected mature live body weight (kg), BW = current body weight, and WG = weight gain.

*Pregnancy* The developing fetus requires a negligible amount of calcium until the last trimester of pregnancy (after day 190 of pregnancy), when the fetal skeleton begins to become calcified. Fetal skeletal calcification is especially great in the last weeks before parturition. The absorbed calcium required to meet the demands of the uterus and conceptus is best described by the exponential equation of House and Bell (House and Bell, 1993) for any given day of gestation beyond day 190 as:

$$\text{Ca (g/day)} = 0.02456\ e^{(0.05581 - 0.00007\ t)t} - 0.02456\ e^{(0.05581 - 0.00007(t-1))(t-1)}$$

where t = day of gestation.

*Lactation* The amount of calcium/kg milk produced varies slightly with the amount of protein in the milk which in turn varies with breed. The absorbed calcium required/kg milk produced is 1.22 g for Holstein cows, 1.45 g for Jersey cows, and 1.37 g for other breeds. Cows require about 2.1 g absorbed Ca/kg of colostrum produced.

### CALCIUM ABSORPTION COEFFICIENT

The amount of calcium that must be fed to meet the requirement for absorbed calcium is dependent on the availability of calcium from the feedstuffs and inorganic calcium sources in the diet, and the efficiency of intestinal calcium absorption in the animal being fed. The amount of calcium absorbed from the diet will generally equal the requirement of the body for calcium if the diet contains enough available calcium. The proportion of dietary calcium absorbed will decrease as dietary calcium increases above requirement of the tissues for absorbed calcium. To truly determine the efficiency of absorption of calcium from a feedstuff, the animals being tested should be fed less total dietary calcium than the amount of absorbed calcium required to meet their needs. This will ensure that intestinal calcium absorption mechanisms are fully activated so that the animal will absorb all the calcium from the feedstuff that it possibly can. Few studies fulfill this requirement; thus, it is likely that the published data have underestimated the availability of calcium in many cases. Previous National Research Council (1978, 1989) publications have determined a single efficiency of absorption of dietary calcium regardless of the source of calcium. This absorption coefficient was 0.38 in the 1989 *Nutrient Requirements of Dairy Cattle* and 0.45 in the 1978 *Nutrient Requirements of Dairy Cattle* based on the average proportion of calcium absorbed during a variety of trials. The coefficient was reduced in the 1989 *Nutrient Requirements of Dairy Cattle* partly in response to reports that cows in early lactation were less able to utilize dietary calcium (Van't Klooster, 1976; Ramberg, 1974) making use of a lower coefficient for calcium absorption more prudent. The decision to utilize 0.38 as the calcium absorption coefficient was based largely on a summary of 11 experiments with lactating dairy cows in which the average percentage of dietary calcium absorbed was 38 (Hibbs and Conrad, 1983). In the majority of these 11 experiments, the cows were fed diets supplying calcium well in excess of their needs placing the cows in positive calcium balance by as much as 20 to 40 g/day. In 3 of the experiments, the cows were in negative calcium balance and the percentage of dietary calcium absorbed was still below 40 percent. In those experiments, alfalfa and/or brome hay were supplying the dietary calcium. The French Institut National de la Recherche Agronomique (1989) used 30 to 35 percent as an estimate of efficiency of absorption for dietary calcium using similar logic. The 1996 *Nutrient Requirements of Beef Cattle* utilized 50 percent as the calcium absorption coefficient. The 1980 United Kingdom Agricultural Research Council (Agricultural Research Council, 1980) chose 68 percent as the coefficient of absorption for calcium; a coefficient considerably higher than the estimate of other groups that had examined dietary calcium requirements of cattle. This number is based on a model that predicts calcium is absorbed by dairy cattle according to need. Using data from a variety of balance studies in which a substantial number of lactating cows was included, the observed efficiency of absorption of calcium (diets utilizing feedstuff and mineral sources of calcium) reached a plateau of about 68 percent. Concern over the validity of this coefficient prompted the Agricultural Research Council (1980) to form a second committee to review the 1980 recommendation for calcium. This technical committee agreed with the use of 68 percent as an estimate of the absorption coefficient to be used in calculating dietary calcium requirements of cattle (AFRC, 1991).

A single coefficient is inappropriate and in this model the coefficient for calcium absorption will be based on the sources of calcium used in the diet. Unfortunately, our knowledge of the efficiency of absorption of calcium from individual feedstuffs is limited. Martz et al. (1990) fed lactating dairy cows two diets with no added mineral sources of calcium in which alfalfa supplied nearly all of the dietary calcium. One diet was 33 percent alfalfa, 39 percent hominy grits and 21.5 percent corn cobs; the second diet was 24 percent alfalfa, 41.5 percent corn silage and 29 percent hominy grits. The diets contained more calcium than suggested by the 1978 National Research Council *Nutrient Requirements of Dairy Cattle* publication and less than suggested by the 1989 National Research Council *Nutrient Requirements of Dairy Cattle*. True absorption of calcium from alfalfa, corrected for endogenous fecal calcium loss, was 25 percent; whereas, from the alfalfa-corn silage ration 42 percent of calcium was truly absorbed. Ward et al. (1972) estimated the efficiency of absorption of calcium from alfalfa ranged from 31 to 41 percent. About 20 to 30 percent of calcium within plants is bound to oxalate which is relatively unavailable to the ruminant (Ward et al., 1979). Studies of Hibbs and Conrad (1983) where cows were in negative calcium balance and were fed only alfalfa or alfalfa/brome diets fit the criteria of determining calcium absorption in animals that are being fed less calcium than they require and in these studies the efficiency of absorption of calcium from alfalfa ranged from 8 to 37 percent. Because alfalfa is a major contributor of calcium in dairy rations, absorption of calcium from alfalfa is used as an estimate of efficiency of absorption of calcium from forages in general. An efficiency of absorption of 30 percent is used in the model for calcium from forages.

Availability of calcium from grains and concentrates has not been determined in ruminants. In nonruminant animals, the availability of calcium from concentrates generally is less than the availability of calcium from an inorganic source such as calcium carbonate (Soares, 1995). The presence of phytate is felt to be a factor impairing absorption in nonruminants. This is not a factor in ruminants. Because oxalate is not as likely in concentrate feedstuffs the proportion of calcium available should be greater than 30 percent. It is possible that it may be comparable to that of the mineral sources of calcium. However the current model uses 60 percent as a conservative estimate of the proportion of calcium available from concentrate feedstuffs based in part on an assumption that the availability is not as high as from calcium carbonate. Efficiency of absorption of calcium from feedstuffs that are not forages (e.g., concentrates) was set at 60 percent.

Most non-forage feedstuffs will contain only small amounts of calcium. However, a notable exception is the calcium soap of palm oil fatty acids, which can be 7 to 9 percent calcium. The fat of this product is approximately 80 percent digestible, and digestion can only occur following dissociation of the calcium from the palmitate in the small intestine. This also implies that 80 percent of the calcium in this feed ingredient is available for absorption. This is in contrast to the work of Oltjen (1975) which suggested that formation of calcium soaps within the rumen impaired calcium absorption necessitating an increase in diet calcium when fat was added to a ration. No effect of added fat on apparent absorption of calcium was observed in the experiments of Rahnema et al. (1994). The model does not include a factor to increase dietary calcium when fat is added to the diet. There may be a need to increase diet magnesium when fat is added to the diet as magnesium must be soluble in the rumen to be absorbed. Since hypomagnesemia can affect calcium metabolism (see Chapter 9) there is an effect of diet fat on calcium metabolism but it is not overcome by adding calcium to the ration.

Calcium within mineral supplements is generally more available than calcium in forages and common feedstuffs (Hansard et al., 1957). Theoretically the factor limiting mineral calcium absorption is the solubility of the calcium from the mineral source. Calcium chloride represents a source of highly soluble calcium. When $^{45}$CaCl was used as a source of radioactive tracer for calcium absorption studies it was absorbed with >95 percent efficiency in young calves (Hansard et al., 1954). Calcium chloride is assigned an efficiency of absorption coefficient of 95 percent. Estimates of the efficiency of absorption of calcium from calcium carbonate range from 40 percent or 51 percent (Hansard et al., 1957) or up to 85 percent (Goetsch and Owens, 1985). Unfortunately, these studies were conducted using steers, with very low requirements for absorbed calcium. The studies of Hansard et al. (1957) demonstrate that calcium chloride is between 1.2 and 1.32 times more absorbable than calcium carbonate. Therefore, the efficiency of absorption of calcium from calcium carbonate is designated to be 75 percent. The absorption of calcium from various mineral sources is often compared to the efficiency of absorption of calcium from calcium carbonate. Table 15-4 lists a number of common mineral sources of calcium (including bone meal) and an estimate of the efficiency of absorption of calcium in each source, using data summarized by Soares (1995a) and based on the efficiency of absorption relative to calcium carbonate. The calcium from limestone generally is slightly less available than from pure calcium carbonate and has been assigned an efficiency of absorption coefficient of 70 percent.

#### EFFECTS OF PHYSIOLOGIC STATE

The amount of available calcium that will actually be absorbed varies with the physiologic state of the animal. Hansard et al. (1954) and Horst et al. (1978) reported that the efficiency of absorption of calcium decreases as animals age. Young animals absorb calcium very efficiently and very old animals absorb calcium poorly. As animals age, there is a decline in vitamin D receptors in the intestinal tract (Horst et al., 1990), which is thought to reduce the ability to respond to 1,25-dihydroxyvitamin D. From the data of Hansard et al. (1954), the difference in efficiency of calcium absorption in beef steers from 1 to 6 years of age is nearly negligible. Age was not included as a factor to adjust dietary calcium requirement in cattle >200 kg body weight. The absorption coefficient for calcium from diets normally fed to calves is high and will be considered to be 90 percent for all calves <100 kg body weight (see calf section, Chapter 10).

In early lactation nearly all cows are in negative calcium balance (Ellenberger et al., 1931; Ender et al. 1971; Ramberg, 1974). As feed intake increases and calcium intake increases most cows go into positive calcium balance about 6 to 8 weeks into lactation (Hibbs and Conrad, 1983; Ellenberger et al., 1931). Cows in the first 10 days of lactation are at greatest risk of being in negative calcium balance (Ramberg, 1974) and some are subclinically hypocalcemic throughout this period (Goff et al., 1996). Ramberg (1974) reported that the rate of entry of calcium into the extracellular fluid pool from the intestine increased about 1.55-fold from the day before parturition until 10 days in milk. Thereafter, the rate of entry of calcium into the extracellular pool from the intestine was not increased any further. Van't Klooster (1976) demonstrated that calcium absorption increased from 22 percent in late gestation to 36 percent by day 8 of lactation after which it remained relatively constant. This represented a 1.6-fold increase in efficiency of calcium absorption over this 8-day period. Regression analysis of data of Ward et al. (1972) predicted that cows need to be fed 5 g Ca/kg milk in early lactation to avoid negative calcium balance. However, there was no evidence to demonstrate that negative calcium balance in early lactation was detrimental to the cow provided the concentration of calcium in plasma remained normal, i.e., lactational osteoporosis ensures adequate entry of calcium from bone into the extracellular calcium pool. During lactational osteoporosis, data of Ellenberger et al. (1931) suggest 800 to 1300 g of calcium are removed from bone to support milk production during early lactation and this calcium is restored to bone during the last 20 to 30 weeks of lactation and the dry period. This could increase the requirement for absorbed calcium in later lactation by as much as 8 g/d to rebuild bone lost during early lactation. No calcium requirement for rebuilding bone is included in the model.

The effects of calcium-to-phosphorus ratio on absorption of calcium and phosphorus was once felt to be important but recent data suggest that the calcium: phosphorus ratio is not critical, unless the ratio is >7:1 or <1:1 (Miller, 1983a; Agricultural Research Council, 1980).

#### CALCIUM DEFICIENCY

A deficiency of dietary calcium in young animals leads to a failure to mineralize new bone and contributes to retarded growth. Rickets is more commonly caused by a deficiency of vitamin D or phosphorus but a deficiency of calcium can contribute to rickets as well. In older animals a deficiency of dietary calcium forces the animal to withdraw calcium from bone for homeostasis of the extracellular fluids. This causes osteoporosis and osteomalacia in the bones, which makes the bone prone to spontaneous fractures. The concentration of calcium in milk is not altered even during a severe dietary deficiency of calcium (Becker et al., 1933).

#### EXCESS DIETARY CALCIUM

Feeding excessive dietary calcium is generally not associated with any specific toxicity. Dietary concentrations of calcium >1 percent have been associated with reduced DMI and lower performance (Miller, 1983a) but diets as high as 1.8 percent calcium have been fed with no apparent problems for nonlactating dairy cows (Beede et al., 1991). Feeding excessive calcium could interfere with trace mineral absorption (especially zinc) and replaces energy or protein the animal might better utilize for increased production. Feeding calcium in excess of requirements has been suggested to improve performance, especially when cows are fed corn silage diets. Because calcium is a strong cation, addition of calcium carbonate to diets above that required to meet absorbed calcium needs may be providing a rumen alkalinizing effect to enhance performance.

### *Phosphorus*

Of all dietary essential mineral elements for dairy animals, phosphorus represents the greatest potential risk if excess is released into the environment contaminating surface waters and causing eutrophication. Accurate and precise management of phosphorus nutrition is crucial to optimize performance and health of dairy animals, and to minimize phosphorus excretion.

PHYSIOLOGIC ROLES

Phosphorus has more known biologic functions than any other mineral element. About 80 percent of phosphorus in the body is found in bones and teeth. It is present in bone, along with calcium, principally as apatite salts, and as calcium phosphate. It is located in every cell of the body and almost all energy transactions involve formation or breaking of high-energy bonds that link oxides of phosphate to carbon or to carbon-nitrogen compounds (such as adenosine triphosphate, ATP). Phosphorus also is intimately involved in acid-base buffer systems of blood and other bodily fluids, in cell differentiation, and is a component of cell walls and cell contents as phospholipids, phosphoproteins, and nucleic acids.

Phosphorus concentrations in blood plasma normally are 1.3 to 2.6 mmol/L (4 to 8 mg/dl; 6 to 8 mg/dl for growing cattle and 4 to 6 mg/dl for adult animals). About 1 to 2 g circulate as inorganic phosphate in blood plasma of a 600-kg animal. Because of greater concentrations in erythrocytes, whole blood contains 6 to 8 times as much phosphorous as plasma. About 5 to 8 g are present in the extracellular pool of a 600-kg cow. The intracellular concentration of phosphorus is about 25 mmol/L (78 mg/dl), and total intracellular phosphorus is about 155 g in a 600-kg cow (Goff, 1998a).

Phosphorus also is required by ruminal microorganisms for digestion of cellulose (Burroughs et al., 1951) and synthesis of microbial protein (Breves and Schroder, 1991). Durand and Komisarczuk (1988) recommended that available phosphorus (from dietary sources and salivary recycling) within the rumen should be at least 5 g/kg of organic matter digested to optimize degradation of cell walls from feeds by microbes. When cattle were fed 0.12 percent dietary phosphorus, ruminal fluid concentration was over 200 mg phosphorus/L, considerably greater than the 20 to 80 mg of phosphorus/L needed for maximum cellulose digestion *in vitro* (Hall et al., 1961; Chicco et al., 1965). This concentration typically is achieved in cattle by salivary recycling of phosphorus and from diets adequate to meet the animal's requirement.

PHOSPHORUS UTILIZATION AND HOMEOSTASIS

Net absorption of phosphorus occurs mainly in the small intestine (Grace et al., 1974; Reinhardt et al., 1988). Only small amounts are absorbed from the rumen, omasum, and abomasum. However, little is known about mechanisms and regulation of absorption anterior to the small intestine (Breves and Schroder, 1991). Absorption is thought to occur mainly in the duodenum and jejunum (Care et al., 1980; Scott et al., 1984). Unlike absorption of calcium, absorption of phosphorus is in direct relation to supply of potentially absorbable phosphorus in the lumen of the small intestine (Care et al., 1980). Presumably, as in nonruminants, absorption occurs via two distinct mechanisms. A saturable vitamin D-dependent active transport system, separate and distinct from the active transport mechanism for Ca, is operative when animals are fed low phosphorus-containing diets. Synthesis of 1,25-dihydroxyvitamin D can be stimulated when blood phosphorus is very low resulting in more efficient absorption (Horst, 1986). Passive absorption predominates when normal to large amounts of potentially absorbable phosphorus are consumed, and absorption is related directly to the amount in the lumen of the small intestine and to concentrations in blood plasma (Wasserman and Taylor, 1976).

Absorbed phosphorus may be retained or secreted (e.g., in milk) for productive functions or secreted into the lumen of the digestive tract for reabsorption or excretion in feces. Homeostasis of phosphorus is maintained predominantly by salivary recycling and endogenous fecal excretion, which are related directly to the amount of dietary phosphorus consumed and absorbed. Concentration of phosphorus in saliva can be 4 to 5 times of that in blood plasma. In cows, between 30 and 90 g of phosphorus is secreted daily into saliva (Reinhardt et al., 1988; Scott, 1988). Almost all phosphorus in saliva is inorganic (Reinhardt et al., 1988), and the amount secreted appears to be regulated by parathyroid hormone (Wasserman, 1981). Inorganic salivary phosphorus is absorbed across the intestine with equal or greater efficiency than dietary phosphorus (Challa et al., 1989).

REQUIREMENT FOR ABSORBED PHOSPHORUS

For the model, the requirement for absorbed phosphorus was factorially derived by summing estimates of true requirements for maintenance, growth, pregnancy, and lactation.

*Maintenance* Typically, 95 to 98 percent of total phosphorus excretion is in feces. Three fractions are present—that of dietary origin unavailable for absorption or not absorbed, that of endogenous origin which is inevitably excreted (inevitable fecal loss), and that of endogenous origin which is excreted to maintain homeostasis (representing phosphorus absorbed by the intestine in excess of the need to maintain normal blood phosphorus). By definition, the maintenance requirement of phosphorus is the endogenous fecal loss (inevitable fecal loss) when phosphorus supply is just below or just meets the true requirement. In the past, the maintenance requirement was expressed as a function of body weight (National Research Council, 1989a), based on fecal phosphorus excretion data extrapolated to zero phosphorus intake (Agricultural Research Council, 1980). This was later determined to be an inappropriate approach (Agricultural and Food Research Council, 1991). Other workers suggested that inevitable fecal loss in ruminants was a function of total fecal dry matter (DM) excretion (Conrad et al., 1956; Preston and Pfander, 1964), which reflects the role of the salivary glands in phosphorus metabolism. It follows, therefore, that inevitable fecal loss of phosphorus also is related to DMI. The Agricultural and Food Research Council (1991) hypothesized that inevitable fecal loss of phosphorus is determined mainly by DMI, and not by live body weight. New research was available with cattle illustrating that a conceptually more sound and repeatable approach than expression as a function of body weight is to express maintenance requirement as a function of DMI when, by definition, dietary phosphorus is fed and absorbed very near the true requirement.

Part of the maintenance requirement for absorbed phosphorus of the animal is the inevitable fecal loss associated with microbial cells of the digestive tract which contain phosphorus and are excreted in feces. It is estimated that about half of the inevitable fecal loss of phosphorus is associated with microbial debris, and purines and pyrimidines of nucleic acids. This fraction can vary depending upon fermentability (fermented organic matter) of the diet. However, sufficient data are lacking to quantify this relationship accurately (Kirchgessner, 1993).

Klosch et al. (1997) fed growing bulls (228 or 435 kg BW) diets low (50 percent) or high (80 percent) in concentrates and total phosphorus balance was determined. Net phosphorus retention was <1 g/animal per day, and fecal phosphorus excretion was not influenced by digestibility of organic matter consumed, or body weight. Total fecal phosphorus excretion (phosphorus of dietary origin not absorbed plus that of endogenous origin that was inevitably excreted) averaged 1.0 g/kg of DMI. The absorption coefficient of total dietary phosphorus was assumed to be about 80 percent in the study of Klosch et al. (1997). Therefore, the absorbed phosphorus requirement for maintenance of growing animals was set at 0.8 g/kg of DMI in the current model. An additional 0.002 g/kg BW (Agricultural Research Council, 1980) of endogenous phosphorus loss from urine was considered part of the maintenance requirement for absorbed phosphorus in the model.

Spiekers et al. (1993) fed a low phosphorus (0.21 percent) diet to two groups of lactating dairy cows of similar BW, but differing in daily milk yield (stage of lactation effect) and feed intake. For the two groups total phosphorus intakes were 37 and 21.5 g/day, respectively; and, phosphorus balance was similar and slightly negative, indicating that animals were fed below or very near the true requirement. Total excretion of fecal phosphorus differed between groups (20.3 versus 13.3 g/cow per day) and was 51 percent greater per kg of body weight for cows at high versus low dietary phosphorus. However, calculated as a function of DMI, excretion of fecal phosphorus was 1.20 and 1.22 g/kg DMI per day for the high and low intake groups, respectively. It is estimated that the absorption coefficient of total dietary phosphorus for cows fed very close to the true requirement is 80 percent. Therefore, in the current model the maintenance requirement for nonlactating pregnant and lactating cows was set at 1.0 g/kg of dietary dry matter consumed. A small amount of endogenous phosphorus is inevitably excreted in urine. To account for this, an additional 0.002 g/kg BW (Agricultural Research Council, 1980) is considered as part of the maintenance requirement for absorbed phosphorus in the model.

*Growth* The requirement for growth is the sum of the amount of absorbed phosphorus accreted in soft tissues plus that deposited in skeletal tissue. An accretion of 1.2 g of phosphorus/kg soft tissue gain was estimated by Agricultural Research Council (1980) and data of Grace (1983) from lambs confirmed this value. However, the majority of phosphorus deposition in growing animals is associated with new bone (hydroxyapatite) growth. Bone contains 120 g of calcium/kg and the theoretic accretion ratio of calcium-to-phosphorus is about 2.1 g calcium-to-1.0 g phosphorus (1.6 mol per 1.0 mol). Using this relationship and the accretion rate in soft tissues, the Agricultural and Food Research Council (1991) developed an allometric equation from data in the literature with growing cattle to describe the requirement for absorbed phosphorus for growth (g/kg average daily gain):

$$P\ (g/day) = (1.2 + (4.635 \times MW^{0.22})(BW^{-0.22}))) \times WG$$

where MW = expected mature live body weight (kg), BW = current body weight, and WG = weight gain.

Because bone is an early maturing component of the body, the allometric equation reflects declining requirement for absorbed phosphorus for growing animals. This equation was used to define the absorbed phosphorus requirement for growing dairy cattle. For example in the model, for an animal with M = 681 kg, the absorbed phosphorus requirements (g/kg average daily gain) ranges from 8.3 g at 100 kg live BW (C) to 6.2 g at 500 kg.

*Pregnancy* Quantitatively the requirement for phosphorus for pregnancy is low until the last trimester. New information on accretion of phosphorus in conceptuses (fetus, fetal fluids and membranes, placentomes and uterine tissues) of 18 multiparous Holstein cows slaughtered at varying times from 190 to 270 days of gestation was available (House and Bell, 1993). Changes in fetal mass and phosphorus content across the sampling period were similar to earlier data (Ellenberger et al., 1950). Therefore, the requirement for absorbed phosphorus to meet demands of the conceptus for any day beyond 190 days of gestation is described in the model by the exponential equation:

$$\text{absorbed phosphorus (g/d)} = 0.02743e^{(0.05527 - 0.000075\ t)t} - 0.02743e^{(0.05527 - 0.000075\ (t-1))(t-1)};$$

where t = day of gestation (House and Bell, 1993).

Estimates of rates of phosphorus accretion in conceptuses of Holstein cows increase from 1.9 g/d at 190 to 5.4 g/d at 280 days of gestation, respectively. This equation should not be used to predict phosphorus accretion of the conceptus prior to 190 days of gestation. The phosphorus requirement of the conceptus at <190 days of gestation is very small and was set to zero in the model.

*Lactation* The requirement for absorbed phosphorus (g per day) for lactation is equal to daily milk yield multiplied by the percentage of phosphorus in milk. The phosphorus content of milk ranged from 0.083 to 0.085 percent (Wu et al., 2000), 0.087 to 0.089 percent (Spiekers et al., 1993), and 0.090 to 0.100 percent (Flynn and Power,1985). The value of 0.090 percent (0.90 g of phosphorus per kg of milk) was used to compute requirements for absorbed phosphorus in the model. This is the same as that used by the working groups in Scotland and the United Kingdom (Agricultural and Food Research Council, 1991), France (Gueguen et al., 1989), and Germany (Kirchgener, 1993). In the last edition of this publication (National Research Council, 1989), the requirement of phosphorus for lactation was adjusted depending upon fat content of milk. However, the phosphorus in cows' milk is distributed as: 20 percent esterified to casein; 40 percent as colloidal inorganic calcium phosphate; 30 percent as phosphate ions in solution; and, only about 10 percent associated with the lipid fraction (Jenness and Patton, 1959; Renner, 1983). Therefore, an adjustment based on milk fat content is not of major quantitative and practical significance in defining the phosphorus requirement for lactation of dairy cows.

DIETARY REQUIREMENT AND EFFICIENCY OF ABSORPTION

The dietary requirement is the sum of the requirements for absorbed phosphorus for maintenance, growth, pregnancy, and lactation divided by the absorption coefficient(s) for phosphorus from the diet. The absorption coefficient in the denominator of the factorial equation potentially has more influence on the final computed dietary requirement than any of the single or combined requirement values for absorbed phosphorus. The smaller the absorption coefficient, the greater will be the calculated dietary requirement. In the last edition, an overall absorption coefficient of 50 percent was used (National Research Council, 1989b). Other working groups established overall values of 58 percent (Agricultural and Food Research Council, 1991), 60 percent (NRLO, 1982), 60 percent (Gueguen et al., 1989), and 70 percent (Kirchgessner, 1993). As with calcium, a single overall absorption coefficient was not considered appropriate for all types of feedstuffs, supplemental mineral sources, or diets fed to various classes of dairy animals because of the known variation in absorption coefficients. The model evaluates the absorbable phosphorus content of the diet by determining the phosphorus available for absorption from each ingredient of the diet and comparing the sum of total phosphorus in the diet with the requirement for absorbed phosphorus of the animal.

To accurately determine the true absorption coefficient from a particular feedstuff or mineral source, phosphorus must be fed in an amount less than the animal's true requirement. This is to insure maximum efficiency of absorption of all potentially absorbable phosphorus from that particular source. Also, especially with phosphorus, the amount of endogenous phosphorus recycled via saliva must be taken into account. This is most appropriately done experimentally by quantifying recycling with a tracer (e.g., $P^{32}$). Most studies do not satisfy these experimental specifications. Thus, the true absorption coefficient is generally unknown and the value given is an underestimation of true absorption. Apparent absorption of phosphorus (or apparent digestibility) determined in many studies is lower (largely because of copious endogenous fecal excretion) and not equivalent to the true absorption coefficient. If apparent absorption estimates are used to compute a dietary requirement, gross over-estimation results.

Based on available data, absorption coefficients of phosphorus used in the model for most feedstuffs commonly fed to cattle of various physiologic states were: 90 percent for calves consuming milk or milk replacer; 78 percent for young ruminating calves 100 to 200 kg body weight. True absorption coefficients for phosphorus from alfalfa hay or corn silage were 67 percent or 80 percent, respectively, for lactating cows yielding about 33.6 kg of 3.5 percent fat-corrected milk and consuming 21.7 kg DM daily (Martz et al., 1990). Using a tracer technique, Lofgreen and Kleiber (1953, 1954) reported the true absorption coefficient of phosphorus in alfalfa hay fed to lambs ranged from 0.81 to 0.96. In the model, absorption coefficients of 64 percent and 70 percent were used for forages and concentrates, respectively.

More complete data are available to estimate absorption coefficients of various potential supplemental mineral sources (Table 15-4). These values were tabulated from Soares (1995b) and Peeler (1972), and other sources in the literature and used in the model. Those values determined with ruminants, and especially with cattle, were given preference whenever possible in tabulation.

Dicalcium phosphate (calcium phosphate dibasic) with a true absorption coefficient of 75 percent in cattle (Tillman and Brethour, 1958; Challa and Braithwaite, 1988), phosphoric acid with true absorption coefficient of 90 percent in cattle (Tillman and Brethour, 1958), and monosodium phosphate with a true absorption coefficient of 90 percent in sheep (Tillman and Brethour, 1958) were taken as reference standards. The absorption coefficients of phosphorus in other mineral sources were set based on these reference standards and data where relative differences in phosphorus absorption among these and other sources were estimated in various experiments (Soares, 1995b).

Because sufficient studies with appropriate tracers are not available to estimate true absorption coefficients for most feedstuffs fed to lactating dairy cattle, an alternate approach would be useful. One such approach involves utilizing experimentally derived phosphorus balance data and the assumption that an accurate estimate of the maintenance requirement for absorbed phosphorus is 1.0 g/kg of DMI (Spiekers et al., 1993) plus endogenous urine output (0.002 g/kg BW; Agricultural Research Council, 1980). A calculated absorption coefficient can be derived as: [true requirement for maintenance (g per day) plus milk phosphorus output (g per day) plus phosphorus balance (g per day)] divided by total phosphorus intake (g per day). The fecal output value from the actual balance determination is ignored because it represents unabsorbed dietary phosphorus plus excess endogenous phosphorus which has been recycled to the digestive tract via saliva and excreted in feces. Using this approach, the calculated absorption coefficients of phosphorus in mixed diets fed to lactating cows ranged from 67 to 100 percent (Morse et al., 1992b; Spiekers et al., 1993; Brintrup et al., 1993; Wu et al., 2000). In each study, two or three different concentrations of dietary phosphorus were fed. Within each study the calculated absorption coefficient declined as the dietary phosphorus concentration increased, as would be expected (Challa et al., 1989). Also, among three studies in which dietary phosphorus concentrations (0.39 to 0.42 percent) most closely supplied the requirement of lactating cows, the calculated absorption coefficients [67 percent, Brintrup et al. (1993); 74 percent, Morse et al. (1992b); 72 percent, Wu et al. (2000)] were similar to the overall absorption coefficient (70 percent) set by the German working group (Kirchgessner, 1993). In the case of Spiekers et al. (1993), in which lactating cows were fed diets with 0.21 percent phosphorus (phosphorus-deficient diet which resulted in slightly negative phosphorus balance) the calculated absorption coefficient was about 100 percent, as would be expected. This relationship is corroborated by regression of the calculated absorption coefficients on dietary phosphorus concentrations ranging from 15 to 62 percent, dry basis. Regression analysis (adjusted for number of experimental observations per treatment mean) was performed with a data set of 71 treatment means from 20 phosphorus balance trials (Hibbs and Conrad, 1983; Martz et al., 1990; Morse et al., 1992b; Spiekers et al., 1993; Brintrup et al., 1993; Wu et al., 2000; Rodriguez, 1998). The regression equation is: calculated absorption coefficient = 1.86696 − 5.01238 (dietary phosphorus percent) + 5.12286 (dietary phosphorus percent)$^2$; ($r^2$ = 0.70). Based on the regression equation, the calculated absorption coefficient was 1.0 with 0.22 percent phosphorus and declined to a minimum absorption coefficient of 0.64 with 0.49 percent dietary phosphorus. All of these calculated absorption coefficients are greater than that (0.5) used by the National Research Council (1989).

Efficiency of absorption of phosphorus depends upon a number of factors: age (or body weight) of the animal; physiologic state (e.g., nonlactating versus lactating); amount of DM or phosphorus intake; calcium-to-phosphorus ratio; dietary concentrations of aluminum, calcium, iron, magnesium, manganese, potassium, and fat; intestinal pH; and, source of phosphorus (e.g., forages, concentrates, inorganic mineral supplements, and salivary phosphorus) (Irving, 1964; Peeler, 1972; Agricultural and Food Research Council, 1991; Soares, 1995b).

#### EFFECT OF INTAKE OF PHOSPHORUS

Efficiency of absorption of phosphorus declines as intake of phosphorus increases in cattle (Challa et al., 1989) and in sheep (Field et al., 1977). However, over a considerable range of phosphorus intakes within recommended amounts the efficiency of absorption (absorption coefficient) from inorganic sources remained high and relatively constant in cattle (83 percent; Challa et al., 1989) and in sheep (74 percent; Braithwaite, 1986). Because salivary phosphorus typically supplies appreciably more (e.g., at least two-fold greater amounts) phosphorus to the lumen of the small intestine than does dietary phosphorus, the efficiency of absorption of salivary phosphorus is important. Salivary phosphorus is in the form of inorganic phosphate salts with sodium and potassium. Over a considerable range of phosphorus intakes in tracer studies, the absorption coefficient of salivary endogenous phosphorus recycled to the small intestine was 68 percent to 81 percent in bull calves (Challa et al., 1989). Excessive dietary phosphorus relative to the requirement reduced the efficiency of absorption of inorganic or salivary phosphorus (Braithwaite, 1983, 1986; Challa et al., 1989).

#### EFFECT OF DIETARY CALCIUM

Effect of increasing dietary calcium on phosphorus absorption was investigated where dietary calcium-to-phosphorus ratios ranged from 0.6 to 3.6 (Field et al., 1983). Efficiency of absorption of phosphorus in sheep was reduced by 18 percent with increasing amounts of calcium;

amounts of calcium and phosphorus were within those amounts recommended by Agricultural Research Council (1980). At higher than recommended supplemental calcium, greater depression of phosphorus absorption would be expected (Agricultural and Food Research Council, 1991). Phosphorus deficiency was exacerbated in lambs fed diets supplying 1.5 times daily requirements for calcium (Sevilla and Ternouth, 1981), likely a result of reduced soluble phosphorus in the digestive tract (Wan-Zahari et al., 1990).

#### PHYTATE PHOSPHORUS

About two-thirds or more of phosphorus in cereal grains, oilseed meals, and grain by-products is bound organically in phytate; stems and leaves of plants contain very little phytate phosphorus (Nelson et al., 1976). Phytate phosphorus is only slightly available or totally unavailable to nonruminants (Soares, 1995b; National Research Council, 1998). However, inherent phytase activity of ruminal microorganisms renders nearly all of the phytate phosphorus available for absorption (Reid et al., 1947; Nelson et al., 1976; Clark et al., 1986; Morse et al., 1992a; Ingalls and Okemo, 1994; Herbein et al., 1996).

#### VARIATION IN PHOSPHORUS CONTENT OF FEEDS

Phosphorus is the most expensive macromineral element supplemented in diets of dairy cattle. Therefore, laboratory analyses of feeds for phosphorus content is critically important for precise and accurate diet formulation to meet requirements at least cost. There is considerable variation in actual phosphorus content within types of forages and concentrates fed to dairy animals (Adams, 1975; Kertz, 1998). Estimates of variation (standard deviations) in phosphorus content of many commonly used feedstuffs are given in Table 15-1 of this publication.

#### GROWTH AND MILK YIELD RESPONSES TO VARYING DIETARY PHOSPHORUS CONCENTRATIONS

In addition to the factorial approach for deriving the absorbed and dietary requirements, results of feeding trials in which varying dietary concentrations of phosphorus were fed to growing calves and lactating cows were evaluated.

#### GROWING CALVES

Huffman et al. (1933) concluded that 0.20 percent dietary phosphorus was not sufficient for growth of dairy heifers from 3 to 18 months of age. Maximum weight gains of dairy calves from 90 to 125 kg BW occurred when dietary phosphorus content was 0.24 percent, dry basis (Wise et al., 1958). However, bone ash content was greater when dietary phosphorus was 0.33 percent compared with 0.24 percent, but greater phosphorus intake did not improve any other performance variables. Noller et al. (1977) found no differences in BW gain, efficiency of converting feed to gain, or concentrations of phosphorus in blood of Holstein heifers gaining between 0.68 to 0.82 kg/head per day when fed diets containing either 0.22 or 0.32 percent phosphorus. In a second trial, 0.32 percent compared with 0.22 percent dietary phosphorus increased concentrations of phosphorus in serum, but no differences in weight gain or efficiency of feed conversion were observed. Increasing dietary phosphorus from 0.24 to 0.31 percent (dry basis) increased DMI, average daily gain, breaking strength of ribs and tibia, and concentrations of inorganic phosphorus in blood plasma of dairy calves (Teh et al., 1982). Langer et al. (1985) compared 0.24, 0.30, and 0.36 percent dietary phosphorus fed to growing calves and found over the 10-week study that 0.30 percent resulted in maximum feed intake, average daily gain, and concentrations of phosphorus in blood plasma; no additional benefits were detected with 0.36 percent phosphorus. Miller et al. (1987) fed diets containing 0.08, 0.14, 0.20, or 0.32 percent phosphorus and concluded, from concentrations of phosphorus in blood plasma and average daily gains, that at least 0.32 percent phosphorus was needed for heifers to gain 0.75 kg per day. Two sources (monoammonium phosphate and dicalcium phosphate) of phosphorus each used to give three dietary phosphorus concentrations (0.26, 0.34, and 0.41 percent, dry basis) were compared with growing dairy calves (Jackson et al., 1988). Increasing dietary phosphorus from 0.26 to 0.34 percent increased feed intake, body weight gain, concentrations of inorganic phosphorus in blood plasma, and bending moment of the tibia and rib. Body weight gain (0.94 kg/head per day) of calves fed 0.34 percent phosphorus was about 13 percent greater than that of calves fed 0.26 percent dietary phosphorus. Only plasma concentration of phosphorus was increased further with 0.41 percent phosphorus compared with lower concentrations. All responses were similar between sources of supplemental phosphorus. Based on all of these studies, 0.30 to 0.34 percent dietary phosphorus was sufficient for normal blood concentrations of phosphorus in blood, maximum average daily gains, and greater bone strength of growing dairy calves.

#### LACTATING CATTLE

Research literature was reviewed to find all possible results characterizing lactational responses to varying dietary concentrations of phosphorus. Phosphorus is often fed in greater dietary concentrations than needed to meet the requirement established in the current model. Is feeding phosphorus in excess of requirement beneficial?

Nine studies, with dietary phosphorus concentrations ranging from 0.24 to 0.65 percent of dietary dry matter, fed for periods ranging from the first 8 weeks of lactation to as long as three consecutive lactations, with average milk yields ranging from 15 to 40/kg per cow per day were examined to try to answer this question.

Overall, supplying more dietary phosphorus than that calculated to meet the dietary requirement did not increase DMI or milk yield in any of the studies. The study of Kincaid et al. (1981) suggested that increasing dietary phosphorus increased DMI and 3.5 percent fat-corrected milk yield. However, based on the description of the analysis of variance in that paper the data were improperly analyzed, thus invalidating interpretation. In one other study, feed intake and milk yield were lower for cows fed 0.24 versus 0.32 or 0.42 percent phosphorus (Call et al., 1987). Within none of the other studies was DMI or milk yield increased by increasing dietary phosphorus from its lowest concentration to a higher concentration (Stevens et al., 1971; Carstairs et al., 1981; Brodison et al., 1989; Brintrup et al., 1993; Dhiman et al., 1996; Wu and Satter, 2000; Wu et al., 2000).

Milk fat and protein percentages were not affected by concentration of dietary phosphorus in most studies. Milk protein percentage increased as phosphorus increased from 0.32 or 0.42 percent compared with 0.24 percent (Call et al., 1987). Protein content of milk was higher with 0.45 versus 0.35 percent phosphorus in the study of Wu and Satter (2000). Milk fat percentage was higher in year 1 of the study of Brodison et al. (1989) with 0.44 versus 0.35 percent phosphorus, but lower in the study of Brintrup et al. (1993) with 0.33 versus 0.39 percent phosphorus. There were no consistent effects of dietary phosphorus concentration on milk composition among studies.

Concentrations of phosphorus in blood were evaluated in seven of the nine studies. The normal concentrations of inorganic phosphorus in plasma is 4.0 to 6.0 mg/dl for adult cattle (Goff, 1998a). In only one case among all of the studies was phosphorus in blood below the normal range (3.6 mg/dl for cows fed 0.24 percent dietary phosphorus; Call et al., 1987); 0.24 percent did not provide the dietary requirement. In other studies, increasing dietary phosphorus increased the concentration of phosphorus in blood within or above the normal range.

The DMI and milk yield of cows during early lactation were maximized with 0.40 to 0.42 percent dietary phosphorus, and greater concentrations (0.50 to 0.52 percent) did not increase DMI or milk yield (Carstairs et al., 1981; Wu et al., 2000). Milk yield was not affected by the concentration of the phosphorus in the diet during the first month, but from week 5 through 12 of lactation, it tended to be greater with 0.40 percent compared with 0.50 percent phosphorus (Carstairs et al., 1981). For the entire 84-d treatment period, cows fed 0.40 percent phosphorus produced 8 percent more milk than those fed 0.50 percent phosphorus. Feeding 0.42 percent phosphorus to high yielding cows during the first 8 weeks of lactation maximized milk production, and resulted in positive phosphorus balance and normal concentrations of phosphorus concentrations in blood serum (Wu et al., 2000).

Based on results of nine studies, a concentration in the range of 0.32 to 0.42 percent phosphorus for the entire lactation was sufficient, depending upon milk production potential of the cows and nutrition supplied. No benefits on lactational performance of dietary concentrations >0.42 percent phosphorus were reported in any short- or long-term studies which were properly analyzed.

Daily dietary requirement determined by the factorial method is expressed as g per cow per day, and not as a percentage of the diet. Therefore, supplying the requirement requires a reasonably accurate estimate of actual DMI.

### FREE-CHOICE PHOSPHORUS

Coppock et al. (1972, 1975) studied the practice of free-choice feeding of phosphorus-containing supplements to dairy heifers and lactating cows to meet requirements when diets were low or marginally deficient in phosphorus or calcium. With heifers there was little relationship between need for the mineral elements and free-choice consumption of dicalcium phosphate or defluorinated phosphate. For lactating cows offered basal diets providing phosphorus and calcium below requirements for 9 and 12 weeks, there was no evidence that cows consumed dicalcium phosphate to correct the deficiency or that appetite for phosphorus and calcium supplements coincided with the animals' nutritional requirements.

### PHOSPHORUS DEFICIENCY

Detailed description of occurrence, etiology, clinical pathology, diagnosis, treatment, and prevention of phosphorus deficiency in ruminants has been described by Goff (1998a). Signs of deficiency may occur rather quickly if dietary phosphorus is insufficient. Deficiency is most common in cattle grazing forages on soils low in phosphorus or in animals consuming excessively mature forages or crop residues with low phosphorus content (less than 0.25 percent, dry basis). Nonspecific chronic signs of deficiency include unthriftiness, inappetence, poor growth and lactational performance, and unsatisfactory fertility; but signs are often complicated by coincidental deficiencies of other nutrients such as protein or energy. Animals may be chronically hypophosphatemic (low phosphorus in blood plasma—2 to 3.5 mg/dl), but the concentration of phosphorus in milk remains within the normal range. In severe deficiency cases, bone mineral mass is lost, and bones become weak. Severe clinical manifestations of phosphorus deficiency include acute hypophosphatemia, rickets in young growing animals, and osteomalacia in adults.

Acute hypophosphatemia (less than 2 mg phosphorus/dl of plasma) may occur if cows are fed marginally low dietary phosphorus and challenged by extra demand for phosphorus in late pregnancy with accelerated fetal growth, especially with twin fetuses, and with colostrum and milk formation during early lactation. The disease usually is complicated with concurrent hypocalcemia, hypomagnasemia, and possibly hypoglycemia.

Concentrations of phosphorus in plasma often fall below the normal range (4 to 6 mg/dl) in the periparturient period. In other mammals, physiologic correction can occur rather rapidly as phosphorus absorption is responsive to renal production of 1,25-dihydroxyvitamin D which is stimulated by very low phosphorus in the blood (Reinhardt et al., 1988; Goff, 1998a). While presumed similar, this response has not been studied in periparturient dairy cows. However, in some cases correction of hypophosphatemia may not occur and may be further complicated if the cow is developing or has severe hypocalcemia because parathyroid hormone is secreted increasing urinary and salivary losses of phosphorus. Secretion of cortisol around parturition also may depress concentrations of phosphorus in plasma. Intravenous calcium to correct hypocalcemia usually results in a rise in phosphorus in plasma because parathyroid hormone secretion is reduced, reducing urinary and salivary loss of phosphorus. It also stimulates resumption of gut motility, recycling of salivary phosphorus, and absorption. Oral or intravenous administration of a soluble form of phosphorus such as sodium monophosphate can help correct hypophosphatemia. In some cows with severe cases of clinical milk fever, protracted hypophosphatemia (phosphorus in plasma $<1$ mg/dl) occurs with recumbency; even with successful treatment for hypocalcemia, phosphorus in blood remains low. This disorder is not well understood. However, it is unlikely that increasing the amount or concentration of phosphorus in the diet in excess of requirement in late pregnancy or early lactation will correct hypophosphatemia in the periparturient period, as this disorder seems to occur secondary to hypocalcemia.

Rickets results in young growing calves that are fed a deficient diet and have low phosphorus in the blood from a failure of mineralization in osteoid and cartilaginous (growth plate) matrices during bone remodeling. In contrast, osteomalacia occurs over time with phosphorus deficiency (2 to 4 mg/dl in plasma) in mature animals (no active growth plates) with failure of mineralization of the remodeled osteoid matrix. During mineralization phosphate and calcium ions are incorporated into cartilage of physes or the osteoid matrix in a ratio of 6-to-10. If dietary phosphorus is deficient, low concentrations of phosphorus in blood may not allow this process to proceed normally. In the adult, phosphorus in bone released during remodeling is used to maintain concentrations of phosphorus in blood rather than being reincorporated into bone. In young animals, bone cartilage remains unmineralized resulting in bone that can be flexed without breaking.

Animals with a deficiency of phosphorus are not able to detect or sense phosphorus in feeds or supplements (Miller, 1983b). With severe deficiency of phosphorus they can exhibit pica. Clinical signs of phosphorus and copper deficiency are similar, but can be differentiated by concentrations of plasma phosphorus and blood hemoglobin.

### PHOSPHORUS TOXICITY

Long-term feeding of excess phosphorus can cause problems of calcium metabolism, inducing excessive bone resorption and urinary calculi, secondary to the elevated concentrations of phosphorus in blood (National Research Council, 1980). Most often, phosphorus toxicity due to high dietary phosphorus is complicated with low dietary calcium, although ruminants can tolerate a wider ratio of calcium-to-phosphorus than nonruminants, as long as phosphorus and calcium are adequate. Supplemental phosphates given in large oral doses are not considered highly toxic, resulting in mild diarrhea and abdominal distress. Dairy cattle are quite adept at excreting excess absorbed phosphorus to maintain concentrations of phosphorus in blood within a normal range via salivary secretion and fecal excretion (Challa et al., 1989). Urinary excretion of phosphorus also may increase, although its quantitative importance is small relative to fecal excretion. Feeding 0.69 percent phosphorus (dry basis) in the diet of Holstein-Friesian cows for 14 weeks prepartum through 22 weeks of lactation caused no problems or signs of toxicity (De Boer et al., 1981). However, over-feeding can be a concern. High (0.64 percent, dry basis) dietary phosphorus reduced apparent absorption of magnesium compared with 0.22 percent phosphorus in pregnant dairy heifers (Schonewille et al., 1994). Additionally, high phosphorus (greater than 80 g/cow per day) in the diet of late pregnant, nonlactating cows increased phosphorus in blood which apparently inhibits production of the active form of vitamin D (Tanaka and Deluca, 1973), consequently increasing the incidences of milk fever and hypocalcemia at parturition (Barton et al., 1978; Reinhardt and Conrad, 1980). Assuming the presence of adequate calcium in the diet, the maximum tolerable concentration of phosphorus in diets for cattle is estimated to be 1.0 percent, dry basis (National Research Council, 1980).

PHOSPHORUS AND REPRODUCTION

Published research reports from 1923 through 1999 were reviewed to assess the effects of dietary phosphorus on reproductive performance of cattle. In some studies, but not all, severe deficiency of dietary phosphorus caused infertility or reduced reproductive performance of cattle (Alderman, 1963; Morrow, 1969; McClure, 1994). Typically, phosphorus concentration was <0.20 percent of dietary DM, the deficient diet was fed for an extended length of time (1 to 4 years), and where measured, feed intake was depressed, causing coincidental deficiencies of energy, protein, and other nutrients. Low BW generally is considered the main cause of reduced reproductive performance in phosphorus-deficient cows (Holmes, 1981). Palmer et al. (1941) showed that reproductive performance of dairy heifers was compromised much more when both dietary protein and phosphorus were deficient, than phosphorus singularly. Little (1975) demonstrated that deficiencies of phosphorus and protein were additive on failure to exhibit first postpartum estrus in grazing multiparous beef cows. However, there is no evidence to support feeding dietary phosphorus in excess of requirements to improve reproductive performance of dairy cattle.

VIRGIN HEIFERS

In growing virgin heifers, experimentally induced reproductive failure caused by a dietary phosphorus deficiency was very difficult to produce. Huffman et al. (1933) found no reproductive problems in dairy heifers fed a diet with 0.20 percent phosphorus. In two trials with growing dairy heifers, increasing dietary phosphorus from 0.22 to 0.32 percent resulted in no improvement in reproductive performance (Noller et al., 1977). With dairy heifers fed diets with 0.13 to 0.22 versus 0.40 percent phosphorus for 5.5 months no differences in estrus exhibition, services per conception, or pregnancy rates were detected (Hecht et al., 1977). Beginning at 7 months of age, Hereford heifers fed 0.16 or 0.40 percent dietary phosphorus for 2 years had similar pregnancy rates (96 versus 100 percent) and percentages of live calves (91 versus 93 percent) (Call et al., 1978). Hurley et al. (1982) examined intensity of estrus in 12- to 16-month old dairy heifers fed diets containing 73, 138, or 246 percent of National Research Council (1978) requirements for phosphorus. Estrous behavior, ovarian activity, and concentration of progesterone and luteinizing hormone in blood serum were not different among heifers fed different amounts of phosphorus. Because heifers are still growing and bone phosphorus is readily available, they apparently can compensate for a short-term (e.g., <2 years) dietary deficiency, thus reproductive performance is not affected.

LACTATING COWS

With lactating dairy cows, evidence from available research to support feeding phosphorus in excess of requirements to improve reproduction is virtually nonexistent. Results of seven studies can be summarized very succinctly (Stevens et al., 1971; Carstairs et al., 1980; Call et al., 1987; Brodison et al., 1989; Brintrop et al., 1993; Wu and Satter, 2000; Wu et al., 2000). All of the various measures of reproductive performance compared within each study were not different due to concentration of dietary phosphorus with one exception. In the study of Stevens et al. (1971), services per conception were greater in the second year for cows fed 0.40 versus 0.55 percent phosphorus, but not in the first year of study.

Among these seven studies, dietary phosphorus ranged from 0.24 to 0.62 percent of dietary DM, length of feeding different dietary phosphorus concentrations ranged from the first 12 weeks of lactation to as long as three consecutive lactations; and, average milk yields ranged from about 15 to almost 32 kg/cow per day. As long as dietary phosphorus was greater than or equal to 0.32 percent, reproductive performance was normal and not improved with greater concentrations of phosphorus.

Cows in some of the studies would not be considered high producing cows by modern standards. However, with Holstein cows yielding an average of 30.8 and 30.5 kg/cow per day of lactation over two lactations and fed 0.35 or 0.45 percent total dietary phosphorus, respectively, days postpartum to first insemination, days not pregnant, and services per conception were not affected by dietary phosphorus concentration (Wu and Satter, 2000). Pregnancy rates at 120 or 230 days of lactation were not different between cows fed 0.35 or 0.45 percent phosphorus for two lactations.

Overall, evidence from the research literature does not support feeding dietary phosphorus at concentrations in excess of those needed to meet dietary requirements to improve reproductive performance. Additional studies with more, higher yielding cows would be useful.

PHOSPHORUS HOMEOSTASIS OF THE PERIPARTURIENT COW

The periparturient dairy cow represents a unique situation with respect to phosphorus homeostasis. Modulation of calcium homeostasis through endocrine regulation is paramount. During mobilization of 10 ions of calcium from bone, six phosphate ions also are released into blood circulation. Indirectly, this serves to increase the pool of phosphorus in blood. In this physiologic circumstance, increasing the supply of potentially absorbable phosphorus via the diet may be of little benefit. Braithwaite (1983) showed in ewes during late pregnant and early lactation that increasing dietary phosphorus (and calcium) did not increase net retention or utilization of phosphorus. Instead, the increased amount of dietary phosphorus supplied was absorbed with lower efficiency and that which was absorbed appeared as a net increase in salivary phosphorus and endogenous fecal phosphorus, in excess of the animal's requirement. Resorption of phosphorus from bone appeared to occur merely as a consequence of greater demand for calcium in the periparturient period. Because of the high physiologic priority and regulatory mechanisms for calcium homeostasis in the periparturient period, it is doubtful that increasing the supply of dietary phosphorus above that to meet requirements will have any positive benefit. Mineral stores in bone were mobilized during late pregnancy and early lactation, irrespective of rate of phosphorus absorption. These stores were replaced later in lactation as long as intake of phosphorus was sufficient to meet requirements. Similar studies were not found for periparturient dairy cows, but physiologic events are presumed similar.

In the past, the calcium-to-phosphorus ratio was held as an important nutritional consideration in diet formulation and for proper utilization of both elements. This is important only if dietary phosphorus or calcium is deficient. With sufficient dietary phosphorus, wide ranges of the ratio can be tolerated (Agricultural Research Council, 1980; National Research Council, 1980; National Research Council, 1989). This, taken with the fact that the efficiencies of absorption of phosphorus and calcium vary greatly depending upon sources of the elements, provides no support for recommending a specific dietary calcium-to-phosphorus ratio. No differences in milk yield, persistency of milk production, milk composition, or reproductive performance were found in cows during early lactation fed diets with calcium-to-phosphorus ratios of 1-to-1, 4-to-1, or 8-to-1 (Smith et al., 1966), or 3-to-1 or 1.5-to-1 (Stevens et al., 1971). Nonetheless, it is important to insure that dietary requirements of each element are met.

### *Sodium*

Cattle evolved without abundant dietary sodium to meet nutritional needs. Therefore, the body developed a tenacious ability to conserve sodium, via the kidney and efficient absorption from the lower small intestine and large intestine. Dairy cattle utilize dietary sodium very efficiently, but only very small amounts are stored in a form that is readily available for metabolism. Feeding sodium in excess of needs directly results in increased excretion, which may contribute to excess in the environment increasing salinity of water and soil, and toxicity to plants. However, when dietary concentrations of other macromineral electrolyte elements (e.g., chlorine) are fed in excess of requirements, additional dietary sodium improves animal performance.

#### PHYSIOLOGIC ROLES

Sodium, is the primary extracellular cation (Aitken, 1976). Additionally, 30 to 50 percent of total body sodium is in a non-exchangeable fraction in the crystalline structure of bone (Eldman et al., 1954). It, along with chlorine and potassium in proper concentrations and balance, are indispensable for a number of important physiologic functions. The exchangeable fraction of sodium modulates extracellular fluid volume and acid-base equilibrium (McKeown, 1986). Additionally, heart function and nerve impulse conduction and transmission are dependent on the proper balance of sodium and potassium. Sodium also plays an indispensable role in sodium-potassium adenosine triphosphate enzyme (Na-K ATPase) responsible for creating electric gradients for nutrient transport. The Na-K pump is essential for all eukaryotic cells, enabling transport of glucose, amino acids, and phosphate into cells, and hydrogen, calcium, bicarbonate, potassium, and chloride ions out of cells (Lechene, 1988). Sodium also is a major component of salts in saliva to buffer acid from ruminal fermentation (Blair-West et al., 1970).

By regression, the sodium content of cattle was estimated at 2.01 to 1.68 g/kg over the range of 75 to 500 kg empty body weight; about 0.4 percent of bone tissue is sodium (Agricultural Research Council, 1980). Typical concentrations of sodium in blood plasma are 150 meq/L and 160 to 180 meq/L in saliva. Concentration in milk is between 25 and 30 meq/L; it is increased during mastitis when serum leaks into milk, but not affected appreciably by dietary sodium content (Kemp, 1964; Schellner et al., 1971).

#### SODIUM UTILIZATION AND HOMEOSTASIS

Absorption occurs throughout the digestive tract, and dietary sodium generally is assumed to be almost completely available. Absorption occurs by an active transport process in the reticulorumen, abomasum, omasum, and duodenum. Passive absorption also occurs through the intestinal wall so there is a tendency towards equal concentrations in intestinal and fecal fluids. However, substantial active absorption against a sizable concentration gradient also occurs in the lower small intestine and large intestine (Renkema et al., 1962). Consequently, relatively little sodium is excreted in feces, especially in sodium-deficit animals. This mechanism helps ensure that ruminants can subsist on feeds relatively low in sodium content over long periods of time.

Sodium concentrations in blood and tissues are maintained principally via reabsorption and excretion by the kidneys. There is close synchrony between the excretion of sodium, and potassium and chloride. Sodium is the central effector of ion excretion and changes in renal reabsorption are chief determinants of sodium excretion. Endocrine control via tissue receptors and the renin-angiotensin system, aldosterone, and atrial natriuretic factor monitor and modulate sodium concentrations in various tissues, which consequently control fluid volume, blood pressure, potassium concentrations, and renal processing of other ions. Kidneys are tremendously efficient in reabsorbing sodium when dietary sodium is deficient. When cattle are depleted of sodium, salivary glands decrease secretion of sodium in saliva. The decrease in sodium content is replaced reciprocally by nearly the same concentration of potassium (Van Leeuwen, 1970; Morris and Gartner, 1971).

### REQUIREMENT FOR ABSORBED SODIUM

*Maintenance* As with calcium and phosphorus, the factorial method was used to derive the absorbed sodium requirement. By definition, the maintenance requirement for absorbed sodium is equal to the inevitable losses in feces and urine of animals fed very near their true requirement. In the model, the daily maintenance requirement for absorbed sodium for growing cattle and non-lactating pregnant cows was set at 1.5 grams/100 kg body weight based on the estimates of total inevitable losses of 0.015 grams/kg body weight per day as reported by Todd et al. (1984) and Gueguen et al. (1989). During initial model development this value for maintenance also was tested for lactating cows. However, this resulted in diets containing amounts and concentrations of total dietary sodium which are known to result in signs of sodium deficiency (Babcock, 1905; Mallonee et al., 1982a), subnormal lactational performance (Aines and Smith, 1957; Kemp, 1964; Kemp and Geurink, 1966; Mallonee et al., 1982a), and negative sodium balance (Lomba et al., 1969). Therefore, the maintenance requirement for absorbed sodium for lactating cows was adjusted based on consideration of results from feeding experiments (see below). The maintenance requirement of absorbed sodium for lactating cows was set empirically at 0.038 g/kg of body weight per day. A higher maintenance requirement for lactating animals compared with growing and nonlactating animals seems logical due to the greater rate and extent of dynamics of some basic physiologic functions (e.g., ruminal buffering or systemic acid-base balance) during lactation that are not accounted for directly by the simple factorial calculation. Doubtless, more research estimates of inevitable losses of sodium in feces and urine by all classes of dairy animals could prove very useful in setting the maintenance requirements for absorbed sodium. Sweating, for aid in heat balance, includes secretion of sodium (Jenkinson and Mabon, 1973). At environmental temperatures between 25 and 30°C, an additional 0.10 g of sodium per 100 kg body weight was considered part of maintenance. With environmental temperatures >30°C, maintenance requirement was increased an additional 0.40 g of sodium per 100 kg BW for a total of 0.50 g per 100 kg BW (Agricultural Research Council, 1980).

*Growth* In the model, the requirement of absorbed sodium for growth was set at 1.40 g/kg of average daily gain for animals weighing between 150 and 600 kg live body weight (Gueguen et al., 1989).

*Pregnancy* Recent slaughter data are available from 18 multiparous pregnant Holstein cows to quantify the requirement for absorbed sodium of the conceptus during the last trimester (House and Bell, 1993). Quantitative requirements for all mineral elements are negligible to about 190 days of gestation. The sodium requirement of the conceptus is 1.39 g/d from 190 to 270 days of gestation, but should not be used to compute the sodium requirement for days of gestation <190 (House and Bell, 1993).

*Lactation* The average sodium concentration in milk from several studies was 0.63 g/kg (Agricultural Research Council, 1965), and this was taken as the requirement for absorbed sodium for milk yield. This constitutes a large portion of the total absorbed sodium requirement of sodium for lactating cows.

### DIETARY REQUIREMENT AND EFFICIENCY OF ABSORPTION

As with calcium, phosphorus, and magnesium, the dietary requirement for sodium was established by dividing the absorbed sodium requirement by an absorption coefficient. Sodium from typical feeds is solubilized and released in the liquid matrix of digesta and is readily available for absorption. Feedstuffs commonly used in diets for dairy cattle do not contain enough sodium to meet requirements and supplemental sources are typically included. Because fecal excretion of sodium is low, especially when the element is fed below or very near the true requirement, apparent digestibility data are useful to determine the efficiency of absorption. Apparent absorption of sodium by dairy cows fed fresh forages ranged from 77 to 95 percent, with an average of 85 percent (Kemp, 1964). Semipurified diets containing corn silage, solka floc, or corn cobs as the primary fiber sources fed to dairy heifers had apparent absorption coefficients for sodium of 74, 86, and 91 percent, respectively (Martz et al., 1988). Common salts of sodium used in diets for dairy cattle are readily soluble within the digestive tract (Peeler, 1972). Sodium chloride is most often used and the sodium is essentially 100 percent available; efficiency of absorption of sodium from other salts (e.g., sodium bicarbonate) also is considered very high. Agricultural Research Council (1980) estimated that 91 percent of sodium consumed by cattle was absorbed.

Because common feedstuffs contain relatively little sodium, and supplemental inorganic sources with high sodium availability are used, an efficiency of absorption coefficient of 90 percent was used in the model to compute the dietary requirement for sodium with common feedstuffs and mineral sources. However, the sodium in some animal by-product feedstuffs containing bone may be less available as it is tightly bound in the crystalline structure.

### LACTATIONAL RESPONSES TO VARYING DIETARY SODIUM CONCENTRATIONS

Aines and Smith (1957) established that sodium was the limiting nutrient in the diet of dairy cows that contained no supplemental sodium chloride. Furthermore, for dairy cows to produce 20 kg of milk, 30 g of sodium chloride per cow was needed, and 15 g was inadequate. Total sodium requirement at that rate of milk production was estimated to be 21.3 g/d per cow. Kemp (1964) calculated a comparable sodium requirement from balance trials of 23.3 g/d. Kemp and Geurink (1966) reported that 0.14 percent sodium in grazed forage was sufficient to support more than 30 kg of milk production per day. However, feeding lactating dairy cows a diet with no supplemental sodium chloride (0.16 percent sodium, dry basis) resulted in marked depressions in DMI and milk yield after just 1 to 2 weeks of feeding (Mallonee et al., 1982a). Sodium balance always was negative in experiments involving lactating dairy cows fed many different diets with <0.2 percent sodium, or when the diets of adult nonpregnant cows contained <0.1 percent sodium, dry basis (Lomba et al., 1969).

Empirical modeling of data from 15 experiments with lactating cows (1,444 cow-period observations) conducted in either cool or warm seasons showed that DMI and milk yield were improved by dietary concentrations of sodium well above those needed to meet requirements (Sanchez et al., 1994a,b). Dry matter intake and milk yield responses over a range of dietary sodium concentrations (0.11 to 1.20 percent, dry basis) were curvilinear, with maximum performance at 0.70 to 0.80 percent sodium, dry basis. However across all experiments, dietary concentrations for sodium, potassium, chloride, calcium, and phosphorus, ranged from below those needed to meet requirements to concentrations considerably higher (e.g., 0.11 to 1.20 percent sodium; 0.66 to 1.96 percent potassium; 0.15 to 1.62 percent chloride; and, 0.33 to 0.65 percent phosphorus, dry basis). Maximum feed intake and milk yield responses at higher concentrations of sodium than needed to meet requirements likely is due to the higher concentrations of other macromineral elements in the diets. There were interactions of sodium by potassium, sodium by chloride, and sodium by phosphorus on DMI indicating that responses to sodium differed, over the range of dietary concentrations of potassium, chloride, and phosphorus. Additionally, interactions of dietary sodium with potassium, chloride, and phosphorus on DMI differed in experiments conducted in the cool versus warm season. It is unknown if maximum performance responses occurring at 0.7 to 0.8 percent dietary sodium would have occurred if the dietary concentrations of other macromineral elements would have been closer to those needed to provide their requirements, or if the high concentrations of sodium (and other elements) may have affected feed intake and (or) digestive physiology, independent of requirements. In hot weather, milk yield and DMI increased when sodium was supplemented to a basal diet (0.18 percent sodium, dry basis) to 0.55 percent total dietary sodium (dry basis) with either sodium chloride or sodium bicarbonate; chlorine was equalized among diets (Schneider et al., 1986).

Few reports of feeding studies with dairy cattle fed graded concentrations of sodium to determine growth responses were found in the literature. Morris and Gartner (1971) considered 3.1 grams of sodium/day adequate for 300 kg bulls gaining 0.9 kg/day. This is estimated to be about 0.05 percent of dietary dry matter intake.

### FREE-CHOICE FEEDING OF SODIUM CHLORIDE

Cattle consume salt liberally if given the choice. Smith et al. (1953) found that lactating cows consumed more salt when provided free-choice in granular versus block form, but consumption of block was sufficient to meet needs for lactation.

### SODIUM DEFICIENCY

Babcock (1905) fed a diet very low in sodium to dairy cows and described intense craving for salt, licking and chewing various objects, and general pica. Deficiency signs were manifested within 2 to 3 weeks. Sodium deficiency signs may not develop for several weeks to months, depending upon rate of milk production. However, Mallonee et al. (1982a) found when feeding a diet with no supplemental sodium chloride (0.16 percent sodium) that feed intake and milk yield began to decline within 1 to 2 weeks, and pica and drinking of urine of other cows was observed. Although dietary chloride concentration was not measured in the study, potassium chloride was supplemented (1.0 percent total dietary potassium), so chloride deficiency was not the cause of the condition. The condition was reversed as quickly as it was caused by inclusion of sodium chloride in the diet. Other deficiency signs include loss of appetite, rapid loss of body weight; an unthrifty, haggard appearance, lusterless eyes, and rough hair coat (Underwood, 1981). More extreme signs of deficiency include incoordination, shivering, weakness, dehydration, and cardiac arrhythmia leading to death.

SODIUM (SODIUM CHLORIDE) TOXICITY

Dermott et al. (1968) fed lactating cows 4 percent sodium chloride in a grain mix at 1 kg of grain for each 2 kg of 4 percent fat-corrected milk yield for 2 weeks without ill effects on milk yield, body weight, or general health. Although total feed intake was not measured, the sodium concentration of the total diet would have been about 0.8 to 1.0 percent, dry basis. High intake of sodium chloride can increase the incidence and severity of udder edema (Randall et al., 1974). Feeding diets with 0.88 percent sodium from sodium chloride or sodium bicarbonate to mid-lactation Holstein cows did not cause toxicity or reduce feed intake and milk yield compared with 0.55 percent sodium (Schneider et al., 1986).

Drinking water that contained 12,000 to 25,000 mg/L sodium chloride by growing cattle produced toxicosis (Weeth et al., 1960; Weeth and Haverland, 1961). Toxicity signs included severe anorexia, reduced water intake, anhydremia, weight loss, and ultimately physical collapse. However, growing cattle tolerated up to 10,000 mg/L sodium chloride in drinking water without ill effects. Jaster (1978) provided drinking water with 0 or 2,500 mg/L sodium chloride for a 28-day period to lactating cows. No changes were noted in feed intake or digestibility, or in macromineral element concentrations in blood or milk. However, milk yield declined and water consumption increased.

A major factor influencing the degree of exhibition of sodium chloride toxicosis is the availability and quality of drinking water. With an adequate supply of good quality drinking water cattle can tolerate large quantities of dietary sodium chloride. The National Research Council (1980) states that the maximum tolerable dietary concentration of sodium chloride is 4.0 percent for lactating cattle (about 1.6 percent sodium, dry basis); this was the highest level tested (Dermott et al., 1968). For other cattle, the maximum tolerable concentration was set at 9.0 percent of dietary DM based on work of Meyer et al. (1955).

## *Chlorine*

The dietary requirements of chlorine for various classes of dairy cattle are the least studied of any of the macromineral electrolyte elements. Nonetheless, its physiologic roles and interrelationships with sodium and potassium are extremely important. Typically, chlorine is provided in the diet in a salt form which is solubilized, releasing the negatively charged chloride ion for absorption. Chloride is functionally important because of its propensity to accept electrons during metabolism.

PHYSIOLOGIC ROLES

Chloride is the major anion in the body involved in regulation of osmotic pressure, making up more than 60 percent of the total anion equivalents in the extracellular fluid. As a strong anion, it always is dissociated in solution. There is a close relationship between chloride, sodium, and potassium to maintain a strong ion difference (Stewart, 1981), and it is essential for transport of carbon dioxide and oxygen. It also is the chief anion in gastric secretions for protein digestion and is accompanied by hydrogen ions in nearly equivalent amounts. It is needed for activation of pancreatic amylase. Typical concentrations of chloride in blood plasma are between 90 and 110 meq/L, 10 to 30 meq/L in ruminal fluid, and 25 to 30 meq/L in milk. The concentration of chloride in cattle was estimated by regression to be between about 1.2 to 1.4 g/kg over the range of 100 to 500 kg empty-body (Agricultural Research Council, 1980).

UTILIZATION AND HOMEOSTASIS

About 80 percent of the chloride entering the digestive tract arises from digestive secretions in saliva, gastric fluid, bile, and pancreatic juice. Chloride is absorbed throughout the digestive tract. It, like sodium, is absorbed mainly from the upper small intestine by passive diffusion following sodium along an electric gradient. Chloride is transported across the ruminal wall to blood against a wide concentration gradient (Sperber and Hyden, 1952). Martens and Blume (1987) showed that chloride was co-transported actively with sodium across the rumen wall, although the exact mechanism is unclear. Appreciable absorption of chloride from gastric secretions (hydrochloric acid) occurs in the distal ileum and large intestine by exchange with secreted bicarbonate. Therefore, in the short term relatively large day-to-day differences in dietary intake of chloride have little effect on the total chloride entering the digestive tract. Excess chloride is excreted mainly in urine and feces, with smaller amounts in sweat mainly as sodium chloride or potassium chloride.

Regulation of the concentration of chloride in extracellular fluid and its homeostasis is coupled intimately to that of sodium, and is controlled precisely. Typically, it is thought that chloride's role in maintaining ionic and fluid balance is passive to that of sodium and potassium. However, Fettman et al. (1984b) showed that during chloride deficiency the ion functioned independently to mediate chloride conservation. Chloride was conserved by reducing excretion at the kidney, and in feces and milk. Chloride intake in excess of needs was excreted mainly in urine of steers and sheep (Nelson et al., 1955). In lactating cows, a significant amount of chloride was excreted in feces (Coppock, 1986). Normally, anion concentration in extracellular fluid is regulated secondarily to cation concentrations, and when the amount exceeds reabsorption capability of the kidney, excess chloride is excreted in urine (Hilwig, 1976). There is a reciprocal relationship between chloride and bicarbonate ions in the kidney and excretion of each chloride ion is associated with reabsorption of a bicarbonate ion or visa versa, depending upon systemic pH (Fischer et al., 1983). Also, renal excretion of excess sodium is accompanied by excretion of chloride. Chloride excretion also is influenced by bicarbonate ion. If blood bicarbonate rises, a comparable amount of chloride is excreted by the kidneys to maintain systemic acid-base balance. If base or electrolyte cations need to be conserved, chloride excretion is accompanied by ammonium ions.

#### REQUIREMENT FOR ABSORBED CHLORIDE

*Maintenance* The inevitable endogenous losses of chloride in feces and urine are about 50 percent higher than that of sodium (Gueguen et al., 1989). Therefore, 2.25 g/100 kg of body weight was used to set the maintenance requirement for absorbed chlorine in the model. More experimental data from dairy animals in different stages of the production cycle and at different levels of performance could be very useful to establish maintenance requirements.

*Growth* For cattle with live body weights between 150 and 600 kg, the requirement for absorbed chloride for growth was set at 1.0 g/kg of average daily gain (Gueguen et al., 1989).

*Pregnancy* No research was available to directly establish the requirement for absorbed chloride for pregnancy. However, based on consideration of the daily sodium accretion rate of the conceptus and the fetus separately (House and Bell, 1993), and assuming that the relative proportions of chloride and sodium in the fetus and in a new born calf (41.5 percent chloride and 58.5 percent sodium; Agricultural Research Council, 1980) are similar, the requirement was set at 1.0 g/d from 190 days of gestation to parturition.

*Lactation* Average concentration of chloride in milk for several studies was 1.15 g/L (Agricultural Research Council, 1965). Chloride exists in milk almost entirely as the free ion (Holt, 1985). Chloride is highest in colostrum, declines rapidly to average concentrations soon after lactation commences, and increases towards the end of lactation (Flynn and Power, 1985). The concentration in milk is independent of dietary intake, except in severe deficiency, and high environmental temperatures increase the chloride content, whereas cold temperatures have the opposite effect. The requirement for chloride for lactation was calculated as 1.15 g/kg of milk produced.

#### DIETARY REQUIREMENT AND EFFICIENCY OF ABSORPTION

Relatively little research has been done in ruminants to measure the true absorption coefficient for chloride principally due to its widespread commercial availability, good palatability of inorganic sources (e.g., sodium chloride), and relatively low cost. Chloride, like sodium and potassium, from inorganic sources and common feedstuffs is freely released into the liquid phase of the digesta and readily absorbed (Underwood, 1981). Because the main excretory route of excess chloride is in urine, using apparent digestibility data collected from animals fed at or just below their true requirement yields values similar to those representing true absorption. Apparent absorption of chloride in lactating cows fed fresh forages ranged from 71 to 95 percent and averaged 88 percent (Kemp, 1966). This is comparable to other estimates of absorption efficiency of 85 to 91 percent in cattle and sheep fed mixed diets (Agricultural Research Council, 1980). Paquay et al. (1969b) found that apparent digestibility of chloride was not influenced by intake of chloride, but was correlated negatively with intakes of dry matter, energy, and pentosan; and positively correlated with intakes of potassium and nitrogen. Although factors such as lactation, pregnancy, and growth affect the requirement for chloride, these factors do not appear to alter the efficiency of absorption of chloride. The efficiency of absorption of chloride from sodium chloride is considered virtually 100 percent. The relative absorption of chloride from potassium chloride is 95 percent of that from sodium chloride. Overall, the absorption coefficient for chloride in feedstuffs and mineral sources commonly fed to dairy cattle is near or >90 percent (Henry, 1995c). Therefore, in the model an absorption coefficient for chloride of 90 percent was assigned for all types of feedstuffs and common supplemental mineral sources.

#### LACTATIONAL AND GROWTH RESPONSES TO VARYING CONCENTRATIONS OF DIETARY CHLORIDE

Coppock (1986) provided a thorough review of the estimated requirements of dietary chloride for lactating dairy cows. Coppock et al. (1979) compared 0.18 percent with 0.40 percent total dietary chloride fed to primiparous Holstein cows for the first 11 weeks of lactation. Cows fed the diet with 0.18 percent chloride conserved chloride by dramatically reducing excretion of chloride in urine and feces. Chloride in milk also tended to decline. However, intakes of feed and water, and milk yield and composition, did not differ due to dietary concentrations of chloride. One-half of the cows in each treatment group had free access to a trace-mineral salt block and cows fed the diet low in chloride consumed more of the salt block. Fettman et al. (1984b) fed diets containing 0.10, 0.27, and 0.45 percent chloride for the first 8 to 11 weeks of lactation. Cows fed 0.10 percent chloride rapidly exhibited clinical signs of deficiency and poor performance compared with those fed medium and high concentrations of dietary chloride. However, health, feed intake, and yield and composition of milk by cows fed the medium and high concentrations of dietary chloride were similar. Coppock (1986) suggested that 0.2 percent chloride in the diet would approximately meet the requirement of a lactating cow. Meeting the true requirement is complicated by the cow's apparent ability to reduce chloride in milk when a low chloride diet is fed. He also suggested a dietary recommendation of 0.25 percent for a cow near zero energy balance, but emphasized that this was likely too low for a cow in peak milk yield and negative energy balance.

Empirical models with a large data set (1,444 cow-period means) showed that increasing dietary chloride over a range of 0.15 to 1.62 percent decreased DMI and milk yield of midlactation cows (Sanchez et al., 1994a). The negative effects of increasing dietary chloride were much more dramatic in hot summer weather than in winter. This is consistent with the results of Escobosa et al. (1984) showing profound exacerbating effects of high dietary chloride on acid-base balance (metabolic acidosis) and lactational performance during heat stress. Loss of chloride from sweating in response to high ambient temperatures is small, compared with losses of potassium and sodium (Jenkinson and Mabon, 1973), and not of quantitative importance in determining the chloride requirement.

Feeding diets with 0.038 percent chloride for 7 weeks to male Holstein calves did not produce clinical deficiency nor depress feed intake, growth rate, or digestibility of feed compared with calves fed 0.50 percent chloride (Burkhalter et al., 1979). Calves fed the low chloride diet adapted by reducing urinary excretion of chloride, and their water intake and urine output were greater than that of calves fed more chloride. In another study, acid-base status of calves fed a low chloride diet (0.038 percent chloride) was characterized (Burkhalter et al., 1980). Sodium bicarbonate was used to equalize the sodium in the low chloride diet. The low chloride diet resulted in lower chloride and potassium in plasma, and increased blood pH, partial pressure of carbon dioxide and bicarbonate, but had no effect on sodium in plasma. However, the mild alkalosis was not severe enough to affect growth and calves adapted to the low intake of chloride. Results of growth performance to varying intermediate dietary concentrations (e.g., between 0.038 and 0.50 percent) of chloride are not available, and therefore, it is uncertain if a dietary concentration of 0.038 percent is adequate if fed for >7 weeks.

If sodium chloride (common salt) is used to meet the sodium requirement the chloride requirement is met or exceeded. However, if sodium bicarbonate or some other sodium-containing salt is used to supply sodium, it may be necessary to meet the chloride requirement with another supplemental source (e.g., potassium chloride). More research to establish the requirements and appropriate dietary concentrations of chloride (and sodium) considering its interrelationships with other nutrients (Sanchez et al., 1994a,b), could greatly reduce the amount supplemented (e.g., sodium chloride) and excreted. Application of manure from cows fed chloride and sodium in excess of animals' needs can increase soil salinity (Coppock, 1986).

Chloride in drinking water also may make a major contribution to intake of chloride and should be considered.

#### CHLORIDE DEFICENCY

Chloride deficiency was created in young calves (100 kg BW) by feeding 0.063 percent chloride in the diet and removing daily about 600 g of abomasal contents (Neathery et al., 1981). General clinical signs were anorexia, weight loss, lethargy, mild polydipsia, and mild polyuria. In latter stages, severe eye defects and reduced respiration rates occurred, and blood and mucus appeared in feces. Metabolically, chloride deficiency resulted in severe alkalosis and hypochloremia, which manifested secondary hypokalemia, hyponatremia, and uremia. Control calves also had abomasal contents removed daily, but were fed a diet with 0.48 percent chloride, and grew normally and showed no signs of deficiency. During the first 8 to11 weeks of lactation, dairy cows fed low (0.1 percent, dry basis) dietary chloride exhibited dramatic and progressive declines in intakes of feed and water, body weight, milk yield, and electrolyte concentrations in blood serum, saliva, urine, milk, and feces (Fettman et al., 1984b). A significant decline of chloride in blood serum was found within 3 days after switching cows from a diet containing 0.42 percent to a diet with 0.10 percent chloride. Clinical signs of deficiency were manifested as depraved appetite, lethargy, hypophagia, emaciation, hypogalactiae, constipation, and cardiovascular depression. Metabolic alterations were severe primary hypochloremia, secondary hypokalemia, and metabolic alkalosis. Similar deficiency signs were induced by low dietary chloride in other studies (Fettman et al., 1984b, c, d). Chloride deficiency, resulting from an inadequate dietary supply or loss of gastric juices, can lead to alkalosis due to an excess of bicarbonate, because inadequate chloride is partially compensated for by bicarbonate.

#### CHLORIDE TOXICITY

The amount or concentration of chloride in the diet *per se* to cause toxicity has not been determined. However, the previous discussion of sodium chloride toxicosis (sodium section) is of interest. High systemic concentrations of chloride, in the absence of a neutralizing cation, can cause disturbance of normal acid-base equilibrium (Stewart, 1981; Escobosa et al., 1984). The maximum tolerable concentration of chloride per se in diets for dairy cattle has not been established. However, the maximum tolerable concentration of dietary sodium chloride was set at 4.0

percent (dry basis) for lactating dairy cows (National Research Council, 1980), based on the work of Demott et al. (1968) although only about one-half of the total daily intake was as the grain mix containing 4.0 percent sodium chloride. For nonlactating dairy animals a maximum tolerable concentration of sodium chloride of 9.0 percent was suggested (National Research Council, 1980). Less tolerance is evident when calcium is the cation accompanying chloride (Escobosa et al., 1984).

### *Potassium*

Potassium is the third most abundant mineral element in the body. It must be supplied daily in the diet because there is little storage in the body and the animal's requirement for potassium is highest of all the mineral element cations. Absorbed potassium in excess of requirements is excreted mainly in urine. Application of manures or fertilizers rich in potassium to crop land can result in excess potassium in the environment and very high potassium content of forages. This can cause problems with calcium and magnesium metabolism particularly for periparturient dairy cows, and may cause udder edema.

#### PHYSIOLOGIC ROLES

Potassium is involved in osmotic pressure and acid-base regulation, water balance, nerve impulse transmission, muscle contraction, oxygen and carbon dioxide transport; in phosphorylation of creatine, pyruvate kinase activity, as an activator or co-factor in many enzymatic reactions, in cellular uptake of amino acids and synthesis of protein, carbohydrate metabolism, and in maintenance of normal cardiac and renal tissue (National Research Council, 1980; Stewart, 1981; Hemken, 1983). It is the major intracellular electrolyte with concentrations in the range of 150 to 155 meq/L. In contrast to sodium and chloride, extracellular concentrations of potassium are very low (about 5 meq/L). Saliva typically contains $<10$ meq/L, whereas concentrations in ruminal fluid range from 40 to 100 meq/L. Blood plasma contains 5 to 10 meq of potassium per liter. However, the vast majority of potassium in blood is located within red blood cells (Aitken, 1976; Hemken, 1983). Potassium is abundant in soft tissues of the body. The potassium content of cattle from 75 to 500 kg empty body weight estimated by regression ranged between 2.37 and 2.01 g/kg, respectively (Agricultural Research Council, 1980). The concentration of potassium in milk is higher than any other mineral element (about 38 meq/L).

#### POTASSIUM UTILIZATION AND HOMEOSTASIS

Ruminants evolved on natural diets relatively rich in potassium, but deficient in sodium. Potassium is absorbed primarily in the duodenum by simple diffusion, and some absorption occurs in the jejunum, ileum, and large intestine. The main excretory route of excess absorbed potassium is via the kidneys. This route is primarily under regulation by aldosterone, which increases sodium reabsorption in the kidney with the concomitant excretion of potassium. Blood acid-base status also affects urinary excretion of potassium (McGuirk and Butler, 1980). With the onset of an alkalotic condition, intracellular hydrogen protons are exchanged with potassium in blood plasma as part of the regulatory mechanisms to maintain acid-base equilibrium and blood pH, reducing potassium in blood. A large gradient exists between intracellular renal tubule concentrations of potassium and that of luminal fluid (urine). This gradient affects the passage of potassium from the tubular cells into urine. Some endogenous as well as unabsorbed potassium also may be excreted in feces. Endogenous fecal losses of potassium increase with increasing DMI (Agricultural Research Council, 1980). However, Paquay et al. (1969a) using data from nonlactating and lactating dairy cows fed many different types of diets estimated that on average about 2.2 g of potassium/kg of dietary DM was excreted in feces.

#### REQUIREMENT FOR ABSORBED POTASSIUM

*Maintenance* By definition, the maintenance requirement for absorbed potassium is the sum of the endogenous losses in urine and feces when animals are fed very near the true requirement. Estimates of endogenous potassium loss in urine were 0.038 g/kg of body weight and 2.6 g/kg of dietary dry matter in feces in the study of (Gueguen et al., 1989). Therefore, in the model for growing animals and non-lactating pregnant cows the daily maintenance requirement of absorbed potassium was set at 0.038 g/kg of body weight plus 2.6 g/kg of dietary dry matter intake. During model development a value of 2.6 g potassium/kg of dietary dry matter intake was tested as the endogenous fecal loss for lactating cows. However, the computed amount of absorbed potassium for maintenance and the resulting total dietary concentrations and amounts of potassium were too low for optimum feed intake and milk yield based on results of feeding experiments (Dennis et al., 1976; Dennis and Hemken, 1978; Erdman et al., 1980a; Sanchez et al., 1994a,b). Therefore, in the model the maintenance requirement for absorbed potassium of lactating cows was set empirically as 0.038 g/kg body weight (endogenous urinary loss) plus 6.1 g/kg of dietary dry matter (endogenous fecal loss). A higher maintenance requirement for absorbed potassium for lactating cows compared with non-lactating animals is justified based on potassium's role in dynamic processes associated with ruminal function at higher levels of feed intake and maintenance of systemic acid-base balance. Doubtless, more definitive research data certainly would be useful to estimate the maintenance requirement for absorbed potassium of all classes of dairy animals. In addition, thermoregulation by sweating at higher environmental temperatures is part of the true maintenance requirement. At environmental temperatures between 25°C and 30°C, an additional 0.04 g of potassium/100 kg body weight was considered part of maintenance. At environmental temperatures >30°C, an additional 0.36 g of potassium/100 kg body weight for a total of 0.40 g per 100 kg BW was used in the model.

*Growth* In the model, the requirement of absorbed potassium for growth was set at 1.6 g/kg average daily gain based on the estimate of Gueguen et al. (1989) for cattle between 150 and 500 kg live weight.

*Pregnancy* Recent slaughter data are available from 18 multiparous pregnant Holstein cows to quantify the requirement for absorbed potassium for conceptus accretion during the last trimester of pregnancy (House and Bell, 1993). Requirements for all nutrients are negligible up until about 190 days of gestation. The requirement of the conceptus for absorbed potassium is 1.027 g/d from 190 to 270 days of gestation, but should not be used to compute the potassium requirement for days of gestation <190 (House and Bell, 1993).

*Lactation* The concentration of potassium in milk is quite constant even under conditions of widely varying potassium intakes (Sasser et al., 1966). The average concentration in milk is 0.15 percent, which is greater than any other mineral element. Therefore, the requirement for absorbed potassium was computed as 1.5 g/kg of milk produced.

### DIETARY REQUIREMENT AND EFFICIENCY OF ABSORPTION

Because the body does not store potassium, it must be consumed daily. The dietary requirement of potassium was established by dividing the requirement for absorbed potassium by an absorption coefficient. Potassium in feeds exists as simple ions, which typically are released in to the liquid matrix in the lumen of the digestive tract and are readily available for absorption (Emanuele and Staples, 1990, 1991; Ledoux and Martz, 1990). Hemken (1983) indicated that potassium is almost completed absorbed with a true digestibility of 95 percent or greater for most feedstuffs. Because potassium is excreted mainly in urine, urinary excretion and apparent digestibility (apparent absorption) are reliable criteria for estimation of efficiency of absorption. Paquay et al. (1969a) found that the apparent absorption of potassium by dairy cows fed alfalfa silage, clover silage, and cabbage silage ranged from 87 to 94 percent. Apparent absorption was slightly lower in four tropical forages fed to sheep, but efficiency of absorption was not affected by maturity of the forage (Perdomo et al., 1977). Average apparent absorption of potassium in eight forages fed to cattle and sheep was 85 percent (Miller, 1995). Supplemental potassium from inorganic sources such as potassium chloride, potassium carbonate, potassium sulfate, potassium acetate, potassium bicarbonate, dibasic potassium phosphate, and potassium citrate monohydrate are readily available for absorption (Peeler, 1972; Miller, 1995). In the model, an absorption coefficient value of 90 percent for potassium was used for all types of feedstuffs and mineral sources.

### GROWTH AND LACTATIONAL RESPONSES TO VARYING CONCENTRATIONS OF DIETARY POTASSIUM

*Growth* Research delineating the optimum dietary concentration of potassium and requirement of potassium for growing dairy calves is sparse. Growth of dairy calves was maximized with 0.58 percent potassium in the diet and no benefits were noted with higher dietary concentrations (Bigelow et al., 1984). Weil et al. (1988) found no differences in BW gain (average 0.73 kg/calf per day for all dietary potassium concentrations), feed intake, or plasma macromineral concentrations when feeding diets with 0.55, 0.84, 1.02, or 1.32 percent potassium (dry basis) to Holstein and Jersey calves of both sexes starting at 4 weeks of age. In a second study, 16 Holstein calves, blocked by sex, were fed either 0.34 or 0.58 percent dietary potassium from 6 to 14 weeks of age. Average daily gain and feed intake were greater for calves fed 0.58 percent potassium. Weil et al. (1988) concluded that a dietary concentration of potassium between 0.34 and 0.58 percent (dry basis) optimized growth of young dairy calves, but suggested that 0.55 percent be recommended until the potassium requirement is more clearly delineated. Tucker et al. (1991) fed diets with 0.4 or 0.6 percent dietary potassium (supplemented as potassium chloride) and 0 or 2.0 percent sodium bicarbonate (2 by 2 factorial) to growing calves (56 to 70 days of age and 76 kg live BW at initiation of study) and found no effects on feed intake. However, average daily gain increased with higher dietary potassium, and tended to be reduced by addition of sodium bicarbonate. Concentrations of potassium in plasma were increased by higher dietary potassium. Authors suggested that dietary concentrations between 0.4 and 0.55 percent (dry basis) may be optimum for growth of young dairy calves. Feedlot cattle require approximately 0.55 to 0.60 percent potassium (National Research Council, 1996). For cattle under range conditions with slower growth rates than feedlot cattle, 0.3 to 0.4 percent potassium appears adequate.

*Lactation* The secretion of potassium in milk (1.5 g potassium/L) necessitates higher dietary concentrations for lactating cows compared with growing cattle. Early research indicated that 0.75 and 0.70 percent dietary potassium (dry basis) were sufficient to meet requirements of early and mid- to late lactation cows, respectively (Dennis et al., 1976; Dennis and Hemken, 1978; Erdman et al., 1980a). Feed intake increased when cows previously fed 0.45 or 0.55 percent potassium were fed 0.66 percent, dry basis (Dennis et al., 1976). In another trial with midlactation cows (average milk yield = 23.0 kg/cow per day), 0.42 percent dietary potassium reduced DMI and milk yield; however, no differences in DMI or milk yield were noted for cows consuming diets with 0.69 or 0.97 percent potassium, dry basis (Dennis and Hemken, 1978). Similarly, during the first 10 weeks of lactation (average milk yield = 29.2 kg/cow per day), feed intake and milk production were similar with potassium concentrations of 0.75 and 0.99 percent, but feed intake declined with 0.51 percent dietary potassium (dry basis) compared with that of cows fed higher concentrations. The major animal response to marginally low concentrations of dietary potassium in these studies was reduced feed intake.

Empirical modeling of data from 15 experiments with midlactation dairy cows (1,444 cow-period observations) conducted in either cool or warm seasons showed that DMI and milk yield were improved with concentrations of dietary potassium well above those needed to meet requirements (Sanchez et al., 1994a,b). Dry matter intake and milk yield responses over a range of dietary potassium concentrations (0.66 to 1.96 percent, dry basis) were curvilinear, with maximum performance when diets contained 1.50 percent potassium, dry basis, in the cool season. In the warm season, DMI and milk yield increased over the range of dietary potassium concentrations in the data set. However, among all experiments in the data set, dietary concentrations for potassium, sodium, chloride, calcium, and phosphorus, ranged from below those needed to meet requirements to concentrations considerably higher (e.g., 0.66 to 1.96 percent potassium; 0.11 to 1.20 percent sodium; 0.15 to 1.62 percent chloride; 0.50 to 1.34 percent calcium; and, 0.33 to 0.65 percent phosphorus, dry basis). Maximum feed intake and milk yield responses at higher concentrations of potassium than needed to meet requirements likely are associated with the higher concentrations of other macromineral elements in the diets. Interactions of potassium by sodium, potassium by chloride, and potassium by calcium on dry matter intake and milk yield indicated that responses to potassium differed, over the range of dietary concentrations of sodium and chloride. Additionally, interactions of dietary potassium with sodium and chloride on dry matter intake differed in cool versus warm season experiments. It is unknown if maximum performance responses occurring at 1.5 percent potassium or greater would have occurred if the dietary concentrations of other macromineral elements would have been nearer those needed to meet dietary requirements. Or, if the high concentrations of potassium (and other elements) may have affected feed intake and (or) other physiologic functions, independent of true requirements. In a winter study in Florida, Mallonee (1984) found no benefit of increasing dietary potassium from 1.07 to 1.58 percent (dry basis) on feed intake or lactational performance of midlactation Holstein cows when diets contained 0.99 percent calcium, 0.43 percent phosphorus, and 0.28 percent magnesium. However, there were interactions on DMI and milk yield of dietary potassium with varying dietary sodium (0.16, 0.42, and 0.70 percent, dry basis).

Diets containing 1.6, 3.1, or 4.6 percent potassium (via supplemental potassium carbonate) were fed to cows during early lactation (Fisher et al., 1994). Feed intake and milk yield were reduced with the 4.6 percent potassium, and water intake, urinary excretion, and total potassium excretion were increased with increasing concentrations of potassium in the diet.

During heat stress, reduced DMI coupled with the requirement for lactation, increased the requirement for potassium for sweating (Johnson, 1967; Jenkinson and Mabon, 1973; Beede et al., 1983) and acid-base maintenance (Beede and Collier, 1986). Feeding higher concentrations of dietary potassium than needed to meet National Research Council (1989) recommendations of lactating cows in thermoneutral environments (0.8 to 1.0 percent potassium, dry basis), increased feed intake and milk yield compared with cows fed lower dietary concentrations (Beede et al., 1983; Schneider et al., 1984; Mallonee et al., 1985; Schneider et al., 1986; West et al., 1987; Sanchez, 1994a). A dietary potassium concentration of 1.5 percent (dry basis) during heat stress maximized lactational performance (Beede and Shearer, 1991). Many, but not all, diets fed to lactating dairy cattle inherently contain basal concentrations of potassium of 1.5 percent or greater and no additional supplementation is necessary.

#### POTASSIUM DEFICENCY

Signs of severe potassium deficiency were manifested in lactating dairy cattle fed diets with 0.06 to 0.15 percent potassium (Pradhan and Hemken, 1968; Mallonee et al., 1982b). Marked decline in feed and water intake, reduced body weight and milk yield, pica, loss of hair glossiness, decreased pliability of the hide, lower concentrations of potassium in plasma and milk, and higher blood hematocrit readings occurred within a few days to a few weeks after cows were offered the potassium-deficient diets. Rate of occurrence and severity of deficiency signs appear to be related to rate of milk production, with higher yielding cows (secreting more total potassium in milk) affected more quickly and severely than lower yielding cows. With severe potassium deficiency, cows will be profoundly weak or recumbent with overall muscular weakness and poor intestinal tone (Sielman et al., 1997). In this case, hypokalemia syndrome was associated with treatment of ketosis.

When diets contained 0.5 to 0.7 percent potassium the only apparent sign of deficiency in lactating cows was reduced feed intake with corresponding lower milk yield compared with cows fed adequate potassium. Severe potassium deficiency under most natural conditions is rare. However, marginal deficiency can occur if diets contain predominantly low-potassium feedstuffs and are not supplemented.

#### POTASSIUM TOXICITY

The dietary concentration of potassium that leads to toxicity is not well defined (Ward, 1966b). Toxicosis is unlikely to occur under natural conditions, but could occur as a result of excess supplementation. Ward (1966a) described death from 501 g of potassium as potassium chloride given by stomach tube to a cow (475 kg body weight); death was apparently from cardiac arrest. It was pointed out that this amount represented approximately the daily amount consumed by similar cows fed 15 kg of alfalfa, apparently without ill effects. Dennis and Harbaugh (1948) administered 182 and 240 g of potassium as potassium chloride without detectable clinical signs of toxicity, but 393 g by stomach tube to cattle weighing about 300 kg resulted in one death, two that required treatment, and two exhibiting no signs of toxicity. The maximum tolerable concentration in the total diet for ruminants was set at 3.0 percent, dry basis (National Research Council, 1980). However, when 4.6 percent dietary potassium (via supplemental potassium carbonate) was fed to cows during early lactation, feed intake and milk yield were reduced, and water intake, urinary excretion, and total potassium excretion were increased (Fisher et al., 1994). High concentrations of dietary potassium, in excess of those needed to meet requirements, also depressed magnesium absorption. Feeding potassium in excess of that needed to meet requirements, can present metabolic and physiologic challenges to cattle, and can increase excretion of potassium into the environment.

#### DIETARY CATION-ANION DIFFERENCE

Interrelationships of the monovalent macromineral elements—sodium, potassium and chlorine—on dairy cattle performance have been of major interest in recent years. Mongin (1980) reviewed these interrelationships for nonruminants and suggested that the net acid intake could be extrapolated from the difference between macromineral cations (sodium and potassium) and the anion (chloride) in the diet. Considerations are inherently analogous to the strong-ion difference concept of basic acid-base chemistry (Stewart, 1981). In recent years, the dietary cation-anion difference concept has been studied in dairy cattle. More work has addressed diets of late prepartum dairy cows (see Transition Cow section, Chapter 9).

#### LACTATIONAL RESPONSES

A limited evaluation of cation-anion difference in diets of lactating dairy cattle and calves has been done. In studies with lactating dairy cows the dietary cation-anion difference generally has been expressed as: milliequivalents (sodium + potassium − chloride)/kg of dietary DM. Tucker et al. (1988) evaluated this concept in lactating dairy cows fed diets with −100, 0, +100, and +200 meq/kg of dietary DM. Dry matter intake and milk yield increased in cows fed +200 compared with those fed −100 meq/kg of dietary DM, independent of the effects of the individual elements (sodium, potassium, and chloride) used to alter the dietary cation-anion difference.

Because of the abundance of sodium and potassium relative to chloride in typical diets for lactating cows, the dietary cation-anion difference is rarely $<+100$ meq/kg of dietary DM. Sanchez et al. (1994b) used data from 10 separate experiments with midlactation cows to develop an empirical regression model characterizing effects of varying dietary cation-anion difference on feed intake and milk yield. The dietary cation-anion difference in experiments in the data set ranged from +58 to +612 meq/kg of dietary DM, averaging 324 meq. Dry matter intake and milk yield both responded in a curvilinear fashion over the range of dietary cation-anion difference. Both response variables were maximized with +380 meq (sodium + potassium − chloride)/kg of dietary DM. However, magnitude in difference of responses was not large (about 0.25 kg/cow per day) between +200 and +500 meq/kg of dietary DM. Many practical diets have cation-anion differences within this range. However, in the regression model from +380 to +612 meq, DMI declined (about 0.5 kg/cow per day), as did milk yield (about 1.0 kg/cow per day). Milk composition was not affected by varying dietary cation-anion difference. The empirical model was tested with independent data (Tucker et al., 1988; West et al., 1991, 1992) and reasonable agreement was found. Similar evaluations of effects of dietary cation-anion difference on performance during early lactation and with higher yielding cows may prove useful.

Escobosa et al. (1984) found that increasing the dietary cation-anion difference from −144 to +350 meq/kg of dietary DM during heat stress increased DMI and milk yield. Similar results were reported subsequently (West et al., 1991), even when different amounts of sodium or potassium were used to achieve the same dietary cation-anion difference (West et al., 1992).

GROWTH RESPONSES

The influence of dietary cation-anion difference on growth of calves has been examined. Xin et al. (1991) studied the effects of −100 and 200 meq [(sodium + potassium) − (chloride + sulfur)]/kg of dietary DM on feed intake, growth, acid-base status, and potential interactions with dietary copper source. Calves were fed dietary treatments beginning 4 to 11 days through 12 weeks of age. Growth rate increased with 200 compared with −100 meq/kg dietary DM, and blood pH was higher with 200 meq at 8 and 12 weeks of age. Copper source did not affect growth rate. In another study, growing dairy calves [(56 to 70 days of age and 79 kg (28 Holsteins) or 54 kg (4 Jerseys) live body weight at initiation of study)] were fed diets varying in cation-anion difference (sodium + potassium − chloride) of 0, 210, 370, and 520 meq/kg dietary DM (Jackson et al., 1992). Feed intake and average daily gain responded quadratically being greatest at 370 meq and lowest with 0 meq. Authors suggested that an optimal dietary cation-anion difference may exist for young growing ruminants. In a follow-up study, feed intake, growth rate, and calcium metabolism were compared for male and female Holstein calves (56 to 70 days and 72 kg average live body weight at the beginning of the study) fed diets with −180 or 130 meq [(sodium + potassium) − (chloride + sulfur)]/kg of dietary DM factorially with 0.42 and 0.52 percent dietary calcium (Jackson and Hemken, 1994). Feed intake did not differ due to dietary treatments. Calves fed the dietary treatment with 130 meq had greater growth rates than those fed diets with −180 meq; dietary calcium had no effect. Urinary calcium excretion was greater for calves fed diets with −180 meq compared with diets with 130 meq. Breaking strength of the $9^{th}$ rib was greater for calves fed the 130 meq treatment compared with the −180 meq treatment; breaking strength of the $7^{th}$ rib was greater with both diets that contained higher dietary cation-anion difference and higher dietary calcium. These studies indicate that there likely is an optimum dietary cation-anion difference for growing dairy calves and that a low or negative cation-anion difference may be deleterious to bone strength. Additional studies will be useful to elucidate the effects of dietary cation-anion difference on growth, bone metabolism, and acid-base physiology of growing calves.

## *Magnesium*

Magnesium is a major intracellular cation that is a necessary cofactor for enzymatic reactions vital to every major metabolic pathway. Extracellular magnesium is vital to normal nerve conduction, muscle function, and bone mineral formation. The concentration of magnesium in plasma of cows is normally between 0.75 and 1.0 mmol/L or 1.8 and 2.4 mg/dl. In a 500-kg cow, there is about 0.7 g of magnesium in the blood, 2.5 g of magnesium in all extracellular fluids, 70 g of magnesium inside cells, and 170 g of magnesium within bone mineral (Mayland, 1988). Bone is not a significant source of magnesium that can be utilized in times of deficit, as bone resorption occurs in response to calcium homeostasis, not magnesium status. Maintenance of normal concentration of magnesium in plasma is nearly totally dependent on absorption of dietary magnesium.

ABSORPTION

Magnesium is absorbed primarily from the small intestine of young calves. As the rumen and reticulum develop they become the main, and perhaps the only, site for magnesium absorption (Martens and Gabel, 1986; Martens and Rayssiguier, 1980; Pfeffer et al., 1970). In adult ruminants, the small intestine is a site of net secretion of magnesium (Greene et al., 1983). Magnesium absorption from the rumen is dependent on the concentration of magnesium in solution in the rumen fluid (important to both the active and passive transport of magnesium across the ruminal wall) and the integrity of the magnesium transport mechanism. The magnesium transport system is a sodium-linked active transport process (Martens and Gabel, 1986), which is critical if the dietary concentration of magnesium is low. In preparing the equations to describe the requirement for magnesium in this model it is assumed that the mechanism for the active transport of magnesium across the rumen wall is intact and functioning. It should be kept in mind when formulating rations that this is often not the case. The following sections will help to clarify when interference with rumen magnesium transport can be expected.

FACTORS AFFECTING SOLUBLE CONCENTRATION OF MAGNESIUM IN RUMINAL FLUID

*Dietary Magnesium Content* Feeding forages with a low magnesium content and inadequate magnesium supplementation of diets will keep the concentration of soluble magnesium low in the rumen. Cool weather, common in spring and fall when pastures are growing rapidly, reduces uptake of magnesium by plant tissue as does potassium fertilization of pastures (Mayland, 1988). Legumes generally contain more magnesium than grasses. Low DMI associated with high moisture diets can also lead to inadequate magnesium in ruminal fluid.

*pH of the Rumen Fluid and Magnesium Solubility* Magnesium solubility declines sharply as ruminal pH rises above 6.5. Grazing animals tend to have higher ruminal pH because of the high content of potassium in pasture and the stimulation of salivary secretions associated with grazing. Heavily fertilized, lush pastures are often high in nonprotein nitrogen and relatively low in readily fermentable carbohydrates. The ability of the ruminal microbes to incorporate the nonprotein nitrogen into microbial protein is exceeded and ammonia and ammonium ion build up in the rumen increasing ruminal pH. When high grain rations are fed ruminal fluid pH is often below 6.5 and magnesium solubility is generally adequate. This may explain why magnesium in concentrates is generally more available than the magnesium in forages (Miller et al., 1972).

*Forage* Forage can often contain 100 to 200 mmol/kg of unsaturated palmitic, linoleic, and linolenic acids, which can form insoluble magnesium salts. Plants also can contain trans-aconitic acid or citric acid. A metabolite of trans-aconitic acid, tricarballylate can complex magnesium and is resistant to ruminal degradation—but its role in hypomagnesemic tetany is unclear (Schwartz et al., 1988).

#### FACTORS AFFECTING MAGNESIUM TRANSPORT ACROSS THE RUMINAL EPITHELIUM

*Dietary Sodium:Potassium Ratio* Forages and pastures are generally low in sodium. Adding sodium to the diet can improve transport of magnesium across the ruminal wall when dietary sodium is low—though in high amounts it increases urinary excretion of magnesium so that the benefit to the animal may be negated. Dietary potassium in high concentrations can reduce the absorption of magnesium. Newton et al. (1972) fed lambs either a low potassium diet (0.6 percent potassium) or a high potassium diet (4.9 percent potassium) and found about a 50 percent reduction in apparent magnesium absorption. The exact mechanism for this interference by potassium is unknown, though it is thought to interfere with the sodium-linked transport of magnesium across the ruminal wall by depolarizing the apical membrane of the ruminal epithelium reducing the electric force driving magnesium across the rumen epithelial cells (Martens and Kasebieter, 1983; Leonard-Marek and Martens, 1996). The negative effects of a high potassium diet cannot be overcome by adding extra sodium to the diet (Martens, 1988). Increasing magnesium in the diet cannot overcome the effect of the high potassium diet on the sodium-linked active transport of magnesium. However, increasing magnesium in the diet will allow enough transport of magnesium across the ruminal wall by passive absorption to meet the animal's requirement for absorbed magnesium (Ram et al., 1998; Leonard-Marck and Martens, 1996). Feeding ionophores (monensin, lasalocid) can improve activity of the sodium-linked transport system for magnesium in the rumen, increasing magnesium absorption efficiency about 10 percent (Greene et al., 1986). However, ionophores are not approved for use in many of the animals they could benefit.

*Lush High-Moisture Pastures* Lush high-moisture pastures increase the rate of passage of material from the rumen. There is some evidence that this prevents the concentration of magnesium within the ruminal fluid from reaching high enough levels (about 11mmol/L in cows) to fully saturate transport sites for magnesium in the rumen (Martens, 1983).

*Ingestion of High Amounts of Aluminum* Some studies have noted that tetany is more likely when animals ingest large amounts of aluminum as a result of soil contamination of forages. Most studies have found no impairment of magnesium absorption as a result of aluminum ingestion. Aluminum absorbed into the blood can depress parathyroid hormone secretion, which might result in a somewhat reduced concentration of magnesium in plasma. However, aluminum is generally very poorly absorbed from the diet (Fontenot et al., 1989).

*Energy Availability* Several reports have demonstrated increased utilization of orally administered magnesium when administered with oral glucose suggesting that glucose supplied the ruminal epithelium with a source of energy to power active transport of magnesium. It is also possible that the rapid fermentation of oral glucose lowered rumen pH enough to solubilize more of the magnesium. Similarly adding glucose may have increased ammonia incorporation into microbial protein, reducing the inhibitory effect of ammonia on magnesium transport (Mayland, 1988).

#### MAGNESIUM REQUIREMENT

A factorial approach was taken to describe the magnesium requirements of dairy cattle. Fecal loss of endogenous magnesium will be considered to be 3 mg/kg body weight for adult cattle and heifers >100 kg BW, based primarily on the data of Allsop and Rook (1972), and in agreement with the figure adopted by the National Research Council's *Nutrient Requirements of Beef Cattle* (1996) and Agricultural Research Council (1980) publications. Obligate urinary loss of magnesium is negligible. In growing heifers the magnesium content of tissue is 0.45 g/kg body weight gain (Agricultural Research Council, 1980). In pregnant animals, the fetal-placental requirement for magnesium is about 0.181 g/day in Holsteins from day 190 until the end of pregnancy (House and Bell, 1993). Grace (1983), however, estimated the requirement of the fetoplacental unit in late gestation was 0.33 g/day. Considering all the problems associated with hypomagnesemia at parturition it was decided to use the higher figure of 0.33 g/day to describe the fetal requirement for magnesium. Colostrum contains about 0.4 g magnesium/kg (Lyford and Huber, 1988) and milk contains about 0.12 to 0.15 g magnesium/kg.

The efficiency of absorption of magnesium as determined by apparent absorption from natural feedstuffs varies from 11 percent to 37 percent with the majority of values falling between 20 and 30 percent (Agricultural Research Council, 1980; Rook et al., 1958; Forbes et al., 1916; Rook and Campling, 1962; Henry and Benz, 1995). Apparent absorption is considered as an estimate of true absorption because few studies have been conducted to determine true absorption of magnesium. In reviewing literature published before 1980, the Agricultural Research Council (page 204) (1980) determined that the average coefficient for absorption of magnesium from a wide variety of natural feedstuffs fed to ruminants averaged 29.4 percent with a standard deviation of 13.5 percent. Because overestimating the efficiency of absorption of magnesium is potentially detrimental, the coefficient of absorption for magnesium from natural feedstuffs was assigned a value of 16 percent, one standard deviation below the mean, as adopted by the Agricultural Research Council (1980); this approach should provide some margin of safety from magnesium deficiency.

Magnesium oxide is the most widely used inorganic source of magnesium in ruminant diets. Studies with cattle have determined that the coefficient for absorption of magnesium from magnesium oxide is between 28 percent and 49 percent (Moore et al., 1971; Storry and Rook, 1963), though in one study with animals that were on pasture that was associated with hypomagnesemia the coefficient of absorption of magnesium from magnesium oxide was between 5 and 10 percent. Ammerman et al., (1972) working with sheep determined that apparent absorption of magnesium from magnesium oxide was 52 percent and true biologic efficiency of absorption was 51 percent. They also determined that the true biologic efficiency of absorption of magnesium sulfate was 57.6 percent and the biologic efficiency of absorption of commercial magnesite (magnesium carbonate) was essentially zero. Reagent grade magnesium carbonate was 43.7 percent biologically absorbable. Most studies express efficiency of absorption of magnesium from other inorganic sources relative to the absorption from magnesium oxide. Unfortunately, the particle size of the magnesium oxide used can have a large effect on absorption of magnesium (Jesse et al., 1981; Schonewille et al., 1992) with solubility and hence absorption being increased greatly with finely ground magnesium oxide. The coefficient of absorption for magnesium from inorganic sources will be set at 50 percent based on magnesium oxide with a particle size where 99 percent of the material is $<250$ $\mu$m in diameter. Magnesium in magnesite and dolomitic limestone should be considered unavailable when formulating dairy rations. Magnesium sulfate and magnesium chloride are much more soluble and available for absorption.

At least some of the variation in estimates of efficiency of absorption of magnesium from both forages and inorganic sources is a result of the experimental diet fed during the trials. Diets high in potassium and nitrogen would result in lower biologic efficiency of absorption of the magnesium. High moisture diets may also reduce absorption of dietary magnesium by the animal. All three are often present in immature forages, especially when animals are at pasture. Because potassium can have such a large effect on magnesium absorption, the coefficient for absorption of magnesium should be decreased when a high concentration of potassium is present in the diet. Greene et al. (1983) determined that in steers fed a diet that contained 0.1 percent magnesium, and 0.6 percent potassium apparent absorption of magnesium was 28.7 percent. Raising dietary potassium to 2.4 percent and 4.8 percent reduced apparent magnesium absorption to 20.9 percent and 7.9 percent, respectively, or about 5 percent for every 1 percent increase in dietary potassium above the potassium requirement. To overcome this 5 percent reduction in the apparent absorption of magnesium caused by potassium theoretically one would need to increase the final concentration of dietary magnesium by 17 percent (5 percent divided by 28.7 percent times 100) to ensure adequate magnesium absorption. Adjusting the absorption coefficient for dietary magnesium for the effect of dietary potassium has not been incorporated into the diet evaluation section of this model as the data fail to allow an adequate equation to be developed. However the problem appears to be pervasive. Blood magnesium concentration should provide a ready index of the adequacy of diet magnesium supply and absorption (Goff, 1998).

Cattle can excrete large amounts of magnesium in the urine so magnesium toxicity is not a practical problem in dairy cattle, although a maximum tolerable level of 0.4 percent was used in previous National Research Council publications. The negative effects of diets high in magnesium are generally restricted to causing a reduction in feed intake (most magnesium salts are not very palatable, especially magnesium sulfate and magnesium chloride) and/or inducing an osmotic diarrhea. Earlier National Research Council publications listed 0.4 percent magnesium in diets as the maximum tolerable level of magnesium based on earlier work where cows fed 0.39 percent magnesium showed no adverse effects (O'Kelly and Fontenot, 1969). However, diets supplemented with magnesium oxide to bring dietary magnesium to 0.61 percent have been used in high concentrate diets to correct milk fat depression without apparent harm except for occasional diarrhea (Erdman et al., 1980b). Diets for dry cows are commonly supplemented with magnesium sulfate and magnesium chloride to raise dietary anion content and magnesium in an effort to control milk fever. Many of these diets will exceed 0.4 percent magnesium with no adverse effect other than a possible reduction in feed intake (van Mosel et al., 1990).

Young calves fed 1.3 percent magnesium had lower feed intake and weight gain and diarrhea with mucus in feces (Gentry et al., 1978). Steers fed 2.5 or 4.7 percent magnesium exhibited severe diarrhea and a lethargic appearance; 1.4 percent magnesium reduced DM digestibility (Chester-Jones et al., 1989).

### *Sulfur*

#### FUNCTION

About 0.15 percent of the body weight is sulfur. Sulfur is found in the amino acids methionine, cysteine (cystine), homocysteine and taurine; in chondroitin sulfate of cartilage; and in the B-vitamins thiamin and biotin. The disulfide bonds of the sulfur containing amino acids are largely responsible for determining the tertiary structure of proteins. Oxidation of methionine and cysteine causes sulfur to also exist in tissues as the sulfate anion, which influences the acid-base balance status of the animal.

Methionine, thiamin, and biotin cannot be synthesized by cattle tissues. These nutrients must either be supplied in the diet or synthesized by ruminal microbes.

The dietary requirement of sulfur for the cow is primarily to provide adequate substrate to ensure maximal microbial protein synthesis. In general, the sulfur content of feedstuffs is directly related to protein concentration. Corn silage is often low in sulfur (0.05 to 0.10 percent) (Hill, 1985) and protein and is the type of diet in which nonprotein nitrogen and sulfur can be successfully added to enhance microbial protein synthesis. Nonprotein nitrogen, such as urea added to these diets will not be incorporated into microbial protein unless adequate sulfur is present to allow formation of methionine.

Emery (1957a) and Emery et al. (1957b) reported that ruminal microbes produce twice as much cysteine as methionine from inorganic sulfate. Not all bacteria in the rumen utilize all forms of sulfur (Emery et al., 1957a). Bryant (1973) found that the predominant ruminal cellulolytic bacteria, *Fibrobacter succinogenes*, could utilize sulfide or cysteine but not sulfate. Many strains of *Ruminococcus* grew in media containing only sulfide or sulfate sulfur. Elemental sulfur is not well utilized by many ruminal bacteria (Ishimoto et al., 1954).

Sulfur incorporated into microbial protein is absorbed from the small intestine as cysteine and methionine. Some dietary sulfur is absorbed as the sulfate or sulfide anion. Bray and Hemsley, 1969 observed that $^{35}$S-sulfide was absorbed more rapidly and efficiently from the rumen of sheep than was sulfate. Sulfate sulfur is absorbed more efficiently in the small intestine (Bird and Moir, 1971).

#### REQUIREMENT

Growth and production have been used to assess the requirement for dietary sulfur especially in low protein diets where nonprotein nitrogen is utilized. Bouchard and Conrad (1973 a,b) determined that 0.20 percent dietary sulfur, when supplied as inorganic sodium, calcium, potassium, or magnesium sulfate was adequate to sustain maximal sulfur retention (microbial protein synthesis of cystine and methionine) even in midlactation dairy cows producing 30 to 37 kg milk/ day. For efficient utilization of nonprotein nitrogen, the dietary nitrogen:sulfur ratio should be between 10 and 12:1 (Bouchard and Conrad, 1973b). The sulfur requirement is set at 0.20 percent of dietary DM.

#### FACTORS AFFECTING SULFUR REQUIREMENT

The sulfur-containing amino acids provide a major dietary source of sulfur for the cow and the ruminal microbes. Protection of proteins and amino acids from ruminal degradation could result in less sulfur being available for microbial protein synthesis in the rumen. Protection of proteins or amino acids from degradation in the rumen may help the cow obtain amino acids required for her tissues. However, failure of the rumen microbes to obtain adequate protein from rumen degradable sources may reduce the supply of sulfur from feed protein sources reducing ruminal cellulose digestion (Hunt et al., 1954; Spears et al., 1976) and reduce animal performance.

Methionine, methionine analogs, and sulfate salts are utilized equally well in meeting the dietary sulfur requirements of the cow and ruminal microbes (Bouchard and Conrad, 1973a,b; Bull and Vandersall, 1973; Thomas et al., 1951). Elemental sulfur is much less available, probably because it is not very soluble (Fron et al., 1990). Ligninsulfonate is also a poorly utilized source of sulfur (Bouchard and Conrad, 1973a).

#### TOXICITY

Excessive dietary sulfur can interfere with absorption of other elements, particularly copper and selenium (see copper and selenium sections). Acute sulfur toxicity causes neurologic changes, including blindness, coma, muscle twitches, and recumbency (Coghlin, 1944). Post-mortem examination reveals severe enteritis, peritoneal effusion, and petechial hemorrhages in many organs, especially kidneys (Bird, 1972). Often the breath will smell of hydrogen sulfide—which is likely the toxic principal in sulfur toxicosis. Sulfates are less toxic, though they can cause an osmotic diarrhea as the sulfate is only poorly absorbed. Excess sulfate added to rations can reduce feed intake and performance (Kandylis, 1984). Water containing 5,000 mg sodium sulfate/kg (1,100 mg S/kg or 0.11%) reduced feed and water intake resulting in reduced growth of cattle (Weeth and Hunter, 1971). Recent observations in beef cattle have determined that a polioencephalomalacia-like syndrome can be induced with diets containing 0.5 percent sulfur using sulfate salts as supplemental sulfur sources or from drinking water high in sulfates (Beke and Hironaka, 1991; McAllister et al., 1997). The strong reducing environment within the rumen can reduce dietary sulfate, sulfite, and thiosulfate to sulfide within the rumen (Lewis, 1954).

Sulfate anions have been added to rations of dry cows just before calving to decrease the dietary cation-anion difference of the ration to help prevent milk fever (Chapter 9), often to levels above 0.5 percent sulfur. No toxicities have been reported in dairy cows. However, the deleterious effects sulfur can have on copper and selenium absorption, and the recent reports of polioencephalomalacia in beef cattle fed 0.5 percent sulfur rations (Beke and Hironaka, 1991; McAllister et al., 1997) suggest the maximal tolerable level of sulfur should remain at 0.4 percent of dietary DM, as estimated earlier (National Research Council, 1980).

## TRACE MINERALS

### *Cobalt*

#### FUNCTION

Cobalt is a component of vitamin $B_{12}$ (cobalamin). Ruminal microbes can produce all of the vitamin $B_{12}$ required by the cow provided adequate cobalt is available in the diet. As much as 13 percent of the dietary cobalt will be incorporated into vitamin $B_{12}$ when a cobalt insufficient diet is fed, though in general only 3 percent of dietary cobalt is incorporated into vitamin $B_{12}$ (Smith and Marston, 1970). As dietary cobalt increases the ruminal microbes also produce a number of analogs of vitamin $B_{12}$ which are not physiologically active. The presence of these vitamin $B_{12}$ analogs in liver and blood reduces the utility of vitamin $B_{12}$ determination to assess the status of cobalt (Halpin et al., 1984). However, a vitamin $B_{12}$ content of liver below 0.1 μg/g wet weight is considered indicative of cobalt deficiency (Smith, 1987). A portion of dietary cobalt can be absorbed in the cation form (Smith, 1987); however it has no known function and once absorbed does not appear capable of re-entering the rumen so microbes could utilize it. Most is excreted in the urine and a smaller amount exits with the bile (Underwood, 1981).

Cobalt chloride and nitrate, and cobaltous carbonate and sulfate all appear to be suitable sources of cobalt for ruminants. Cobaltous oxide, which is less soluble is somewhat less available (Henry, 1995). Cobaltous oxide pellets and controlled release glass pellets containing cobalt that remain in the rumen-reticulum have been used successfully to supply cobalt over extended periods of time to ruminants on pasture, though regurgitation can cause loss of some types of pellets (Poole and Connolly, 1967).

#### DEFICIENCY

Ruminants appear to be more sensitive to vitamin $B_{12}$ deficiency than nonruminants, largely because they are so dependent on gluconeogenesis for meeting needs of tissues for glucose. A breakdown in propionate metabolism at the point where methylmalonyl-CoA is converted to succinyl-CoA may be a primary defect arising from a deficiency of vitamin $B_{12}$. The appearance of methylmalonic acid in urine may be used as an indicator of a deficiency of vitamin $B_{12}$ (Gawthorne et al., 1971). A deficiency of vitamin $B_{12}$ may limit methionine production and limit nitrogen retention (Gawthorne and Smith, 1974). The advantages and disadvantages of methylmalonic acid and vitamin $B_{12}$ determinations to assess vitamin $B_{12}$ and (or) cobalt status have been reviewed (Mills, 1987). Without cobalt in the diet, production of vitamin $B_{12}$ in the rumen rapidly (within days) declines (Underwood, 1981). Stores of vitamin $B_{12}$ in the liver of adult ruminants are usually sufficient to last several months when they are placed on a cobalt-deficient diet. Young animals are more sensitive to dietary insufficiency of cobalt because they have lower reserves of vitamin $B_{12}$ in the liver. Early signs of a deficiency of cobalt include failure to grow, unthriftiness, and loss of weight (Smith, 1997). More severe signs include fatty degeneration of the liver, anemia with pale mucous membranes (Underwood, 1981), and reduced resistance to infection as a result of impaired neutrophil function (MacPherson et al., 1987; Paterson and MacPherson, 1990).

Although the cow may have adequate stores of vitamin $B_{12}$ to last several months, the ruminal microbes apparently do not. Within a few days of a switch to a diet deficient in cobalt ruminal concentrations of succinate rise. This may be the result of a blockade of microbial conversion of succinate to propionate, or a shift in ruminal bacterial populations toward succinate production rather than propionate production (Kennedy et al., 1996).

#### REQUIREMENT

The dietary requirement for cobalt was estimated to be 0.11 mg/kg of dietary DM (Smith and Loosli, 1957; Ammerman, 1970), and is based on the amount of cobalt that must be supplied to keep tissue concentrations of vitamin $B_{12}$ above 0.3 μg/L (Marston, 1970). The critical concentration of cobalt in the ruminal fluid to allow production of adequate vitamin $B_{12}$ is about 20 ng cobalt/ml. Ruminal fluid normally contains about 40 ng cobalt/ml (Miller et al., 1988).

Plant and animal derived feedstuffs will generally contain between 0.1 and 0.5 mg cobalt/kg DM. Soils along the southeastern Atlantic coast are deficient in cobalt and forages grown on these soils may not meet the animal requirement for cobalt (Ammerman, 1970). Alkaline soils or liming of soils can prevent adequate uptake of cobalt by plants (Mills, 1981).

SPECIAL PROPERTIES OF COBALT

Dietary cobalt may also have some effects independent of its necessity for production of vitamin $B_{12}$. Cobalt fed at 0.25 to 0.35 mg/kg of dietary DM, well above those required for sufficient vitamin $B_{12}$ synthesis, seems to enhance ruminal digestion of feedstuffs, especially lower quality forages (Lopez-Guisa and Satter, 1992; Saxena and Ranjhan, 1978). This effect may be due to selection of certain microbial populations with a higher cobalt requirement or may be a result of the divalent cobalt cation forming crosslinks between negatively charged bacteria and negatively charged forage particles, which allows bacteria to cling to forage particles more efficiently (Lopez-Guisa and Satter, 1992). Copper, calcium, and magnesium are divalent cations that may have some of the same ability to "cross-bridge" bacteria and forage particles (Somers, 1983; Storry, 1961). Addition of cobalt has been reported to increase total anaerobic bacteria in the rumen by 50 percent and increase lactic acid production in the rumen by 86 percent (Young, 1979). These results suggest that ruminal microbes may require more cobalt than previous research that focused on the ruminant's vitamin $B_{12}$ status would suggest. However, these data do not yet justify increasing dietary cobalt above 0.11 mg/kg of dietary DM.

Phalaris staggers, a neurologic syndrome induced by alkaloids in the grass, *Phalarus tuberosa* (Ulvund, 1985), can be prevented by supplemental cobalt. Cobalt inactivates or interferes with the absorption of this neurotoxin (Lee and Kuchel, 1953).

TOXICITY

Cobalt toxicity causes reduced feed intake, loss of body weight, hyperchromemia, and eventually anemia—signs similar to those seen in cobalt deficiency (National Research Council, 1980; Ely et al., 1948; Keener et al., 1949). Though toxicity in these reports occurred when there was about 30 mg cobalt/kg of dietary DM, the maximal tolerable dietary cobalt concentration has previously been set at 10 mg/kg of dietary DM (National Research Council, 1980).

### *Copper*

FUNCTION

Copper is a component of enzymes such as cytochrome oxidase, necessary for electron transport during aerobic respiration; lysyl oxidase, which catalyzes formation of desmosine cross links in collagen and elastin necessary for strong bone and connective tissues; ceruloplasmin, which is essential for absorption and transport of iron necessary for hemoglobin synthesis; tyrosinase, necessary for production of melanin pigment from tyrosine; and superoxide dismutase, which protects cells from the toxic effects of oxygen metabolites, which is particularly important to phagocytic cell function.

COPPER REQUIREMENTS

Endogenous losses of copper are approximately 7.1 μg/kg body weight (Agricultural Research Council, 1980). Copper content of growing tissues, when the liver is included as part of the carcass, is about 1.15 mg/kg based primarily on studies of sheep and cattle (Grace, 1983; Simpson et al., 1981). In liver, where excess absorbed copper is stored, copper concentrations can be much higher depending on diet. Copper content of colostrum is about 0.6 mg/kg (Lyford and Huber, 1988). Copper content of milk is about 0.15 mg/kg though it can be about 0.2 mg/kg when animals are fed a high copper diet (Schwarz and Kirchgessner, 1978). The requirement for absorbed copper during lactation that was used in the model is 0.15 mg copper/kg milk produced. This is a 50 percent increase over the value of 0.10 mg copper/kg milk produced used by the Agricultural Research Council (1980). In early gestation (<100 days) about 0.5 mg copper is incorporated into fetal, placental, and uterine tissue each day, increasing to between 1.5 and 2 mg/day during the last month of gestation (Agricultural Research Council, 1980; House and Bell, 1993). In the model, the requirement for absorbed copper is set at 0.5 mg/day for cows <100 days in gestation, 1.5 mg/day if gestation is between 100 and 225 days, and 2.0 mg/day if gestation is >225 days (Table 6-1).

EFFICIENCY OF COPPER ABSORPTION FROM DIETS

The amount of dietary copper required to supply the copper needed for maintenance, growth, and lactation will vary with the age of the animal, the chemical form of the dietary copper, and the presence of substances in the diet that interfere with absorption of dietary copper. In newborn calves, up to 70 percent of dietary copper is absorbed, similar to nonruminants. Bremner and Dalgarno (1973 a,b) found that 50 to 60 percent of dietary copper (supplied as copper sulfate) was retained in the liver of calves between 3 and 14 weeks of age. During the first 4 weeks of life (before weaning) the coefficient for absorption assigned to copper was 60 percent. With the development of the rumen there is a tremendous decrease in absorption of copper. Only between 1 and 5 percent of dietary copper will be absorbed by adult cattle. The absorption of dietary

TABLE 6-1 Comparison of Estimated Dietary Copper Requirements (mg/d) and Dietary Copper Concentrations (mg/kg of DM) for Cattle in Various Physiologic States

| | | 1989 | | 1980 | | 2000 | |
|---|---|---|---|---|---|---|---|
| Cow Description[a] | Feed Intake (kg DM) | NRC mg/day | NRC mg/kg diet | ARC mg/day | ARC mg/kg diet | NRC mg/day | NRC mg/kg diet |
| 300-kg heifer, ADG = 0.7 kg | 6 | 60 | 10 | 71 | 11.8 | 72.6 | 12 |
| 500-kg heifer, ADG = 0.5 kg, day 250 of gestation | 10 | 100 | 10 | 154 | 15.4 | 152 | 15.2 |
| 650-kg cow, 40 kg of milk per day | 20 | 200 | 10 | 214 | 10.7 | 313 | 15.7 |
| 650-kg cow, day 270 of gestation | 12 | 120 | 10 | 167 | 13.9 | 163.5 | 13.7 |

[a]ADG = average daily gain.

copper is reduced by the presence of sulfur and molybdenum in the diet. Sulfur sources can be converted to sulphide within the rumen leading to formation of copper sulphide precipitates rendering the copper unavailable for absorption (Bird, 1970). Allen and Gawthorne (1987) suggest that sulfur and molybdenum form tetrathiomolybdate in the solid phase of the ruminal digesta. Tetrathiomolybdate binds copper to form a highly insoluble complex that renders the copper unavailable for absorption. Suttle and McLauchlan (1976) developed a nomogram which models the effect of dietary sulfur and molybdenum on the efficiency of absorption of dietary copper (CopperAbsorbable) from a diet based on dietary sulfur (g/kg) and molybdenum (mg/kg) concentrations.

$$\log(\text{CopperAbsorbable}) = -1.153 - 0.076\,(\text{sulfur}) - 0.013\,(\text{sulfur} \times \text{molybdenum})$$

In Table 6-2, the calculated absorption coefficient for copper decreases from 4.6 percent when dietary sulfur is at the required concentration (0.20 percent), to 3.1 percent when dietary sulfur is at the maximum concentration (0.40 percent) in a diet that contains 1 mg molybdenum/kg.

TABLE 6-2 Calculated Copper Absorption Coefficients Across Various Dietary Sulfur and Molybdenum Concentrations

| Dietary Sulfur (g/kg) | Dietary Molybdenum (mg/kg) | Cu absorption coefficient |
|---|---|---|
| 2.0 | 1 | 0.046 |
| 4.0 | 1 | 0.031 |
| 6.0 | 1 | 0.021 |
| 2.5 | 0.5 | 0.043 |
| 2.5 | 1 | 0.042 |
| 2.5 | 2 | 0.039 |
| 2.5 | 5 | 0.0314 |
| 2.5 | 10 | 0.0217 |
| 2.5 | 20 | 0.010 |
| 2.5 | 100 | 0.003 |

Dietary molybdenum concentrations >10 mg/kg present a major obstacle to absorption of copper.

In the model, the assumption was made that molybdenum content of the diet is 1 mg/kg and dietary sulfur is 2.5 g/kg (0.25 percent sulfur). The coefficient of copper absorption utilized in the model was 4 percent. If the dietary molybdenum or sulfur content differs from these values, the user can adjust the amount of dietary copper required by calculating the proper copper coefficient or referring to Table 6-2, based on the work of Suttle and McLauchlan (1976). The required dietary copper would then be 0.04/"copper absorbable" times the requirement determined by the model, where "copper absorbable" is the calculated absorption coefficient of copper. This adjustment to the copper requirement is the adjustment suggested by the 1980 ARC publication.

However as summarized and discussed by Underwood and Suttle (1999), the relationship between copper availability and dietary copper and molybdenum is probably more difficult to predict than the equation of Suttle and McLauchlan (1976) would suggest. The effect of sulfur and molybdenum varies depending on the feedstuff serving as a source of copper. Underwood and Suttle (1999) conclude that the absorbable amount of copper in ensiled grass was not greatly impaired by an increase in dietary molybdenum but was greatly depressed by the addition of sulfur to the ration. When the diet was 0.2 percent sulfur about 5.5 percent of the copper was available, but when the diet was 0.4 percent sulfur the absorbable copper was reduced to about 1.5 percent. In hays, the inhibitory effect of molybdenum is present but relatively small. As sulfur increases from 0.2 to 0.4 percent in hays the percent absorbable copper decreases by 20–30 percent. The percent absorbable copper in fresh grasses is lower than that of hays or ensiled grasses at any given sulfur or molybdenum concentration and the addition of sulfur or molybdenum drastically decreases copper absorbability. The inhibitory effect of increasing diet molybdenum on copper absorption is greatest when dietary molybdenum is low and seems to reach a plateau once diet molybdenum is about 4–5 mg/kg DM. Beyond this point higher dietary molybdenum concentrations do not impair copper absorbability significantly further (Underwood and Suttle, 1999; Gengelbach, 1994).

### OTHER FACTORS KNOWN TO INFLUENCE THE ABSORPTION OF COPPER

*Pasture Grazing* Up to 10 percent of the DMI of pastured animals can be from soil ingested as they graze—especially if pastures are short. Suttle et al. (1975) found that inclusion of soil at 10 percent of DM reduced copper absorption by 50 percent, across several different soil types. The coefficient for absorption of copper for animals at pasture should be decreased by one-half to ensure adequate copper supplementation. This is not included in the model, and the user may decide to adjust requirements for copper accordingly, essentially doubling the copper required, as suggested by the model, when animals are at pasture.

*High Dietary Zinc* Zinc induces increased metallothionein in the intestine. Metallothionein coats the surface of the lumenal side of the intestinal cells and binds and sequesters copper at the lumenal surface. The bound copper is eventually lost to the feces upon desquamation of the intestinal epithelial cells. A fairly strong negative linear relationship was found between dietary zinc and copper retained in the liver of lambs by Bremner et al. (1976). Lambs fed diets with 40 (30 was considered the requirement), 220, or 420 mg zinc/kg retained 4, 2.8, or 1.5 percent of the dietary copper in their liver respectively, suggesting that the coefficient for absorption should be decreased by 16 percent for every 100 mg of zinc per kg diet above 40 mg/kg. However, this adjustment factor was not included in this model. In adult lactating cows, supplementation with 2000 mg of zinc/kg of diet reduced copper in plasma, but 1000 mg of zinc/kg of diet did not (Miller et al., 1989). These data suggest that under practical conditions zinc is not a major factor affecting absorption of copper unless the diet contains at least twenty-fold more zinc that is recommended. In some areas, zinc oxide is fed at $>$ 1000 mg zinc/kg DM in an effort to control facial eczema. However because of the poor solubility of zinc oxide it appears that in most cases this does not induce copper insufficiency (Lee et al., 1991).

*High Dietary Iron* Copper reserves in liver of calves were found to be depleted when calves were fed diets containing 1400 mg of iron/kg of diet, greater than ten-fold the concentration of iron recommended (Agricultural Research Council, 1980). Increasing diet iron from 500 to 800 mg/kg DM dramaticly reduced the liver copper content from 134 to 16 mg copper/kg DM in 8 weeks (Phillippo et al., 1987). There seems to be an interaction between high dietary iron and sulfur as when both are present the inhibition of diet copper absorbability is more pronounced (Underwood and Suttle, 1999). Water containing large amounts of iron also has been implicated as a cause of copper deficiency but no specific recommendation on how iron affects the coefficient of absorption of copper can be made and no adjustment is included in the model.

*High Dietary Calcium* Some studies have suggested a decrease in absorption of copper when calcium was added to the diet (Kirchgessner and Weser, 1965; Dick, 1954). In the study of Kirchgessner (1965) increasing calcium from 0.70 percent to 0.95 percent of the diet reduced copper absorption. However, other studies failed to show an effect of calcium on copper status (Huber and Price, 1971) despite larger changes in dietary calcium content. No adjustment of the absorption coefficient for copper was recommended based on dietary calcium.

*Differences in Breeds* Breed differences exist among cattle that may make some breeds more susceptible to copper toxicity. Jersey cattle fed the same diet as Holstein cattle accumulated more copper in their livers (Du et al., 1996). It is not clear whether this reflects differences in feed intake, efficiency of copper absorption, or biliary excretion of copper. Although these data caution that Jersey cows may be more prone to copper toxicity than Holstein cows, an adjustment of the copper requirement based on breed does not seem warranted at this time.

### SUPPLEMENTAL COPPER ABSORPTION

Copper is usually supplemented in the sulfate, carbonate, or oxide forms. Recent studies indicate that copper oxide is not very available relative to copper sulfate (Langlands et al., 1986; Kegley and Spears, 1993). In early studies, copper carbonate was at least equal to copper (cupric) sulfate (Chapman and Bell, 1963). Various organic forms of copper also are available. In calves fed diets high in molybdenum, copper proteinate was more available than copper sulfate (Kincaid et al., 1986). However, Wittenberg et al. (1990) found similar efficiency of absorption of copper from copper proteinate and copper sulfate in steers fed high-molybdenum diets. Studies that compared copper lysine to copper sulfate have yielded inconsistent results. Ward and Spears (1993) reported that copper lysine and copper sulfate had similar efficiencies of absorption when fed to cattle; however, Rabiansky et al. 1999 and Nockels et al. (1993) found that copper lysine was more available than copper sulfate.

The studies cited above to determine the coefficient of absorption for copper are primarily based on the use of cupric sulfate as the source of copper. The sulfates have the highest biologic efficiency of absorption of the common inorganic sources; the carbonate and oxide forms are of intermediate and low efficiency of absorption, respectively (Ammerman and Miller, 1972). Cupric oxide is nearly insoluble and does not serve as an adequate source of supplemental copper (Xin et al., 1991, Kegley and Spears, 1993). However, cupric oxide needles (oxidized copper wire particles - 24 g/cow) which degrade slowly in the rumen-reticulum have been successfully used to provide long term supplementation (6 to 8 months) to pastured animals (Judson, 1984; Richards, 1985). In general, supplemental forms of copper that are as soluble or exceed the solubility of cupric sulfate are good sources of copper for cattle. In some studies (Kincaid et al., 1986) the efficiency of absorption of copper proteinates has exceeded that of cupric sulfate. However, in most studies (Du et al., 1996; Wittenberg, 1990) the copper proteinates have nearly the same efficiency of absorption as cupric sulfate. Cupric chloride, which is highly soluble, may be up to 20 percent more available than cupric sulfate (Ivan et al., 1990). A chelated copper source demonstrating a specific mechanism for absorption that bypasses normal impediments to copper absorption could improve copper absorbability. However the data supporting this concept have not been reported in a refereed journal.

#### SIGNS OF COPPER DEFICIENCY

An early classic sign of copper deficiency in cattle is loss of hair pigmentation, particularly around the eyes. Scours is a clinical sign of copper deficiency that seems to be unique to ruminants, though the pathogenesis of this lesion is not understood. Anemia (hypochromic macrocytic), fragile bones and osteoporosis, cardiac failure, poor growth, and reproductive inefficiency characterized by depressed estrus also are observed in copper deficiency (Underwood, 1981). An effect of copper deficiency that is not easily observed is reduced immune function. Neutrophils have a reduced ability to kill invading microbes (Boyne, 1981) leading to increased susceptibility to infections. The dietary copper required for optimal immune function may exceed the amount required to prevent the more classic signs of copper deficiency (Xin et al., 1993; Xin et al., 1991; Stabel et al., 1993).

#### ASSESSING COPPER ADEQUACY

Forage concentrations of copper are of limited value in assessing adequacy of copper unless concentrations of copper antagonists in forage such as molybdenum, sulfur, and iron are also considered. Forages vary greatly in content of copper depending on plant species and available copper in the soil (Minson, 1990).

Concentrations of copper in liver <20 mg/kg on a DM basis (5 mg/kg wet weight) or plasma concentrations <0.50 mg/L are definitive of a copper deficiency. Copper concentration in normal liver is between 200 and 300 mg/kg of DM (Underwood, 1981; Ammerman, 1970; Puls, 1994). However, in the presence of high dietary molybdenum and sulfur which promote formation and absorption of thiomolybdates into the blood, copper in liver and plasma may not accurately reflect copper status because the copper can exist in tightly bound forms with the absorbed thiomolybdates, rendering it unavailable for biochemical functions (Suttle, 1991).

#### COPPER TOXICITY

Of all the minerals, copper is the most likely to become toxic if over-supplemented. Copper toxicosis can occur in cattle that consume excessive amounts of supplemental copper or feeds that have been contaminated with copper compounds used for other agricultural or industrial purposes (Underwood, 1977). When cattle consume excessive copper, they may accumulate extremely large amounts of the mineral in the liver before toxicosis becomes evident. Stress or other factors may result in the sudden liberation of large amounts of copper from the liver to the blood, causing a hemolytic crisis. Such crises are characterized by considerable hemolysis, jaundice, methemoglobinemia, hemoglobinuria, generalized icterus, widespread necrosis, and often death (Underwood, 1977; National Research Council, 1980).

Cattle are more tolerant of higher levels of dietary copper than are sheep, perhaps because of their greater capacity to eliminate copper from the body by way of bile. However, chronic copper poisoning is possible in cattle with supplementation of diets at just 4 to 5-fold the "required" amount of copper (Auza, 1999; Bradley, 1993). In most cases of copper intoxication, the concentration of copper in liver will exceed 900 mg/kg on a dry weight basis (Radostits et al., 1994); copper toxicity may occur at concentrations of copper in liver as low as 331 mg/kg liver on a dry weight basis (Auza, 1999). These data suggest the maximal tolerable dietary copper should be reduced to 40 mg/kg, unless dietary molybdenum is elevated greatly.

### *Iodine*

#### FUNCTION

Iodine is necessary for the synthesis of the thyroid hormones thyroxine and triiodothyronine that regulate energy metabolism. The amount of iodine incorporated into thyroid hormones is about 0.4 mg/day in calves weighing 40 kg and increases to 1.3 mg iodine/day in nonpregnant heifers weighing 400 kg. Late gestation cows incorporate about

1.5 mg iodine/day into thyroid hormone. During lactation thyroid hormone production is increased, especially in high producing cows and iodine incorporation into thyroid hormones may reach 4 to 4.5 mg iodine/day (Sorensen, 1962). Thyroid hormone production also is increased during cold weather to stimulate an increase in basal metabolic rate as the animal attempts to remain warm (Goodman and Middlesworth, 1980).

About 80 to 90 percent of dietary iodine is absorbed and most of the iodine not taken up by the thyroid gland is excreted in urine and milk (Miller et al., 1988). Milk normally contains from 30 to 300 μg iodine/L and the iodine content of milk generally increases as dietary iodine increases making the iodine content of milk a reasonable indicator of iodine status (Berg et al., 1988). The availability of thyroid hormone assays provides more accurate assessment of actual thyroid function and the causes of thyroid dysfunction.

When the iodine content of the diet is more than adequate, <20 percent of the dietary iodine will be incorporated into the thyroid gland (Sorensen, 1962). Under conditions where intake of dietary iodine is marginal the thyroid gland will incorporate about 30 percent of the dietary iodine into thyroid hormones (Miller et al., 1975). When severely iodine deficient the hyperplastic thyroid can bind up to 65 percent of the iodine consumed by the cow (Lengemann and Swanson, 1957).

#### REQUIREMENT

*Maintenance* The daily thyroxine production of growing and mature nonlactating cattle is 0.2 to 0.3 mg thyroxine/ 100 kg of body weight, which contains 0.13 to 0.2 mg iodine (Miller et al., 1988). Miller et al. (1988) suggested that about 30 percent of dietary iodine actually was utilized by the thyroid gland to synthesize thyroxine and that 15 percent of the iodine that is used to synthesize thyroxine each day comes from recycling of iodine from the degradation of previously secreted thyroxine. Therefore, about 0.6 mg dietary iodine/ 100 kg of body weight is required to meet the requirement of the body for thyroxine synthesis. Pregnancy does not increase the requirement for iodine for thyroxine production to any significant degree (Miller et al., 1988). Assuming DMI of the 600-kg nonlactating pregnant cow is 1.8 percent of body weight, the diet must contain 3.6 mg of iodine/10.8 kg of dietary DM or 0.33 mg iodine/kg of dietary DM.

*Lactation* The rate of thyroxine production increases about 2.5-fold in heavily lactating cows (Sorenson, 1962). This increases the iodine requirement of lactating cows to 1.5 mg/100 kg body weight. Assuming that DMI of lactating cows is about 3.3 percent of body weight, the diet of a lactating cow should contain 0.45 mg iodine/kg DM.

#### FACTORS AFFECTING IODINE REQUIREMENT

Goitrogens are compounds that interfere with the synthesis or secretion of thyroid hormones and cause hypothyroidism. Goitrogens fall into two main categories. Cyanogenic goitrogens impair iodide uptake by the thyroid gland. Cyanogenic glucosides can be found in many feeds, including raw soybeans, beet pulp, corn, sweet potato, white clover, and millet and once ingested are metabolized to thiocyanate and isothiocyanate. These compounds alter iodide transport across the thyroid follicular cell membrane, reducing iodide retention. This effect is easily overcome by increasing supplemental iodine in the diet. The National Research Council (1989) included a safety factor (set dietary iodine requirement at 0.6 mg/kg dietary DM) to account for possible interference with iodine utilization by protein sources common in diets for lactating cows.

Progoitrins and goitrins found in cruciferous plants (rape, kale, cabbage, turnips, mustard) and aliphatic disulfides found in onions inhibit thyroperoxidase preventing formation of mono- and diiodotyrosine (Ermans and Bourdoux, 1989). With goitrins, especially those of the thiouracil type, hormone synthesis may not be readily restored to normal by dietary iodine supplementation and the offending feedstuff needs to be reduced or removed from the diet.

#### SOURCES OF IODINE

Most sources of iodine are readily available and the iodides of sodium, potassium, and calcium are commonly used. Potassium iodide tends to be easily oxidized and volatilizes before the animal can ingest it. Pentacalcium orthoperiodate and ethylenediamine dihydroiodine (EDDI) are more stable, less soluble, and are commonly used in mineral blocks and salt licks exposed to the weather.

Concentrations of iodine in forage are extremely variable and the concentration depends on the iodine content of the soil. Soil near the oceans tends to provide adequate iodine in plants. However, in the Great Lakes regions and Northwest United States, iodine concentrations in forages are generally low enough to result in a deficiency of iodine unless iodine is supplemented to the diet.

Supplemental iodine should not exceed 0.5 mg/kg diet due to concerns for human health (see toxicity section).

#### DEFICIENCY SYMPTOMS

Iodine deficiency reduces production of thyroid hormones slowing the rate of oxidation of all cells. Often the first indication of iodine deficiency is enlargement of the thyroid (goiter) of newborn calves (Miller et al., 1968). Calves also may be born hairless, weak, or dead. Fetal death can occur at any stage of gestation. Often the cows will appear normal (Hemken, 1970). In adult cattle, iodine deficiency can cause enlarged thyroid glands, reduced fertility (males and females), and increased morbidity. Under conditions of marginal or deficient dietary iodine the maternal thyroid gland becomes extremely efficient in the removal of iodine from the plasma and in the recovery of iodine during the degradation of spent thyroid hormone and thyroglobulin. Unfortunately, this leaves little iodine for the fetal thyroid gland and the fetus becomes hypothyroid. The goiter condition is the hyperplastic response of the thyroid gland to increased stimulation of thyroid growth by thyroid-stimulating hormone produced in the pituitary gland. Under mild iodine deficiency, the hyperplastic thyroid gland can compensate for the reduced absorption of iodine (Hetzel and Wellby, 1997).

#### TOXICITY

Iodine toxicity has been reported in adult dairy cows with dietary intakes of just 50 mg/day (about 5 mg/kg dietary DM). Symptoms included excessive nasal and ocular discharge, salivation, decreased milk production, coughing and dry, scaly coats (Olson et al., 1984). High concentrations of dietary iodine in the diet also increase iodine concentrations in milk, and because humans are much more sensitive to iodine thyrotoxicosis than cows the danger of excess dietary iodine fed to cattle also is a public health issue (Hetzel and Welby, 1997).

Current US Food and Drug Administration Regulations set the maximum limit of iodine supplementation from EDDI at 10 mg/day.

### *Iron*

Iron primarily functions as a component of heme found in hemoglobin and myoglobin. Enzymes of the electron transport chain, cytochrome oxidase, ferredoxin, myeloperoxidase, catalase, and the cytochrome P-450 enzymes also require iron as cofactors.

Iron deficiency results in hypochromic microcytic anemia due to failure to produce hemoglobin. Light colored veal is due to low muscle myoglobin as a result of restricted dietary iron. Anemic calves are listless and have poor feed intake and weight gain (Blaxter et al., 1957; Bremner and Dalgarno, 1973b). Another important aspect of iron deficiency is greater morbidity and mortality associated with depressed immune responses (Mollerberg and Moreno-Lopez, 1975). Increased morbidity was observed before there was an effect of iron deficiency on packed red blood cell volume.

Iron deficiency in adult cattle is very rare—in part because their requirement is reduced, but also because iron is ubiquitous in the environment, and soil contamination of forages (and soil ingested by animals on pasture) generally ensures that iron needs of the adult will be met or exceeded (Underwood, 1981).

#### ABSORPTION

Iron in the ferric form ($Fe^{+3}$) is poorly absorbed from the intestinal tract. Much of the dietary iron exists within feedstuffs in the ferric form. Some of the ferric iron can be reduced to the ferrous ($Fe^{+2}$) form upon reaction with the acid of the abomasum (Wollenberg and Rummel, 1987). During digestion, dietary non-heme iron in the ferrous state usually becomes bound to some chelator such as histidine, mucin, or fructose. These chelators enhance iron absorption by solubilizing iron and protecting it in the ferrous state. Other chelators (e.g., oxalate and phosphate) can inhibit iron absorption. During absorption, the iron binds to specific non-heme iron-binding receptors within the brush border of the enterocyte and is transported into the cell. Once inside the cell the iron can be transported to the basolateral membrane and becomes bound to transferrin for transport within the blood. If iron status of the body is adequate the iron entering the enterocyte is not transported to the basolateral membrane but is instead bound by ferritin, a protein produced by the enterocytes when iron is not needed by the body. Once bound to ferritin, the iron is excreted with the feces when the enterocyte dies and is sloughed (Beard and Dawson, 1997). The amount of dietary iron absorbed can be controlled by up-regulation or down-regulation of ferritin content of enterocytes. How concentrations of ferritin in enterocytes are regulated by iron status of somatic cells is unknown.

#### FACTORIAL REQUIREMENT DETERMINATION

The majority of iron incorporated into tissues is very effectively recovered and recycled so that maintenance requirements for iron are negligible. Milk contains about 1 mg iron/kg (National Research Council, 1989). The iron requirement of the conceptus of the pregnant cow between day 190 of gestation and the day of calving has been estimated to be 18 mg/day (House and Bell, 1993). Estimates of iron content in the body range from 18 to 34 mg/kg body weight of calves (Bremner and Dalgarno, 1973a). The absorbed iron requirement for growth of cattle has been set at 34 mg iron/kg average daily gain.

Matrone et al. (1957) estimated that 60 percent of iron supplemented as ferric chloride was absorbed in calves. In calves that are iron deficient, as assessed by anemia, about 55 percent of the iron in the diet can be retained in the calf's tissues (Miltenberg et al., 1993). Bremner and Dalgarno (1973a,b) using hemoglobin synthesis as their criterion, estimated the iron absorption coefficient in 9 to 12-week-old calves was 72 percent in an iron deficient liquid diet providing just 10 mg iron/kg diet. When ferrous sulfate or ferric citrate were added to the diets to raise total dietary iron to 40 mg/kg diet, the iron absorption coefficient declined to 43 percent; yet these animals were still considered iron deficient as assessed by blood hemoglobin content and muscle pigmentation. At least in calves, the true efficiency of absorption of iron appears to decrease as the concentration of dietary iron increases—even before the absorbed iron requirement for growth has been achieved. An analysis of balance studies done in growing calves presented in the 1980 ARC publication (p. 238) suggests that the availability of soluble iron from liquid diets declines from 0.40 to 0.15 as the diet iron content increases from 40 to 100 mg/kg. Feeding calves <15 weeks of age as little as 39 mg of iron/kg DM will allow calves to grow at a normal rate but the muscles remain pale and the animals remain slightly anemic (Bernier et al., 1984). A recent study by Lindt and Blum (1994) suggests that 50 mg iron/kg diet (which would likely correspond to an absorption coefficient for iron of approximately 0.35) is adequate to support growth but the carcass remains pale. To maximize myoglobin synthesis and strength of the calf the diet must contain more iron.

Once the animal is ruminating the efficiency of iron absorption is considerably lower. In part this is because most forages will supply more than adequate amounts of iron to cattle as a result of soil contamination of the forage. Therefore iron absorption mechanisms tend to be down-regulated to protect the animal from iron toxicity as opposed to maximizing iron absorption. However a second factor is that the form of the iron in the forages is often ferric oxide which is less soluble and poorly absorbed. Studies utilizing radioactive iron determined that iron absorption efficiency was less than 2 percent in adult cattle fed a diet that supplied much more iron to the cows than was needed (Van Bruwaene et al., 1984). Though no data exists for cattle, when pregnant ewes were fed diets that provided adequate but not excessive dietary iron content (20 mg iron/kg diet) the animals were absorbing 21 percent of the dietary iron (Hoskins and Hansard, 1964) Assuming iron absorption in cattle is similar, it may not be desirable to base requirements on maximal iron absorption efficiency. Therefore, the absorption coefficient for dietary iron utilized to determine the requirement for iron in adult animals is set at 0.10 for iron in feedstuffs.

Using this approach a 6-week-old calf gaining 0.8 kg of body weight/day and consuming 0.9 kg dietary DM/day requires 150 mg iron/kg dietary DM. A 12-week-old calf gaining 1.8 kg body weight/day consuming 2.6 kg dietary DM/day requires 118 mg iron/kg dietary DM. A cow producing 25 kg of milk/day at 205 days of gestation and consuming 20 kg/day of DM requires just 24 mg iron/kg DM. Most feedstuffs will contain adequate iron to meet the iron requirements of adult cattle. Milk-fed calves are the only group of cattle that ordinarily require iron supplementation. Ferrous sulfate and ferric chloride are good iron supplements. Ferric oxide and ferrous carbonate are poorer iron sources (Henry and Miller, 1995).

#### TOXICITY

*Concerns about Excessive Dietary Iron* Iron can interfere with the absorption of other minerals, primarily copper and zinc. As little as 250 to 500 mg of iron/kg dietary DM has been implicated as a cause of copper depletion in cattle (Bremner et al., 1987; Phillippo et al., 1987).

If absorption of dietary iron exceeds the binding capacity of transferrin and lactoferrin in blood and tissues, free iron may increase in tissues. Free iron is very reactive and can cause generation of reactive oxygen species, lipid peroxidation, and free radical production leading to "oxidative stress," increasing anti-oxidant requirements of the animal (Halliwell, 1987). Free iron also is required by bacteria for their growth and excessive dietary iron can contribute to bacterial infection (Baynes et al., 1986). Iron toxicity is associated with diarrhea, reduced feed intake, and weight gain. The National Research Council (1980) recommended that dietary iron not exceed 1000 mg/kg DM.

Water containing more than 0.3 mg iron/L is considered unacceptable for human consumption by the US Environmental Protection Agency. Livestock can tolerate higher levels but iron in water will be much more available and therefore more toxic than iron in feedstuffs.

### *Manganese*

Manganese deficiency can cause impaired growth, skeletal abnormalities (shortened and deformed), disturbed or depressed reproduction, and abnormalities of the newborn (including ataxia—due to failure of the inner ear to develop) (Underwood, 1977). The skeletal changes are related to loss of galactotransferase and glycosyltransferase enzymes that are vital to production of cartilage and bone ground substance mucopolysaccharides and glycoproteins. Manganese super oxide dismutase works in concert with other anti-oxidants to minimize accumulation of reactive forms of oxygen, which could damage cells. Manganese is found in highest concentrations within the mitochondria of cells. It also accumulates in the inorganic matrix of bone.

#### MANGANESE HOMEOSTASIS

The majority of the dietary manganese that is absorbed is removed from the portal circulation by the liver and is excreted into the bile. A small portion is bound to transferrin within the liver and released into the circulation for transport to the tissues. Some of the absorbed manganese is bound to 2-macroglobulin and albumen and remains in the circulation. The proportion of manganese absorbed from the diet is <4 percent and generally is closer to 1 percent. A mechanism to enhance the efficiency of absorption of manganese during a deficiency of manganese does not appear to exist (Gibbons et al., 1976). The major homeostatic control for manganese appears to be regulation of biliary excretion of manganese absorbed in excess of tissue needs. Enterohepatic circulation of manganese also may be a factor in manganese homeostasis (Miller, 1978). Almost no manganese is excreted in urine.

Most of the manganese in the body is found in the skeleton, liver, and hair. Manganese accumulates in the liver in direct proportion to dietary manganese providing a more precise index of manganese status (Black, 1985), with an adequate concentration of manganese in liver being 10 to 24 mg/kg on a DM basis (Puls, 1994). The liver and perhaps other tissues have a limited ability to store manganese that can be mobilized, which may satisfy needs for several weeks during times of manganese deficiency (Lassiter and Morton, 1968).

#### MANGANESE REQUIREMENTS

There are no precise data on maintenance requirements for manganese in dairy cattle. However, manganese deficiency has been reported when diets contained 16 to 17 mg of dietary manganese/kg of DM. Assuming maintenance intakes of these diets did not exceed 2 percent of body weight and that <1 percent of ingested manganese was absorbed, we can estimate that the maintenance requirement for absorbed manganese of cattle is <0.002 mg/kg body weight or about 1 mg in a 500 kg cow. House and Bell (1993) determined that the fetus and placenta in cows at 190 days in gestation take up nearly 0.3 mg manganese/day. Colostrum contains 0.16 mg/kg and milk contains 0.03 mg/kg (Lyford and Huber, 1988). The concentration of manganese in carcasses of calves averages about 2.5 mg/kg of total carcass on a DM basis (Suttle, 1979). Assuming the carcasses used in these experiments were 27 percent DM, the manganese requirement for growth can be estimated to be 0.7 mg manganese/kg of body weight gain.

The coefficient for absorption of manganese from most diets is about 1 percent (Sansom, 1978; Gibbons, 1976) though Vagg (1976) found that just 0.5 percent of 54Mn was absorbed from the diet. For this model, the coefficient for absorption of manganese was set at 0.75 percent.

High concentrations of dietary calcium, potassium, or phosphorus increase excretion of manganese in the feces, presumably by reducing absorption of manganese (Lassiter, 1972; Hartmans, 1974). Excessive dietary iron depresses retention of manganese in calves (Ho, 1984).

In one experiment, all calves born from cows fed 16–17 mg/kg of dietary DM for 12 months had neonatal deformities (Dyer et al., 1965). The deformities included weak legs and pasterns, enlarged joints, stiffness, twisted legs, general weakness, and reduced bone strength. Heifers and cows that are fed low-manganese diets are slower to exhibit estrus, are more likely to have "silent heats," and have a lower conception rate than cows with sufficient manganese in their diet. Cows that were fed 7 to 10 mg of dietary manganese/kg of dietary DM for extended periods exhibited abscessed livers and had practically no bile in their gall bladders (Bentley and Phillips, 1951).

The National Research Council's *Nutrient Requirements of Beef Cattle* (1996) lists the requirement for manganese as 20 mg of manganese/kg dietary DM for growing cattle and 40 mg/kg dietary DM for breeding cattle. The Agricultural Research Council (1980) recommends 10 mg of manganese/kg dietary DM for growth of cattle increasing to 20 to 25 mg manganese/kg dietary DM to maintain normal reproduction. The National Research Council's *Nutrient Requirements of Dairy Cattle* (1989b) suggests that 40 mg of manganese/kg dietary DM should be adequate for all classes of cattle, though a requirement was not actually determined.

Using the factorial approach, a more precise determination of the manganese requirement can be made (Table 6-3). For example, a 500 kg heifer in late gestation gaining 0.5 kg body weight/d would require 1.65 mg absorbed manganese to meet her requirements. Assuming the coefficient of manganese absorption is 0.75 percent, then the diet must provide 220 mg manganese. If the heifer is consuming 10 kg DM/d, then the concentration of manganese would need to be 22 mg/kg.

The manganese content of feedstuffs is quite variable and is influenced by soil types, soil pH, fertilization, and plant species. Manganese sulfate is commonly used to supplement diets as it is a fairly soluble source of manganese. Other mineral sources of manganese and their efficiency of absorption relative to manganese sulfate are manganese carbonate (30 percent), manganese dioxide (35 percent), manganese monoxide (60 percent), and manganese methionine (125 percent) (Henry, 1995).

Manganese toxicity in ruminants is unlikely to occur, and there are few documented incidences with adverse effects limited to reduced feed intake and growth (Jenkins and Hidiroglou, 1991). These negative effects began to appear when dietary manganese exceeded 1000 mg/kg. The maximum tolerable amount of manganese, as given by the National Research Council (1980), is 1,000 mg/kg.

### *Molybdenum*

#### FUNCTION AND REQUIREMENT

Molybdenum is a component of xanthine oxidase, sulfide oxidase, and aldehyde oxidase, enzymes found in milk and

TABLE 6-3 Comparison of Estimated Dietary Manganese Requirements (mg/d) and Dietary Manganese Concentrations (mg/kg of DM) for Cattle in Various Physiologic States

| Cow Description[a] | Feed intake (kg of DM) | 1989 NRC mg/day | 1989 NRC mg/kg of diet | 1980 ARC mg/day | 1980 ARC mg/kg of diet | 2000 NRC mg/day | 2000 NRC mg/kg of diet |
|---|---|---|---|---|---|---|---|
| 300-kg heifer, ADG = 0.7 kg | 6 | 240 | 40 | 60 | 10 | 145 | 24.2 |
| 500-kg heifer, ADG = 0.5 kg, day 250 of gestation | 10 | 400 | 40 | 200–250 | 20–25 | 220 | 22.0 |
| 650-kg cow, 40 kg milk per day | 20 | 800 | 40 | 400–500 | 20–25 | 333 | 16.7 |
| 650-kg cow, day 270 gestation | 12 | 480 | 40 | 240–300 | 20–25 | 213 | 17.8 |

[a]ADG = average daily gain.

many tissues (Mills and Davis, 1987). Concentrations of molybdenum in milk and plasma increase as dietary molybdenum increases (Underwood, 1981). Lesperance et al. (1985) determined that molybdenum in plasma of cows fed 3 mg molybdenum/kg diet were <0.1 g/ml. In animals fed 100 mg molybdenum/kg diet for 11 months, the plasma concentration of molybdenum had increased to 2.5 g/ml. A molybdenum deficiency in cattle has been difficult to reproduce. Shariff et al. (1990) observed that addition of 10 mg molybdenum/kg of a high forage diet containing 1.7 mg molybdenum/kg of diet increased the rate of in situ DM disappearance from the rumen of cattle, but adding molybdenum to a ground barley-based diet containing just 1.0 mg molybdenum/kg had no effect. Studies with lambs also were unable to define the dietary requirement for molybdenum (Ellis and Pfander, 1970; Ellis et al., 1958). It is not suggested to supplement molybdenum as it would seem very unlikely that dairy cattle would develop a deficiency of molybdenum when fed practical diets.

#### TOXICITY

Dietary molybdenum becomes a practical concern because it antagonizes the absorption of copper (and to a lesser extent phosphorus). Molybdenum toxicosis signs are essentially those associated with copper deficiency. Molybdenum and sulfate interact within the digestive tract to form a thiomolybbdate complex that has a high affinity for copper. Copper bound to this molybbdate is unavailable for absorption (see section on copper). The toxicity of molybdenum can be overcome by increased copper supplementation and copper toxicity can be reduced by molybdenum supplementation.

The maximal tolerable dietary concentration of molybdenum is suggested to be 10 mg/kg diet (National Research Council, 1980). However, as little as 5 mg Mo/kg diet has been demonstrated to cause copper depletion in heifers (Bremner et al., 1987; Phillippo et al., 1987).

### *Selenium*

#### FUNCTIONS AND ANIMAL RESPONSE

The best understood function of selenium is as a component of the enzyme, glutathione peroxidase (GSH-px) (Rotruck et al., 1973). This enzyme converts hydrogen peroxide to water and is an important component of the cellular antioxidant system. More recently, selenium was identified as a component of Type I iodothyronine-5′-deiodinase (Berry et al., 1991); the enzyme that converts $T_4$ to $T_3$. Selenium is also found in other proteins but the functions of those proteins remain unclear (Deagen et al., 1991; Yeh et al., 1997).

White muscle disease or nutritional muscular dystrophy is caused by selenium deficiency. Clinical signs of this disease include leg weakness and stiffness, flexion of the hock joints, and muscle tremors (National Research Council, 1983). Cardiac and skeletal muscles have chalky striations and necrosis. Animals often die from cardiac failure. Marginal or short term deficiencies of selenium have been related to poor growth, general unthriftiness, and diarrhea (Andrews et al., 1968). In several studies, the prevalence of retained fetal membranes was reduced when supplemental selenium was fed or injected into dairy cows during late gestation (Harrison et al., 1984; Miller et al., 1993). The prevalence of retained fetal membranes was not reduced when injections of selenium were given to animals reared in areas of the country with adequate concentrations of selenium in feeds (Schingoethe et al., 1982). Other problems that have responded to supplementation of selenium include metritis, cystic ovaries (Harrison et al., 1984), and udder edema (Miller et al., 1993).

Selenium is involved with metabolism of arachadonic acid via GSHpx (Maddox et al., 1991). This relationship probably is one reason supplementation of selenium improves the killing ability of neutrophils (Hogan et al., 1993) and reduces the prevalence and severity of mastitis in dairy cattle (Smith et al., 1984; Erskine et al., 1989;

Maddox et al., 1991). Those experiments were conducted in areas where basal ingredients had low concentrations of selenium (<0.08 mg/kg) and supplementation consisted of either an injection of selenium (50 mg/cow) or supplementation of 0.2 to 0.3 mg of dietary selenium/kg of diet.

### SOURCES

The concentrations of selenium in plant material are highly correlated with those in the soil. Fertilization of soil with selenium increases selenium concentrations in plants. Because of the strong relationship between concentrations of selenium in soils and plants, accurate maps have been developed that depict expected concentrations of selenium in feeds (National Research Council, 1983). In general, feeds grown in the central plains of the U.S. and Canada contain more than 0.1 mg selenium/kg of DM, and feeds grown east of the Mississippi river and west of the Rocky mountains typically contain <0.1 mg selenium/kg of DM. The leaves of forage plants contain 1.5 to 2 times more selenium than do stems (Harada et al., 1989; Gupta, 1991). When soils contain low concentrations of selenium, seeds and vegetative matter generally have similar concentrations of selenium, but as selenium in soil increases, concentrations of selenium in seeds increase more than do those in the vegetative matter (Harada et al., 1989; Stephen et al., 1989). Plant genetics also may influence concentrations of selenium in forages (McQuinn et al., 1991).

Most animal byproducts with the exception of milk products tend to have high concentrations of selenium. Fish meal often contains more than 1 mg selenium/kg of DM. However, the efficiency of absorption of selenium by nonruminants from these products, especially from fish meal, is low (Meltzer et al., 1993); comparative data for ruminants are not available.

Based on current regulations of the U.S. FDA (1997), the only two forms of inorganic selenium that can be added legally to diets in the United States are sodium selenite and sodium selenate at levels not to exceed 0.3 mg of supplemental selenium/kg of DM. Slow release ruminal boluses that contain selenium (from sodium selenite) also are available. Other sources of supplemental selenium include calcium selenite, selenium dioxide, and selenium enriched yeast.

### EFFICIENCY OF ABSORPTION

The literature on the efficiency of absorption of selenium is not extensive for ruminants. Extrapolation of data collected from nonruminants should be done with caution because of extensive ruminal metabolism of selenium. Apparent digestibility of selenium in forages and concentrates is between 30 and 60 percent for sheep, goats, and nonlactating dairy cows (Harrison and Conrad, 1984a; Harrison and Conrad, 1984b; Aspila, 1988; Koenig et al., 1997). Limited data suggest that the true digestibility of selenium from feeds is between 40 and 65 percent for ruminants (Harrison and Conrad, 1984b; Aspila, 1988). The selenium from sodium selenate, sodium selenite, and Se-enriched yeast had apparent digestibilities by ruminants in the range of 40 to 50 percent (Harrison and Conrad, 1984b; Aspila, 1988; Koenig et al., 1997), but one study (Koenig et al., 1991) found that the apparent digestibility of selenium from sodium selenite fed to dairy cows was <4 percent.

Comparative absorption of different sources of selenium can be assessed by concentrations of selenium in tissue and blood and by activity of GSHpx. Overall, few differences have been found among the different inorganic sources of selenium or between dietary supplementation and ruminal boluses based on concentrations in tissue or blood of dairy cattle (Podoll et al., 1992; Gibson et al., 1993; Grace et al., 1995). Feeding organic sources of selenium (including Se-enriched yeast and feedstuffs with high concentrations of selenium) to ruminants usually increases concentrations of selenium in blood and tissues and the activity of GSHpx more than feeding inorganic sources of selenium (Conrad and Moxon, 1979; Johansson et al., 1990; Nicholson et al., 1991a, b).

### REQUIREMENTS AND FACTORS AFFECTING REQUIREMENTS

The 6th revised edition (National Research Council, 1989b) defined the selenium requirement as 0.3 mg/kg of dietary DM for all classes of dairy cattle. No new data are available to dispute this requirement. However, the majority of data supporting this requirement were generated from experiments in which 0.3 mg of supplemental selenium/kg of dietary DM (DM basis) was fed so that total dietary selenium ranged from 0.35 to 0.40 mg/kg. Proper selenium nutrition of dairy animals in late gestation is important for preventing some periparturient disorders and also for ensuring that the calf is born with adequate selenium. Selenium efficiently passes through the placenta and calves born from dams receiving adequate selenium are in better selenium status than calves from dams not fed adequate selenium (Van Saun et al., 1989). The concentration of selenium in milk is increased when cows are fed additional selenium (Grace et al., 1997). Increased concentrations of selenium in milk may have positive effects on calf and human health.

Establishing requirements for selenium using the factorial approach is difficult because the deposition of selenium in body tissues, conceptus, and milk is dependent on selenium intake. As cows consume more selenium, the concentrations of selenium in milk and in the conceptus increase. Assuming a cow is fed a diet with approximately 0.3 mg of selenium/kg of dietary DM, the conceptus will accumulate approximately 0.055 mg of selenium/day during the last trimester of gestation (House and Bell, 1994). Selenium concentration of milk ranges from 0.01 to 0.025 mg/kg (Conrad and Moxon, 1979; Lean et al., 1990; Van Dael et al., 1991). Endogenous fecal losses of selenium in dairy cattle range from 0.011 to 0.019 mg/kg of dry matter intake (Harrison and Conrad, 1984b; Koenig et al., 1991 a, b; Ivancic, 1999). Urinary excretion is dependent on Se intake (Ivancic, 1999). For lactating cows consuming approximately 2.5 mg of Se/day, urinary Se losses averaged 0.5 mg/d (Ivancic, 1999). Similar values were reported for dry cows fed similar amounts of Se (Harrison and Conrad, 1984b). Therefore, for a nonlactating cow in the last trimester of gestation that consumed 10 kg of DM/day, the requirement for absorbed selenium is approximately 0.7 mg/day. Assuming an absorption coefficient of 40 percent, the dietary requirement would be 1.75 mg/d. For a lactating cow producing 30 kg/d of milk, the requirement for absorbed selenium would be approximately 1.7 mg/day and the dietary requirement would be 4 mg/day. In agreement with those calculations, dry cows fed approximately 1.4 mg of Se/d (Harrison and Conrad, 1984b), and lactating cows fed approximately 4.2 mg/d (Ivancic, 1999) were in slightly positive Se balance. However, based on blood concentrations and prevalence of mastitis and retained fetal membranes, the calculated requirements are not adequate. Maus et al. (1980) reported that plasma concentrations of selenium in lactating dairy cows reached a plateau when selenium intake was 6 mg/day.

Current FDA regulations limit selenium supplementation to 0.3 mg/kg of diet (FDA, 1997) and in most situations, that amount of supplemental selenium will maintain dairy cattle in good selenium status. Based on the effect of selenium on mastitis, concentrations of selenium in whole blood should be greater than about 0.18 μg/ml or approximately 0.08 μg/ml for plasma (Jukola et al., 1996). Intake of approximately 6 mg/day of selenium should maintain those blood concentrations (Maus et al., 1980). Based on available data, the selenium requirement was maintained at 0.3 mg/kg of dietary DM.

Certain nutrients affect the absorption and metabolism of selenium and can alter the requirement for selenium. The requirements for vitamin E and selenium are clearly interdependent, but the relationship has not been quantified. Dairy cattle that are marginal in either selenium or vitamin E will require additional amounts of the other nutrient. The apparent digestibility of selenium is reduced when cows are fed diets with high (ca. 1.3 percent) or low (ca. 0.5 percent) concentrations of calcium (Harrison and Conrad, 1984a). Increased consumption of sulfur may increase the requirement for selenium. In sheep, increasing dietary sulfur (from sulfate) from 0.05 percent to 0.24 percent decreased selenium absorption (Pope et al., 1979) but had no effect on metabolism of selenium when dietary sulfur was increased from 0.28 to 0.78 percent (Paulson et al., 1966). In contrast, true digestibility of selenium by lactating dairy cows was reduced from about 56 percent to 46 percent when dietary sulfur was increased from 0.2 percent to 0.4 or 0.7 percent (from calcium and magnesium sulfate) (Ivancic, 1999). Supplementation of sulfur from anionic salts for the last three weeks of gestation did not influence selenium status of nonlactating cows (Gant et al., 1998). With beef cattle, long term feeding of diets that contained approximately 0.2 or 0.5 percent total sulfur did not affect concentrations of selenium in whole blood or the activity of GSHpx in red blood cells (Khan et al., 1987). A relationship between dietary copper and selenium also may occur. In sheep fed a diet with >0.3 mg/kg of selenium, increasing dietary copper from about 7 mg/kg of DM to 21 mg/kg of DM increased the selenium concentrations in liver but decreased the concentration of selenium in muscle (Hartmann and van Ryssen, 1997). An isotope study found similar results when sheep were fed low selenium diets (<0.1 mg/kg) (White et al., 1989). Koenig et al. (1991b) reported no effect of feeding diets with 0 or 16 mg of supplemental copper/kg on selenium balance in dairy cows (diets contained 0.2 mg of selenium/kg of DM). Increasing the amount of zinc in diets fed to rats from 5 to 20 mg/kg reduced absorption of selenium by 25 percent (House and Welch, 1989). Data concerning the effects of zinc with ruminants are lacking.

#### TOXICITY

Historic concerns regarding selenium were not about providing adequate selenium to cows, but rather about toxicity. Alkali disease and blind staggers result from selenium toxicity. Clinical signs include sloughing of hooves, lameness, loss of hair, and emaciation (National Research Council, 1983). Most cases of selenium toxicity have been related to consumption of selenium accumulating plants (e.g., *Astragalus* sp.). Chronic toxicity can occur when cattle are fed diets with 5 to 40 mg of selenium/kg for a period of several weeks or months (National Research Council, 1983). Acute toxicity can occur when cows are fed 10 to 20 mg of Se/kg of body weight. An injection of about 0.5 mg of Se/kg of body weight to young cattle (ca. 200 kg) resulted in a 67 percent mortality rate (National Research Council, 1983). The recommendation for dietary selenium is approximately 16 times less than the lowest dietary level that has been related to chronic toxicity.

### *Zinc*

#### FUNCTION

Zinc is a component of many metalloenzymes such as copper-zinc superoxide dismutase, carbonic anhydrase, alcohol dehydrogenase, carboxypeptidase, alkaline phosphatase, and RNA polymerase, which affects metabolism of carbohydrates, proteins, lipids, and nucleic acids. Zinc regulates calmodulin, protein kinase C, thyroid hormone binding, and inositol phosphate synthesis. Zinc deficiency alters prostaglandin synthesis, which may affect luteal function (Graham, 1991). Zinc is a component of thymosin, a hormone produced by thymic cells that regulates cell-mediated immunity.

ABSORPTION

Intestinal absorption of zinc occurs primarily in the small intestine (Flagstad, 1976). In animals that are zinc deficient, zinc readily enters the enterocytes and is transported across the cell by an intestinal protein (CRIP) that is rich in cysteine and is released into the portal circulation to be carried primarily by transferrin (Evans and Winter, 1975) and albumin. In animals that are zinc replete, metallothionein, a second protein rich in cysteine, is found in the mucosal cells and this metallothionein competes with the cysteine rich protein for zinc transported across the brush border membrane. Zinc bound to metalothionein will remain in the enterocyte and be excreted with the feces when the enterocyte dies and is sloughed (Chesters, 1997). By up-regulating or down-regulating metallothionein in mucosal enterocytes the amount of dietary zinc that is absorbed can be regulated. How the status of zinc regulates the concentration of intestinal metallothionein is unknown, but it requires days to weeks for the concentration of metallothionein in the intestine to adjust to a low zinc diet (Taylor et al., 1991).

About 50 percent of the zinc in milk is absorbed by calves (Miller and Cragle, 1965). Adding soybean protein to a milk diet adds phytic acid and reduces the efficiency of zinc absorption by more than one-half (Miller et al., 1967). In ruminating calves weighing 70 to 150 kg, efficiency of zinc absorption ranged from 16 percent to 51 percent, depending on the level of supplementation in one study (Miller et al., 1968) and was about 20 percent in another (Miller and Cragle, 1965). In adult cattle, only 12 to 14 percent of dietary zinc was absorbed in the study of Miller and Cragle (1965). Total zinc in the diet was not reported. In a study by Hansard et al. (1968), about 22 percent of dietary zinc was absorbed in adult cows fed a diet containing 28 mg zinc/kg diet, which was probably not greatly in excess of the needs of the animals. Animals that were adapted to a low zinc diet with no inhibitors of zinc absorption can absorb nearly 50 percent of dietary zinc (Kirchgessner and Schwarz, 1976). However, optimal zinc absorption is neither likely, nor desirable and a coefficient of zinc absorption of 15 percent is used for all ruminating animals, based on the results of Miller and Cragle (1965) with adult cattle. This approach might be too conservative. The Agricultural Research Council (1980) reviewed the literature on efficiency of zinc absorption and concluded that pre-ruminant calves absorb about 50 percent of dietary zinc, growing ruminants absorb 30 percent of dietary zinc, and adult ruminants absorb 20 percent of dietary zinc. Since intrinsic zinc from feedstuffs is apparently absorbed to about the same extent as added inorganic zinc (Stuart et al., 1986), no correction was made for zinc from inorganic or organic sources. The poor solubility of zinc oxide suggests that it may not be as well absorbed as zinc sulfate. However, when zinc oxide was added to diets to raise dietary zinc, it was comparable to other forms of zinc in preventing signs of zinc deficiency in most studies (Miller et al., 1967; Miller et al., 1970; Kincaid, 1979; Kincaid et al., 1997). Unfortunately, these studies used large amounts of zinc (200 to 600 mg/kg diet) in basal diets. A comparison of efficiency of absorption of zinc sources at dietary concentrations closer to or slightly below the metabolic needs of the animals remains to be done in ruminants.

DIETARY ZINC REQUIREMENT

A factorial approach was taken to determine the dietary requirement for zinc. The daily endogenous fecal loss of zinc is approximately 0.033 mg zinc/kg body weight and the obligate urinary loss of zinc has been estimated as 0.012 mg zinc/kg body weight for a total maintenance requirement for zinc of 0.045 mg zinc/kg body weight (Hansard et al., 1968). During gestation, the fetus and uterus retain about 12 mg zinc/day (House and Bell, 1993) between day 190 of gestation and the end of gestation and nearly double that estimated by Agricultural Research Council (1980). The zinc content of milk is about 4 mg/kg (range 3.4 to 5.8 mg) (Osis et al., 1972; Schwarz and Kirchgessner, 1975). The lactational requirement for zinc can be very large. The amount of zinc retained during growth of body tissues is estimated to be 24 mg zinc/kg average daily gain (range 16 to 31 mg) (Kirchgessner and Neesse, 1976; Miller, 1970). Using these values, the requirement for the amount of zinc that must be absorbed from the diet can be estimated. This requirement divided by the efficiency of absorption of dietary zinc, which is estimated to be 15 percent, is the total amount of zinc the diet must supply each day.

A comparison of the requirement for dietary zinc of cattle in various physiologic states estimated by the National Research Council (1989b), the Agricultural Research Council (1980), and the current model are presented in Table 6-4. The National Research Council (1989b) may have underestimated the dietary zinc required to support lactation. Kirchgessner and Weigand (1982) utilized semi-purified diets that contained between 6 and 436 mg of zinc/kg to derive a dose response relationship

TABLE 6-4 Comparison of Estimated Dietary Zinc Requirements (mg/d) and Dietary Zinc Concentrations (mg/kg of DM) for Cattle in Various Physiologic States

| Cow Description | Feed intake (kg of DM) | 1989 NRC mg/day | 1989 NRC mg/kg of diet | 1980 ARC mg/day | 1980 ARC mg/kg of diet | 2000 NRC mg/day | 2000 NRC mg/kg of diet |
|---|---|---|---|---|---|---|---|
| 300-kg heifer, ADG = 0.7 kg | 6 | 240 | 40 | 151 | 25 | 202 | 33 |
| 500-kg heifer, ADG = 0.5 kg day 250 gestation | 10 | 400 | 40 | 204 | 20.4 | 310 | 31 |
| 650-kg cow, 40 kg milk/d | 20 | 800 | 40 | 946 | 47.3 | 1261 | 63 |
| 650-kg cow, day 270 gestation | 12 | 480 | 40 | 178 | 14.8 | 274 | 22.8 |

between dietary zinc and the concentration of zinc in serum or milk or serum alkaline phosphatase. They reported that diets containing 35 mg zinc/kg were sufficient to provide 90 percent of the maximal response for zinc in serum, milk, and serum alkaline phosphatase activity during lactation. Semi-purified diets may not be an adequate indication of expected results in practical feeding situations where chelation may reduce the availability of dietary zinc.

#### FACTORS AFFECTING ZINC REQUIREMENTS

Two major dietary factors that can modify the efficiency of absorption of dietary zinc are interactions of zinc with other metal ions and the presence of organic chelating agents in the diet.

Zinc and copper are antagonistic to one another. In most cases, zinc interferes with absorption of copper to cause a deficiency of copper, if copper availability is marginal, but when dietary copper-to-zinc ratios are very high (50:1), copper could interfere with absorption of zinc, although this is unlikely in cattle (Van Campen, 1969). Excessive dietary iron can interfere with absorption of zinc in man and other species. In rats, a deficiency of iron enhanced both absorption of iron and zinc suggesting iron and zinc share a common absorption mechanism (Flanagan et al., 1980). In man, the effect of excess iron is evident when the iron-to-zinc ratio is >2:1 (Solomons, 1986). No data exist for the interaction between dietary iron and absorption of zinc in ruminants. Under practical conditions dietary iron is often well in excess of requirements for iron by the cow.

Cadmium is antagonistic to the absorption of both zinc and copper and also interferes with tissue metabolism of zinc and copper in the liver and kidneys (see cadmium section). Lead competitively inhibits absorption of zinc and also interferes with the function of zinc during heme synthesis (Finelli et al., 1975). Tin also may interfere with absorption of zinc (Johnson and Greger, 1984).

High dietary concentrations of calcium interfere with absorption of zinc in nonruminants, perhaps because the effect of phytate is exaggerated by dietary calcium (O'Dell et al., 1958). In cattle supplementation of calcium was associated with a reduction of zinc in serum of yearling steers and calves (Mills et al., 1967; Perry et al., 1968). Studies with sheep did not demonstrate a deleterious effect of increased dietary calcium on metabolism of zinc or growth (Pond and Oltjen, 1988; Pond and Wallace, 1986).

Organic chelators of zinc can increase or decrease efficiency of absorption of zinc. Those that interfere with absorption tend to form insoluble complexes with zinc. Phytate commonly binds zinc in plants and greatly diminishes absorption of zinc in calves and nonruminant animals. However, ruminal microbes metabolize most of the dietary phytate so it is not a factor affecting absorption of zinc in ruminating animals.

Deficiency symptoms for zinc were not observed in ruminating calves fed semi-synthetic rations containing as little as 8 mg zinc/kg DM. Most of these rations utilized urea to supply some of the nitrogen required by the animals (Agricultural Research Council, 1980, Table 6.13, p. 257) (Mills et al., 1967). However, a deficiency of zinc has been reported numerous times in calves of similar age fed natural diets supplying at least 8 and as much as 30 mg zinc/kg diet (Demertzis, 1973; Agricultural Research Council, 1980—Table 6.16, p. 261). These data raise suspicions that unknown organic factors found in common feed ingredients interfere with absorption of zinc by ruminants and other species.

Some naturally occurring chelators of zinc improve absorption of zinc. Scott and Ziegler (1963) demonstrated with chicks that adding distillers dried solubles and liver extract to soybean protein based diets improved the efficiency of absorption of the dietary zinc, though the factor remained unknown. Peptides and amino acids can form complexes with zinc and both cysteine and histidine bind zinc strongly and improve efficiency of absorption of zinc in chicks (Nielsen et al., 1966; Hortin et al., 1991). At the alkaline pH found in the intestine, it is likely that little free zinc cation exists in solution. One action of beneficial chelates is to form soluble zinc complexes within the small intestine permitting soluble zinc to reach the brush border membrane for absorption.

DEFICIENCY

Cattle that are deficient for zinc quickly exhibit reduced feed intake and growth rate. With a more prolonged deficiency the animals exhibit reduced growth of testes, weak hoof horn, and perakaratosis of the skin on the legs, head (especially nostrils), and neck. On necropsy thymic atrophy and lymphoid depletion of the spleen and lymph nodes are evident (Brummerstedt et al., 1974; Mayland et al., 1980; Miller and Miller, 1962; Mills et al., 1967). A genetic defect that greatly reduces absorption of zinc has been identified in Dutch-Friesan cattle. These animals become severely deficient in zinc unless fed extremely large amounts of dietary zinc (Flagstad, 1976).

Concentrations of zinc in serum are normally between 0.7 and 1.3 μg/ml. Concentrations of zinc in serum below 0.4 μg/ml are often considered deficient. However, stress or disease can cause a rapid redistribution of zinc out of extracellular fluids causing concentrations of zinc in serum to fall into the "deficient" range even when dietary zinc is adequate (Hambridge et al., 1986; Goff and Stabel, 1990). Concentrations of zinc in the liver are more reliable and should be 100 to 400 mg/kg on a dry weight basis (Puls, 1994). However, responsive conditions to zinc have been seen in cattle with concentrations of zinc in liver above 100 mg/kg because zinc in liver does not serve as a readily mobilizable source of zinc during times of dietary insufficiency of zinc (Miller, 1978). Thus, it is difficult to certify adequacy of zinc by concentrations of zinc in liver but it is possible to diagnose zinc deficiency when zinc in liver is below 100 mg/kg dry weight. Carbonic anhydrase and alkaline phosphatase activities in blood have been used to assess the status of zinc but these determinations are difficult to interpret because concurrent disease can affect these enzymes as much as a deficiency of zinc. A promising indicator of the status of zinc is metallothionein in plasma or urine. This protein is induced by zinc in tissues and released into blood (Garvey, 1984) and may be a better indication of the status of zinc in tissues.

TOXICITY

A large amount of dietary zinc is fairly well tolerated by cattle, however zinc toxicity was observed in cattle fed 900 mg zinc/kg diet (Ott et al., 1966). Very high levels of zinc have a negative effect on absorption and metabolism of copper (Miller et al., 1989), and it is for this reason primarily that dietary zinc should be limited. The maximal tolerable level of dietary zinc is suggested to be 300 to 1000 mg/kg diet. However very high levels of zinc oxide, providing more than 1000 mg Zn/kg DM are routinely fed to cattle in some areas to combat facial eczema with no sign of zinc intoxication.

### *Chromium*

Chromium is primarily found in tissues as an organometallic molecule composed of $Cr^{+3}$, nicotinic acid, glutamic acid, glycine, and cysteine known as glucose tolerance factor (Toepfer et al., 1977). Without $Cr^{+3}$ the glucose tolerance factor is inactive. Glucose tolerance factor can potentiate the effect of insulin on tissues, either by stabilizing the insulin molecule (Govindaraju et al., 1989), or by facilitating the interaction of insulin with its receptor in tissues (Mertz, 1993). Studies in rats have determined that chromium is absorbed primarily from the small intestine (Chen et al., 1973). Inorganic forms of $Cr^{+3}$ ($CrCl_3$, $Cr_2O_3$) are very poorly absorbed (hence the utility of $Cr_2O_3$ as a marker for digestion studies). Complexing $Cr^{+3}$ with organic compounds greatly increases the absorption of chromium. Chromium nicotinate and chromium picolinate are usually considered the most available sources of supplemental chromium. Chromium from naturally occurring sources such as brewer's yeast also is efficiently absorbed with as much as 10 to 25 percent absorbed by rats (Underwood, 1977a).

The essentiality of chromium as a required element necessary for normal glucose metabolism in the diet of humans is well accepted and it is recommended that the diet of adult humans supply from 50 to 200 μg chromium/day (National Research Council, 1989a). The role of chromium in animal nutrition recently was reviewed by the National Research Council (1997). Several studies in cattle have demonstrated a favorable response to chromium supplementation, especially if the animals are under some physiologic stress. These positive studies examined the effects of supplementation of chromium during the peripartuient period in dairy cattle. The positive findings included improved humoral and possibly cell mediated immune response (Burton et al., 1993), improved energy status (reduced liver triglyceride accumulation), DMI, and milk production (Besong et al., 1996), and increased milk production in primiparous cows but not multiparous cows (Yang et al., 1996). In these studies the basal rations generally contained <1.6 mg chromium/kg diet and diets were supplemented with 0.5 to 10 mg chromium/kg diet. Together with reports of reduced morbidity of stressed feedlot calves supplemented with chromium (Moonsie-Shageer and Mowat, 1993), these studies suggest that cattle require chromium in their diets. Unfortunately, the amount of chromium required in the diet for optimal performance is unclear and the literature does not support a general recommendation for supplementation of chromium of typical cattle diets. Additional research on the bioavailable chromium contained in common feedstuffs and the effects of diets deficient in chromium on performance of dairy cows will be required, including appropriate titration studies, before a dietary requirement for chromium can be established (National Research Council, 1997).

It is generally accepted that trivalent chromium added to diets is safe and non-toxic. Chromium toxicity is primarily associated with exposure to hexavalent $Cr^{+6}$ (chromium trioxide, chromates, bichromates). Hexavalent chromium passes into the interior of cells much more readily than trivalent chromium (Jennette, 1979) and is able to depress mitochondrial oxygen consumption by inhibiting alpha-ketoglutarate dehydrogenase (Ryberg and Alexander, 1990). If significant amounts reach the cell nucleus there can be a variety of pathologic changes in the DNA (Alexander, 1993). For livestock the maximum tolerable concentration of chromium in the diet is set at 3000 mg/kg for the oxide form and 1000 mg/kg for the chloride form of the trivalent forms of chromium. Hexavalent forms of chromium are at least five times more toxic (National Research Council, 1997).

*Aluminum, Arsenic, Nickel, Silica, Tin, and Vanadium*

These elements can be found in minute amounts in the tissues of animals. When removed from the diet of laboratory rodents, some of these elements have been demonstrated to be essential for these species. Data on essentiality in dairy cattle are non-existent and practical diets would not be expected to result in deficiency of any of these elements. Most of these elements can be toxic when provided in large amounts and this is occasionally a problem in dairy cattle.

Our current understanding of metabolism does not include any specific role for aluminum, arsenic, silica, tin, or vanadium. Nickel is required for activity of urease.

Aluminum is the third most common element in the earth's crust. It is found in only trace amounts in plants and animals. Animals on pasture can consume up to 10 percent of their total DMI as soil. Most of the aluminum ingested is not absorbed, and the majority of the small amount that is absorbed is rapidly excreted in urine. Bone and other tissues will accumulate aluminum, especially if renal function is compromised (Thurston et al., 1972).

Aluminum binds phosphate, which reduces absorption of phosphorus. In animals, aluminum toxicosis is primarily associated with malabsorption of phosphorus and other minerals (Allen, 1984). The maximum tolerable dietary aluminum is 1000 mg/kg of diet (National Research Council, 1980; Bailey, 1977; Valdivia et al., 1978).

A deficiency of arsenic has been reported in goats and mini-pigs fed diets containing <50 mg arsenic/kg of diet (Anke et al., 1976). Deficiency signs consisted of impaired reproductive performance and lower weight gains in second generation animals.

Organic arsenicals have been used in swine and poultry for their antibiotic and anti-coccidial properties (Frost et al., 1955). They have not been used in cattle. However, organic arsenicals, as well as inorganic forms of arsenic are well absorbed and can cause toxicosis when feedstuffs are accidentally contaminated with arsenic. Arsenic released from copper and lead smelters can contaminate soil and forages (Lillie, 1970). Unfortunately, sheep and cattle do not find arsenic unpalatable and may even develop a taste for it (Clarke and Clarke, 1975). Insecticides, wood preservatives, and herbicides containing arsenic also have been sources of contamination.

Arsenic binds to sulfhydryl groups of proteins interfering with their function. Inorganic arsenicals are more toxic than organic arsenicals. Cattle fed poultry manure containing 18 mg/kg organic arsenic/kg of diet exhibited no signs of toxicity (Calvert and Smith, 1972). The maximal tolerable dietary arsenic was set at 50 mg/kg and 100 mg/kg for inorganic and organic forms, respectively, per kg of diet (National Research Council, 1980).

Deficiencies of nickel have been produced in chicks, pigs, goats, and rats (Nielsen and Ollerich, 1974; Nielsen and Sandstead, 1974) and in lambs (Spears and Hatfield, 1978). Lambs fed a diet low in nickel had lower ruminal urease activity than lambs fed 5 mg of nickel/kg of DM (Spears, 1984). Nickel deficiency is associated with reduced growth, which is perhaps the result of pathologic changes in the liver (Nielsen et al., 1975). Nickel is relatively non-toxic with maximal tolerable dietary concentrations of 50 mg/kg for cattle (National Research Council, 1980). The main adverse affect of nickel is reduced feed intake.

Silicon is the second most abundant element on earth but is found in only very trace amounts in animal tissues. In chicks and rats, a deficiency in silicon has been demonstrated using carefully purified diets. A deficiency in silicon is associated with disturbances of bone formation and depression in growth rate (Carlisle, 1974).

Silicon is primarily found combined with oxygen to form silica. Silica is only poorly absorbed. Contamination of forages with soil makes a deficiency of silicon very unlikely in ruminants. Silicon in forages is more likely to present a problem as it can depress DM digestibility in ruminants (Van Soest and Jones, 1968).

While primarily a clinical problem in males, urinary calculi of ruminants often contain silica. Although urinary calculi in grazing steers has been associated with the silica content of forages (Parker, 1957), there is evidence that low dietary intake of magnesium is the main dietary factor associated with increased formation of silica containing uroliths (Schneider et al., 1952; Parker, 1957). The maximal tolerable silicon concentration was set at 0.2 percent of the diet, based primarily on the negative affects of silicon on dietary organic matter digestibility (National Research Council, 1980).

Tin has been demonstrated to be essential for growth in rats (Schwartz et al., 1970). However, because tin is so commonly used for production of "tin cans" and alloys, the greater concern is that tin will contaminate feedstuffs. Inorganic forms of tin are poorly absorbed and dietary levels as high as 150 mg/kg were considered safe (deGroot, 1973). Organic forms of tin may be more toxic (National Research Council, 1980).

Vanadium at 0.1 mg/kg of diet optimizes growth in rats (Schwartz and Milne, 1971) and calves (Drebickas, 1966). How it acts is unknown. Less than 1 percent of dietary vanadium is absorbed in sheep (Hansard, 1975).

Vanadium toxicity is associated with inhibition of enzyme activity, particularly the Na-K ATPases (Cantley et al., 1977). The maximum tolerable vanadium was suggested to be 50 mg/kg of diet (National Research Council, 1980). However, ruminal function (DM digestibility) in lambs was disrupted with just 7 mg vanadium/kg of diet (Williams, 1973). Rock phosphates can contain up to 6,000 mg of vanadium/kg, which could be a potentially toxic source of vanadium (Romoser et al., 1960).

## TOXIC MINERALS

### *Cadmium*

Cadmium is a heavy metal that accumulates within the body, particularly the kidney, to cause renal damage. It is cleared from the body very poorly and very slowly. It is of particular concern to humans because of our long life span and because cadmium has become so commonly distributed in the environment. The Joint FAO/WHO Expert Committee on Food Additives (1972) established a provisional maximum tolerable intake of cadmium at 57 to 71 μg/day. Ryan et al. (1982) estimated that men and women consume 33 and 26 μg cadmium/day respectively. The maximal tolerable cadmium in the diet of cattle was set at 0.5 mg/kg in an effort to avoid adding cadmium to the diet of humans consuming products primarily derived from dairy cattle (National Research Council, 1980).

Cadmium is antagonistic to zinc and copper, and to a lesser degree iron. Diets containing from 5 to 30 mg cadmium/kg of diet generally decrease animal performance by interfering with copper and zinc absorption, resulting in symptoms usually associated with copper and zinc deficiency. Diets containing more than 5 mg of cadmium/kg can cause copper concentrations in liver to decline (Smith, 1986). Cadmium binds to metallothionein very tightly, which competitively decreases absorption of copper and to a lesser degree absorption of zinc. Liver and kidney contain metallothionein proteins (Kagi et al., 1974) that accumulate cadmium throughout the life of animals. Ruminant diets containing more than 30 mg of cadmium/kg have produced anorexia, reduced growth, decreased milk production, and abortion (Doyle et al., 1974; Wright et al., 1977).

Cadmium is a contaminant of the zinc sulfides used to galvanize iron to prevent corrosion. It is a component of nickel-cadmium batteries and is used as a stabilizer in polyvinylchloride plastics. Waste from zinc smelting operations and zinc plating operations have been sources of contamination that have resulted in cadmium intoxication. Urban sewage sludge contains significant amounts of cadmium and should not be used as fertilizer on farmland growing crops intended for consumption by humans or food animals. Some phosphate fertilizers can also contain significant amounts of cadmium (National Research Council, 1980).

High concentrations of cadmium (up to 10 mg/kg) have been found in forages grown in fields near industrial zinc-plating sites and where urban sludge has been used as a fertilizer (Smith, 1986). In most areas of the country, cadmium toxicosis is not a concern because most feeds and forages contain <0.50 mg/kg (National Research Council, 1980).

Less than 1 percent of dietary cadmium is absorbed by ruminants (Neathery et al., 1974). Intestinal metallothionein binds cadmium tightly and limits the absorption of cadmium. Cadmium can be detected in small amounts in milk but the mammary gland limits cadmium transport and the concentration of cadmium in milk is not increased by high dietary concentrations of cadmium (Sharma et al., 1979; Smith, 1986; Van Bruwaene et al., 1982). Concentrations of cadmium in muscle are much lower than in kidney (Sharma et al., 1979). However, significant accumulation in muscle has been reported after prolonged feeding of diets high in cadium to cattle (Smith, 1986).

### *Fluorine*

Although fluorine in very small amounts can increase the strength of bones and teeth, it is generally not regarded as an essential dietary component (National Research Council, 1980). Fluorine is generally regarded as a toxic element with regards to domestic livestock because in large amounts fluorine will accumulate in bone to an extent that actually weakens bone, increasing lameness and increasing wear of teeth (Shupe, 1980; Crissman et al., 1980). The teeth of cattle intoxicated with fluorine become mottled and stained, and are eroded or pitted.

Soluble forms of fluoride, such as sodium fluoride, are rapidly and nearly completely absorbed by cattle (Perkinson Jr. et al., 1955). About 50 percent of fluorine in undefluorinated phosphates of bone meal is absorbed. Dietary calcium, aluminum, sodium chloride, and fat can reduce fluorine absorption (National Research Council, 1980). Fluorine does not pass readily into milk and fluorine in milk does not increase markedly with increased dietary fluorine (Greenwood et al., 1964).

Minor morphologic lesions can occur in young cattle receiving as little as 20 mg of fluorine/kg of diet when teeth are developing rapidly, but the relationship between these minor lesions and animal performance is unknown

(National Research Council, 1980). The maximal tolerable dietary content of fluorine was set at 40 mg/kg of diet (National Research Council, 1980).

Rock phosphates from Florida [fluorapatite, $Ca_{10}F_2(PO_4)_6$] can contaminate cattle when used in feed or when applied as a fertilizer without first being defluorinated. To qualify as defluorinated, feed grade phosphates can contain no more than 1 part of fluorine to 100 parts of phosphorus (AAFCO, 1977). Other potential sources of fluorine include bone meal, deep well water, and soil near volcanoes and fumaroles. Fluorine in the form of hydrofluoric acid, silicon tetrafluoride, or fluoride containing particulates can be released from industrial sites associated with aluminum or phosphate processing. These emissions can contaminate water, soil, and plants near these sites, resulting in fluorine intoxicosis in animals grazing in the areas (Bunce, 1985).

*Lead*

Lead is the most common cause of toxicoses in domestic livestock (Neathery and Miller, 1975). Lead halides and lead bromochloride, which were once added to gasoline as engine valve lubricants were emitted from automobile exhaust during combustion and continue to contaminate much of the American landscape. Lead based pigments were common until restrictions were imposed and paint chips from older structures remain a significant source of lead contamination in cattle. Lead intoxication also has occurred in cattle consuming lead from batteries, putty from window glazing, linoleum, asphalt roofing, and used engine or crankcase oil. From 3 to 10 percent of ingested lead is absorbed by adult ruminants (Fick et al., 1976). Elevated dietary calcium, phosphorus, iron, zinc, fat, and protein decrease the absorption and retention of lead (Mahaffey, 1983; White et al., 1985). Lead accumulates in bone (Schroeder and Tipton, 1968). Lead readily passes into milk so that increasing dietary concentrations of lead results in increased lead concentration in milk (Murthy et al., 1967; Lopez et al., 1985; Underwood, 1977).

Clinical intoxicosis interferes with normal metal-dependent enzyme functions. Lead causes derangements in porphyrin and heme synthesis, interferes with protein synthesis, basophilic stippling of erythrocytes, and causes microcytic hypochromic anemia (National Research Council, 1980).

Chronic exposure to low levels of lead is not associated with clinical symptoms in cattle because bones sequester lead and release it gradually to the blood for excretion. In humans, low exposure to lead is associated with a loss of cognitive powers—this is not generally detected in cattle. Acute intoxication with lead causes impaired neurologic function resulting in blindness and irritability (Radostits et al., 1994). Lead toxicity also causes intestinal pain and colic, and abortion. Lead accumulates in the kidney cortex and renal tubular inclusion bodies suggest impaired renal function. In cattle that have died from lead poisoning, lead in the kidney cortex is often >50 mg/kg and in the liver is often >20 mg/kg (fresh tissue) (Allcroft and Blaxter, 1950).

Whereas cattle can tolerate up to 100 mg of lead/kg in their diet without noticeable effects the maximum tolerable dietary lead was set at 30 mg/kg (National Research Council, 1980). A single dose of 200 mg lead/kg body weight is lethal to cattle (Allcroft and Blaxter, 1950). Young animals tend to be more susceptible to lead intoxication than adults because they have a higher rate of absorption of lead (90 percent versus 10 percent) and are more likely to exhibit pica (eating non-food substances).

*Mercury*

Mercury toxicity is uncommon. Most cases have been associated with ingestion of seed grain coated with an organic mercury fungicide (Radostits et al., 1994). Fish meal protein concentrates also have accidentally caused mercury poisoning. Fish concentrate methyl mercury that might be in the water (Annett et al., 1975). The organic mercury compounds, especially methyl mercury, are more toxic than the inorganic forms of mercury (Potter et al., 1972; Ansari et al., 1973; Sell and Dawson, 1973). Organic mercury compounds are more efficiently absorbed and are retained longer (Ansari et al., 1973). Because they are more lipophilic, they tend to cross the blood-brain barrier easier resulting in greater neurologic problems. Little organic or inorganic mercury is secreted into milk (Sell and Dawson, 1973; Potter et al., 1972; Neathery et al., 1974).

Inorganic mercury compounds are very caustic and cause acute gastroenteritis when ingested. Low doses of inorganic mercury ingested over time cause depression, anorexia, and a stiff-legged gait followed by paresis. Alopecia, pruritus, scabby lesions around the anus and vulva, shedding of teeth, and diarrhea are typical of later stages of inorganic mercury poisoning (Radostits et al., 1994). The primary cause of death is acute renal failure (Bulger and Siegel, 1975).

The organic mercury compounds (alkyl mercuries) primarily affect the nervous system and clinical signs are similar to those seen in calves with polioencephalomalacia: listlessness, incoordination, progressive blindness, and convulsions. However, animals poisoned by organic mercury compounds do not respond to thiamin (Oliver and Platonow, 1960; Herigstad et al., 1972; Davis et al., 1965).

A single 8-g dose of mercuric chloride was toxic to cattle (Radostits et al., 1994). Calves fed a diet of milk containing 10 mg of mercury from methyl mercury/kg of milk died in 36 to 81 days, whereas calves receiving 2 to 4 mg of mercury as methyl mercury /kg of milk remained clinically normal (Herigstad et al., 1972). The suggested maximum tolerable concentration of dietary mercury in organic or inorganic form is 2 mg/kg (National Research Council, 1980).

## REFERENCES


Adams, R. S. 1975. Variability in mineral and trace element content of dairy cattle feeds. J. Dairy Sci. 58:1538–1548.

Agricultural and Food Research Council. 1991. Technical Committee on Responses to Nutrients, Report 6. A reappraisal of the calcium and phosphorus requirements of sheep and cattle. Nutr. Abstr. and Rev. (Series B). 61:573–612.

Agricultural Research Council. 1965. The nutrient requirements of farm livestock. No. 2. Ruminants. London.

Agricultural Research Council. 1980. The Nutrient Requirements of Ruminant Livestock. Slough, England: Commonwealth Agricultural Bureaux.

Aines, P. D., and S. E. Smith. 1957. Sodium versus chloride for the therapy of salt-deficient dairy cows. J. Dairy Sci. 40:682–688.

Aitken, F. C. 1976. Sodium and potassium nutrition of mammals. Tech. Comm. No. 26. Commonwealth Agricultural Bureaux of Nutrition. Bucksburn, Aberdeen, U.K.

Alderman, G. 1963. Mineral nutrition and reproduction in cattle. Vet. Record. 75:1015–1018.

Alexander, J. 1993. Toxicity versus essentiality of chromium. Scand. J. Work. Environ. Health 19(S1):126–127.

Allcroft, R., and K. L. Baxter. 1950. Lead as a nutritional hazard to farm livestock. V. The toxicity of lead to cattle and sheep and an evaluation of the lead hazard under farm conditions. J. Comp. Pathol. 60:209–218.

Allen, V. G. 1984. Influence of dietary aluminum on nutrient utilization in ruminants. J. Anim. Sci. 59:836–844.

Allen, J. D., and J. M. Gawthorne. 1987. Involvement of the solid phase of rumen digesta in the interochan between copper, molybdenum and sulfur in sheep. Br. J. Nutr. 58:265.

Allsop, T. F. and Rook, J. A. F. 1972. The effect of diet and blood-plasma magnesium concentration on the endogenous faecal loss of magnesium in sheep. J. Ag. Sci., Cambridge 92, 403–408.

Ammerman, C. B. 1970. Recent developments in cobalt and copper in ruminant nutrition: A review. J. Dairy Sci. 53:1097–1107.

Ammerman, C. B., and S. M. Miller. 1972. Biological availability of minor mineral ions: a review. 35:681–694.

Ammerman, C. B., C. F. Chico, P. E. Loggins, and L. R. Arrington. 1972. Availability of different inorganic salts of magnesium to sheep. J. Anim. Sci. 34:122–126

Andrews, E. D., W. J. Hartley, and A. R. Grant. 1968. Selenium-responsive disease of animals in New Zealand. N.Z. Vet. J. 16:3–17.

Anke, M., A. Hennig, M. Grun, M. Partschefeld, B. Groppel, and H. Ludke. 1976. Arsenic—a new essential trace element. Arch. Tierernahr. 26(10):742–743.

Annett, C. S., F. M. D'Itri, J. R. Ford, and H. H. Prince. 1975. Mercury in fish and waterfowl from Lake Ball, Ontario. J. Environ. Qual. 4:219–222.

Ansari, M. S., W. J. Miller, R. P. Gentry, M. W. Neathery, and P. E. Stake. 1973. Tissue 203Hg distribution in young Holstein calves after single tracer oral doses in organic and inorganic forms. J. Anim. Sci. 36:414–419.

Aspila, P. 1988. Metabolism of selenite, selenomethionine, and feed-incorporated selenium in lactating goats and dairy cows. J. Ag. Sci. Finland.

Association of American Feed Control Officials (AAFCO). 1977. Official Publication of the Association of American Feed Control Officials, Inc. Baton Rouge, LA: Association of American Feed Control Officials, Inc.

Auza, N. J., W. G. Olson, M. J. Murphy, and J. G. Linn. 1999. Diagnosis and treatment of copper toxicosis in ruminants. J. Am. Vet. Med. Assoc. 214:1624–1628.

Babcock, S. M. 1905. The addition of salt to the ration of dairy cows. Pp. 129–156 in Wisc. Exp. Stn. 22nd Annu. Rep. Madsion: University of Wisconsin.

Bailey, C. B. 1977. Influence of aluminum hydroxide on the solubility of silicic acid in rumen fluid and the absorption of silicic acid from the digestive tract of ruminants. Can. J. Anim. Sci. 57:239–244.

Barton, B. A., N. A. Jorgensen, R. L. Horst, and H. F. DeLuca. 1978. Influence of dietary phosphorus level on the concentration of 1, 25-dihydroxyvitamin D, 24, 25-dihydroxyvitamin D, calcium and phosphorus in plasma of aged dairy cows. J. Dairy Sci. 61:145 (Abstr.).

Baynes, R., W. Bezwoda, T. Bothwell, Q. Khan, and N. Mansoor. 1986. The non-immune inflammatory response:serial changes in plasma iron, iron-binding capacity, lactoferrin, ferritin and C-reactive protein. Scand. J. Clin. Lab. Invest. 46:695–704.

Beard, J. L., and H. D. Dawson. 1997. Iron. Pp. 278–284 in Handbook of Nutritionally Essential Mineral Elements, B. L. O'Dell and R. A. Sunde, eds. New York: Marcel Dekker, Inc.

Becker, R., W. Neal, and A. L. Shealy. 1933. Effect of calcium-deficient roughage upon milk production and welfare of dairy cows. Fla. Agric. Exp. Stn. Tech. Bull. #262. Gainesville: University of Florida.

Beede, D. K., and J. K. Shearer. 1991. Nutritional management of dairy cattle during hot weather. Agri-Prac. 12:5–12.

Beede, D. K., and R. J. Collier. 1986. Potential nutritional strategies for intensively managed cattle during thermal stress. J. Anim. Sci. 62:543–554.

Beede, D. K., C. Wang, G. A. Donovan, L. F. Archbald, and W. K. Sanchez. 1991. Dietary cation-anion difference (electrolyte balance) in late pregnancy. Pp. 1–6 in Florida Dairy Production Conference Proceedings. Gainesville: University of Florida.

Beede, D. K., P. G. Mallonee, P. L. Schneider, C. J. Wilcox, and R. J. Collier. 1983. Potassium nutrition of heat-stressed lactating dairy cows. S. Afr. J. Anim. Sci. 13:198–200.

Beke, G. J., and R. Hironaka. 1991. Toxicity to beef cattle of sulfur in saline well water: A case study. Sci. Total Env. 101:281–290.

Bentley, O. G., and P. H. Phillips. 1951. The effect of low manganese rations upon dairy cattle. J. Dairy Sci. 34:396–403.

Berg, J. N., D. Padgitt, and B. McCarthy. 1988. Iodine concentrations in milk of dairy cattle fed various amounts of iodine as ethylenediamine dihytroiodide. J. Dairy Sci. 71:3283–3291.

Bernier, J. F., F. J. Filion, and G. J. Brisson. 1984. Dietary fibers and supplemental iron in a milk replacer for veal calves. J. Dairy Sci. 67:2369–2379.

Berry, M. J., L. Banu, and P. R. Larsen. 1991. Type I iodothyronine deiodinase is a selenocysteine-containing enzyme. Nature. 349:438–440.

Besong, S., J. Jackson, S. Trammell, and D. Amaral-Phillips. 1996. Effect of supplemental chromium picolinate on liver triglycerides, blood metabolites, milk yield, and milk composition in early-lactation cows. J. Dairy Sci. 79(Suppl. 1):97. (Abstr.)

Bigelow, A. C., R. W. Hemken, and R. J. Harmon. 1984. Potassium requirement of the dairy calf. J. Dairy Sci. 67(Suppl. 1):104.

Bird, P. R. 1972. Sulfur metabolism and excretion studies in ruminants. X. Sulfide toxicity in sheep. Aust. J. Biol. Sci. 25:1087–1098.

Bird, P. R., and R. J. Moir. 1971. Sulphur metabolism and excretion studies in ruminants. I. The absorption of sulfate in sheep after intraruminal or intraduodenal infusions of sodium sulfate. Austr. J. Biol. Sci. 24:1319–1328.

Bird, P. R. 1970. Sulphur metabolism and excretion studies in ruminants. III. The effect of sulphur intake on the availability of copper in sheep. Proceedings of the Australian Society of Animal Production 8:212–218.

Black, J. R., C. B. Ammerman, and P. R. Henry. 1985. Effects of high dietary manganese as manganese oxide or manganese carbonate in sheep. J. Anim. Sci. 60:861–866.

Blair-West, J. R., J. P. Coghlan, D. A. Denton, and R. D. Wright. 1970. Factors affecting sodium and potassium metabolism. Pp. 350–361 in Physiology of Digestion in the Ruminant. A. T. Phillipson (ed.)., Newcastle upon Tyne, UK: Oriel Press Limited.

Blaxter, K. L., G. A. M. Sarman, and A. M. MacDonald. 1957. Iron-deficiency anemia in calves. Br. J. Nutr. 11:234–246.

Bouchard, R., and H. R. Conrad. 1973a. Sulfur requirement of lactating dairy cows. II. Utilization of sulfates, molasses, and lignin-sulfonate. J. Dairy Sci. 56:1429–1434.

Bouchard, R., and H. R. Conrad. 1973b. Sulfur requirement of lactating dairy cows. I. Sulfur balance and dietary supplementation. J. Dairy Sci. 56:1276–1282.

Bradley, C. H. 1993. Copper poisoning in a dairy herd fed a mineral supplement. Can. Vet. J. 34:287–292.

Braithwaite, G. D. 1983. Calcium and phosphorus requirements of the ewe during pregnancy and lactation. 2. Phosphorus. Br. J. Nutr. 50:723–736.

Braithwaite, G. D. 1986. Phosphorus requirements of ewes in pregnancy and lactation. J. Ag. Sci. 106:271–278.

Bray, A. C., and J. A. Hemsley. 1969. Sulfur metabolism of sheep. IV. The effect of a varied dietary sulfur content on some fluid sulfate levels and on the utilization of a urea-supplemented roughage diet by sheep. Aust. J. Ag. Res. 20:759–773.

Bremner, I., and A. C. Dalgarno. 1973a. Iron metabolism in the veal calf. 2. Iron requirements and the effect of copper supplementation. Br. J. Nutr. 30:61–76.

Bremner, I., and A. C. Dalgarno. 1973b. Iron metabolism in the veal calf. The availability of different iron compounds. Br. J. Nutr. 29:229–243.

Bremner, I., W. R. Humphries, M. Phillippo, M. J. Walker, and P. C. Morrice. 1987. Iron-induced copper deficiency in calves: Dose-response relationships and interactions with molybdenum and sulfur. Anim. Prod. 45:403–414.

Bremner, I., Young, B.W., and Mills, C. F. 1976. Protective effect of zinc supplementation agaisnt copper toxicosis in sheep. Br. J. Nutr. 36:551–561.

Breves, G., and B. Schroder. 1991. Comparative aspects of gastrointestinal phosphorus metabolism. Nutr. Res. Rev. 4:125–140.

Brintrup, R., T. Mooren, U. Meyer, H. Spiekers, and E. Pfeffer. 1993. Effects of two levels of phosphorus intake on performance and faecal phosphorus excretion of dairy cows. J. Anim. Physiol. Anim. Nutr. 69:29–36.

Brodison, J. A., E. A. Goodall, J. D. Armstrong, D. I. Givens, F. J. Gordon, W. J. McCaughey, and J. R. Todd. 1989. Influence of dietary phosphorus on the performance of lactating dairy cattle. J. Agric. Sci. Camb. 112:303–311.

Bronner, F. 1987. Intestinal calcium absorption: Mechanisms and applications. J. Nutr. 117:1347–1352.

Brummerstedt, E. E. Andresen, A. Basse, and T. Flagstad. 1974. Lethal trait A 46 in cattle. Immunological investigations. Nord. Vet. Med. 26:279–293.

Bryant, M. P. 1973. Nutritional requirements of the predominant rumen cellulytic bacteria. Fed. Proc. 32:1809–1813.

Bulger, R. E., and F. L. Siegel. 1975. Alterations of the renal papilla during mercuric chloride-induced acute tubular necrosis. Lab. Invest 33:712–719.

Bull, L. S., and J. H. Vandersall. 1973. Sulfur source for in vitro cellulose digestion and in vivo ration utilization, nitrogen metabolism, and sulfur balance. J. Dairy Sci. 56:106–112.

Bulter, G. W., and D. I. H. Jones. 1973. Pg. 127 in Mineral Biochemistry of Herbage, Vol 2. G. W. Butler and R. W. Bailey, eds. New York: Academic Press.

Bunce, H. W. F. 1985. Fluoride in air, grass, and cattle. J. Dairy Sci. 68:1706–1711.

Burkhalter, D. L., M. W. Neathery, W. J. Miller, R. H. Whitlock, and J. C. Allen. 1979. Effects of low chloride intake on performance, clinical characteristics, and chloride, sodium, potassium, and nitrogen metabolism in dairy calves. J. Dairy Sci. 62:1895–1901.

Burkhalter, D. L., M. W. Neathery, W. J. Miller, R. H. Whitlock, J. C. Allen, and R. P. Gentry. 1980. Influence of a low chloride practical diet on acid-base balance and other factors of blood in young dairy calves. J. Dairy Sci. 63:269–276.

Burroughs, W., A. Latone, P. DePaul, P. Gerlaugh, and R. M. Bethke. 1951. Mineral influences upon urea utilization and cellulose digestion by rumen microorganisms using the artificial rumen technique. J. Anim. Sci. 10:693–697.

Burton, J., B. Mallard, and D. Mowat. 1993. Effects of supplemental chromium on immune responses of periparturient and early-lactation dairy cows. J. Anim. Sci. 71:1532–1539.

Call, J. W., J. E. Butcher, J. L. Shape, R. C. Lamb, R. L. Woman, and A. E. Olson. 1987. Clinical effects of low dietary phosphorus concentrations in feed given to lactating cows. Am. J. Vet. Res. 48:133–136.

Call, J. W., J. E. Butcher, J. T. Blake, R. A. Smart, and J. L. Shape. 1978. Phosphorus influence on growth and reproduction of beef cattle. J. Anim. Sci. 47:216–225.

Calvert, C. C., and L. W. Smith. 1972. Arsenic in milk and blood of cows fed organic arsenic compounds. J. Dairy. Sci. 55:706–714.

Cantley, L. C. Jr., L. Josephson, R. Warner, M. Yanagisawa, C. Lechene, and G. Guidotti. 1977. Vanadate is a potent (Na, K)-ATPase inhibitor found in ATP derived from muscle. J. Biol. Chem. 252:7421–7423.

Care, A. D., J. P. Bartlet, and H. M. Abdel-Hafeez. 1980. Calcium and phosphate homeostasis in ruminants and its relationship to the aetiology and prevention of parturient paresis. Pp. 429–446 in Digestive Physiology and Metabolism in Ruminants, Y. Ruckebusch and P. Thivend, eds. Lancaster, England: MTP Press.

Carlisle, E. M. 1974. Silicon as an essential element. Fed. Proc. 33:1758 (Abstr).

Carstairs, J. A., D. A. Morrow, and R. S. Emery. 1980. Postpartum reproductive function of dairy cows as influenced by energy and phosphorus status. J. Anim. Sci. 51:1122–1130.

Carstairs, J. A., R. R. Neitzel, and R. S. Emery. 1981. Energy and phosphorus status as factors affecting postpartum performance and health of dairy cows. J. Dairy Sci. 64:34–41.

Challa, J., and G. D. Braithwaite. 1988. Phosphorus and calcium metabolism in growing calves with special emphasis on phosphorus homeostasis. 1. Studies of the effect of changes in the dietary phosphorus intake on phosphorus and calcium metabolism. J. Ag. Sci., Camb. 110:573–581.

Challa, J., G. D. Braithwaite, and M. S. Dhanoa. 1989. Phosphorus homoeostasis of growing calves. J. Agric. Sci., Camb. 112:217–226.

Chapman, H. L. and M. C. Bell. 1963. Relative absorption and excretion by beef cattle of copper from various sources. J. Anim. Sci. 22:82.

Chen, N., A. Tsai, and I. Dyer. 1973. Effect of chelating agents on chromium absorption in rats. J. Nutr. 103:1182–1186.

Chester-Jones, H., J. P. Fontenot, H. P. Veit, and K. E. Webb, Jr. 1989. Physiological effects of feeding high levels of magnesium to sheep. J. Anim. Sci. 67:1070.

Chesters, J. 1997. Zinc. Pp. 185–231 in Handbook of Nutritionally Essential Mineral Elements, B. L. O'Dell and R. Sunde, eds. New York: Marcel Dekker, Inc.

Chicco, C. F., C. B. Ammerman, J. E. Moore, P. A. Van Walleghen, L. R. Arlington, and R. L. Shirley. 1965. Utilization of inorganic ortho-, meta-, and pyrophosphates by lambs and by cellulolytic rumen microorganisms *in vitro*. J. Anim. Sci. 24:355–363.

Clark, W. D. Jr., J. E. Wohlt, R. L. Gilbreath, and P. K. Zajac. 1986. Phytate phosphorus intake and disappearance in the gastrointestinal tract of high producing dairy cows. J. Dairy Sci. 69:3151–3155.

Clarke, E. G. C., and M. L. Clarke. 1975. Veterinary Toxicology, 3rd Ed. Baltimore: Williams & Wilkins, Co.

Coghlin, C. L. 1944. Hydrogen sulfide poisoning in cattle. Can. J. Comp. Med. 8:111–113.

Conrad, H. R., and A. L. Moxon. 1979. Transfer of dietary selenium to milk. J. Dairy Sci. 62:404–411.

Conrad, H. R., S. L. Hansard, and J. W. Hibbs. 1956. Studies on milk fever. V. Excretion and retention of calcium and phosphorus. J. Dairy Sci. 39:1697–1705.

Coppock, C. E. 1986. Mineral utilization by the lactating cow—chlorine. J. Dairy Sci. 69:595–603.

Coppock, C. E., R. A. Aguirre, L. E. Chase, G. B. Lake, E. A. Oltenacu, R. E. McDowell, M. J. Fettman, and M. E. Woods. 1979. Effect of low chloride diet on lactating cows. J. Dairy Sci. 62:723–731.

Coppock, C. E., R. W. Everett, and R. L. Belyea. 1975. Effect of low calcium and low phosphorus diets on free choice consumption of dicalcium phosphate by lactating cows. J. Dairy Sci. 59:571–580.

Coppock, C. E., R. W. Everett, and W. G. Merrill. 1972. Effect of ration on free choice consumption of calcium-phosphorus supplements by dairy cattle. J. Dairy Sci. 55:245–256.

Coppock. C. E., and M. J. Fettman. 1977. Chloride as a required nutrient for lactating dairy cows. Pg. 43 in Proc. Cornell Nutr. Conf., Ithaca, NY.

Crissman, J. W., G. A. Maylin, and L. Krook. 1980. New York state and U. S. federal fluoride pollution standards do not protect cattle health. Cornell Vet. 70:183–192.

Davis, E. T., A. H. Phil, D. F. Collings, J. A. J. Venn, and G. D. Bridges. 1965. Cerebrocortical necrosis in calves. Vet. Rec. 77:2 90–96.

De Boer, G., J. G. Buchanan-Smith, G. K. MacLead, and J. S. Walton. 1981. Responses of dairy cows fed alfalfa silage supplemented with phosphorus, copper, zinc, and manganese. J. Dairy Sci. 64:2370–2377.

Deagen, J. T., M. A. Beilstein, and P. D. Whanger. 1991. Chemical forms of selenium in selenium containing proteins from human plasma. J. Inorg. Biochem. 41:261–268.

deGroot, A. P. 1973. Subacute toxicity of inorganic tin as influenced by dietary levels of iron and copper. Food Cosmet. Toxicol. 11:955–962.

DeLuca, H. F. 1979. The vitamin D system in the regulation of calcium and phosphorus metabolism. Nutr. Rev. 37:161–193.

Demertzis, P. N. 1973. Oral zinc therapy in the control of infectious pododermatitis in young bulls. Vet. Rec. 93:219–222.

Demott, B. J., S. A. Hinton, E. W. Swanson, and J. T. Miles. 1968. Influence of added sodium chloride in grain ration on the freezing point of milk. J. Dairy Sci. 51:1363–1365.

Dennis, J., and F. G. Harbaugh. 1948. The experimental alteration of blood potassium and calcium levels in cattle. Am. J. Vet. Res. 9:20–25.

Dennis, R. J., and R. W. Hemken. 1978. Potassium requirement of dairy cows in early and mid-lactation. J. Dairy Sci. 61:757–761.

Dennis, R. J., R. W. Hemken, and D. R. Jacobson. 1976. Effect of dietary potassium percent for lactating dairy cows. J. Dairy Sci. 59:324–328.

Dhiman, T. R., L. D. Satter, and R. D. Shaver. 1996. Milk production and blood phosphorus concentrations of cows fed low and high dietary phosphorus. Pp. 105–106 in U.S. Dairy Forage Res. Center 1995 Res. Summaries, Madison, WI.

Dick, A. T. 1954. Studies on the assimilation and storage of copper in crossbred sheep. Aust. J. Agric. Res. 5:511.

Doyle, J. J., W. H. Pfander, S. E. Grebing, and J. O. D. Pierce. 1974. Effect of dietary cadmium on growth, cadmium absorption, and cadmium tissue levels in growing lambs. J. Nutr. 104:160–166.

Drebickas, V. 1966. Effect of additions of vanadium and titanium salts on some physiological indexes of calves. Liet. TSR Aukst. Mokykly Mokslo Darbia, Biol. 6:71–75.

Du, Z., R. W. Hemken, and R. J. Harmon. 1996. Copper metabolism of Holstein and Jersey cows and heifers fed diets high in cupric sulfate or copper proteinate. J. Dairy Sci. 79:1873–1880.

Durand, M., and S. Komisarczuk. 1988. Influence of major minerals on rumen microbiota. J. Nutr. 118:249–260.

Dyer, I. A., and M. A. Rojas. 1965. Manganese requirements and functions in cattle. J. Am. Vet. Med. Assoc. 147:1393–1396.

Eldman, I. S., A. H. James, H. Boden, and F. D. Moore. 1954. Electrolyte composition of bone and the penetration of radiosodium and deuterium oxide into dog and human bone. J. Clin. Invest. 33:122–131.

Ellenberger, H. B., J. A. Newlander, and C. H. Jones. 1950. Composition of the bodies of dairy cattle. Univ. Vermont Agric. Exp. Stn. Bull. No. 558, Burlington.

Ellenberger, H., J. Newlander, and C. H. Jones. 1931. Calcium and phosphorus requirements of dairy cows: Weekly balances through lactation and gestation periods. Vermont Agricultural Experiment Station Bulletin 10:245–260.

Ellis, W. C., and W. H. Pfander. 1970. Further studies on molybdenum as a possible component of the "alfalfa ash factor" for sheep. J. Anim. Sci. 19:1260 (abstr.).

Ellis, W. C., W. H. Pfander, M. E. Muhrer, and E. E. Pickett. 1958. Molybdenum as a dietary essential for lambs. J. Anim. Sci. 17:180–188.

Ely, R. E., K. M. Dunn, and C. F. Huffman. 1948. Cobalt toxicity in calves resulting from high oral administration. J. Anim. Sci. 7:239–243.

Emanuele, S. M., and C. R. Staples. 1990. Ruminal release of minerals from six forage species. J. Anim. Sci. 6:2052–2060.

Emanuele, S. M., C. R. Staples, and C. J. Wilcox. 1991. Extent and site of mineral release from six forage species incubated in mobile dacron bags. J. Anim. Sci. 69:801–810.

Emery, R. S., C. K. Smith, and L. Fai To. 1957a. Utilization of inorganic sulfate by rumen microorganisms. II. The ability of single strains of bacteria to utilize inorganic sulfate. App. Microbiol. 5:363–367.

Emery, R. S., C. K. Smith, and C. F. Huffman. 1957b. Utilization of inorganic sulfate by rumen microorganisms. I. Incorporation of inorganic sulfate into amino acids. App. Microbiol. 5:360–363.

Ender, F., I. W. Dishington, and I. W. Helegebostad. 1971. Calcium balance studies in dairy cows under experimental induction and prevention of hypocalcaemic paresis puerperalis. The solution of the aetiology and the prevention of milk fever by dietary means. Zeitschrift fuer Tierphysiologie Tierernaehrung und Futtermittelkunde. 28:233–256.

Erdman, R. A., R. W. Hemken, and L. S. Bull. 1980a. Effects of dietary calcium and sodium on potassium requirement for lactating dairy cows. J. Dairy Sci. 63:538–544.

Erdman, R. A., R. L. Botts, R. W. Hemken, and L. S. Bull. 1980b. Effect of dietary sodium bicarbonate and magnesium oxide on production and physiology in early lactation. J. Dairy Sci. 63:923–930.

Ermans, A., and P. Bourdoux. 1989. Antithyroid sulfurated compounds. Pp. 15 in Environmental Goitrogenesis, G. E., ed. Boca Raton, FL: CRC Press.

Erskine, R. J., R. J. Eberhart, P. J. Grasso, and R. W. Scholz. 1989. Induction of Escherichia coli mastitis in cows fed selenium-deficient or selenium-supplemented diets. Amer. J. Vet. Res. 50:2093–2100.

Escobosa, A., C. E. Coppock, L. D. Rowe, Jr., W. L. Jenkins, and C. E. Gates. 1984. Effects of dietary sodium bicarbonate and calcium chloride on physiological responses of lactating dairy cows in hot weather. J. Dairy Sci. 67:574–584.

Evans, G., and T. Winter. 1975. Zinc transport by transferrin in rat portal blood plasma. Biochem. Biophys. Res. Commun. 66:1218–1224.

Fettman, M. J., L. E. Chase, J. Bentinck-Smith, C. E. Coppock, and S. A. Zinn. 1984a. Restricted dietary chloride with sodium chloride supplementation for Holstein cows in early lactation. J. Dairy Sci. 67:1457–1467.

Fettman, M. J., L. E. Chase, J. Bentinck-Smith, C. E. Coppock, and S. A. Zinn. 1984b. Nutritional chloride deficiency in early lactation Holstein cows. J. Dairy Sci. 67:2321–2335.

Fettman, M. J., L. E. Chase, J. Bentinck-Smith, C. E. Coppock, and S. A. Zinn. 1984c. Effects of dietary chloride restriction in lactating cows. JAVMA 185:167–172.

Fettman, M. J., L. E. Chase, J. Bentinck-Smith, C. E. Coppock, and S. A. Zinn. 1984d. Restricted dietary chloride and sodium bicarbonate supplementation in early lactation Holstein cows: Cerebrospinal fluid electrolyte alterations. Am. J. Vet. Res. 45:1403–1408.

Fick, K. R., C. B. Ammerman, S. M. Miller, C. F. Simpson, and P. E. Loggins. 1976. Effect of dietary lead on performance, tissue mineral composition and lead absorption in sheep. J. Anim. Sci. 42:515–523.

Field, A. C., C. S. Munro, and N. F. Suttle. 1977. Dried poultry manure as a source of phosphorus for sheep. J. Ag. Sci. 89:599–604.

Field, A. C., J. Kamphues, and J. A. Woolliams. 1983. The effect of dietary intake of calcium and phosphorus on the absorption and excretion of phosphorus in chimaera-derived sheep. J. Ag. Sci. 101:597–602.

Finelli, V. N., D. S. Klauder, M. A. Karaffa, and H. G. Petering. 1975. Interaction of zinc and lead on delta-aminolevulinate deydratase. Biochem. Biophys. Res. Commun. 65:303–312.

Fischer, J. L., R. F. Husted, and P. R. Steinmetz. 1983. Chloride dependence of the bicarbonate exit step in urinary acidification by the turtle bladder. Am. J. Physiol. 254:F564–568.

Fisher, L. J., N. Dinn, R. M. Tait, and J. A. Shelford. 1994. Effect of level of dietary potassium on the absorption and excretion of calcium and magnesium by lactating dairy cows. Can. J. Anim. Sci. 74:503–509.

Flagstad, T. 1976. Lethal trait A46 in cattle intestinal zinc absorption. Nord. Vet. Med. 28:160–169.

Flanagan, P. R., J Haist, and L. S. Valberg. 1980. Comparative effects of iron deficiency induced by bleeding and a low-iron diet on the intestinal absorptive interactions of iron, cobalt, manganese, zinc, lead, and cadmium. J. Nutr. 110:1754–1763.

Flynn, A., and P. Power. 1985. Nutritional aspects of minerals in bovine and human milks. Pp. 183–215 in Developments in Dairy Chemistry-3: Lactose and Minor Constituents, P. F. Fox, ed. New York: Elsevier Applied Science Publishers,

Fontenot, J. P., V G. Allen, G. E. Bunce, and J. P. Goff. 1989. Factors influencing magnesium absorption and metabolism in ruminants. J. Anim. Sci. 67:3445–3455.

Food and Drug Administration. 1997. Food additives permitted in feed and drinking water of animals; selenium. Federal Register. (Aug. 25)62:44892–44894.

Forbes, E. B., F. M. Beegle, C. M. Fritz, L. E. Morgan, and S. N. Rhue. 1916. The mineral metabolism of the milk cow. First paper. Ohio Agric. Exp. Stat. Bull. 295:323.

Fron, M. J., J. A. Bling, L. P. Bush, and K. A. Dawson. 1990. Sulfur and nitrogen metabolism in the bovine fed different forms of supplemental sulfur. J. Anim. Sci. 68:543–552.

Frost, D. V., L. R Overby, and H. C. Spruth. 1955. Studies with arsanilic acid and related compounds. J. Ag. Food Chem. 3:235–243.

Gant, R G., W. Sanchez, and R.L. Kincaid. 1998. Effect of anionic salts on selenium metabolism in nonlactating, pregnant dairy cows. J. Dairy Science 81:1637–1642.

Garvey, J. S. 1984. Metallothionein: Structure/antigenicity and detection-quantitation in normal physiological fluids. Env. Health Persp. 54:117–127.

Gawthorne, J. M., and R. M. Smith. 1974. Folic acid metabolism in vitamin $B_{12}$-deficient sheep. Effects of injected methionine on methotrexate transport and the activity of enzymes associated with folate metabolism in liver. Biochem. J. 142:119–126.

Gawthorne, J. M., J. Waston, and E. L. Stokstad. 1971. Automated methylmalonic acid assay. Anal. Biochem. 42:555–559.

Gengelbach, G. P. 1994. PhD thesis, Department of Animal Science and Interdepartmental Nutrition Program, North Carolina State University, Raleigh, NC.

Gentry, R. P., W. J. Miller, D. G. Pugh, M. W. Neathery, and J. B. Bynoum. 1978. Effects of feeding high magnesium to young dairy calves. J. Dairy Sci. 61:1750–1754.

Gibbons, R. A., S. N. Dixon, K. Hallis, A. M. Russell, B. F. Sansom, and H. W. Symonds. 1976. Manganese Metabolism in cows and goats. Biochim. Biophys. Acta. 444(1):1–10.

Gibson, C. D., F. H. Coe, R. G. Ellis, H. D. Stowe, P. C. Bartlett, and P. E. Naasz. 1993. Field trial to evaluate the effects of different forms of oral selenium supplementation on production in lactating Holstein cows. Agri-Prac. 14:14–19.

Goetsch, A., and F. Owens. 1985. Effects of calcium source and level on site of digestion and calcium levels in the digestive tract of cattle fed high concentrate diets. J. Anim. Sci. 61:995–1003.

Goff, J. P. 1998a. Phosphorus deficiency. Pp. 218–220 in Current Veterinary Therapy 4: Food Animal Practice. J. L. Howard, and R. A. Smith, eds. Philadelphia: W. B. Saunders, Co.

Goff, J. P. 1998b. Ruminant Hypomagnesemic Tetanies. Pp. 215–218 in Current Veterinary Therapy 4:Food Animal Practice, J. L. Howard and R. A. Smith, eds. Philadelphia: W.B. Saunders Co.

Goff, J. P., and J. R. Stabel. 1990. Decreased plasma retinol, alpha-tocopherol, and zinc concentration during the periparturient period: Effect of milk fever. J. Dairy Sci. 73:3195–3199.

Goff, J. P., and R. L. Horst. 1993. Oral administration of calcium salts for treatment of hypocalcemia in cattle. J. Dairy Sci. 76:101–108.

Goff, J. P., R. L. Horst, P. W. Jardon, C. Borelli, and J. Wedam. 1996. Field trials of an oral calcium propionate paste as an aid to prevent milk fever in periparturient dairy cows. J. Dairy Sci. 79:378–383.

Goodman, H., and L. Middlesworth. 1980. The thyroid gland. Pp. 1495–1518 in Medical Physiology, Vol. 2, V. Mountcastle, ed. St. Louis: C.V. Mosby Co.

Govindaraju, K., T. Ramasami, and D. Ramaswamy. 1989. Chromium (III)-insulin derivatives and their implication in glucose metabolism. J. Inorg. Biochem. 35:137–147.

Grace, N. D. 1983. Amounts and distribution of mineral elements associated with fleece-free body weight gains in grazing sheep. N.Z. J. Ag. Res. 26:59–70.

Grace, N. D., J. Lee, R. A. Mills, and A. F. Death. 1997. Influence of Se status on milk Se concentrations in dairy cows. N.Z. J. Ag. Res. 40:75–78.

Grace, N. D., M. J. Ulyatt, J. C., and MacRae. 1974. Quantitative digestion of fresh herbage by sheep. 3. Movement of Mg, Ca, P, K, and Na in digestive tract. J. Ag. Sci. 82:321–330.

Grace, N. D., M. Venning, A. R. Mills, and A. F. Death. 1995. The efficacy of selenium dioxide as a selenium supplement for dairy cattle. N.Z. Vet. J. 43:77–78.

Graham, T. W. 1991. Trace element deficiencies in cattle. Vet. Clin. N. Am. Food Anim. Pract. 7:153–215.

Greene, L. W., G. T. Schelling, and F. M. Byers. 1986. Effects of dietary monensin and potassium on apparent absorption of magnesium and other macroelements in sheep. J. Anim. Sci. 63:1960–1967.

Greene, L. W., J. P. Fontenot, and K. E. Webb, Jr. 1983. Site of magnesium and other macromineral absorption in steers fed high levels of potassium. J. Anim. Sci. 57:503–510.

Greenwood, D. A., J. L. Shupe, G. E. Stoddard, L. E. Harris, H. M. Nielson, and L. E. Olson. 1964. Fluorosis in Cattle. Utah Ag. Exp. Stn. Spec. Rep. 17:36–38.

Gueguen, L., M. Lamand, and F. Meschy. 1989. Mineral requirements. Pp. 49–56 in Ruminant Nutrition:Recommended Allowances and Feed Tables, R. Jarrige, ed. Institut National de la Recherche Agronomique,

Gupta, U. C. 1991. Boron, molybdenum and selenium status in different plant parts in forage legumes and vegetable crops. J. Plant Nutr. 14:613–621.

Hall, O. G., H. D. Baxter, and C. S. Hobbs. 1961. Effect of phosphorus in different chemical forms on *in vitro* cellulose digestion by rumen microorganisms. J. Anim. Sci. 20:817–819.

Halliwell, B. 1987. Oxidants and human disease: Some new concepts. FASEB J. 1:358–64.

Halpin, C. G., D. J. Harris, I. W. Caple, and D. S. Petterson. 1984. Contribution of cobalamin analogues to plasma vitamin $B_{12}$ concentrations in cattle. Res. Vet. Sci. 37:249–251.

Hambridge, K. M., C. C. Casey, and N. F. Krebs. 1986. Zinc. Pp. 1–137 in Trace Elements in Human and Animal Nutrition, Vol. 2, W. Mertz, ed. New York: Academic Press.

Hansard, S. L. 1975. Toxicity and physiological movement of vanadium in the sheep and rat. Ph.D. (Thesis) University of Florida. 190.

Hansard, S. L., C. L. Comar, and G. K. Davis. 1954. Effects of age upon the physiological behavior of calcium in cattle. Amer. J. Physiol. 177:383–389.

Hansard, S., A. Mohammed, and J. Turner. 1968. Gestation age effects upon maternal-fetal zinc utilization in the bovine. J. Anim. Sci. 27:1097–1102.

Hansard, S., H. Crowder, and W. A. Lyke. 1957. The biological availability of calcium in feeds for cattle. J. Anim. Sci. 16:437–443.

Harada, I., I. Shinohara, and S. Sato. 1989. The absorption characteristics of selenious acid applied to corn (Zea mys L.). J. Rakuno gakuen Univ. 14:49–55.

Harrison, J. H., and H. R. Conrad. 1984a. Effect of calcium on selenium absorption by the nonlactating dairy cow. J. Dairy Sci. 67:1860–1864.

Harrison, J. H., and H. R. Conrad. 1984b. Effect of selenium intake on selenium utilization by the nonlactating dairy cow. J. Dairy Sci. 67:219–223.

Harrison, J. H., D. D. Hancock, and H. R. Conrad. 1984. Vitamin E and selenium for reproduction of the dairy cow. J. Dairy Sci. 67:123–132.

Hartmann, F., and J. B. J. van Ryssen. 1997. Metabolism of selenium and copper in sheep with and without sodium bicarbonate supplementation. J. Ag. Sci. (Camb.) 128:357–364.

Hartmans, J. 1974. Tracing and treating mineral disorders in cattle under field conditions. Pp. 261–273 in Trace Element Metabolism in Animals—2, W. G. Hoekstra, J. W. Suttie, H. E. Ganther, W. Merttz, eds. Baltimore: University Park Press.

Hecht, D., M. E. Wells, L. J. Bush, and G. D. Adams. 1977. Effects of dietary phosphorus levels on reproductive efficiency in dairy heifers. Anim. Sci. Res. Rep., Okla Ag. Exp. Stn 101:126–129.

Hemken, R. W. 1970. Iodine. J. Dairy Sci. 53:1138–1143.

Hemken, R. W. 1983. Potassium in ruminant nutrition. Page 1 in Sodium and potassium in ruminant nutrition. West Des Moines: National Feed Ingredients Association, IA.

Henry, P. R. 1995a. Cobalt bioavailability. Pp. 119–126 in Bioavailability of Nutrients for Animals, C. B. Ammerman, D. H. Baker, and A. J. Lewis, eds. San Diego: Academic Press.

Henry, P. R. 1995b. Manganese bioavailability. Pp. 239–256 in Bioavailability of Nutrients for Animals, C. B. Ammerman, D. H. Baker, and A. J. Lewis, eds. San Diego: Academic Press.

Henry, P. R. 1995c. Sodium and chlorine bioavailability. Pp. 337–348 in Bioavailability of Nutrients for Animals. C. B. Ammerman, D. H. Baker, and A. J. Lewis, eds. New York: Academic Press.

Henry, P. R., and E. R. Miller. 1995. Iron bioavailability. Pp. 169–201 in Bioavailability of Nutrients for Animals, C. B. Ammerman, D. H. Baker, and A. J. Lewis, eds. San Diego: Academic Press.

Henry, P. R., and S. A. Benz. 1995. Magnesium Bioavailability. Pg. 201 in Bioavailability of Nutrients for Animals, C. B. Ammerman, D. H. Baker, and A. J. Lewis, eds. San Diego: Academic Press.

Herbein, J. H., J. D. Cox, M. M. Weisbarth, and W. A. Wark. 1996. Phosphorus retention in lactating cows fed inorganic or organic forms of supplemental dietary phosphorus. J. Dairy Sci. 79(Suppl. 1):229.

Herigstad, R. R., C. K. Whitehair, N. Beyer, O. Mickelson, and M. J. Zabik. 1972. Chronic methylmercury toxicosis in calves. J. Am. Vet. Med. Assoc. 160:173–182.

Hetzel, B., and M. Welby. 1997. Iodine. Pp. 557–581 in Handbook of Nutritionally Essential Mineral Elements, B. L. O'Dell and R. A. Sunde, eds. New York: Marcel Dekker, Inc.

Hibbs, J. W., and H. R. Conrad. 1983. The relationship of calcium and phosphorus intake and digestion and the effects of vitamin D feeding on the utilization of calcium and phosphorus by lactating dairy cows. Pp. 1–23 in Research Bulletin 1150, Ohio State University, Ohio Agr. Res. & Dev. Center, Wooster, Ohio.

Hill, G. M. 1985. The relationship between dietary sulfur and nitrogen metabolism in the ruminant. Pp. 37 in Georgia Nutrition Conference. Athens, Georgia.

Hilwig, R. V. 1976. Excretion and renal regulation of neutrality. Pg. 19 in Buffers in Ruminant Physiology and Metabolism, M. S. Weinberg and A. L. Sheffner, eds. New York: Church and Dwight, Inc.

Ho, S. Y., W. J. Miller, R. P. Gentry, M. W. Neathery, and D. M. Blackmon. 1984. Effects of high, but nontoxic dietary manganese and iron on their metabolism by calves. J. Dairy Sci. 67(7):1489–1495.

Hogan, J. S., W. P. Weiss, and K. L. Smith. 1993. Role of vitamin E and selenium in host defense against mastitis. J. Dairy Sci. 76:2795–2803.

Holmes, J. H. G. 1981. Phosphate deficiency in cattle on the sepik plains, Papua New Guinea. Trop. Anim. Health Prod. 13:169–176.

Holt, C. 1985. The milk salts: Their secretion, concentrations and physical chemistry. Pp. 143–181 in Developments in Dairy Chemistry-3:Lactose and Minor Constituents, P. F. Fox, ed. New York: Elsevier Applied Science Publishers.

Horst, R. L. 1986. Regulation of calcium and phosphorus homeostasis in the dairy cow. J. Dairy Sci. 69:604–616.

Horst, R. L., H. F. DeLuca, and N. A. Jorgensen. 1978. The effect of age on calcium absorption and accumulation of 1,25-dihydroxyvitamin $D_3$ in intestinal mucosa of rats. Metabolic Bone Disease & Related Research. 1:29–33.

Horst, R. L., J. P. Goff, and T. A. Reinhardt. 1990. Advancing age results in reduction of intestinal and bone 1,25-dihydroxyvitamin D receptor. Endocrinol. 126:1053–1057.

Hortin, A. E., P. J. Bechtel, and D. H. Baker. 1991. Efficacy of pork loin as a source of zinc and effect of added cysteine on zinc bioavailability. J. Food Sci. 56:1505–1507.

Hoskins, F. H. and Hansard, S. L. 1964. *In* Agricultureal Research Council. 1980. p. 239.

House, W. A., and A. W. Bell. 1993. Mineral accretion in the fetus and adnexa during late gestation in Holstein Cows. J. Dairy Sci. 76:2999–3010.

House, W. A., and A. W. Bell. 1994. Sulfur and selenium accretion in the gravid uterus during late gestation in Holstein cows. J. Dairy Sci. 77:1860–1869.

House, W. A., and R. M. Welch. 1989. Bioavailability of and interactions between zinc and selenium in rats fed wheat grain intrinsically labeled with $^{65}$Zn and $^{75}$Se. J. Nutr. 119:916–921.

Huber, J. T. and N. O. Price. 1971. Influence of high dietary calcium and phosphorus and Ca:P ratio on liver copper and iron stores in lactating cows. J. Dairy Sci. 54:429–432.

Huffman, C. F., C. S. Robinson, C. W. Duncan, L. W. Lamb, and M. F. Mason. 1933. Study of the phosphorus requirement of dairy cattle. I. Phosphorus requirement for growth and reproduction from three months of age to first calving. J. Dairy Sci. 16:203–223.

Hunt, C. H., O. G. Bentley, T. V. Hershberger, and J. H. Cline. 1954. The effect of carbohydrates and sulfur on B-vitamins synthesis, cellulose digestion, and urea utilization by rumen microorganisms in vitro. J. Anim. Sci. 13:570–575.

Hurley, W. L., L. A. Edgerton, D. Olds, and R. W. Hemken. 1982. Estrous behavior and endocrine status of dairy heifers with varied intakes of phosphorus. J. Dairy Sci. 65:1979–1986.

Ingalls, J. R., and R. C. Okemo. 1994. The bioavailability of phosphorus from canola meal as measured by Holstein calves and mobile bag technique. Anim. Feed Sci. Tech. 47:321–334.

Institut National de la Recherche Agronomique. 1989. Ruminant Nutrition: Recommended allowances and feed tables. R. Jarrige (ed.)., John Libbey Eurotext, Paris-London Rome. p. 54–55.

Irving, J. T. 1964. Dynamics and functions of phosphorus. Pg. 149 in Mineral Metabolism, vol. 2. C. L. Comar and F. Bonner, Eds. Academic Press, NY.

Ishimoto, M. J., J. Koyama, T. Omura, and Y. Nagai. 1954. Biochemical studies on sulfate reducing bacteria. III. Sulfate reduction by cell suspension. J. Biochem. 41:537–546.

Ivan, M., J. G. Proulx, R. Morales, H. C. V. Codagnone and M. de S. Dayrell. 1990. Copper accumulation in the liver of sheep and cattle fed diets supplemented wth copper sulfate or copper chloride. Can. J. Anim. Sci. 70:727.

Ivancic, J. Jr, and W. P. Weiss. 2001. Effect of dietary sulfur and selenium concentrations on selenium balance of lactating dairy cows. J. Dairy Sci. 84 (In press).

Jackson, J. A., Jr., and R. W. Hemken. 1994. Calcium and cation-anion balance effects on feed intake, body weight gain, and humoral response of dairy calves. J. Dairy Sci. 77:1430–1436.

Jackson, J. A., Jr., D. L. Langer, and R. W. Hemken. 1988. Evaluation of content and source of phosphorus fed to dairy calves. J. Dairy Sci. 71:2187–2192.

Jackson, J. A., Jr., D. M. Hopkins, Z. Xin, and R. W. Hemken. 1992. Influence of cation-anion balance on feed intake, body weight gain, and humoral response of dairy calves. J. Dairy Sci. 75:1281–1286.

Jaster, E. H., J. D. Schuh, and T. N. Wegner. 1978. Physiological effects of saline drinking water on high producing cows. J. Dairy Sci. 61:66–71.

Jenkins, K. J., and M. Hidiroglou. 1991. Tolerance of the preruminant calf for excess manganese or zinc in milk replacer. J. Dairy Sci. 74:1047–1053.

Jenkinson, D. M., and R. M. Mabon. 1973. The effect of temperature and humidity on skin surface pH and the ionic composition of skin secretions in Ayrshire cattle. Br. Vet. J. 129:282–283.

Jenness, R., and S. Patton. 1959. Principles of Dairy Chemistry. New York, John Wiley and Sons.

Jennette, K. W. 1979. Chromate metabolism in liver microsomes. Biol. Trace Elem. Res. 1:55–62.

Jesse, B. W., J. W. Thomas, and R. S. Emery. 1981. Availability of magnesium from magnesium oxide particles of differing sizes and surfaces. J Dairy Sci. 64:197–205.

Johansson, E., S. O. Jacobsson, J. Luthman, and U. Lindh. 1990. The biological response of selenium in individual erythrocytes and GSH-px in lambs fed sodium selenite or selenium yeast. J. Vet. Med. Assoc. 37:463–470.

Johnson, H. D. 1967. Climate effects on physiology and productivity of cattle. In Ground Level Climatology, R. H. Shaw, ed. Amer. Assoc. Adv. Sci. Pub. 86. Washington, D.C.

Johnson, M. A., and J. L. Greger. 1984. Absorption, distribution, and endogenous excretion of zinc by rats fed various dietary levels of inorganic tin and zinc. J. Nutr. 114:1843–1852.

Joint FAO/WHO Expert Committee on Food Additives. 1972. Evaluation of certain food additives and the contaminants mercury, lead, and cadmium. WHO Tech Rep. Ser. # 505:20, 32. World Health Organization.

Judson, G. J., C. L. Trengove, M. W. Langman, and R. Vandergraaff. 1984. Copper supplementation of sheep. Aust. Vet. J. 61:40.

Jukola, E., J. Hakkarainen, H. Saloniemi, and S. Sankari. 1996. Blood selenium, vitamin E, vitamin A, and B-carotene concentrations and udder health, fertility treatments and fertility. J. Dairy Sci. 79:838–845.

Kagi, J. H., S. R. Himmelhoch, P. D. Whanger, J. L. Bethune, and B. L. Vallee. 1974. Equine hepatic and renal metallothioneins. Purification, molecular weight, amino acid composition, and metal content. J. Biol. Chem. 249:3537–3542.

Kandylis, K. 1984. Toxicology of sulfur in ruminants. J. Dairy Sci. 67:2179–2187.

Keener, H. A., G. P. Percival, and K. S. Marrow. 1949. Cobalt tolerance in young dairy cattle. J. Dairy Sci. 32:527.

Kegley, E. B. and J. W. Spears. 1993. Bioavailability of feed grade copper sources (oxide, sulfate or lysine) in growing cattle. J. Anim. Sci. 71 (Suppl. 1):27 [Abstract].

Kemp, A. 1964. Sodium requirement of milking cows: Balance trials with cows on rations of freshly mown herbage and on winter rations. Neth. J. Ag. Sci. 12:263–280.

Kemp, A. 1966. Mineral balance in dairy cows fed on grass, with special reference to magnesium and sodium. Pg. 411 in Proc. of the X International Grassland Congress.

Kemp, A., and J. M. Geurink. 1966. Further investigation on the sodium supply of lactating cows. Tijdschr. Diergeneeskd. 91:580–589.

Kemp, A., and J. R. Todd. 1970. Prevention of hypomagnesaemia in cows: The use of magnesium alloy bullets. Vet. Rec. 86:463–464.

Kennedy, D. G., S. Kennedy, and P. B. Young. 1996. Effects of low concentrations of dietary cobalt on rumen succinate concentration in sheep. Int. J. Vitam. Nutr. Res. 66:86–92.

Kercher, C. J., and S. E. Smith. 1955. The response of cobalt-deficient lambs to orally administered vitamin $B_{12}$. J. Anim. Sci. 14:458–464.

Kertz, A. 1998. Variability in delivery of nutrients to lactating dairy cows. J. Dairy Sci. 81:3075–3084.

Khan, A. A., D. Lovejoy, A. K. Sharma, R. M. Sharma, M. G. Prior, and L. E. Lillie. 1987. Effects of high dietary sulphur on enzyme activities, selenium concentrations and body weights of cattle. Can. J. Vet. Res. 51:174–180.

Kincaid, R. L. 1979. Biological availability of zinc from inorganic sources with excess dietary calcium. J. Dairy Sci. 62:1081–1085.

Kincaid, R. L., J. K. Hillers, and J. D. Cronrath. 1981. Calcium and phosphorus supplementation of rations for lactating cows. J. Dairy Sci. 64:754–758.

Kincaid, R. L., R. M. Blauwiekel and J. D. Conrath. 1986. Supplementation of copper as copper sulfate or copper proteinate for growing calves fed forages containing molybdenum. J. Dairy Sci 69:160.

Kincaid, R. L., B. P. Chew, and J. D. Cronrath. 1997. Zinc oxide and amino acids as sources of dietary zinc for calves: Effects on uptake and immunity. J. Dairy Sci. 80:1381–1388.

Kirchgessner, M. 1993. Mitteilungen des ausschusses für bedarfsnormen der gesellschaft für ernährungsphysiologie. Überarbeitete empfehlungen zur versorgung von milchkühen mit calcium und phosphor. (translation: Communications of the working group for requirement standards of the Society of Nutrition Physiology. Revised recommendations for supply of calcium and phosphorus to dairy cows.). Proc. Soc. Nutr. Physiol. 42:108–113.

Kirchgessner, M., and K. R. Neesse. 1976. [Copper, manganese, and zinc contents in the whole body and in individual parts of veal calves at different weights (author's transl)]. Z. Lebensm. Unfers. Forsch. 161:1–6.

Kirchgessner M., and W. A. Schwarz. 1976. [Effect of zinc deficiency and varying zinc supplements on absorption and retention in dairy cows (translation from German)]. Arch. Tierernahr. 26(1):3–16.

Kirchgessner, M., and E. Weigand. 1982. [Optimal zinc requirement of lactating dairy cows based on various dose-response relationships (translation from German)]. Arch. Tierernahr. 32(7–8):569–578.

Kirchgessner, M., and U. Weser. 1965. Complex-stability and copper absorption. 4. On the dynamics of copper absorption. Z. Tierphysiol Tiererenahr Futtermittelkd. 20:44–49.

Klosch, M., G. H. Richter, A. Schneider, G. Flachowsky, and E. Pfeffer. 1997. Influence of feeding on fecal phosphorus excretion of growing bulls varying in body weight. Arch. Anim. Nutr. 50:163–172.

Koenig, K. M., L. M. Rode, L. M. Cohen, and W. T. Bucklet. 1997. Effects of diet and chemical form of selenium on selenium metabolism in sheep. J. Anim. Sci. 75:817–827.

Koenig, K. M., W. T. Buckley, and J. A. Shelford. 1991a. Measurement of endogenous fecal excretion and true absorption of selenium in dairy cows. Can J Anim Sci 71:167–174.

Koenig, K. M., W. T. Buckley, and J. A. Shelford. 1991b. True absorption of selenium in dairy cows: Stable isotope tracer methodology and effect of dietary copper. Can. J. Anim. Sci. 71:175–183.

Langer, D. L., J. A. Jackson, Jr., R. W. Hemken, and R. J. Harmon. 1985. Effect of level and source of phosphorus fed to dairy calves. J. Dairy Sci. 68(Suppl. 1):136.

Langlands, J. P., J. E. Bowles, C. E. Donald, and A. J. Smith. 1986. Trace element nutrition of grazing ruminants. II. Hepatic copper storage in young and adult sheep and cattle given varying quantities of oxidized copper particles and other copper supplements. Aust. J. Agric. Res. 37:189.

Lassiter, J. W., and J. D. Morton. 1968. Effects of low manganese diet on certain bovine characteristics. J. Anim. Sci. 27:776–779.

Lassiter, J. W., W. J. Miller, F. M. Pate, and R. P. Gentry. 1972. Effect of dietary calcium and phosphorus on $^{54}$Mn metabolism following single tracer intraperitoneal and oral doses in rats. Proc. Soc. Exp. Biol. Med. 139:345–348.

Lean, L. J., H. F. Troutt, H. Boermans, G. Moller, G. Webster, and M. Tracy. 1990. An investigation of bulk tank milk selenium levels in the San Joaquin Valley of California. Cornell Vet 80:41–51.

Lechene, C. 1988. Physiological role of the Na-K pump. Pg. 171 in The Na, K-pump, part B: Cellular Aspects. Alan R. Liss, Inc.

Ledoux, D. R., and F. A. Martz. 1990. Ruminal solubilization of selected macrominerals from forages and diets. J. Dairy Sci. 74:1654–1661.

Lee, H. J., and R. E. Kuchel. 1953. The aetiology of Phalaris staggers in sheep. 1. Preliminary observations on the preventive role of cobalt. Aust. J. Agr. Res. 4:88–99.

Lee, J., N. Grace, and D., Martell, S. 1991. Effect of high and sustained zinc supplements on trace element metabolism in sheep. Proceedings of the New Zealand Society of Animal Production. 51:173–177.

Lengemann, F. W., and E. W. Swanson. 1957. A study of the secretion of iodine in milk of dairy cows, using daily oral doses of $^{131}$I. J. Dairy Sci. 40:215–222.

Leonard-Marek, S., and H. Martens. 1996. Effects of potassium on magnesium transport across rumen epithelium. Am. J. Physiol. 271, G1034–8.

Lesperance, A. L., V. R. Bohman, and J. E. Oldfield. 1985. Interaction of molybdenum, sulfate and alfalfa in the bovine. J. Anim. Sci. 60:791–802.

Lewis, D. 1954. The reduction of sulfate in the rumen of the sheep. Biochem. J. 56:391–399.

Lillie, R. J. 1970. Arsenic. Air pollutants affecting the performance of domestic animals—A literature review. Agricultural Handbook No. 380, Government Printing Office, U.S. Department of Agriculture, Washington, D.C.

Lindt, F., and J. W. Blum. 1994. Growth performance, haematological traits, meat variables, and effects of treadmill and transport stress in veal calves supplied different amounts of iron. Zentralbl Veterinarmed A 41:333–342.

Little, D. A. 1975. Effects of dry season supplements of protein and phosphorus to pregnant cows on the incidence of first postpartum estrus. Aust. J. Exp. Agric. Anim. Husb. 15:25–31.

Lofgreen, G. P., and M. Kleiber. 1953. The availability of the phosphorus in alfalfa hay. J. Anim. Sci. 12:366–731.

Lofgreen, G. P., and M. Kleiber. 1954. Further studies on the availability of phosphorus in alfalfa hay. J. Anim. Sci. 13: 258–264.

Lomba, F., R. Paquay, V. Bienfet, and A. Lousse. 1969. Statistical research on the fate of dietary mineral elements in dry and lactating cows. VI. Sodium. J. Ag. Sci. 73: 453–458.

Lopez, A., W. F. Collins, and H. L. Williams. 1985. Essential elements, cadmium, and lead in raw and pasteurized cow and goat milk. J. Dairy Sci. 68:1878–1886.

Lopez-Guisa, J. M., and L. D. Satter. 1992. Effect of copper and cobalt addition on digestion and growth in heifers fed diets containing alfalfa silage or corn crop residues. J. Dairy Sci. 75:247–256.

Lyford, S. J., and J. T. Huber. 1988. Digestion, Metabolism and nutrient needs in pre-ruminants. Pg. 416 in The Ruminant Animal: Digestive Physiology and Nutrition, D. C. Church, ed. Prospect Heights, IL: Waveland Press, Inc.

MacPherson, A., D. Gray, G. B. Mitchell, and C. N. Taylor. 1987. Ostertagia infection and neutrophil function in cobalt-deficient and cobalt-supplemented cattle. Br. Vet. J. 143:348–353.

Maddox, J. F., C. C. Reddy, R. J. Eberhart, and R. W. Scholz. 1991. Dietary selenium effects on milk eicosanoid concentration in dairy cows during coliform mastitis. Prostaglandins. 42:369–378.

Mahaffey, D. R. 1983. Biotoxicity of lead: Influence of various factors. Fed. Proc. 42:1730–1734.

Mallonee, P. G. 1984. Potassium and sodium nutrition and metabolism in lactating dairy cows. M.S. Thesis, Univ. Florida, Gainesville.

Mallonee, P. G., D. K. Beede, and C. J. Wilcox. 1982a. Lactational and physiological responses of dairy cows to varying potassium and sodium quantities and ratios in complete mixed diets. J. Dairy Sci. 65(Suppl. 1):212 (Abstr.).

Mallonee, P. G., D. K. Beede, P. L Schneider, S. J. Caputo, and C. J. Wilcox. 1982b. Acute response of lactating Holstein cows to dietary potassium deficiency. J. Dairy Sci. 65(Suppl. 1):112.

Mallonee, P. G., D. K. Beede, R. J. Collier, and C. J. Wilcox. 1985. Production and physiological responses of dairy cows to varying dietary potassium during heat stress. J. Dairy Sci. 68:1479–1487.

Marston, H. R. 1970. The requirement of sheep for cobalt or for vitamin $B_{12}$. Br. J. Nutr. 24:615–33.

Martens, H. 1983. Saturation kinetics of magnesium efflux across the rumen wall in heifers. Br. J. Nutr. 49:153–158.

Martens, H., and I. Blume. 1987. Studies on the absorption of sodium and chloride from the rumen of sheep. Comp. Biochem. Physiol. 86A:653–656.

Martens, H., and G. Gabel. 1986. Pathogenesis and prevention of grass tetany from the physiologic viewpoint. DTW Dtsch Tierarztl Wochenschr 93:170–177.

Martens, H., and H. Kasebieter. 1983. In vitro studies of the effect of sodium and potassium ions on magnesium transport across the isolated rumen mucosa of sheep. Zentralbl Veterinarmed [A] 30:1.

Martens, H., and Y. Rayssiguier. 1980. Magnesium metabolism and hypomagnesemia. Pg. 447 in Digestive Physiology and Metabolism in Ruminants. Y. Ruckebusch and P. Thivend, eds. Lancaster, England: MTP Press.

Martens, H., G. Heggermann, and K. Regier. 1988. Studies on the effects of K, NO, $NH_4^+$) VFA and $CO_2$ on the net absorption of magnesium from the temporarily isolated rumen of heifers. J. Vet. Med. A 35:73.

Martz, F. A., A. T. Belo, M. F. Weiss, R. L. Belyea, and J. P. Goff. 1990. True absorption of calcium and phosphorus from alfalfa and corn silage when fed to lactating cows. J. Dairy Sci. 73:1288–1295.

Martz, F. A., R. Nieto Ordax, M. F. Weiss, and R. L. Belyea. 1988. Mineral balance for growing dairy heifers fed semipurified diets. Nutr. Rep. Int. 38:665–673.

Matrone, G., C. Conley, G. H. Wise, and R. K. Wangh. 1957. A study of iron and copper requirements of dairy calves. J. Dairy Sci. 40:1437–1439.

Maus, R. W., F. A. Martz, R. L. Belyea, and M. F. Weiss. 1980. Relationship of dietary selenium to selenium in plasma. J. Dairy Sci. 63:532–539.

Mayland, H. 1988. Grass tetany. Pg. 511 in The Ruminant Animal: Digestive Physiology and Nutrition, D. Church, ed. Prospect Heights, Illinois: Waveland Press, Inc.

Mayland, H. F., R. C. Rosenau, and A. R. Florence. 1980. Grazing cow and calf responses to zinc supplementation. J. Anim. Sci. 51:966–974.

McAllister, M. M., D. H. Gould, M. F. Raisbeck, B. A. Cummings, and G. H. Loneragan. 1997. Evaluation of ruminal sulfide concentrations and seasonal outbreaks of polioencephalomalacia in beef cattle in a feedlot. J. Am. Vet. Med. Assoc. 211:1275–1279.

McClure, T. J. 1994. Nutritional and metabolic infertility in the cow. Oxon, UK: CAB International. p. 49.

McGuirk, S. M., and D. G. Butler. 1980. Metabolic alkalosis with paradoxic aciduria in cattle. JAVMA. 177:551–558.

McKeown, J. W. 1986. Disorders of Na metabolism. Page 63 in Fluids and electrolytes. J. P. Kakko and R. L. Tannen, eds. Philadelphia: W. P. Saunders Co.

McQuinn, S. D., D. A. Sleper, H. F. Mayland, and G. F. Krause. 1991. Genetic variation for selenium content in tall fescue. Crop Sci. 31:617–620.

Meltzer, H. M., K. Bibow, I. T. Paulsen, H. H. Mundal, G. Norheim, and H. Holm. 1993. Different bioavailabilities in humans of wheat and fish selenium as measured by blood platelet response to increased dietary Se. Biol. Trace Min. Res. 36:229–241.

Mertz, W. 1993 Chromium in human nutrition: A review. J. Nutr. 123:626–633.

Meyer, J. H., R. R. Grunert, R. H. Grummer, P. H. Phillips, and G. Bohstedt. 1950. Sodium, potassium, and chlorine contents of feedstuffs. J. Anim. Sci. 153–156.

Meyer, J. H., W. C. Weir, N. R. Ittner, and J. D. Smith. 1955. The influence of high sodium chloride intakes by fattening sheep and cattle. J. Anim. Sci. 14:412–418.

Miller, E. R. 1995. Potassium bioavailability. Pp. 295–301 in Bioavailability of Nutrients for Animals. C. B. Ammerman, D. H. Baker, and A. J. Lewis, eds. New York: Academic Press.

Miller, J. K., and R. G. Cragle. 1965. Gastrointestinal site of absorption and endogenous secretion of zinc in dairy cattle. J. Dairy Sci. 48:370–373.

Miller, J. K., and W. J. Miller. 1962. Experimental zinc deficiency and recovery of calves. J. Nutr. 76:467–474.

Miller, J. K., B. R. Moss, E. W. Swanson, P. W. Aschbacher, and R. G. Cragle. 1968. Calcium iodate and pentacalcium orthoperiodate as sources of supplemental iodine for calves. J. Dairy Sci. 51:1831–1836.

Miller, J. K., E. Brzezinska-Slebodzinska, and F. C. Madsen. 1993. Oxidative stress, antioxidants, and animal function. J. Dairy Sci. 76:2812–2823

Miller, J. K., E. W. Swanson, and G. E. Spalding. 1975. Iodine absorption, excretion, recycling, and tissue distributions in the dairy cow. J. Dairy Sci. 58:1578–1593.

Miller, J. K., N. Ramsey, and F. C. Madsen. 1988. The trace elements. Pp. 342–400 in The Ruminant Animal: Digestive Physiology and Nutrition, D.C. Church, ed. Englewood Cliffs, NJ: Prentice-Hall, Inc.

Miller, W. J. 1970. Zinc nutrition of cattle: A review. J. Dairy Sci. 53:1123–1135.

Miller, W. J. 1978. Dairy Cattle Feeding and Nutrition. New York: Academic Press.

Miller, W. J. 1983a. Using mineral requirement standards in cattle feeding programs and feed formulations. Pp. 69–74 Georgia Nutrition Conference for the Feed Industry. Athens: University of Georgia.

Miller, W. J. 1983b. Phosphorus nutrition, biochemistry, metabolism ad requirements in ruminants. Paper presented at the meeting of the National Feed Ingredients Association, Chicago, Illinois, April 5–7.

Miller, W. J., D. M. Blackmon, J. M. Hiers, Jr., P. R. Fowler, C. M. Clifton, and R. P. Gentry. 1967. Effects of adding two forms of supplemental zinc to a practical diet on skin regeneration in Holstein heifers and evaluation of a procedure for determining rate of wound healing. J. Dairy Sci. 50:715–721.

Miller, W. J., D M. Blackmon, R. P. Gentry, and F. Pate. 1970. Effects of high but nontoxic levels of zinc in practical diets on 65Zinc and zinc metabolism in Holstein calves. J. Nutr. 100:893–902.

Miller, W. J., H. E. Amos, R. P. Gentry, D. M. Blackmon, R. M. Durrance, C. T. Crowe, A. S. Fielding, and M. W. Neathery. 1989. Long term feeding of high zinc sulfate diets to lactating and gestating dairy cows. J. Dairy Sci. 72:1499–1508.

Miller, W. J., M. W. Neatherly, D. M. Gentry, C. T. Blackmon, C. T. Crowe, G. O. Watt, and A. S. Fielding. 1987. Bioavailability of phosphorus from defluorinated and dicalcium phosphate and phosphorus requirements of calves. J. Dairy Sci. 70:1885–1892.

Miller, W. J., W. M. Britton, and M. S. Ansari. 1972. Magnesium in livestock nutrition. Pp. 109–130 *in* Magnesium in the Environment, J. B. Jones, Jr., M. C. Blount, and S. R. Wilkinson, eds. Reynolds, GA.: Taylor County Printing.

Miller, W. J., Y. G. Martin, R. P. Gentry, and D. M. Blackmon. 1968. 65Zn and stable zinc absorption, excretion and tissue concentrations as affected by type of diet and level of zinc in normal calves. J. Nutr. 94:391–401.

Mills, C. F. 1981. Cobalt deficiency and cobalt requirements of ruminants. Pp. 129–141 in Recent Advances in Animal Nutrition, W. Haresign, ed. Boston: Butterworths Publishing.

Mills, C. F. 1987. Biochemical and physiological indicators of mineral status in animals: Copper, cobalt and zinc. J. Anim. Sci. 65:1702–1711.

Mills, C. F., and G. K. Davis. 1987. Molybdenum. Pp. 429–463 in Trace Elements in Human and Animal Nutrition, Vol. 1, W. Mertz, ed. New York: Academic.

Mills, C. F., A. C. Dalgarno, R. B. Williams, and J. Quarterman. 1967. Zinc deficiency and the zinc requirements of calves and lambs. Br. J. Nutr. 21:751–768.

Miltenburg, G. A., T. Wensing, H. J. Bruekink, and J. J. Marx, 1993 Mucosal uptake, mucosal transfer and retention of iron in veal calves. Vet Res Commun 17:209–217

Minson, D. J. 1990. Copper. In: Forage in Ruminal Nutrition. Academic Press, Sydney, pp. 316–324.

Mollerberg, L., and J. Moreno-Lopez. 1975. The response of normal and iron anemic calves to nasal infection with an attenuated strain of parainfluenza-3 virus. Acta. Vet. Scand. 16:186–196.

Mongin, P. 1980. Electrolytes in nutrition: review of basic principles and practical application in poultry and swine. Pg. 1 in Proc. Int. Min. Chem. Corp., Mundelein, IL.

Moonsie-Shageer, S., and D. N. Mowat. 1993. Effect of level of supplemental chromium on performance, serum constituents, and immune status of stressed feeder calves. J. Anim. Sci. 71:232–238.

Moore, W. F., J. P. Fontenot, and R. E. Tucker. 1971. Relative effects of different supplemental magnesium sources on apparent digestibility in steers. J. Anim. Sci. 33:502.

Morris, J. G., and R. J. W. Gartner. 1971. The sodium requirements of growing steers given an all-sorghum ration. Br. J. Nutr. 25:191–205.

Morrow, D. A. 1969. Phosphorus deficiency and infertility in dairy heifers. JAVMA 154:761–768.

Morse, D., H. H. Head, and C. J. Wilcox. 1992a. Disappearance of phosphorus in phytate from concentrates in vitro from rations fed to lactating dairy cows. J. Dairy Sci. 75:1979–1986.

Morse, D., H. H. Head, C. J. Wilcox, H. H. VanHorn, C. D. Hissem, and B. Harris, Jr. 1992b. Effects of concentration of dietary phosphorus on amount and route of excretion. J. Dairy Sci. 75:3039–3049.

Murthy, G. K., U. Rhea, and J. T. Peeler. 1967. Rubidium and lead content of market milk. J. Dairy Sci. 50:651–655.

National Research Council. 1978. Nutrient Requirements of Dairy Cattle. 5th rev. ed. Washington, D.C.: National Academy Press.

National Research Council. 1980. Mineral Tolerance of Domestic Animals. Washington, D.C.: National Academy Press.

National Research Council. 1983. Selenium in nutrition. 2nd rev. ed. Natl. Acad. Sci., Washington, DC.

National Research Council. 1989a. Recommended Dietary Allowances, 10th edition. Washington, D.C.: National Academy Press.

National Research Council. 1989b. Nutrient Requirements of Dairy Cattle. 6th rev. ed. Natl. Acad. Sci., Washington, DC.

National Research Council. 1996. Nutrient Requirements of Beef Cattle. 7th edition Washington, D.C.: National Academy Press.

National Research Council. 1997. The Role of Chromium in Animal Nutrition. Washington, D.C.: National Academy Press.

National Research Council. 1998. Nutrient Requirements of Swine. $10^{th}$ rev. ed. Natl. Acad. Sci., Washington, DC.

Nationale Raad voor Landbouwkundig Onderzoek. 1982. Handleiding mineralenonderzoek bij rundvee in de praktijk. Nationale Raad voor Landbouwkundig Onderzoek's Gravenhage, Neth.

Neathery, M. W., and W. J. Miller. 1975. Metabolism and toxicity of cadmium, mercury, and lead in animals: A review. J. Dairy Sci. 58:1767–1781.

Neathery, M. W., D. M. Blackmon, W. J. Miller, S. Heinmiller, S. McGuire, J. M. Tarabula, R. P. Gentry, and J. C. Allen. 1981. Chloride deficiency in Holstein calves from a low chloride diet and removal of abomasal contents. J. Dairy Sci. 64:2220–2233.

Neathery, M. W., W. J. Miller, R. P. Gentry, P. E. Stake, and D. M. Blackmon. 1974. Cadmium-109 and methyl mercury-203 metabolism, tissue distribution, and secretion into milk of cows. J. Dairy Sci. 57:1177–1183.

Nellans, H. N. 1988. Contributions of cellular and paracellular pathways to transepithelial intestinal calcium transport. Pg. 269 in Cellular calcium and phosphate transport in health and disease. F. Bronner and M. Peterlik. New York: Alan R. Liss, Inc.

Nelson, A. B., R. W. MacVicar, Jr., and J. C. Meiske. 1955. Effect of a high salt intake on the digestibility of ration constituents and on nitrogen, sodium, and chloride retention by steers and wethers. J. Anim. Sci. 14:825–830.

Nelson, T. S., L. B. Daniels, J. R. Hall, and L. G. Shields. 1976. Hydrolysis of natural phytate phosphorus in the digestive tract of calves. J. Anim. Sci. 42:1509–1512.

Newton, G. L., J. P. Fontenot, R. E. Tucker, and C. E. Polan. 1972. Effects of high dietary potassium intake on the metabolism of magnesium by sheep. J. Anim. Sci. 35:440.

Nicholson, J. W., A. M. S. Laurent, R. E. McQueen, and E. Charmley. 1991a. The effect of feeding organically bound selenium and a-tocopherol to dairy cows on susceptibilty of milk to oxidation. Can J. Anim. Sci. 71:135–143.

Nicholson, J. W., R. E. McQueen, and R. S. Bush. 1991b. Response of growing cattle to supplementation with organically bound or inorganic sources of selenium or yeast cultures. Can. J. Anim. Sci. 71:803–811.

Nielsen, F. H., and D. A. Ollerich. 1974. Nickel: A new essential trace element. Fed. Proc. 33:1767–1772.

Nielsen, F. H., and H. H. Sandstead. 1974. Are nickel, vanadium, silicon, fluorine, and tin essential for man? Am. J. Clin. Nutr. 27:515–522.

Nielsen, F. H., D. R. Myron, S. H. Givand, and D. A. Ollerich. 1975. Nickel deficiency and nickel-rhodium interaction in chicks. J. Nutr. 105:1607–1619.

Nielsen, F. H., M. L. Sunde, and W. G. Hoekstra. 1966. Effect of dietary synthetic and natural chelating agents on the zinc-deficiency syndrome in the chick. J. Nutr. 89:35–42.

Nockels, C. F., J. DeBonis, and J. Torrent. 1993. Stress induction affects copper and zinc balance in calves fed organic and inorganic copper and zinc sources. J. Anim. Sci. 71:2539–2545.

Noller, C. H., A. G. Castro, W. E. Wheeler, D. L. Hill, and N. J. Moeller. 1977. Effect of phosphorus supplementation on growth rate, blood minerals, and conception rate of dairy heifers. J. Dairy Sci. 60:1932–1940.

Nutrients, A.T.C.o.R.t. 1991. A reappraisal of the calcium and phosphorus requirements of sheep and cattle. Nutr. Abstr. Rev. Ser. B 61:573–612.

O'Dell, B. L., P. M. Newberne, and J. E. Savage. 1958. Significance of dietary zinc for the growing chicken. J. Nutr. 65:303–312.

O'Kelley, R. E., and J. P. Fontenot. 1969. Effects of feeding different magnesium levels o drylot-fed lactating beef cows. J. Anim. Sci. 29:994–1000.

Oliver, W. T., and N. Platonow. 1960. Studies on the pharmacology of the N-(ethyl mercuri)-p-toluenesulfonanilide. Am. J. Vet. Res. 21:906–916.

Olson, W., J. Stevens, J. Anderson, and D. W. Haggard. 1984. Iodine toxicosis in six herds of dairy cattle. J. Am. Vet. Med. Assoc. 184:179–179.

Oltjen, R. 1975. Fats for ruminants-utilization and limitations, including value of protected fats. Proc. Ga. Nutr. Conf. Athens: University of Georgia.

Osis, D., L. Kramer, E. Wiatrowski, and H. Spencer. 1972. Dietary zinc intake in man. Am. J. Clin. Nutr. 25:582–588.

Ott, E. A., W. H. Smith, R. B. Harrington, and W. M. Beeson. 1966. Zinc toxicity in ruminants. II. Effect of high levels of dietary zinc on gains, feed consumption and feed efficiency of beef cattle. J. Anim. Sci. 25:419–423.

Palmer, T. W., T. W. Gullickson, W. L. Boyd, C. P. Fitch, and J. W. Nelson. 1941. The effect of rations deficient in phosphorus and protein on ovulation, estrous, and reproduction of dairy heifers. J. Dairy Sci. 24:199–210.

Paquay, R, F. Lomba, A. Lousse, and V. Bienfet. 1969a. Statistical research on the fate of dietary mineral elements in dry and lactating cows. V. Potassium. J. Ag. Res. 73:445–452.

Paquay, R., F. Lomba, A. Lousse, and V. Bienfet. 1969b. Statistical research on the fate of dietary mineral elements in dry and lactating cows. IV. Chloride. J. Ag. Sci. 73:223–229.

Parker, G. 1957. "Water-belly" (urolithiasis) in range steers in relation to some characteristics of rangeland. J. Range Manag. 10:105–108.

Paterson, J. E., and A. MacPherson. 1990. The influence of a low cobalt intake on the neutrophil function and severity of Ostertagia infection in cattle. Br. Vet. J. 146:519–530.

Paulson, G. D., C. A. Baumann, and A. L. Pope. 1966. Fate of a physiological dose of selenate in the lactating ewe: effect of sulfate. J. Anim. Sci. 25:1054–1058.

Peeler, H. T. 1972. Biological availability of nutrients in feeds: Availability of major mineral ions. J. Anim. Sci. 35:695–712.

Perdomo, J. T., R. L. Shirley, and C. R. Chicco. 1977. Availability of nutrient minerals in four tropical forages fed freshly chopped to sheep. J. Anim. Sci. 45:1114–1119.

Perkinson, Jr., J. D., I. B. Whitney, R. A. Monroe, W. E. Lotz, and C. L. Comar. 1955. Metabolism of fluorine-18 in domestic animals. Am. J. Physiol. 182:383–389.

Perry, T. W., W. M. Beeson, W. H. Smith, and M. T. Mohler. 1968. Value of zinc supplementation of natural rations for fattening beef cattle. J. Anim. Sci. 27:1674–1677.

Pfeffer, E., A. Thompson, and D. Armstrong. 1970. Studies on intestinal digestion in sheep. 3. Net movement of certain inorganic elements in the digestive tract on rations containing different proportions of hay and rolled barley. Br. J. Nutr. 24:197–204.

Phillippo, M., W. R. Humphries, and P. H. Garthwaite. 1987. The effect of dietary molybdenum and iron on copper status and growth in cattle. J. Ag. Sci. Camb. 109:315–320.

Podoll, K. L., J. B. Bernard, D. E. Ullrey, S. R. DeBar, P. K. Ku, and W. T. Magee. 1992. Dietary selenate versus selenite for cattle, sheep, and horses. J. Anim. Sci. 70:1965–1970.

Pond, W. G., and R. R. Oltjen. 1988. Response of large and medium frame beef steers to protein and zinc supplementation of a corn silage-corn finishing diet. Nutr. Rep. Int. 38:737–743.

Pond, W. G., and M. H. Wallace. 1986. Effects of gestation-lactation diet calcium and zinc levels and of parental vitamin A, D and E during gestation on ewe body weight and lamb weight and survival. J. Anim. Sci. 63:1019–1025.

Poole, D. B. R., and J. F. Connolly. 1967. Some observations on the use of the cobalt heavy pellet in sheep. Irish J. Ag. Res. 6:281–284.

Pope, A. L., R. J. Moir, M. Somers, E. J. Underwood, and C. L. White. 1979. The effect of (dietary) sulphur on $^{75}$Se (selenium isotope) absorption and retention in sheep. J. Nutr. 109:1448–1455.

Potter, G. W., D. R. McIntyre, and G. M. Vattuone. 1972. Metabolism of $^{203}$Hg administered as $HgCl_2$ in the dairy cow and calf. Health Phys. 22:103–106.

Pradhan, K., and R. W. Hemken. 1968. Potassium depletion in lactating dairy cows. J. Dairy Sci. 51:1377–1381.

Preston, R. L., and W. H. Pfander. 1964. Phosphorus metabolism in lambs fed varying phosphorus intakes. J. Nutr. 83:369–378.

Puls, R. 1994. Mineral Levels in Animal Health: Diagnostic Data. Clearbrook: Canada Sherpa International.

Rabiansky, P. A., L. R. McDowell, J. Velasquez-Pereira, N. S. Wilkinson, S. S. Percival, F. G. Martin, D. B. Bates, A. B. Johnson, T. R. Batra, and E. Salgado-Madriz. 1999. J. Dairy Sci. 82:2642–2650.

Radostits, O., D. Blood, and C. Gay. 1994. Veterinary Medicine, Eight edition/Ed. London: Bailliere Tindall.

Rahnema, S., Z. Wu, O. A. Ohajuruka, W. P. Weiss, and D. L. Palmquist. 1994. Site of mineral absorption in lactating cows fed high-fat diets. J. Anim. Sci. 72:229–235.

Ram, L., J. T. Schonewille, H. Martens, A. T. van't Klooster, and A. C. Beynen. 1998. Magnesium absorption by wethers fed potassium bicarbonate in combination with different dietary magnesium concentrations. J. Dairy Sci. 81:2485–2492.

Ramberg, C. F., Jr. 1974. Kinetic analysis of calcium metabolism in the cow. Fed. Proc. 33:183–187.

Randall, W. E., R. W. Hemken, L. S. Bull, and L. W. Douglas. 1974. Effect of dietary sodium and potassium on udder edema in Holstein heifers. J. Dairy Sci. 57:472–475.

Reid, R. L., M. C. Franklin, and E. G. Hallsworth. 1947. The utilization of phytate phosphorus by sheep. Aust. Vet. J. 23:136–139.

Reinhardt, T. A., and H. R. Conrad. 1980. Mode of action of pharmacological doses of cholecalciferol during parturient hypocalcemia in dairy cows. J. Nutr. 110:1589–1596.

Reinhardt, T. A., R. L. Horst, and J. P. Goff. 1988. Calcium, phosphorus, and magnesium homeostasis in ruminants. In: Metabolic Diseases of Ruminant Livestock. Veterinary Clinics of North America: Food Animal Practice. 4:331–350.

Renkema, J. A., T. Senshu, B. D. E. Gaillard, and E. Brouwer. 1962. Regulation of sodium excretion and retention by the intestine in cows. Nature. 195:389–390.

Renner, E. 1983. Milk and Dairy Products in Human Nutrition. Volkswirtschaftlicher, Verlag, Munchen.

Richards, D. H., G. R. Hewett, J. M. Parry, and C. H. Yeoman. 1985. Bovine copper deficiency: Use of copper oxide needles. Vet. Rec. 116:618.

Robinson, D. L., L. C. Kappel, and J. A. Boling. 1989. Management practices to overcome the incidence of grass tetany. J. Anim. Sci. 67:3470–3484.

Rodriguez, L. A. 1998. Periparturient responses of cows fed varying dietary cation-anion differences and calcium contents prepartum. Ph.D. Diss., Michigan State University, East Lansing.

Romoser, G. L., L. Loveless, L. J. Machlin, and R. S. Gordon. 1960. Toxicity of vanadium and chromium for the growing chicken. Poult. Sci. 39:1288–1293.

Rook, J. A. F., and R. C. Campling. 1962. Magnesium metabolism in the dairy cow. IV. The availability of the magnesium in various feeding stuffs. J. Agric. Sci. 59:225.

Rook, J. A. F., C. C. Balch, and C. Line. 1958. Magnesium metabolism in the dairy cow. I. Metablism on stall rations. J. Agric. Sci. 51:189.

Rotruck, J. T., A. L. Pope, H. E. Ganther, A. B. Swanson, D. G. Hafeman, and W. G. Hoekstra. 1973. Selenium: biochemical role as a component of glutathione peroxidase. Science 179:588–590.

Ryan, J. A., H. R Pahren, and J. B. Lucas. 1982. Controlling cadmium in the human food chain: A review and rationale based on health effects. Env. Res. 28:251–302.

Ryberg, D., and J. Alexander. 1990. Mechanism of chromium toxicity in mitochondria. Chemic-Biol. Interact. 75:141–151.

Sanchez, W. K., D. K. Beede, and M. A. DeLorenzo. 1994b. Macromineral element interrelationships and lactational performance: Empirical models from a large data set. J. Dairy Sci. 77:3096–3001.

Sanchez, W. K., M. A. McGuire, and D. K. Beede. 1994a. Macromineral nutrition by heat stress interactions in dairy cattle: Review and original research. J. Dairy Sci. 77:2051–2079.

Sansom, B. F., E. W. Symonds, and M. J. Vagg. 1978. The absorption of dietary manganese by dairy cows. Res. Vet. Sci. 24:366–369.

Sasser, L. B., G. M. Ward, and J. E. Johnson. 1966. Variations in potassium concentration of cow's milk. J. Dairy Sci. 49:893–895.

Schellner, G., M. Anke, H. Ludke, and A. Henning. 1971. Die Abhangigkeit der Milcheistung und Milchzusammensetzung von der Natriumversorgung. Arch. Exp. Vet. Med. 5:823–827.

Schingoethe, D. J., C. A. Kirkbride, I. S. Palmer, M. J. Owens, and W. L. Tucker. 1982. Response of cows consuming adequate selenium to vitamin E and selenium supplementation prepartum. J. Dairy Sci. 65:2338–2344.

Schneider, B. H., E. D. Tayson, and W. E. Ham. 1952. Urinary calculi in male farm animals. Wash. Ag. Exp. Stn. Circ. 203.

Schneider, P. L., D. K. Beede, C. J. Wilcox, and R. J. Collier. 1984. Influence of dietary sodium and potassium bicarbonate and total potassium on heat-stressed dairy cows. J. Dairy Sci. 67:2546–2553.

Schneider, P. L., D. K. Beede, and C. J. Wilcox. 1986. Responses of lactating cows to dietary sodium source and quantity and potassium quantity during heat stress. J. Dairy Sci. 69:99–110.

Schonewille, J. T., A. T. Van't Klooster, and M. van Mosel. 1992. A comparative study of the invitro solubility and availability of magnesium from various sources for cattle. Tidschr. Diergeneeskd. 117:105–108.

Schonewillie, J. T., A. T. Van't Klooster, and A. C. Beynen. 1994. High phosphorus intake depresses apparent absorption of magnesium absorption in pregnant heifers. J. Anim. Physiol. Anim. Nutr. 71:15–21.

Schroeder, H. A., and I. H. Tipton. 1968. The human body burden of lead. Arch. Environ. Health. 17:965–978.

Schwarz, F. J., and M. Kirchgessner. 1978. Copper and zinc contents in milk and plasma of cows after high nutritional copper supplements. Z. Lebensm Unters Forsch. 166:5–8.

Schwarz, K., and D. B. Milne. 1971. Growth effects of vanadium in rats in a trace element controlled environment. Fed. Proc. 30:462 (Abstr.).

Schwarz, K., D. B. Milne, and E. Vinyard. 1970. Growth effects of tin compounds in rats maintained in a trace element-controlled environment. Biochem. Biophys. Res. Commun. 40:22–29.

Schwartz, W. A., and M. Kirchgessner. 1975. Experimental zinc deficiency in lactating dairy cows. Vet. Med. Rev. 1:19–23.

Schwartz, R., Topley, M., and J. B. Russell. 1988. Effect of tricarballylic acid, a nonmetabolizable rumen fermentation product of trans-aconitic acid on Mg, Ca, and Zn utilization of rats. J. Nutr. 118:183–188.

Scott, D. 1988. Control of phosphorus balance in ruminants. Pp. 156–174 in Aspects of Digestive Physiology in Ruminants, A. Dobson and M. J. Dobson, eds. Cornell University Press: Comstock Publishing Associates.

Scott, D., A. F. McLean, and W. Buchan. 1984. The effect of variation in phosphorus uptake on net intestinal phosphorus absorption, salivary phosphorus secretion and pathway of excretion in sheep fed roughage diets. Q. J. Exp. Physiol. 69:439–452.

Scott, M. L., and T. R. Ziegler. 1963. Evidence for natural chelates which aid in the utilization of zinc by chicks. J. Ag. Food Chem. 11:123–125.

Sell, J. L., and K. L. Dawson. 1973. Mercury-203 in milk and tissues of cow and goat following intraruminal injection of methyl mercuric (labeled 203) chloride. J. Dairy Sci. 56:671 (Abstr.).

Sevilla, C. C., and J. H. Ternouth. 1981. Effects of dietary levels of calcium and phosphorus in sheep. Proc. Australian Society Animal Proc. 13:449–452.

Shariff, M. A., R. J. Boila, and K. M. Wittenberg. 1990. Effect of dietary molybdenum on rumen dry matter disappearance in cattle. Can. J. Anim. Sci. 70:319–323.

Sharma, R. P., J. C. Street, M. P. Verma, and J. L. Shupe. 1979. Cadmium intake from feed and its distribution to food products of livestock. Environ. Health Perspect. 28:59–66.

Shenk, J. S., and M. O. Westerhaus. 1994. The application of near infrared reflectance spectroscopy (NIRS) to forage analysis. Pp. 406–449 in Forage Quality, Evaluation, and Utilization. Am. Soc. Agronomy, Crop Sci. Soc. Am., and Soil Sci. Soc. Am., Madison, WI.

Shupe, J. L. 1980. Clinico pathologic features of fluoride toxicosis in cattle. J. Anim. Sci. 51:746–758.

Sielman, E. S., R. W. Sweeney, R. H. Whitlock, and R. Y. Reams. 1997. Hypokalemia syndrome in dairy cows: 10 cases (1992–1996). JAVMA. 210:240–243.

Simpson, A. M., C. F. Mills, and I. McDonald. 1981 Tissue copper retention or loss in young growing cattle. IN Howell, J. McC., Gawthorne, JM, and White, CL (eds.) Proceedings of the Fourth International Symposium on Trace Element Metabolism in Man and Animals. Australian Academy of Sciences, Canberra, pp. 133–136.

Smith, A. M., G. L. Holck, and H. B. Spafford. 1966. Re-evaluation of nutrient allowances for high-producing cows. Calcium, phosphorus, and vitamin D. J. Dairy Sci. 49:239–246.

Smith, K. L., J. H. Harrison, D. D. Hancock, D. A. Todhunter, and H. R. Conrad. 1984. Effect of vitamin E and selenium supplementation on incidence of clinical mastitis and duration of clinical symptoms. J. Dairy Sci. 67:1293–1300.

Smith, R. M. 1986. Effects of long-term, low-level oral cadmium on performance, blood parameters, and tissue and milk mineral concentrations of dairy cattle through first gestation and subsequent lactation. Ph.D. dissertation. Pennsylvania State University.

Smith, R. M. 1987. Cobalt. in Trace Elements in Human Health and Disease, Vol. 1, W. Mertz, ed. San Diego: Academic Press.

Smith, R. M. 1997. Cobalt. Pp. 357–387 in Handbook of Nutritionally Essential Mineral Elements, B. O'Dell and R. Sunde, eds. New York: Marcel Dekker, Inc.

Smith, R. M., and H. R. Marston. 1970. Production, absorption, distribution, and excretion of vitamin $B_{12}$ in sheep. Br. J. Nutr. 24:857–877.

Smith, S. E., and J. K. Loosli. 1957. Cobalt and vitamin $B_{12}$ in ruminant nutrition: A review. J. Dairy Sci. 40:1215–1220.

Smith, S. E., F. W. Lengemann, and J. T. Reid. 1953. Block vs. loose salt consumption by dairy cattle. J. Dairy Sci. 36:762–765.

Soares, J. 1995a. Calcium bioavailability. Pp. 95–113 in Bioavailability of Nutrients for Animals. C. B. Ammerman, D. H. Baker, and A. J. Lewis, eds. New York: Academic Press, Inc.

Soares, J. H. 1995b. Phosphorus bioavailability. Pp. 257–294 in Bioavailability of Nutrients for Animals. C. B. Ammerman, D. H. Baker, and A. J. Lewis, eds. New York: Academic Press, Inc.

Solomons, N. W. 1986. Competitive interaction of iron and zinc in the diet: Consequences for human nutrition. J. Nutr. 116:927–935.

Somers, G. F. 1973. The affinity of onion cell walls for calcium ions. Am. J. Bo. 60:987–990.

Sorensen, P. 1962. Studies of thyroid function in cattle and pigs. Pg. 455 in Use of Radioisotopes in Animal Biology and Medical Sciences, Vol. 1. New York: Academic Press.

Spears, J. 1984. Nickel as a "new trace element" in the nutrition of domestic animals. J. Anim. Sci. 59:823–835.

Spears, J. W., and E. E. Hatfield. 1978. Nickel depletion in the growing bovine. Nutr. Rep. Int. 18:621–629.

Spears, J. W., D. G. Ely, L. P. Bush, and R. C. Buckner. 1976. Sulfur supplementation and in vitro digestion of forage cellulose by rumen microorganisms. J. Anim. Sci. 43:513–517.

Sperber, I., and S. Hyden. 1952. Transport of chloride through the ruminal mucosa. Nature. 169:587–593.

Spiekers, H., R. Bintrup, M. Balmelli, and E. Pfeffer. 1993. Influence of dry matter intake on faecal phosphorus losses in dairy cows fed rations low in phosphorus. J. Anim. Physiol. Anim. Nutr. 69:37–43.

Stabel J. R., J. W. Spears, and T. T. Brown Jr. 1993. Effect of copper deficiency on tissue, blood characteristics, and immune function of calves challenged with infectious bovine rhinotracheitis virus and Pasteurella hemolytica. J Anim Sci. 71:1247–55.

Stephen, R. C., D. J. Saville, and J. H. Watkinson. 1989. The effects of sodium selenate applications on growth and selenium concentration in wheat. N.Z. J. Crop Hort. Sci. 17:229.

Stevens, B. J., L. J. Bush, J. D. Stout, and E. I. Williams. 1971. Effects of varying amounts of calcium and phosphorus in rations for dairy cows. J. Dairy Sci. 54:655–661.

Stewart, P. A. 1981. How to understand acid-base: A quantitative acid-base primer for biology and medicine. New York: Elsevier North Holland, Inc.

Storry, J. E. 1961. Studies on calcium and magnesium in the alimentary tract of sheep. II. The effect of reducing the acidity of abomasal digesta in vitro on the distribution of calcium and magnesium. J. Ag. Sci. (Camb.) 57:103–105.

Storry, J. E., and J. A. F. Rook. 1963. Magnesium metabolism in the dairy cow. V. Experimental observations with a purified diet low in magnesium. J. Agric. Sci. 61:167.

Stowe, H. D., and T. H. Herdt. 1992. Clinical assessment of selenium status of livestock. J. Anim. Sci. 70:3928–3933.

Stuart, S. M., S. M. Ketelsen, C. M. Weaver, and J.W. Erdman , Jr. 1986. Bioavailability of zinc to rats as affected by protein source and previous dietary intake. J. Nutr. 116:1423–1431.

Stuedemann, J. A., S. R. Wilkinson, and R. S. Lowrey. 1984. Efficacy of a large magnesium alloy rumen bolus in the prevention of hypomagnesemic tetany in cows. Am. J. Vet. Res. 45:698–702.

Suttle, N. F. 1991. The interactions between copper, molybdenum and sulphur in ruminant nutrition. Annual Review of Nutrition 11:121–140.

Suttle, N. F. 1979. Copper, iron, manganese and zinc concentrations in the carcasses of lambs and calves and the relationship to trace elements required for growth. Br. J. Nutr. 42:89–96.

Suttle, N. F. 1975. Effects of age and weaning on the apparent availability of dietary copper to young lambs. J. Agric. Sci. 84:255–261.

Suttle, N. F., and M. McLauchlin. 1976. Predicting the effects of dietary molybdenum and sulphur on the availability of copper to ruminants. Proc. Nutr. Soc. 35:22A–23A.

Tanaka, Y., and H. F. DeLuca. 1973. The control of 25-hydroxyvitamin D metabolism by inorganic phosphorus. Arch. Biochem. Biophys. 154:566–574.

Taylor, C., J. Bacon, P. Aggett, and I. Bremner. 1991. Homeostatic regulation of zinc absorption and endogenous losses in zinc-deprived men. Am. J. Clin. Nutr. 53:755–763.

Teh, T. H., R. W. Hemken, and L. S. Bull. 1982. Evaluation of urea ammonium polyphosphate as a phosphorus source for dairy calves. J. Anim. Sci. 55:174–179.

Thomas, W. E., J. K. Loosli, H. H. Williams, and L. A. Maynard. 1951. The utilization of inorganic sulfates and urea nitrogen by lambs. J. Nutr. 43:515–523.

Thurston, H., G. R. Glimore, and J. D. Swales. 1972. Aluminum retention and toxicity in chronic renal failure. The Lancet. 1:881–883.

Tillman, A. D., and J. R. Brethour. 1958. Dicalcium phosphate and phosphoric acid as phosphorus sources for beef cattle. J. Anim. Sci. 17:100–103.

Todd, J. R. 1984. Mineral, trace element and vitamin allowances for ruminant livestock. MAFF, DAFS, DANI, UKASTA, BVA working party report. Pp. 113–133 in Recent Advances in Animal Nutrition, W. Haresign, and D. J. A. Cole, eds. London: Butterworths.

Toepfer, E., W. Mertz, M. Polansky, E. Roginski, and W. Wolf. 1977. Preparation of chromium-containing material of glucose tolerance factor activity from brewer's yeast extracts and by synthesis. J. Ag. Food Chem. 25:162–166.

Tucker, W. B., G. A. Harrison, and R. W. Hemken. 1988. Influence of dietary cation-anion balance on milk, blood, urine, and rumen fluid in lactating dairy cattle. J. Dairy Sci. 71:346–354.

Tucker, W. B., J. A. Jackson, D. M. Hopkins, and J. F. Hogue. 1991. Influence of dietary sodium bicarbonate on the potassium metabolism of growing calves. J. Dairy Sci. 74:2296–2302.

Ulvund, M. J. 1985. Chronic poisoning in a lamb grazing Phalaris arundinacea. Acta Vet. Scand. 26:286–288.

Underwood, E. 1977a. Chromium. Pp. 258–270 in Trace Elements in Human and Animal Nutrition, E. J. Underwood, ed. New York: Academic Press.

Underwood, E. J. 1977b. Trace Elements in Human and Animal Nutrition. Fourth ed. New York: Academic Press.

Underwood, E. J. 1981. The Mineral Nutrition of Livestock. 2nd Ed. Slough, England: Commonwealth Agricultural Bureaux.

Underwood, E. J. and N. F. Suttle. 1999. Copper. In The Mineral Nutrition of Livestock, 3rd edition. CABI Publishing, New York. pp. 283–342.
Vagg, M. J. 1976. Assessment of trace element metabolism in farm animals. Pro. Roy. Soc. Med. 69:473–474.
Valdivia, R., C. B. Ammerman, C. J. Wilcox, and P. R. Henry. 1978. Effect of dietary aluminum on animal performance and tissue mineral levels in growing steers. J. Anim. Sci. 47:1351–1356.
Van Bruwaene, R., G. B. Gerber, R. Kirchmann, J. Colard, and J. van Kerkom. 1984 Metabolism of $^{51}Cr$, $^{54}Mn$, $^{59}Fe$ and $^{60}Co$ in lactating dairy cows. Health Phys. 46:1069–1082.
Van Bruwaene, R., G. B. Gerber, R. Kirchmann, and J. Colard. 1982. Transfer and distribution of radioactive cadmium in dairy cows. Intern. J. Environ. Stud 19:47–51.
Van Campen, D. R. 1969. Copper interference with intestinal absorption of Zn-65 by rats J. Nutr. 97:104–108.
Van Dael, P., G. Vlaemynck, R. V. Renterghem, and H. Deelstra. 1991. Selenium content of cow's milk and its distribution in protein fractions. Z Lebensm Unters Forsch 192:422–426.
Van Leeuwen, J. M. 1970. Physiological aspects of the supplementation of sodium chloride in rations with low and normal sodium contents. Keukenzout in de Rundveevoeding. Versl. Landbouwkd. Onderz. 737. Instituut voor Veevoedingsonderzoek "Hoorn."
van Mosel, M., T. van't Klooster, and A. Malestein. 1990. Effects of an inadequate dietary intake of magnesium on osteogenesis in dairy cows during the dry period. Research in Veterinary Science 48:280–287.
Van Saun, R. J., T. H. Herdt, and H. D. Stowe. 1989. Maternal and fetal selenium concentrations and their interrelationships in dairy cattle. J. Nutr. 119:1128–1137.
Van Soest, P. J., and L. H. P. Jones. 1968. Effect of silica in forages upon digestibility. J. Dairy Sci. 51:1644–1649.
van't Klooster, A. T. 1976. Adaptation of calcium absorption from the small intestine of dairy cows to changes in the dietary calcium intake and at the onset of lactation. Zeitschrift fuer Tierphysiology. 37:169–182.
Visek, W. J., R. A. Monroe, E. W. Swanson, and C. L. Comar. 1953. Determination of endogenous fecal calcium in cattle by a simple isotope dilution method. J. Nutr. 50:23–33.
Wan-Zahari, M., J. K. Thompson, D. Scott, and W. Buchan. 1990. The dietary requirements of calcium and phosphorus for growing lambs. Anim. Prod. 50 301–308.
Ward, G. M. 1966a. Oral potassium chloride fatal to a cow. JAVMA. 148:543–544.
Ward, G. M. 1966b. Potassium metabolism of domestic ruminants. A review. J. Dairy Sci. 49:268–276.
Ward, J. D., and J. W. Spears. 1993. Comparison of copper lysine and copper sulfate as copper sources for ruminants using in vitro methods. J. Dairy Sci. 76:2994–2998.
Ward, G., L. H. Harbers, and J. J. Blaha. 1979. Calcium-containing crystals in alfalfa: Their fate in cattle. J. Dairy Sci. 62:715–722.
Ward, G., R. C. Dobson, and J. R. Dunham. 1972. Influences of calcium and phosphorus intakes, vitamin D supplement, and lactation on calcium and phosphorus balances. J. Dairy Sci. 55:768–776.
Wasserman, R. H. 1981. Intestinal absorption of calcium and phosphorus. Fed. Proc. 40:68–72.
Wasserman, R. H., and A. N. Taylor. 1976. Gastrointestinal absorption of calcium and phosphorus. Pp. 137–155 in Handbook of Physiology. Sect. 7: Endocrinology. Vol. VII, Parathyroid Gland. G. D. Aubach, ed. Washington, D.C.: Am. Physiol. Soc.
Weeth, H. J., and J. E. Hunter. 1971. Drinking of sulfate-water by cattle. J. Anim. Sci. 32:277–281.
Weeth, H. J., and L. H. Haverland. 1961. Tolerance of growing cattle for drinking water containing sodium chloride. J. Anim. Sci. 20:518–521.
Weeth, H. J., L. H. Haverland, and D. W. Cassard. 1960. Consumption of sodium chloride water by heifers. J. Anim. Sci. 19:845–851.
Weil, A. B., W. B. Tucker, and R. W. Hemken. 1988. Potassium requirement of dairy calves. J. Dairy Sci. 71:1868–1872.
West, J. W., B. G. Mullinix, and T. G. Sandifer. 1991. Changing dietary electrolyte balance for dairy cows in cool and hot environments. J. Dairy Sci. 74:1662–1674.
West, J. W., C. E. Coppock, K. Z. Milam, D. H. Nave, J. M. LaBore, and L. D. Rowe, Jr. 1987. Potassium carbonate as a potassium source and dietary buffer for lactating Holstein cows during hot weather. J. Dairy Sci. 70:309–320.
West, J. W., K. D. Haydon, B. G. Mullinix, and T. G. Sandifer. 1992. Dietary cation-anion balance and cation source effects on production and acid-base status of heat-stressed cows. J. Dairy Sci. 75:2776–2786.
White, C. L., T. K. Cadwalader, W. G. Hoekstra, and A. L. Pope. 1989. The metabolism of $^{75}Se$-selenomethionine in sheep given supplementary copper and molybdenum. J. Anim. Sci. 67:2400–2408.
White, F., M. W. Neathery, R. P. Gentry, W. J. Miller, Logner. K. R., and Blackmon. D. M. 1985. The effects of different levels of dietary lead on zinc metabolism in dairy calves. J. Dairy Sci. 68:1215–1225.
Williams, D. L. 1973. Biological value of vanadium for rats, chickens, and sheep. Ph.D., Purdue University.
Wise, M. B., S. E. Smith, and L. L. Barnes. 1958. The phosphorus requirement of calves. J. Anim. Sci. 17:89–99.
Wittenberg, K. M., R. J. Boila, and M. A. Shariff. 1990. Comparison of copper sulfate and copper proteinate as copper sources for copper-depleated steers fed high molybdenum diets. Can. J. Anim. Sci. 70:895.
Wollenberg, P., and W. Rummel. 1987. Dependence of intestinal iron absorption on the valency state of iron. Naunyn Schmiedebergs Arch. Pharmacol. 336:578–582.
Wright, F., J. Palmer, J. Riner, M. Haufler, J. Miller, and C. McBeth. 1977. Effects of feeding on organocadmium to cattle and sheep. J. Ag. Food Chem. 25:293–297.
Wu, Z., and L. D. Satter. 2000. Milk production and reproductive performance of dairy cows fed two concentrations of phosphorus for two years. J. Dairy Sci. 83:1052–1063.
Wu, Z., L. D. Satter, and R. Sojo. 2000. Milk production, reproductive performance, and fecal excretion of phosphorus by dairy cows fed three amounts of phosphorus. J. Dairy Sci. 83:1028–1041.
Xin Z., D. F. Waterman, R. W. Hemken, and R. J. Harmon. 1993. Copper status and requirement during the dry period and early lactation in multiparous Holstein cows. J. Dairy Sci. 76:2711–6.
Xin Z., D. F. Waterman, R. W. Hemken, and R. J. Harmon. 1991. Effects of copper status on neutrophil function, superoxide dismutase, and copper distribution in steers. J. Dairy Sci. 74:3078–85.
Xin, Z., D. F. Waterman, R. W. Hemken, R. J. Harmon, and J. A. Jackson. 1991. Effects of copper sources and dietary cation-anion balance on copper availability and acid-base status in dairy calves. J. Dairy Sci. 74:3167–3173.
Yang, W., D. Mowat, A. Subiyatno, and R. Liptrap. 1996. Effects of chromium supplementation on early-lactation performance of Holstein cows. Can. J. Anim. Sci. 76:221–230.
Yeh, J. Y., Q. P. Gu, M. A. Beilstein, N. E. Forsberg, and P. D. Whanger. 1997. Selenium influences tissue levels of selenoprotein W in sheep. J. Nutr. 127:394–402.
Young, R. 1979. Cobalt in biology and biochemistry. London: Academic Press.

# 7 Vitamins

Vitamins are classified as either fat-soluble or water-soluble. Vitamins A, D, E, and K are fat-soluble and the B-vitamins and vitamin C are water-soluble. Vitamins have diverse functions including involvement in many metabolic pathways, immune cell function, and gene regulation. A clinical deficiency of a vitamin results in a specific deficiency disease such as rickets when vitamin D is deficient. Subclinical deficiencies may occur in which clinical signs of the deficiency are not evident but performance or overall animal health is less than optimal.

## FAT-SOLUBLE VITAMINS

Dairy cattle require vitamins A, D, E, and K; however, vitamins A and E are the only ones with an absolute dietary requirement. Vitamin K is synthesized by ruminal and intestinal bacteria. Vitamin D is synthesized by ultraviolet radiation of the skin. Many natural feedstuffs contain vitamin A precursors and vitamin E, and under certain situations these will not need to be supplemented. However, relying solely on vitamins contained within feedstuffs and on synthesis of vitamin D via exposure to sunlight has risk because of the large variability in vitamin concentrations in feeds and exposure to sunlight. As management systems for dairy cattle trend toward more confinement with less exposure to sunlight and fresh forages, there is an increased need to add supplemental sources of vitamins A, D, and E.

### *Vitamin A*

#### SOURCES

Vitamin A activity is defined in retinol equivalents. An IU of vitamin A corresponds to 0.3 μg of all-*trans* retinol (0.344 μg of all-*trans* retinyl acetate or 0.550 μg of all-*trans* palmitate). Retinol is not found in plants, but many feeds contain β-carotene (provitamin A). Other carotenoids can be converted to vitamin A by animals, but conversion efficiency appears to be poor and most common feeds do not contain substantial amounts of those carotenoids. Most of the β-carotene in plants is found in vegetative material; therefore, forages can contain substantial amounts of β-carotene but most grains and grain byproducts are practically void of β-carotene (corn gluten meal contains moderate concentrations of β-carotene). Beta-carotene concentrations decrease as forages mature (Park et al., 1983). Beta-carotene is easily oxidized and once plants are cut, concentrations decrease quickly so that stored forages (silage and hay) have significantly lower concentrations of β-carotene than do fresh forage (Bruhn and Oliver, 1978; Park et al., 1983). The length of time forages are stored is negatively correlated with β-carotene concentrations (Bruhn and Oliver, 1978). Even when known sources of variation are considered, the β-carotene concentrations in feedstuffs are highly variable.

The common forms of supplemental vitamin A used in the United States are all-*trans* retinyl acetate and all-*trans* retinyl palmitate. When these forms of vitamin A are stored properly, vitamin A activity is relatively stable with losses of about 1 percent/month. When these retinyl esters are stored in combination with minerals or other feedstuffs or are pelleted, storage losses increase to 5 to 9 percent/month (Coelho, 1991).

#### BIOAVAILABILITY

Studies on the bioavailability of various forms of vitamin A and β-carotene for dairy cattle are extremely limited. Bioavailability of vitamin A is dependent upon the degree of ruminal destruction and on absorption efficiency by the small intestine. In addition to those factors, the bioavailability of β-carotene also depends on the efficiency of converting it to retinol. Beta-carotene is converted to retinol by enzymes located in intestinal mucosal cells. Dairy cattle also absorb and store β-carotene. Blood and milk of Guernsey and Jersey cattle contain more β-carotene than that from other breeds because they are either more efficient at absorbing β-carotene or less efficient at converting β-carotene to retinol. The vitamin A activity of β-carotene for cattle is defined as 1 mg of β-carotene = 400 IU of vitamin A (equivalent to 120 μg of retinol), and is much lower for cattle than for rats (1 mg β-carotene = 1800 IU of vitamin A). The defined activity of β-carotene for cattle is based largely on experiments using lambs fed corn silage (Martin et al., 1968).

Ruminal destruction of vitamin A can be extensive. Approximately 60 percent of supplemental vitamin A was destroyed in the rumen of steers fed hay and corn grain diets (Warner et al., 1970). Similar values have been obtained using in vitro rumen systems (Rode et al., 1990; Weiss et al., 1995). In vitro data suggest that ruminal destruction of vitamin A was approximately 20 percent when cattle were fed high forage diets, but it increased to about 70 percent when cattle were fed diets with 50 to 70 percent concentrate. Limited studies with β-carotene suggest that between 0 and 35 percent of dietary β-carotene is destroyed in the rumen (Potanski et al., 1974). Essentially no reliable data are available on the intestinal absorption of retinyl esters in cattle. Data collected from humans and rats suggest 20 to 60 percent of dietary retinyl esters are absorbed (Blomhoff et al., 1991). Absorption in those species is dependent on the amount and type of dietary fat. Apparent digestibility of β-carotene from a variety of forages averaged 77 percent in dairy steers (Wing, 1969), but Cohen-Fernandez et al. (1976) reported that fecal recovery (indigestibility) of radiolabeled β-carotene was about 90 percent in sheep.

### FUNCTIONS AND ANIMAL RESPONSES

Vitamin A (retinaldehyde) is necessary for the production of rhodopsin (a vision pigment) that is necessary for low light vision. Vitamin A also is needed for normal growth and development (including fetal growth), spermatogenesis, and for maintenance of skeletal tissue and epithelial tissue. Abortions, increased prevalence of retained fetal membranes, and increased calf morbidity and mortality are indicators of vitamin A deficiency in gestating cows. Ross and Ternus (1993) reported that retinoic acid indirectly regulates gene expression which may explain the many diverse functions of vitamin A. Vitamin A also increases disease resistance and has stimulatory effects on cell-mediated immunity (Chew, 1987; Bendich, 1993). A deficiency of vitamin A often results in increased prevalence of infectious diseases. Beta-carotene, independent of its provitamin A function, is an antioxidant and can enhance the killing ability of neutrophils (Chew, 1993). In some (Chew, 1987) but not all (Michal et al., 1994) studies, supplementing between 150,000 and 250,000 IU/day of vitamin A or feeding 300 to 600 mg of β-carotene/day reduced the incidence of intramammary gland infections and mastitis. These studies were conducted with cows at dry-off or peripartum cows.

Vitamin A is clearly needed for good reproduction and some data suggests that β-carotene also may be involved with reproduction. In a review, Hurley and Doane (1989) reported that supplemental β-carotene (usually at 300 to 400 mg/day) improved some measure of reproductive efficiency in 12 of 22 studies. When studies conducted only in North America were summarized, β-carotene had no effect on reproduction in 4 of 5 studies.

### FACTORS THAT AFFECT REQUIREMENTS

Since the actual β-carotene content of diets is highly variable and almost never known in commercial situations, the vitamin A requirements presented in this publication are for supplemental vitamin A, not total dietary vitamin A. Fresh forage (e.g., pasture) has relatively high concentrations of β-carotene. Therefore the amount of supplemental vitamin A needed when fresh forage is fed will be less than for cattle consuming conserved forages. The requirements presented below assume conserved forages are fed and are probably in excess of requirements for grazing cattle.

Based on a reevaluation of older data, the vitamin A requirement for growing dairy animals was increased to 80 IU/kg of body weight (BW). In the previous *Nutrient Requirements of Dairy Cattle* (National Research Council, 1989), the requirement for vitamin A of growing dairy animals was 42 IU/kg of BW. That requirement for growing cattle was based on the amount of vitamin A needed to maintain cerebrospinal fluid pressure below 120 mm Hg in calves (Rousseau et al., 1954). Other data (Rousseau et al., 1954; Eaton et al., 1972) using different criteria (i.e., a statistically significant increase in cerebrospinal fluid pressure or the presence of papillary edema of the eye) suggests that the vitamin A requirement for growing dairy animals was between 60 and 100 IU/kg of BW. The subcommittee decided that rather than discounting these studies, a compromise using all the data was appropriate.

The vitamin A requirement for adult dairy cattle has been increased to 110 IU/kg of BW. In *Nutrient Requirements of Dairy Cattle* (National Research Council, 1989), the vitamin A requirement for adult animals (76 IU/kg of BW) was based largely on a long-term reproduction study (Ronning et al., 1959). The sole source of vitamin A in that study was β-carotene, and cows were fed low concentrate diets. The previous requirement (National Research Council, 1989) also was based on data from a study (Swanson et al., 1968) that indicated the amount of vitamin A deemed adequate by Ronning et al. (1959) was adequate to maintain milk production. In that study, cows produced approximately 3500 kg of milk during a 40-week lactation. Mean milk production is currently about twice as high and many herds have mean milk production that is more than four times higher. Furthermore, in a more recent study, milk production increased from about 35 kg/day to 40 kg/day when cows in early lactation were fed diets that provided approximately 280 IU of vitamin A/kg of BW compared with cows fed approximately 75 IU/kg of BW (Oldham et al., 1991). The new requirement for lactating cows (110 IU/kg of BW) was based on data used by the previous *Nutrient Requirements of Dairy Cattle* (National Research Council, 1989) and on data showing that the bioavailability of vitamin A (retinyl esters) may be as much as 50 percent less than that of β-carotene when fed in high concentrate diets because of ruminal destruction. Dry cows are typically fed diets with lower amounts of concentrate and bioavailability of vitamin A should be higher than for lactating cows. The previous National Research Council requirement for dry cows (76 IU/kg of BW) may be adequate, but in light of potential improvements in mammary gland health and data showing increased milk production after dry cows were supplemented with vitamin A in amounts greater than National Research Council (1989) requirements, the vitamin A requirement for dry cows was kept the same as that for lactating cows (110 IU/kg of BW).

Presently available data are not adequate to define a specific requirement for β-carotene for any class of dairy cattle. Conditions that may warrant additional supplementation of vitamin A include:

- low forage diets (more ruminal destruction and less consumption of β-carotene);
- diets that contain larger amounts of corn silage and smaller amounts of haycrops (lower concentrations of β-carotene and potentially lower bioavailability of basal β-carotene);
- diets that contain lower quality forages (lower basal concentrations of β-carotene);
- increased exposure to infectious pathogens (increased demands on the immune system); and
- times when immunocompetence maybe reduced (peripartum period).

Vitamin A toxicosis should not be a problem under most practical situations. The presumed safe limit for vitamin A is 66,000 IU/kg of diet for both lactating and nonlactating cattle (National Research Council, 1987).

### *Vitamin D*

#### PHYSIOLOGY

Vitamin D is a pro-hormone, a necessary precursor for the production of the calcium regulating hormone 1,25-dihydroxyvitamin D. Vitamin D can be produced within the skin of most mammals, including cattle, as a result of the photochemical conversion of 7-dehydrocholesterol to vitamin $D_3$. In plants, ultraviolet irradiation causes photochemical conversion of ergosterol to vitamin $D_2$. Vitamin D, supplied by the skin or the diet, is rapidly transported to and sequestered by the liver. The rapid removal of vitamin D from circulation prevents concentrations of vitamin D in blood from becoming very high; the normal concentration is 1 to 2 ng vitamin D/ml plasma (Horst and Littledike, 1982). Within the liver, vitamin D can be converted to 25-hydroxyvitamin D by vitamin D 25-hydroxylase and released into the blood. The production of 25-hydroxyvitamin D within the liver is dependent on the vitamin D content of the diet. Thus plasma 25-hydroxyvitamin D concentration is the best indicator of vitamin D status of an animal (Horst et al., 1994).

The 25-hydroxyvitamin D then circulates to the kidney where it can be converted to the hormone 1,25-dihydroxyvitamin D. This hormone acts to increase the active transport of calcium and phosphorus across the intestinal epithelial cells, and potentiates the action of parathyroid hormone to increase bone calcium resorption. Both functions are vital for calcium and phosphorus homeostasis. In addition to calcium and phosphorus homeostasis, 1,25-dihydroxyvitamin D is involved in maintaining immune function (Reinhardt and Hustmyer, 1987); generally it promotes $Th_2$ (humoral) immunity while inhibiting $Th_1$ (cell mediated) immunity (Daynes et al., 1995).

Renal production of 1,25-dihydroxyvitamin D is tightly regulated. The 25-hydroxyvitamin D-1-α-hydroxylase activity of the kidney is stimulated by parathyroid hormone, which is released in response to declining concentrations of calcium in blood (DeLuca, 1979). In the absence of parathyroid hormone, when an animal is in positive Ca balance, 25-hydroxyvitamin D can be hydroxylated in the kidney to 24,25-dihydroxyvitamin D as a primary step in the inactivation and catabolism of vitamin D. The vitamin D catabolic enzymes also function to deactivate 1,25-dihydroxyvitamin D. These catabolic enzymes exist in tissues throughout the body. In these tissues the catabolic pathway is generally stimulated by 1,25-dihydroxyvitamin D as a negative feedback to reduce high concentrations of 1,25-dihydroxyvitamin D in plasma (Goff et al., 1992; Reinhardt and Horst, 1989).

A low concentration of phosphorus in blood also can enhance renal production of 1,25-dihydroxyvitamin D, even when the concentration of calcium in plasma is normal or above normal (Tanaka and DeLuca, 1973; Gray and Napoli, 1983). Also, higher than normal concentrations of phosphorus in blood can inhibit renal production of 1,25-dihydroxyvitamin D, which can be a factor contributing to milk fever in the periparturient cow (Barton et al., 1987). Pharmacologic doses of vitamin D have been utilized with limited success to prevent milk fever. This is discussed in the section on milk fever (Chapter 9).

Vitamin $D_2$, the form associated with plants, and vitamin $D_3$, the form associated with vertebrates are both used for supplementation of diets. The biologic activity of the two forms is generally considered equal in cattle; however Horst and Littledike (1982) demonstrated an apparent discrimination against the vitamin $D_2$ form in cattle. Presumably this discrimination is the result of reduced binding of vitamin $D_2$ metabolites to vitamin D-binding proteins in blood leading to more rapid clearance of vitamin $D_2$ metabolites from plasma. However, the subcommittee does not recommend adjusting the vitamin D requirement based on the form of vitamin D used as a supplement.

Vitamin D deficiency reduces the ability to maintain calcium and phosphorus homeostasis, resulting in a decline for phosphorus and less often a decrease for calcium in plasma. This eventually causes rickets in young animals and osteomalacia in adults; both are bone diseases in which the primary lesion is failure to mineralize the organic matrix of bone. In young animals rickets causes enlarged and painful joints; the costochondral joints of the ribs are often readily palpated. In adults, lameness and pelvic fracture are a common sequelae of vitamin D deficiency.

### REQUIREMENT

The amount of dietary vitamin D required to provide adequate substrate for production of 1,25-dihydroxyvitamin D is difficult to define. Animals exposed to sunlight at the lower latitudes may not require any dietary vitamin D. Sun-cured hay also may provide enough vitamin D to prevent symptoms of vitamin D deficiency (Thomas and Moore, 1951).

The movement away from pasture feeding systems and toward confinement and feeding of stored feeds and by-products has increased the need for dietary supplementation of vitamin D for dairy cows. As a general rule, the contribution of sunlight and forage to the supply of vitamin D for the cow is not considered when describing the vitamin D requirement. The vitamin D requirement in this publication will consider the "requirement" to be the amount of supplemental vitamin D that should be added to the diet.

Horst et al. (1994) determined that plasma 25-hydroxyvitamin D concentrations below 5 ng/ml are indicative of vitamin D deficiency and concentrations of 200 to 300 ng/ml would indicate vitamin D toxicosis. Normal cows have concentrations of 25-hydroxyvitamin D in plasma between 20 and 50 ng/ml.

Dry, pregnant cows housed indoors and fed a corn silage based diet had plasma concentrations of 25-hydroxyvitamin D in plasma of 19 ng/ml at 14 days prior to parturition and 10.5 ng/ml at 35 days into lactation. Supplementation of the diet with 5,000 (7.5 IU vitamin D/kg BW) or 10,000 IU vitamin D (15 IU vitamin D/kg BW) maintained plasma concentrations between 25 and 31 ng/ml throughout the dry period and early lactation (Vinet et al., 1985).

Ward et al. (1971) reported that cows fed an alfalfa hay-concentrate diet receiving 300,000 IU vitamin $D_3$ once each week ($\approx$ 43,000 IU/day) returned to estrus 16 days earlier than cows given no supplement. Ward et al. (1972) also demonstrated that cows receiving 300,000 IU vitamin $D_3$/week had improved absorption of dietary calcium. Hibbs and Conrad (1983) summarized the results of several Ohio State University trials and concluded that cows supplemented with 40,000 IU vitamin $D_2$/day (50 to 70 IU vitamin D/kg BW) produced more milk and generally ate more than cows fed the same diets with no vitamin D supplementation or supplemented with 80,000 or more IU vitamin D/day. Reduced milk production, which could be interpreted as the beginning of vitamin D intoxicosis, was observed when cows were fed 80,000 IU vitamin D/day (120–140 IU/kg BW).

McDermott et al. (1985) fed an orchard grass-corn silage based ration supplemented with 0, 10,000, 50,000, or 250,000 IU vitamin $D_3$/day to Holstein cows in late gestation and for the first 12 weeks of lactation. Cows had no access to sunlight from 2 weeks before calving until 4 days postpartum. Thereafter they were outside and exposed to sunlight 1 to 2 h/day. Plasma 25-hydroxyvitamin D concentrations in unsupplemented cows were below 20 ng/ml during late gestation and the first 4 weeks of lactation. Plasma 25-hydroxyvitamin D concentrations in cows receiving 10,000 or 50,000 IU vitamin $D_3$/day (16–80 IU/kg) were similar (between 30 and 45 ng 25-hydroxyvitamin D/ml). Cows receiving 250,000 IU vitamin D/day had elevated plasma 25-hydroxyvitamin D concentrations (60–80 ng/ml). The rapid changes in plasma concentrations of 25-hydroxyvitamin D, 24,25-dihydroxyvitamin D, and vitamin D suggested that at 250,000 IU/day the capacity of the liver to store vitamin D had been exceeded, which was interpreted as excessive vitamin D supplementation though no outward clinical signs of vitamin D intoxication were noted.

Under most circumstances 10,000 IU/day (16 IU vitamin D/kg BW) should provide adequate vitamin D for dairy cows during late gestation. Astrup and Nedkvitne (1987) reported that lactating cows producing about 20 kg of milk/day required about 10 IU vitamin D/kg body weight to maintain normal concentrations of calcium and phosphorus in blood. These studies were conducted in Norway in winter and spring when effective sunlight exposure should have been minimal.

The 1989 *Nutrient Requirements of Dairy Cattle* (National Research Council, 1989) requirement for vitamin D for adult dairy cows was set at 30 IU/kg body weight. This is more vitamin D than many studies suggest is necessary for maintenance of normal plasma concentrations of 25-hydroxyvitamin D (17 IU/kg BW) (McDermott et al.,

1985) or calcium and phosphorus (10 IU/kg BW) (Astrup and Nedkvitne, 1987) in plasma. However, Ward et al. (1971, 1972) and Hibbs and Conrad (1983) suggested that milk production and reproductive and health benefits were potentially improved when diets were supplemented with as much as 70 IU/kg BW. Based on all available data, the requirement of 30 IU/kg BW established previously (National Research Council, 1989) seems justified.

TOXICITY

The maximum tolerable amount of vitamin D is inversely related to dietary concentrations of calcium and phosphorus. The studies of McDermott et al. (1985) suggest that 50,000 IU $D_3$/day (80 IU/kg BW) is well tolerated while 250,000 IU vitamin $D_3$/day (400 IU/kg BW) is not. Hibbs and Conrad (1983) reported a slight decline in milk production when cows were fed 80,000 IU $D_2$/day ($\approx$ 160 IU/kg BW). The 1987 National Research Council committee on vitamin tolerance of animals (National Research Council, 1987) suggested the maximal tolerable level of vitamin D is 2,200 IU/kg diet when fed for long periods (more than 60 days) and 25,000 IU/kg diet when fed for short periods of time. Vitamin D intoxication is associated with reduced feed intake, polyuria initially followed by anuria, dry feces, and reduced milk production. Upon necropsy calcification of kidneys, aorta, abomasum, and bronchioles is evident (Littledike and Horst, 1980).

Some of the dietary vitamin D is degraded in the rumen by bacteria to inactive metabolites (Sommerfeldt et al., 1983; Gardner et al., 1988). Injection of vitamin D avoids this problem; however, the maximal tolerable dose of parenterally administered vitamin D is at least 100-fold lower than the maximal tolerable oral dose and repeated injections can be especially toxic (Littledike and Horst, 1980).

## *Vitamin E*

SOURCES

Vitamin E is a generic name for a series of lipid-soluble compounds called tocopherols and tocotrienols. The most biologically active form of vitamin E is $\alpha$-tocopherol; it is also the most common form of vitamin E found in feedstuffs. Eight different stereoisomers of $\alpha$-tocopherol can exist, and the isomer that has the highest biologic activity is *RRR*-$\alpha$-tocopherol. The vitamin E content of feedstuffs is highly variable (coefficients of variation are often 50 percent). Depending on species and maturity (Tramontano et al., 1993; Jukola et al., 1996), fresh forage plants contain between 80 and 200 IU of vitamin E/kg of DM. Alpha-tocopherol concentrations in forages decrease quickly after the plant is cut; prolonged exposure to oxygen and sunlight exacerbates the loss in vitamin E activity (Thafvelin and Oksanen, 1966). Silage and hay contain 20 to 80 percent less $\alpha$-tocopherol than does fresh forage. In general, concentrations of vitamin E in concentrates are low; possible exceptions are raw whole soybeans and whole cottonseeds. Heat treatment of whole soybeans destroys essentially all the $\alpha$-tocopherol (Weiss, unpublished). Alpha-tocopherol concentrations in feeds generally decrease as storage time increases.

The commercial form of supplemental vitamin E usually fed to dairy cows is all-*rac*-$\alpha$-tocopheryl acetate (previously designated DL-$\alpha$-tocopheryl acetate). The esterified form of the vitamin is more stable than the alcohol form; expected losses in biologic activity from premixes containing all-*rac*-$\alpha$-tocopheryl acetate are less than 1 percent per month under most storage conditions, but extruded products containing all-*rac*-$\alpha$-tocopheryl acetate may have storage losses of 6 percent per month (Coelho, 1991). *RRR*-$\alpha$-tocopherol is available commercially but is not commonly fed to ruminants.

BIOAVAILABILITY

Early data (Alderson et al., 1971) suggested that significant amounts of supplemental vitamin E were destroyed in the rumen and that destruction increased as the amount of concentrate in the diet increased. More recent studies (Leedle et al., 1993; Weiss et al., 1995) found that vitamin E (all-*rac*-$\alpha$-tocopheryl acetate) was not destroyed during in vitro fermentation. The authors of these studies suggested that poor extraction of tocopherol from digesta was the reason early reports indicated that vitamin E was destroyed by ruminal fermentation. Based on the new data using better analytic techniques, ruminal metabolism of vitamin E appears minimal.

The USP defines 1 IU of vitamin as equal to 1 mg of all-*rac*-$\alpha$-tocopheryl acetate, and 1.49 IU of vitamin E is equal to 1 mg of *RRR*-$\alpha$-tocopherol. Those conversion factors are based largely on research with laboratory animals. Data from cows comparing bioavailability of various tocopherol stereoisomers is contradictory. Hidiroglou et al. (1988, 1989) reported no or only slight differences in concentrations of $\alpha$-tocopherol in plasma and tissue between cows and heifers fed similar IU amounts of vitamin E as all-*rac*-$\alpha$-tocopherol or all-*rac*-$\alpha$-tocopheryl acetate. Concentrations of $\alpha$-tocopherol in tissue and plasma were 20 to 60 percent higher in beef cows fed *RRR*-$\alpha$-tocopherol than those fed all-*rac*-$\alpha$-tocopheryl acetate (Hidiroglou et al., 1988). Based on that study 1 mg of *RRR*-$\alpha$-tocopherol would be equal to 1.8 to 2.4 IU of vitamin E. Different formulations of all-*rac*-$\alpha$-tocopheryl acetate (silica adsorbate, oil, or a microencapsulated form) did not greatly affect concentrations of $\alpha$-tocopherol in plasma suggesting equivalent bioavailability (Baldi et al., 1997). Insufficient consistent data are available currently to warrant changing IU conversion factors for vitamin E for ruminants. The current USP factors will be used for describing vitamin E requirements in this publication.

### FUNCTIONS AND ANIMAL RESPONSES

The best understood function of vitamin E is as a lipid-soluble cellular antioxidant (Hogan et al., 1993). Via this function and perhaps other functions, vitamin E is involved in maintenance of cellular membranes, arachadonic acid metabolism, immunity, and reproductive function.

White muscle disease is a classic sign of a clinical deficiency of vitamin E. White muscle disease was prevented in preweaned calves when 50 IU of vitamin E/day (all-*rac*-∝-tocopheryl acetate) were supplemented to a vitamin E-free diet based on skim milk (Blaxter et al., 1952). Presumably those data were used to formulate the vitamin E requirements for all classes of dairy cattle in the last *Nutrient Requirements of Dairy Cattle* (National Research Council, 1989). More recent experiments with vitamin E have focused on its relationship with reproductive disorders, mastitis and immune function.

Dietary or parenteral supplementation of vitamin E to dairy cows during the peripartum period has consistently improved the function of neutrophils and macrophages (Hogan et al., 1990, 1992; Politis et al., 1995, 1996). In those studies the amount of supplemental vitamin E fed per day during the prepartum period was either 1000 IU/day or 3000 IU/day. In three of those studies (Hogan et al., 1992; Politis et al., 1995, 1996) vitamin E also was injected (3000 or 6000 IU on approximately day 7 prepartum). During the postpartum phase, cows were fed either 500 or 3000 IU/day of supplemental vitamin E. Cows in all studies were fed stored forages.

Clinical studies have been conducted to evaluate the effect of supplemental vitamin E on prevalence of retained fetal membranes, intramammary infections, and clinical mastitis. Feeding approximately 1000 IU/day of supplemental vitamin E (usually all-*rac*-∝-tocopheryl acetate) to dry cows when adequate selenium was supplemented reduced the prevalence of retained fetal membranes in some (Harrison et al., 1984; Miller et al., 1993) but not all (Wichtel et al., 1996) studies. When vitamin E was injected (usually in combination with selenium) rather than fed, about half the time there was no effect for prevalence of retained fetal membranes and about half the time there was a positive response (Miller et al., 1993). The typical treatment was a single injection of approximately 700 IU of vitamin E and 50 mg of selenium given about 3 weeks before calving. Relative to the amount of vitamin E normally consumed, 700 IU of vitamin E over 21 days is trivial. Most likely, selenium, not vitamin E, was the nutrient responsible for the positive effect.

Two clinical studies conducted in Ohio (Smith et al., 1984; Hogan et al., 1993) reported that feeding supplemental vitamin E significantly reduced the incidence and duration of intramammary gland infections and clinical mastitis. In those studies, approximately 1000 IU/day of supplemental vitamin E was fed during the 60-day prepartum period and 500 IU/day was fed during lactation. Conversely, a study conducted in Canada (Batra et al., 1992) found that similar amounts of supplemental vitamin E did not reduce the incidence of clinical mastitis. Based on the concentrations of selenium in the plasma (<35 ng/ml), cows in that study (Batra et al., 1992) were deficient in selenium. Another study (Weiss et al., 1997) using diets low in total selenium (0.15 ppm) but with animals in better selenium status (plasma selenium >50 ng/ml) than cows in the Batra et al. (1992) study found that feeding 1000 IU/day of vitamin E during the dry period reduced clinical mastitis at calving by 30 percent but did not affect prevalence of intramammary gland infections. In that same study, feeding 4000 IU of supplemental vitamin E/day during the last 2 weeks of the dry period resulted in an 80 percent reduction in clinical mastitis at calving and a 60 percent reduction in intramammary gland infections (Weiss et al., 1997).

### REQUIREMENTS AND FACTORS THAT AFFECT REQUIREMENTS

The vitamin E requirement (15 IU/kg of DMI) in the previous *Nutrient Requirements of Dairy Cattle* (National Research Council, 1989) was for total, not supplemental, vitamin E and the basis for that requirement was not given. The previous vitamin E requirement should prevent classic signs of vitamin E deficiency. The vitamin E content of the basal diet is highly variable and will not be known in most situations; therefore, vitamin E requirements in this edition are presented for supplemental vitamin E. The requirements presented assume that cattle are consuming conserved forages. Because fresh forage is an excellent source of vitamin E the requirements for supplemental vitamin E for grazing cattle are probably substantially less than those presented for cattle fed conserved forages. Because titration studies are lacking, a specific requirement cannot be defined. The subcommittee concluded that there were adequate data available on the effect of vitamin E on mastitis and reproductive disorders to justify an increase in the vitamin E requirement. Based on health and immune function in cows, plasma concentrations of ∝-tocopherol in peripartum cows should be approximately 3 μg/ml (Weiss et al., 1994, 1997). To maintain these blood values, dry cows and heifers fed stored forages during the last 60 days of gestation require approximately 1.6 IU of supplemental vitamin E/kg of body weight (approximately 80 IU/kg of DMI). An additional benefit on calf health may be observed by increasing vitamin E intake by cows and heifers in late gestation. Only minor amounts of vitamin E can pass the placenta (Van Saun et al., 1989); hence newborn calves rely on colostrum for vitamin E. Increased intake of vitamin E during the prepartum period significantly elevates vitamin E in colostrum. For lactating cows, the recommended amount of vitamin E (supplemental) was changed to 0.8 IU/kg of body weight (approximately 20 IU/kg of DMI) when stored forages are fed. This recommendation is based on a reduction in mastitis. The difference between the recommendations for vitamin E for the two classes of cattle is mainly caused by expected differences in intake of vitamin E from basal feedstuffs and perhaps reduced absorption of vitamin E by cows fed conventional dry cow diets. Based on typical feed intakes and average vitamin E concentrations in feedstuffs, the recommended amount of total vitamin E (supplemental plus vitamin provided by feedstuffs) is approximately 2.6 IU/kg of body weight during late gestation and for lactating dairy cows. Of that amount, the basal diet will provide on average about 1.8 IU/kg of body weight for lactating cows (ranges from about 0.8 for cows fed diets based on severely weathered hay to about 2.8 IU/kg of body weight for cows fed diets based on pasture) and about 1 IU/kg body weight (ranges from 0.5 to about 2.3 IU/kg of body weight) for dry cows.

Although several factors are known to influence vitamin E requirements, limited data make quantifying the necessary adjustments difficult. The amount of supplemental vitamin E fed may need to be changed during the following situations:

- When fresh forage is fed there should be less need for supplemental vitamin E. A diet based on fresh forage (ca. 50 percent of dietary DM) would require about 67 percent less supplemental vitamin E to meet the cows requirements compared with a diet that contained a similar amount of stored forage. Requirements for supplemental vitamin E is reduced 67 percent in the accompanying software when animals are fed pasture.
- The amount of supplemental vitamin E probably should be increased when low forage diets are fed (forages typically have more vitamin E than do concentrates). The requirements listed above were generated from studies using diets with 50 to 60 percent forage (lactating cows) and 60 to 80 percent forage (animals in late gestation).
- Cows in suboptimal selenium status probably require more vitamin E.
- Milk is not a major excretion route for $\alpha$-tocopherol (0.4 to 0.6 $\mu$g/ml) but colostrum contains high concentrations of $\alpha$-tocopherol (3 to 6 $\mu$g/ml). Additional vitamin E may be useful during colostralgenesis.
- Intake of polyunsaturated fatty acids increases the vitamin E requirement of nonruminants. As methods for protecting fats from biohydrogenation in the rumen improve, additional vitamin E may be required when protected unsaturated fats are fed.
- Additional vitamin E may be useful during periods of immunosuppression (peripartum period).
- Large amounts of supplemental vitamin E (>1000 IU/day) can reduce oxidative flavors in milk (St.-Laurent et al., 1990).

#### TOXICITY

Vitamin E is one of the least toxic vitamins due in part to its relatively low absorption. Toxicity studies have not been conducted with ruminants but data from rats suggest an upper limit of approximately 75 IU/kg of body weight per day (National Research Council, 1987).

### *Vitamin K*

Vitamin K is a generic term used to describe a group of quinone compounds exhibiting antihemorrhagic effects. The basic form of vitamin K is 2-methyl-1,4-naphthoquinone. Isomers of vitamin K differ in the length and nature of the side chain (Frye et al., 1991). The three most common isomers or vitamers of K are: phylloquinone (vitamin $K_1$), menaquinones (vitamin $K_2$) and menadione (vitamin $K_3$). The phylloquinones are commonly found in the chloroplast of green plants and have side chains consisting of several isoprenoid units. Menaquinones are synthesized by bacteria flora and have isoprene side chains containing double bonds. Menadione (2-methyl-1,4-napthoquinone without a side chain) does not exist naturally. Menadione and its derivatives are the synthetic forms of vitamin K used in feed supplements (Combs, 1992).

Cattle require vitamin K for the synthesis of at least a dozen proteins. Among these are four blood clotting factors; prothrombin (factor II), and factors VII, IX and X. These vitamin K dependent protein factors are components of a complex system that functions to prevent hemorrhage by activation of thrombin and ultimately clot formation (Combs, 1992).

Because large quantities of menaquinones are synthesized by ruminal bacteria and ruminant diets generally contain green forages and/or pasture plants high in phylloquinones, a deficiency of vitamin K rarely occurs. The only reported deficiencies have occurred when moldy sweet clover hay was fed (National Research Council, 1989). Dicoumarol is a fungal metabolite produced from substances in sweet clover that inhibits the synthesis of clotting factors. Holstein calves were shown to develop dicoumarol toxicosis when fed sweet clover hay containing 18 mg/kg of dicoumarol for two weeks or longer (Yamini et al., 1995). Early signs of vitamin K deficiency include stiffness and/or lameness and hematoma of tissues. Prolonged feeding of dicoumarol leads to uncontrolled bleeding. Dicoumarol can pass placental barriers resulting in the fetus or newborn animals being affected (Frye et al., 1991). Vitamin $K_3$ was found to be ineffective in preventing the anticoagulant effects of dicoumarol (Casper et al., 1989).

Toxicity data for either naturally occurring or synthetic forms of vitamin K are extremely limited. For humans and laboratory animals the presumed upper safe level for oral ingestion of menadione ($K_3$) is 1,000 times the dietary requirement (National Research Council, 1987), but toxicity data for cattle are not available.

## WATER-SOLUBLE VITAMINS

Ruminal microorganisms synthesize most water-soluble vitamins (biotin, folic acid, niacin, pantothenic acid, pyridoxine, riboflavin, thiamin, and vitamin $B_{12}$) and common feedstuffs generally contain high concentrations of most of those vitamins. Vitamin C is synthesized by ruminant animals. True deficiencies of these vitamins are rare in animals with a functional rumen. To date, a limited amount of research has been conducted on most water-soluble vitamins (niacin is the exception) for adult cattle; however, research in this area has increased during the past few years. Adequate data to quantify bioavailability, ruminal synthesis, and requirements for most water-soluble vitamins are not available. Deficiency diseases for most B vitamins can be induced when preruminant calves are fed synthetic diets but are rare when calves are fed milk. Milk replacers should be supplemented with B vitamins as described in Chapter 10.

## B-VITAMINS

### *Biotin*

Biotin acts as a cofactor for many enzymes involved in carboxylation reactions. Ruminal bacteria normally synthesize biotin and concentrations of the vitamin may exceed 9 μg/L of strained ruminal fluid (Briggs et al., 1964). Biotin is not extensively metabolized in the rumen and increased intake of dietary biotin results in elevated concentrations of biotin in serum and milk (Frigg et al., 1993; Midla et al., 1998). Unpublished epidemiologic data suggest a negative relationship between serum concentrations of biotin and the incidence of clinical lameness in dairy cattle. In controlled long-term field studies, feeding approximately 20 mg/day of supplemental biotin statistically improved measures of hoof health (Bergsten et al., 1999; Fitzgerald et al., 2000; Midla et al., 1998). However, insufficient data are available at this time to quantify the requirement for biotin of dairy cattle.

### *Folic Acid*

Folic acid containing coenzymes are involved in movement of one-carbon units in biochemical pathways. Methionine also serves as a methyl donor; therefore, folic acid may spare methionine. Folic acid is necessary for the synthesis of nucleic acids. Growth rate and hematologic responses have been used to access adequacy in animal studies. Microbial degradation of supplemental folic acid can be extensive (Zinn, 1987). Consequently, parenteral administration of folic acid is usually used to examine responses to supplemental folic acid.

Weekly intramuscular injections of 40 mg folic acid from 45 days after mating until 6 weeks after parturition did not alter blood parameters or influence calf birth weight, therefore, dietary folic acid and microbial synthesis of this vitamin appear to supply sufficient amounts to prevent deficiency symptoms in adult dairy cattle (Girard et al., 1995). Young calves that do not have a completely developed ruminal microflora may be most susceptible to folic acid deficiency. Calves given weekly intramuscular injections of 40 mg of folic acid from 10 days of age until 16 weeks of age increased average daily gain by 8 percent during the 5 weeks following weaning (approximately 7 to 12 weeks of age; Dumoulin et al., 1991). Treatment also increased serum folates, blood hemoglobin, and packed cell volume suggesting that folic acid may be deficient in young calves.

Parenteral supplementation of 160 mg of folic acid each week from 45 days of gestation until 6 weeks postpartum tended to increase milk and milk protein production during mid to late lactation of primi- and multiparous cows. After calving, milk protein percentage was increased in multiparous cows only during the first 6 weeks of lactation (Girard et al., 1995). Milk production during days 1 to 200 of lactation was increased linearly for multiparous cows but not for primiparous cows when 0, 2, or 4 mg folate/kg BW were fed (Girard and Matte, 1998). Blood folates were increased indicating that some dietary folic acid escaped ruminal degradation. Deficiency symptoms for folate have not been observed in lactating dairy cattle. The increased milk production observed when supplemental folate was fed may be a direct response to the vitamin or may be an indirect response caused by sparing methionine. Insufficient data are currently available to quantify the folic acid requirement of cattle.

### *Inositol*

Inositol is an important nutrient in the metabolism and transport of lipids, and is a constituent of phospholipids, and has lipotropic activity. Myo-inositol is found in feeds as a component of phytic acid (Gerloff et al., 1984). Because phytic acid can be degraded in the rumen, deficiencies of inositol are not likely to occur. However, during periods of hepatic lipidosis or fatty liver syndrome where feed intakes may be low, supplementation of inositol has been investigated as an aid to help minimize triglyceride accumulation in the liver. Gerloff et al. (1984) in a field study involving 80 multiparious cows reported that the lipid content of liver was not decreased by feeding 17 grams of nonphytate myo-inositol for one month pre- and postpartum. Similarly, Grummer et al. (1987) indicated that neither milk production nor milk fat percentage were increased with abomasal infusion of 37 grams of myo-inositol.

Dietary requirements for inositol have not been demonstrated in dairy animals with normal rumen activity. Bacterial synthesis in the rumen and/or the amounts in feeds apparently supply adequate amounts to meet metabolic requirements. The previous edition of *Nutrient Requirements of Dairy Cattle,* (National Research Council, 1989) cited research from 1940 and 1950 showing deficiencies in calves after several weeks when fed purified or semi-purified diets. Because dairy products are generally good sources of these vitamins (Combs, 1992) and milk replacers are fortified with additional amounts (Tomkins and Jaster, 1991), deficiencies are unlikely to occur under typical calf raising practices.

### *Niacin*

Niacin is a generic name for pyridine 3-carboxylic acids and their derivatives that demonstrate activity similar to the amide form (i.e., nicotinamide). Niacin functions as a coenzyme for the pyridine nucleotide electron carriers NAD(H) and NADP(H). Consequently, niacin plays a critical role in mitochondrial respiration and the metabolism of carbohydrates, lipids, and amino acids.

Net synthesis of niacin in the rumen is likely because supply of niacin to the intestine exceeds intake when unsupplemented diets are fed to cattle (Zinn et al., 1987). Rate of niacin synthesis may be inversely related to level of supplementation (Abdouli and Schaefer, 1986b). During supplementation, the amount of niacin reaching the intestine may be less than that fed, indicating niacin degradation or absorption from the rumen (Zinn et al., 1987). Niacin absorption from the rumen appears to be low, particularly for nicotinic acid (Erickson et al., 1991). Feeding supplemental niacin increases concentrations in ruminal and duodenal fluid, which suggests that some supplemental niacin reaches the small intestine (Zinn et al., 1987; Campbell et. al., 1994). Estimates are that 17 to 30 percent of supplemental niacin reaches the small intestine (Harmeyer and Kollenkirchen, 1989; Campbell et al., 1994). Nicotinamide is rapidly converted to nicotinic acid in the reticulorumen (Harmeyer and Kollenkirchen, 1989; Campbell et al., 1994).

Niacin may increase microbial protein synthesis (Shields et al., 1983; Riddell et al., 1980, 1981); however, several studies indicate no effects (Hannah and Stern, 1985; Abdouli and Schaefer, 1986a; Doreau and Ottou, 1996). Differences between these studies, all of which utilized in vitro systems, may reflect the amount and availability of niacin in the unsupplemented diet, the niacin status of the microbes, or both. When niacin was fed in combination with other B-vitamins to feedlot calves (Zinn et al., 1987), or nicotinic acid or nicotinamide was fed to lactating cows (Doreau and Ottou, 1996), there were no treatment effects on microbial flow to the intestine.

Niacin is required in the diet of preweaned calves. Calves fed synthetic milk that was deficient in niacin developed scours within 48 hours (Hopper and Johnson, 1955). Immediate improvement was observed on the day following oral (6 mg/head/day) or intramuscular (10 mg/head/day) nicotinic acid administration. Niacin supplementation did not improve growth rates of heifers that began on trial at approximately 110 or 370 kg (Riddell et al., 1981).

A total of 30 treatment comparisons from peer reviewed literature (Fronk et al., 1980; Kung et al., 1980; Riddell et al., 1981; Dufva et al., 1983; Jaster et al., 1983a,b; Horner et al., 1986, 1988; Muller et al., 1986; Skaar et al., 1989; Driver et al., 1990; Erickson et al., 1990, 1992; Martinez et al., 1991; Lanham et al., 1992; Zimmerman et al., 1992; Bernard et al., 1995; Ottou et al., 1995; Madison-Anderson et al., 1997; Minor et al., 1998) were summarized to examine niacin effects on lactation; a significant increase or decrease was declared if $P < 0.05$. One comparison indicated a significant increase in milk production and 29 comparisons indicated no significant change in milk production. For the fourteen comparisons in which niacin administration began prepartum or prior to two weeks postpartum, none indicated a positive response. The absence of a response in many trials may be the consequence of inadequate replication. The only positive milk yield response was from one of the two field trials that have utilized large animal numbers (Muller et al., 1986). The numbers of significant positive, neutral, or significant negative responses were 3, 26, and 1 for milk fat percentage and 5, 20, and 2 for milk protein percentage.

A similar summary by Erdman (1992) indicated that average milk yield response was 0.3 kg/day; 0.4 kg/day if studies were restricted to those in which niacin supplementation began prepartum. A summary of 23 to 30 treatment comparisons by Drackley (1992) indicated that average milk production was increased by 0.62 kg/day and milk fat and protein were increased by 0.033 and 0.002 percentage units when supplemental niacin was fed. Summaries by Erdman (1992) or Drackley (1992) indicated that milk production was decreased 1.1 or 0.42 kg/day when niacin was added to diets that contained supplemental fat. However, there have been no significant ($P < 0.05$) interactions between fat and niacin for milk yield in the eight studies that have tested for interactions (Horner et al., 1986; Skaar et al., 1989; Driver et al., 1990; Martinez et al., 1991; Erickson et al., 1992; Lanham et al., 1992; Ottou et al., 1995; Madison-Anderson et al., 1997).

Niacin is antilipolytic and has been examined closely as a feed additive to prevent or treat fatty liver and ketosis. Early studies indicated that small (12 g/day until negative milk acetone test; Fronk and Schultz, 1979) or large (160 grams over 8 hours; Waterman et al., 1972) pharmacologic doses of niacin reduced blood ketones in ketotic cows. In these studies, there were no ketotic cows assigned to a control (no niacin) treatment. Consequently, niacin effects were confounded with time. A slug dose of 12 or 120 grams of niacin decreased plasma concentrations of nonesterified fatty acids but not beta-hydroxybutyrate (Jaster et al., 1983a). A summary of 14 treatment comparisons in which niacin was fed (Fronk et al., 1980; Dufva et al., 1983; Jaster et al., 1983a; Skaar et al., 1989; Driver et al., 1990; Erickson et al., 1990; Martinez et al., 1991; Erickson et al., 1992; Zimmerman et al., 1992; Bernard et al., 1995; Chilliard and Ottou, 1995; Ottou et al., 1995; Minor et al., 1998) indicated plasma nonesterified fatty acids were significantly reduced once, increased twice, and not altered 11 times. If restricted to studies in which niacin was fed prepartum or within two weeks postpartum, plasma nonesterified fatty acids were significantly reduced once, increased twice, and not altered 8 times. In 10 comparisons (9 of which niacin treatment began prepartum or prior to two weeks postpartum) plasma ketones were significantly reduced 4 times and not affected 6 times. However, three of the four comparisons in which significant reductions were observed were from a single experiment and corresponded to contrasts between three different doses of niacin to a control treatment (Dufva et al., 1983). Initiating the feeding of niacin prepartum did not reduce the amount of fat in liver of cows at 1 to 2 days or 28 to 35 days postpartum (Skaar et al., 1989; Minor et al., 1998).

Niacin requirements for dairy cattle are not known. Supplemental niacin may be required by calves fed milk replacer (Hopper and Johnson, 1955) but not by post weaned growing heifers (Riddell et al., 1981). Data summarized from more than 25 trials does not support routine use of niacin to enhance lactation performance of dairy cattle. Data also do not support the routine use of niacin to minimize the risk of lipid-related metabolic disorders such as ketosis and fatty liver.

### *Pantothenic Acid*

Pantothenic acid is a constituent of coenzyme A and is therefore essential for several fundamental reactions in metabolism including fatty acid oxidation, amino acid catabolism and acetylcholine synthesis (Smith and Song, 1996). No dietary requirement for pantothenic acid has been established as synthesis of pantothenic acid by ruminal microorganisms appears to be 20 to 30 times more than dietary amounts. Net microbial synthesis of pantothenic acid in the rumen of steer calves has been estimated to be 2.2 mg/kg of digestible organic matter consumed per day and degradation of dietary pantothenic acid in the rumen is estimated to be 78 percent (Zinn et al., 1987). Supplementation of pantothenic acid at five to 10 times theoretic requirements did not improve performance of feedlot cattle (Cole et al., 1982; Zinn et al., 1987). Deficiency symptoms are very diverse and nonspecific. In nonruminants, some generally reported symptoms include: disorders of the nervous, gastrointestinal, and immune systems, reduced growth rate, decreased food intake, skin lesions and changes in hair coat, alterations in lipid and carbohydrate metabolism and death (Smith and Song, 1996).

### *Riboflavin ($B_2$)*

Riboflavin is a constituent of several enzyme systems associated with intermediary metabolism. No dietary requirement for ruminants has been established. Tissue requirements are apparently met through microbial synthesis of the vitamin in the rumen as destruction of dietary riboflavin in the rumen is nearly 100 percent (Zinn et al., 1987). Miller et al. (1986) reported ruminal synthesis of riboflavin to be 148 percent of intake with apparent absorption from the small intestine averaging 23 percent. Synthesis of riboflavin in the rumen and flow to the small intestine was unaffected by concentrate content of the diet fed to steers. Zinn et al. (1987) estimated the flow of riboflavin from the rumen at 15.2 mg/kg of digestible organic matter consumed per day and a net absorption from the small intestine of 25 percent.

### *Thiamin ($B_1$)*

Thiamin is a water-soluble vitamin, which in pure form is white in color, and has a sulfurous odor. It functions as an important coenzyme in several energy metabolism pathways and has a role, although not well defined, in nerve and brain function (Combs, 1992). Sources of thiamin include grains, grain by-products, soybean meal, and brewers yeast. Amounts of thiamin synthesized daily in the rumen (28 to 72 mg) have been reported to equal or exceed dietary intake (Breves et al., 1981).

A dietary requirement for thiamin has not been established for healthy animals with a functional rumen. The combination of thiamin in feeds and synthesis of thiamin in the rumen meet or exceed metabolic requirements even with an estimated 48 percent destruction of dietary thiamin in the rumen (Zinn et al., 1987). Thiamin is generally nontoxic as the upper safe feeding level for most nonruminants is 1,000 times the requirement (National Research Council, 1987). An upper safe feeding level has not been established for ruminants.

Deficiencies of thiamin have been found when thiaminases associated with either feeds or produced from altered ruminal fermentation destroy thiamin or produce an antimetabolite of thiamin, which blocks thiamin dependent reactions. Bracken ferns and some raw fish products have been found to contain thiaminases. Feeding diets high in sulfate (Gould et al., 1991) or those which cause a sudden drop in ruminal pH (Zinn et al., 1987) can result in a thiamin deficiency. Because thiamin is intricately involved in several of the energy producing Krebs cycle reactions and because of the importance of glucose as an energy supply for the brain, any deficiency of thiamin results in a central nervous system disorder. Polioencephalomalacia (PEM), is the most common thiamin deficiency disorder. Symptoms of PEM include a profuse, but transient diarrhea, listlessness, circling movements, opisthotonus (head drawn back over neck), and muscle tremors. If treated promptly by parenteral injection of thiamin (2.2 mg/kg of body weight), the condition can be reversed (National Research Council, 1996).

### *Vitamin $B_{12}$*

Vitamin $B_{12}$ is a cofactor for two major enzymes; methylmalonyl coenzyme A mutase necessary for conversion of propionate to succinate, and tetrahydrofolate methyl transferase which catalyzes transfer of methyl groups from 5-methyltetrahydrofolate to homocysteine to form methionine and tetrahydrofolate. Vitamin $B_{12}$ is not found in the tissues of plants. Microbes are the only natural source of vitamin $B_{12}$. Ruminal microbes can produce all of the vitamin $B_{12}$ required by the cow provided adequate available cobalt is in the diet (see section on cobalt, Chapter 6).

Vitamin $B_{12}$ deficiency has been demonstrated in calves when fed diets devoid of animal protein (Lassiter et al., 1953) demonstrating that vitamin $B_{12}$ is a required nutrient in dairy cattle. Based on this work, it was suggested that the vitamin $B_{12}$ requirement for dairy cattle was between 0.34 and 0.68 μg/kg of live weight. Vitamin $B_{12}$ deficiency is the principle manifestation of cobalt deficiency (See section on cobalt).

Significant quantities of vitamin $B_{12}$ are synthesized in the rumen. Vitamin $B_{12}$ activity in the rumen tends to be greater in animals either grazing or fed high forage diets compared with animals fed high concentrate diets (Sutton and Elliot, 1972; Walker and Elliot, 1972). Data from beef cattle (Zinn et al., 1987) suggest more than adequate synthesis of vitamin $B_{12}$ to meet expected requirements for lactating dairy cows (Erdman, 1992), although exact requirements have not been established.

In the mature ruminant, vitamin $B_{12}$ is of interest because of its roles in propionate metabolism (gluconeogenesis) and in methionine synthesis. It was suggested that inadequate $B_{12}$ may be related to the low-milk fat syndrome in cows fed high grain diets (Frobish and Davis, 1977). Studies using both supplemental (Elliot et al., 1979) and injected (Croom et al., 1981) vitamin $B_{12}$ failed to show any response in fat test from cows fed high grain diets. There is no evidence that lactating dairy cows fed adequate amounts of cobalt will respond to dietary or intramuscular injections of vitamin $B_{12}$.

Vitamin $B_{12}$ also is required as part of the enzyme complex methionine synthase in which methionine is synthesized from S-adenosylhomocysteine and 5-methyl tetrahydrofolate. Methionine is used as a methyl donor for synthesis of choline , carnitine, and others compounds; therefore, a deficiency of vitamin $B_{12}$ is likely to affect methionine and methyl donor metabolism. Methyl donor requirements are not defined in ruminants and again it is unlikely that vitamin $B_{12}$ deficiency is of practical significance except during cobalt deficiency.

### *B-Vitamins—General*

In general, B-vitamin requirements can be met through synthesis by ruminal microorganisms and escape of dietary sources from the rumen. Table 7-1 illustrates potential requirements extrapolated from swine requirements and average vitamin concentrations found in milk. Based on these estimated requirements and limited research on B-vitamins of Miller et al. (1986) and Zinn et al. (1987) only folic acid and pantothenic acid appear to be limiting based on ruminal synthesis and escape of these vitamins occurring naturally in feeds. In contrast, some studies have demonstrated production and/or health benefits to dairy cows when diets have been supplemented with B-vitamins, most notably niacin, biotin, and folic acid. At the present time, almost no research is available on requirements of B complex vitamins for gestation, health, and milk production of high producing dairy cows.

## VITAMIN C

Vitamin C or ascorbic acid is synthesized from L-gulonic acid within the cells of ruminants. Calves cannot synthesize ascorbic acid until approximately 3 weeks of age (Cummins and Brunner, 1991). Therefore, vitamin C is not considered an essential nutrient for healthy cattle that are older than about 3 weeks. Some studies, however, have reported beneficial responses when supplemental vitamin C is administered to cattle, particularly calves. Ascorbic acid functions as a water-soluble cellular antioxidant. Specifically, ascorbic acid is thought to be involved in regulation of steroid synthesis and the concentration of ascorbic acid is high in

TABLE 7-1 Estimated Absorption of Selected B-vitamins From the Small Intestine Compared with Estimated Requirements for Tissue and Milk Synthesis of a 650-kg Cow Producing 35 kg of 4 Percent Fat-Corrected Milk/Day

| Vitamin | Daily Estimated Requirement Tissue[a] (mg/day) | Milk[b] (mg/day) | Total (mg/day) | Ruminal Synthesis[c,d] (mg/day) | Ruminal Escape[d] from diet (%) |
|---|---|---|---|---|---|
| Biotin | 5 | 1 | 6 | 14 | 100 |
| Folic acid | 33 | 2 | 35 | 7 | 3 |
| Niacin | 256 | 33 | 289 | 1804 | 6 |
| Pantothenic acid | 304 | 121 | 425 | 38 | 22 |
| Riboflavin | 95 | 61 | 156 | 261 | 1 |
| Thiamin | 26 | 15 | 41 | 143 | 52 |
| $B_6$ | 26 | 22 | 48 | 96 | 100 |
| $B_{12}$ | 0.4 | 0.2 | 0.6 | 70 | 10 |

[a] Based on lactating sow (175 kg) requirements (NRC, 1998) adjusted to 650 kg lactating cow weight.
[b] Adapted from Jenness (1985) and adjusted to 35 kg milk production.
[c,d] Adapted from Miller et al. (1986)[c] and Zinn et al. (1987)[d] and adjusted to digestible organic matter intake of 17.2 kg/day (total DM intake 22.9 kg/day).

steroid secreting cells. Plasma concentrations of ascorbic acid were lower in calves (Cummins and Brunner, 1991) and growing steers (Hidiroglou et al., 1977) reared under stressful (i.e., slatted floors, cold stress) conditions than animals housed in better environments. That effect may be mediated by cortisol. Oral supplementation of 1 or 2 grams of vitamin C/day to preruminant calves elevated plasma concentrations of ascorbic acid compared with no supplemental vitamin C (Hidiroglou et al., 1995). The 2 grams supplementation rate tended to increase plasma concentrations of ascorbic acid above the 1 gram rate but the difference was not statistically consistent during the 35 day experiment. Data are lacking on the effect of oral supplementation of vitamin C with cattle. Most orally ingested ascorbic acid is destroyed in the rumen, but newer formulations of vitamin C may provide some protection from ruminal metabolism. With sheep, oral supplementation of 4 g/day of various forms of vitamin C for 28 days significantly increased plasma ascorbic acid concentrations (Hidiroglou et al., 1997).

No growth response has been reported when calves were supplemented with vitamin C. Because of its antioxidant function, most research has concentrated on the effects of vitamin C on immune function. Immunoglobulin titers in calves were generally not affected by vitamin C supplementation (Cummins and Brunner, 1989; Hidiroglou et al., 1995). Steers injected subcutaneously with 20 mg of ascorbic acid/kg of BW had improved neutrophil function compared with uninjected controls (Roth and Kaeberle, 1985). In the same study, an injection of 40 mg of ascorbic acid/kg of BW counteracted the negative effects on neutrophil function induced by dexamethasone. Current data do not support routine supplementation of vitamin C to calves or adult cattle.

## CHOLINE

Choline is not a vitamin in a traditional sense because it is not a part of an enzyme system, and is required in gram rather than milligram amounts as for true vitamins. Johnson et al. (1951) produced a choline deficiency in week-old dairy calves using synthetic milk replacer diets containing 15 percent casein. Choline requirements estimated from that experiment were 260 mg/L of milk replacer (1733 mg/kg DM). Current estimates of requirements for the calf are 1000 mg/kg dry matter (DM) (Chapter 10). The predominant sign of choline deficiency in most animals is fatty liver. In calves, reported deficiency signs included muscular weakness, fatty infiltration of the liver, and renal hemorrhage; similar to those observed in other species.

Both naturally occurring choline in feeds, predominantly found in phospholipids (lecithin) and dietary choline from supplements such as choline chloride have been shown to be extensively degraded in the rumen (Neil et al., 1979; Sharma and Erdman, 1988a,b, 1989b). Microbial degradation of choline in the rumen results in the production of acetaldehyde and trimethylamine. Methyl group carbon from trimethylamine is subsequently degraded to methane (Neil et al., 1978). Supplementation of dietary choline in an unprotected form is useless because of extensive ruminal degradation (Erdman, 1992).

Because of extensive degradation of dietary choline, methyl group requirements for synthesis of methyl-containing metabolites in the dairy cow are presumably produced via methylation pathways involving methionine and the enzyme, S-adenosylmethionine methyl transferase. Sources of methyl groups for ruminants would include dietary methionine, betaine resulting from degradation of choline, and de novo synthesized methyl groups produced through 5-methyl tetrahydrofolate. Approximately one-third of the methionine methyl groups were transferred to choline in studies with lactating dairy goats (Emmanuel and Kennelly, 1984). Intravenous infusion of choline and carnitine reduced the irreversible loss of methionine by 18 to 25 percent in sheep suggesting that methionine could be spared with the addition of methyl-group-containing metabolites (Lobley et al., 1996).

Choline content of whole milk varies substantially (43 to 285 mg/L; Hartman and Dryden, 1974) with about 25 mg/L in the form of phospholipids. More recently, Deuchler et al. (1998) found that the concentration of choline in milk ranged from 70 to 90 mg/L with an average secretion rate of choline into milk of between 2 to 3 g/day. Secretion of choline into milk was increased by either postruminal infusion of choline chloride (Aliev and Burkova, 1987; Deuchler et al., 1998) or by dietary supplementation of rumen-protected choline. This suggests that secretion of choline into milk could be used as a qualitative indicator of postruminal choline supply.

Choline requirements for lactating dairy cows have not been established. As a ruminant animal, the dairy cow has evolved under circumstances where intestinally absorbed choline is almost nonexistent because of extensive ruminal degradation of dietary choline. Experiments where choline has been supplemented either by feeding in a rumen-protected form or by postruminal infusion of choline chloride have produced variable results. Milk production increased 0 to 3 kg/day in experiments where 15 to as much as 90 grams of choline chloride were infused postruminally (Grummer et al., 1987; Erdman and Sharma, 1991; Sharma and Erdman, 1989a). In an experiment where methyl transfer from methionine was inhibited but choline was provided, 4 percent FCM production was increased by 3.4 kg/day suggesting the importance of methionine in methyl group metabolism in the dairy cow (Sharma and Erdman, 1988b).

Lactational responses to choline are likely to be affected by methionine supply. Dairy cows that are fed diets that supply adequate amounts of intestinally absorbed methionine are less likely to respond to supplemental choline than when methionine is limiting. Because of the relationship between fatty liver and ketosis, it has been speculated that choline could play a role in ketosis treatment and prevention, but there is no direct evidence to date to support this theory (Erdman, 1992). The establishment of a choline requirement, either for the lactating dairy cow, or for the transition cow in the late dry period and in early lactation, will require more extensive feeding experiments than were available at the time of this publication.

## REFERENCES


Abdouli, H., and D. M. Schaefer. 1986a. Impact of niacin and length of incubation on protein synthesis, soluble to total protein ratio and fermentative activity of ruminal microorganisms. J. Anim. Sci. 62:244–253.

Abdouli, H., and D. M. Schaefer. 1986b. Effects of two dietary niacin concentrations on ruminal fluid free niacin concentration, and of supplemental niacin and source of inoculum on in vitro microbial growth, fermentative activity and nicotinamide adenine dinucleotide pool size. J. Anim. Sci. 62:254–262.

Alderson, N. E., Jr., G. E. Mitchell, C. O. Little, R. E. Warner, and R. E. Tucker. 1971. Preintestinal disappearance of vitamin E in ruminants. J. Nutr. 101:655–660.

Aliev, A. A., and L. M. Burkova. 1987. Effect of choline chloride on the metabolism of nitrogen and choline in the stomach and intestines of lactating cows. Skh. Biol. 4:80–85.

Astrup, H. N., and J. J. Nedkvitne. 1987. Effects of vitamin D supplement on cows and sheep. Norw.. J. Agric. Sci. 1:87–95.

Baldi, A., V. Bontempo, F. Cheli, S. Carli, C. S. Rossi, and V. Dell'Orto. 1997. Relative bioavailability of vitamin E in dairy cows following intraruminal administration of three different preparations of DL-α-tocopheryl acetate. Vet. Res. 28:1–8.

Barton, B. A., N. A. Jorgensen, and H. F. DeLuca. 1987. Impact of prepartum dietary phosphorus intake on calcium homeostasis at parturition. J. Dairy Sci. 70:1186–1191.

Batra, T. R., M. Hidiroglou, and M. W. Smith. 1992. Effect of vitamin E on incidence of mastitis in dairy cattle. Can. J. Anim. Sci. 72:287–297.

Bendich, A. 1993. Physiological role of antioxidants in the immune system. J. Dairy Sci. 76:2789–2794.

Bergsten, C., P. R. Greenough, J. M. Gay, R. C. Dobson, and C. C. Gay. 1999. A controlled field trial of the effects of biotin supplementation on milk production and hoof lesions. J. Dairy Sci. 82 (Suppl. 1):34 (Abstr.).

Bernard, J. K., J. D. Quigley, H. H. Dowlen, and K. C. Lamar. 1995. Supplemental niacin and heat-treated whole soybeans for Jersey cows during early lactation. J. Dairy Sci. 78:2016–2023.

Blaxter, K. L., P. S. Watts, and W. A. Woods. 1952. The nutrition of the young Ayrshire calf. 8. Muscular dystrophy in the growing calf. Br. J. Nutr. 6:125–169.

Blomhoff, R., M. H. Green, J. B. Green, T. Berg, and K. Norum, R. 1991. Vitamin A metabolism: new perspectives on absorption, transport, and storage. Physiological Reviews 71:951–990.

Breves, G., M. Brandt, H. Hoeller, and K. Rohr. 1981. Flow of thiamin to the duodenum in dairy cows fed different rations. J. Agric. Sci. Cambridge 96:587–591.

Briggs, M. H., T. W. Heard, A. Whitcroft, and M. L. Hogg. 1964. Studies on urea-fed cattle. 2. Rumen levels of B vitamins and related coenzymes. Life Sci. 3:11–14.

Bruhn, J. C., and J. C. Oliver. 1978. Effect of storage on tocopherol and carotene concentrations in alfalfa hay. J. Anim. Sci. 61:980–982.

Campbell, J. M., M. R. Murphy, R. A. Christensen, and T. R. Overton. 1994. Kinetics of niacin supplements in lactating cows. J. Dairy Sci. 77:566–575.

Casper, H. H., A. D. Alstad, D. B. Tacke, L. J. Johnson, and W. E. Lloyd. 1989. Evaluation of vitamin $K_3$ feed additive for the prevention of sweet clover disease. J. Vet. Diagn. Invest. 1:116–119.

Chew, B. P. 1987. Vitamin A and β-carotene in host defense. J. Dairy Sci. 70:2732–2743.

Chew, B. P. 1993. Role of carotenoids in the immune response. J. Dairy Sci. 76:2804–2811.

Chilliard, Y., and J. F. Ottou. 1995. Duodenal infusion of oil in midlactation cows. 7. Interaction with niacin on responses to glucose, insulin, and β-agonist challenges. J. Dairy Sci. 78:2452–2463.

Coelho, M. B. 1991. Vitamin stability in premixes and feeds: a practical approach. Pp. 56–71. BASF Tech. Symp. Bloomington, MN.

Cohen-Fernandez, S., P. Budowski, I. Ascarelli, H. Neumark, and A. Bondi. 1976. Low utilization of carotene by sheep. Int. J. Vit. Nutr. Res. 46:446–453.

Cole, N. A., J. B. McLaren, and D. P. Hutcheson. 1982. Influence of preweaning and B-vitamin supplementation of the feedlot receiving diet on calves subjected to marketing and transit stress. J. Anim. Sci. 54:911–917.

Combs, Jr., G. F. 1992. The Vitamins: Fundamental Aspects in Nutrition and Health. Academic Press Inc.

Croom, W. J., A. H Rakes, A. C. Linnerud, G. A. Ducharme, and J. M. Elliot. 1981. Vitamin $B_{12}$ administration for milk fat synthesis in lactating dairy cows fed a low fiber diet. J. Dairy Sci. 64:1555–1560.

Cummins, K. A., and C. J. Brunner. 1989. Dietary ascorbic acid and immune response in dairy calves. J. Dairy Sci. 72:129–134.

Cummins, K. A., and C. J. Brunner. 1991. Effect of calf housing on plasma ascorbate and endocrine and immune function. J. Dairy Sci. 74:1582–1588.

Daynes, R. A., B. A. Araneo, J. Hennebold, E. Enioutina, and H. H. Mu. 1995. Steroids as regulators of the mammalian immune response. J. Invest. Dermatol. 105:14S–19S.

DeLuca, H. F. 1979. The vitamin D system in the regulation of calcium and phosphorus metabolism. Nutr. Rev. 37:161–193.

Deuchler, K. N., L. S. Piperova, and R. A. Erdman. 1998. Milk choline excretion as an indirect indicator of post-ruminal choline supply. J. Dairy Sci. 81:238–242.

Doreau, M., and J. F. Otto. 1996. Influence of niacin supplementation on in vivo digestibility and ruminal digestion in dairy cows. J. Dairy Sci. 79:2247–2254.

Drackley, J. K. 1992. Niacin and carnitine in the nutrition of dairy cows. Page 8 in Proc Pacific Northwest Nutr. Conf. Tech. Symp., October 20, Lonza Inc. ed., Spokane, WA.

Driver, L. S., R. R. Grummer, and L. H. Schultz. 1990. Effects of feeding heat-treated soybeans and niacin to high producing cows in early lactation. J. Dairy Sci. 73:463–469.

Dufva, G. S., E. E. Bartley, A. D. Dayton, and D. O. Riddell. 1983. Effect of niacin supplementation on milk production and ketosis of dairy cattle. J. Dairy Sci. 66:2329–2336.

Dumoulin, P. G., C. L. Girard, J. J. Matte, and G. J. St-Laurent. 1991. Effects of a parenteral supplement of folic acid and its interaction with level of feed intake of young dairy heifers. J. Anim. Sci. 69:1657–1666.

Eaton, H. D., J. E. Rousseau, Jr., R. C. Hall, Jr., H. I. Frier, and J. J. Lucas. 1972. Reevaluation of the minimum vitamin A requirement of Holstein male calves based upon elevated cerebrospinal fluid pressure. J. Dairy Sci. 55:232–237.

Elliot, J.M., E. P. Barton, and J. A. Williams. 1979. Milk fat as related to vitamin $B_{12}$ status. J. Dairy Sci. 62:642–645.

Emmanual, B., and J. J. Kennelly. 1984. Kinetics of methionine and choline and their incorporation into plasma lipids and milk components in lactating goats. J. Dairy Sci. 67:1912–1919.

Erdman, R. A. 1992. Vitamins. Pp. 297–308 in Large Dairy Herd Management. H. H. Van Horn and C. J. Wilcox, eds. American Dairy Science Association, Champaign, IL.

Erdman, R. A., and B. K. Sharma. 1991. Effect of dietary rumen-protected choline in lactating dairy cows. J. Dairy Sci. 74:1641–1647.

Erickson, P. S., M. R. Murphy, and J. H. Clark. 1992. Supplementation of dairy cow diets with calcium salts of long-chain fatty acids and nicotinic acid in early lactation. J. Dairy Sci. 75:1078–1089.

Erickson, P. S., A. M. Trusk, and M. R. Murphy. 1990. Effects of niacin source on epinephrine stimulation of plasma nonesterified fatty acid and glucose concentrations, on diet digestibility and on rumen protozoal numbers in lactating dairy cows. J. Nutr. 120:1648–1653.

Erickson, P. S., M. R. Murphy, C. S. McSweeney, and A. M. Trusk. 1991. Niacin absorption from the rumen. J. Dairy Sci. 74:3492–3495.

Fitzgerald, T., B. W. Norton, R. Elliott, H. Podlich, and O. L. Svendsen. 2000. The influence of long-term supplementation with biotin on the prevention of lameness in pasture fed dairy cows. J. Dairy Sci. 83:338–344.

Frigg, M., O. C. Straub, and D. Hartmann. 1993. The bioavailability of biotin in cattle. Internat. J. Vit. Nutr. Res. 63:122–128.

Frobish, R. A., and C.L. Davis. 1977. Theory involving propionate and vitamin $B_{12}$ in the low-fat milk syndrome. J. Dairy Sci. 60:268–276.

Fronk, T. J., and L. H. Schultz. 1979. Oral nicotinic acid as a treatment for ketosis. J. Dairy Sci. 62:1804–1807.

Fronk, T. J., L. H. Schultz, and A. R. Hardie. 1980. Effect of dry period overconditioning on subsequent metabolic disorders and performance of dairy cows. J. Dairy Sci. 63:1080–1090.

Frye, T. M., S. N. Williams, and T. W. Graham. 1991. Vitamin deficiencies in cattle. Veterinary Clinics of North America: Food Animal Practice. 7:217– 275.

Gardner, R.M., T. A. Reinhardt, and R.L. Horst. 1988. The biological assessment of vitamin $D_3$ metabolites produced by rumen bacteria. J. Ster. Biochem. 29:185–189.

Gerloff, B. J., T. H. Herdt, R. S. Emery, and W. W. Wells. 1984. Inositol as a lipotropic agent in dairy cattle diets. J. Anim. Sci. 59:806–812.

Girard, C. L., and J. J. Matte. 1998. Dietary supplements of folic acid during lactation: effects on performance of dairy cows. J. Dairy Sci. 81:1412–1419.

Girard, C. L., J. J. Matte, and G. F. Tremblay. 1995. Gestation and lactation of dairy cows: A role for folic acid? J. Dairy Sci. 78:404–411.

Goff, J. P., T. A. Reinhardt, G. W. Engstrom, and R. L. Horst. 1992. Effect of dietary calcium or phosphorus restriction and 1,25-dihyroxyvitamin D administration on rat intestinal 24-hydroxylase. Endocrinology 131:101–104.

Gould, D. H., M. M. McAllister, J. C. Savage, and D. W. Hamar. 1991. High sulfide concentrations in rumen fluid associated with nutritionally induced polioencephalomalacia in calves. Am. J. Vet. Res. 52:1164–1167.

Gray, R. W., and J. L. Napoli. 1983. Dietary phosphate deprivation increases 1,25-dihydroxyvitamin $D_3$ synthesis in rat kidney in vitro. J. Biol. Chem. 258:1152–1155.

Grummer, R. R., L. E. Armentano, and M. S. Marcus. 1987. Lactation response to short-term abomasal infusion of choline, inositol, and soy lecithin. J. Dairy Sci. 70:2518–2524.

Hannah, S. M., and M. D. Stern. 1985. Effect of supplemental niacin or niacinamide and soybean source on ruminal bacterial fermentation in continuous culture. J. Anim. Sci. 61:1252–1263.

Hartman and Dryden. 1974. The vitamins in milk and milk products. *In: Fundamentals of Dairy Chemistry*, 2nd ed. B. H. Webb, A. H. Johnson, and J. A. Alford (Editors) AVI Publishing Co. Westport, CT.

Harmeyer, J., and U. Kollenkirchen. 1989. Thiamin and niacin in ruminant tissues. Nutr. Res. Rev. 2:201–225.

Harrison, J. H., D. D. Hancock, and H. R. Conrad. 1984. Vitamin E and selenium for reproduction of the dairy cow. J. Dairy Sci. 67:123–132.

Hibbs, J. W., and H. R. Conrad. 1983. The relation of calcium and phosphorus intake on digestion and the effects of vitamin D feeding on the utilization of calcium and phosphorus by lactating dairy cows. Rep. No. 1150. Ohio State University.

Hidiroglou, M., T. R. Batra, and X. Zhoa. 1997. Comparison of vitamin C bioavailability after multiple or single oral dosing of different formulations in sheep. Reprod. Nutr. Dev. 37:443–448.

Hidiroglou, M., M. Ivan, and J. R. Lessard. 1977. Effect of ration and inside versus outside housing on plasma levels of ascorbic acid, lactic acid, glucose, and cholesterol in Hereford steers wintered under practical conditions. Can. J. Anim. Sci. 57:519–529.

Hidiroglou, N., L. R. McDowell, and O. Balbuena. 1989. Plasma tocopherol in sheep and cattle after ingesting free or acetylated tocopherol. J. Dairy Sci. 72:1793–1799.

Hidiroglou, N., L. F. Laflamme, and L. R. McDowell. 1988. Blood plasma and tissue concentrations of vitamin E in beef cattle as influenced by supplementation of various tocopherol compounds. J. Anim. Sci. 66:3227–3234.

Hidiroglou, M., T. R. Batra, M. Ivan, and F. Markham. 1995. Effects of supplemental vitamins E and C on the immune response of calves. J. Dairy Sci. 78:1578–1583.

Hogan, J. S., K. L. Smith, W. P. Weiss, D. A. Todhunter, and W. L. Shockey. 1990. Relationships among vitamin E, selenium, and bovine blood neutrophils. J. Dairy Sci. 73:2372–2378.

Hogan, J. S., W. P. Weiss, and K. L. Smith. 1993. Role of vitamin E and selenium in host defense against mastitis. J. Dairy Sci. 76:2795–2803.

Hogan, J. S., W. P. Weiss, D. A. Todhunter, K. L. Smith, and P. S. Schoenberg. 1992. Bovine neutrophil responses to parenteral vitamin E. J. Dairy Sci. 75:399–405.

Hopper, J. H., and B. C. Johnson. 1955. The production and study of an acute nicotinic acid deficiency in the calf. J. Nutr. 56:303–310.

Horner, J. L., C. E. Coppock, G. T. Schelling, J. M. Labore, and D. H. Nave. 1986. Influence of niacin and whole cottonseed on intake, milk yield and composition, and systematic responses of dairy cows. J. Dairy Sci. 69:3087–3093.

Horner, J. L., L. M. Windle, C. E. Coppock, J. M. Labore, J. K. Lanhan, and D. H. Nave. 1988. Effects of whole cottonseed, niacin, and niacinamide on in vitro rumen fermentation and on lactating Holstein cows. J. Dairy Sci. 71:3334–3344.

Horst, R. L., and E. T. Littledike. 1982. Comparison of plasma concentrations of vitamin D and its metabolites in young and aged domestic animals. Comp. Biochem. Physiol. [B] 73:485–489.

Horst, R. L., J. P. Goff, and T. A. Reinhardt. 1994. Calcium and vitamin D metabolism in the dairy cow. J. Dairy Sci. 77:1936–1951.

Hurley, W. L., and R. M. Doane. 1989. Recent developments in the roles of vitamins and minerals in reproduction. J. Dairy Sci. 72:784–804.

Jaster, E. H., D. F. Bell, and T. A. McPherron. 1983a. Nicotinic acid and serum metabolite concentrations of lactating dairy cows fed supplemental niacin. J. Dairy Sci. 66:1039–1045.

Jaster, E. H., G. F. Hartnell, and M. F. Hutjens. 1983b. Feeding supplemental niacin for milk production in six dairy herds. J. Dairy Sci. 66:1046–1051.

Jennes, R. 1985. Biochemical and nutritional aspects of milk and colostrum. In: Lactation. P. 164, B. L. Larson, ed., Iowa State Press, Ames IA.

Johnson, B. C., H. H. Mitchell, and A. Pinkos. 1951. Choline deficiency in the calf. J. Nutr. 43:37–48.

Jukola, E., J. Hakkarainen, H. Saloniemi, and S. Sankari. 1996. Effect of selenium fertilization on selenium in feedstuffs and selenium, vitamin E, and B-carotene concentrations in blood of cattle. J. Dairy Sci. 79:831–837.

Kung Jr., L., K. Gubert, and J. T. Huber. 1980. Supplemental niacin for lactating cows fed diets of natural protein or nonprotein nitrogen. J. Dairy Sci. 63:2020–2025.

Lanham, J. K., C. E. Coppock, K. N. Brooks, D. L. Wilks, and J. L. Horner. 1992. Effects of whole cottonseed or niacin or both on casein synthesis by lactating Holstein cows. J. Dairy Sci. 75:184–192.

Lassiter, C. A., G. M. Ward, C. F. Huffman, C. W. Duncan, and H. D. Welester. 1953. Crystalline vitamin $B_{12}$ requirements of the young dairy calf. J. Dairy Sci. 36:997–1004.

Leedle, R. A., J. A. Leedle, and M. D. Butine. 1993. Vitamin E is not degraded by ruminal microorganisms: assessment with ruminal contents from a steer fed a high-concentrate diet. J. Anim. Sci. 71:3442–3450.

Littledike, E. T., and R. L. Horst. 1980. Problems with vitamin D injections for prevention of milk fever: toxicity of large doses and increased incidence of small doses. J. Dairy Sci. 63(Supp. 1):89.

Lobley, G. E., A. Connell, and D. Revell. 1996. The importance of transmethylation reaction to methionine metabolism in sheep: Effects of supplementation with creatine and choline. Brit. J. Nutr. 75:47–56.

Madison-Anderson, R. J., D. J. Schingoethe, M. J. Brouk, R. J. Baer, and M. R. Lentsch. 1997. Response of lactating cows to supplemental unsaturated fat and niacin. J. Dairy Sci. 80:1329–1338.

Martin, F. H., D. E. Ullrey, H. W. Newland, and E. R. Miller. 1968. Vitamin A activity of carotenes in corn silage fed to lambs. J. Nutr. 96:269–274.

Martinez, N., E. J. DePeters, and D. L. Bath. 1991. Supplemental niacin and fat effects on milk composition of lactating Holstein cows. J. Dairy Sci. 74:202–210.

McDermott, C. M., D. C. Beitz, E. T. Littledike, and R. L. Horst. 1985. Effects of dietary vitamin $D_3$ on concentrations of vitamin D and its metabolites in blood plasma and milk of dairy cows. J. Dairy Sci. 68:1959–1967.

Michal, J. J., L. R. Heirman, T. S. Wong, B. P. Chew, M. Frigg, and L. Volker. 1994. Modulatory effects of dietary β-carotene on blood and mammary leukocyte function in periparturient dairy cows. J. Dairy Sci. 77:1408–1421.

Midla, L. T., K. H. Hoblet, W. P. Weiss, and M. L. Moeschberger. 1998. Supplemental dietary biotin for prevention of lesions associated with aseptic clinical laminitis (Pododermatitis aseptica diffusa) in primiparous Holsteins. Am. J. Vet. Res. 59:733–738.

Miller, B. L., J. C. Meiske, and R. D. Goodrich. 1986. Effects of grain and concentrate level on B-vitamin production and absorption in steers. J. Anim. Sci. 62:473–483.

Miller, J. K., E. Brzezinska-Slebodzinska, and F. C. Madsen. 1993. Oxidative stress, antioxidants, and animal function. J. Dairy Sci. 76:2812–2823.

Minor, D. J., S. L. Trower, B. D. Strang, R. D. Shaver, and R. R. Grummer. 1998. Effects of nonfiber carbohydrate and niacin on periparturient metabolic status and lactation of dairy cows. J. Dairy Sci. 81:189–200.

Muller, L. D., A. J. Heinrichs, J. B. Cooper, and Y. H. Atkin. 1986. Supplemental niacin for lactating cows during summer feeding. J. Dairy Sci. 69:1416–1420.

National Research Council. 1996. Nutrient Requirements of Beef Cattle, Seventh Revised Ed. Washington, D.C.: National Academy Press.

National Research Council. 1987. Vitamin Tolerance of Domestic Animals. Washington, D.C.: National Academy Press.

National Research Council. 1989. Nutrient Requirements of Dairy Cattle. 6th rev. ed. Washington, D.C.: National Academy Press.

National Research Council. 1998. Nutrient requirements of Swine. 10th revised edition. National Academy Press, Washington, DC.

Neil, A. R., D. W. Grime, and R. M. C. Dawson. 1978. Conversion of choline methyl groups through trimethyl amine into methane in the rumen. Biochemical J. 170:529–535.

Neil, A. R., D. W. Grime, A. M. Snoswell, A. J. Northrop, D. B. Lindsay, and R. M. C. Dawson. 1979. The low availability of dietary choline for the nutrition of the sheep. Biochem. J. 180:559–565.

Oldham, E. R., R. J. Eberhart, and L. D. Muller. 1991. Effects of supplemental vitamin A and B-carotene during the dry period and early lactation on udder health. J. Dairy Sci. 74:3775–3781.

Ottou, J. F., M. Doreau, and Y. Chilliard. 1995. Duodenal infusion of rapeseed oil in midlactation cows. 6. Interaction with niacin on dairy performance and nutritional value. J. Dairy Sci. 78:1345–1352.

Park, Y. W., M. J. Anderson, J. L. Walters, and A. W. Mahoney. 1983. Effects of processing methods and agronomic variables on carotene contents in forages and predicting carotene in alfalfa hay with near-infrared-reflectance spectroscopy. J. Dairy Sci. 66:235–245.

Politis, I., M. Hidiroglou, T. R. Batra, J. A. Gilmore, R. C. Gorewit, and H. Scherf. 1995. Effects of vitamin E on immune function of dairy cows. Am. J. Vet. Res. 56:179–184.

Politis, I., N. Hidiroglou, J. H. White, J. A. Gilmore, S. N. Williams, H. Scherf, and M. Frigg. 1996. Effects of vitamin E on mammary and blood leukocyte function, with emphasis on chemotaxis, in periparturient dairy cows. Am. J. Vet. Res. 57:468–471.

Potanski, A. A., R. E. Tucker, G. E. Mitchell Jr., and G. T. Schelling. 1974. Pre-intestinal losses of carotene in sheep fed high-starch or high-cellulose diets. Int. J. Vit. Nutr. Res. 44:

Reinhardt, T. A., and R. L. Horst. 1989. Self-induction of 1,25-dihydroxyvitamin $D_3$ metabolism limits receptor occupancy and target tissue responsiveness. J. Biol. Chem. 264:15917–15921.

Reinhardt, T. A., and F. G. Hustmyer. 1987. Role of vitamin D in the immune system. J. Dairy Sci. 70:952–962.

Riddell, D. O., E. E. Bartley, and A. D. Dayton. 1980. Effect of nicotinic acid on rumen fermentation in vitro and in vivo. J. Dairy Sci. 63:1429–1436.

Riddell, D. O., E. E. Bartley, and A. D. Dayton. 1981. Effect of nicotinic acid on microbial protein synthesis in vitro and on dairy cattle growth and milk production. J. Dairy Sci. 64:782–791.

Rode, L. M., T. A. McAllister, and K. J. Cheng. 1990. Microbial degradation of vitamin A in rumen fluid from steers fed concentrate, hay or straw diets. Can. J. Anim. Sci. 70:227–233.

Ronning, M. E., R. Berousek, J. R. Griffiths, and W. D. Gallop. 1959. Carotene requirement of dairy cattle. Pp. 30. Okla. Agric. Exp. Tech. Bull. No. T-76 Stillwater, OK.

Ross, C., and M. E. Ternus. 1993. Vitamin A as a hormone: recent advances in understanding the actions of retinol, retinoic acid and beta carotene. J. Am. Diet. Assoc. 93:1285–1290.

Roth, J. A., and M. L. Kaeberle. 1985. In vivo effect of ascorbic acid on neutrophil function in healthy and dexamethasone-treated cattle. Am. J. Vet. Res. 46:2434-2436.

Rousseau Jr., J. E , H. D. Eaton, C. F. Helmbolt, E. L. Hunghers, S. A. Robrish, G. Beall, and L. A. Moore. 1954. Relative value of carotene and vitamin A from a dry carrier fed at minimum levels to Holstein calves. J. Dairy Sci. 37:889–899.

Sharma, B. K., and R. A. Erdman. 1988a. Abomasal infusion of choline and methionine with or without 2-amino-2-methyl-1-propanol for lactating dairy cows. J. Dairy Sci. 71:2406–11.

Sharma, B. K., and R. A. Erdman. 1988b. Effect of high levels of dietary choline supplementation on duodenal choline flow and production responses of dairy cows. J. Dairy Sci. 71: 2670–76.

Sharma, B. K., and R. A. Erdman. 1989a. Effects of dietary added and abomasally infused choline on milk production responses of lactating dairy cows. J. Nutr. 119:248–254.

Sharma, B. K., and R. A. Erdman. 1989b. In vitro degradation of choline from selected feedstuffs and choline supplements. J. Dairy Sci. 72:2771–2776.

Shields, D. R., D. M. Schaefer, and T. W. Perry. 1983. Influence of niacin supplementation and nitrogen source on rumen microbial fermentation. J. Anim. Sci. 57:1576–1583.

Skaar, T. C., R. R. Grummer, M. R. Dentine, and R. H. Stauffacher. 1989. Seasonal effects of prepartum and postpartum fat and niacin feeding on lactation performance and lipid metabolism. J. Dairy Sci. 72:2028–2038.

Smith, C. M. and W. O. Song. 1996. Comparative nutrition of pantothenic acid. Nutr. Biochem. 7:312–321.

Smith, K. L., J. H. Harrison, D. D. Hancock, D. A. Todhunter, and H. R. Conrad. 1984. Effect of vitamin E and selenium supplementation on incidence of clinical mastitis and duration of clinical symptoms. J. Dairy Sci. 67:1293–1300.

Sommerfeldt, J. L., J. L. Napoli, E. T. Littledike, D. C. Beitz, and R. L. Horst. 1983. Metabolism of orally administered [$^3$H] ergocalciferol and [$^3$H] cholecalciferol by dairy calves. J. Nutr. 113:2595–2600.

St.-Laurent, A. M., M. Hidiroglou, M. Snoddon, and J. W. Nicholson. 1990. Effect of α-tocopherol supplementation to dairy cows on milk and plasma α-tocopherol concentrations and on spontaneous oxidized flavor in milk. Can. J. Anim. Sci. 70:561–570.

Sutton, A. L., and J. M. Elliot. 1972. Effect of ratio of roughage to concentrate and level of feed intake on ovine ruminal vitamin $B_{12}$ production. J. Nutr. 102:1341–1346.

Swanson, E. W , G. G. Martin, F. E. Pardue, and G. M. Gorman. 1968. Milk production of cows fed diets deficient in vitamin A. J. Anim. Sci. 57:541–548.

Tanaka, Y., and H. F. DeLuca. 1973. The control of 25-hydroxyvitamin D metabolism by inorganic phosphorus. Arch. Biochem. Biophys. 154:566–574.

Thafvelin, B., and H. E. Oksanen. 1966. Vitamin E and linolenic acid content of hays as related to different drying conditions. J. Dairy Sci. 49:282–286.

Thomas, J. W., and L. A. Moore. 1951. Factors affecting the antirachitic activity of alfalfa and its ability to prevent rickets in young calves. J. Dairy Sci. 34:916–928.

Tomkins, T., and E. H. Jaster. 1991. Preruminant calf nutrition. Vet. Clinics of North Am.: Food Anim. Pract. 7:557–576.

Tramontano, W. A., D. Ganci, M. Pennino, and E. S. Dierenfeld. 1993. Distribution of α-tocopherol in early foliage samples in several forage crops. Phytochem. 34:389–390.

Van Saun, R. J., T. H. Herdt, and H. D. Stowe. 1989. Maternal and fetal vitamin E concentrations and selenium-vitamin E interrelationships in dairy cattle. J. Nutr. 119:1156–1164.

Vinet, C., H. R. Conrad, T. A. Reinhardt, and R. L. Horst. 1985. Minimal requirements for vitamin D in lactating cows. Fed. Proc. 28:549 (Abstr.).

Walker, C. K., and J. M. Elliot. 1972. Lactational trends in vitamin $B_{12}$ status on conventional and restricted roughage rations. J. Dairy Sci. 55:474–482.

Ward, G., R. C. Dobson, and J. R. Dunham. 1972. Influences of calcium and phosphorus intakes, vitamin D supplement, and lactation on calcium and phosphorus balances. J. Dairy Sci. 55:768–776.

Ward, G., G. B. Marion, C. W. Campbell, and J. R. Dunham. 1971. Influences of calcium intake and vitamin D supplementation on reproductive performance of dairy cows. J. Dairy Sci. 54:204–206.

Warner, R. L., G. E. Mitchell, Jr., C. O. Little, and N. E. Alderson. 1970. Pre-intestinal disappearance of vitamin A in steers fed different levels of corn. International J. Vitamin Research 40:585–588.

Waterman, R., J. W. Schwalm, and L. H. Schultz. 1972. Nicotinic acid treatment of bovine ketosis I. Effects on circulatory metabolites and interrelationships. J. Dairy Sci. 55:1447–1453.

Weiss, W. P., J. S. Hogan, and K. L. Smith. 1994. Use of α-tocopherol concentrations in blood components to assess vitamin E status of dairy cows. Agri-Practice 15 (7):5–8.

Weiss, W. P., J. S. Hogan, D. A. Todhunter, and K. L. Smith. 1997. Effect of vitamin E supplementation in diets with a low concentration of selenium on mammary gland health of dairy cows. J. Dairy Sci. 80:1728–1737.

Weiss, W. P., K. L. Smith, J. S. Hogan, and T. E. Steiner. 1995. Effect of forage to concentrate ratio on disappearance of vitamins A and E during in vitro ruminal fermentation. J. Dairy Sci. 78:1837–1842.

Wichtel, J. J., A. L. Craigie, K. G. Thompson, and N. B. Williamson. 1996. Effect of selenium and α-tocopherol supplementation on postpartum reproductive function of dairy heifers at pasture. Theriogenology 46:491–502.

Wing, J. M. 1969. Effect of source and season on apparent digestibility of carotene in forage by cattle. J. Dairy Sci. 52:479–483.

Yamini, B., R. H. Poppenga, W. E. Braselton, Jr. and L. J. Judge. 1995. Dicoumarol (moldy sweet clover) toxicosis in a group of Holstein calves. J. Vet. Diagn. Invest. 7:420–422.

Zimmerman, C. A., A. H. Rakes, T. E. Daniel, and B. A. Hopkins. 1992. Influence of dietary protein and supplemental niacin on lactational performance of cows fed normal and low fiber diets. J. Dairy Sci. 75:1965–1978.

Zinn, R. A., F. N. Owen, R. L. Stuart, J. R. Dunbar, and B. B. Norman. 1987. B-Vitamin supplementation of diets for feedlot calves. J. Anim. Sci. 65:267–277.

# 8 Water

Water is the most important nutrient for dairy cattle. It is required for all of life's processes—transport of nutrients and other compounds to and from cells; digestion and metabolism of nutrients; elimination of waste materials (urine, feces, and respiration) and excess heat (perspiration) from the body; maintenance of a proper fluid and ion balance in the body; and provision of a fluid environment for the developing fetus (Houpt, 1984; Murphy, 1992). A loss of 20 percent of the body water is fatal (Houpt, 1984).

The total body water content of dairy cattle is 56 to 81 percent of their body weight (Murphy, 1992). Physiologic stage and body composition affect the body's water content. Cows in early lactation have more body weight in water (69.0 percent) than cows in late lactation (62.4 percent) with late-gestation dry cows intermediate in body water content (64.7 percent) (Andrew et al., 1995). Fat cows have a lower water content than thin lactating cows, and younger, leaner animals have a higher water content than older animals (Murphy, 1992).

Body water is divided into intracellular and extracellular compartments. Intracellular water is the largest compartment, accounting for about two-thirds of the water in the body. The extracellular fluid comprises water around cells and connective tissue, water in plasma, and transcellular water or water in the gastrointestinal tract. Intestinal water accounts for 15-35 percent of body weight (Odwongo et al., 1985; Woodford et al., 1984). Cows in early lactation had about 15 percent of their body weight in gastrointestinal water, while cows in late lactation and in gestation had 10 to 11 percent (Andrew et al., 1995). Resident time of a water molecule in the rumen was estimated to be 61 minutes in sheep (Faichney and Boston, 1985) and 62 minutes in lactating dairy cattle (Woodford et al., 1984).

Loss of water from the body occurs through milk production, urine excretion, fecal excretion, sweat, and vapor loss from the lungs. Water losses through milk of cows producing 33 kg/day were about 34 percent (Holter and Urban, 1992), 29 percent (Dado and Allen, 1994), and 26 percent (Dahlborn et al., 1998) of total water intake (feed plus free water consumed). Fecal water losses are similar to those of milk (30 to 35 percent of total water intake), and urine losses are about half of fecal losses (15 to 21 percent) in lactating cows (Holter and Urban, 1992; Dahlborn et al., 1998). Factors that affect fecal water loss include dry matter intake (DMI), dry matter (DM) content of the diet being fed, and digestibility of the diet (Murphy, 1992). Dahlborn et al. (1998) reported that fecal DM percentage did not change with changing dietary DM, but water loss via feces increased with increasing dietary forage content. Urinary water excretion in cattle is variable at 4.5 to 35.4 L/day in cows producing an average of 34.6 kg/day of milk and 5.6 to 27.9 L/day in dry cows (Holter and Urban, 1992). Urinary water excretion was related positively to water availability, amount of water absorbed from the intestinal tract (total intake minus fecal loss), urinary nitrogen, and urinary potassium excretion and negatively related to dietary DM content (Murphy, 1992). Increasing forage in the diet increased urinary water loss (Dahlborn et al., 1998). Sweat, salivary, and evaporative losses combined account for about 18 percent of water loss (Holter and Urban, 1992).

## WATER INTAKE

Cattle require large amounts of water every day. They meet this requirement via three sources: drinking or free water intake (FWI), ingestion of water contained in feed, and water produced by the body's metabolism of nutrients. Metabolic water is an insignificant source compared with the water ingested freely or in feed. The sum of FWI and the water ingested in feed is the total water intake (TWI).

Several factors that affect the amount of FWI of dairy cows each day have been identified. Of studies in which equations were developed to predict daily FWI, DMI was included as a variable in four (Holter and Urban, 1992; Little and Shaw, 1978; Murphy et al., 1983; Stockdale and King, 1983), daily milk production in five (Castle and Thomas, 1975; Dahlborn et al., 1998; Holter and Urban, 1992; Little and Shaw, 1978; Murphy et al., 1983), DM content of the diet (DM percent of diet) in four (Castle and Thomas, 1975; Dahlborn et al., 1998; Holter and Urban, 1992; Stockdale and King, 1983), temperature or environmental factors in two (Holter and Urban, 1992; Murphy et al., 1983) and sodium intake in one (Murphy et al., 1983). Equations for predicting FWI, (kg/day) of lactating dairy cows are shown below:

$$-15.3 + 2.53 \times \text{milk, kg/d} + 0.45 \times \text{DM\% of diet.} \quad \text{(Castle and Thomas, 1975)} \quad (8\text{-}1)$$

$$14.3 + 1.28 \times \text{milk, kg/d} + 0.32 \times \text{DM\% of diet.} \quad \text{(Dahlborn et al., 1998)} \quad (8\text{-}2)$$

$$-32.39 + 2.47 \times \text{DMI, kg/d} + 0.6007 \times \text{milk, kg/d} + 0.6205 \times \text{DM\% of diet} + 0.0911 \times \text{Julian Day(JD)} - 0.000257 \times \text{JD}^2 \quad \text{(Holter and Urban, 1992)} \quad (8\text{-}3)$$

$$12.3 + 2.15 \times \text{DMI, kg/d} + 0.73 \times \text{milk, kg/d} \quad \text{(Little and Shaw, 1978)} \quad (8\text{-}4)$$

$$15.99 + 1.58 \times \text{DMI, kg/d} + 0.90 \times \text{milk, kg/d} + 0.05 \times \text{Na intake g/d} + 1.20 \times \text{min temp C} \quad \text{(Murphy et al., 1983)} \quad (8\text{-}5)$$

$$-9.37 + 2.30 \times \text{DMI, kg/d} + 0.053 \times \text{DM\% of diet} \quad \text{(Stockdale and King, 1983)} \quad (8\text{-}6)$$

Winchester and Morris (1956) indicated that 0.87 kg of water per kilogram of milk was an expected requirement for water based on milk being 87 percent water. The 0.90 coefficient of Murphy et al. (1983) is close to this coefficient with the lower coefficients of 0.73 and 0.6007 reported by Little and Shaw (1978) and Holter and Urban (1992). Thus, because the milk coefficient in the Murphy et al. (1983) equation is biologically closest to the water content of milk (87 percent) and other variables in the equation have been shown to affect water intake, this equation is recommended for predicting FWI.

In studies in which milk production was 33–35 kg/d, FWI was 2.0 kg (Holter and Urban, 1992), 2.3 kg (Dado and Allen, 1994), and 2.7 kg (Murphy et al., 1983) per kilogram of milk produced. Total water intake was 3.0 kg (Dado and Allen, 1994; Murphy et al., 1983) and 2.6 kg (Holter and Urban, 1992) per kilogram of milk produced. In studies (Dahlborn et al., 1998; Little and Shaw, 1978; Castle and Thomas, 1975) with lower milk production (less than 26 kg/d), both FWI (2.6–3.0 kg/kg of milk) and TWI (3.3–4.2 kg/kg of milk) were higher.

Results of seven studies (Castle and Thomas, 1975; Dado and Allen, 1994; Dahlborn et al., 1998; Holter and Urban, 1992; Little and Shaw, 1978; Murphy et al., 1983; Nocek and Braun, 1985) indicated that an average of 83 percent (range, 70–97 percent) of the total water consumed by lactating cows was by drinking. DM content of the diet is one of the major factors affecting FWI. Holter and Urban (1992) reported no difference in FWI of cows fed diets that contained 50 to 70 percent DM, but FWI decreased by 33 kg/d when diets decreased from 50 to 30 percent DM. That observation is supported by other studies (Castle and Thomas, 1975; Dahlborn et al., 1998) and the research of Stockdale and King (1983), in which cattle grazing pasture consumed only 38 percent of their TWI by drinking.

Diets high in salt, sodium bicarbonate, or protein appear to stimulate water intake (Holter and Urban, 1992; Murphy, 1992). Sodium intake alone was found to increase water intake by 0.05 kg/day per gram of sodium intake (Murphy et al., 1983). High-forage diets might also increase water requirements by increasing the loss of water in feces and urine (Dahlborn et al., 1998)

Water is an especially important nutrient during periods of heat stress. The physical properties of water, thermal conductivity and latent heat of vaporization, are important for the transfer of heat from the body to the environment. During periods of cold stress, the high heat capacity of body water acts as insulation conserving body heat. As air temperature increases above the thermal neutral zone, shifts in the amount of water consumed and how water is lost from the body occur. McDowell (1967) reported that increasing temperatures from 18 to 30°C increased water consumption by 29 percent, decreased fecal water loss by 33 percent, but increased water loss via urine, sweating, and respiration by 15, 59, and 50 percent, respectively. The equations of Murphy et al. (1983) and Holter and Urban (1992) contain an environmental variable. Murphy et al. (1983) included a variable associated with minimal daily temperature that increased FWI by about 25 percent as minimal temperatures increased from 0 to 25°C. Holter and Urban (1992) included Julian days in their FWI equation and going from 1 to peak intake at 178 days, increased FWI by about 10 percent. Besides air temperature, the effect of exposure to direct sunlight has been shown to affect FWI. During summer months, cows provided with no shade consumed 18 percent more water per day than cows provided shade (Muller et al., 1994).

### *Dry Cows*

Holter and Urban (1992) developed the following equation to predict FWI of dry cows:

$$\text{FWI, kg/d} = -10.34 + .2296 \times \text{DM\% of diet} + 2.212 \times \text{DMI kg/d} + 0.03944 \times (\text{CP\% of diet})^2 \quad (8\text{-}7)$$

where CP = crude protein.

The major factors affecting FWI of dry cows are DMI and the percentage of DM in the diet. Increasing dietary DM from 30 to 60 percent increased FWI, but increasing dietary DM content above 60 percent had only a minor effect on either FWI or TWI. The increased FWI of dry cows caused by increasing crude protein content of the diet is a physiologic response to dilute and excrete nitrogen in excess of needs.

### *Calves and Heifers*

During the liquid feeding stage, calves receive most of their water via milk or milk replacer. It is recommended water be provided free choice to calves receiving liquid diets to enhance growth and DMI. Kertz et al. (1984) reported calves offered water free choice in addition to the liquid diet gained faster and consumed dry feed quicker than calves provided water only in their liquid diet. Water intakes increased from about 1 kg/day during the first week of life to over 2.5 kg/d during the fourth week of life; with most of the increase occurring during the fourth week.

### *Drinking Behavior*

Water consumption occurs several times per day and is generally associated with feeding or milking. Nocek and Braun (1985) reported that the relationship between feeding frequency and voluntary water intake was not significant; however, cows fed once per day consumed slightly less DM and water than cows fed eight times per day. Peak hourly water intakes were associated with peak hourly intakes of DM. Dado and Allen (1994) reported that lactating cows housed in tie stalls drank an average of 14 times per day. Water intake was correlated positively with both total DMI and number of eating bouts per day. In loose housing with water bowls, lactating cows consumed water an average of 6.6 times per day (Andersson, 1985). Nocek and Braun (1985) and Castle and Watson (1973) indicated that most water is consumed during daylight hours.

Reported rates of water intake vary from 4 to 15 kg/minute (Dado and Allen, 1994; Castle and Thomas, 1975). On the basis of the farm studies of Castle and Thomas (1975), the length of water troughs should be 5 cm/cow with an optimal height of 90 cm. A minimum of one water bowl per 10 cows was recommended.

The temperature of drinking water has only a slight effect on drinking behavior and animal performance. Cooling of drinking water to 10°C had a transient effect on reducing body temperature but did not affect milk production relative to production when water was at 27.7°C (Stermer et al., 1986). In other studies, the chilling of drinking water to 10°C increased milk production (Milam et al., 1986; Wilks et al., 1990) and DMI (Baker et al., 1988; Stermer et al., 1986; Wilks et al., 1990). Responses to chilling of water under most conditions would not warrant the additional cost of cooling water. Given a choice of water temperature, cows prefer to drink water with moderate temperatures (17–28°C) rather than cold or hot water (Andersson, 1987; Lanham et al., 1986; Wilks et al., 1990).

## WATER QUALITY

Water quality is an important issue in the production and health of dairy cattle. The five criteria most often considered in assessing water quality for both humans and livestock are: organoleptic properties (odor and taste), physiochemical properties (pH, total dissolved solids, total dissolved oxygen, and hardness), presence of toxic compounds (heavy metals, toxic minerals, organophosphates, and hydrocarbons), presence of excess minerals or compounds (nitrates, sodium, sulfates, and iron), and presence of bacteria. Research information on water contaminants and their effects on cattle performance is sparse. The following attempts to define some common water-quality problems in relation to cattle performance.

*Salinity, total dissolved solids (TDS), and total soluble salts (TSS)* are measures of constituents soluble in water. Sodium chloride is the first consideration in this category, but other components associated with salinity, TDS, or TSS are bicarbonate, sulfate, calcium, magnesium, and silica (National Research Council, 1974). A secondary group of constituents, found in lower concentrations than the major constituents, consists of iron, nitrate, strontium, potassium, carbonate, phosphorus, boron, and fluoride. Guidelines for TSS in water for dairy cattle are in Table 8-1.

Research at Arizona (Ray, 1986; Wegner and Schuh, 1986) has evaluated the effects of saline water on feedlot

TABLE 8-1 Guidelines for Total Soluble Salts (TSS) in Water for Cattle

| TSS (mg/L) | Comments |
|---|---|
| <1,000 | Safe and should pose no health problems. |
| 1,000–2,999 | Generally safe but may cause a mild temporary diarrhea in animals not accustomed to the water. |
| 3,000–4,999 | Water may be refused when first offered to animals or cause temporary diarrhea. Animal performance may be less than optimum because water intake is not maximized. |
| 5,000–6,999 | Avoid these waters for pregnant or lactating animals. May be offered with reasonable safety to animals where maximum performance is not required. |
| 7,000 | These waters should not be fed to cattle. Health problems and/or poor production will result. |

SOURCE: National Research Council (1974).

steers and lactating dairy cows. Feedlot cattle drinking saline water (TDS, 6,000 mg/L) had lower weight gains than cattle drinking normal water (1,300 mg/L) when energy content of the ration was low and during heat stress. High-energy rations and the cold of the winter months negated the detrimental effects of high-saline water consumption. Likewise, milk production of dairy cows drinking high saline water (TDS, 4,400 mg/L) was not different from that of cows drinking normal water during cool months but was significantly lower during summer months. Cows offered the salty water drank more water per day (136 vs 121 kg/cow) over a 12-month period than cows drinking normal water.

The performance of dairy cows consuming high-saline waters has been variable. In a study that compared water with dissolved solids from sodium chloride at 196 mg/L and 2,500 mg/L, lactating cows consuming water with the high salt content increased water intake by 7 percent and exhibited a tendency for less milk yield and DMI compared with cows consuming low-saline water (Jaster et al., 1978). An Israeli study (Solomon et al., 1995) with Holstein cows producing milk at over 30 kg/day showed that cows consuming desalinated water consumed 11 kg more water per day and produced 2.2 kg more milk per day than cows consuming salty water. Also, both milk protein percentage (2.89 vs 2.84 percent) and lactose percentage (4.50 vs 4.44 percent) were higher for cows consuming the desalinated water. Similar results were observed by Challis et al. (1987) under hot desert conditions. They reduced the TDS of water from about 4,400 to 440 mg/L and obtained a greater than 20 percent increase in milk production, water intake, and feed intake. Cooling of the desalinated water resulted in a small additional increase in milk production. Bahman et al. (1993) offered cows natural water that contained TDS at 3,574 mg/L and desalinated water at 449 mg/L and observed no differences in milk production. The equation of Murphy et al. (1983), which considers sodium intake, predicted intake of high-saline water better than the equations of Holter and Urban (1992).

Sanchez et al. (1994) indicated that high intakes of chloride and sulfate are detrimental to milk production during summer months. Saline water generally contains high concentrations of chloride and sulfate and so would contribute to high intakes of these elements. Likewise, saline waters are high in sodium, but feeding high amounts of sodium does not reduce milk production or lactation performance (Sanchez et al., 1994). The cation-anion differences (CAD, mEq/L) of the high-saline water in studies in which milk production or water intake reductions were observed was −1.9 (Solomon et al., 1995) and −4.4 (Challis et al., 1987). Reductions in milk production or water consumption were not observed in the study of Bahman et al. (1993) when brackish well water with a CAD of −3.0 mEq/L was offered for 196 days.

*Hardness* is generally expressed as the sum of calcium and magnesium reported in equivalent amounts of calcium carbonate. Other cations in water—such as zinc, iron, strontium, aluminum, and manganese—can contribute to hardness but are usually in very low concentrations compared with calcium and magnesium. Hardness categories are listed in Table 8-2. The hardness of water had no effect on animal performance or water intake (Graf and Holdaway, 1952; Blosser and Soni, 1957).

*Nitrate* can be used in the rumen as a source of nitrogen for synthesis of bacterial protein, but reduction to nitrite also occurs. When absorbed into the body, nitrite reduces the oxygen-carrying capacity of hemoglobin and in severe cases results in asphyxiation. Symptoms of acute nitrate or nitrite poisoning are asphyxiation and labored breathing, rapid pulse, frothing at the mouth, convulsions, blue muzzle and bluish tint around eyes, and chocolate-brown blood. More moderate levels of nitrate poisoning have been incriminated in poor growth, infertility problems, abortions, vitamin A deficiencies, and general unhealthiness, but research has not always substantiated these claims (Crowley et al., 1974; Stuart and Oehme, 1982).

The general safe concentration of nitrate-nitrogen ($NO_3$-N) in water is less than 10 mg/L and of nitrate less than 44 mg/L (Table 8-3). In evaluating potential nitrate problems, feeds also should be analyzed for nitrate in that the effects of feed and water nitrate are additive.

*Sulfate* guidelines for water are not well defined, but general recommendations are less than 500 mg/L for calves and less than 1,000 mg/L for adult cattle. When sulfate exceeds 500 mg/L, the specific salt form of sulfate or sulfur

TABLE 8-2 Water Hardness Guidelines

| Category | Hardness (mg/L)[a] |
|---|---|
| Soft | 0–60 |
| Moderately hard | 61–120 |
| Hard | 121–180 |
| Very hard | >180 |

[a] 1 grain/gal = 17.1 mg/L.
SOURCE: National Research Council (1980).

TABLE 8-3 Nitrate in Water

| Nitrate ($NO_3$) (mg/L) | Nitrate Nitrogen ($NO_3$-N) (mg/L) | Guidelines |
|---|---|---|
| 0–44 | 0–10 | Safe for consumption by ruminants |
| 45–132 | 10–20 | Generally safe in balanced diets with low nitrate feeds |
| 133–220 | 20–40 | Could be harmful if consumed over long periods |
| 221–660 | 40–100 | Cattle at risk; and possible death |
| 661 | 100 | Unsafe—possible death; should not be used as a source of water |

SOURCE: National Research Council (1974).

should be identified. The form of sulfur is an important determinant of toxicity (National Research Council, 1980). Hydrogen sulfide is the most toxic form, and concentrations as low as 0.1 mg/L can reduce water intake. Common forms of sulfate in water are calcium, iron, magnesium, and sodium salts. All are laxative, but sodium sulfate is the most potent. Cattle fed water that is high in sulfates (2,000–2,500 mg/L) show diarrhea initially but appear to become resistant to the laxative effect. Iron sulfate was reported by Horvath (1985) to be a more potent depressor of water intake than other forms of sulfate.

Research from Nevada (Digesti and Weeth, 1976; Weeth and Capps, 1972; Weeth and Hunter, 1971) has shown that cattle can tolerate sulfate at up to 2,500 mg/L in water for short periods (less than 90 days) with no major metabolic problems. At 2,500 mg/L, heifers increased renal filtration of sulfate by 37 percent compared with heifers drinking water that contained 110 mg/L. Heifers also rejected water that contained 2,500 mg/L if lower-sulfate water was available. Research from Canada (Smart et al., 1986) has shown that beef cows drinking water that contained sulfate at 500 mg/L had lower concentrations of copper in plasma and liver than cows consuming water that contained 42 mg/L. No significant differences in health, reproduction, weight changes of cows, or birth weight of calves were reported, but calves of cows that received the high-sulfate water had lower weaning weights than calves of cows that received low-sulfate water. Water and feed with high sulfate contents have been linked to polioencephalomalacia in beef calves (Hibbs and Thilsted, 1983; Gould, 1998).

*pH* guidelines of water for dairy cattle have not been established. The EPA (1997) recommendation for the pH of human drinking water is between 6.5 and 8.5. No information was found in the scientific literature as to what effects the pH of water has on water intake, animal health, animal production, or the microbial environment in the rumen.

*Other nutrients and contaminants* are sometimes found in water and can pose a health hazard to cattle. For safe consumption, water contaminants should not exceed the guidelines in Table 8-4. However, many dietary, physiologic, and environmental factors affect these guidelines and make it impossible to determine precisely the concentrations at which problems will occur.

*Microbiologic analysis* of water for coliform bacteria and other microorganisms is necessary to determine sanitary quality. A common microbiologic analysis is for total coliforms, not specific coliforms. Results from the assay are usually reported as a most probable number (MPN), which is an index of the number of coliforms present (0 MPN = satisfactory; 1–8 MPN = unsatisfactory; over 9 MPN = unsafe). A more specific analysis for contamination is a fecal-coliform test. Coliforms found in human and animal feces can be determined directly, and information as to the source of contamination can be obtained. The effect of coliforms in water on health of cattle or ruminal microorganisms is unknown.

TABLE 8-4 Generally Considered Safe Concentrations of Some Potentially Toxic Nutrients and Contaminants in Water for Cattle

| Item | Upper-limit guideline |
|---|---|
| | (mg/L or ppm) |
| Aluminum | 0.5 |
| Arsenic | 0.05 |
| Boron | 5.0 |
| Cadmium | 0.005 |
| Chromium | 0.1 |
| Cobalt | 1.0 |
| Copper | 1.0 |
| Fluorine | 2.0 |
| Lead | 0.015 |
| Manganese | 0.05 |
| Mercury | 0.01 |
| Nickel | 0.25 |
| Selenium | 0.05 |
| Vanadium | 0.1 |
| Zinc | 5.0 |

SOURCE: National Research Council (1974, 1980); Environmental Protection Agency (1997).

## SUMMARY

Water availability and quality are extremely important for animal health and productivity. Limiting water availability to cattle will depress production rapidly and severely.

Some water contaminants—such as nitrates, sodium chloride, and sulfates—have been reported to affect animal performance and health. However, most water contaminants have an unknown effect on animal performance. That is particularly true for water that has low concentrations of contaminants and is consumed over a long period.

On the basis of the scientific literature, no widespread specific beef cattle or dairy cattle production problems have been caused by consumption of water of low quality. Water quality might cause poor production or nonspecific diseases and should be one aspect of the procedures used to investigate such problems.

## REFERENCES

Andersson, M. 1985. Effects of drinking water temperatures on water intake and milk yield of tied-up dairy cows. Livest. Prod. Sci. 12:329–338.

Andersson, M. 1987. Effects of number and location of water bowls and social rank on drinking behaviour and performance of loose-housed dairy cows. Livest. Prod. Sci. 17:19–31.

Andrew, S. M., R. A. Erdman, and D. R. Waldo. 1995. Prediction of body composition of dairy cows at three physiological stages from deuterium oxide and urea dilution. J. Dairy Sci. 78:1083–1095.

Bahman, A. M., J. A. Rooke, and J. H. Topps. 1993. The performance of dairy cows offered drinking water of low or high salinity in a hot arid climate. Anim. Prod. 57:23–28.

Baker, C. C., C. E. Coppock, J. K. Lanham, D. H. Nave, J. M. Labore, C. F. Brasington, and R. A. Stermer. 1988. Chilled drinking water effects on lactating Holstein cows in summer. J. Dairy Sci. 71:2699–2708.

Blosser, T. H., and B. K. Soni. 1957. Comparative influence of hard and soft water on milk production of dairy cows. J. Dairy Sci. 40:1519–1524.

Castle, M. E., and T. P. Thomas. 1975. The water intake of British Friesian cows on rations containing various forages. Anim. Prod. 20:181–189.

Castle, M. E., and J. N. Watson. 1973. The intake of drinking water by grazing dairy cows; the effect of water availability. J. Br. Grassland Soc. 28:203–207.

Challis, D. J., J. S. Zeinstra, and M. J. Anderson. 1987. Some effects of water quality on the performance of high yielding dairy cows in an arid climate. Vet. Rec. 120:12–15.

Crowley, J. W., N. A. Jorgensen, L. W. Kahler, L. D. Satter, W. J. Tyler, and M. F. Finner 1974. Effect of nitrate in drinking water on reproductive and productive efficiency of dairy cattle. Tech. Rep. 74-06. Univ. of Wisconsin-Madison.

Dado, R. G., and M. S. Allen. 1994. Variation in and relationships among feeding, chewing, and drinking variables for lactating cows. J. Dairy Sci. 77:132–144.

Dahlborn, K., M. Akerlind, and G. Gustafson. 1998. Water intake by dairy cows selected for high or low milk-fat percentage when fed two forage to concentrate ratios with hay or silage. Swedish J. Agric. Res. 28:167–176.

Digesti, R. D., and H. J. Weeth. 1976. A defensible maximum for inorganic sulfate in drinking water of cattle. J. Anim. Sci. 42:1498–1502.

Environmental Protection Agency. 1997. Current drinking water standards (Human). Office of Ground Water and Drinking Water. U.S. Environ. Protection Agency. Wash., DC. EPA 815-k-97-002

Faichney, G. J., and R. C. Boston. 1985. Movement of water within the body of sheep fed at maintenance under thermoneutral conditions. J. Biol. Sci. 38:85–94.

Gould, D. H. 1998. Polioencephalomalacia. J. Animal Sci. 76:309–314.

Graf, G. C., and C. W. Holdaway. 1952. A comparison of hard and commercially softened water in the ration of lactating dairy cows. J. Dairy Sci. 35:998–1000.

Hibbs, C. M., and J. P. Thilsted. 1983. Toxicosis in cattle from contaminated well water. Vet. and Human Toxicol. 25:253–254.

Holter, J. B., and W. E. Urban, Jr. 1992. Water partitioning and intake in dry and lactating Holstein cows. J. Dairy Sci. 75:1472–1479.

Horvath, D. 1985. The transparent nutrient. Water: Its quality and importance in production and health. Proc., 14th Biennial Ruminant Health Conf. Syracuse, NY.

Houpt, T. R. 1984. Water balance and excretion. In: Duke's Physiology of Domestic Animals. 10th Edition. M. J. Swenson, Ed. Comstock Publishing Co., NY.

Jaster, E. H., J. D Schuh, and T. N. Wegner. 1978. Physiological effects of saline drinking water on high producing dairy cows. J. Dairy Sci. 61:66–71.

Kertz, A. F., L. F. Reutzel, and J. H. Mahoney. 1984. Ad libitum water intake by neonatal calves and its relationship to calf starter intake, weight gain, feces score, and season. J. Dairy Sci. 67:2964–2969.

Lanham, J. K., C. E. Coppock, K. Z. Milam, J. M. Labore, D. H. Nave, R. A. Stermer, and C. F. Brasington. 1986. Effects of drinking water temperature on physiological responses of lactating Holstein cows in summer. J. Dairy Sci. 69:1004–1012.

Little, W., and S. R. Shaw. 1978. A note on the individuality of the intake of drinking water by dairy cows. Anim. Proc. 26:225–227.

McDowell, R. E. 1967. Water exchange of cattle under heat stress. Biometerology 2:414.

Milam, K. Z., C. E. Coppock, J. W. West, J. K. Lanham, D. H. Nave, J. M. Labore, R. A. Stermer, and C. F. Brasington. 1986. Effects of drinking water temperature on production responses in lactating Holstein cows in summer. J. Dairy Sci. 69:1013–1019.

Muller, C. J. C., J. A. Botha, and W. A. Smith. 1994. Effect of shade on various parameters of Friesian cows in a Mediterranean climate in South Africa. 1. Feed and water intake, milk production and milk composition. S. Afr. J. Anim. Sci. 24(2):49–55.

Murphy, M. R., C. L. Davis, and G. C. McCoy. 1983. Factors affecting water consumption by Holstein cows in early lactation. J. Dairy Sci. 66:35–38.

Murphy, M. R. 1992. Water metabolism of dairy cattle. J. Dairy Sci. 75:326–333.

National Research Council. 1974. Nutrients and Toxic Substances in Water for Livestock and Poultry. Washington, DC: National Academy Press.

National Research Council. 1980. Mineral Tolerance of Domestic Animals. Washington, DC: National Academy Press.

Nocek, J. E., and D. G. Braun. 1985. Effect of feeding frequency on diurnal dry matter and water consumption, liquid dilution rate, and milk yield in first lactation. J. Dairy Sci. 68:2238–2247.

Odwongo, W. O., H. R. Conrad, A. E. Staubus, and J. H. Harrison. 1985. Measurement of water kinetics with deuterium oxide in lactating dairy cows. J. Dairy Sci. 68:1155–1164.

Ray, D. E. 1986. Water salinity and performance of feedlot cattle. Proc., Southwest Nutr. Conf. Univ. of Arizona.

Sanchez, W. K., M. A. McGuire, and D. K. Beede. 1994. Macromineral nutrition by heat stress interactions in dairy cattle: Review and original research. J. Dairy Sci. 77:2051–2079.

Smart, M. E., R. Cohen, D. A. Christensen, and C. M. Williams. 1986. The effects of sulphate removal from drinking water on the plasma and liver copper and zinc concentrations of beef cows and their calves. Can. J. Anim. Sci. 66:669–680.

Solomon, R., J. Miron, and D. Ben-Ghedalia. 1995. Performance of high producing cows offered drinking water of high and low salinity in the Arava desert. J. Dairy Sci. 78:620–624.

Stermer, R A., C. F. Brasington, C. E. Coppock, J. K. Lanham, and K. Z. Milam. 1986. Effect of drinking water temperature on heat stress of dairy cows. J. Dairy Sci. 69:546–551.

Stockdale, C. R., and K. R. King. 1983. A note on some of the factors that affect the water consumption of lactating dairy cows at pasture. Anim. Prod. 36:303–306.

Stuart, L. D., and F. W. Oehme. 1982. Environmental factors in bovine and porcine abortion. Vet. and Human Toxicol. 24:435–441.

Weeth, H. J., and D. L. Capps. 1972. Tolerance of growing cattle for sulfate-water. J. Anim. Sci. 34:256–260.

Weeth, H. J., and J. E. Hunter. 1971. Drinking of sulfate-water by cattle. J. Anim. Sci. 32:277–281.

Wegner, T., and J. Schuh. 1986. Water quality and animal performance—lactating dairy cows. Proc., Southwest Nutr. Conf. Univ. of Arizona.

Wilks, D. L., C. E. Coppock, J. K. Lanham, K. N. Brooks, C. C. Baker, W. L. Bryson, R. G. Elmore, and R. A. Stermer. 1990. Responses of lactating Holstein cows to chilled drinking water in high ambient temperatures. J. Dairy Sci. 73:1091–1099.

Winchester, C. F., and M. J. Morris. 1956. Water intake rates of cattle. J. Anim. Sci. 15:722–740.

Woodford, S. T., M. R. Murphy, and C. L. Davis. 1984. Water dynamics of dairy cattle as affected by initiation of lactation and feed intake. J. Dairy Sci. 67:2336–2343.

# 9 Unique Aspects of Dairy Cattle Nutrition

## TRANSITION COWS AND NONLACTATING COWS

### *Nutritional and Physiologic Status of the Transition Cow*

Fetal dry weight increases exponentially during gestation (House and Bell, 1993; National Research Council, 1996). Bell et al. (1995) indicated linear or nonlinear regression models were more suitable than exponential models for describing increases in fetal dry weight, fresh weight, and crude protein (CP) and energy accretion during the final trimester of pregnancy. They speculated that exponential models might be more appropriate when describing fetal growth for the entire gestation (i.e., including periods when fetal size is very small). Because conceptus growth approaches linearity during the final stages of gestation, exponential models developed from data obtained throughout pregnancy may overestimate growth during late gestation. Fetal sex does not influence growth rates (Ferrell et al., 1982; House and Bell, 1993). Fetal tissue accounts for 45 percent of the uterine dry weight at day 190 of pregnancy and 80 percent at day 270 of pregnancy (Bell et al., 1995).

The dry period, in particular the transition period, is characterized by dramatic changes in endocrine status. These changes prepare the cow for parturition and lactogenesis. Plasma insulin decreases and growth hormone increases as the cow progresses from late gestation to early lactation, with acute surges in plasma concentrations of both hormones at parturition (Kunz et al., 1985). Plasma thyroxine (T4) concentrations gradually increase during late gestation, decrease approximately 50 percent at calving, and then begin to increase (Kunz et al., 1985). Similar but less pronounced changes occur with 3, 5, 3′-triiodothyronine (T3). Estrogen, primarily estrone of placental origin, increases in plasma during late gestation but decreases immediately at calving (Chew et al., 1979). Progesterone concentrations during the dry period are elevated for maintenance of pregnancy but decline rapidly, approximately 2 days before calving (Chew et al., 1979). Glucocorticoid and prolactin concentrations increase on the day of calving and return to near prepartum concentrations the following day (Edgerton and Hafs, 1973).

Changes in endocrine status and decreases in dry matter intake (DMI) during late gestation influence metabolism and lead to mobilization of fat from adipose tissue and glycogen from the liver. Plasma nonesterified fatty acids (NEFA) increase two-fold or more between 2 to 3 weeks prepartum and 2 to 3 days prepartum, at which time the concentration increases dramatically until completion of parturition (Bertics et al., 1992; Vazquez-Anon, 1994; Grum et al., 1996). How much of the initial increase in plasma NEFA can be accounted for by changing endocrine status compared with energy restriction resulting from decreased DMI is not known. Force feeding cows during the prefresh transition period reduced the magnitude of NEFA increase, but did not completely eliminate it (Bertics et al., 1992). These observations indicate at least part of the prepartum increase in plasma NEFA is hormonally induced. The rapid rise in NEFA on the day of calving is presumably due to the stress of calving. Plasma NEFA concentrations decrease rapidly after calving, but concentrations remain higher than they were before calving.

Plasma glucose concentrations remain stable or increase slightly during the prefresh transition period, increase dramatically at calving, and then decrease immediately postpartum (Kunz et al., 1985; Vazquez-Anon et al., 1994). The transient increase at calving may result from increased glucagon and glucocorticoid concentrations that promote depletion of hepatic glycogen stores. Although the demand for glucose by mammary tissue for lactose synthesis continues after calving, hepatic glycogen stores begin to replete and are increased by day 14 postpartum (Vazquez-Anon et al., 1994). This probably reflects an increase in gluconeogenic capacity to support lactation.

Blood calcium decreases during the last few days prior to calving due to the loss of calcium for the formation of colostrum (Goff and Horst, 1997b). Plasma Ca concentrations are controlled by the coordinated actions of parathyroid hormone and 1, 25-dihydroxyvitamin $D_3$. These hormones act on the intestine, kidney, and bone to increase blood calcium during the periparturient period. Adaptation of the intestine, kidney, and bone to higher demands for calcium takes several days so that blood calcium typically does not return to normal concentrations until several days postpartum (Goff and Horst, 1997b).

As cows initiate and terminate the dry period, there are changes in rumen dynamics. These alterations are nutritionally induced rather than physiologically induced. Changing from a diet that is high in concentrate to a diet that is high in fiber causes alterations in the microbial population and characteristics of the rumen epithelium. High concentrate diets favor starch utilizing bacteria that enhance propionate and lactate production; high fiber diets favor cellulolytic bacteria and methane production and discriminate against bacteria that produce propionate and utilize lactate. End products of fermentation influence papillae growth in the rumen (Dirksen et al., 1985). Papillae are responsible for the absorption of volatile fatty acids. Increasing grain in the diet and propionate concentration in the rumen favors elongation of papillae; diets high in fiber cause the papillae to shorten. As much as 50 percent of the absorptive area in the rumen may be lost during the first 7 weeks of the dry period and elongation of papillae after reintroduction of concentrate takes several weeks (Dirksen et al., 1985). Consequently, sudden introduction of grain immediately postcalving has several deleterious consequences. Lactate production increases prior to the re-establishment of lactate utilizing bacteria. Lactate is more potent in reducing ruminal pH than other volatile fatty acids and volatile fatty acids are absorbed at a faster rate when pH is low (Goff and Horst, 1997b). Rumen papillae will not have had sufficient time to elongate, therefore, volatile fatty acid absorption is limited.

During the transition period, the immunologic status of the cow is compromised. Neutrophil and lymphocyte function is depressed and plasma concentrations of other components of the immune system are decreased (Goff and Horst, 1997b). It is not known why immune function is suppressed but it may be related to the nutritional and physiologic status of the cow. Estrogen and glucocorticoids are immunosuppressive agents and they increase in plasma as parturition approaches (Goff and Horst, 1997b). Intake of vitamin A and E and other nutrients essential for immune function may be decreased as DMI is reduced during the periparturient period.

### *Nutrient Requirements for Pregnancy*

Dry cows require nutrients for maintenance, growth of the conceptus, and perhaps growth of the dam. Estimation of the nutrient requirements for pregnancy by the factorial method requires knowledge of the rates of nutrient accretion in conceptus tissues (fetus, placenta, fetal fluids, and uterus) and the efficiency with which dietary nutrients are utilized for conceptus growth. There are limited data for dairy cattle.

Estimates of CP, energy, and most mineral requirements for gestation during the last two months of pregnancy are from House and Bell (1993) and Bell et al. (1995). Rates of growth and chemical composition were measured in multiparous Holstein cows that were serially slaughtered from 190 to 270 days of pregnancy. Requirements derived from these studies and equations used for the model are discussed in chapters 2 (energy), 5 (protein), and 6 (minerals).

Other estimates for energy and crude protein requirements are available, but they were obtained from beef cattle, dairy breeds other than Holsteins, or from research conducted more than 25 years ago. However, estimates from Bell et al. (1995) do not vary greatly from previous estimates and thus are supportive of requirements published in *Nutrient Requirements of Dairy Cattle* (National Research Council, 1989). Additionally, by using the data from Bell et al. (1995) energy, protein, and mineral requirements for pregnancy were all derived from the same study.

A quadratic regression equation best described protein and energy accretion in the gravid uterus. Estimates of CP and energy requirements to support pregnancy were derived from cows with a mean body weight of 714 kg that carried a single fetus. They are a function of day of gestation, but an adjustment to accommodate differences in calf birth weight was added to the equations derived from Bell et al. (1995). Crude protein requirements for gestation were obtained by assuming an efficiency of 0.33 for conversion of metabolizable protein (MP) to conceptus protein and efficiency of 0.7 for conversion of dietary CP to MP (Bell et al., 1995). The efficiency of conversion of MP to conceptus protein has been reduced from 0.5 used in the previous edition (National Research Council, 1989). The efficiency of conversion of metabolizable energy to conceptus net energy (NE) was assumed to be 0.14 (Ferrell et al., 1976). The low efficiency most likely reflects the high cost of maintaining the fetus.

### *Nutrient Intake*

Intake of nutrients is a function of DMI and nutrient density of the diet. Dry matter intake during the final 21 days of gestation was described (Hayirli et al., 1998) by an exponential function: $y = a + p \times e^{k \times t}$ where y = DMI as a percentage of body weight, a = the asymptotic intercept at time = $-\infty$ (minus infinity), p = the magnitude of intake depression (kg) from the asymptotic intercept until parturition, and $e^{k \times t}$ describes the shape of the curve. Time (t) is expressed as: days pregnant − 280. Following evaluation of the model (mean square predicted error = 0.06 percent $BW^2$, mean bias = 0.01 percent BW when plotting mean daily observed DMI versus mean daily predicted DMI), the original data set and the data set used for evaluation were combined to generate the following prediction equations for DMI during the final 21 days of gestation:

$$\text{Heifers:}\quad \text{DMI (\% of BW)} = 1.71 - 0.69e^{0.35t} \qquad (9\text{-}1)$$
$$\text{Cows:}\quad \text{DMI (\% of BW)} = 1.97 - 0.75e^{0.16t} \qquad (9\text{-}2)$$

These equations were from a data set that included 172 heifers and 527 cows used in 16 experiment treatments that were conducted at 8 universities and involved 49 treatments.

Factors that influence prepartum DMI are not well established. Zamet et al. (1979a) reported lower prepartum DMI for cows diagnosed with fat cow syndrome compared with "normal" cows that did not have postpartum complications. Hayirli et al. (1998) indicated that over conditioned cows experience a gradual decline in DMI during the prefresh transition period whereas thin cows maintain DMI longer prior to experiencing a more abrupt decrease in DMI shortly before calving. However, a relationship between body condition and prepartum DMI does not imply cause and effect. Categorization of cows on the basis of body condition may also categorize cows into groups that have many genetic, physiologic, and biochemical differences.

Ration composition and nutrient content may influence prepartum DMI. Increasing energy (Coppock et al., 1972; Hernandez-Urdaneta et al., 1976; Minor et al., 1998) or energy and protein (VandeHaar et al., 1999) content of the diet during the prefresh transition period resulted in higher dry matter (DM) and energy intake. In contrast, replacement heifers fed 35 percent concentrate during the final 5 months before first calving had lower DMI (but similar energy intake) during the final 10 days prepartum than did cows fed 6 percent concentrate during the same period (Grummer et al., 1995).

The blood concentrations of many hormones increase or decrease dramatically at parturition and may be potent modifiers of DMI. For example, plasma estrogen of placental origin (specifically estrone) increases in blood as parturition approaches. Exogenous estrogen administration inhibits DMI (Grummer et al., 1990). Reduced DMI during estrus and late pregnancy may reflect greater endogenous estrogen production.

Development of metabolic disorders during the transition period may cause a reduction in DMI. Cows with hypocalcemia have lower prepartum DMI (Goff and Horst, 1997b). Hypocalcemia may cause loss of muscle tone that could adversely affect rumen function, intestinal peristalsis, and passage rate of digesta. Slower passage rates may have a negative effect on DMI.

### *Energy and Protein Density for Dry Cow Diets*

Table 6-5 of *Nutrient Requirements of Dairy Cattle* (National Research Council, 1989) listed one set of nutrient density recommendations for dry, pregnant cows. In the current edition, separate nutrient density guidelines have been developed for far-off dry cows and prefresh transition cows (Chapter 14). This gives greater recognition to DMI depression prior to calving and the unique physiologic and nutritional changes that are associated with late pregnancy, parturition, and lactogenesis. Formulation of a unique diet for prefresh transition cows should reduce the risk of metabolic disorders during early lactation and improve lactation performance.

Nutrient density guidelines for dairy cattle can be obtained by dividing nutrient requirements as determined by the factorial method by predicted DMI. While this approach is appropriate for most classes of cattle, it is problematic for prefresh transition dairy cows because DMI and nutrient requirements are changing relatively rapidly during late gestation. Clearly it is not practical to constantly reformulate diets on a daily basis as cows progress through the prefresh transition period. Additionally, animal physiology at parturition, microbial ecology of the rumen, and pharmacologic effects of nutrients also must be considered when deriving nutrient density recommendations for transition cows. Unique considerations for feeding protein and energy are described below; discussion of adjustments for other nutrients can be found in appropriate sections within this chapter (e.g., selenium/retained placenta, calcium/milk fever).

#### PROTEIN

Results obtained by dividing CP requirements for maintenance, growth (heifers only), and gestation (Bell et al., 1995; data in this edition) by predicted DMI are shown by the solid lines in Figure 9-1. Using this approach, it appears that CP content could be 12 percent or slightly less for mature cows during all but the last few days of the dry period. The previous edition established a minimum of 12 percent CP for diets of dry cows (National Research Council, 1989). Justification for establishing a minimum of 12 percent was absent. Presumably this was based on a minimum amount of CP believed to be necessary to optimize some aspect of ruminal function (e.g., microbial protein synthesis or fiber digestion) (Sahlu et al., 1995). In this revision, it has been established that prefresh transition diets should not be formulated to contain less than 12 percent CP. Feeding a diet containing 12 percent CP provides a margin of safety in the event that DMI would be lower for low protein diets. Chew et al. (1984) fed approximately 9 or 11 percent CP during the entire dry period and observed higher prepartum DMI and higher milk yields when feeding the higher protein diet. Feeding diets with 12 percent CP at predicted DMI is insufficient to meet protein requirements for heifers during the transition period (Figure 9-1). Heifers have lower DMI as a

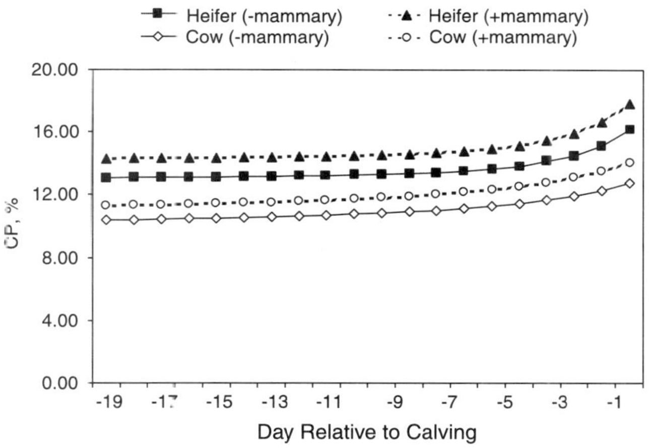


FIGURE 9-1 Dietary concentrations of crude protein needed in diets fed to transition cows to meet requirements. Values were calculated assuming dry matter intakes as predicted by the exponential model described in the text. Solid lines represent calculations using estimates of CP requirements for maintenance, growth, and gestation (from this edition) for a 740 kg mature cow or a 615 kg replacement heifer. Dotted lines represent calculations using estimates of requirements for maintenance, growth, gestation (from this edition), and mammary growth (130 g/d, see text). Body condition score = 3.3, calf birth weight = 45 kg, and heifer growth rate = 300 g/d (without conceptus). Diet consisted of 35 percent corn silage, normal; 34 percent grass silage, C-3, mid-maturity; 10 percent corn grain, ground high moisture; 8 percent soybean meal, solvent, 48 percent CP and 13 percent beet sugar pulp.

percentage of body weight and have additional nutrient requirements for growth. A preliminary report (Santos et al., 1999a,b) indicated that primiparous but not multiparous cows have improved lactation performance when the CP in prepartum diets is increased from 12.7 to 14.7 percent by the addition of animal proteins.

Crude protein requirements for mammary growth were not included in the model. Insufficient data for mammary parenchymal growth rates, mammary composition, and efficiency of conversion of MP to net protein during late gestation were available to accurately predict requirements for mammary growth. However, as outlined by VandeHaar and Donkin (1999), if mammary parenchymal mass increases by 460 g/d during the transition period (Capuco et al., 1997), mammary parenchymal tissue is 10 percent crude protein (Ferrell et al., 1976; Swanson and Poffenbarger, 1979), and efficiencies of conversion of dietary CP to MP and MP to tissue net protein are 0.7 and 0.5 (National Research Council, 1996), then additional CP for mammary growth would be approximately 130 g/d. This would increase the dietary CP needed to meet requirements by approximately one percentage unit (dotted lines, Figure 9-1). Additional research is needed to determine protein and amino acid requirements for mammary growth.

Several research trials have been conducted to examine the effects of dietary CP during the prefresh transition period on health and productivity of postpartum dairy cows. Increasing dietary CP beyond 12 percent during the dry period by addition of feeds that are high in ruminally undegradable protein improved reproductive performance of first lactation cows (Van Saun et al., 1993) and reduced the incidence of ketosis in multiparous cows (Van Saun and Sniffen, 1995). Increasing dietary CP by 2 to 4 percentage units above 12 to 13 percent CP during the prefresh transition period has reduced postpartum feed intake (Crawley and Kilmer, 1995; Van Saun et al., 1995; Greenfield et al., 1998; Hartwell et al., 1999; Putnam et al., 1999) or milk yield (Crawley and Kilmer, 1995; Greenfield et al., 1988). Most studies have shown that milk yield is not influenced by protein content of prepartum diets (Van Saun et al., 1993, Van Saun and Sniffen, 1995; Wu et al., 1997; Putnam and Varga, 1998; Huyler et al., 1999; Putnam et al., 1999; VandeHaar et al., 1999). Although not observed in the majority of studies, milk protein yield (Moorby et al., 1996) and percentage (Van Saun et al., 1993; Moorby et al., 1996) have been increased when feeding additional ruminally undegradable protein prepartum. Cows fed diets containing 10.5, 12.6, or 14.5 percent CP were all in positive nitrogen balance during the prefresh transition period and had similar lactation performance when fed identical diets postpartum (Putnam and Varga, 1998). Strategic supplementation of limiting amino acids may prove to be more successful than increasing total CP or ruminally undegradable protein; however, amino acid requirements for pregnancy have not been defined. A preliminary report (Chalupa et al., 1999) did not indicate a benefit of feeding ruminally protected amino acids during the prefresh transition period; milk and protein yields were increased when supplementation occurred during the postpartum or prepartum and postpartum period.

Although some positive results have been noted when increasing CP beyond 12 percent by feeding additional ruminally undegradable protein, the results have been inconsistent and sometimes negative (e.g., reduced feed intake). The capacity of the cow to detoxify ammonia may be limited during the periparturient period (Strang et al., 1998). Feeding excess protein may be detrimental to the environment. At this time, there is insufficient evidence to support feeding diets with more than 12 percent CP to mature cows during the prefresh transition period. Therefore, the recommendation of 12 percent CP for dry cow diets that was made in the last edition (National Research Council, 1989) has been retained for mature cows (Table 14-11). Heifers may benefit from feeding higher amounts of CP. According to Figure 9-1, average CP density needed in prefresh transition diets to meet requirements at predicted feed intakes would be 14.2 percent if an adjustment is made for mammary growth. Therefore, it is recommended that heifers be fed diets containing 15 percent CP during the prefresh transition period (Table 14-10). Further research is required to more clearly define protein and amino acid requirements during the prefresh transition period.

ENERGY

The recommended energy density for diets fed to dry cows was 1.25 Mcal $NE_L$/kg DM in Table 6-5 of *Nutrient Requirements of Dairy Cattle* (National Research Council, 1989). Assuming DMI as predicted above, 1.25 Mcal $NE_L$/kg DM appears adequate for meeting the energy requirements of cows during the far-off dry period but becomes inadequate during the final one to two weeks of the prefresh transition period depending on whether an adjustment has been made for mammary growth (Figure 9-2). Heifers have lower DMI and additional energy requirements for growth, therefore, 1.25 Mcal $NE_L$/kg DM is inadequate during the entire prefresh transition period.

The recommendation for energy density in diets fed to prefresh transition cows and heifers is 1.62 Mcal $NE_L$/kg DM (Tables 14-10, 14-11). At predicted dry matter intakes, 1.62 Mcal $NE_L$/kg DM will not provide sufficient energy to meet requirements of heifers during a significant portion

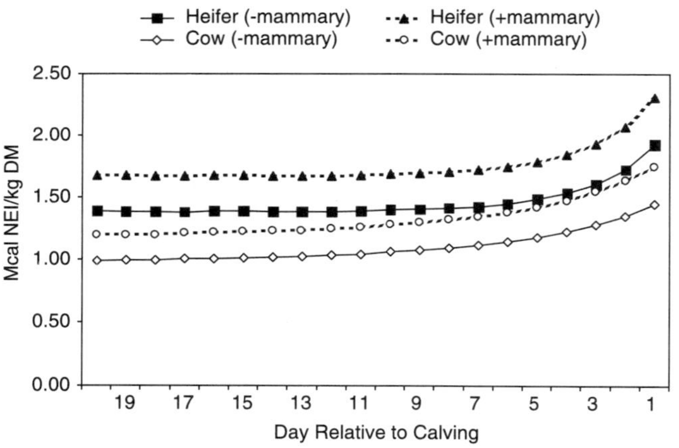


FIGURE 9-2 Dietary concentrations of $NE_L$ needed in diets fed to transition cows to meet requirements. Values were calculated assuming dry matter intakes as predicted by the exponential model described in the text. Solid lines represent calculations using estimates of $NE_L$ requirements for maintenance, growth, and gestation (from this edition) for a 740 kg mature cow or a 615 kg replacement heifer. Dotted lines represent calculations using estimates of requirements for maintenance, growth, gestation (from this edition), and mammary growth (3Mcal/d, VaneHaar et al., 1999). Body condition score = 3.3, calf birth weight = 45 kg, and heifer growth rate = 300 g/d (without conceptus). Diet consisted of 35 percent corn silage, normal; 34 percent grass silage, C-3, mid-maturity; 10 percent corn grain, ground high moisture; 8 percent soybean meal, solvent, 48 percent CP and 13 percent beet, sugar pulp.

of the prefresh transition period and possibly of mature cows during the final few days prior to calving. However, it is recommended not to feed diets with greater than 1.62 Mcal $NE_L$/kg DM (Tables 14-10, 14-11) because feeding more energy dense diets may increase intake of rapidly fermentable carbohydrate too quickly and adversely affect ruminal fermentation and DMI. Feeding diets with 1.62 Mcal $NE_L$/kg DM will probably provide more energy than required for maintenance and gestation for the majority of the prefresh transition period for cows in the 2nd or greater gestation. However, there are several reasons why feeding diets that high in energy could be beneficial. Increasing energy density by increasing nonfiber carbohydrate will allow ruminal microorganisms to adapt to the high concentrate diets that will be fed postpartum. Greater volatile fatty acid production in the rumen will stimulate papillae growth and increase the capacity for acid to be absorbed from the rumen when additional grain is fed postpartum (Dirksen et al., 1985). Increased propionate formation may trigger an insulin response, which can act to reduce fatty acid mobilization from adipose tissue and lipid-related metabolic disorders (Grummer, 1993; Grummer, 1995). Finally, energy requirements for mammary growth have not been described and were not considered when determining total energy requirements for prefresh transition cows. Feeding diets with 1.62 Mcal $NE_L$/kg DM would probably accommodate energy requirements for maintenance, pregnancy, and mammary growth in mature cows (VandeHaar et al., 1999) except for the final few days prior to calving.

## ETIOLOGY AND NUTRITIONAL PREVENTION OF METABOLIC DISORDERS

### *Fatty Liver and Ketosis*

Fatty liver and ketosis are most likely to occur during periods when blood NEFA concentrations are elevated. The most dramatic elevation occurs at calving when plasma concentrations often exceed 1000 μeq/L (Bertics et al., 1992; Vazquez-Anon et al., 1994; Grum et al., 1996). Uptake of NEFA by liver is proportional to NEFA concentrations in blood (Bell, 1979). Extensive reviews on regulation of hepatic lipid metabolism and its relation to fatty liver and ketosis have been published recently (Emery et al., 1992; Grummer, 1993; Bauchart et al., 1996; Drackley, 1999; Hocquette and Bauchart, 1999) and will not be detailed here. Briefly, nonesterified fatty acids taken up by the liver can either be esterified or oxidized in the mitochondria or peroxisomes (Drackley, 1999). The primary esterification product is triglyceride. Triglyceride can either be exported as part of a very low density lipoprotein or be stored. In ruminants, export of triglyceride occurs at a very slow rate relative to many other species (Kleppe et al., 1988; Pullen et al., 1990). Therefore, under conditions of elevated hepatic NEFA uptake (e.g., low blood glucose and insulin) fatty acid esterification and triglyceride accumulation occurs. The cause for the slow rate of triglyceride export from the liver of ruminants is not known. Complete oxidation of NEFA leads to the formation of $CO_2$; incomplete oxidation yields ketones, primarily acetoacetate and beta-hydroxybutyrate. Ketone formation is also favored when blood glucose and insulin concentrations are low, partially because of greater fatty acid mobilization from adipose tissue. Low insulin probably enhances fatty acid oxidation by decreasing hepatocyte malonyl-CoA concentrations and sensitivity of carnitine palmitoyltransferase-1 to malonyl-CoA (Emery et al., 1992). Carnitine palmitoyltransferase-1 is responsible for translocating fatty acids from the cytosol to the mitochondria for oxidation and is inhibited by malonyl-CoA. Propionate is antiketogenic. The antiketogenic properties of propionate are likely due to indirect effects as an insulin secretegogue as well as direct effects on hepatic metabolism (Grummer, 1993). Ketonemia is common at calving during the sudden surge in NEFA, when energy requirements for milk production far exceed energy intake, and as a secondary disorder to others that may cause DMI depression and elevated NEFA.

Elevated liver triglyceride concentration is common in cows immediately after parturition suggesting that measures to prevent fatty liver take place during the prefresh transition period (Grummer, 1993). Fatty liver can be a secondary complication to any disorder that causes a cow to experience negative energy balance. Because of the slow rate of triglyceride export as lipoprotein, once fatty liver has developed, it will persist for an extended period of time. Depletion usually commences when the cow reaches positive energy balance and may take several weeks until completion. Ketosis usually occurs 2 to 4 weeks postpartum; reasons for the lag period between fatty liver and ketosis are not known. However, cows with elevated liver triglyceride and depressed glycogen are most susceptible to ketosis, and fatty liver preceded ketosis when ketosis was experimentally induced (Veenhuizen et al., 1991). Fatty acid oxidation and ketogenesis are likely the major routes of depletion of excess fat from the liver. Ketones may inhibit fatty acid mobilization from adipose tissue and ultimately reduce hepatic fatty acid uptake and triglyceride accumulation (Emery et al., 1992).

Reducing severity and duration of negative energy balance is crucial in the prevention of fatty liver and ketosis. The critical time for the prevention of fatty liver is approximately one week prior to calving through one week after parturition (Grummer, 1993). This is when the cow is most susceptible to development of fatty liver, which is an indicator of ketosis. Maximizing DMI during the week prior to and after calving may be achieved by avoiding overconditioned cattle, rapid diet changes, unpalatable feeds, periparturient diseases, and environmental stress. Effects of body condition score on health and productivity are variable; however, extremely thin or overconditioned cows should be avoided. Thin cows (body condition score $\leq 3$) can be fed additional energy during the dry period to replenish condition without causing fatty liver because the liver is not a lipid depot during positive energy balance. Over conditioned cattle (body condition score $\geq 4$) should not be feed restricted as this will promote fat mobilization from adipose tissue and elevate blood NEFA and liver triglyceride.

Compounds to decrease fatty acid mobilization from adipose tissue or increase lipoprotein export from the liver have been suggested for prevention of fatty liver and ketosis. Feeding 3 to 12 g niacin per day may reduce blood ketones (Dufva et al., 1983) but a beneficial effect on liver triglyceride concentration has not been observed (Skaar et al., 1989; Minor et al., 1998). Glucose or compounds that can be converted to glucose may decrease blood ketones following intravenous administration (Hamada et al., 1982). The response is presumably mediated via insulin, which suppresses fatty acid mobilization from adipose tissue. Propylene glycol is a glucose precursor that can be given as an oral drench to reduce blood nonesterified fatty acids and the severity of fatty liver at calving (Studer et al., 1993) or blood ketones postcalving (Sauer et al., 1973). Salts of propionic acid are also a glucose precursor and may be effective in lowering blood ketones when fed (Schultz, 1958). There is insufficient evidence to support the use of compounds that are known to be lipotropic agents in nonruminants (e.g., choline, inositol, and methionine) to prevent or treat fatty liver or ketosis (Grummer, 1993).

### *Udder Edema*

Udder edema is a periparturient disorder characterized by excessive accumulation of fluids in the intercellular tissue spaces of the mammary gland. In severe cases, edema and congestion occur in the udder and umbilical area, and may be prominent in the vulva and brisket. Typically the incidence and severity are greater in pregnant heifers than in cows (Zamet et al., 1979; Erb and Grohn, 1988), and tend to be more severe in older than younger heifers (Hays and Albright, 1966). Udder edema can be a major discomfort to the animal and causes management problems such as difficulty with milking machine attachment, increased risk of teat and udder injury, and mastitis. Severe udder edema may reduce milk production and cause a pendulous udder (Dentine and McDaniel, 1984).

The exact cause(s) of udder edema is unknown, more likely it is a multi-factorial condition. Restriction or stasis of venous and lymph flow from the udder in late pregnancy due to fetal pressure in the pelvic cavity, or increased blood flow to the udder without the concomitant increase in flow from the udder, causing increased venous pressure may be contributing factors (Vestweber and Al-Ani, 1983; Al-Ani and Vestweber, 1986). Changes in amounts and relative proportions of steroid hormones during late pregnancy may be involved, but are not well understood (Mavlen et al., 1983; Miller et al., 1993). Reduced concentrations of proteins and especially globulins in blood, suggesting an increase in vascular permeability as animals approach calving, were associated with greater incidences of udder edema (Vestweber and Al-Ani, 1984). Other potential causes such as inheritance and dietary factors have been associated with the condition (Al-Ani and Vestweber, 1986). The remaining discussion focuses on possible contributing nutritional factors.

#### HIGH CONCENTRATE (GRAIN) FEEDING PREPARTUM

Many early studies showed no effects of concentrate feeding prepartum on udder edema regardless of parity (Fountaine et al., 1949; Greenhalgh and Gardner, 1958; Schmidt and Schultz, 1959). However, Hathaway et al. (1957) and Hemken et al. (1960) reported increased severity of edema in cows fed greater amounts of concentrate before parturition. Emery et al. (1969) found increased udder edema in pregnant heifers fed 7 to 8 kg of concentrate/head per day compared with no concentrate during the last 3 weeks of gestation. Udder edema was not found in multiparous cows. Greenhalgh and Gardner (1958) observed no increase in the severity of udder edema in heifers fed 4 kg of concentrate/head per day. Effects of prepartum concentrate feeding on udder edema in multiparous cows are less well documented. In one study, cows fed diets composed primarily of corn and alfalfa silages (88 percent of diet, dry basis) plus 12 percent high moisture corn, or 53.5 percent silages plus 46.5 percent high moisture corn had more edema and mastitis than cows fed an all hay diet for 30 days prepartum (Johnson and Otterby, 1981). Overall, the degree of influence of concentrate feeding on udder edema is unclear and a biologic mechanism(s) has not been elucidated. The possibility of influence of other nutrients (e.g., minerals) present in some concentrate mixes should not be overlooked.

Obese cows may be more predisposed to udder edema (Vigue, 1963). Different concentrations of dietary protein, fed for the last 60 days of gestation did not affect incidence of udder edema, but the severity was greater in heifers than in cows (Wise et al., 1946).

#### MINERALS

It was suggested that increased edema observed in heifers in the study of Emery et al. (1969) resulted from 1 percent trace mineralized salt in the grain mix rather than increased concentrate feeding. Excessive intakes of sodium and potassium were implicated as causative agents in udder edema (Randall et al., 1974; Conway et al., 1977; Sanders and Sanders, 1981; Jones et al., 1984). Restriction of sodium chloride and water intakes reduced the severity and incidence of udder edema in pregnant heifers (Hemken et al., 1969). Lower incidence and severity of udder edema were found when diets contained no supplemental salts of sodium or potassium (Randall et al., 1974). In a field study of two commercial dairy herds, potassium fertilization to improve alfalfa production was implicated as the cause of increased udder edema (Sanders and Sanders, 1981). Cows consumed about 450 g of potassium/head per day. In an earlier controlled study, consumption of 454 g of a combination of sodium and potassium chlorides increased the incidence and severity of udder edema (Randall et al., 1974). In a second study, the incidence and severity of udder edema were compared in pregnant heifers fed a grain mix containing 1 percent sodium chloride versus a grain mix with 4 percent supplemental potassium chloride plus 1 percent sodium chloride for 20 days with ad libitum intake of alfalfa hay. The mix with potassium chloride had no influence on the severity of udder edema (Randall et al., 1974). Chronic udder edema also was associated with anemia and hypomagnasemia (Hicks and Pauli, 1976).

Overall, evidence supports the idea that excessive intake of the chloride salts of sodium or potassium increases the severity of udder edema, especially in late pregnant heifers. Intake of these salts typically can be controlled in the peripartum period. Evaluation of other salts of sodium (e.g., sodium bicarbonate) as they might affect the severity of udder edema was not reported. However, Nestor et al. (1988) reported that the severity of udder edema was greater when pregnant heifers were fed additional potassium bicarbonate (0 versus 272 g/head per day) or sodium chloride (23 versus 136 g/head per day) separately, but not when both salts were fed together. Utilizing forages and other feeds that contain low basal concentrations of potassium and sodium would be prudent if udder edema is prevalent.

Tucker et al. (1992) and Lema et al. (1992) studied the effects of calcium chloride, a so-called anionic salt with diuretic properties, on incidence and severity of udder edema. Calcium chloride was used to reduce the cation-anion difference of the prepartum diet of primiparous and multiparous cows. In one study, udder edema was not reduced by supplementation of calcium chloride in the prepartum period, but edema tended to regress more quickly in the early postpartum period, especially in primiparous cows compared with multiparous cows. In a second study, pregnant heifers were fed similar basal diets supplemented with either calcium chloride (1.5 percent, dry basis) or calcium carbonate (2.17 percent) for 3 weeks prepartum. Calcium chloride reduced udder edema most during the first week of feeding. The effect was less but still evident the last 2 weeks before calving. Onset and development of edema were more gradual in heifers fed calcium chloride prepartum. When animals were fed the same calcium chloride supplemented diet after parturition (without prepartum feeding of calcium chloride), udder edema was greater at 2 weeks postpartum for heifers fed calcium chloride versus calcium carbonate fed prepartum.

#### OXIDATIVE STRESS

Oxidative stress of mammary tissues resulting from reactive oxygen metabolites may play a role in udder edema (Mueller et al., 1989a; Miller et al., 1993; Mueller et al., 1998). Excessive reactive oxygen metabolites (e.g., superoxide and hydrogen peroxide) generated from increased metabolic activity, or for example, excessive exposure to aflatoxins, can initiate abnormal oxidative reactions causing peroxidation of lipids; damage to proteins, polysaccharides, and DNA; degeneration of integrity of cell walls and contents; and tissue damage. Reactive oxygen molecules by themselves are not reactive enough to cause peroxidative chain reactions, but conversion to even more reactive free radicals can be triggered by transition elements such as iron (a pro-oxidant). Release of catalytic iron occurs under conditions of stress, trauma, or nutritional imbalance. Zinc may protect against the catalytic action of iron.

Sources of endogenous molecules (e.g., transferrin, lactoferrin, ceruloplasmin, serum albumin, antioxidant enzymes, and glutathione) and exogenous antioxidants (e.g., β-carotene and α-tocopherol) are important to reduce excessive oxidation. Presumably the diet must supply adequate α-tocopherol (vitamin E) as a chain-breaking antioxidant, copper, zinc, and manganese for superoxide dismutase, selenium for glutathione peroxidase, zinc to displace catalytic iron, and magnesium and zinc to stabilize membranes and maintain cellular integrity.

Mueller et al. (1989b) evaluated the effectiveness of supplemental vitamin E to reduce severity of udder edema in pregnant heifers. Udder edema during the first week after calving was less in heifers supplemented for 6 weeks before calving with 1000 IU vitamin E/head per day versus none. In another study, late pregnant heifers were fed factorial combinations of vitamin E [0 or 1000 IU/head per day], zinc [0 or 800 mg/head per day (about 90 mg/kg)], and iron [0 or 12 g/head per day (about 1300 mg/kg)]. When effects were compared regardless of dietary iron concentration, supplemental vitamin E reduced severity of udder edema, but zinc did not. However, when iron was excessive, vitamin E was ineffective in reducing the severity of udder edema, but zinc was somewhat effective. It is believed that vitamin E and zinc may complement each other in antioxidant function.

Nutritional defense against oxidative stress likely is supplied by supplementation of dietary antioxidants fed to meet nutrient requirements (Mueller et al., 1998). More research evaluating effects of oversupply of pro-oxidants in the diet and (or) supplementation of antioxidants in excess of nutrient requirements would be helpful to understand the effects of oxidative stress on udder edema and potential for its prevention.

### *Milk Fever*

#### OCCURRENCE

Milk fever affects about 6 percent of the dairy cows in the United States each year, according to the 1996 National Animal Health Monitoring Survey (USDA, 1996). In these cows the calcium homeostatic mechanisms, which normally maintain blood calcium concentration between 9 and 10 mg/dl, fail and the lactational drain of calcium causes blood calcium concentration to fall below 5 mg/dl. This hypocalcemia impairs muscle and nerve function to such a degree that the cow is unable to rise. Intravenous calcium treatments are used to keep the cow with milk fever alive long enough for intestinal and bone calcium homeostatic mechanisms to adapt. Although milk fever is relatively easy to treat, cows that have had milk fever are more susceptible to other disorders such as mastitis (especially coliform), displaced abomasum, retained placenta, and ketosis (Curtis et al., 1983). Though milk fever affects only a small percentage of cows, nearly all cows experience some decrease in blood calcium (hypocalcemia) during the first days after calving, while their intestines and bones adapt to the calcium demands of lactation. This sub-clinical hypocalcemia contributes to inappetance in the fresh cow and predisposes the cow to develop other diseases such as ketosis, retained placenta, displacement of the abomasum, and mastitis. Efforts made to raise the concentration of calcium in the blood of the fresh cow can benefit milk production even in herds that do not seem to have a milk fever problem (Beede et al., 1991).

#### ETIOLOGY AND PATHOGENESIS

Milk fever is characterized by and the result of severe hypocalcemia (Oetzel and Goff, 1998). Hypophosphatemia (see phosphorus section in chapter 6) and hypomagnesemia also can be present and can be complicating factors in some cases. The degree of hypocalcemia experienced will depend on the amount of calcium leaving the extracellular calcium pool and the rate at which the calcium homeostasis system can replace that calcium loss. The adaptation to the onset of lactation during the critical first days of lactation is accomplished by release of parathyroid hormone (PTH), which reduces urinary calcium losses, stimulates bone calcium resorption, and increases 1,25-dihydroxyvitamin D synthesis to enhance active intestinal transport of calcium. All three must be operational if hypocalcemia is to be minimized. Milk fever risk factors reduce the efficiency of one or more of these homeostatic mechanisms.

An important determinant of the risk for milk fever is the acid-base status of the cow at the time of parturition (Craige, 1947; Ender et al., 1971). Metabolic alkalosis impairs the physiologic activity of PTH so that bone resorption and production of 1,25-dihydroxyvitamin D are impaired reducing the ability to successfully adjust to the calcium demands of lactation (Block, 1984; Block, 1994; Gaynor et al., 1989; Goff et al., 1991; Phillippo et al., 1994). Evidence suggests that metabolic alkalosis induces conformational changes in the PTH receptor, which prevents tight binding of PTH to its receptor. Cows fed diets that are relatively high in potassium or sodium are in a relative state of metabolic alkalosis, which increases the likelihood that they will not successfully adapt to the calcium demands of lactation and will develop milk fever. The parathyroid glands recognize the onset of hypocalcemia and secrete adequate PTH. However, the tissues respond poorly to the PTH, leading to inadequate osteoclastic bone resorption and renal 1,25-dihydroxyvitamin D production (Goff et al., 1991; Phillippo et al., 1994). This is particularly evident in cows that have been treated for milk fever and require further treatments due to reappearance (relapse) of milk fever signs. These cows have very high blood PTH concentrations but produce little 1,25-dihydroxyvitamin D at parturition. Full recovery from milk fever occurs only after the cow has responded to the PTH by producing 1,25-dihydroxyvitamin D. Production of 1,25-dihydroxyvitamin D can be delayed for 24 to 48 hours in some cows (Goff et al., 1989).

### MILK FEVER RISK FACTORS

*Age* Heifers almost never develop milk fever. The risk of a cow developing milk fever increases with age. Heifers generally produce less colostrum than older cows, which may reduce the calcium stress they experience at calving. More importantly, the bones of heifers are still growing. Growing bones have large numbers of osteoclasts present, which can respond to parathyroid hormone more readily than the bones of mature cows. Aged cows have fewer intestinal vitamin D receptors (Horst et al., 1990).

*Breed* The Jersey and, to a lesser extent, the Swedish Red and White and Norwegian Red breeds are well known to have a higher incidence of milk fever. The reasons remain unclear. Colostrum and milk of Jersey cows have a higher content of calcium than that produced by Holsteins, which may place a relatively large calcium stress on the Jersey cows. In one study, Jersey cows had significantly fewer intestinal receptors for 1,25-dihydroxyvitamin D than did Holsteins (Goff et al., 1995). Fewer receptors may impair the ability of Jersey cows to maintain calcium homeostasis.

### NUTRITIONAL CONSIDERATIONS

*Dietary Cation-Anion Difference.* Because metabolic alkalosis is an important factor in the etiology of milk fever it is important to prevent metabolic alkalosis. The reason the cow's blood is alkaline is because of high dietary cations, especially potassium. Cations are minerals with a positive charge and include potassium, sodium, calcium, and magnesium. If the cations in the feed are absorbed into the blood they cause the blood to become more alkaline. If dietary cations are not absorbed they do not affect blood pH (Stewart, 1983). Nearly all of the potassium and sodium in the diet is absorbed by cows, making these two elements very powerful alkalinizing cations. Calcium and magnesium are poorly absorbed from the diet of the dry cow so these cations are not strong alkalinizing agents. Dry cow diets that are high in potassium, sodium, or both alkalinize the cow's blood and increase the susceptibility for milk fever. Addition of potassium or sodium to the prepartal ration of dairy cows will increase the incidence of milk fever. Adding calcium (from 0.5 to 1.5 percent) to practical prepartal diets does not increase the incidence of milk fever (Goff and Horst, 1997a).

*Hypomagnesemia.* A second common cause of hypocalcemia and milk fever in the periparturient cow is hypomagnesemia (van de Braak et al., 1987; Allen and Davies, 1981; Barber et al., 1983; Sansom et al., 1983). Low magnesium in blood can reduce PTH secretion from the parathyroid glands; and can alter the responsiveness of tissues to PTH by inducing conformational changes in the PTH receptor and G-stimulatory protein complex (Rude et al., 1985; Rude et al., 1978; Littledike et al., 1983). Cows fed adequate dietary magnesium in the prepartal ration will be slightly hypermagnesemic the day after parturition. Blood magnesium concentrations below 2.0 mg/dl within 24 h after calving suggest inadequate dietary magnesium absorption (Goff, 1998b).

### PREVENTION OF MILK FEVER

*Adjustment of Dietary Cation-Anion Difference (DCAD)* Equations to describe DCAD include $(Na^+ + K^+) - (Cl^- + S^{-2})$ (Ender et al., 1971), $(Na^+ + K^+ - Cl^-)$ (Mongin, 1981), and $(Na^+ + K^+ + 0.15\ Ca^{+2} + 0.15\ Mg^{+2}) - (Cl^- + 0.6\ S^{-2} + 0.5\ P^{-3})$ (Goff et al., 1997). The last equation assigns coefficients to the major dietary cations and anions based on their acidifying or alkalinizing potential. To achieve a low DCAD prepartal ration to prevent hypocalcemia, the following adjustments are recommended:

*Reduce Dietary Sodium and Potassium* Removing potassium from the ration can present a problem as alfalfa, other legumes, and many grasses accumulate potassium within their tissues to concentrations that are well above that required for optimal growth of the plant if soil potassium is high. Corn, a warm season grass, is less likely to accumulate potassium and corn silage is often a practical feedstuff to use to reduce DCAD (Beede, 1992). Other agronomic options to reduce dietary potassium have recently been reviewed (Horst et al., 1997; Thomas, 1999).

*Add Anions to Induce Mild (Compensated) Metabolic Acidosis* Landmark studies (Ender et al., 1971; Ender and Dishington, 1967; Block, 1984) demonstrated that addition of anions to the prepartal diet could prevent milk fever. Ammonium, calcium, and magnesium salts of chloride and sulfate have been successfully used as acidifying anion sources. Chloride salts are more acidogenic than sulfate salts (Goff et al., 1997; Oetzel, 1991; Tucker et al., 1991). Hydrochloric acid also has been successfully utilized as a source of anions for prevention of milk fever and is the most potent of the anion sources available (Ender and Dishington, 1967; Goff and Horst, 1998). Monitoring urine pH of cows during the week before parturition has proven an effective means of assessing effectiveness of anion addition to the prepartal ration. In Holstein cows effective anion addition reduces urine pH to between 6.2 and 6.8 (Gaynor et al., 1989; Jardon, 1995; Oetzel and Goff, 1998). Using the equation favored by most nutritionists, $(Na^+ + K^+) - (Cl^- + S^{-2})$ it is common to attempt to bring DCAD below zero mEq/kg diet to achieve proper acidification of the cow. These targets are not well defined and anions should be added in small increments to the dry cow ration until the proper urine pH is achieved. Urine pH can be assessed as quickly as 48 to 72 hours after a DCAD adjustment.

Feeding 0.35 to 0.40 percent magnesium in prepartal rations prevents a decline in the concentration of magnesium in the blood at parturition. These levels ensure that there is adequate magnesium in the rumen to utilize the passive absorption mechanism for magnesium across the rumen wall and not be reliant on active transport of magnesium across the rumen wall, a process that may be inhibited by dietary potassium (Oetzel and Goff, 1998). Because there is no readily labile body store of magnesium, the daily intake of dietary magnesium must supply needs. These higher levels are needed to accommodate the decline in DMI occurring in the periparturient period (Goff, 1998b; Horst and Goff, 1997). Phosphorus requirements are met by feeding 40 to 50 g of phosphorus/cow/day. Less than 25 g/cow/day may lead to hypophosphatemia and the downer cow syndrome (Julien et al., 1977; Goff, 1998a; Cox, 1998). More than 80 g of phosphorus/cow/day may induce milk fever (Barton et al., 1987).

The optimal prepartal dietary calcium concentration is not well defined. In one study, the incidence of milk fever was not different in cows fed 0.5 or 1.5 percent calcium in diets (Goff and Horst, 1997a). Other studies have successfully utilized diets providing more than 150 g of calcium/cow/day along with anionic salts to prevent hypocalcemia (Oetzel, 1988; Beede et al., 1991). Very high concentrations of dietary calcium (>1.0 percent calcium) may reduce DMI and animal performance (Miller, 1983).

*Very Low Calcium Diets to Prevent Milk Fever* Diets providing less than 15 g calcium/cow/day and fed for at least 10 days before calving will reduce the incidence of milk fever (Goings et al., 1974; Boda, 1954). This concentration of calcium places the cow in negative calcium balance, stimulating parathyroid hormone secretion prior to calving. This activates bone osteoclasts stimulating bone calcium resorption and activates renal tubules to resorb urinary calcium and begin producing 1,25-dihydroxyvitamin D prior to calving (Green et al., 1981). Thus at the onset of lactation these homeostatic mechanisms for calcium are active, preventing a severe decline in the concentration of calcium in the plasma of cows. In the United States, it is nearly impossible to formulate this type of diet. Diets consisting of as little as 35 to 45 g of calcium/day will meet the calcium requirement of cows and will not stimulate the parathyroid glands adequately and will not effectively prevent milk fever.

*Oral Calcium Drenches at Calving* Oral administration of calcium at calving reduces the incidence of milk fever but carries a slight risk of inducing aspiration pneumonia (Jonsson and Pehrson, 1970; Hallgren, 1955; Oetzel, 1993; Goff et al., 1996), and can be labor intensive.

*Exogenous Vitamin D and Parathyroid Hormone* Earlier literature often recommended feeding or injecting massive doses (up to 10 million units) of vitamin D 10 to 14 days prior to calving to prevent milk fever (Hibbs and Pounden, 1955; Littledike and Horst, 1980). This will increase intestinal absorption of calcium and can help prevent milk fever. Unfortunately, the dose of vitamin D that effectively prevents milk fever is very close to the level that causes irreversible metastatic calcification of soft tissues. Lower doses may actually induce milk fever because the high levels of 25-OH D and 1,25-dihydroxyvitamin D suppress PTH secretion and renal synthesis of endogenous 1,25-dihydroxyvitamin D (Littledike and Horst, 1980).

Treatment with 1,25-dihydroxyvitamin D and its analogues or parathyroid hormone prior to calving can be effective but the effective dose is close to the toxic dose and problems with timing of administration, withdrawal from treatment, and expense have not made these treatments practical (Bar et al., 1985; Goff and Horst, 1990; Goff et al., 1986).

*Grass Tetany*

Hypomagnesemic tetany is most often associated with cows in early lactation (milk production removes 0.15 g magnesium from the blood for each liter of milk produced) grazing lush pastures high in potassium and nitrogen and low in magnesium and sodium (Littledike et al., 1983). This is the most common situation and it is often referred to as Grass Tetany, Spring Tetany, Grass Staggers, or Lactation Tetany. The clinical signs in affected cows will depend on the severity of the hypomagnesemia. The disease will progess more rapidly and tends to be more severe if accompanied by hypocalcemia, which is often the case. Dairy cows are usually affected 1 to 3 weeks into lactation especially if they are on pasture. Moderate hypomagnesemia (between 0.5 and 0.75 mmol/L or 1.1 and 1.8 mg/dl) is associated with reduced DMI, nervousness, and reduced production of milk fat and total milk. This can be a chronic problem in some dairy herds that often goes unnoticed. It also can predispose these animals to milk fever (Goff, 1998).

Despite the importance of magnesium there is no hormonal mechanism concerned principally and directly with magnesium homeostasis. Factors affecting magnesium transport across the rumen epithelium have been discussed in the section on magnesium requirements.

PREVENTION

If hypomagnesemic tetany has occurred in one cow in a herd, steps should be taken immediately to increase intake of magnesium to prevent further losses. Getting an additional 10 to 15 g of magnesium into each pregnant cow and 30 g of magnesium into each lactating dairy cow each day will usually prevent further hypomagnesemic tetany cases. The problem with prevention is getting the extra magnesium into the animal (Goff, 1998b).

Most magnesium salts are unpalatable. Magnesium oxide is the most palatable, most concentrated, least expensive, and, unfortunately, least soluble source of magnesium. Magnesium is readily acceptable in grain concentrates. Including 60 g of magnesium oxide in just 0.5 to 1 kg of grain will be effective. However the expense of the grain and the problems associated with feeding concentrates to pastured cattle often make this option difficult to implement (Goff, 1998b).

Feeding ionophores (monensin, lasalocid) can improve activity of the sodium-linked magnesium transport system in the rumen, increasing magnesium absorption efficiency about 10 percent. However, ionophores are not approved for use in many of the animals they could benefit. Rumen boluses that release ionophores for up to 150 days have been developed to make delivery of ionophores to animals at pasture practical.

Pasture foliage can be dusted with magnesium oxide (500 g of magnesium oxide/cow or 50 kg magnesium oxide/hectare or 50 lb/acre) weekly during the period when cows are tetany prone. Adding 2.5–5 g/L or 10 to 20 lb/500 gal magnesium sulfate $7H_2O$ (epsom salts) or magnesium chloride $6H_2O$ to the drinking water can be an economic means of supplementing magnesium if cows have access to no other water supply as the addition of the salts can reduce palatability. Unfortunately cows grazing lush high moisture pasture rarely drink enough water to make this method effective on tetany prone pastures. Molasses licks and mineral blocks containing magnesium oxide and salt can help supply magnesium to animals at pasture if made readily available and if the animals learn to use the licks prior to parturition. A problem with many of these methods is that some cows in the herd may not voluntarily consume enough of the magnesium supplement and on some tetanogenic pastures cows that do not receive supplementation are often found dead (Goff, 1998b).

Intraruminal magnesium releasing boluses and bullets have been developed, which remain in the reticulum and release low levels of magnesium (1 to 1.5 g) each day for periods of up to 90 days. A 100 g magnesium alloy rumen "bullet" that is 86 percent magnesium has been developed and releases about 1 g of magnesium/day. Some producers administer 2 to 4 bullets per cow. These devices do not supply enough magnesium to raise magnesium in the blood subsantially, though there may be situations where they prove successful despite the low supplementation achieved.

*Retained Placenta and Metritis*

Retained placenta (retained fetal membranes) is defined as failure of the fetal membranes to be expelled within 12 to 24 hours after parturition. Metritis, an inflammation or infection of the uterus, is often associated with retained placenta. In path analysis, retained placenta was associated directly with increased days to first service and risk of metritis when compared with cows that expelled their placentas within 24 hours. Also, retained placenta was associated indirectly with the greater occurrence of cystic ovaries, lower milk yield, and greater culling; all were mediated through metritis (Erb et al., 1985).

Multiple physiologic and nutritional factors have been associated with or implicated as causes of retained placenta and metritis (Maas, 1982; Miller et al., 1993; Goff and Horst, 1997b). Dystocia in heifers increased the risk of retained placenta and metritis by 3 to 4 times (Erb et al.,

1985). Other predisposing or associated factors include: twinning; various stressors; short dry periods; exposure to toxins such as mycotoxins or nitrates; heredity; milk fever; abnormally low prostaglandin $F_2$ concentrations in placentomes, caruncles, and cotyledons; and, other atypical peripartum profiles of steroid, pituitary, and adrenal hormones in blood (Pelissier, 1976; Chew et al., 1977; Leidl et al., 1980; Maas, 1982). Immunosuppression in the peripartum period has been implicated as a possible contributing factor (Goff and Horst 1997b). Several dietary essential nutrients are involved in immune function. However, the exact mechanisms of action and nutrient needs to promote periparturient immunocompetence have not been elucidated fully.

NUTRITIONAL FACTORS

Nutritional causes of retained placenta are due primarily to the diet fed the last 6 to 8 weeks before calving. During this time, dietary deficiencies or imbalances of energy; protein; phosphorus; calcium; selenium; iodine; vitamins A, D, and E; and excesses of dietary energy, protein, and calcium all have been associated with or implicated as causes of retained placenta and metritis (Maas, 1982; Weaver, 1987; Goff and Horst, 1997b).

*Energy and Protein* Extreme deficiency of dietary energy, protein or both can result in retained placenta because cows are weak, and coupled with the stress of parturition lack strength to expel the placenta (Mass, 1982). Cows fed diets for the entire dry period low in dietary crude protein (8 percent) had a higher incidence (50 percent) of retained placenta compared with cows fed 15 percent crude protein (20 percent incidence) (Julien et al., 1976a). Fat cow syndrome (hepatic lipidosis), resulting from excessive energy intake prepartum, also frequently is associated with increased incidences of retained placenta and metritis (Morrow, 1976).

*Phosphorus* The rate of retained placenta was associated with imbalances in calcium and phosphorus metabolism (Noorsdsy et al., 1973; Pelissier, 1976). However, Julien et al. (1977) found no influence of prepartum dietary phosphorus content (0.30 versus 0.70 percent, dry basis) on rate of retention of placentas, and the correlation between phosphorus intake and incidence of retained placenta was low. Dietary concentrations of calcium were similar among treatments, and rate of calcium intake was not correlated with retained placenta.

*Calcium* The association between hypocalcemia (either clinical or subclinical) in the peripartum period and retained placenta has been known for some time (Pelissier, 1976; Greunert, 1980). Excess of calcium and phosphorus in the diet, and a deficiency of vitamin $D_3$ all affect calcium metabolism in the periparturient period and can result in hypocalcemia. Path analyses showed that multiparous cows having milk fever were 2 times more likely to have retained placenta and metritis than cows without milk fever (Erb et al., 1985). In another study, multiparous cows having milk fever were 4 times more likely to have placental retention (Curtis et al., 1985). Hypocalcemia results in loss of muscle tone in the uterus, which may contribute to the increased incidence of retained placenta (Goff and Horst, 1997b). Decreasing the dietary cation-anion difference of the prepartum diet by supplementation of ammonium sulfate and ammonium chloride reduced hypocalcemia and reduced the incidence of retained placenta (Oetzel et al., 1988). Other details about prevention of hypocalcemia are discussed in the milk fever and transition cow sections of this publication. Harrison et al. (1984) reported that apparent absorption of selenium from natural feeds by nonlactating pregnant cows was lower with low (0.4 percent) or high (1.4 percent) dietary calcium, and maximal with about 0.8 percent calcium, dry basis; calcium intake ranged from about 30 to 200 g/cow per day. Even though large amounts of dietary calcium reduced selenium absorption, feeding 1.32 percent calcium with supplemental anions plus 3 mg of selenium/cow per day by oral bolus to pregnant Holstein cows for 14 to 21 days before calving did not negatively affect peripartum selenium status of cows or newborn calves compared with that of cows receiving 1.08 percent dietary calcium, no supplemental anions, and 3 mg of oral selenium (Gant et al., 1998).

*Selenium and Vitamin E* An excess of highly reactive oxygen metabolites (e.g., peroxides and superoxide) can cause peroxidative damage of cell membranes and other cellular components, and interfere with normal metabolic function, including normal steroidogenesis (Miller et al., 1993). Nutrient antioxidants (e.g., selenium and vitamin E) are needed to reduce peroxidation. Cows with retained placenta had lower total antioxidants in blood plasma during the 2 weeks before calving than cows without retained placenta (Miller et al., 1993). Supplementation of diets with antioxidants to meet requirements is crucial especially during the periparturient period (Weiss et al., 1990), when blood $\alpha$-tocopherol (vitamin E) concentrations are the lowest of the entire lactation cycle (Goff and Stabel, 1990; Weiss et al., 1990).

However, supplementation with selenium and vitamin E reduced the incidence of retained placenta and improved reproduction of dairy cows in some (Trinder et al., 1969, 1973; Julien et al., 1976b,c; Harrison et al., 1984; Mueller et al., 1988, 1989b,c; Thomas et al., 1990), but not all (Gwazdauskas et al., 1979; Schnigoethe et al., 1982; Ishak et al., 1983; Kappel et al., 1984; Hidiroglou et al., 1987; Stowe et al., 1988) comparisons. In cows fed selenium-deficient diets (0.05 to 0.07 mg/kg), supplemental selenium substantially reduced the incidence of retained placenta (Julien et al., 1976 b,c). Administration of selenium and vitamin E in combination was more effective in reducing retained placenta than either antioxidant alone. Trinder et al. (1973) reported in a summary of three experiments involving 171 parturitions that injection 28 days before expected calving of 15 mg of selenium as potassium selenate alone was slightly less effective (10 percent incidence) for reducing retained placenta than the combination of selenium (15 mg) plus vitamin E (680 IU) (2 percent incidence). The incidence rate was 39 percent with no selenium or vitamin E injection. Basal diets contained between 0.025 and 0.047 mg/kg of selenium, dry basis. Segerson et al. (1981) found that the incidence of retained placenta was reduced by a combination of selenium and vitamin E injection in the prepartum period of cows marginally deficient in blood serum selenium concentrations (14.9 versus 25.4 percent incidences with and without selenium and vitamin E), but not in cows either adequate or very deficient in selenium. With prepartum diets having basal concentrations of 0.035 to 0.109 mg/kg of selenium, one injection of selenium (2.3 to 23 mg) alone about 3 weeks before expecting calving was as effective in reducing retained placenta as a selenium-vitamin E combination (Eger et al., 1985). Low doses of selenium (2.3 to 4.6 mg given 3 weeks before calving) tended to be more effective than higher doses. In some studies, 50 mg of selenium plus 680 IU of vitamin E were injected intramuscularly 3 weeks before expected calving of Holstein cows (Segerson et al., 1981; Julien et al., 1976 b, c). This amount of selenium was adequate to reduce retained placenta as long as adequate vitamin E also was administered; however, given alone neither nutrient was very effective for reducing retained placenta or metritis.

Retained placenta and days to conception were not reduced by 1000 IU of vitamin E/cow per day given orally in cows fed diets with less than 0.06 mg/kg of selenium, unless cows also were injected intramuscularly with 0.1 mg of selenium/kg live weight 3 weeks before expected calving (Harrison et al., 1984). When the diet contained at least 0.12 mg/kg of selenium, 1000 IU of dietary vitamin E/cow per day reduced the incidence of retained placenta compared with cows not receiving supplemental vitamin E (Mueller et al., 1988, 1989b,c; Thomas et al., 1990; Brzezinska-Slebodzinska and Miller, 1992). Miller et al. (1993) noted that preventive (e.g., selenium) and chain breaking antioxidants (e.g., vitamin E and β-carotene) work in concert, and effectiveness of the total antioxidant system is impaired if one or more of the antioxidant components is inadequate, and the supplemented antioxidant may be less effective if another antioxidant is limiting.

Schingoethe et al. (1982) and Ishak et al. (1983) found no reduction in incidence of retained placenta by intramuscular injection of selenium, vitamin E, or a combination of the two given in the feed, if diets already contained 0.1 to 2.0 mg/kg of selenium. Data are not available on the effect of supplementing more than 0.3 mg selenium/kg of feed (dry matter basis) and (or) more than 1000 IU of vitamin E per day on the incidence of retained placenta. The legal upper limit for selenium supplementation of complete diets for cattle is 0.3 mg/kg (Food and Drug Administration, 1997).

*Vitamin A and β-Carotene* Avitaminosis was shown to increase the incidence of retained placenta (Ronning et al., 1953; Roberts, 1961; Nicholson and Cunningham, 1965). Ronning et al., (1953) demonstrated a decrease in the incidence of retained placenta with increased intake of carotene. Dairy cows fed 600 mg/cow per day of β-carotene for 4 weeks before calving had reduced incidence of retained placenta compared with cows fed an equivalent amount of pre-formed vitamin A (240,000 IU/day) (Michal et al., 1990).

*Iodine* Controlled studies on the effects of iodine deficiency on the incidence of retained placenta and metritis are lacking. Some case studies indicate that iodine deficiency was associated with retained placenta (Moberg, 1959; McDonald et al., 1961; Hemken and Vandersall, 1967). However, in a later field study with 1,572 cows in an iodine-deficient area of Finland, retained placenta was not reduced with supplementary iodine (Moberg, 1961). An association between retained placenta and goiter in calves was reported (Maas, 1982).

### *Displacement of the Abomasum*

Displacement of the abomasum is a disease of increasing importance as milk production increases in the United States. A survey of high producing herds found that on average 3.3 percent of cows developed displaced abomasum (Jordan and Fourdraine, 1993). The transition period from 3 weeks before calving until 4 weeks postpartum is the major risk period for development of displaced abomasum. About 85 percent of cases involve displacement to the left side of the cow.

#### ABOMASAL PHYSIOLOGY

In the nonpregnant cow, the abomasum occupies the ventral portion of the abdomen, very nearly on the midline, with the pylorus extending to the right side of the cow caudal to the omasum. As pregnancy progresses, the growing uterus occupies an increasing amount of the abdominal cavity. The uterus begins to slide under the caudal aspects of the rumen, reducing rumen volume by one third at the end of gestation. This also forces the abomasum forward and slightly to the left side of the cow, although the pylorus continues to extend across the abdomen to the right side of the cow (Habel, 1981). After calving, the uterus retracts back toward the pelvic inlet which, under normal conditions, allows the abomasum to return to its original position. During left displacement of the abomasum, the pyloric end of the abomasum slides completely under the rumen to the left side of the cow. Three factors are believed to be responsible for allowing the abomasum to move to the left side of the cow. First, the rumen must fail to take up the void left by the retracting uterus. If the rumen moved into its normal position on the left ventral floor of the abdomen, the abomasum would not be able to slide under it. Second, the omentum attached to the abomasum must have been stretched to permit movement of the abomasum to the left side. These two factors constitute opportunity for displacement. A third factor necessary to cause abomasal displacement is abomasal atony. Normally, gases produced in the abomasum (from fermentation of feedstuffs or $CO_2$ released when bicarbonate from the rumen meets the HCl of the abomasum) are expelled back into the rumen as a result of abomasal contractions. It is felt that these contractions are impaired in cows developing left displacement of the abomasum (Goff and Horst, 1997b; Breukink, 1991; Hull and Wass, 1973). The cause of abomasal atony is less clear.

A decline in the concentration of calcium in plasma around parturition linearly decreases abomasal contractility, which is suspected to lead to atony and distension of the abomasum (Massey et al., 1993; Hull and Wass, 1973; Curtis et al., 1983). At a concentration of 5 mg/dl calcium in plasma, abomasal motility was reduced by 70 percent and strength of contractions is reduced by 50 percent as compared to when plasma calcium is normal (9 to 10 mg/dl). At a concentration of 7.5 mg/dl calcium in plasma, the motility and strength of abomasal contractions were reduced by 30 percent and 25 percent, respectively (Daniel, 1983). Clinical signs of milk fever (down cows) often are not seen until calcium is about 4 mg/dl. In a recent study of plasma calcium concentrations in periparturient Holstein and Jersey cows, 10 to 50 percent of cows remained subclinically hypocalcemic (plasma calcium <7.5 mg/dl) up to 10 days after calving, depending on herd efforts to combat milk fever (Goff et al., 1986). Oetzel (1996) reported that administration of oral calcium chloride at calving to reduce subclinical hypocalcemia resulted in a significant decrease in the incidence of displacement of the abomasum.

Decreasing the forage to concentrate ratio of the diet fed in late gestation and early lactation will increase the incidence of displaced abomasum (Coppock et al., 1972). Volatile fatty acids within the abomasum have been demonstrated to reduce abomasal contractility (Breukink, 1991); however, ruminal VFA concentrations are not highly correlated with the concentration of VFA in the abomasum (Breukink and de Ruyter, 1976). A high grain, low forage diet can promote the appearance of VFA in the abomasum by reducing the depth of the ruminal mat or raft (made up primarily of the long fibers of forages). Physical reduction of forage particle length by chopping forages too finely prior to ensiling or overzealous use of mixer wagons also can contribute to loss of rumen raft (Shaver, 1997). The ruminal raft captures grain particles so that they are fermented at the top of the ruminal fliud. The VFA produced at the top of the ruminal fliud are generally absorbed from the rumen with little VFA entering the abomasum. In cows with an inadequate ruminal raft, grain particles fall to the ventral portion of the rumen and reticulum where they are fermented or pass on to the abomasum (where they can then be fermented to some extent). The VFA produced in the ventral rumen can pass through the rumenoreticular orifice to enter the abomasum before the rumen can absorb them. A thick ruminal raft is generally present during the dry period when cows are fed a high forage diet, but the depth of the ruminal raft is rapidly reduced in early lactation; especially if the cow experiences a pronounced decline in DMI. Since the ruminal raft also stimulates regurgitation of the cud and mastication, the release of saliva, which promotes rumen buffering, is decreased when cows are fed a higher grain ration. Also, early in lactation, the underdeveloped ruminal papillae allow more of the VFA produced in the ventral rumen to escape the rumen than would a highly absorptive ruminal mucosa typical of later lactation (Dirksen, 1985).

Cows dried off with high body condition scores are at increased risk of left displaced abomasum as a result of poor DMI around parturition (Cameron et al., 1998).

The amount of effective fiber determines the consistency and depth of the rumen raft and stimulates rumen contractility. Guidelines are poorly defined, but readers are referred to Chapter 4 of this report and recent reviews that discuss methods for evaluating the amount of effective fiber needed in the diet (Armentano and Pereira, 1997; Firkins, 1997; Grant, 1997; Allen, 1997; Mertens, 1997).

TMR that are easily sorted by cows may affect the ratio of forage to concentrate of total feed consumed by individual cows and will contribute to displaced abomasum (Shaver, 1997). When a TMR is not fed, grain intake after calving should be increased slowly (0.2 to 0.25 kg/day) until peak grain intake is achieved. Grain fed to cows should be divided into at least 3 meals per day (Shaver, 1997).

### *Rumen Acidosis and Laminitis*

Acids produced during fermentation of grains generally keep rumen pH slightly below neutral or 7.0. How far below neutral is dependent on the rate of production and total amount of acid produced, the rate of absorption of acids out of the rumen, and the amount of salivary secretion released to neutralize the acids. High forage diets produce acids only slowly and stimulate release of large amounts of saliva as they stimulate mastication. Rumen pH tends to be higher on forage diets. Rumen acidosis is associated with the feeding of diets with higher amounts of grain in them and the acidosis commonly occurs in the first month of lactation (Nocek, 1997). Upon dry-off, the cow is fed a high forage ration that is less energy dense and higher in neutral detergent fiber than the lactation ration. This affects rumen function in two ways. The bacterial population shifts away from the lactate producers (bacteria such as *Streptococcus bovis*, and the lactobacilli) as a result of the decrease in readily fermentable starches in the diet (Yokoyama and Johnson, 1988) Therefore, the population of those bacteria (primarily *Megasphaera elsdenii* and *Selenomonas ruminantium*) capable of converting lactate to acetate, propionate, or long chain fatty acids useful to the cow declines. Another effect of the lower energy diet of the early dry period is a reduction in the papillae length and volatile fatty acid (VFA) absorptive capacity of the ruminal mucosa. As much as 50 percent of the absorptive area may be lost during the first 7 weeks of the dry period (Dirksen et al., 1985). If the fresh cow is now abruptly switched to a high energy lactation diet, she is at risk of developing rumen acidosis because the lactate producers will respond rapidly to the higher starch diets and produce high amounts of lactate. The lactate converting bacterial population responds only slowly to a change in diet, requiring 3 to 4 wk to reach levels that will effectively prevent lactate from building up in the rumen. Lactate is a stronger acid ($pK_a = 3.86$) than propionate ($pK_a = 4.87$), acetate ($pK_a = 4.76$), or butyrate ($pK_a = 4.82$), so that its presence has a slightly larger effect on rumen pH than the VFA especially as the rumen pH falls below 6.0. Also, lactate and the other VFA are absorbed by rumen epithelium when in the undissociated acid state only. As the pH of the rumen decreases more of the VFA exists in the undissociated acid state. Because the $pK_a$ of lactate is lower than the VFA, it is absorbed more slowly than acetate, propionate, or butyrate from the rumen (Merchen, 1988).

Normally, only a small amount of lactate is produced within the rumen and it is all in the L-lactate form. An early hypothesis on the etiology of the "grain overload" syndrome attached a great deal of significance to the observation that under conditions of grain engorgement, D-lactate is produced in very high amounts by the lactobacilli. The theory contended that D-lactate was not absorbed from the rumen as well as L-lactate, and also was metabolized only slowly by body tissues once it was absorbed. However D-lactate is absorbed from the rumen (Huntington and Britton, 1979) and metabolized by tissues (Harmon et al., 1983) at the same rate as L-lactate.

Much of the research conducted on the etiology of rumen acidosis was performed using the feedlot steer as a model. In this model it appears that lactic acid production is an important aspect of the development of rumen acidosis. However recent research with dairy cattle suggests that rumen acidosis observed in early and mid-lactation cows is more closely related to total VFA production within the rumen and build-up of VFA. High rumen fluid lactic acid concentrations may not play as prominent a role in dairy "rumen acidosis" as it does in feedlot cattle (Oetzel et al., 1999).

The lactic acid, and the endotoxins and histamine released as the rumen flora die, are absorbed systemically, and affect the microvasculature of the growing hoof wall, which can then result in clinical laminitis (Radostits et al., 1994) Metabolic acidosis will follow rumen acidosis if the amount of organic acid absorbed into the blood exceeds the ability of the liver and other tissues to metabolize these anions.

The scientific name for laminitis is pododermatitis aseptic diffusa, which is an inflammation of the dermal layers inside the foot. Incidence rate of laminitis from surveys ranged from 5.5 to 30 percent (Nocek, 1997). Laminitis has a multifaceted etiology and is thought to be associated with several, largely independent factors. Nutritional management has been identified as a key component in the development of laminitis, particularly the feeding of diets high in fermentable carbohydrates, which can result in an acidotic state. Manson and Leaver (1988) compared diets containing 60:40 or 40:60 concentrate to silage fed to cows during weeks 3 to 26 of lactation. The 60:40 diet increased the number and incidences of clinical lameness, and decreased hoof hardness. Other nutritional factors including adequate effective fiber to stimulate salivation and presence of mycotoxins have been suggested to predispose animals to the development of laminitis (Vermunt and Greenough, 1994). Metabolic and digestive disorders can predispose the cow to laminitis. Supplementary biotin may improve hoof strength and provide greater resistance to laminitis (Midla et al., 1998).

Infectious diseases, such as mastitis, metritis, and foot rot, can cause specific endotoxic insults (Maclean, 1971). Factors related to the environment, such as hard surfaces, lack of or little use of bedding, and lack of or excessive exercise on undesirable surfaces, can separately or in combination predispose animals to mechanical damage (Bergsten, 1994). Bergsten (1995) found a higher prevalence of solar hemorrhages in cows kept in tie stalls with concrete floors as compared with cows housed in tie stalls that had been fitted with rubber mats.

Other factors such as excess body condition, heavy body weight, and poor feet and leg structure (Greenough, 1991), can increase the weight load and stress on feet, exacerbating the internal mechanical damage that is associated with laminitis (Nocek, 1997).

### *Milk Fat Depression*

Diet has a significant impact on both the yield and concentration of fat in milk of the dairy cow. Fat is the milk component on which diet has the greatest influence (Sutton, 1989), principally by reducing fat content. Requirements for NDF and effective fiber are driven in part, by the need to maintain milk fat (Erdman, 1988). Several dietary factors are known to depress milk fat including high levels of concentrate, finely chopped forages, and diets containing high amounts of polyunsaturated fatty acids such as those contained in either marine or vegetable oils. Under extreme dietary circumstances, milk fat concentration can be reduced by as much 50 to 60 percent from normal levels.

#### PREVIOUS THEORIES

The influence of diet and the dietary factors that alter milk fat has been known for a long time. Van Soest (1994) cited work of Boussingault in 1845 that documented low milk fat in cows fed a low fiber and high starch diet of beets. Petersen (1932) demonstrated that feeding cod liver oil markedly reduced milk fat. Shaw and Ensor (1959) confirmed the response to feeding cod liver oil and also found that inclusion of vegetable oils containing high levels of polyunsaturated fatty acids (PUFA) in the diet, also depressed milk fat content. Powell (1939) in a series of experiments showed that feeding high grain diets or feeding diets with ground or pelleted hay reduced milk fat and he concluded that the factors, which caused the fat depression, were related to changes in rumen fermentation. Finally, Emery and Brown (1961) demonstrated the importance of rumen pH in milk fat depression where the addition of dietary buffers partially corrected the reduction in milk fat content in cows fed high concentrate diets.

Most previously proposed mechanisms by which diet influences milk fat concentration have been related to changes in rumen volatile fatty acids (VFA) and the subsequent changes in metabolism associated with altered rumen VFA (Van Soest, 1994). Where milk fat depression is caused by feeding either high grain diets or diets where the forage particle size is too small, the molar percentage of acetate declines and propionate increases. Tyznick and Allen (1951) suggested that because of the reduced rumen acetate concentrations, the reduction in milk fat was caused by a deficiency in acetate, a precursor for de novo fatty acid synthesis in the mammary gland.

Because of the acetate deficiency theory, rumen acetate: propionate molar ratios have frequently been used as an indicator of fermentation changes associated with fat depressing diets. The importance of rumen VFA patterns was reinforced by the work of Emery and Brown (1961) and Emery et al. (1964). Based on the observation that rumen pH was reduced when cows were fed low forage diets, it was correctly hypothesized that addition of buffer to the diet would increase rumen pH and milk fat production. These experiments also showed increased rumen acetate: propionate ratios with buffer addition that reinforced the concept that changes in rumen VFA patterns were the cause of milk fat depression. However, Bauman and Davis (1970) using radioisotopes to measure actual VFA production in the rumen, showed that acetate production did not decrease with fat depressing diets, but rather, propionate production increased causing decreased acetate: propionate molar ratios. This indicated that acetate did not become deficient during milk fat depression.

Other theories related to changes in rumen VFA patterns included a deficiency in beta-hydroxy butyrate (Van Soest and Allen, 1959), increased uptake of acetate by adipose caused by elevated blood insulin (McClymont and Valence, 1962) and vitamin $B_{12}$ deficiency (Frobish and Davis, 1977). Intramuscular injections of vitamin $B_{12}$ had no effect on milk fat percentage in cows that were fed fat depressing diets (Croom et al., 1981). McGuire et al. (1995) using a hyperinsulinemic-euglycemic clamp where circulating insulin levels were increased 5-fold while blood glucose was held constant, failed to show any effect of insulin on milk fat synthesis.

#### ROLE OF TRANS FATTY ACIDS

Research conducted during the last 10 years strongly suggests that milk fat depression is the result of changes in the rumen biohydrogenation process and not changes in rumen VFA patterns. Rumen biohydrogenation is the process by which polyunsaturated fatty acid (PUFA) present in dietary fat, are hydrogenated (saturated) by rumen bacteria. Under normal conditions, very few unsaturated fatty acids reach the small intestine even when large amounts of PUFA are fed because of rumen biohydrogenation. The predominant PUFA in dairy cow diets are linoleic (C 18:2) and linolenic (C 18:3) acids in plant lipids whereas eicosapentaenoic (C 20:5), docosapentaenoic (C 22:5) and docosahexaenoic (C 22:6) acids are common PUFA in marine oils. The biohydrogenation process is one of the principle reasons that ruminant animals generally have both milk and tissue fatty acids that are highly saturated (Christie, 1981).

The steps in rumen fatty acid biohydrogenation include: hydrolysis of triglycerides to glycerol and free fatty acids; isomerization of PUFA to trans double bond containing dienes such as conjugated linoleic acid (CLA) (cis-9, trans-11 C-18), hydrogenation of CLA to vaccenic acid (trans-11, C-18:1) and finally hydrogenation of vaccenic acid to stearic acid (C 18:0) (Harfoot and Hazlewood, 1987). Although the steps outlined above are typically thought of as the most common pathways of rumen biohydrogenation, many different CLA and trans 18:1 isomers are created as the result of rumen biohydrogenation. Although trans-11 is the most common, positional isomers ranging from trans-3 to trans-16 have been identified in rumen contents (Katz and Keeney, 1966; Griinari et al., 1998; Piperova et al., 2000). The numbers of individual CLA isomers produced are even greater including both positional and geometric (cis versus trans) variation in the double bonds (Yurawecz et al., 1998; Piperova et al., 2000).

During milk fat depression, trans fatty acids (TFA) in milk are increased. Storry and Rook (1965) first reported increased TFA in milk of cows fed high concentrate restricted forage diets. Teter et al. (1990) found a significant negative correlation between milk TFA content and milk fat percent ($r = -0.53$). Wonsil et al. (1994) found that the change in fat concentration in milk was negatively related to TFA content in milk fat. Postruminal infusion of TFA isomers resulted in milk fat depression (Gaynor et al., 1994; Romo et al., 1996). High concentrate diets result in increased TFA in milk (Kalscheur et al., 1997a; Griinari et al., 1998). The addition of buffers in the diet decreased both duodenal flow of TFA and TFA content in milk fat but increased milk fat percent (Kalscheur et al., 1997a).

The trans double bond in TFA and CLA's in milk fat can originate only from bacterial (rumen) fermentation and not from metabolism of the cow. Milk TFA can increase substantially in cows fed diets that are high in PUFA without depressing milk fat percent if diets contain adequate forage (Griinari, et al., 1998; Kalscheur et al., 1997b). The specific positional isomer of the TFA double bond produced during rumen fermentation is important. Griinari et al. (1998) reported that milk fat depression occurred only when trans-10 (C18:1) isomer was increased compared with normal situations where trans-11 (C18:1) isomer was the most abundant. In this experiment, cows fed high concentrate diets with the addition of vegetable fat had reduced milk fat which corresponded to increased trans-10 (C18:1) whereas, feeding vegetable fat in a high forage diet resulted in increased trans-11 (C18:1) isomer but did not result in milk fat depression.

Conjugated linoleic acid can directly decrease milk fat content. Chouinard et al. (1999) showed that postruminal infusion of 50 to 150 grams per day of CLA mixtures decreased milk fat by more than 50 percent. More recent experiments (Baumgard et al., 2000; Chouinard et al., 1999) using mixtures where the proportion of cis-9, trans-11 CLA versus trans-10, cis-12 CLA are altered showed that trans-10 containing CLA inhibit milk fat synthesis while trans-11 CLA have no effect on milk fat synthesis. The amounts of trans-10 containing CLA required to reduce milk fat are small (10 grams or less) compared to the amounts of TFA reaching the duodenum (50–300 g/day). At present, the amounts of trans-10 containing CLA that reach the duodenum for absorption are not known. The fact that postruminal infusion of either trans-10 containing C18:1 fatty acids or CLA decrease milk fat suggest that both probably play a role in diet induced milk fat depression. Although there is strong evidence that cis-9, trans-11 CLA can be synthesized in the mammary gland from absorbed trans-11 (C18:1) fatty acids (Griinari et al., 2000), the source of trans-10 containing CLA is presumed to be the result of rumen fermentation because a delta-10 desaturase enzyme has not been reported.

The short chain fatty acids ($C<16$) are the fatty acids in milk fat that are decreased most during milk fat depression. This suggests that the mechanism by which trans containing fatty acids reduce overall fat synthesis is by a reduction in de novo fatty acid synthesis. Acetyl CoA carboxylase (ACC) has been demonstrated to be the rate limiting enzyme for fatty acid synthesis in the mammary gland (Mellenberger et al. 1973). Measured enzyme activities along with mRNA for ACC, fatty acid synthase, and stearolyl CoA desaturase in the mammary gland of cows have been reported to be markedly reduced in cows fed fat depressing diets (Loor et al., 1998; Piperova et al., 2000).

Milk fat percent and yield can be altered by diet formulation and ingredient selection. Two factors, dietary PUFA and dietary fiber are important. Dietary polyunsaturated fatty acids are required as substrates for production of CLA and TFA. Inadequate dietary fiber results in low rumen pH. Low rumen pH influences the proportion of trans-10 fatty acids produced as a result of rumen biohydrogenation and potentially inhibits the complete saturation of trans 18:1 fatty acids to stearate. Griinari et al. (1998) found that increased trans-10 fatty acid in milk fat and milk fat depression occurred only when low forage diets (low rumen pH) supplemented with vegetable oil (PUFA source) were fed. The direct effect of rumen pH was shown by Kalscheur et al. (1997a) where addition of buffers to high concentrate diets reduced duodenal TFA flow, decreased milk TFA content, and increased milk fat percent. Diets that cause mean rumen pH to fall below 6.0 appear to be required to cause milk fat depression, and addition of dietary buffers to correct milk fat depression is effective as a means to increase rumen pH and milk fat percent in those circumstances (Erdman, 1988). Addition of high levels of polyunsaturated fatty acids failed to cause milk fat depression in diets with normal amounts of forage (Kalscheur et al., 1997b; Griinari et al., 1998). Sources of dietary PUFA can include those from direct addition of marine or vegetable oils, indirectly from feedstuffs that are relatively high in fat such as fish meal or oilseeds, or to a lesser extent, those naturally contained in cereal grains and forages. Diet formulations that result in adequate amounts of effective fiber needed to maintain adequate rumen pH, and those that also restrict the amounts of dietary PUFA as potential sources of TFA, should result in normal milk fat percent.

## PERFORMANCE MODIFIERS

### *Mineral Salts and Their Role as Buffers*

Compounds such as sodium bicarbonate, sodium sesquicarbonate, calcium carbonate, or magnesium oxide are added to diets in an effort to reduce digestive upsets or to maintain milk fat percentage when diets high in grain and carbohydrate fermentability or low in effective fiber are fed to lactating dairy cows. Efficacy of dietary buffers for dairy cows is well-documented (Davis, 1979; Emery, 1976; Erdman, 1988; Muller, 1979). Sodium bicarbonate has been shown to increase DMI (Erdman et al., 1982; Staples et al., 1986; Vicini et al., 1988; West et al., 1987), milk yield (Erdman et al., 1980; Kilmer et al., 1981; Rogers et al., 1985; Solorzano et al., 1989; Thomas et al., 1984), and milk fat yield (Rogers et al., 1985; Soloranzo et al., 1989; Staples et al., 1986) in some studies. In other studies (DePeters et al., 1984; Rogers et al., 1985) there was no response to dietary buffers.

Erdman (1988) reported that the relationship between ruminal pH and the percentage of fat in milk from dairy cows fed alfalfa haylage-based rations was not significant. Additionally, relationships between dietary sodium bicarbonate or magnesium oxide and blood or urine pH, blood $pCO_2$, or blood bicarbonate concentrations were not found to be significant (Erdman, 1988). Aslam et al. (1991) indicated there was no difference in ruminal pH or volatile fatty acid concentrations for a period of 6 hours after the addition of sodium bicarbonate to the rumen. Two sodium bicarbonate buffers fed to dairy cows resulted in no differences in ruminal pH or organic acids; however, milk fat percentage was increased for some diets (Xu et al., 1994). Tucker et al. (1994) evaluated the use of 0 or 1 percent sodium sesquicarbonate in lactating dairy cows for 308 days postpartum. The buffer did not affect milk yield or composition the first 56 days of lactation. In midlactation (56 to 252 days postpartum), buffer increased milk protein content only. During 252 to 308 days postpartum, fat and protein contents in milk increased with buffer supplementation. Xin et al. (1989) observed that 0.4 percent MgO increased milk fat content without increasing milk yield. Sodium sesquicarbonate increased milk fat percentage and 4 percent FCM (Cassida et al., 1988). A buffer containing KCl, NaCl, and Mg and Na bicarbonates increased 4 percent FCM without modifying DMI (Soloranzo et al., 1989; Staples et al., 1986).

Staples and Lough (1989) summarized 41 experiments involving supplemental feeding of 0.4 to 1.7 percent sodium bicarbonate to dairy cows consuming diets that contained 57 percent concentrate. When corn silage was the main dietary forage, cows receiving supplemented diets produced an average of 0.8 kg/day more milk with 0.22 percentage units higher milk fat resulting in 1.6 kg/day more 4 percent FCM. When a grass and legume silage- or hay-based diet was fed, results were inconsistent with sodium bicarbonate feeding. Little response in production to sodium bicarbonate was obtained when feeding cottonseed hull-containing diets.

In general it is recommended that buffers will be of greatest benefit to the cow: 1) during early lactation; 2) when large amounts of rapidly fermentable carbohydrates are fed; 3) when cows are fed at infrequent intervals; 4) when fermented forage, primarily corn silage is the major forage source; 5) when concentrates and forages are fed separately; 6) when particle size of the total dietary DM has been reduced to the extent that chewing activity is reduced; 7) when milk fat content is low and when low dry matter intake problems are encountered (Davis and Clark, 1983); and 8) when NDF of the ration is below minimum recommendations (Chapter 4). It is recommended that buffers be fed at 0.6 to 0.8 percent of DMI or 1.2 to 1.6 percent of a concentrate mixture.

Lack of a strong relationship between feeding buffers and metabolic or physiologic variables of acid-base status does not support the idea that these compounds function as ruminal or metabolic buffers. Russell and Chow (1993) concluded that physiologically it was unlikely that dietary buffers could have much of an effect on ruminal fluid pH relative to the predominant effect of transfer of $CO_2$ from blood. They proposed that the mechanism of action of sodium bicarbonate is to increase water consumption, increase dilution of ruminal fluid, and therefore increase the amount of starch that escapes fermentation. Kohn and Dunlap (1998) however demonstrated that when the impact of ruminal bicarbonate under carbon dioxide pressure is considered, pH is predicted to decrease from dilution rather than increase. Dilution would result in an increase in the effective volume of the liquid. Additional liquid in the rumen enables more carbon dioxide to be converted to bicarbonate with the release of more protons, thereby pH would be reduced by dilution with water. These researchers indicate that the effect of sodium bicarbonate on raising ruminal pH may not completely be explained by dilution effects alone.

### *Ionophores*

Ionophores are antibiotics produced by a variety of actinomycetes, most often Streptomyces spp. Ionophores alter the flux of ions across biological membranes. Gram negative bacteria contain a complex outer membrane and are usually unaffected by ionophores. Gram positive bacteria lack the outer membrane and are more sensitive to ionophores. Addition of ionophores to the diet decreases the proportion of gram positive bacteria and increases the proportion of gram negative bacteria. As a result, there is a shift in fermentation end-products. Methane production is decreased and the molar proportion of acetate and butyrate are decreased while the molar proportion of propionate is increased. Propionate production may increase 50 to 75 percent depending on the basal diet (Van Maanen et al., 1978) and methane production may be reduced by 30 percent (Schelling, 1984; Mackintosh, et al., 1997). Consequently, the net energy content of feeds is increased when ionophores are fed. Several ionophores have been approved for cattle in the United States. At the time of this writing, ionophores had not been approved for lactating cattle in the United States. Claims for use in nonlactating cattle include increased feed efficiency, prevention of coccidiosis, and increased rate of gain. In countries where ionophores have been approved for lactating cattle (e.g., Australia, Mexico, and Brazil) claims include increased milk production, prevention of ketosis, bloat reduction, and increased milk protein production.

Lasalocid and monensin are approved for prevention and control of coccidiosis. Reduction in the severity of coccidiosis was demonstrated when ionophores were fed to calves that were naturally (Heinrichs and Bush, 1991) or experimentally (Quigley et al., 1997) exposed to coccidia oocysts. Young calves (<4 weeks of age) are at risk of infection, but low DMI of calf starter may preclude consumption of sufficient ionophore to control coccidiosis. Inclusion of ionophore in milk or milk replacer may provide greater control than feeding in calf starters only (Eicher-Pruiett et al., 1992; McMeniman and Elliot, 1995; Quigley et al., 1997). Body weight gains have been improved by the inclusion of ionophores in milk or milk replacer when calves were experimentally exposed to coccidia (Quigley et al., 1997) or when coccidia were not present (Ilan et al., 1981). Eicher-Pruiett et al. (1992) indicated that lasalocid is most effective when delivered at greater than 1 mg/kg body weight.

Almost all of the growth studies with ionophores have been done with beef cattle. Feeding ionophores typically increases the efficiency of feed utilization. In general, when high-concentrate diets were fed, feed intake was decreased and average daily gain was not altered. In contrast when high forage diets were fed, feed intake was not affected but rate of gain was increased (National Research Council, 1996). Very few studies have examined the effects of ionophores on growth of dairy heifers. Feed intake was not significantly reduced by ionophore supplementation (Baile et al., 1982; Meinert et al., 1992; Steen et al., 1992). Average daily gain or efficiency of feed utilization by heifers has been increased by ionophore supplementation, but the differences have not always been significant (Bartley et al., 1979; Baile et al., 1982; Meinert et al., 1992; Chester-Jones et al., 1997). Studies utilizing large numbers of animals will be required to detect quantitative growth responses by dairy heifers to ionophores. Ionophore supplementation may improve reproductive performance of growing heifers. A reduction in days to first estrus (Snyder et al., 1981), days to conception (Baile et al., 1982), or age at first breeding and age at first calving (Meinert et al., 1992) have been reported. Ionophore supplementation had no effects on first lactation milk yield (Baile et al., 1982).

Ionophore effects on ruminal fermentation may influence lactation performance. Increasing propionate production at the expense of acetate, butyrate, and methane will increase energy that is potentially available for milk synthesis. Increased propionate production may enhance glucose synthesis by the animal, which could influence milk production directly by providing a precursor for the synthesis of lactose. Indirect effects of additional glucose production include sparing of amino acids for gluconeogenesis and alteration of hormonal status, which could influence the partitioning of nutrients and milk components. Milk yield is often increased during ionophore supplementation; as much as 3 kg/d when cows received pasture (Moshen et al., 1981; Lean and Wade, 1997; Beckett et al., 1998; Van Der Werf et al., 1998). Pasture fed cows may benefit from bloat reduction. Duffield et al. (1997) indicated an interaction between body condition score and milk production; milk yield responses to ionophore supplementation were greater as body condition score was increased. Milk yield responses of Holsteins may be greater than Jerseys, and Holsteins with high breeding value for milk protein and fat production may be more responsive than those with low breeding value (Van Der Werf et al., 1998). Milk fat percentage is usually decreased by 0.1 percentage units or more (Kennelly and Lien, 1997) and the response in milk protein percentage is variable (Kennelly and Lien, 1997). The effect of ionophore to depress milk fat was alleviated as forage to concentrate ratio was increased (Phipps et al., 1995). Potential mechanisms for depressed milk fat percentage include less acetate and butyrate for fatty acid synthesis, endocrine changes resulting in the partitioning of nutrients away from mammary tissue, or depressed biohydrogenation resulting in greater production of TFA (Fellner et al., 1997).

Effects of ionophores on DMI have been variable; most studies indicate no effects or a decrease in intake (Johnson et al., 1988; Sauer et al., 1989; Weiss and Amiet, 1990). A preliminary report (Symanowski et al., 1999) from a large multi-university trial employing 858 cows and examining 0, 8, 16, and 24 mg/kg dietary monensin indicated that DMI is modestly decreased (< 1 kg/d), solids-corrected milk yield is modestly increased (< 1 kg/d), and efficiency of solids-corrected milk production is increased. The same study indicated that cows fed monensin lost less body condition during early lactation and maintained a higher body condition score (Wagner et al., 1999). Reductions in DMI and greater body weight gain during mid to late lactation might be expected if cows are in positive energy balance, and ionophores cause an increase in the NE content of the diet. Knowlton et al. (1996a) observed a slight increase in DMI when feeding lasalocid. Ionophores could have a positive influence on DMI if cows are fed high concentrate diets and lactate production in the rumen is decreased (Nagaraja et al , 1981); however, lactate concentration was increased in the study of Knowlton et al. (1996b).

Reproductive performance of lactating cows grazing pasture was not improved by ionophore supplementation in two large field trials (Abe et al., 1994; Lean et al., 1994; Hayes et al., 1996). Phipps et al. (1997b) indicated that reproductive performance was not improved during the first lactation but was improved when cows were fed ionophores for a second lactation.

Feeding ionophores may improve animal health. Increased propionate production and gluconeogenesis may spare amino acid catabolism and reduce fat mobilization from adipose tissue and ketone production by the liver. An increase in plasma glucose, decrease in plasma nonesterified fatty acids, decrease in blood beta-hydroxybutyrate, or combinations of the above have been attributed to ionophore feeding on several occasions (Sauer et al., 1989; Lean and Wade, 1997; Phipps et al., 1997a; Duffield et al., 1998a; Green et al., 1999). Lower nonesterified fatty acids and beta-hydroxybutyrate in blood probably reflect less body condition loss when feeding ionophores (Knowlton et al., 1996a; Erasmus et al., 1997; Wagner et al., 1999). The prevalence and incidence of subclinical ketosis was reduced by 50 percent when monensin was delivered by a sustained-release intraruminal device beginning at 3 weeks precalving (Duffield et al., 1998b). A lower incidence of bloat when feeding ionophores (Lowe et al., 1991) is probably attributed to less gas production. As previously indicated, ionophores may have a role in the prevention of subclinical acidosis by reducing lactate formation in the rumen and stabilizing rumen pH.

### *Direct Fed Microbials*

Direct fed microbials (DFM), traditionally referred to as "probiotics" are live or viable naturally occurring organisms supplemented to animals. Direct fed microbials have generally been supplemented to animals during periods of stress or low DMI with the assumption that establishment of a beneficial microorganism population in the digestive tract will decrease or prevent pathogenic organism establishment. The DFM have been fed continuously to attempt to enhance production performance, alter ruminal fermentation, or improve nutrient utilization. The most common DFM are fungal cultures (*Aspergillus oryzae* and *Saccharomyces cerevisiae*), and the lactic acid bacteria *Lactobacillus* or *Streptococcus*. Other bacterial species such as *Bifidobacterium* spp., *Bacillus* spp., and *Propionibacterium* spp. are found in DFM, but to a lesser extent than lactic acid bacteria. Yoon and Stern (1995) in a review found that multiple modes of action have been proposed in which DFM may elicit responses, but none are clearly understood or well defined. They categorized mode of actions into the following:

- stimulation of desirable microbial growth in the rumen,
- stabilization of rumen pH,
- altered ruminal fermentation pattern and end product production,
- increased nutrient flow postruminally,
- increased nutrient digestibility, and
- alleviation of stress through enhanced immune response.

### *Fungal Cultures*

Production responses to the addition of fungal cultures to diets of lactating dairy cows have been variable. Yoon and Stern (1995) reported significant increases in DMI in 2 of 10 studies and significant increases in milk production in 3 of 11 studies with supplementation of *S. cerevisiae*. In more recent studies, supplementation of *S. cerevisiae* increased DMI and milk production in three studies (Adams et al., 1995; Putman et al., 1997; Wohlt et al., 1998), but not in two others (Robinson, 1997; Kung et al., 1997). *Aspergillus oryzae* increased DMI in 1 of 8 studies and milk production in 6 of 14 studies summarized by Yoon and Stern (1995). In more recent studies with supplementation of *A. oryzae* to lactating cow diets, no increase in milk production was reported in one study (Bertrand and Grimes, 1997) and mixed, but an overall positive increase in milk production was reported in 46 commercial dairy herds (McGilliard and Stallings, 1998).

Stimulation of the growth and activities of both total and certain specific groups of ruminal bacteria have been the most consistent reproducible modes of action for fungal cultures (Yoon and Stern, 1995, 1996; Beharka and Nagaraja, 1998; Newbold et al., 1996). Cellulose digesting and lactic acid utilizing bacteria are the most commonly enhanced ruminal bacteria groups by fungal supplementation (Callaway and Martin, 1997). Why and how fungal cultures increase bacterial numbers is not understood, but one proposed mechanism is that the respiratory activity of yeast protects anaerobic rumen bacteria from damage by oxygen (Newbold et al., 1996).

Dietary composition and forage source are significant factors affecting production responses to fungal cultures. High concentrate diets (60:40 concentrate to forage ratio) resulted in greater milk production response to fungal culture supplementation than lower concentrate diets (Williams et al., 1991), and ruminal digestion of NDF in alfalfa was increased more than that of NDF in corn silage or other sources of NDF by fungal culture supplementation (Miranda et al., 1996; Adams et al., 1995). Total volatile fatty acid (VFA) production or ratios of VFA are generally not affected by additions of fungal cultures (Yoon and Stern, 1995, 1996; Beharka and Nagaraja, 1998). Passage of essential amino acids or the ratio of microbial to feed nitrogen that passed to the small intestine was not increased with yeast supplementation (Putman et al., 1997) nor was overall total tract digestibility (Yoon and Stern, 1995).

LACTOBACILLUS

Considerably less research has been conducted to determine the effects of lactic acid bacteria on production responses or ruminal fermentation changes than with fungal cultures. Supplementation of lactic acid bacteria to diets has primarily been for a "probiotic" effect where ingestion of beneficial organisms colonize the intestinal tract preventing pathogen proliferation, compete with enterotoxin-producing organisms for absorption sites in the intestine, and possibly enhance digestion of nutrients in the small intestine (Yoon and Stern, 1995). In the review by Yoon and Stern (1995), only two studies were found where *Lactobacillus acidophilus* was fed to lactating dairy cattle. In both studies, milk production increased by feeding *L. acidophilus*. Cruywagen et al. (1996) reported supplementing *L. acidophilus* in milk replacer resulted in calves losing less weight the initial two weeks of life, but over a six-week period had no affect on weight gain, feed intake, or diarrhea occurrence. The addition of *L. acidophilus* or *Bifidobacterium animalis* to a milk replacer containing an antibiotic increased growth rate and efficiency of feed utilization by calves during the milk replacer feeding period (first 35 days of life) and the next 21 days postweaning (Abe et al., 1995).

*Bovine Somatotropin*

Bovine somatotropin (BST) is a naturally-occurring protein hormone produced in the pituitary gland of dairy cattle. It is a major regulator of growth and milk production. This hormone can be produced in commercial quantity using recombinant DNA technology. BST was approved for use in lactating dairy cows by the Food and Drug Administration in November 1993. Because of a 90-day moratorium passed by the U.S. Congress, BST could not be sold for commercial use until February 1994.

Supplementation of BST to growing and lactating animals affects many physiologic processes (Peel and Bauman, 1987; Bauman et al., 1989a; National Research Council, 1994). Metabolic adaptations that partition increased quantities of absorbed nutrients to the required tissue for optimum growth or milk production is the principle effect of BST in growing and lactating dairy cattle. Supplementation of BST to growing or lactating dairy cattle does not affect digestibilities of DM, energy, or protein (Bauman et al., 1989a; Boyd and Bauman, 1989; Chalupa and Galligan, 1989) nor does BST affect energy utilization for maintenance or the partial efficiency of milk synthesis (Tyrrell et al., 1988; Sechen et al., 1989; Kirchgessner et al., 1991). However, the efficiency of overall nutrient utilization for milk production by cows is improved because a smaller proportion of the nutrient intake is needed to fulfill the maintenance requirements.

The effects of BST on milk yield have been reviewed (Peel and Bauman, 1987; Chilliard, 1989; McBride et al., 1988; Chalupa and Galligan, 1989; Peel et al., 1989; Crooker and Otterby, 1991; Hartnell et al., 1991; McGuffey and Williamson, 1991; Bauman, 1992; National Research Council, 1994; Bauman et al., 1999). Increases in milk yield to varying doses of BST (5 to 50 mg/cow/day) range from about 3 to 6 kg of milk/cow/day (National Research Council, 1994). Persistency of lactation also is improved. Supplementation of BST has increased milk yield in all breeds of dairy cattle studied and in animals of different parity and genetic potential (National Research Council, 1994). The magnitude of the increased milk yield will be affected by the quality of management, especially nutrition management (Bauman, 1987).

Nutritional status, diet composition, environment, season, stage of lactation, genetics, and age affect the concentration of fat and protein in milk (Linn, 1988; Sutton, 1989). These factors also affect the composition of milk from cows supplemented with BST. The nutritional status of cows both before and during supplementation of BST determines the effect of BST on the concentration of fat and protein in milk (Peel and Bauman, 1987; McBride et al., 1988; Bauman et al., 1989a; Chalupa and Galligan, 1989; van den Berg, 1991; Dell'Orto and Savoini, 1991; Barbano et al., 1992; Lynch et al., 1992; Laurent et al., 1992). Short-term changes in milk composition when BST is supplemented may occur because of increased milk synthesis and because of increased mobilization of energy and protein from body reserves to meet the increased nutrient demands for synthesis of milk and milk components. However, when BST was supplemented for a complete lactation the concentration of fat and protein in milk was not different for control and BST cows (Bauman et al., 1989b). BST did not affect milk composition during long-term supplementation, because cows, within a few weeks after the start of BST administration, increased nutrient intake to meet requirements for synthesis of milk and milk components and to replenish body reserves (Peel and Bauman, 1987; Chalupa and Galligan, 1989; Chilliard, 1989). High quality feeds and excellent nutrition management are required to attain maximum response from cows supplemented with BST (Bauman, 1987, 1992).

Nutrition of dairy cows supplemented with BST has been discussed in several papers (Bauman, 1987; Chalupa and Galligan, 1989; Chilliard, 1989; Crooker and Otterby, 1991; Kirchgessner et al., 1991; McGuffey and Wilkinson, 1991; Muller, 1992; Collier et al., 1992; National Research Council, 1994). Nutrient requirements are identical for BST supplemented cows and unsupplemented cows if they are producing the same amount of milk with an identical composition, have the same body size and weight, and are losing or gaining the same body weight. Diet formulation and feeding strategies should be the same for BST supplemented and unsupplemented cows of the same size and weight that are producing the same amount of milk and milk components. Current recommendations are that cows supplemented with BST should be fed and managed like unsupplemented cows at similar levels of production.

## REFERENCES


Abe, F., N. Ishibashi, and S. Shimamura. 1995. Effect of administration of bifidobacteria and lactic acid bacteria to newborn calves and piglets. J. Dairy Sci. 78:2838–2845.

Abe, N., I. J. Lean, A. Rabiee, J. Porter, and C. Graham. 1994. Effects of sodium monensin on reproductive performance of dairy cattle. II. Effects on metabolites in plasma, resumption of ovarian cyclicity and oestrus in lactating cows. Aust. Vet. J. 71:277–282.

Adams, A. L., B. Harris, Jr., H. H. Van Horn, and C. J. Wilcox. 1995. Effects of varying forage types on milk production responses to whole cottonseed, tallow and yeast. J. Dairy Sci. 78:573–581.

Al-Ani, F. K., and J. G. E. Vesteweber. 1986. Udder edema: An updated review. Vet. Bull. 56:763–769.

Allen, M. S. 1997. Relationship between fermentation acid production in the rumen and the requirements for physically effective fiber. J. Dairy. Sci. 80:1447–1462.

Allen, W. M., and D. C. Davies. 1981. Milk fever, hypomagnesaemia, and the 'downer cow' syndrome. Br. Vet. J. 137:435–441.

Anderson, K. L., T. G. Nagaraja, J. L. Morrill, P. G. Reddy, T. B. Avery, and N. V. Anderson. 1988. Performance and ruminal changes of early-weaned calves fed lasalocid. J. Anim. Sci. 66:806–813.

Armentano, L., and M. Pereira. 1997. Measuring the effectiveness of fiber by animal response trials. J. Dairy Sci. 80:1416–1425.

Aslam, M., W. B. Tucker, J. F. Hogue, R. K. Vernon, and G. D. Adams. 1991. Controlled ruminal infusion of sodium bicarbonate. 2. Effects of dietary and infused buffer on ruminal milieu. J. Dairy Sci. 74:3496–3504.

Baile, C. A., C. L. McLaughlin, W. V. Chalupa, D. L. Snyder, L. C. Pendlum, and E. L. Potter. 1982. Effects of monensin fed to replacement dairy heifers during the growing and gestation period upon growth, reproduction, and subsequent lactation. J. Dairy Sci. 65:1941–1944

Bar, A., R. Perlman, and M. Sachs. 1985. Observation on the use of 1-alpha-hydroxyvitamin D3 in the prevention of bovine parturient paresis: The effect of a single injection on plasma 1-alpha-hydroxyvitamin D3, 1,25-dihydroxyvitamin D3, calcium, and hydroxyproline. J. Dairy Sci. 68:1952–1958.

Barbano, D. M., J. M. Lynch, D. E. Bauman, G. F. Hartnell, R. L. Hintz, and M. A. Nemeth. 1992. Effect of a prolonged-release formulation of N-methionyl bovine somatotropin (sometribove) on milk composition. J. Dairy Sci. 75:1775–1793.

Barber, D. M., C. L. Wright, and W. MacLennan. 1983. Hypomagnesaemia in periparturient dairy cows. Vet. Rec. 112:35–36.

Bartley, E. E., E. L. Herod, R. M. Bechtle, D. A. Sapienza, and B. E. Brent. 1979. Effect of monensin or lasalocid, with and without niacin or amicloral, on rumen fermentation and feed efficiency. J. Anim. Sci. 49:1066–1075.

Barton, B. A., N. A. Jorgensen, and H. F. DeLuca. 1987. Impact of prepartum dietary phosphorus intake on calcium homeostasis at parturition. J. Dairy Sci. 70:1186–91.

Bauchart, D., D. Gruffat, and D. Durand. 1996. Lipid absorption and hepatic lipid metabolism. Proc. Nutr. Soc. 55:39–47.

Bauman, D. E. 1987. Bovine somatotropin: The Cornell experience. Pp. 46 in National Invitational Workshop on Bovine Somatotropin. Washington, D.C.: U.S. Department of Agriculture Extension Service.

Bauman, D. E. 1992. Bovine somatotropin: Review of an emerging animal technology. J. Dairy Sci. 75:3432–3451.

Bauman, D. E., B. A. Corl, and L. H. Baumgard. 1998. Trans fatty acids, conjugated linoleic acid and milk fat synthesis. Proceeding 1998 Cornell Nutrition Conference. p. 95.

Bauman, D. E., F. R. Dunshea, Y. R. Biosclair, M. A. McGuire, D. M. Harris, and K. L. Houseknecht. 1989a. Regulation of nutrient partitioning: Homeostasis, homeorhesis and exogenous somatotropin. Pp. 306–323 in Seventh International Conference on Production Diseases in Farm Animals, F. A. Kallfelz, ed. Ithaca, NY: Cornell University.

Bauman, D. E., R. W. Everett, W. H. Weiland, and R. J. Collier. 1999. Production responses to bovine somatotropin in northeast dairy herds. J. Dairy Sci. 82:2564–2573.

Bauman, D. E., D. L. Hard, B. A. Crooker, M. S. Partridge, K. Garrick, L. D. Sandles, H. N. Erb, S. E. Franson, G. F. Hartnell, and R. L. Hintz. 1989b. Long-term evaluation of prolonged-release formulation of N-methionyl bovine somatotropin in lactating dairy cows. J. Dairy Sci. 72:642–651.

Baumgard, L. H., B. A. Corl, D. A. Dwyer, A. Saeb, and D. E. Bauman. 2000. Identification of the conjugated linoleic acid isomer that inhibits milk fat synthesis. Am. J. Physiol. 278:R179–184.

Beckett, S., I. Lean, R. Dyson, W. Tranter, and L. Wade. 1998. Effects of monensin on the reproduction, health, and milk production of dairy cows. J. Dairy Sci. 81:1563–1573.

Beede, D. K. 1992. Dietary cation-anion difference: Preventing milk fever. Feed Management 43:28–31.

Beede, D. K., C. Wang, G. A. Donovan, L. F. Archbald, and W. K. Sanchez. 1991. Dietary cation-anion difference (electrolyte balance) in late pregnancy. Florida Dairy Production Conf. Proc., April 10, 1991. pp. 1–6.

Beharka, A. A., and T. G. Nagaraja. 1998. Effect of *Aspergillus oryzae* extract alone or in combination with antimicrobial compounds on ruminal bacteria. J. Dairy Sci. 81:1591–1598.

Bell, A. W. 1979. Lipid metabolism in the liver and selected tissues and in the whole body of ruminant animals. Prog. Lipid Res. 18:117–164.

Bell, A. W. 1995. Regulation of organic nutrient metabolism during transition from late pregnancy to early lactation. J. Anim. Sci. 73:2804–2819.

Bell, A. W., G. Slepetis, and R. A. Ehrhardt. 1995. Growth and accretion of energy and protein in the gravid uterus during late pregnancy in Holstein cows. J. Dairy Sci. 78:1954–1961.

Bergsten, C. 1994. Hemorrhages of the sole horn of dairy cows as a retrospective indicator of laminitis: An epidemiological study. Acta Vet. Scand. 35:55–66.

Bergsten, C. 1995. Digital disorders in dairy cattle with special reference to laminitis and heel erosion: The influence of housing, management and nutrition. Dissertation. Skara, Sweden.

Bertics, S. J., R. R. Grummer, C. Cadorniga-Valino, and E. E. Stoddard. 1992. Effect of prepartum dry matter intake on liver triglyceride concentration and early lactation. J. Dairy Sci. 75:1914–1922.

Bertrand, J. A., and L. W. Grimes. 1997. Influence of tallow and *Aspergillus oryzae* fermentation extract in dairy cattle rations. J. Dairy Sci. 80:1179–1184.

Block, E. 1984. Manipulating dietary anions and cations for prepartum dairy cows to reduce incidence of milk fever. J. Dairy Sci. 67:2939–2948.

Block, E. 1994. Manipulation of dietary cation-anion difference on nutritionally related production diseases, productivity and metabolic responses of dairy cows. J. Dairy Sci. 77:1437–1450

Boda, J. M., and H. H. Cole. 1954. The influence of dietary calcium and phosphorus on the incidence of milk fever in dairy cattle. J. Dairy Sci. 37:360–372.

Boyd, R. D., and D. E. Bauman. 1989. Mechanisms of action for somatotropin in growth. Pp. 257–293 in Current Concepts of Animal Regulation, D. R. Campion, G. J. Hausman, and R. J. Martin, eds. New York: Plenum.

Breukink, H. J. 1991. Abomasal displacement, etiology, pathogenesis, treatment and prevention. Bovine Practitioner 26:148–153.

Breukink, H. J., and T. de Ruyter. 1976. Abomasal displacement in cattle: Influence of concentrates in the ration on fatty acid concentrations in ruminal, abomasal, and duodenal contents. Am. J. Vet. Res. 37:1181–1184.

Brzezinska-Slebodzinska, E., and J. K. Miller. 1992. Antioxidant status of dairy cows supplemented prepartum with vitamin E and selenium. Fed. Am. Soc. Exp. Biol. J. 6:A1953 (Abstr.).

Callaway, E. S., and S. A. Martin. 1997. Effects of a *Saccharomyces cerevisiae* culture on ruminal bacteria that utilize lactate and digest cellulose. J. Dairy Sci. 80:2035–2044.

Cameron, R. E., P. B. Dyk, T. H. Herdt, J. B. Kaneene, R. Miller, H. F. Bucholtz, J. S. Liesman, M. J. Vandehaar, and R. S. Emery. 1998. Dry cow diet, management, and energy balance as risk factors for displaced abomasum in high producing dairy herds. J. Dairy Sci. 81:132–139.

Campling, R. C., M. Freer, and C. C. Balch. 1962. Factors affecting the voluntary intake of food by cows. Brit. J. Nutr. 16:115–124.

Capuco, A. V., R. M. Akers, and J. J. Smith. 1997. Mammary growth in Holstein cows during the dry period: Quantification of nucleic acids and histology. J. Dairy Sci. 80:447–487.

Cassida, K. A., L. D. Muller, and T. F. Sweeney. 1988. Sodium sesquicarbonate for early lactation dairy cows fed corn silage-based diets. J. Dairy Sci. 71:381–387.

Chalupa, W., and D.T. Galligan. 1989. Nutritional implications of somatotropin for lactating cows. J. Dairy Sci. 72:2510–2524.

Chalupa, W., C. J. Sniffen, W. E. Julien, H. Sato, T. Fujieda, T. Ueda, and H. Suzuki. 1999. Lactation response of cows in a commercial dairy to rumen protected methionine and lysine. J. Dairy Sci. 82(Suppl. 1): 121. (Abstr.).

Chester-Jones, H., J. G. Linn, D. M. Ziegler, and M. Engstrom. 1997. Determination of the caloric equivalency of an ionophore in dairy heifer diets. J. Dairy Sci. 80(Suppl. 1):216 (Abstr.).

Chew, B. P., F. R. Murdock, R. E. Riley, and J. K. Hillers. 1984. Influence of prepartum dietary crude protein on growth hormone, insulin, reproduction, and lactation of dairy cows. J. Dairy Sci 67:270–275.

Chew, B. P., H. F. Keller, R. E. Erb, and P. V. Malven. 1977. Periparturient concentrations of prolactin, progesterone, and estrogen in blood plasma of cows retaining or not retaining fetal membranes. J. Anim. Sci. 44:1055–1060.

Chew, B. P., R. E. Erb, J. F. Fessler, C. J. Callahan, and P. V. Malven. 1979. Effects of ovariectomy during pregnancy and of prematurely induced parturition on progesterone, estrogens, and calving traits. J. Dairy Sci. 62:557–566.

Chilliard, Y. 1989. Long-term effects of recombinant bovine somatotropin (rbST) on dairy cow performances: A review. Pp. 61–87 in Use of Somatotropin in Livestock Production, K. Sejrsen, M. Vestergaard, and A. Neimann-Sorensen, eds. New York: Elsevier Applied Science.

Chouinard, P. Y., L. Corneau, A. Sb, and D. E. Bauman. 1999a. Milk yield and composition during abomasal infusion of conjugated linoleic acid. J. Dairy Sci. 82:2737–2745.

Chouinard, P. Y., L. Corneau, D. M. Barbano, I. E. Metzger, and D. E. Bauman. 1999b. Conjugated linoleic acids alter milk fatty acid composition and inhibit milk fat secretion in dairy cows. J. Nutr. 129:1579–1584.

Christie, W. W. 1981. The effects of diet and other factors on the lipid composition of ruminant tissues and milk. *In* Lipid metabolism in ruminant animals. Ed. W. W. Christie, Pergamon Press.

Collier, R. J., J. L. Vicini, C. D. Knight, C. L. McLaughlin, and C. A. Baile. 1992. Impact of somatotropins on nutrient requirements in domestic animals. J. Nutr. 122:855–866.

Conway, J. F., H. H. Olson, and G. C. McGoy. 1977. Effects of sodium chloride supplementation on the incidence and severity of mammary edema and on serum sodium levels in pre-parturient cows and heifer. J. Dairy Sci. 60(Suppl.1):110 (Abstr.).

Coppock, C. E., C. H. Noller, S. A. Wolfe, C. J. Callahan, and J. S. Baker. 1972. Effect of forage-concentrate ratio in complete feeds fed ad libitum on feed intake prepartum and the occurrence of abomasal displacement in dairy cows. J. Dairy Sci. 55:783–789.

Cox, V. S. 1998. Downer cow syndrome. Pp. 215–218 in Current Veterinary Therapy 4: Food Animal Practice, J. L. Howard and R. A. Smith, eds. Philadelphia: W.B. Saunders Co.

Craige, A. H., and I.V. Stoll. 1947. Milk fever (parturient paresis) as a manifestation of alkalosis. Am. J. Vet. Res. 8:168–172.

Crawley, D. D., and L. H. Kilmer. 1995. Effects of level and source of rumen degradable protein fed prepartum on postpartum performance of dairy cattle. J. Dairy Sci. 78(Suppl.1):266 (Abstr.).

Crooker, B. A., and D. E. Otterby. 1991. Management of the dairy herd treated with bovine somatotropin. Food Anim. Prac. 7:417–437.

Croom, W. J., A. H. Rakes, A. C. Linnerud, G. A. Ducharme, and J. M. Elliot. 1981. Vitamin $B_{12}$ administration for milk fat synthesis in lactating dairy cows fed a low fiber diet. J. Dairy Sci. 64:1555–1560.

Cruywagen, C. W., I. Jordaan, and L. Venter. 1996. Effect of *Lactobacillus acidophilus* supplementation of milk replacer on preweaning performance of calves. J. Dairy Sci. 79:483–486.

Curtis, C. R., H. N. Erb, C. J. Sniffen, R. D. Smith, and D. S. Kronfeld. 1985. Path analysis of dry period nutrition, postpartum metabolic and reproductive disorders, and mastitis in Holstein cows. J. Dairy Sci. 68:2347–2360.

Curtis, C. R., H. N. Erb, C. J. Sniffen, R. D. Smith, P. A. Powers, M. C. Smith, M. E. White, R. B. Hillman, and E. J. Pearson. 1983. Association of parturient hypocalcemia with eight periparturient disorders in Holstein cows. JAVMA 183:559–561.

Daniel, R. C. W. 1983. Motility of the rumen and abomasum during hypocalcaemia. Can. J. Comp. Med. 47:276–280.

Davis, C. L. 1979. The use of buffers in the rations of lactating cows. Pp. 51–64 in Regulation of Acid-Base Balance, W. H. Hale and P. Meinhardt, eds. Church and Dwight, Co. Inc.

Davis, C. L., and J. H. Clark. 1983. Response of dairy cattle to buffers. Proc. Buffers, Neutralizers and Electrolytes Symp. West Des Moines, Iowa: National Feed Ingredients Association.

Dell'Orto, V., and G. Savoini. 1991. Recombinant bovine somatotropin (rbST) treatment in dairy cows: Effect on ruminal activity and milk properties. Microbiol. Aliments Nutr. 9:121–132.

Dentine, M. R., and B. T. McDaniel. 1984. Association of subjective udder edema scores and description trait codes for udder types. J. Dairy Sci. 67:208–215.

DePeters, E. J., A. H. Fredeen, D. L. Bath, and N. E. Smith. 1984. Effect of sodium bicarbonate addition to alfalfa hay-based diets on digestibility of dietary fractions and rumen characteristics. J. Dairy Sci. 67:2344–2355.

Drackley, J. K. 1999. Biology of dairy cows during the transition period: the final frontier? J. Dairy Sci. 82:2259–2273.

Dirksen, G. U., H. G. Liebich, and E. Mayer. 1985. Adaptive changes of the ruminal mucosa and their functional and clinical significance. Bovine Pract. 20:116–120.

Duffield, T. F., D. Sandals, K. E. Leslie, K. Lissemore, B. W. McBride, J. H. Lumsden, P. Dick, and R. Bagg. 1998a. Effect of prepartum administration of monensin in a controlled-release capsule on postpartum energy indicators in lactating cows. J. Dairy Sci. 81:2354–2361.

Duffield, T. F., D. Sandals, K. E. Leslie, K. Lissemore, B. W. McBride, J. H. Lumsden, P. Dick, and R. Bagg. 1998b. Efficacy of monensin for the prevention of subclinical ketosis in lactating dairy cows. J. Dairy Sci. 81:2866–2873.

Duffield, T. F., K. E. Leslie, D. Sandals, K. Lissemore, B. McBride, and J. H. Lumsden. 1997. Effect of monensin on cow health and milk production. J. Dairy Sci. 80(Suppl. 1):167 (Abstr.).

Dufva, G. S., E. E. Bartley, A. D. Dayton, and D. O. Riddell. 1983. Effect of niacin supplementation on milk production and ketosis of dairy cattle. J. Dairy Sci. 66:2329–2336.

Edgerton, L. A., and H. D. Hafs. 1973. Serum luteinizing hormone, prolactin, glucocorticoid, and progestin in dairy cows from calving to gestation. J. Dairy Sci. 56:451–458.

Eger, S., D. Drori, I. Kadoori, N. Miller, and H. Schindler. 1985. Effects of selenium and vitamin E on incidence of retained placenta. J. Dairy Sci. 68:2119–2122.

Eicher-Pruiett, S. D., J. L. Morrill, T. G. Nagaraja, J. J. Higgins, N. V. Anderson, and P. G. Reddy. 1992. Response of young dairy calves with lasalocid delivery varied in feed sources. J. Dairy Sci. 75:857–862.

Emery, R. S. 1976. High energy feeds for milk production. Pp. 149–159 in Buffers in Ruminant Physiology and Metabolism, M. S. Weinberg, and A. L. Sheffner, eds. Church and Dwight Co., Inc.

Emery, R. S. and L. D. Brown. 1961. Effect of feeding sodium and potassium bicarbonate on milk fat, rumen pH, and volatile fatty acid production. J. Dairy Sci. 44:1899–1902.

Emery, R. S., L. D. Brown, and J. W. Thomas. 1964. Effect of sodium bicarbonate and calcium carbonates on milk production and composition of milk, blood, and rumen contents of cows fed grain ad libitum with restricted roughage. J. Dairy Sci. 47:1325.

Emery, R. S., H. D. Hafs, D. Armstrong, and W. W. Snyder. 1969. Prepartum grain feeding effects on milk production, mammary edema, and incidence of diseases. J. Dairy Sci. 52:345–351.

Emery, R. S., J. S. Liesman, and T. H. Herdt. 1992. Metabolism of long chain fatty acids by rumimant liver. J. Nutr. 122:832–837.

Ender, F., and I. W. Dishington. 1967. Comparative studies on calcium balance levels in parturient cows fed diets inducing and preventing milk fever. Pp. 557A in XVIII[th] World Veterinary Congress, Vol. II. Paris.

Ender, F., I. W. Dishington, and A. Helgebostad. 1971. Calcium balance studies in dairy cows under experimental induction and prevention of hypocalcaemic paresis puerperalis. The solution of the aetiology and the prevention of milk fever by dietary means. Z. Tierphysiol. 28:233–256.

Erasmus, L. J., A. Muller, I. Smith, and D. O'Hagan. 1997. Effect of lasalocid on performance of lactating dairy cows. J. Dairy Sci. 80(Suppl. 1):208 (Abstr.).

Erb, H. N., and Y. T. Grohn. 1988. Epidemiology of metabolic disorders in the periparturient dairy cow. J. Dairy Sci. 71:2557–2571.

Erb, H. N., R. D. Smith, P. A. Oltenaw, C. L. Guard, R. B. Hillman, P. A. Powers, M. C. Smith, and M. E. White. 1985. Path model of reproductive disorders and performance, milk fever, mastitis, milk yield, and culling in Holstein cows. J. Dairy Sci. 68:3337–3349.

Erdman, R. A. 1988. Dietary buffering requirements of the lactating dairy cow. J. Dairy Sci. 71:3246–3266.

Erdman, R. A., R. W. Hemken, and L. S. Bull. 1982. Dietary sodium bicarbonate and magnesium oxide for early post partum lactating dairy cows: effects on production, acid-base metabolism, and digestion. J. Dairy Sci. 65:712–731.

Erdman, R. A., R. L. Botts, R. W. Hemken, and L. S. Bull. 1980. Effect of sodium bicarbonate and magnesium oxide on production and physiology in early lactation. J. Dairy Sci. 63:923–930.

Fellner, V., F. D. Sauer, and J. K. G. Kramer. 1997. Effect of nigericin, monensin, and tetronasin on biohydrogenation in continuous flow-through ruminal fermenters. J. Dairy Sci. 80:921–928.

Ferrell, C. L., W. N. Garrett, and N. Hinman. 1976. Growth, development and composition of the udder and gravid uterus of beef heifers during pregnancy. J. Anim. Sci. 42:1477–1489.

Ferrell, C. L., D. B. Laster, and R. L. Prior. 1982. Mineral accretion during prenatal growth of cattle. J. Anim. Sci. 54:618–624.

Ferrell, C. L., W. N. Garrett, N. Hinman, and G. Grichting. 1976. Energy utilization by pregnant and nonpregnant heifers. J. Anim. Sci. 42:937–950.

Firkins, J. L. 1997. Effects of feeding nonforage fiber sources on site of fiber digestion. J. Dairy Sci. 80:1426–1437.

Food and Drug Administration. 1997. Food additives permitted in feed and drinking water of animals; selenium. Federal Register (Aug. 25) 62:44892–44894.

Fountaine, F. C., D. B. Parrish, and F. W. Atkeson. 1949. Comparison of the incidence and severity of mammary edema of cows fed roughages alone or roughages plus grain during the dry period. J. Dairy Sci. 32:721 (Abstr.).

Frobish, R. A., and C. L. Davis. 1977. Theory involving propionate and vitamin $B_{12}$ in the low-fat milk syndrome. J. Dairy Sci. 60:268–273.

Gant, R. G., W. Sanchez, and R. L. Kincaid. 1998. Effects of anionic salts on selenium metabolism in nonlactating, pregnant dry cows. J. Dairy Sci. 81:1637–1642.

Gaynor, P. J., F. J. Mueller, J. K. Miller, N. Ramsey, J. P. Goff, and R. L. Horst. 1989. Parturient hypocalcemia in Jersey cows fed alfalfa haylage-based diets with different cation to anion ratios. J. Dairy Sci. 72:2525–2531.

Gaynor, P. J., R. A. Erdman, B. B. Teter, J. Sampugna, A. V. Capuco, D. R. Waldo and M. Hamosh. 1994. Milk fat yield and composition during abomasal infusion of cis or trans octadecenoates in Holstein cows. J. Dairy Sci. 77:157–165.

Goff, J. P. 1998a. Phosphorus deficiency. Pp. 218–220 in Current Veterinary Therapy 4: Food Animal Practice, J. L. Howard and R. A. Smith, eds. Philadelphia: W.B. Saunders Co.

Goff, J. P. 1998b. Ruminant hypomagnesemic tetanies. Pp. 215–218 in Current Veterinary Therapy 4: Food Animal Practice, J. L. Howard and R. A. Smith, eds. Philadelphia: W.B. Saunders Co.

Goff, J. P. 2000. Pathophysiology of calcium and phosphorus disorders. Vet Clin North Am Food Animal Pract. 16:319–337.

Goff, J. P., and R. L. Horst. 1990. Effect of subcutaneously released 24F-1,25-dihydroxyvitamin D3 on incidence of parturient paresis in dairy cows. J. Dairy Sci 73:406–412.

Goff, J. P., and R. L. Horst. 1997a. Effects of the addition of potassium or sodium, but not calcium, to prepartum rations on milk fever in dairy cows. J. Dairy Sci. 80:176–186.

Goff, J. P., and R. L. Horst. 1997b. Physiological changes at parturition and their relationship to metabolic disorders. J. Dairy Sci. 80:1260–1268.

Goff, J. P., and R. L. Horst. 1998. Use of hydrochloric acid as a source of anions for prevention of milk fever. J. Dairy Sci. 81: 2874–2880.

Goff, J. P., and J. R. Stabel. 1990. Decreased plasma retinal, alpha-tocopherol, and zinc concentration during the periparturient period: effect on milk fever. J. Dairy Sci. 73:3195–3199.

Goff, J. P., E. T. Littledike, and R. L. Horst. 1986. Effect of synthetic bovine parathyroid hormone in dairy cows: Prevention of hypocalcemic parturient paresis. J. Dairy Sci. 69:2278–2289.

Goff, J. P., T. A. Reinhardt, and R. L. Horst. 1989. Recurring hypocalcemia of bovine parturient paresis is associated with failure to produce 1,25-dihydroxyvitamin D. Endocrinol. 125:49–53.

Goff, J. P., R. L. Horst, F. J. Mueller, J. K. Miller, G. A. Kiess, and H. H. Dowlen. 1991. Addition of chloride to a prepartal diet high in cations increases 1,25-dihydroxyvitamin D response to hypocalcemia preventing milk fever. J. Dairy Sci. 74:3863–3871.

Goff, J. P., T. A. Reinhardt, D. C. Beitz, and R. L. Horst. 1995. Breed affects tissue vitamin D receptor concentration in periparturient dairy cows: A milk fever risk factor? J. Dairy Sci. 78(Suppl. 1):184.

Goff, J. P., R. L. Horst, P. W. Jardon, C. Borelli, and J. Wedam. 1996. Field trials of an oral calcium propionate paste as an aid to prevent milk fever in periparturient dairy cows. J. Dairy Sci. 79:378–383.

Goff, J. P., R. Ruiz, and R. L. Horst. 1997. Relative acidiogenic activity of commonly used anionic salts—re-thinking the dietary cation-anion difference equations. J. Dairy Sci. 80(Suppl. 1):169.

Goings, R. L., N. L. Jacobson, D. C. Beitz, E. T. Littledike, and K. D. Wiggers. 1974. Prevention of parturient paresis by a prepartum, calcium-deficient diet. J. Dairy Sci. 57:1184–1188.

Grant, R. J. 1997. Interactions among forages and nonforage fiber sources. J. Dairy Sci. 80:1438–1446.

Green, B. L., B. W. McBride, D. Sandals, K. E. Leslie, R. Bagg, and P. Dick. 1999. The impact of a monensin controlled-release capsule on subclinical ketosis in the transition dairy cow. J. Dairy Sci. 82:333–342.

Green, H. B., R. L. Horst, D. C. Beitz, and E. T. Littledike. 1981. Vitamin D metabolites in plasma of cows fed a prepartum low-calcium diet for prevention of parturient hypocalcemia. J. Dairy Sci. 64:217–226.

Greenfield, R., S. S. Donkin, M. J. Cecava, and T. R. Johnson. 1998. Protein requirements of transition dairy cows. J. Dairy Sci. (Midwest Section Abstr.):79.

Greenhalgh, J. F. D., and K. E. Gardner. 1958. Effects of heavy concentrate feeding before calving upon lactation and mammary gland edema. J. Dairy Sci. 41:822–829.

Greenough, P. R., and J. J. Vermunt. 1991. Evaluation of subclinical laminitis in a dairy herd and observations on associated nutritional and management factors. Vet. Rec. 128:11–17.

Greunert, E. 1980. Etiology of retained bovine placenta. In: Current Therapy in Theriogenology, D. A. Morrow (ed.). W. B. Saunders Co., Philadelphia, pp. 180–186.

Griinari, J. M., B. A. Corl, S. H. Lacy, P. Y. Chouinard, K. V. V. Nurmela, and D. E. Bauman. 2000. Conjugated linoleic acid is synthesized endogenously in lactating dairy cows by 9-desaturase. J. Nutr. 130:2285–2291.

Griinari, J. M., D. A. Dwyer, M. A. McGuire, D. E. Bauman, D. L. Palmquist, and K. V. V. Nurmela. 1998. Trans-octadecaenoic acids and milk fat depression in lactating dairy cows. J. Dairy Sci. 81:1251–1261.

Grohn, Y., L. A. Lindberg, M. L. Bruss, and T. B. Farver. 1983. Fatty infiltration of liver in spontaneously ketotic dairy cows. J. Dairy Sci. 66:2320–2328.

Grum, D. E., J. K. Drackley, R. S. Younker, D. W. LaCount, and J. J. Veenhuizen. 1996. Nutrition during the dry period and hepatic lipid metabolism of periparturient cows. J. Dairy Sci. 79:1850–1864.

Grummer, R. R. 1993. Etiology of lipid-related metabolic disorders in periparturient dairy cows. J. Dairy Sci. 76:3882–3896.

Grummer, R. R. 1995. Impact of changes in organic nutrient metabolism on feeding the transition dairy cow. J. Anim. Sci. 73:2820–2833.

Grummer, R. R., P. C. Hoffman, M. L. Luck, and S. J. Bertics. 1995. Effect of prepartum and postpartum dietary energy on growth and lactation of primiparous cows. J. Dairy Sci. 78:172–180.

Grummer, R. R., S. J. Bertics, D. W. LaCount, J. A. Snow, M. R. Dentine, and R. H. Stauffacher. 1990. Estrogen induction of fatty liver in dairy cattle. J. Dairy Sci. 73:1537–1543.

Gwazdanskas, F. C., T. L. Bibb, T. L. McGilliard, and J. A. Lineweaver. 1979. Effect of selenium -vitamin E injection on time for placenta to pass and on reproductive functions. J. Dairy Sci. 62:978–981.

Habel, R. E. 1981. Stomach. Pp. 230 in Applied Veterinary Anatomy, Robert E. Habel, Ithaca, NY.

Hallgren, W. 1955. Studies on parturient paresis in dairy cows. Nord. Vet. Med. 7:433–463.

Hamada, T., T. Ishii, and S. Taguchi. 1982. Blood changes of spontaneously ketotic cows before and four hours after administration of glucose, xylitol, 1,2-propanediol, or magnesium propionate. J. Dairy Sci. 65:1509–1513.

Harfoot, C. G., and G. P. Hazlewood. 1987. Lipid Metabolism in the rumen. Page 285 in The Rumen Microbial Ecosystem. P. N. Hobson Ed. Elsevier Science Publishers, LTD, Essex, England.

Harmon, D. L., R. A. Britton, and R. L. Prior. 1983. Influence of diet on glucose turnover and rates of gluconeogenesis, oxidation, and turnover of $D_{(-)}$ lactate in the bovine. J. Nutr. 113:1842–1850.

Harrison, J. H., and H. R. Conrad. 1984. Effect of dietary calcium on selenium absorption by the nonlactating dairy cow. J. Dairy Sci. 67:1860–1664.

Harrison, J. H., D. D. Hancock, and H. R. Conrad. 1984. Vitamin E and selenium for reproduction of the dairy cow. J. Dairy Sci. 67:123–132.

Hartnell, G. F., S. E. Franson, D. E. Bauman, H. H. Head, J. T. Huber, R. C. Lamb, K. S. Madsen, W. J. Cole, and R. L. Hintz. 1991. Evaluation of sometribove in a prolonged-release system in lactating dairy cows production responses. J. Dairy Sci. 74:2645–2663.

Hartwell, J. H., M. J. Cecava, B. Miller, and S. S. Donkin. 1999. Rumen protected choline and dietary protein for transition cows. J. Dairy Sci. 82(Suppl. 1):125. (Abstr.).

Hathaway, H. D., W. J. Brakel, W. J. Tyznik, and H. E. Kaeser. 1957. The effect of concentrate intake at calving time on physiological activities with special emphasis on ketosis. J. Dairy Sci. 40:616 (Abstr.).

Hayes, D. P., D. U. Pfeiffer, and N. B. Williamson. 1996. Effect of intraruminal monensin capsules on reproductive performance and milk production of dairy cows fed pasture. J. Dairy Sci. 79:1000–1008.

Hayirli, A., R. R. Grummer, E. Nordheim, P. Crump, D. K. Beede, M. J. VandeHaar, and L. H. Kilmer. 1998. A mathematical model for describing dry matter intake of transition cows. J. Dairy Sci. 81(Suppl. 1): 296 (Abstr.).

Hays, R. L., and J. L. Albright. 1966. Udder edema: Its incidence and severity as affected by certain management practices. Illinois Res. 8:6.

Heinrichs, A. J., and G. J. Bush. 1991. Evaluation of decoquinate or lasalocid against coccidiosis from natural exposure in neonatal dairy calves. J. Dairy Sci. 74:3223–3227.

Hemken, R. W., and J. H. Vandersall. 1967. Feasibility of an all silage forage program. J. Dairy Sci. 50:417–422.

Hemken, R. W., E. Gainer, and R. F. Davis. 1960. Effect of kind and level of concentrates on udder edema. J. Dairy Sci. 43:887-888.

Hemken, R. W., W. H. Choate, and R. D. Plowman. 1969. Salt and water intakes as related to udder edema. J. Anim. Sci. 28:874 (Abstr.).

Hernandez-Urdaneta, A., C. E. Coppock, R. E. McDowell, D. Gianola, and N. E. Smith. 1976. Changes in forage-concentrate ratio of complete feeds for dairy cows. J. Dairy Sci. 59:695–707.

Hibbs, J. W., and W. D. Pounden. 1955. Studies on milk fever in dairy cows. IV. Prevention by short-time, prepartum feeding of massive doses of vitamin D. J. Dairy Sci. 38:65–72.

Hicks, J. D., and J. V. Pauli. 1976. Chronic udder edema: Clinical aspects of the syndrome and its connection with hypomagnasemia and anemia. New Zealand Vet. J. 24:225–228.

Hidiroglou, M., A. J. McAllister, and C. J. Williams. 1987. Prepartum supplementation of selenium and vitamin E to dairy cows: Assessment of selenium status and reproductive performance. J. Dairy Sci. 70:1281–1288.

Hocquette, J. F., and D. Bauchart. 1999. Intestinal absorption, blood transport, and hepatic muscle metabolism of fatty acids in preruminant and ruminant animals. Reprod. Nutr. Dev. 39:27–48.

Horst, R. L., and J. P. Goff. 1997. Milk fever and dietary potassium. Pp. 181–189 in 1997 Cornell Nutrition Conference. Rochester, N.Y.: Cornell University.

Horst, R. L., J. P. Goff, and T. A. Reinhardt. 1990. Advancing age results in reduction of intestinal and bone 1,25-dihydroxyvitamin D receptor. Endocrinol. 126:1053–1057.

Horst, R. L., J. P. Goff, T. A. Reinhardt, and D. R. Buxton. 1997. Strategies for preventing milk fever in dairy cattle. J. Dairy Sci. 80:1269–1280.

House, W. A., and A. W. Bell. 1993. Mineral accretion in the fetus and adnexa during late gestation in Holstein cows. J. Dairy Sci. 76:2999–3010.

Hull, B. L., and W. M. Wass. 1973. Abomasal displacement. 2. Hypocalcemia as a contributing causative factor. Vet. Med. Small Anim. Clin. 68:412–417.

Huntington, G. B., and R. Britton. 1979. Effect of dietary lactic acid content and energy level on rumen lactate metabolism in sheep. J. Anim. Sci. 47:241–246.

Huyler, M. T., R. L. Kincaid, and D. F. Dostal. 1999. Metabolic and yield responses of multiparous Holstein cows to prepartum rumen-undegradable protein. J. Dairy Sci. 82:527–536.

Ilan, D., A. Bne-Asher, Z. Holzer, Z. Nitsan, I. Nir, and D. Levy. 1981. Effect of monensin supplementation on growth, feed digestibility and utilization in young calves. Anim. Prod. 32:125–131.

Ishak, M. A., L. L. Larson, F. G. Owen, S. R. Lowry, and E. D. Erickson. 1983. Effects of selenium, vitamins, and ration fiber on placental retention and performance of dairy cattle. J. Dairy Sci. 66:99–106.

Jardon, P. W. 1995. Using urine pH to monitor anionic salt programs. Compend. Contin. Educ. Pract. Vet. 17:860–862.

Johnson, D. G., and D. E. Otterby. 1981. Influence of dry period diet on early postpartum health, feed intake, milk production, and reproductive efficiency of Holstein cows. J. Dairy Sci. 64:290–295.

Johnson, J. C., F. R. Utley, B. G. Mullinix, Jr., and A. Merrill. 1988. Effects of adding fat and lasalocid to diets of dairy cows. J. Dairy Sci. 71:2151–2165.

Jones, T. O., R. Knight, and R. K. Evans. 1984. Chronic udder edema in milking cows and heifers. Vet. Record 115:218–219.

Jonsson, G., and B. Pehrson. 1970. Trials with prophylactic treatment of parturient paresis. Vet. Rec. 87:575–583.

Jordan, E. R., and R. H. Fourdraine. 1993. Characterization of the management practices of the top milk producing herds in the country. J. Dairy Sci. 76:3247–3256.

Julien, W. E., H. R. Conrad, and D. R. Redman. 1976a. Influence of dietary protein on susceptibility to alert downer syndrome. J. Dairy Sci. 60:210–215.

Julien, W. E., H. R. Conrad, J. E. Jones, and A. L. Moxon. 1976b. Selenium and vitamin E and incidence of retained placenta in parturient dairy cows. J. Dairy Sci. 59:1954–1959.

Julien, W. E., H. R. Conrad, J. E. Jones, and A. L. Moxon. 1976c. Selenium and vitamin E and incidence of retained placenta in parturient dairy cows. II. Prevention in commercial herds with prepartum treatment. J. Dairy Sci. 59:1960–1962.

Julien, W. E., H. R. Conrad, J. W. Hibbs, and W. L. Crist. 1977. Milk fever in dairy cows. VIII. Effect of injected vitamin $D_3$ and calcium and phosphorus intake on incidence. J. Dairy Sci. 60:431–436.

Kalscheur, K. F., B. B. Teter, L. S. Piperova, and R. A. Erdman. 1997a. Effect of dietary forage level and buffer addition on milk trans fatty acids and duodenal trans fatty acid flow in lactating dairy cows. J. Dairy Sci. 80:2104–2114.

Kalscheur, K. F., B. B. Teter, L. S. Piperova, and R. A. Erdman. 1997b. Effect of fat source on trans fatty acid flow and milk fat production in lactating dairy cows. J. Dairy Sci. 80:2115–2126.

Kappel, L. C., R. H. Ingraham, E. D. Morgan, J. M. Dixon, L. Zeringue, D. Wilson, and D. K. Babcock. 1984. Selenium concentrations in feeds and effect of treating pregnant cows with selenium and vitamin E on blood selenium values and reproductive performance. Am. J. Vet. Res. 45:691–694.

Katz, I., and M. Keeney. 1966. Characterization of the octadecaenoic acids in rumen digesta and rumen bacteria. J. Dairy Sci. 49:962.

Kennelly, J. J., and K. A. Lien. 1997. Effect of ionophore supplementation on milk components from lactating cows. Pp. 40-49 in Proceedings of a symposium: Usefulness of ionophores in lactating dairy cattle. Ontario Veterinary College. June 25–26, 1997.

Kilmer, L. H., L. D. Muller, and T. J. Snyder. 1981. Addition of sodium bicarbonate to rations of postpartum dairy cows: physiological and metabolic effects. J. Dairy Sci. 64:2357–2369.

Kirchgessner, M., W. Windisch, W. Schwab, and H. L. Muller. 1991. Energy metabolism of lactating dairy cows treated with prolonged-release bovine somatotropin or energy deficiency. J. Dairy Sci. 74(Suppl. 2):35–43.

Kleppe, B. B., R. J. Aiello, R. R. Grummer, and L. E. Armentano. 1988. Triglyceride accumulation and very low density lipoprotein secretion by rat and goat hepatocytes in vitro. J. Dairy Sci. 71:1813–1822.

Knowlton, K. F., M. S. Allen, and P. S. Erickson. 1996a. Lasalocid and particle size of corn grain for dairy cows in early lactation. 1. Effect on performance, serum metabolites, and nutrient digestibility. J. Dairy Sci. 79:557–564.

Knowlton, K. F., M. S. Allen, and P. S. Erickson. 1996b. Lasalocid and particle size of corn grain for dairy cows in early lactation. 2. Effect on ruminal measurements and feeding behavior. J. Dairy Sci. 79:566–574.

Kohn, R. A., and T. F. Dunlap. 1998. Calculation of the buffering capacity of bicarbonate in the rumen and in vitro. J. Anim. Sci. 76(6):1702–1709.

Kung, L., Jr., E. M. Kreck, R. S. Tung, A. O. Hession, A. C. Sheperd, M. A. Cohen, H. E. Swain and J. A. Z. Leedlet. 1997. Effects of a live yeast culture and enzymes on in vitro ruminal fermentation and milk production of dairy cows. J. Dairy Sci. 80:2045–2051.

Kunz, P. L., J. W. Blum, I. C. Hart, H. Bickel, and J. Landis. 1985. Effects of different energy intakes before and after calving on food intake, performance and blood hormones and metabolites in dairy cows. Anim. Prod. 40:219–231.

Laurent, F., B. Vignon, D. Coomans, J. Wilkinson, and A. Bonnel. 1992. Influence of bovine somatotropin on the composition and manufacturing properties of milk. J. Dairy Sci. 75:2226–2234.

Lean, I. J., M. Curtis, R. Dyson, and B. Lowe. 1994. Effects of sodium monensin on reproductive performance of dairy cattle. I. Effects of conception rates, calving-to-conception intervals, calving-to-heat and milk production in dairy cows. Aust. Vet. J. 71:273–277.

Lean, I. J., and L. Wade. 1997. Effects of monensin on metabolism, production, and health of dairy cattle. Pp. 50–70 in Proceedings of a symposium: Usefulness of ionophores in lactating dairy cattle. Ontario Veterinary College. June 25–26, 1997.

Leidl, W., D. Hegner, and P. Rockel. 1980. Investigations on the $PGF_2$ concentration in maternal and feotal cotyledons of cows with and without retained fetal membranes. Zbl. Vet. Med. A. 27:691–696.

Lema, M., W. B. Tucker, M. Aslam, I. S. Shin, P. Le Ruyet, and G. D. Adams. 1992. Influence of calcium chloride fed prepartum on severity of edema and lactational performance of dairy heifers. J. Dairy Sci. 75:2388–2393.

Linn, J. G. 1988. Factors affecting the composition of milk from dairy cows. Pp. 224–241 in Designing Foods: Animal Product Options in the Marketplace. Washington, D.C.: National Academy Press.

Littledike, E. T., and R. L. Horst. 1980. Problems with vitamin D injections for prevention of milk fever: Toxicity of large doses and increased incidence of small doses. J. Dairy Sci. 63(Suppl. 1):89.

Littledike, E. T., J. A. Stuedemann, S. R. Wilkinson, and R. L. Horst. 1983. Grass tetany syndrome. Pp. 173–195 in Role of Magnesium in Animal Nutrition, J. P. Fontenot, G. E. Bunce, K. E. Webb, V. G. Allen, eds. Blacksburg, VA: Virginia Polytechnic Inst. and State Univ.

Loor, J. J., and J. H. Herbein. 1998. Exogenous conjugated linoleic acid isomers reduce bovine milk fat concentration and yield by inhibiting de novo synthesis. J. Nutr. 128:2411–2419.

Lowe, L. B., G. J. Ball, V. R. Carruthers, R. C. Dobos, G. A. Lynch, P. J. Moate, P. R. Poolse, and S. C. Valentine. 1991. Monensin controlled-release intraruminal capsule for control of bloat in pastured dairy cows. Aust. Vet. J. 68:17–20.

Lynch, J. M., D. M. Barbano, D. E. Bauman, G. F. Hartnell, and M. A. Nemeth. 1992. Effects of prolonged-release formulation of N-methionyl bovine somatotropin (sometribove) on milk fat. J. Dairy Sci. 75:1794–1809.

Maas, J. P. 1982. Prevention of retained fetal membranes in dairy cattle. Compend. Contin. Educ. 4:S519–S527.

Mackintosh, E. D., R. H. Phipps, J. D. Sutton, and J. I. D. Wilkinson. 1997. The effects of monensin and diet composition on methane production using the *in vitro* semi-continuous rumen simulation technique (Rusitec). J. Dairy Sci. 80(Suppl. 1):208 (Abstr.).

Maclean, C. W. 1971. The histopathology of laminitis in dairy cows. J. Comp. Pathol. 81:563–570.

Malven, P. V., R. E. Erb, M. F. D'Amico, T. S. Stewart, and B. P. Chew. 1983. Factors associated with edema of the mammary gland in primigravid dairy heifers. J. Dairy Sci. 66:246–252.

Manson, F. J., and J. D. Leaver. 1988. The influence of concentrate amount on locomotion and clinical lameness in dairy cattle. Anim. Prod. 47:185–190.

Massey, C. D., C. Wang, G. A. Donovan, and D. K. Beede. 1993. Hypocalcemia at parturition as a risk factor for left displacement of the abomasum in dairy cows. J. Am. Vet. Med. Assoc. 203:852–853.

McBride, B. W., J. L. Burton, and J.H. Burton. 1988. The influence of bovine growth hormone (somatotropin) on animals and their products. Res. Dev. Agric. 5:1–21.

McClymont, G. L., and S. Valence. 1962. Depression in blood glycerides and milk fat synthesis by glucose infusion. Proc. Nutr. Soc. 21:xli.

McDonald, R. J., G. W. McKay, and J. D. Thompson. 1961. The use of organic iodine in the treatment of repeat breeder cows. Proc. 4th Int. Congr. Anim. Reprod. 3:679–681.

McGilliard, M. L., and C. C. Stallings. 1998. Increase in milk yield of commercial dairy herds fed a microbial and enzyme supplement. J. Dairy Sci. 81:1353–1375.

McGuffey, R. K., and J. I. D. Wilkinson. 1991. Nutritional implications of bovine somatotropin for the lactating dairy cow. J. Dairy Sci. 74(Suppl. 2):63–71.

McGuire, M. A., J. M. Griinari, D. A. Dywer, and D. E. Bauman. 1995. Role of insulin in the regulation of mammary synthesis of fat and protein. J. Dairy Sci. 78:816–824.

McMeniman, N. P., and R. Elliot. 1995. Control of coccidia in young calves using lasalocid. Aust. Vet. J. 72:7–9

Meinert, R. A., C. M. J. Yang, A. J. Heinrichs, and G. A. Varga. 1992. Effect of monensin on growth, reproductive performance, and estimated body composition in Holstein heifers. J. Dairy Sci. 75:257–261.

Mellenberger, R. W., D. E. Bauman, and D. E. Nelson. 1973. Fatty acid and lactose synthesis in cow mammary tissue. Biochem J. 136:741–748.

Merchen, N. R. 1988. Digestion, absorption and excretion in ruminants. In The Ruminant Animal: Digestive Physiology and Nutrition, D. C. Church editor, Waveland Press, Prospect Heights, IL. pp. 176–177.

Mertens, D. R. 1997. Creating a system for meeting the fiber requirements of dairy cows. J. Dairy Sci. 80:1463–1481.

Michal, J. J., B. P. Chew, T. S. Wong, L. R. Heirman, and F. E. Sandaert. 1990. Effects of supplemental β-carotene on blood and mammary phagocyte function in peripartum dairy cows. J. Dairy Sci. 73(Suppl. 1): 149.(Abstr.).

Midla, L. T., K. H. Hoblet, W. P. Weiss, and M. L. Moeschberger. 1998. Supplemental dietary biotin for prevention of lesions associated with aseptic subclinical laminitis (pododermatitis aseptica diffusa) in primiparous cows. Am. J. Vet. Res. 59:733–738.

Miller, J. K., E. Brzezinska-Slebodzinska, and F. C. Madsen. 1993. Oxidative stress, antioxidants, and animal function. J. Dairy Sci. 76:2812–2823.

Minor, D. J., S. L. Trower, B. D. Strang, R. D. Shaver, and R. R. Grummer. 1998. Effects of nonfiber carbohydrate and niacin on periparturient metabolic status and lactation of dairy cows. J. Dairy Sci. 81:189–200.

Miranda, R. L. A., M.G. D. Mendoza, J. R. Barcena-Gama, M. S. S. Gonzalez, R. Ferrara, C. M. E. Ortega, and P.M. A. Cobos. 1996. Effect of *Saccharomyces cerevisiae* or *Aspergillus oryzae* cultures and NDF level on parameters of ruminal fermentation. Anim. Feed Sci. Tech. 63:289–296.

Moberg, R. 1959. Possible influences of iodine deficiency in reproductive performance in cattle with special reference to retained placenta. Proc. 3rd World Congress on Fertility and Sterility, Amsterdam.

Moberg, R. 1961. Possible influences of supplementary iodine, administered by evaporation, on reproductive performances in cattle. Proc. 4th Int. Congr. Anim. Reprod. 3:682–685.

Mongin, P. 1981. Recent advances in dietary anion-cation balance: Applications in poultry. Proc. Nutr. Soc. 40:285–295.

Moorby, J. M., R. J. Dewhrst, and S. Marsden. 1996. Effect of increasing digestible undegraded protein supply to dairy cows in late gestation on the yield and composition of milk during the subsequent lactation. Anim. Sci. 63:201–213.

Morrow, D. A. 1976. Fat cow syndrome. J. Dairy Sci. 59:1625–1629.

Moshen, M. K., F. El-Keraby, and M. S. El-Safty. 1981. Effect of monensin on milk yield, milk composition and reproductive performance of Friesian cows. Agric. Res. Rev. 59:15–27.

Mueller, F. J., J. K. Miller, M. H. Campbell, and F. C. Madsen. 1998. Prevention of udder edema in dairy cows. Proc. Tri-State Dairy Nutr. Conf. pp. 79–95, Fort Wayne, IN.

Mueller, F. J., J. K. Miller, N. Ramsey, R. C. DeLost, and F. C. Madsen. 1989a. Reduced udder edema in heifers fed vitamin E prepartum. J. Dairy Sci. 72:2211 (Abstr.).

Mueller, F. J., J. K. Miller, N. Ramsey, R. C. Delost, and F. C. Madsen. 1989b. Effects of vitamin E and excess iron on placental retention and subsequent milk yield in dairy cows. J. Dairy Sci. 72(Suppl. 1):564 (Abstr.).

Mueller, F. J., J. K. Miller, N. Ramsey, R. C. Delost, F. C. Madsen, and T. D. Mayers. 1988. Effects of vitamin E and excess iron on placental retention in dairy cows. J. Dairy Sci. 71(Suppl. 1):157 (Abstr.).

Muller, L. D. 1979. Buffers in rations for dairy calves and pre- and postpartum dairy cows. Pp. 125–156 in Regulation of Acid-Base Balance, W. H. Hale and P. Meinhardt, eds. Church and Dwight, Co. Inc.

Muller, L. D. 1992. BST and dairy cow performance. Pp. 53–72 in Bovine Somatotropin and Emerging Issues—An Assessment. M.C. Halberg, ed. Westview Press, Boulder, CO.

Nagaraja, T. G., T. B. Avery, E. E. Bartley, S. J. Galitzer, and A. D. Dayton. 1981. Prevention of lactic acidosis in cattle by lasalocid or monensin. J. Anim. Sci. 53:206–215.

National Research Council. 1989. Nutrient requirements of dairy cattle, sixth revised ed. Washington, D.C.: National Academy Press.

National Research Council. 1994. Metabolic modifiers: Effects on the nutrient requirements of food-producing animals. Washington, D.C.: National Academy Press.

National Research Council. 1996. Nutrient Requirements of Beef Cattle, Seventh Revised Ed. Washington, D.C.: National Academy Press.

Nestor, K. E., Jr., R. W. Hemken, and R. J. Harmon. 1988. Influence of sodium chloride and potassium bicarbonate on udder edema and selected blood parameters. J. Dairy Sci. 71:366–372.

Newbold, C. J., R. J. Wallace and F. M. McIntosh. 1996. Mode of action of the yeast *Saccharomyces cerevisiae* as a feed additive for ruminants. Brit. J. Nutr. 76:249–261.

Nicholson, J. W. G., and H. M. Cunningham. 1965. Retained placenta, abortion, and abnormal calves from beef cows fed all barley rations. Can. Vet. J. 6:275–281.

Nocek, J. E. 1997. Bovine acidosis: Implications on laminitis. J. Dairy Sci. 80:1005–1028.

Noorsdsy, J. L., H. W. Leipold, D. L. Carmahan, R. A. Frey, J. Vestweber, M. G. Robl, G. Kennedy, J. R. Dunham, T. E. Chapin, and W. E. Moore. 1973. Metabolic disturbances in the dairy cow influenced by managerial practices: Case reports and epidemiological studies. Rumen Function Conf., Chicago, IL.

Oetzel G. R. 1996. Effect of calcium chloride gel treatment in dairy cows on incidence of periparturient diseases. J Am Vet Med. Assoc. 209:958–961.

Oetzel, G. R. 1993. Effects of prophylactic treatment with a calcium chloride gel on serum calcium concentration at calving, milk fever, and displaced abomasum in Holstein cows. J. Dairy Sci. 76(Suppl 1): 304 (Abstr.).

Oetzel, G. R., and J. P. Goff. 1998. Milk fever (parturient paresis) in cows, ewes, and doe goats. Pp. 215–218 in Current Veterinary Therapy 4: Food Animal Practice, J. L. Howard and R. A. Smith, eds. Philadelphia: W. B. Saunders Co.

Oetzel, G. R., J. D. Olson, C. R. Curtis, and M. J. Fettman. 1988. Ammonium chloride and ammonium sulfate for prevention of parturient paresis in dairy cows. J. Dairy Sci. 71:3302–3309.

Oetzel, G. R., M. J. Fettman, D. W. Hamar, and J. D. Olson. 1991. Screening of anionic salts for palatability, effects on acid-base status and urinary calcium excretion in dairy cows. J. Dairy Sci. 74:965–971.

Oetzel, G. R., K. V. Nordlund, and E. F. Garrett. 1999. Effect of ruminal pH and stage of lactation on ruminal lactate concentrations in dairy cows J. Dairy Sci. 82(Suppl. 1):38.

Peel, C. J., and D. E. Bauman. 1987. Somatotropin and lactation. J. Dairy Sci. 70:474–486.

Peel, C. J., D. L. Hard, K. S. Madsen, and G. de Kerchove. 1989. Bovine somatotropin: Mechanism of action and experimental results from different world areas. Pp. 9–18 in Meeting the Challenges of New Technology. Proceedings of the Monsanto Technical Symposium, Animal Science Division, St. Louis, MO: Monsanto Agricultural Company.

Pelissier, C. L. 1976. Dairy cattle breeding problems and their consequences. Theriogenology 6:575–583.

Petersen, W. E. 1932. The effects of cod liver oil in the ration upon the quantity and quality of cow's milk. J. Dairy Sci. 15:283.

Phillippo, M., G. W. Reid, and I. M. Nevison. 1994. Parturient hypocalcaemia in dairy cows: Effects of dietary acidity on plasma minerals and calciotrophic hormones. Res. Vet. Sci. 56:303–309.

Phipps, R. H., B. A. Jones, J. I. D. Wilkinson, and M. E. Tarrant. 1995. Effect of monensin on milk production of Friesian dairy cows in the United Kingdom. J. Dairy Sci. 78(Suppl. 1):268 (Abstr.).

Phipps, R. H., B. A. Jones, J. I. D. Wilkinson, and M. E. Tarrant. 1997a. The influence of monensin on milk production of Friesian dairy cows in the United Kingdom. J. Dairy Sci. 80(Suppl. 1):208 (Abstr.).

Phipps, R. H., J. I. D. Wilkinson, A. K. Jones, L. J. Jonker, M. Tarrant, E. D. Mackintosh, and A. M. Cocker. 1997b. A study over two lactations: The effect of monensin on milk production, health, and reproduction in lactating dairy cows. Pp. 26–39 in Proceedings of a symposium: Usefulness of ionophores in lactating dairy cattle. Ontario Veterinary College. June 25–26, 1997.

Piperova, L. S., B. B. Teter, I. Bruckental, J. Sampagna, S. E. Mills, M. P. Yurawecz, J. Fritsche, K. Ku, and R. A. Erdman. 2000. Mammary lipogenic enzyme activity, trans fatty acids and conjugated linoleic acid isomers during milk fat depression in lactating dairy cows. J. Nutr. 130:2568–2574.

Powell, E. B. 1939. Some relations of the roughage intake to composition of milk. J. Dairy Sci. 22:452.

Pullen, D. L., J. S. Liesman, and R. S. Emery. 1990. A species comparison of liver slice synthesis and secretion of triacylglycerol from nonesterified fatty acid in the media. J. Anim. Sci. 68:1395–1399.

Putnam, D. E., and G. A. Varga. 1998. Protein density and its influence on metabolite concentration and nitrogen retention by Holstein cows in late gestation. J. Dairy Sci. 81:1608–1618.

Putnam, D. E., C. G. Schwab, M. T. Socha, N. L. Whitehouse, N. A. Kierstead, and B. D. Garthwaite. 1997. Effect of yeast culture in the diets of early lactation dairy cows on ruminal fermentation and passage of nitrogen fractions and amino acids to the small intestine. J. Dairy Sci. 80:374–384.

Putnam, D. E., G. A. Varga, and H. M. Dann. 1999. Metabolic and production responses to dietary protein and exogenous somatotropin in late gestation dairy cows. J. Dairy Sci. 82:982–995.

Quigley III, J. D., J. J. Drewry, L. M. Murray, and S. J. Ivey. 1997. Effects of lasalocid in milk replacer or calf starter on health and performance of calves challenged with *eimeria* species. J. Dairy Sci. 80:2972–2976.

Radostits, O. M., D. C. Blood, and C. C. Gay. 1994. Page 1618 *in* Veterinary Medicine. Bailliere Tindall, Philadelphia, PA.

Ramanzin, M., L. Bailoni, S. Schiavon, and G. Bittante. 1997. Effect of monensin on milk production and efficiency of dairy cows fed two diets differing in forage to concentrate ratios. J. Dairy Sci. 80:1136–1142.

Randall, W. E., R. W. Hemken, L. S. Bull, and L. W. Douglas. 1974. Effect of dietary sodium and potassium on udder edema in Holstein heifers. J. Dairy Sci. 57:472–475.

Roberts, S. J. 1961. Page 225 *in* Veterinary obstetrics and genital diseases. Edwards Bros., Ann Arbor, MI.

Robinson, P. H. 1997. Effect of yeast culture (*Saccharomyces cerevisiae*) on adaptation of cows to diets postpartum. J. Dairy Sci. 80:1119–1125.

Rogers, J. A., L. D. Muller, C. L. Davis, W. Chalupa, D. S. Kronfeld, L. F. Karcher, and K. R. Cummings. 1985. Response of dairy cows to sodium bicarbonate and limestone in early lactation. J. Dairy Sci. 68:646–660.

Rogers, J. A., L. D. Muller, T. J. Snyder, and T. L. Maddox. 1985. Milk production, nutrient digestion, and rate of digesta passage in dairy cows fed long or chopped alfalfa hay supplemented with sodium bicarbonate. J. Dairy Sci. 68:868–880.

Romo, G. A., D. P. Casper, R. A. Erdman, and B. B. Teter. 1996. Abomasal infusion of cis or trans fatty acid isomers and energy metabolism of lactating dairy cows. J. Dairy Sci. 79:2005–2015.

Ronning, M., E. R. Berousek, A. H. Kuhman, and W. D. Gallap. 1953. The carotene requirements for reproduction in Guernsey cattle. J. Dairy Sci. 36:52–56.

Rude, R. K., J. S. Adams, E. Ryzen, D. B. Endres, H. Niimi, R. L. Horst, J. G. Haddad, Jr., and F. R. Singer. 1985. Low serum concentrations of 1,25-dihydroxyvitamin D in human magnesium deficiency. J. Clin. Endo. Met. 61:933–940.

Rude, R. K., S. B. Oldham, C. F. Sharp, Jr., and F. R. Singer. 1978. Parathyroid hormone secretion in magnesium deficiency. J. Clin. Endocrin. Metab. 47:800–806.

Russell, J. B., and J. M. Chow. 1993. Another theory for the action of ruminal buffer salts: Decreased starch fermentation and propionate production. J. Dairy Sci. 76:826–830.

Sahlu, T., S. P. Hart, T. Le-Trong, Z. Jia, L. Dawson, T. Gipson, and T. H. Teh. 1995. Influence of prepartum protein and energy concentrations for dairy goats during pregnancy and early lactation. J. Dairy Sci. 78:378–387.

Sanders, D. E., and J. A. Sanders. 1981. Chronic udder edema in dairy cows. J. Am. Vet. Med. Assoc. 178:1273–1274.

Sansom, B. F., R. Manston, and M. J. Vagg. 1983. Magnesium and milk fever. Vet. Rec. 112:447–449.

Santos, J. E. P., E. J. DePeters, P. W. Jaron, and J. T. Huber. 1999a. Effect of prepartum crude protein level on performance of multiparous Holstein cows. J. Dairy Sci. 82(Suppl.1):120 (Abstr.).

Santos, J. E. P., E. J. DePeters, P. W. Jaron, and J. T. Huber. 1999b. Effect of prepartum crude protein level on performance of primiparous Holstein cows. J. Dairy Sci. 82(Suppl.1):120 (Abstr.).

Satter, L. D., and L. L. Slyter. 1974. Effect of ammonia concentration on rumen microbial protein production in vitro. Brit. J. Nutr. 32:199–208.

Sauer, F. D., J. D. Erfle, and L. J. Fisher. 1973. Propylene glycol and glycerol as a feed additive for lactating dairy cows: An evaluation of blood metabolite parameters. Can. J. Anim. Sci. 53:265–271.

Sauer, F. D., J. K. G. Kramer, and W. J. Cantwell. 1989. Antiketogenic effects of monensin in early lactation. J. Dairy Sci. 72:436–442.

Schelling, G. T. 1984. Monensin mode of action in the rumen. J. Anim. Sci. 58:1518–1527.

Schingoethe, D. J., C. A. Kirkbride, I. S. Palmer, M. J. Owens, and W. L. Tucker. 1982. Response of cows consuming adequate selenium to vitamin E and selenium supplementation prepartum. J. Dairy Sci. 65:2338–2344.

Schmidt, G. H., and L. H. Schultz. 1959. Effect of three levels of grain feeding during the dry period on the incidence of ketosis, severity of udder edema, and subsequent milk production of dairy cows. J. Dairy Sci. 42:170–179.

Schultz, L. H. 1958. Use of sodium propionate in the prevention of ketosis in dairy cattle. J. Dairy Sci. 41:160.

Sechen, S. J., D. E. Bauman, H. F. Tyrrell, and P. J. Reynolds. 1989. Effect of somatotropin on kinetics of nonesterified fatty acids and partition of energy, carbon, and nitrogen in lactating dairy cows. J. Dairy Sci. 72:59–67.

Segerson, E. C., G. J. Riviere, H. L. Dalton, and M. D. Whitacre. 1981. Retained placenta of Holstein cows treated with selenium and vitamin E. J. Dairy Sci. 64:1833–1836.

Shaver, R. D. 1997. Nutritional risk factors in the etiology of left displaced abomasum in dairy cows: A review. J. Dairy Sci. 80:2449–2453.

Shaw, J. C., and W. L. Ensor. 1959. Effect of feeding cod liver oil and unsaturated fatty acids on ruminal volatile fatty acids and milk fat content. J. Dairy Sci. 42:1238.

Skaar, T. C., R. R. Grummer, M. R. Dentine, and R. H. Stauffacher. 1989. Seasonal effects of pre- and postpartum fat and niacin feeding on lactation performance and lipid metabolism. J. Dairy Sci. 72:2028–2038.

Snyder, D. L., R. K. McGuffey, L. C. Pendlum, and E. L. Potter. 1981. Growth and reproduction of Holstein heifers fed monensin. J. Dairy Sci. 64(Suppl. 1):127 (Abstr.).

Solorzano, L. D., L. E. Armentano, R. S. Emery, and B. R. Schricker. 1989. Effects of Rumen-Mate on lactational performance of Holsteins fed a high grain diet. J. Dairy Sci. 72:1831–1841.

Staples, C. R., S. M. Emanuele, M. Ventura, D. K. Beede, and B. Schricker. 1986. Effects of a new multielement buffer on production, ruminal environment and blood minerals of lactating dairy cows. J. Dairy Sci. 71:1573–1586.

Steen, T. M., J. D. Quigley III, R. N. Heitman, and J. D. Gresham. 1992. Effects of lasalocid and undegradable protein on growth and body composition of Holstein heifers. J. Dairy Sci. 75:2517–2523.

Stewart, P. A. 1983. Modern quantitative acid-base chemistry. Can. J. Physiol. Pharmacol. 61:1444–1461.

Storry, J. E., and J. A. F. Rook. 1965. The effects of a diet low in hay and high in flaked maize on milk-fat secretion and on the concentrations of certain constituents in the blood plasma of the cow. Brit. J. Nutr. 19:101.

Stowe, H. D., J. W. Thomas, T. Johnson, J. V. Marateniuk, D. A. Morrow, and D. E. Ullrey. 1988. Responses of dairy cattle to long-term and short-term supplementation with oral selenium and vitamin E. J. Dairy Sci. 71:1830–1839.

Strang, B. D., S. J. Bertics, R. R. Grummer, and L. E. Armenatno. 1998. Effect of long-chain fatty acids on triglyceride accumulation, gluconeogenesis, and ureagenesis in bovine hepatocytes. J. Dairy Sci. 81:728–739.

Studer, V. A., R. R. Grummer, and S. J. Bertics. 1993. Effect of prepartum propylene glycol administration on periparturient fatty liver in dairy cows. J. Dairy Sci. 76:2931–2939.

Sutton, J. D. 1989. Altering milk composition by feeding. J. Dairy Sci. 72:2801–2814.

Swanson, E. W., and J. I. Poffenbarger. 1979. Mammary gland development of dairy heifers during their first gestation. J. Dairy Sci. 62:702–714.

Symanowski, J. T., H. B. Green, J. R. Wagner, J. I. D. Wilkinson, J. S. Davis, M. R. Himstedt, M. S. Allen, E. Block, J. J. Brennen, H. H. Head, J. J. Kennelly, J. N. Nielsen, J. E. Nocek, J. J. Vand Der List, and L. W. Whitlow. 1999. Milk production and efficiency of cows fed monensin. J. Dairy Sci. 82(Suppl. 1):75 (Abstr.).

Teter, B. B., J. Sampugna, and M. Keeney. 1990. Milk fat depression in C57B1/6J mice consuming partially hydrogenated fat. J. Nutr. 120:818.

Thomas, D. G., J. K. Miller, F. J. Mueller, C. R. Holmes, and F. C. Madsen. 1990. Daily supplementation of dairy cows with 1,000 IU vitamin E for 6 weeks before calving reduced placental retention by almost 60 percent. J. Dairy Sci. 73(Suppl. 1):166 (Abstr.).

Thomas, E. D. 1999. A new look at managing potassium levels in grasses. Hoard's Dairyman. Jan. 29th:53.

Thomas, J. W., R. S. Emery, J. K. Breaux, and J. S. Liesman. 1984. Response of milking cows fed a high concentrate, low roughage diet plus sodium bicarbonate, magnesium oxide, or magnesium hydroxide. J. Dairy Sci. 67:2532–2545.

Trinder, N., C. D. Woodhouse, and C. P. Renton. 1969. The effect of vitamin E and selenium on the incidence of retained placentae in dairy cows. Vet. Rec. 85:550–553.

Trinder, N., R. J. Hall, and C. P. Renton. 1973. The relationship between the intake of selenium and vitamin E on the incidence of retained placentae in dairy cows. Vet. Rec. 93:641–643.

Tucker, W. B., I. S. Shin, J. F. Hougue, G. D. Aslam, M. T. Van Koevering, R. K. Vernon, and K. R. Cummings. 1994. Natural sodium sesquicarbonate fed for an entire lactation: Influence on performance and acid-base status of dairy cows. J. Dairy Sci. 77:3111–3117.

Tucker, W. B., J. F. Hogue, D. F. Waterman, T. S. Swenson, Z. Xin, R. W. Hemken, J. A. Jackson, G. D. Adams, and L. J. Spicer. 1991. Role of sulfur and chloride in the dietary cation-anion balance equation for lactating dairy cattle. J. Anim. Sci. 69:1205–1213.

Tucker, W. B., J. F. Hogue, G. D. Adams, M. Aslam, I. S. Shin, and G. Morgan. 1992. Influence of dietary cation-anion balance during the dry period on the occurrence of parturient paresis in cows fed excess calcium. J. Anim. Sci. 70:1238–1250.

Tyrrell, H. F., A. C. G. Brown, P. J. Reynolds, G. L. Haaland, D. E. Bauman, C. J. Peel, and W. D. Steinhour. 1988. Effect of bovine somatotropin on metabolism of lactating dairy cows: Energy and nitrogen utilization as determined by respiration calorimetry. J. Nutr. 118:1024–1030.

Tyznick W., and N. N. Allen. 1951. The relation of roughage intake to the fat content of the milk and the level of fatty acids in the rumen. J. Dairy Sci. 34:493.

U.S. Department of Agriculture, Animal and Plant Health Inspection Service. 1996. Part I: Reference of 1996 Dairy Management Practices. Fort Collins, CO: Centers for Epidemiology and Animal Health.

Van de Braak, A. E., A. T. van't Klooster, and A. Malestein. 1987. Influence of a deficient supply of magnesium during the dry period on the rate of calcium mobilisation by dairy cows at parturition. Res. Vet. Sci. 42:101–108.

Van den Berg, G. 1991. A review of quality and processing suitability of milk from cows treated with bovine somatotropin. J. Dairy Sci. 74(Suppl. 2):2–11.

Van Der Werf, J. H. J., L. J. Jonker, and J. K. Oldenbroek. 1998. Effect of monensin on milk production by Jersey cows. J. Dairy Sci. 81:427–433.

Van Maanen, R. W., J. H. Herbein, A. D. McGilliard, and J. W. Young. 1978. Effects of monensin on in vivo rumen propionate production and blood glucose kinetics in cattle. J. Nutr. 108:1002–1007.

Van Soest. P. J. 1994. pp. 334–336 In Nutritional Ecology of the Ruminant. Cornell University Press, Ithaca, New York.

VandeHaar, M. J., and S. S. Donkin. 1999. Protein nutrition of dry cows. Proc. Tri-State Dairy Nutr. Conf., M. L. Eastridge, ed. April 20, Ft. Wayne, IN, pages 113–130. The Ohio State University, Columbus.

VandeHaar, M. J., G. Yousif, B. K. Sharma, T. H. Herdt, R. S. Emery, M. S. Allen, and J. S. Liesman. 1999. Energy and protein density of prepartum diets alters fat and protein metabolism of dairy cows in the periparturient period. J. Dairy Sci. 82:1282–1295.

VanSaun, R. J., and C. J. Sniffen. 1995. Effects of undegradable protein fed prepartum on lactation, reproduction, and health in dairy cattle. J. Dairy Sci. 78:265 (Abstr.).

VanSaun, R. J., S. C. Idleman, and C. J. Sniffen. 1993. Effect of undegradable protein amount fed prepartum on postpartum production in first lactation Holstein cows. J. Dairy Sci. 76:236–244.

Vazquez-Anon, M., S. Bertics, M. Luck, R. R. Grummer, and J. Pinheiro. 1994. Peripartum liver triglyceride and plasma metabolites in dairy cows. J. Dairy Sci. 77:1521–1528.

Veenhuizen, J. J., J. K. Drackley, M. J. Richard, T. P. Sanderson, L. D. Miller, and J. W. Young. 1991. Metabolic changes in blood and liver during development and the early treatment of experimental fatty liver and ketosis in cows. J. Dairy Sci. 74:4238–4253.

Vermunt, J. J., and P. R. Greenough. 1994. Predisposing factors of laminitis in cattle. Brit. Vet. J. 150:151–164.

Vestweber, J. G. E., and F. K. Al-Ani. 1983. Udder edema in cattle. Compendium Continuing Education Practicing Vet. 5:S5–S12.

Vestweber, J. G. E., and F. K. Al-Ani. 1984. Udder edema: Biochemical studies in Holstein cows. Cornell Vet. 74:366–372.

Vicini, J. L., W. S. Cohick, J. H. Clark, S. N. McCutcheon, and D. E. Bauman. 1988. Effects of feed intake and sodium bicarbonate on milk production and concentration of hormones and metabolites in plasma of cows. J. Dairy Sci. 71:1232–1238.

Vigue, R. F. 1963. Management of udder edema in cattle. Can. Vet. J. 4:236–241.

Wagner, J. R., H. B. Green, J. T. Symanowski, J. I. D. Wilkinson, J. S. Davis, M. R. Himstedt, M. S. Allen, E. Block, J. J. Brennen, H. H. Head, J. J. Kennelly, J. N. Nielsen, J. E. Nocek, J. J. Vand Der List, and L. W. Whitlow. 1999. Effect of monensin on feed intake, body weight, and body condition in dairy cows. J. Dairy Sci. 82(Suppl. 1): 75 (Abstr.).

Weaver, L. D. 1987. Effects of nutrition on reproduction in dairy cows. Vet. Clin. North Am. [Food Anim. Pract.] 3:513–531.

Weiss, W. P., and B. A. Amiet. 1990. Effect of lasalocid on performance of lactating dairy cows. J. Dairy Sci. 73:153–162.

Weiss, W. P., J. S. Hogan, K. L. Smith, and K. H. Hoblet. 1990. Relationships among selenium, vitamin E and mammary gland health in commercial diary herds. J. Dairy Sci. 73:381–390.

West, J. W., C. E. Coppock, D. H. Nave, J. M. Labore, and L. W. Greene. 1987. Effects of potassium carbonate and sodium bicarbonate on rumen function in lactating Holstein cows. J. Dairy Sci. 70:81–90.

Williams, P. E. V., C. A. G. Tait, G. M. Innes, and C. J. Newbold. 1991. Effects of the inclusion of yeast culture (*Saccharomyces cerevisiae* plus growth medium) in the diet of dairy cows on milk yield and forage degradation and fermentation patterns in the rumen of steers. J. Anim. Sci. 69:3016–3026.

Wise, G. H., F. W. Atkeson, M. J. Caldwell, and J. S. Hughes. 1946. Effect of level of protein in the prepartum ration of dairy heifers and cows on the degree of mammary edema. J. Anim. Sci. 5:397 (Abstr.).

Wohlt, J. E., T. T. Corcione, and P.K. Zajac. 1998. Effect of yeast on feed intake and performance of cows fed diets based on corn silage during early lactation. J. Dairy Sci. 81:1345–1352.

Wonsil, B. J., J. H. Herbein, and B. A. Watkins. 1994. Dietary and ruminally derived trans-18:1 fatty acids alter bovine milk lipids. J. Nutr. 124:556–565.

Wu, Z., R. J. Fisher, C. E. Polan, and C. G. Schwab. 1997. Lactational performance of cows fed low or high ruminally undegradable protein prepartum and supplemental methionine and lysine postpartum. J. Dairy Sci. 80:722–729.

Xin, Z., W. B. Tucker, and R. W. Hemken. 1989. Effect of reactivity rate and particle size of magnesium oxide on magnesium availability, acid-base balance, mineral metabolism, and milking performance of dairy cows. J. Dairy Sci. 72:462–470.

Xu, S., J. H. Harrison, R. E. Riley, and K. A. Loney. 1994. Effect of buffer addition to high grain total mixed rations on rumen pH, feed intake, milk production, and milk composition. J. Dairy Sci. 77:782–788.

Yokoyama, M. T., and K. A. Johnson. 1988. Microbiology of the rumen and intestine. Page 125 *in* The Ruminant Animal: Digestive Physiology and Nutrition. D. C. Church, ed. Waveland Press, Inc., Prospect Heights, IL.

Yoon, I. K., and M. D. Stern. 1995. Influence of direct-fed microbials on ruminal microbial fermentation and performance of ruminants: A review. Austral. Asian J. Anim. Sci. 8:533–555.

Yoon, I. K., and M. D. Stern. 1996. Effects of *Saccharomyces cerevisiae* and *Aspergillus oryzae* cultures on ruminal fermentation in dairy cows. J. Dairy Sci. 79:411–417.

Yurawecz, M. P., J. A. G. Roach, N. Sehat, M. M. Mossoba, J. K. G. Kramer, J. Fritsche, H. Steinhart, and K. Ku. 1998. A new conjugated linoleic acid isomer, 7 trans, 9 cis-octadecadienoic acid, in cow milk, cheese, beef and human milk and adipose tissues. Lipids 33:803–809.

Zamet, C. N., V. F. Colenbrander, C. J. Callahan, B. P. Chew, R. E. Erb, and N. J. Moeller. 1979a. Variables associated with peripartum traits in dairy cows. I. Effect of dietary forages and disorders on voluntary intake of feed, body weight and milk yield. Theriogenology 11:229–244.

Zamet, C. N., V. F. Colenbrander, R. E. Erb, C. J. Callahan, B. P. Chew, and N. J. Moeller. 1979b. Variables associated with peripartum traits in dairy cows. II. Interrelationships among -disorders and their effects on intake of feed and on reproductive efficiency. Theriogenology 11:245–260.

# 10 Nutrient Requirements of the Young Calf

From birth until weaning to dry feed, the calf undergoes tremendous physiologic and metabolic changes (Toullec and Guilloteau, 1989). During the preruminant stage, digestion and metabolism are similar to those of nonruminant animals in many respects. Thus, dietary requirements are best met with high-quality liquid diets formulated from sources of carbohydrates, proteins, and fats that are digested efficiently. The most critical period is the first 2-3 wk of life, during which time the calf's digestive system is immature but developing rapidly with regard to digestive secretions and enzymatic activity (Toullec and Guilloteau, 1989; Davis and Drackley, 1998).

Calves raised for purposes other than veal production should be encouraged to consume dry feed at an early age to stimulate development of a functional rumen. Development of the ruminal epithelial tissue that is responsible for absorption of volatile fatty acids (VFA) depends on the presence of the VFA, particularly butyrate (Sander et al., 1959). The chemical composition and physical form of the starter feed are important characteristics (Warner, 1991). The starter should be relatively high in readily fermentable carbohydrates but adequate in digestible fiber to support the fermentation necessary for proper ruminal tissue growth (Brownlee, 1956; Flatt et al., 1958; Williams and Frost, 1992; Greenwood et al., 1997). The rumen and its microbial population are immature at this stage (Anderson et al., 1987a,b) and ruminal cellulose digestibility is limited (Williams and Frost, 1992). Consequently, long hay is not as effective as concentrates in developing a functional rumen and limits metabolizable energy intake in young calves (Stobo et al., 1966). Long hay should not be fed to calves until after weaning (Quigley, 1996a; Davis and Drackley, 1998). Nevertheless, adequate particle size of starter feed—whether pelleted, ground, or texturized—is important to prevent abnormal development and keratinization of ruminal papillae and to prevent impaction of fine particles between papillae (McGavin and Morrill, 1976; Greenwood et al., 1997; Beharka et al., 1998).

With respect to the nutrient requirements of the calf, three phases of development related to digestive function are recognized (Davis and Clark, 1981):

- Liquid-feeding phase. All or essentially all the nutrient requirements are met by milk or milk replacer. The quality of these feeds is preserved by a functional esophageal groove, which shunts liquid feeds directly to the abomasum and so avoids microbial breakdown in the reticulo-rumen (Orskov, 1972).
- Transition phase. Liquid diet and starter both contribute to meeting the nutrient requirements of the calf.
- Ruminant phase. The calf derives its nutrients from solid feeds, primarily through microbial fermentation in the reticulo-rumen.

This chapter discusses nutrient requirements of calves in each of those phases.

## ENERGY REQUIREMENTS OF CALVES

Energy requirements of calves, like those of other ages and classes of cattle, can be expressed in numerous ways (see Chapter 2). Regardless of the system preferred, it is imperative to understand where the major losses of energy occur as the energy-yielding components of the diet undergo digestion and metabolism. If the efficiencies of conversion of gross energy to digestible energy or metabolizable energy and of conversion of metabolizable energy to net energy (both $NE_M$ and $NE_G$) are known, users can select the system that best fits their needs.

In this edition, the energy requirements of calves have been derived on the basis of metabolizable energy; however, requirements and feed composition also are given in units of net energy and digestible energy for those who prefer to use those systems.

Data on energy requirements are organized around replacement calves fed only milk or milk replacer (Table 10-1); calves fed milk and starter feed or milk replacer and

TABLE 10-1 Daily Energy and Protein Requirements of Young Replacement Calves Fed Only Milk or Milk Replacer

| | | | Energy | | | | Protein | | |
|---|---|---|---|---|---|---|---|---|---|
| Live Weight (kg) | Gain (g) | Dry Matter Intake[a] (kg) | $NE_M$[b] (Mcal) | $NE_G$[c] (Mcal) | ME[d] (Mcal) | DE[e] (Mcal) | ADP[f] (g) | CP[g] (g) | Vitamin A[h] (IU) |
| 25 | 0 | 0.24 | 0.96 | 0 | 1.12 | 1.17 | 18 | 20 | 2,750 |
| | 200 | 0.32 | 0.96 | 0.26 | 1.50 | 1.56 | 65 | 70 | 2,750 |
| | 400 | 0.42 | 0.96 | 0.60 | 2.00 | 2.08 | 113 | 121 | 2,750 |
| 30 | 0 | 0.27 | 1.10 | 0 | 1.28 | 1.34 | 21 | 23 | 3,300 |
| | 200 | 0.36 | 1.10 | 0.28 | 1.69 | 1.76 | 68 | 73 | 3,300 |
| | 400 | 0.47 | 1.10 | 0.65 | 2.22 | 2.31 | 115 | 124 | 3,300 |
| 40 | 0 | 0.34 | 1.37 | 0 | 1.59 | 1.66 | 26 | 28 | 4,400 |
| | 200 | 0.43 | 1.37 | 0.31 | 2.04 | 2.13 | 73 | 79 | 4,400 |
| | 400 | 0.55 | 1.37 | 0.72 | 2.63 | 2.74 | 120 | 129 | 4,400 |
| | 600 | 0.69 | 1.37 | 1.16 | 3.28 | 3.41 | 168 | 180 | 4,400 |
| 45 | 0 | 0.37 | 1.49 | 0 | 1.74 | 1.81 | 28 | 30 | 4,950 |
| | 200 | 0.46 | 1.49 | 0.32 | 2.21 | 2.30 | 76 | 81 | 4,950 |
| | 400 | 0.59 | 1.49 | 0.75 | 2.82 | 2.94 | 123 | 132 | 4,950 |
| | 600 | 0.74 | 1.49 | 1.21 | 3.50 | 3.64 | 170 | 183 | 4,950 |
| 50 | 0 | 0.40 | 1.62 | 0 | 1.88 | 1.96 | 31 | 33 | 5,500 |
| | 200 | 0.45 | 1.62 | 0.34 | 2.37 | 2.47 | 78 | 84 | 5,500 |
| | 400 | 0.63 | 1.62 | 0.77 | 3.00 | 3.13 | 125 | 135 | 5,500 |
| | 600 | 0.78 | 1.62 | 1.26 | 3.70 | 3.86 | 173 | 185 | 5,500 |

[a] Dry matter intake necessary to meet ME requirements for calves fed milk replacer composed primarily of milk proteins and containing ME at 4.75 Mcal/kg of dry matter.
[b] $NE_M$ (Mcal) = 0.086 $LW^{0.75}$, where LW is live weight in kilograms.
[c] $NE_G$ (Mcal) = ($0.84\ LW^{0.355} \times LWG^{1.2}$) × 0.69, where LW and LWG (live weight gain) are in kilograms.
[d] ME (Mcal) = 0.1 $LW^{0.75}$ + ($0.84\ LW^{0.355} \times LWG^{1.2}$), where LW and LWG are in kilograms.
[e] DE (Mcal) = ME/0.96.
[f] ADP (apparent digestible protein, g/d) = 6.25 [1/BV(E + G + M × D) − M × D]. BV (biologic value) is assumed to be 0.8. E (endogenous urinary nitrogen) is 0.2 $LW^{0.75}$/d, where LW is in kilograms. M (metabolic fecal nitrogen) is 1.9 g/kg of dry matter intake (D). G (nitrogen in live weight gain) is 30 g/kg of LWG.
[g] CP (crude protein) = ADP/0.93. The digestibility of undenatured milk proteins is assumed to be 93 percent.
[h] Vitamin A (IU) = 110 IU/kg of LW. See Chapter 7.

starter feed (Table 10-2); calves reared for veal on only milk or milk replacers (Table 10-3); and weaned replacement calves to 100 kg of body weight fed starter or grower diets (Table 10-4). The amount of liquid feed (milk or milk replacer) offered to replacement calves is restricted to encourage intake of dry feed (starter), but calves reared for veal are fed milk or milk replacer at near ad libitum intakes.

### *Young Replacement Calves Fed Milk or Milk Replacer Only*

The energy requirements of young calves fed only milk or milk replacer and weighing 25-50 kg are given in Table 10-1. On the basis of available data, $NE_M$ is set at 0.086 Mcal/kg$^{0.75}$ of live weight (LW) daily as in the previous edition of this publication (National Research Council, 1989). This equates reasonably well with estimates of fasting metabolism of young milk-fed calves that are limited in activity (see chapter 4 of Davis and Drackley, 1998). The efficiency of use of metabolizable energy (ME) from milk or milk replacer to meet maintenance requirements is set at 86 percent. Consequently, maintenance ME is defined as 0.100 Mcal/kg$^{0.75}$ daily. The values for ME and efficiency of ME use for maintenance are within the range of values in the scientific literature (Van Es et al., 1969; Johnson and Elliott, 1972a,b; Holmes and Davey, 1976; Okamoto et al., 1986; Arieli et al., 1995; Gerrits et al., 1996). The Agricultural Research Council (ARC) specified an ME requirement of 0.102 Mcal/kg$^{0.75}$ daily, with an efficiency of use of ME for maintenance of 85 percent (Agricultural Research Council, 1980).

Requirements for ME were calculated with the equation derived by Toullec (1989) as follows:

$$\text{ME requirement (Mcal/d)} = 0.1\ LW^{0.75} + (0.84\ LW^{0.355})(LWG^{1.2}), \qquad (10\text{-}1)$$

where LW and daily liveweight gain (LWG) are in kilograms. The first portion of the equation sets the ME required for maintenance at 100 kcal/kg$^{0.75}$ per day. The second portion of the equation is used to derive the ME required for LWG, which is a function of both body size (LW) and rate of gain (LWG). This equation was derived on the basis of an efficiency of conversion of ME to $NE_G$ of 69 percent for calves fed only milk or milk replacer, which is consistent with most published values (Gonzalez-Jimenez and Blaxter, 1962; Van Es et al., 1969; Johnson and Elliott, 1972a,b; Vermorel et al., 1974; Webster et al., 1975; Donnelly and Hutton, 1976a,b; Holmes and Davey, 1976; Neergard, 1976; Toullec, 1989; Gerrits et al., 1996). The energy content of LWG predicted by equation 10-1 is 1556 kcal/kg LWG for a 40-kg calf gaining 200 g/d, and 2567 kcal/kg LWG for a 75-kg calf gaining 800 g/d. Values

TABLE 10-2 Daily Energy and Protein Requirements of Calves Fed Milk and Starter or Milk Replacer and Starter

| | | | Energy | | | | Protein | | |
|---|---|---|---|---|---|---|---|---|---|
| Live Weight (kg) | Gain (g) | Dry Matter Intake[a] (kg) | $NE_M$[b] (Mcal) | $NE_G$[c] (Mcal) | ME[d] (Mcal) | DE[e] (Mcal) | ADP[f] (g) | CP[g] (g) | Vitamin A[h] (IU) |
| 30 | 0 | 0.32 | 1.10 | 0 | 1.34 | 1.43 | 23 | 26 | 3,300 |
| | 200 | 0.42 | 1.10 | 0.28 | 1.77 | 1.89 | 72 | 84 | 3,300 |
| | 400 | 0.56 | 1.10 | 0.65 | 2.33 | 2.49 | 122 | 141 | 3,300 |
| 35 | 0 | 0.36 | 1.24 | 0 | 1.50 | 1.61 | 25 | 29 | 3,850 |
| | 200 | 0.47 | 1.24 | 0.30 | 1.96 | 2.09 | 75 | 87 | 3,850 |
| | 400 | 0.61 | 1.24 | 0.68 | 2.55 | 2.73 | 125 | 145 | 3,850 |
| 40 | 0 | 0.40 | 1.37 | 0 | 1.66 | 1.78 | 25 | 33 | 4,400 |
| | 200 | 0.51 | 1.37 | 0.31 | 2.14 | 2.29 | 78 | 90 | 4,400 |
| | 400 | 0.66 | 1.37 | 0.72 | 2.76 | 2.95 | 128 | 148 | 4,400 |
| | 600 | 0.83 | 1.37 | 1.16 | 3.44 | 3.68 | 178 | 205 | 4,400 |
| 45 | 0 | 0.44 | 1.49 | 0 | 1.81 | 1.94 | 31 | 36 | 4,950 |
| | 200 | 0.56 | 1.49 | 0.32 | 2.31 | 2.47 | 80 | 93 | 4,950 |
| | 400 | 0.71 | 1.49 | 0.75 | 2.96 | 3.16 | 130 | 151 | 4,950 |
| | 600 | 0.88 | 1.49 | 1.21 | 3.67 | 3.93 | 180 | 209 | 4,950 |
| 50 | 0 | 0.47 | 1.62 | 0 | 1.96 | 2.10 | 33 | 38 | 5,500 |
| | 200 | 0.60 | 1.62 | 0.34 | 2.48 | 2.65 | 83 | 96 | 5,500 |
| | 400 | 0.76 | 1.62 | 0.77 | 3.15 | 3.37 | 133 | 154 | 5,500 |
| | 600 | 0.94 | 1.62 | 1.26 | 3.89 | 4.17 | 183 | 212 | 5,500 |
| | 800 | 1.13 | 1.62 | 1.78 | 4.69 | 5.02 | 233 | 270 | 5,500 |
| 55 | 0 | 0.51 | 1.74 | 0 | 2.11 | 2.25 | 36 | 41 | 6,050 |
| | 200 | 0.63 | 1.74 | 0.35 | 2.64 | 2.83 | 85 | 99 | 6,050 |
| | 400 | 0.80 | 1.74 | 0.80 | 3.33 | 3.57 | 135 | 157 | 6,050 |
| | 600 | 0.99 | 1.74 | 1.30 | 4.10 | 4.39 | 185 | 215 | 6,050 |
| | 800 | 1.18 | 1.74 | 1.84 | 4.93 | 5.27 | 236 | 273 | 6,050 |
| 60 | 0 | 0.54 | 1.85 | 0 | 2.25 | 2.41 | 38 | 44 | 6,600 |
| | 200 | 0.67 | 1.85 | 0.36 | 2.80 | 3.00 | 88 | 102 | 6,600 |
| | 400 | 0.84 | 1.85 | 0.83 | 3.51 | 3.76 | 138 | 159 | 6,600 |
| | 600 | 1.04 | 1.85 | 1.34 | 4.31 | 4.61 | 188 | 217 | 6,600 |
| | 800 | 1.24 | 1.85 | 1.90 | 5.16 | 5.52 | 238 | 275 | 6,600 |

[a]These data apply to calves fed milk replacer (MR) plus starter. MR contains ME at 4.75 Mcal/kg of DM and starter ME at 3.28 Mcal/kg. It is assumed that MR provided 60 percent and starter 40 percent of dry matter intake; thus, dry matter consumed contained ME at 4.16 Mcal/kg. The DMI here is the total necessary to meet ME requirements and is not intended to predict voluntary intake.

[b]$NE_M$ (Mcal) = 0.086 $LW^{0.75}$, where LW is live weight in kilograms.

[c]$NE_G$ (Mcal) = (0.84 $LW^{0.355}$ × $LWG^{1.2}$) × 0.69, where LW and LW gain (LWG) are in kilograms.

[d]ME (Mcal) was computed as follows:

ME (maintenance) = $NE_M$/0.825. Efficiency of use of ME for maintenance (0.825) was computed as average of efficiencies of 0.86 for MR and 0.75 for starter, weighted according to proportions of ME supplied by each feed.

ME (gain) = $NE_G$/0.652. Efficiency of use of ME for gain (0.652) was computed as weighted average of efficiencies of 0.69 and 0.57 for MR and starter, respectively.

[e]DE (Mcal) = ME/0.934. Efficiency of conversion of DE to ME is assumed to be 0.96 for MR and 0.88 for starter.

[f]ADP (apparent digestible protein, g/d) = 6.25 [1/BV(E + G + M × D)- M × D]. BV (biologic value) = 0.764 (weighted average of MR = 0.8 and starter = 0.70); E (endogenous urinary nitrogen, g ) = 0.2$LW^{0.75}$; G (nitrogen content of gain, g) = 30 g/kg gain; M (metabolic fecal nitrogen, g/d) = 2.46 × dry matter intake, D, kg). Metabolic fecal nitrogen for MR assumed to be 1.9 g/kg of DMI and for starter 3.3 g/kg of DMI.

[g]CP (crude protein, g) = ADP/0.8645. Digestibility of protein was assumed to be weighted average of 93 percent for MR and 75 percent for starter; MR was assumed to contain 21 percent CP and starter 18 percent CP.

[h]Vitamin A (IU) = 110 IU/kg of LW. See Chapter 7.

predicted by this equation are similar to those in the 1989 edition of this publication for smaller calves at low rates of gain (1460 kcal/kg LWG for a 40-kg calf gaining 200 g/d) but are substantially higher than the 1989 edition for larger calves at higher rates of gain (1869 kcal/kg LWG for a 75-kg calf gaining 800 g/d). Values predicted by the present equation agree well with available experimental data on body composition of dairy calves (Webster et al., 1975; Donnelly and Hutton, 1976b; Holmes and Davey, 1976; Neergard, 1976; Gerrits et al., 1996). Data for composition of LWG for dairy calves of current genotypes would be useful for future refinement of requirements for growth.

The ME requirements given in Table 10-1 for calves weighing 30-60 kg and gaining at different rates are in close agreement with most published data. The digestible energy (DE) values in Table 10-1 are calculated from ME, assuming an efficiency of 96 percent for conversion of DE to ME (Neergard, 1976; National Research Council, 1989; Toullec, 1989; Gerrits et al., 1996). Users that desire requirements for higher rates of gain than included in Table 10-1 for calves fed milk or milk replacer only should refer to Table 10-3.

Users should be aware that ME requirements for maintenance may be underestimated for calves during the first week of life because of the high and variable basal meta-

TABLE 10-3 Daily Energy and Protein Requirements of Veal Calves Fed Only Milk or Milk Replacer

| | | | Energy | | | | Protein | | |
|---|---|---|---|---|---|---|---|---|---|
| Live Weight (kg) | Gain (g) | Dry Matter Intake[a] (kg) | $NE_M$[b] (Mcal) | $NE_G$[c] (Mcal) | ME[d] (Mcal) | DE[e] (Mcal) | ADP[f] (g) | CP[g] (g) | Vitamin A[h] (IU) |
| 40 | 0 | 0.34 | 1.37 | 0 | 1.59 | 1.66 | 26 | 28 | 4,400 |
| | 300 | 0.49 | 1.37 | 0.51 | 2.32 | 2.42 | 97 | 104 | 4,400 |
| | 600 | 0.69 | 1.37 | 1.16 | 3.28 | 3.41 | 168 | 180 | 4,400 |
| 50 | 0 | 0.40 | 1.62 | 0 | 1.88 | 1.96 | 31 | 33 | 5,500 |
| | 300 | 0.56 | 1.62 | 0.55 | 2.67 | 2.79 | 102 | 109 | 5,500 |
| | 600 | 0.78 | 1.62 | 1.26 | 3.71 | 3.86 | 172 | 185 | 5,500 |
| | 900 | 1.02 | 1.62 | 2.05 | 4.85 | 5.05 | 244 | 262 | 5,500 |
| 60 | 0 | 0.45 | 1.85 | 0 | 2.16 | 2.25 | 35 | 38 | 6,600 |
| | 300 | 0.63 | 1.85 | 0.58 | 3.00 | 3.13 | 106 | 114 | 6,600 |
| | 600 | 0.86 | 1.85 | 1.34 | 4.10 | 4.27 | 177 | 190 | 6,600 |
| | 900 | 1.12 | 1.85 | 2.18 | 5.32 | 5.54 | 248 | 267 | 6,600 |
| 70 | 0 | 0.51 | 2.08 | 0 | 2.42 | 2.52 | 39 | 42 | 7,700 |
| | 300 | 0.70 | 2.08 | 0.62 | 3.32 | 3.45 | 110 | 119 | 7,700 |
| | 600 | 1.94 | 2.08 | 1.42 | 4.48 | 4.66 | 181 | 195 | 7,700 |
| | 900 | 1.21 | 2.08 | 2.31 | 5.76 | 6.01 | 253 | 272 | 7,700 |
| | 1,200 | 1.50 | 2.08 | 3.26 | 7.14 | 7.44 | 324 | 348 | 7,700 |
| 80 | 0 | 0.56 | 2.30 | 0 | 2.68 | 2.79 | 44 | 47 | 8,800 |
| | 300 | 0.76 | 2.30 | 0.65 | 3.61 | 3.76 | 115 | 123 | 8,800 |
| | 600 | 1.02 | 2.30 | 1.49 | 4.83 | 5.03 | 186 | 200 | 8,800 |
| | 900 | 1.30 | 2.30 | 2.42 | 6.18 | 6.44 | 257 | 276 | 8,800 |
| | 1,200 | 1.61 | 2.30 | 3.42 | 7.63 | 7.95 | 328 | 353 | 8,800 |
| 90 | 0 | 0.62 | 2.51 | 0 | 2.92 | 3.04 | 48 | 51 | 9,900 |
| | 300 | 0.82 | 2.51 | 0.68 | 3.90 | 4.06 | 119 | 128 | 9,900 |
| | 600 | 1.09 | 2.51 | 1.55 | 5.17 | 5.39 | 190 | 204 | 9,900 |
| | 900 | 1.38 | 2.51 | 2.55 | 6.62 | 6.85 | 263 | 283 | 9,900 |
| | 1,200 | 1.70 | 2.51 | 3.56 | 8.09 | 8.42 | 332 | 357 | 9,900 |
| 100 | 0 | 0.67 | 2.72 | 0 | 3.16 | 3.29 | 52 | 55 | 11,000 |
| | 300 | 0.88 | 2.72 | 0.70 | 4.18 | 4.35 | 122 | 132 | 11,000 |
| | 600 | 1.16 | 2.72 | 1.61 | 5.50 | 5.72 | 194 | 208 | 11,000 |
| | 900 | 1.46 | 2.72 | 2.62 | 6.96 | 7.25 | 265 | 285 | 11,000 |
| | 1,200 | 1.80 | 2.72 | 3.70 | 8.52 | 8.88 | 336 | 362 | 11,000 |
| | 1,500 | 2.14 | 2.72 | 4.84 | 10.17 | 10.59 | 408 | 438 | 11,000 |
| 110 | 0 | 0.72 | 2.92 | 0 | 3.40 | 3.54 | 55 | 60 | 12,100 |
| | 300 | 0.94 | 2.92 | 0.72 | 4.45 | 4.63 | 126 | 136 | 12,100 |
| | 600 | 1.22 | 2.92 | 1.66 | 5.81 | 6.05 | 198 | 212 | 12,100 |
| | 900 | 1.54 | 2.92 | 2.71 | 7.32 | 7.63 | 269 | 289 | 12,100 |
| | 1,200 | 1.88 | 2.92 | 3.83 | 8.94 | 9.32 | 340 | 366 | 12,100 |
| | 1,500 | 2.24 | 2.92 | 5.00 | 10.65 | 11.09 | 412 | 443 | 12,100 |
| 120 | 0 | 0.76 | 3.12 | 0 | 3.63 | 3.78 | 59 | 64 | 13,200 |
| | 300 | 0.99 | 3.12 | 0.75 | 4.71 | 4.91 | 130 | 140 | 13,200 |
| | 600 | 1.29 | 3.12 | 1.72 | 6.12 | 6.39 | 201 | 217 | 13,200 |
| | 900 | 1.62 | 3.12 | 2.80 | 7.68 | 8.00 | 273 | 293 | 13,200 |
| | 1,200 | 1.97 | 3.12 | 3.69 | 9.34 | 9.74 | 329 | 353 | 13,200 |
| | 1,500 | 2.34 | 3.12 | 5.16 | 11.10 | 11.56 | 416 | 447 | 13,200 |
| 130 | 0 | 0.81 | 3.31 | 0 | 3.85 | 4.01 | 63 | 67 | 14,300 |
| | 300 | 1.05 | 3.31 | 0.77 | 4.97 | 5.17 | 134 | 144 | 14,300 |
| | 600 | 1.35 | 3.31 | 1.77 | 6.41 | 6.68 | 205 | 220 | 14,300 |
| | 900 | 1.69 | 3.31 | 2.88 | 8.02 | 8.35 | 276 | 297 | 14,300 |
| | 1,200 | 2.05 | 3.31 | 4.06 | 9.74 | 10.14 | 348 | 374 | 14,300 |
| | 1,500 | 2.43 | 3.31 | 5.31 | 11.54 | 12.02 | 420 | 451 | 14,300 |
| 140 | 0 | 0.86 | 3.50 | 0 | 4.07 | 4.24 | 66 | 71 | 15,400 |
| | 300 | 1.10 | 3.50 | 0.79 | 5.22 | 5.43 | 137 | 148 | 15,400 |
| | 600 | 1.41 | 3.50 | 1.82 | 6.70 | 6.98 | 209 | 224 | 15,400 |
| | 900 | 1.76 | 3.50 | 2.95 | 8.35 | 8.70 | 280 | 301 | 15,400 |
| | 1,200 | 2.13 | 3.50 | 4.17 | 10.11 | 10.53 | 352 | 378 | 15,400 |
| | 1,500 | 2.52 | 3.50 | 5.45 | 11.97 | 12.45 | 423 | 455 | 15,400 |
| 150 | 0 | 0.90 | 3.69 | 0 | 4.29 | 4.46 | 70 | 75 | 16,500 |
| | 300 | 1.15 | 3.69 | 0.81 | 5.46 | 5.69 | 141 | 152 | 16,500 |
| | 600 | 1.47 | 3.69 | 1.86 | 6.98 | 7.27 | 212 | 228 | 16,500 |
| | 900 | 1.82 | 3.69 | 3.02 | 8.67 | 9.03 | 284 | 305 | 16,500 |
| | 1,200 | 2.21 | 3.69 | 4.27 | 10.48 | 10.91 | 355 | 382 | 16,500 |
| | 1,500 | 2.61 | 3.69 | 5.58 | 12.38 | 12.90 | 427 | 459 | 16,500 |

[a] The DMI necessary to meet ME requirements when veal calves are fed a milk replacer containing ME at 4.75 Mcal/kg of DM.
[b] $NE_M$ (Mcal) = 0.086 $LW^{0.75}$, where LW is live weight in kilograms.
[c] $NE_G$ (Mcal) = $(0.84\ LW^{0.355} \times LWG^{1.2}) \times 0.69$, where LW and LW gain (LWG) are in kilograms.
[d] ME (Mcal) = $0.1\ LW^{0.75} + (0.84\ LW^{0.355} \times LWG^{1.2})$, where LW and LWG are in kilograms.
[e] DE (Mcal) = ME/0.93.
[f] ADP (apparent digestible protein, g/d) = 6.25 [1/BV(E + G + M × D) − M × D]. BV (biologic value) is assumed to be 0.8. E (endogenous urinary nitrogen) is 0.2 $LW^{0.75}$/d, where LW is in kilograms. M (metabolic fecal nitrogen) is 1.9 g/kg of dry matter intake (D). G (nitrogen in live weight gain) is 30 g/kg LWG.
[g] CP (crude protein) = ADP/0.93. The digestibility of undenatured milk proteins is assumed to be 93 percent.
[h] Vitamin A (IU) = 110 IU/kg of LW. See Chapter 7.

TABLE 10-4 Daily Energy and Protein Requirements of Weaned (Ruminant) Calves[a]

| | | | Energy | | | | Protein | | |
|---|---|---|---|---|---|---|---|---|---|
| Live Weight (kg) | Gain (g) | Dry Matter Intake (kg) | $NE_M$[b] (Mcal) | $NE_G$[c] (Mcal) | ME[d] (Mcal) | DE[e] (Mcal) | ADP[f] (g) | CP[g] (g) | Vitamin A[h] (IU) |
| 50 | 0 | 0.70 | 1.62 | 0 | 2.16 | 2.58 | 40 | 53 | 5,500 |
| | 400 | 1.13 | 1.62 | 0.77 | 3.51 | 3.92 | 151 | 201 | 5,500 |
| | 500 | 1.27 | 1.62 | 1.01 | 3.93 | 4.35 | 179 | 238 | 5,500 |
| | 600 | 1.86 | 1.62 | 1.26 | 4.36 | 4.77 | 207 | 276 | 5,500 |
| 60 | 0 | 0.80 | 1.85 | 0 | 2.47 | 2.89 | 46 | 61 | 6,600 |
| | 400 | 1.26 | 1.85 | 0.83 | 3.92 | 4.33 | 156 | 209 | 6,600 |
| | 500 | 1.41 | 1.85 | 1.08 | 4.36 | 4.77 | 185 | 246 | 6,600 |
| | 600 | 1.56 | 1.85 | 1.34 | 4.83 | 5.23 | 213 | 284 | 6,600 |
| | 700 | 1.71 | 1.85 | 1.62 | 5.31 | 5.70 | 241 | 322 | 6,600 |
| | 800 | 1.87 | 1.85 | 1.90 | 5.80 | 6.19 | 269 | 359 | 6,600 |
| 70 | 0 | 0.90 | 2.08 | 0 | 2.77 | 3.19 | 51 | 68 | 7,700 |
| | 400 | 1.39 | 2.08 | 0.87 | 4.31 | 4.71 | 163 | 217 | 7,700 |
| | 500 | 1.54 | 2.08 | 1.14 | 4.77 | 5.17 | 191 | 254 | 7,700 |
| | 600 | 1.70 | 2.08 | 1.42 | 5.26 | 5.66 | 219 | 292 | 7,700 |
| | 700 | 1.86 | 2.08 | 1.71 | 5.77 | 6.16 | 247 | 330 | 7,700 |
| | 800 | 2.03 | 2.08 | 2.00 | 6.29 | 6.67 | 275 | 367 | 7,700 |
| 80 | 0 | 0.99 | 2.30 | 0 | 3.07 | 3.48 | 57 | 75 | 8,800 |
| | 400 | 1.51 | 2.30 | 0.92 | 4.67 | 5.07 | 168 | 224 | 8,800 |
| | 500 | 1.66 | 2.30 | 1.20 | 5.16 | 5.56 | 196 | 262 | 8,800 |
| | 600 | 1.83 | 2.30 | 1.49 | 5.68 | 6.07 | 225 | 300 | 8,800 |
| | 700 | 2.00 | 2.30 | 1.79 | 6.21 | 6.59 | 253 | 337 | 8,800 |
| | 800 | 2.18 | 2.30 | 2.10 | 6.75 | 7.13 | 281 | 375 | 8,800 |
| 90 | 0 | 1.16 | 2.51 | 0 | 3.35 | 3.76 | 62 | 82 | 9,900 |
| | 600 | 2.09 | 2.51 | 1.55 | 6.07 | 6.46 | 231 | 309 | 9,900 |
| | 700 | 2.28 | 2.51 | 1.87 | 6.62 | 7.00 | 260 | 346 | 9,900 |
| | 800 | 2.48 | 2.51 | 2.19 | 7.19 | 7.57 | 288 | 385 | 9,900 |
| | 900 | 2.68 | 2.51 | 2.52 | 7.78 | 8.15 | 317 | 423 | 9,900 |
| 100 | 0 | 1.25 | 2.72 | 0 | 3.63 | 4.04 | 68 | 90 | 11,000 |
| | 600 | 2.22 | 2.72 | 1.61 | 6.45 | 6.83 | 237 | 316 | 11,000 |
| | 700 | 2.42 | 2.72 | 1.94 | 7.02 | 7.40 | 265 | 354 | 11,000 |
| | 800 | 2.63 | 2.72 | 2.27 | 7.62 | 7.99 | 294 | 392 | 11,000 |
| | 900 | 2.84 | 2.72 | 2.62 | 8.22 | 8.59 | 323 | 430 | 11,000 |

[a] These data apply to small-breed female calves from 50 to 80 kg gaining 0.4 to 0.5 kg/d and large-breed calves from 60 to 100 kg gaining from 0.6 to 0.9 kg/d.

[b] $NE_M$ (Mcal) = $0.086\ LW^{0.75}$ (NRC 1989), where LW is live weight in kilograms.

[c] $NE_G$ (Mcal) = $(0.84\ LW^{0.355} \times LWG^{1.2}) \times 0.69$, where LW and LW gain (LWG) are in kilograms.

[d] ME, maintenance (Mcal) = $NE_M/0.75$. ME values of diets (Mcal/kg of DM) are 3.10 for calves weighing 60, 70, and 80 kg and 2.90 for calves weighing 90 and 100 kg. ME, gain (Mcal) = $NE_G/0.57$.
Sum of ME values for maintenance plus gain equals total ME requirement.

[e] DE (Mcal) = (ME + 0.45) /1.01 (see Chapter 2).

[f] ADP (apparent digestible protein, g/d) as follows: ADP (g/d) = $6.25\ [1/BV(E + G + M \times D) - M \times D]$ where BV is biologic value set at 0.70; E (endogenous urinary nitrogen) = $0.2LW^{0.75}$; G is nitrogen content of gain, assuming 30 g/kg of gain ; and M is metabolic fecal nitrogen computed as 3.3 g/kg of dry matter consumed (D).

[g] CP (crude protein) calculated as ADP/0.75.

[h] Vitamin A (IU) = 110 IU/kg of LW. See Chapter 7.

bolic rate observed during this time (Roy et al., 1957; Vermorel et al., 1983; Okamoto et al., 1986; Schrama et al., 1992; Ortigues et al., 1994; Arieli et al., 1995). Furthermore, because the digestive tract is immature and developing rapidly, the metabolizability of diets may be lower during this time (Schrama et al., 1992; Arieli et al, 1995), thereby overestimating dietary energy supply. The net result of these effects is that LWG of calves during the first week of life may be considerably less than the predicted energy-allowable gains shown in Table 10-1. As more data become available it may become possible in future editions to model these effects.

Energy requirement values for young calves in this edition represent several improvements over the previous edition (National Research Council, 1989). First, tabulated values in this edition are derived directly from the equations presented, in contrast with values given in the tables of the 1989 edition that could not be calculated from the information provided. Second, as discussed above, values for the energy content of body weight gain ($NE_G$) in this edition agree more closely with available data on calves derived from slaughter experiments; values in the 1989 edition were too low (see Davis and Drackley, 1998). Third, the equations used to derive the $NE_M$ and $NE_G$ values for milk or milk replacers in the previous edition were those of Garrett (see National Research Council, 1989) established for feedlot cattle fed diets with ME content of 2.19-2.86 Mcal/kg of dry matter (DM). Those equations result in erroneously low NE values for diets of milk or milk-derived products. Garrett (1980) cautioned against using the established equations to derive NE values for feedstuffs with ME values outside the range stated above. A different approach has been taken in this edition to derive the NE values for liquid diets and starter.

### *Young Replacement Calves Fed Milk and Starter Feed or Milk Replacer and Starter Feed*

Under good management on dairy farms, calves should be consuming appreciable nutrients from starter feed by the second week of life. To encourage early consumption of calf starter, calves should be given free access to water and a nutritious, highly palatable starter feed from the first week of life until they are weaned. Consumption of starter feed is critical to development of an active, functioning rumen. Fermentation products, principally butyrate, from fermentation of solid feeds in the developing rumen are responsible for development of functional ruminal epithelial tissue (Sander et al., 1959).

Deriving the energy requirements of calves fed a combination diet (liquid plus dry feed) requires the application of basic knowledge from related areas because there are few data on the subject. Only one study, which used three calves per treatment, has examined this question directly by using calorimetry (Holmes and Davey, 1976). The maintenance requirement and efficiency of use of ME by calves did not differ appreciably between an all-milk diet and a diet consisting of milk and dry feed.

Regardless of the diet fed, the NE required for maintenance and gain should not change. Efficiencies of utilization of ME for maintenance and gain will be somewhat lower for starter feeds than for milk or milk replacer (National Research Council, 1978). As described for Table 10-1, calves use the ME from milk or milk replacer with efficiencies of 86 percent and 69 percent for maintenance and gain, respectively. Efficiency of ME use from milk or milk replacer is assumed not to change when starter also is consumed. The previous edition of this publication (National Research Council, 1989) used the equations of Garrett (1980) to derive the efficiencies of utilization of ME (percent) from starter for maintenance ($k_m$) and gain ($k_g$):

$$k_m = 51.045\ ME - 10.836\ ME^2 + 0.754\ ME^3 - 7.35 \quad (10\text{-}2)$$

$$k_g = 76.149\ ME - 15.755\ ME^2 + 1.062\ ME^3 - 69.7 \quad (10\text{-}3)$$

where ME is expressed as Mcal/kg DM.

However, these data were for older growing cattle fed feedlot diets and are not appropriate for young calves. For example, the Garrett (1980) equations yield efficiencies of ME use for maintenance and gain of 69.4 and 46.4 percent, respectively, for a starter containing 3.1 Mcal ME/kg DM. These efficiencies are lower than those calculated from experimental data (Holmes and Davey, 1976) and used in other systems (Agricultural Research Council, 1980). Furthermore, the Garrett (1980) equations were developed using ME values calculated as 0.82 DE (National Research Council, 1989). Because methane production is minimal even in young calves consuming 44 percent of their ME from concentrates (Holmes and Davey, 1976), these derived ME values are too low when compared with experimental data (Spanski et al., 1997). Consequently, the use of the Garrett (1980) equations for young calves has been discontinued in this edition.

The Agricultural Research Council (1980) calculated efficiencies of ME use for maintenance and gain as a function of the metabolizability (ME/GE, or "q") of the diet. Over the range of ME concentrations expected for calf starters and growers (2.5–3.4 Mcal/kg), the efficiency of ME use for maintenance would vary from only about 72 to 77 percent, and that for gain from 50 to 59 percent. In this edition, efficiencies of ME use from dry feeds for maintenance and gain were fixed at 75 and 57 percent, respectively. The efficiency of use of ME from the total diet is then calculated as the average of individual efficiencies for milk and starter, weighted according to their contribution to the total ME in the diet.

In the example given in Table 10-2, it was assumed that a calf at about 2 wk of age would consume on the average a diet in which 60 percent of DM intake (DMI) is derived from milk replacer (ME at 4.75 Mcal/kg of DM) and 40 percent from starter (ME at 3.28 Mcal/kg of DM). In this diet, milk-replacer supplies 68 percent of the total ME, and starter supplies 32 percent. Consequently, the overall efficiencies for use of ME in the combined diet (milk replacer plus starter) are 82.5 and 65.2 percent for maintenance and gain, respectively, calculated as the weighted average (weighted by contribution to the total ME supply) of the individual efficiencies. The computer model included with this edition calculates these values for varied proportions of DMI from milk and starter or milk replacer and starter.

A comparison of the ME requirement of a 50-kg calf gaining 400 g/d when fed only milk or milk replacer (see Table 10-1) with the ME requirement of the same calf fed milk and starter or milk replacer and starter (Table 10-2) reveals a relatively small difference (3.00 vs 3.15 Mcal/d). The ME requirements given here for calves consuming both starter and milk or milk replacer are markedly lower than those given in the 1989 edition (5.90 Mcal/d) but are similar to those given by Roy (1980). A comparison of LWG predicted by this model with actual performance of calves receiving both milk or milk replacer and starter in 16 published research studies reveals good agreement (Stewart and Schingoethe, 1984; Jenny et al., 1991; Jaster et al., 1992; Reddy et al., 1993; Akayezu et al., 1994; Quigley et al., 1994a; Abdelgadir and Morrill, 1995; Quigley et al.,

1995; Abdelgadir et al., 1996a, b; Quigley, 1996b; Quigley and Bernard, 1996; Quigley and Welborn, 1996; Terui et al., 1996; Quigley et al., 1997b; Lammers et al., 1998).

Table 10-2 also presents requirements for energy in units of DE. Values for DE were calculated as ME/0.934, representing the weighted average of conversion of DE to ME for milk or milk replacer (0.96) and starter (0.88). The conversion from ME to DE for starter was calculated as (ME + 0.45)/1.01 (National Research Council, 1989), as described in Chapter 2 (also see later discussion on energy values for feeds).

The DMI listed in Tables 10-1 through 10-4 have been computed as the amount of DM necessary to provide the ME requirement. Consequently, these should not be construed to be predictions of voluntary feed intake. An analysis of literature data presented elsewhere (see chapter 16 of Davis and Drackley, 1998) predicts that intake of DM from starter increases from about 0.8–1.0 percent of BW at 3 wk of age to about 2.8–3.0 percent of BW at 8 wk of age.

### *Veal Calves*

The calculations used to derive the ME requirements for veal calves (Table 10-3) are the same as those for milk-fed replacement calves (Table 10-1). Veal calves are fed essentially for ad libitum intake, so rates of gain will be higher than those of limit-fed replacement calves. The ME and DM requirements given here agree closely with those reported by Webster et al. (1975) on the basis of an energy-balance study with veal calves.

### *Ruminant Calves (Large-Breed and Small-Breed Females) from Weaning to Body Weight of 100 Kilograms*

In the previous edition of *Nutrient Requirements of Dairy Cattle*, (National Research Council, 1989) no information was given on the nutrient requirements of calves from weaning to 100 kg of body weight even though this is a critical period in the life of the replacement calf. Similar to calves consuming milk and starter, very few research data determined by calorimetry or comparative slaughter studies exist for this class of cattle. However, the subcommittee believes that estimates should be made. Methods used in this edition to establish requirements for growth of heifers from 100 to 500 kg of body weight could not be extrapolated accurately to calves weighing less than 100 kg. Given the paucity of data on tissue growth and nutrient use for this class of calves, estimated requirements have been derived using the same methodology as described already for younger calves. Users will note that requirements for ruminant calves weighing less than 100 kg do not merge smoothly into requirements for larger calves.

Energy-allowable LWG was predicted using this model from LW and estimated ME intakes from 25 treatments in 19 published studies (Stewart and Schingoethe, 1984; Beharka et al., 1991; Chester-Jones et al., 1991; Jenny et al., 1991; Quigley et al., 1991; Quigley et al., 1992; Reddy et al., 1993; Akayezu et al., 1994; Jackson and Hemken, 1994; Kuehn et al., 1994; Maiga et al., 1994; Quigley et al., 1994a; Abdelgadir and Morrill, 1995; Abdelgadir et al., 1996a,b; Quigley, 1996b; Terui et al., 1996; Kincaid et al., 1997). Comparisons were expressed as predicted/observed; the mean was 1.04. Twelve predicted values were greater than observed, twelve were less than observed, and one was equal. As more research information becomes available, future editions of this publication may be better able to define requirements for this group of calves. However, in comparing requirements established here with literature data on average daily gains, the methodology presented in this edition adequately predicts gains of large-breed calves up to 100 kg and small-breed calves to 80 kg.

Table 10-4 shows the requirements of weaned calves weighing 50–100 kg and gaining at various rates. Calves weighing 50–80 kg were assumed to be fed a starter containing ME at 3.1 Mcal of ME per kg of DM, and those weighing 90–100 kg a starter or grower containing ME at 3.0 Mcal per kg of DM. Given the paucity of data, no distinction is made between large and small breed calves. Similarly, no distinction is made between male and female calves since differences are negligible before about 100 kg LW (National Research Council, 1978).

### *Effects of Environmental Temperature on Energy Requirements of Young Calves*

The calf is born with limited body energy reserves and only modest insulation afforded by hair coat and body fat. A newborn calf is estimated to have enough body energy stores in the form of fat and glycogen to last no more than about 1 d under very cold conditions (Alexander et al., 1975; Okamoto et al., 1986; Rowan, 1992).

Energy standards are based on the premise that the animal is in a thermoneutral environment during measurements of energy transformations. In such an environment, the animal is not required to elicit specific heat-conserving or heat-dissipating mechanisms to maintain core body temperature (National Research Council, 1981). The thermoneutral zone shifts depending on many factors, the more important factors being age, amount of feed intake, amount of subcutaneous fat, and length and thickness of hair coat. The thermoneutral zone in very young calves ranges from 15–25°C. Thus, when the environmental temperature drops below 15°C, which is referred to as the lower critical temperature, the calf must expend energy to maintain its body temperature. In practical terms, the maintenance energy requirement is increased. For older calves and calves at greater feed intakes, the lower critical temperature may be as low as −5 to −10°C (Webster et al., 1978).

Data in Table 10-5 illustrate the effects of a decrease in environmental temperature below the lower critical temperature of the calf on energy requirements for maintenance. The values were calculated from research data of Schrama (1993). Note in the example given in Table 10-5 that if the lower critical temperature is 10°C and the effective ambient temperature is 0°C, the maintenance energy requirement is increased by 27 percent. This calculation agrees with experimental findings (Scibilia et al., 1987). Effects of cold stress in increasing maintenance requirements have been incorporated into the computational model provided with this publication.

It is clear from these and other data that calves, especially very young calves, should be fed extra energy during cold weather to satisfy the increase in maintenance energy requirements. That can be accomplished by increasing the amount of liquid diet being fed, by adding additional milk solids to the liquid diet, or by incorporating additional fat into the liquid diet (Schingoethe et al., 1986; Scibilia et al., 1987; Jaster et al., 1990). However, additional fat in milk replacer or starter decreases starter intake (Kuehn et al., 1994), which negates at least a portion of the increased energy density from fat supplementation. If additional solids are fed, the DM concentration of milk replacer should not exceed 20 percent to avoid problems with excessive mineral intake (Jenny et al., 1978; Ternouth et al., 1985), and supplemental water should be provided. The availability of free water is critically important to starter intake (Kertz et al., 1984); provision of warm water 2-3 times daily during cold weather may help to stimulate starter feed intake, which also would help to counteract cold stress.

## PROTEIN REQUIREMENTS OF CALVES

In contrast with the 1978 edition of *Nutrient Requirements of Dairy Cattle* (National Research Council, 1978), the 1989 edition provided little information on the protein requirements of young calves weighing less than 100 kg. The tabular data given for protein requirements in the 1989 edition could not be reproduced with information provided (see chapter 9 of Davis and Drackley, 1998). The present edition computes the protein requirement of calves weighing up to 100 kg with the factorial method of Blaxter and Mitchell (1948).

The requirement is partitioned into components of maintenance and gain. Maintenance constitutes obligatory nitrogen (N) losses in urine and feces, whereas gain pertains to N stored in tissues. The protein requirement is expressed in terms of apparent digestible protein (ADP, g/d) and is computed as follows:

$$\text{ADP, g/d} = 6.25\,[1/\text{BV}\,(E + G + M \times D) - M \times D] \qquad (10\text{-}4)$$

where BV = biological value (discussed below). Endogenous urinary N (E, g/d) is computed as $0.2\text{LW}^{0.75}$ (Agricultural Research Council, 1980), where live weight (LW) is in kilograms. This value is somewhat higher than that ($0.165\ \text{LW}^{0.75}$) computed with the formula (2.75 g of net protein per kilogram $\text{LW}^{0.5}$) given in the 1989 National Research Council publication; however, both are within the range of values in the scientific literature (Blaxter and Wood, 1951; Cunningham and Brisson, 1957; Roy, 1970). The amount of N in gain (G) is assumed to be constant at 30 g N/kg LWG, which is in the range of values reported by others (Blaxter and Wood, 1951; Roy, 1970; Donnelly and Hutton, 1976b; National Research Council, 1978; Davis

TABLE 10-5 Effect of Environment on Energy Requirement of Young Calves[a]

| Environmental Temperature | | Increase in Maintenance Energy Requirement (kcal of $NE_M$/day) | | Maintenance Energy Requirement (kcal of ME/day)[b] | | Increase in ME Required for Maintenance | |
|---|---|---|---|---|---|---|---|
| °F | °C | Birth to 3 wk of age[c] | >3 wk of age[d] | Birth to 3 wk of age[c] | >3 wk of age[d] | Birth to 3 wk of age[c] | >3 wk of age[d] |
| 68 | 20 | 0 | 0 | 1,735 | 1,735 | 0 | 0 |
| 59 | 15 | 187 | 0 | 1,969 | 1,735 | 13 | 0 |
| 50 | 10 | 373 | 0 | 2,203 | 1,735 | 27 | 0 |
| 41 | 5 | 560 | 187 | 2,437 | 1,969 | 40 | 13 |
| 32 | 0 | 746 | 373 | 2,671 | 2,205 | 54 | 27 |
| 23 | −5 | 933 | 568 | 2,905 | 2,437 | 68 | 40 |
| 14 | −10 | 1,119 | 746 | 3,139 | 2,671 | 86 | 54 |
| 5 | −15 | 1,306 | 933 | 3,373 | 2,905 | 94 | 68 |
| −4 | −20 | 1,492 | 1,119 | 3,607 | 3,139 | 108 | 81 |
| −13 | −25 | 1,679 | 1,306 | 3,834 | 3,373 | 121 | 94 |
| −22 | −30 | 1,865 | 1,492 | 4,066 | 3,607 | 134 | 107 |

[a] Calculated for calf weighing 45.35 kg (100 lbs; 17.35 $\text{kg}^{0.75}$). Extra heat production = 2.15 $\text{kcal/kg}^{0.75}$ per day for each degree decrease in environmental temperature (°C) below lower critical temperature (Schrama, 1993). Because heat production is in terms of net energy (NE), metabolizable energy (ME) was computed as ME = NE/0.8.
[b] Maintenance energy requirement 100 $\text{kcal/kg}^{0.75}$ per day.
[c] Calves from birth to 3 wk of age have lower critical temperature in range of 15–25 °C. Data above were calculated on basis of lower critical temperature 20° C.
[d] Data for calves older than 3 wk of age were calculated on basis of lower critical temperature 10° C.

and Drackley, 1998). Insufficient data were available to describe changes in N content of LW gain as a function of increasing growth rate. Metabolic fecal N (M) is set as 1.9 g/kg of dry matter consumed (D) from milk or milk replacer and 3.3 g/kg of starter DM consumed (Roy, 1980); these values are additive for calves fed both milk and starter.

Loss of N in scurf (hair and skin) is ignored in the present edition. The 1989 edition calculated the loss as 0.032 g of N/kg of $LW^{0.6}$, which equates to a daily loss of 0.33 g of N for a 50-kg calf. In practice, this loss is compensated by the higher endogenous N losses predicted in the present edition (3.76 g of N for a 50-kg calf) than in the 1989 edition (3.10 g of N).

The biological value (BV) of milk proteins, equated to the efficiency of N use for growth above maintenance, is assigned a value of 0.80 (Donnelly and Hutton, 1976a). The same factor is assumed to apply for efficiency of use of dietary protein for maintenance functions. This value was determined at limiting protein intakes and assumes that the diet being fed is properly balanced for all essential nutrients and that energy intake is sufficient to support protein synthesis. Protein intake must not be in excess of that required for the targeted gain allowed by energy intake. The BV decreased as protein intake was increased in the studies of Donnelly and Hutton (1976a). The 1978 National Research Council publication used a value of 0.77. Recent studies by Terosky et al. (1997) found that apparent BV for milk replacers containing 21 percent CP from skim milk protein, whey protein concentrate, or mixtures of the two ranged from 0.692 to 0.765. Estimates of true biological value (corrected for endogenous N loss and metabolic fecal N) from that study are in excess of 0.80.

The conversion of CP to ADP was assumed to be 93 percent for milk proteins (Agricultural Research Council, 1980), which is slightly higher than the value for conversion of dietary CP to absorbable amino acids (91 percent) used in an earlier edition of this publication (National Research Council, 1978). Users should note that requirements for ADP and crude protein (CP) have been established on the basis of diets containing milk proteins with high digestibility and BV; calves might not use alternative, nonmilk proteins in milk replacers at these high efficiencies, and appropriate adjustments may need to be made when such protein sources are used to ensure adequate supply of amino acids for growth (Davis and Drackley, 1998). Furthermore, because digestion of even high-quality milk proteins is immature during the first 2–3 weeks of age (Arieli et al., 1995; Terosky et al., 1997), the value of milk proteins may be overestimated during the early liquid-feeding period. Similar to the situation for energy requirements, however, the subcommittee concluded that information was insufficient to model increasing CP digestibility in the young calf.

The BV of absorbed proteins supplied by starter is set at 0.70 (National Research Council, 1978). Calves fed milk plus starter and weaned calves (fed starter only) derive a portion of their protein needs from microbial protein produced in the rumen. However, insufficient data were available to allow calculations of the amounts of rumen-degradable protein (RDP) or rumen-undegradable protein (RUP) supplied with any degree of confidence; thus, the factorial approach using ADP was adopted for calves weighing up to 100 kg. Requirements also are presented in terms of CP. The conversion of CP to ADP is assumed to be 75 percent for starter and grower feeds (Agricultural Research Council, 1980). Quigley et al. (1985) found that an average of 58 percent of the protein reaching the abomasum of weaned calves was of microbial origin; flows of N to the abomasum were not reported. Assuming that N flow to the abomasum approximated N intake, that microbial CP is 80 percent true protein that is 80 percent digestible (National Research Council, 1989), and that undegraded feed proteins are 80 percent digestible (National Research Council, 1989) leads to a conversion of CP to ADP of about 71 percent; adoption of the slightly higher value of 75 percent from Agricultural Research Council (1980) leads to better agreement with literature data. The BV and conversions of ADP to CP for calves fed starter and milk or starter and milk replacer are assumed to be additive on the basis of the relative amounts of CP supplied by starter and milk (or milk replacer).

Examples of requirements for ADP and CP for calves fed milk or milk replacer only, milk replacer plus starter, veal calves, and weaned (ruminant) calves are found in Tables 10-1, 10-2, 10-3, and 10-4, respectively.

## MINERAL AND VITAMIN REQUIREMENTS OF CALVES

Detailed information on the specific roles of mineral elements and vitamins in the nutrition and metabolism of dairy cattle is presented in Chapters 6 and 7. Since the last edition (National Research Council, 1989), there have been few definitive studies of and few problems associated with the field application of the previous recommendations that warrant making major changes in recommendations for most mineral elements or vitamins in diets of young calves. Changes that have been made in the recommendations are discussed below.

### *Minerals*

The recommended dietary concentrations of mineral elements and vitamins are shown in Table 10-6. For calcium and phosphorus recommended concentrations in milk-replacer diets were increased compared with those

TABLE 10-6 Mineral and Vitamin Concentrations Recommended for Diets of Young Calves, Compared with Average for Fresh Whole Milk (DM basis)

| Nutrient[a] | Milk Replacer[b] | Starter Feed | Grower Feed | Whole Milk |
|---|---|---|---|---|
| *Minerals* | | | | |
| Ca (%) | 1.00 | 0.70 | 0.60 | 0.95 |
| P (%) | 0.70 | 0.45 | 0.40 | 0.76 |
| Mg (%) | 0.07 | 0.10 | 0.10 | 0.10 |
| Na (%) | 0.40 | 0.15 | 0.14 | 0.38 |
| K (%) | 0.65 | 0.65 | 0.65 | 1.12 |
| Cl (%) | 0.25 | 0.20 | 0.20 | 0.92 |
| S (%) | 0.29 | 0.20 | 0.20 | 0.32 |
| Fe (mg/kg) | 100[c] | 50 | 50 | 3.0 |
| Mn (mg/kg) | 40 | 40 | 40 | 0.2–0.4 |
| Zn (mg/kg) | 40 | 40 | 40 | 15–38 |
| Cu (mg/kg) | 10 | 10 | 10 | 0.1–1.1 |
| I (mg/kg) | 0.50 | 0.25 | 0.25 | 0.1–0.2 |
| Co (mg/kg) | 0.11 | 0.10 | 0.10 | 0.004–0.008 |
| Se (mg/kg) | 0.30 | 0.30 | 0.30 | 0.02–0.15 |
| *Vitamins* | | | | |
| A (IU/kg of DM) | 9,000 | 4,000 | 4,000 | 11,500 |
| D (IU/kg of DM) | 600 | 600 | 600 | 307 |
| E (IU/kg of DM) | 50 | 25 | 25 | 8 |

[a] B-complex vitamins are necessary only in milk-replacer diets. Required concentrations (mg/kg of DM): thiamin, 6.5; riboflavin, 6.5; pyridoxine, 6.5; pantothenic acid, 13.0; niacin, 10.0; biotin, 0.1; folic acid, 0.5; $B_{12}$, 0.07; choline, 1,000.

[b] Required concentrations specified for milk replacer fed at 0.53 kg of DM per day to 45-kg calf. Assuming ME content of 4.75 Mcal/kg, this amount of milk replacer would provide energy-allowable growth of 0.3 kg/d. Concentrations of minerals and vitamins specified will provide adequate daily amounts of minerals and vitamins as defined in Chapters 6 and 7 and in text of this chapter. User is cautioned that feeding larger or smaller amounts of milk replacer, or same amount of milk replacer to larger or smaller calf, changes expected growth and, consequently, requirements for many vitamins and minerals.

[c] For veal calves, decrease to less than 50 mg/kg of DM.

of National Research Council (1989), from 0.7 to 1.0 percent for calcium and from 0.6 to 0.7 percent for phosphorus. Recommended concentrations are closer to those found in whole milk (see Table 10-6). Previous calcium recommendations were made considering a fat content in milk replacer of 10 percent, whereas a majority of commercial milk replacers today contain fat at 18–22 percent. Higher dietary fat results in increased loss of calcium in the feces because of soap formation between calcium and long-chain fatty acids in the gut (Toullec et al., 1980).

The recommended content of sodium in milk replacer was increased from 0.10 to 0.40 percent and from 0.20 to 0.25 percent for chloride (Table 10-6). The committee is unaware of any problems in young calves posed by the previous recommendations for sodium and chloride, but whole milk and most milk replacers that contain milk products usually are substantially higher in sodium and chloride than even the new recommendations, thus making practical deficiencies unlikely. As stated earlier, the solids content of milk replacers should be maintained less than 20 percent and free drinking water should be available to avoid problems with excessive intakes of sodium and chloride.

The potassium requirement was left unchanged at 0.65 percent of DM for milk-replacer, starter, and grower diets. Weil et al. (1988) compared dietary potassium concentrations of 0.55, 0.84, 1.02, and 1.32 percent of DM for calves from 4 to 14 wk of age. They detected no differences in feed intake, average daily gain, or mineral status among treatments. In a second trial, Weil et al. (1988) compared dietary potassium concentrations of 0.34 and 0.58 percent for calves from 6 to 14 wk of age. Feed intake and live weight gain were greater for calves fed 0.58 percent potassium. The authors concluded that potassium requirement of growing dairy calves was "within the range of 0.34 to 0.58 percent," but no concentrations between 0.58 and 0.84 percent were tested. Consequently, the subcommittee concluded that there was insufficient evidence to decrease the requirement from the current value of 0.65 percent of DM.

Requirements for most of the trace minerals are unchanged from the previous edition of *Nutrient Requirements of Dairy Cattle* (National Research Council, 1989). The required concentrations of iodine were increased from 0.25 mg/kg to 0.50 mg/kg on the basis of information described in Chapter 6, although, as in the situation with sodium and chloride, no indication of deficiency has been noted under practical conditions. The content of cobalt was increased slightly, from 0.10 to 0.11 mg/kg, to be consistent with requirements for other classes of cattle (Chapter 6). Recommended contents of most macromineral elements in milk replacer and starters are close to those of whole milk, whereas recommendations for many of the trace mineral elements are higher than those found in milk, to prevent deficiencies. Caution should be exercised in making drastic changes in dietary concentrations of a specific mineral element without being aware of the possible effects of such changes on the status of other mineral elements (McDowell, 1992).

### *Vitamins*

#### VITAMIN A

The subcommittee has markedly increased requirements for vitamin A in all classes of dairy cattle for reasons discussed in Chapter 7. The requirement for vitamin A in calves was increased from 42.4 (National Research Council, 1989) to 110 IU/kg of LW in the present edition. Eaton et al. (1972) suggested, on the basis of changes in cerebrospinal fluid pressure, that the requirement for vitamin A should be 96.7 IU/kg of LW for growing Holstein calves. In the *Nutrient Requirements of Dairy Cattle* (National Research Council, 1989), these data were discussed, but the requirement was not increased; the subcommittee stated that "if substantial evidence for a higher vitamin A requirement is forthcoming, the requirement should be raised." Data from Swanson et al. (2000) demonstrated that an intake of about 134 IU/kg of LW (9,000 IU/kg of DM) maintained liver vitamin A stores in male Holstein calves fed milk replacer, whereas 93 IU/kg or less resulted in decreases in liver concentrations of vitamin A. Calves in that study had received adequate colostrum after birth, were healthy, and were housed under nonstressful environmental conditions throughout the study. No clinical measures were affected in that study, even at vitamin A intake (34 IU/kg of LW) less than the previous requirement. However, the liver concentration of vitamin A is believed to be a much more sensitive indicator of vitamin A status than measures used previously to establish requirements. The new requirement was set to be the same as for other classes of cattle and is between the estimates made by Eaton et al. (1972) and Swanson et al. (2000). Required concentrations have been increased to 9,000 IU/kg of DM for milk replacer and 4,000 IU/kg of DM for starter and grower diets in the present edition. The concentration recommended here for starter or grower feeds will provide required amounts of vitamin A for weaned calves weighing less than 100 kg and gaining 400–900 g/d (Table 10-4).

The presumed safe limit for vitamin A is 66,000 IU/kg of dietary DM for lactating and nonlactating cattle (National Research Council, 1987), but safe limits specifically for young calves have not been established. Supplementation levels of several times the requirement established in the present edition are common in commercial milk replacers (Tomkins and Jaster, 1991). Data to firmly support such a practice are not available. Eicher et al. (1994) found improved fecal consistency in calves fed milk replacer that contained vitamin A at 87,000 IU/kg, with no effect on vitamin E status. In contrast, several studies have reported adverse effects of high vitamin A on vitamin E status and on other measures of calf health and growth (see Nonnecke et al., 1999). Calves fed a milk replacer containing vitamin A at 44,000 IU/kg of DM rapidly accumulated vitamin A in liver but showed no signs of toxicity during 28 days of feeding (Swanson et al., 2000). Supplementation with vitamin A in amounts greater than recommended in the present edition cannot be justified on the basis of available data. In particular, caution should be observed in formulation of milk replacers for veal calves and for replacement calves in accelerated-growth schemes to avoid potential problems with excessive vitamin A intake.

#### VITAMIN E

The requirement for vitamin E for calves continues to be debated. Requirements for vitamin E were increased substantially for lactating and dry cows in the present edition (Chapter 7). The subcommittee has increased the requirement for vitamin E for calves by 25 percent, from 40 IU/kg of dietary DM to 50 IU/kg. The decision to increase the vitamin E requirement represents a compromise until more-definitive data are available. The increase is based on two main factors. First, although 40 IU/kg of DM is adequate to prevent classic signs of deficiency, such as muscular dystrophy or retardation of growth of calves in controlled systems, calves under conditions of stress more typical in practice might require higher intakes of vitamin E to augment the immune system. Vitamin E supplementation improved immune-system responses, as measured by lymphocyte stimulation indexes, IgM concentrations, serum cortisol concentrations, and antibody response to a booster vaccine (Reddy et al., 1986, 1987b). Indicators of cell-membrane damage (serum creatine kinase, glutamic oxalacetic transaminase, and lactic acid dehydrogenase) suggested that Vitamin E supplementation protected membranes from oxidative damage (Reddy et al., 1986, 1987b). Vitamin E functions as an antioxidant and interacts with selenium to maintain the structural integrity of tissues (Combs, 1992; McDowell, 1992).

Reddy et al. (1987a) suggested—on the basis of a study in which calves were supplemented with 125, 250, or 500 IU of vitamin E per day—that the requirement was about 2.4 IU/kg of body weight. However, no supplementation levels lower than 125 IU/d were tested, and numbers of animals were insufficient to determine clinical responses. The subcommittee felt that, in the absence of large-scale dose-response studies to determine clinical responses, such a large increase was not justified. Furthermore, increased requirements for dry cows should increase concentrations of vitamin E in colostrum (Quigley and Drewry, 1998), which could provide more vitamin E to calves than was consumed by calves in the Kansas State University studies.

Second, the relationship of vitamin E with other dietary nutrients must be considered. For the young calf, dietary vitamin E should be balanced with the content of essential fatty acids (1.5–2.5 IU of vitamin E per gram of linoleic acid; Stobo, 1983) to prevent oxidative stress from increased intake of polyunsaturated fatty acids, as in young nonruminant animals. With typical daily intakes of 10–15 g of linoleic acid from milk replacers, 15–38 IU of vitamin E daily would be necessary, according to guidelines of Stobo (1983). To supply adequate vitamin E to meet this guideline for a calf fed 600 g of milk-replacer DM daily, vitamin E content would need to be 25–63 IU/kg of DM.

Some evidence suggests that increased vitamin A in the diet decreases the bioavailability of vitamin E (see Nonnecke et al., 1999). Consequently, the moderate increase in the vitamin E requirement also is justified because of the substantially increased vitamin A requirement. Diarrhea and gut infections decrease fat digestion and hence lower the absorption of the fat-soluble vitamins A, D, and E. Given the widespread occurrence of digestive disturbances in young calves before weaning, the increases in recommendations for both vitamin A and vitamin E should be beneficial in practical situations. The subcommittee recognizes that the requirement for vitamin E might need to be adjusted in future editions if data from large-scale dose-response studies become available.

#### VITAMIN D AND WATER-SOLUBLE VITAMINS

Requirements for vitamin D were not changed from the 1989 edition (Table 10-6). Water-soluble vitamins must be included in the milk-replacer diet of calves (see Table 10-6). Once the calf is weaned to dry feed, there is no evidence that these vitamins need to be supplemented to the diet, inasmuch as the microorganisms in the digestive tract synthesize ample amounts to meet the needs of the calf.

## FEED-COMPOSITION DATA WITH APPLICATION TO DIET FORMULATIONS FOR CALVES

Values for digestible energy and metabolizable energy for feedstuffs for calves in the National Research Council (1989) are realistic compared with known gross energy and digestibility data and agree closely with values assigned by other sources. However, as pointed out earlier in this chapter, the $NE_M$ and $NE_G$ values for milk, milk byproducts, and milk replacers given in the 1989 edition were too low according to reported efficiencies of use of ME by young milk-fed calves (see chapter 9 in Davis and Drackley, 1998). The problem arose from the inappropriate use of the equations derived by Garrett (1980) from growth studies with feedlot cattle to derive the net energy of liquid diets for nonruminant calves. A different approach has been taken in the present edition to establish the net energy values for calf diets.

Gross energy (GE) values have been calculated from data on composition and heat of combustion. For milk and milk-derived ingredients used in milk replacers,

$$\text{GE (Mcal/kg)} = 0.057\ \text{CP\%} + 0.092\ \text{fat\%} + 0.0395\ \text{lactose\%}, \qquad (10\text{-}5)$$

where lactose was calculated as 100 − CP% − fat% − ash%; all components are expressed on a DM basis. For whole milk, milk replacers, and milk-derived ingredients, DE was calculated as 0.97 GE. For all milk and milk products, including milk replacers, ME was calculated as 0.96 DE. Values calculated by these methods agree closely with those in the previous edition of this publication (National Research Council, 1989).

The $NE_M$ values for milk , milk-derived ingredients, and milk replacers is calculated as 0.86 ME, consistent with the $NE_M$ requirements discussed earlier. This is similar to the value of 0.85 used by the Agricultural Research Council (1980). The approach used to derive values for $NE_G$ for milk and milk-derived ingredients is based on the relationship between the metabolizability (q) of the diet (ME/GE) and the efficiency of use of ME for maintenance and gain (Agricultural Research Council, 1980). The $NE_G$ values for milk-based diets can then be estimated as follows (Agricultural Research Council, 1980):

$$NE_G = (0.38q + 0.337)\ \text{ME} \qquad (10\text{-}6)$$

Values for q have been computed and are included in Table 10-7, which provides composition data for ingredients used in milk replacers. The values for $NE_M$ and $NE_G$ calculated by these methods agree well with efficiencies of use of ME of 80 and 69 percent for maintenance and gain, respectively, determined by others (Roy, 1980; Toullec, 1989).

A slightly different procedure was used to calculate $NE_M$ and $NE_G$ values for ingredients used in starter and grower diets. For all nonmilk ingredients,

$$\text{GE (Mcal/kg)} = 0.057\ \text{CP\%} + 0.094\ \text{ether extract (EE)\%} + 0.0415\ \text{carbohydrate\%} \qquad (10\text{-}7)$$

where carbohydrate was calculated as 100 − CP% − fat% − ash%. The DE values were calculated as the sum of the products of digestible CP, EE, and carbohydrates multiplied by their heats of combustion; this is the approach described in Chapter 2 to calculate energy values for feeds fed to other classes of dairy cattle in this edition. Values for ME were calculated with the approach in the previous edition (National Research Council, 1989), except that the equation was corrected to reflect increased efficiency of use of fat:

TABLE 10-7 Energy, Protein, Calcium, and Phosphorus Concentrations in Feedstuffs Commonly Used in Formulation of Milk Replacers for Young Calves[a]

| Feed | International Feed Number | DM (%) | GE (Mcal/kg of DM) | DE (Mcal/kg of DM) | ME (Mcal/kg of DM) | ME/GE (q) | $NE_M$ (Mcal/kg of DM) | $NE_G$ (Mcal/kg of DM) | CP (% of DM) | EE (% of DM) | Ca (% of DM) | P (% of DM) | Ash (% of DM) |
|---|---|---|---|---|---|---|---|---|---|---|---|---|---|
| Whole milk | 5-01-168 | 12.5 | 5.76 | 5.59 | 5.37 | 0.93 | 4.62 | 3.70 | 25.4 | 30.8 | 1.00 | 0.75 | 6.3 |
| Skim milk, fresh | 5-01-170 | 10 | 4.31 | 4.19 | 4.02 | 0.93 | 3.46 | 2.77 | 35.5 | 0.3 | 1.35 | 1.02 | 6.9 |
| Skim milk, powder | 5-01-175 | 94 | 4.38 | 4.25 | 4.08 | 0.93 | 3.51 | 2.82 | 37.4 | 1.0 | 1.29 | 1.08 | 6.9 |
| Whey-powder | 4-01-182 | 93 | 3.92 | 3.80 | 3.65 | 0.93 | 3.14 | 2.52 | 13.5 | 1.0 | 0.76 | 0.68 | 8.1 |
| Whey protein concentrate | — | 93 | 4.48 | 4.35 | 4.17 | 0.93 | 3.59 | 2.88 | 37.1 | 2.2 | 0.54 | 0.60 | 6.0 |
| Whey, fresh | 4-08-134 | 7 | 3.89 | 3.78 | 3.62 | 0.93 | 3.12 | 2.50 | 14.2 | 0.7 | 0.73 | 0.65 | 8.7 |
| Whey, delactosed | 4-01-186 | 93 | 3.65 | 3.54 | 3.40 | 0.93 | 2.92 | 2.34 | 17.9 | 0.7 | 1.71 | 1.12 | 16.5 |
| Whey permeate | — | 98 | 3.66 | 3.55 | 3.41 | 0.93 | 2.93 | 2.35 | 3.7 | 0 | 1.77 | 0.97 | 9.0 |
| Casein | 5-01-162 | 91 | 5.45 | 5.29 | 5.08 | 0.93 | 4.37 | 3.50 | 92.7 | 0.7 | 0.40 | 0.35 | 4.0 |

[a]Data from NRC (1989); Toullec (1989); Tomkins and Jaster (1991). Calculations are described in text.

$$ME = (1.01 \times DE - 0.45) + 0.0046\,(EE - 3) \qquad (10\text{-}8)$$

where ME and DE are Mcal/kg and EE is percent of dietary DM. These ME values are analogous to ME values at maintenance for older cattle (Chapter 2) and are more consistent with known efficiencies of conversion of DE to ME, given that methane production in young calves is extremely low (Gonzlalez-Jimenez and Blaxter, 1962; Holmes and Davey, 1976). Values for $NE_M$ and $NE_G$ were calculated as described in the section on energy requirements earlier in this chapter. For $NE_M$ and $NE_G$, ME as calculated above was multiplied by the respective efficiencies of 0.75 for maintenance and 0.57 for gain. These efficiencies are similar to those estimated by others from the metabolizability (q) of ingredients. For example, Agricultural Research Council (1980) calculated $NE_M$ as $(0.287q + 0.554)ME$ and $NE_G$ as $(0.78q + 0.006)ME$. For a calf starter with $q = 0.70$, efficiencies for maintenance and gain would be 75 and 55 percent when calculated with the Agricultural Research Council equations.

Table 10-8 presents composition data on examples of three typical milk replacers, a starter diet, and a grower diet for calves. The values presented for $NE_M$ and $NE_G$ content are considerably higher for all feeds than those calculated with the previous methods (National Research Council, 1989). The computer model automatically calculates ME, $NE_M$, and $NE_G$ concentrations for feeds used for young calves. Users are cautioned that the requirements and feed values are designed to be used together. Use of $NE_M$ and $NE_G$ values from previous editions with the present growth model, or vice versa, will result in erroneous predictions.

Values for total digestible nutrients (TDN) are not given for calf requirements or feeds in this edition. If desired, TDN can be calculated as described for feeds for other classes of cattle (see Chapter 2). For milk, milk replacer, and milk ingredients,

$$TDN = 0.93\,CP + (EE \times 2.25) + 0.98\,(100 - CP - EE - Ash) - 7 \qquad (10\text{-}9)$$

## OTHER ASPECTS OF CALF NUTRITION

### *Fetal Nutrition*

Although severe undernutrition can impair normal fetal development (National Research Council, 1968), the developing fetal calf is afforded a high priority for maternal nutrients. Moderate underfeeding of either protein or energy did not result in measurable changes in calf birth weight, viability, or health (Davis and Drackley, 1998; Quigley and Drewry, 1998). Prolonged restriction of protein or energy during gestation decreased thermogenic abilities of beef calves at birth (Carstens et al., 1987; Ridder et al., 1991).

Maternal deficiencies of phosphorus, manganese, cobalt, copper, zinc, and selenium can result in deficiencies in the fetus and newborn calf (National Research Council, 1968). The fetus has the ability to concentrate some of these minerals, particularly copper (Hidiroglou and Knipfel, 1981) and selenium (Van Saun et al., 1989a), providing some protection against marginal deficiencies in the mother. Selenium supplementation of pregnant cows increased selenium reserves in the newborn calves (Abdelrahman and Kincaid, 1995). Placental transfer of vitamin E to the developing fetus is low, although the fetal calf appears to have some ability to concentrate vitamin E from the dam (Van Saun et al., 1989b). The calf is born with a low vitamin E status and is highly dependent on intake of colostrum and then milk or milk replacer to obtain needed vitamin E during early postnatal life. If diets for pregnant cows are balanced to meet recommendations for pregnancy and maternal growth (see Chapters 6 and 7), as well as for optimal transition success (see Chapter 9), nutrient supply should be adequate for normal growth and development

TABLE 10-8 Energy, Protein, Fiber, and Mineral Composition of Three Milk Replacers (MR), a Starter Feed, and a Grower Feed for Young Calves

| Feed | GE[a] (Mcal/kg DM) | DE[a] (Mcal/kg of DM) | ME[a] (Mcal/kg of DM) | $NE_M$ (Mcal/kg of DM) | $NE_G$ (Mcal/kg of DM) | CP (%) | EE (%) | ADF (%) | NDF (%) | Ca (%) | P (%) |
|---|---|---|---|---|---|---|---|---|---|---|---|
| MR-1 | 4.61 | 4.47 | 4.29 | 3.69[b] | 2.96[c] | 22 | 10 | — | — | 1.0 | 0.70 |
| MR-2 | 5.10 | 4.95 | 4.75 | 4.09[b] | 3.28[c] | 20 | 20 | — | — | 1.0 | 0.70 |
| MR-3 | 5.07 | 4.91 | 4.72 | 4.06[b] | 3.26[c] | 18 | 20 | — | — | 1.0 | 0.70 |
| Starter | 4.49 | 3.69 | 3.28 | 2.46[d] | 1.78[e] | 18 | 3 | 11.6 | 12.8 | 0.7 | 0.45 |
| Grower | 4.36 | 3.65 | 3.24 | 2.43[d] | 1.61[e] | 16 | 3 | 8.0 | 18.0 | 0.6 | 0.40 |

[a]Energy values calculated as follows:
Gross energy (GE) is calculated from composition and heat of combustion. For milk replacers, GE (kcal/kg) = 0.057 CP + 0.092 fat + 0.0395 lactose. For starter and grower, GE (kcal/kg) = 0.057 CP + 0.092 EE + 0.0415 carbohydrate.
For MR, digestible energy (DE) = 0.97 GE. For starter and grower, DE is calculated as sum of digestible protein, fat, and carbohydrates, each multiplied by heat of combustion.
For MR, metabolizable energy (ME) calculated as 0.93 GE (ME/GE of whole milk has been measured at 0.93; Roy, 1980). For starter and grower feeds, ME = (1.01 × DE − 0.45) + (0.0046EE − 3) (see text and Chapter 2).
[b]$NE_M$ = 0.86 ME. See text for details.
[c]$NE_G$ = (0.38q + 0.337) × ME. Based on q of 0.93 yielding an efficiency of 0.69 for ME use (ARC, 1980).
[d]$NE_M$ = ME × 0.75.
[e]$NE_G$ = ME × 0.57.

of the fetal calf (Davis and Drackley, 1998; Quigley and Drewry, 1998).

### *Colostrum*

Calves are born with negligible circulating concentrations of immunoglobulins (McCoy et al., 1970). Early provision of high-quality colostrum in amounts sufficient to provide at least 100 g of IgG is critical to calf survival and well-being (Davis and Drackley, 1998; Quigley and Drewry, 1998). The immunoglobulin content of colostrum is highly variable (Pritchett et al., 1991); therefore, to maximize the likelihood of obtaining sufficient IgG, it is recommended that calves be fed at least 3 L of colostrum from multiparous cows within an hour after birth. Holstein calves can be administered as much as 3.8 L of colostrum in a single feeding after birth to ensure delivery of sufficient IgG (Besser et al., 1991; Hopkins and Quigley, 1997).

In addition to disease protection, early provision of colostrum is important as a source of nutrients (Davis and Drackley, 1998; Quigley and Drewry, 1998). Because supplies of endogenous fuels are exhausted within hours without feed (Okamato et al., 1986; Rowan, 1992), the carbohydrate, fat, and protein in colostrum are essential as fuels for the newborn. Most of the essential minerals and vitamins are substantially more concentrated in colostrum than in milk (Foley and Otterby, 1978). Consumption of adequate amounts of colostrum by the newborn calf, followed by consumption of milk or milk replacer that is adequate in mineral and vitamin content, is important to compensate for any maternal inadequacies during gestation. Increasing evidence in calves and other species indicates that colostrum also provides a number of hormones and growth factors necessary to stimulate growth and development of the digestive tract and other organ systems (Hammon and Blum, 1998).

Commercial products containing immunoglobulins may be useful to supplement poor-quality colostrum (Garry et al., 1996; Morin et al., 1997; Arthington et al., 2000). Other products are designed to be injected to increase serum immunoglobulins in calves (Quigley and Welborn, 1996). At present, none of the commercially available supplements or substitutes can completely replace colostrum in providing passive immunity to calves (Arthington et al., 2000). High-quality colostrum should be provided whenever possible; supplements are of little additional value when sufficient amounts of high-quality colostrum are administered (Hopkins and Quigley, 1997). Development of products that can deliver sufficient biologically active immunoglobulins to the newborn calf might be increasingly important for use in biosecurity programs to control contagious diseases, such as Johne's disease, in which it would be desirable to avoid the feeding of any colostrum or whole milk to calves. Although the nutritional aspects of colostrum probably could be replaced by a properly formulated milk replacer, the consequences of the absence of the growth factors and hormones normally consumed in colostrum are not known.

### *Water and Electrolytes*

Water is the most important nutrient and, although essential, is often overlooked. Too often, it is assumed that if a calf is being fed a liquid diet, its needs for water will be satisfied. Fresh water, in addition to water consumed as part of the diet, is essential for optimal growth and consumption of dry feed (Leaver and Yarrow, 1972; Kertz et al., 1984).

Aside from constituting 70–75 percent of the weight of the calf, water plays important roles as a solvent for nutrients, a thermoregulator, and an osmoregulator (Davis and Drackley, 1998). Calves, because of their greater propensity to develop digestive disturbances (diarrhea), experience greater problems with water balance than do older animals.

During incidents of diarrhea, 10–12 percent of body weight can be lost as water. The water loss in feces carries with it major losses of the electrolytes sodium, chloride, and potassium (Lewis and Phillips, 1978; Phillips, 1985). Such losses of water and electrolytes result in severe dehydration and electrolyte imbalances, which if not rapidly corrected will result in death. In fact most deaths associated with diarrhea occur from these phenomena rather than directly from infectious agents (Booth and Naylor, 1987). Recent evidence indicates that electrolyte disturbances are more important than dehydration itself in causing death from diarrhea (Walker et al., 1998).

At the first signs of diarrhea, a calf should be started on oral rehydration (Davis and Drackley, 1998). Current information suggests that the calf should continue to receive a portion of, if not all, its regular feeding of milk or milk replacer with the oral electrolyte product (McGuirk, 1992; Garthwaite et al., 1994) as long as it is alert and willing to drink. Calves that are severely dehydrated, recumbent, or acidemic will require intravenous fluid therapy for recovery.

### *Milk Replacers*

Milk replacers are used on a majority of dairy farms in the United States (Heinrichs et al., 1995). Substantial changes in milk-replacer formulation have occurred since the last edition of this publication (National Research Council, 1989). Increases in market prices for dried skim milk, coupled with development of low-temperature ultrafiltration techniques for preparation of high-quality whey protein concentrates, have led to the almost complete replacement of dried skim milk with whey-derived products (Davis and Drackley, 1998). Milk-replacer formulations generally are classified as all-milk protein or as alternative protein. Milk replacers of all-milk protein contain whey protein concentrate, dried whey, and delactosed whey as protein sources. Many alternative-protein formulations are available, in which portions of the milk proteins (typically 50 percent) are replaced with lower-cost ingredients, such as soy protein concentrate, soy protein isolates, animal plasma or whole-blood proteins, and modified wheat gluten (Davis and Drackley, 1998). Examples of formulations and a review of recent research can be found in chapter 14 of Davis and Drackley (1998). Aspects of milk replacer use also have been reviewed by Heinrichs (1994, 1995).

The ability of these protein sources to supply an adequate amount and profile of amino acids for growth of preruminant calves depends on the amino acid profile of the protein, the quality of the manufacturing process, and the ability of the calf to digest the protein. High temperatures during drying can damage proteins and lessen their biologic value (Wilson and Wheelock, 1972). Furthermore, antinutritional factors present in some protein sources can decrease efficiency of amino acid use (Huisman, 1989; Lallès, 1993). Whey protein concentrate is digested and utilized as least as well as skim milk protein by young calves (Terosky et al., 1997; Lammers et al., 1998).

The proteolytic digestive system of the young calf is immature at birth, and until the age of about 3 weeks the calf is less able to digest most nonmilk proteins (Toullec and Guilloteau, 1989). Therefore, for optimal growth during the first 3 weeks of life, it is recommended that milk replacers containing only milk proteins be used. Older calves are able to use formulations that contain nonmilk proteins.

Milk replacers typically contain tallow, choice white grease, or lard as a fat source. The degree of homogenization is critical for high digestibility (Raven, 1970). Emulsifiers, such as lecithin and monoglycerides, often are added to enhance mixing characteristics and fat digestibility. In general, vegetable oils and fat sources that contain large amounts of free fatty acids are poorly used by calves (Jenkins et al., 1985). Research data on optimal concentrations of fat in milk replacers are conflicting, with little definitive evidence that a fat content beyond 10–12 percent is needed, at least in moderate environments (Heinrichs, 1995).

### *Feed Additives*

A variety of feed additives have been examined for inclusion in milk replacers or dry feeds (Heinrichs, 1993). The addition of medications to milk replacers in the US is regulated by the Food and Drug Administration. Antibiotics such as oxytetracycline and neomycin are widely used in milk replacers (Heinrichs et al., 1995). Antibiotics consistently improve growth rates and feed efficiency and decrease incidence and severity of scouring of calves (Morrill et al., 1977; Quigley et al., 1997a), although the mode of action still is poorly understood. Benefits of antibiotic inclusion may be more evident for calves raised intensively in large numbers, for shipped-in calves originating from different farms, and for calves raised under conditions of stress (Morrill et al., 1977; Morrill et al., 1995; Davis and Drackley, 1998).

Lasalocid and decoquinate added to feeds are effective in control of coccidiosis (Hoblet et al., 1989; Heinrichs et al., 1990; Heinrichs and Bush, 1991; Eicher-Pruiett et al., 1992; Quigley et al., 1997b). Supplementation in calf starter requires adequate feed intake to achieve effective dosages, but infection with coccidia often occurs before starter intake is sufficient (Quigley et al., 1997b). Bacterial probiotic products have shown some benefit in improving calf health and performance (Jenny et al., 1991; Higginbotham and Bath, 1993; Morrill et al., 1995; Abe et al., 1995; Cruywagen et al., 1996) although responses have been variable and inconsistent (Morrill et al., 1977). Experimental results from additions of fungal (Beharka et al., 1991) or yeast (Quigley et al., 1992) culture products to starter diets have been inconclusive.

Sodium bicarbonate increased starter intake and growth of young calves in one study (Curnick et al., 1983) but did not affect intake or calf performance in another study (Quigley et al., 1992).

*Practical Feeding Considerations*

As mentioned in the introduction to this chapter, female calves in the United States destined for herd replacements should be fed restricted amounts of milk or milk replacer (typically 8–10 percent of birth weight) to encourage early consumption of calf starter (National Research Council, 1989). Development of early starter intake is inversely proportional to the amount of liquid fed (Hodgson, 1971). Growth rates of young calves during the liquid feeding period thus are much lower than the maximal growth rates of calves (Khouri and Pickering, 1968; Hodgson, 1971), and feed efficiency is lower than that in the young of other farm animals that consume milk ad libitum (Khouri and Pickering, 1968; Davis and Drackley, 1998). Nevertheless, restricted liquid feeding encourages earlier starter intake and ruminal development, which in turn allows for earlier weaning and more economic body weight gains. Ad libitum or increased liquid feeding programs researched to date have resulted in greater growth rates and improved feed efficiency during the liquid feeding period, but lower consumption of dry feed and variable effects on calf health (Khouri and Pickering, 1968; Hodgson, 1971; Huber et al., 1984; Nocek and Braund, 1986; Richard et al., 1988). Methods to capitalize on the early growth potential are being researched in the context of accelerated rearing programs for heifers that encompass all stages of growth from birth to first calving. However, these programs are still under development and evaluation, and cannot yet be recommended at this time.

During the early liquid feeding period, growth of calves fed milk or milk replacer is directly proportional to the amount of liquid provided (Khouri and Pickering, 1968; Hodgson, 1971; Huber et al., 1984). In contrast, in restricted liquid feeding programs, growth rates are directly proportional to the amount of calf starter consumed (Kertz et al., 1979, 1984). Users should be aware that typical milk replacers contain 10–20 percent less energy than comparable volumes of whole milk because of the lower fat content of milk replacers. A 40-kg calf fed milk replacer at 9 percent of body weight would consume 454 g of DM. If the milk replacer contains ME at 4.7 Mcal/kg of DM, the calf would consume enough energy for maintenance and a body weight gain of 234 g/d under thermoneutral conditions. According to the model presented in this edition, feeding the same volume of whole milk would support a gain of 331 g/d. In contrast, if the same calf is housed at 20°C below its lower critical temperature, 454 g/d of milk replacer powder is insufficient even for maintenance. Increasing evidence suggests that these low feeding rates also are inadequate to support optimal health and function of the immune system, especially under adverse environmental conditions (Williams et al., 1981; Griebel et al., 1987; Pollock et al., 1993, 1994).

High intakes of milk or milk replacer are important for veal production. The effects of increasing intake of whole milk and milk replacer for a 40-kg calf are illustrated in Figure 10-1. Note that the difference in growth performance predicted between whole milk and milk replacer fed at equal amounts is accounted for entirely by the 13 percent greater ME content of whole-milk solids versus the milk replacer solids. Gains predicted here agree closely with literature studies with high rates of milk feeding (Khouri and Pickering, 1968; Hodgson, 1971).

Large-breed calves can be weaned easily when consuming at least 0.68 kg of a good-quality starter daily for 3

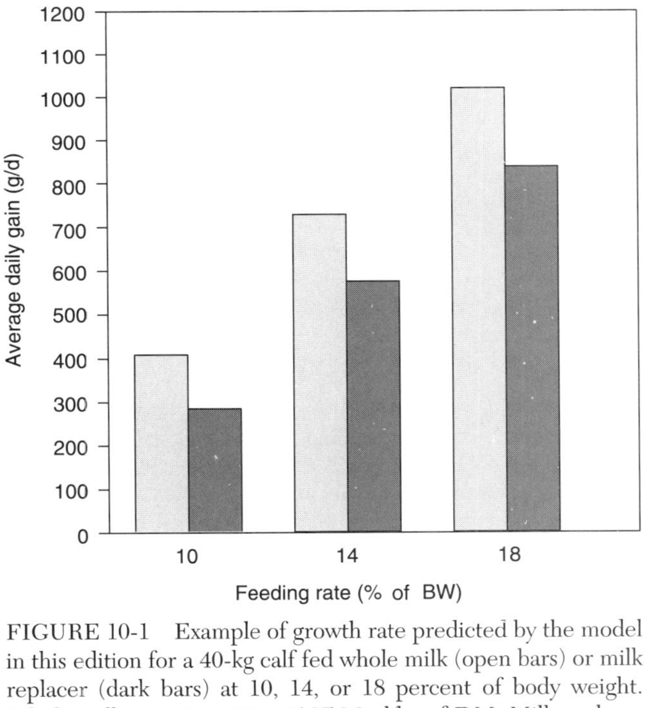


FIGURE 10-1 Example of growth rate predicted by the model in this edition for a 40-kg calf fed whole milk (open bars) or milk replacer (dark bars) at 10, 14, or 18 percent of body weight. Whole milk contains ME at 5.37 Mcal/kg of DM. Milk replacer contains ME at 4.75 Mcal/kg of DM and is assumed to be reconstituted to 12.5 percent solids, similar to total solids content of whole milk.

consecutive days. Under good management, with restricted milk or milk replacer feeding this can occur as early as the age of 4 weeks (Kertz et al., 1979, 1984). More aggressive milk-feeding programs will delay development of starter intake and weaning age (Hodgson, 1971; Huber et al., 1984). Other factors important for early development of dry-feed intake include free access to supplemental water; provision of palatable starter feeds (generally of coarse texture rather than finely ground); keeping feeds fresh, dry, and free of mold; and good health of calves. A major metabolic factor could be the establishment of stable ruminal fermentation with pH greater than 5.5 (Williams and Frost, 1992).

## REFERENCES

Abdelgadir, I. E. O., and J. L. Morrill. 1995. Effect of processing sorghum grain on dairy calf performance. J. Dairy Sci. 78:2040–2046.

Abdelgadir, I. E. O., J. L. Morrill, and J. J. Higgins. 1996a. Effect of roasted soybeans and corn on performance and ruminal and blood metabolites of dairy calves. J. Dairy Sci. 79:465–474.

Abdelgadir, I. E. O., J. L. Morrill, and J. J. Higgins. 1996b. Ruminal availabilities of protein and starch: effects on growth and ruminal and plasma metabolites of dairy calves. J. Dairy Sci. 79:283–290.

Abdelrahman, M. M., and R. L. Kincaid. 1995. Effect of selenium supplementation of cows on maternal transfer of selenium to fetal and newborn calves. J. Dairy Sci. 78:625–630.

Abe, F., N. Ishibashi, and S. Shimamura. 1995. Effect of administration of bifidobacteria and lactic acid bacteria to newborn calves and piglets. J. Dairy Sci. 78:2838–2846.

Agricultural Research Council. 1980. The Nutrient Requirements of Ruminant Livestock. Farnham Royal, Slough, England: Commonwealth Agricultural Bureaux.

Akayezu, J. M., J. G. Linn, D. E. Otterby, W. P. Hansen, and D. G. Johnson. 1994. Evaluation of calf starters containing different amounts of crude protein for growth of Holstein calves. J. Dairy Sci. 77:1882–1889.

Alexander, G., J.W. Bennett, and R.T. Gammell. 1975. Brown adipose tissue in the newborn calf (Bos Taurus). J. Physiol. 244: 223–234.

Anderson, K. L., T. G. Nagaraja, and J. L. Morrill. 1987a. Ruminal metabolic development in calves weaned conventionally or early. J. Dairy Sci. 70:1000–1005.

Anderson, K. L., T. G. Nagaraja, J. L. Morrill, T. B. Avery, S. J. Galitzer, and J. E. Boyer. 1987b. Ruminal microbial development in conventionally or early weaned calves. J. Anim. Sci. 64:1215–1226.

Arieli, A., J. W. Schrama, W. Van Der Hel, and M. W. A. Verstegen. 1995. Development of metabolic partitioning of energy in young calves. J. Dairy Sci. 78:1154–1162.

Arthington, J. D., M. B. Cattell, and J. D. Quigley, III. 2000. Effect of dietary IgG source (colostrum, serum, or milk-derived supplement) on the efficiency of Ig absorption in newborn Holstein calves. J. Dairy Sci. 83:1463–1467.

Beharka, A. A., T. G. Nagaraja, and J. L. Morrill. 1991. Performance and ruminal function development of young calves fed diets with Aspergillus oryzae fermentation extract. J. Dairy Sci. 74:4326–4336.

Beharka, A. A., T. G. Nagaraja, J. L. Morrill, G. A. Kennedy, and R. D. Klemm. 1998. Effects of form of the diet on anatomical, microbial, and fermentative development of the rumen of neonatal calves. J. Dairy Sci. 81:1946–1955.

Besser, T. E., C. C. Gay, and L. Pritchett. 1991. Comparison of three methods of feeding colostrum to dairy calves. J. Am. Vet. Med. Assoc. 198:419–422.

Blaxter, K. L. and H. H. Mitchell. 1948. The factorization of the protein requirements of ruminants and of the protein value of feeds, with particular reference to the significance of the metabolic fecal nitrogen. J. Anim. Sci. 7: 351–372.

Blaxter, K. L., and W. A. Wood. 1951. The nutrition of the young Ayrshire calf. 4. Some factors affecting the biological value of protein determined by nitrogen balance methods. Br. J. Nutr. 5:55–67.

Booth, A. J., and J. M. Naylor. 1987. Correction of metabolic acidosis in diarrheal calves by oral administration of electrolyte solutions with or without bicarbonate. J. Am. Vet. Med. Assoc. 191: 62–68.

Brownlee, A. 1956. The development of rumen papillae in cattle fed on different diets. Br. Vet. J. 112:369–375.

Carstens, G. E., D. E. Johnson, M. D. Holland, and K. G. Odde. 1987. Effects of prepartum protein nutrition and birth weight on basal metabolism in bovine neonates. J. Anim. Sci. 65:745–51.

Chester-Jones, H., D. M. Ziegler, and J. C. Meiske. 1991. Feeding whole or rolled corn with pelleted supplement to Holstein steers from weaning to 190 kilograms. J. Dairy Sci. 74:1765–1771.

Combs, G. F., Jr. 1992. The Vitamins: Fundamental Aspects in Nutrition and Health. San Deigo, CA: Academic Press, Inc.

Cruywagen, C. W., I. Jordaan, and L. Venter. 1996. Effect of Lactobacillus acidophilus supplementation of milk replacer on preweaning performance of calves. J. Dairy Sci. 79:483–486.

Cunningham, H. M., and G. J. Brisson. 1957. The endogenous urinary and metabolic fecal nitrogen excretions of newborn dairy calves. Can. J. Anim. Sci. 37:152–156.

Curnick, K. E., L. D. Muller, J. A. Rogers, T. J. Snyder, and T. F. Sweeney. 1983. Addition of sodium bicarbonate to calf starter rations varying in protein percent. J. Dairy Sci. 66:2149–2160.

Davis C. L., and J. H. Clark. 1981. Ruminant digestion and metabolism. Dev. Ind. Microbiol. 22:247–259.

Davis, C. L. and J. K. Drackley. 1998. The Development, Nutrition, and Management of the Young Calf. Iowa State University Press, Ames, Iowa.

Donnelly, P. E., and J. B. Hutton. 1976a. Effects of dietary protein and energy on the growth of Friesian bull calves. I. Food intake, growth, and protein requirements. N.Z. J. Agric. Res. 19: 289–297.

Donnelly, P. E., and J. B. Hutton. 1976b. Effects of dietary protein and energy on the growth of Friesian bull calves. II. Effects of level of feed intake and dietary protein content on body composition. N.Z. J. Agric. Res. 19: 409–414.

Eaton, H. D., J. E. Rousseau, Jr., R. C. Hall, Jr., H. I. Frier, and J. J. Lucas. 1972. Reevaluation of the minimum vitamin A requirement of Holstein male calves based upon elevated cerebrospinal fluid pressure. J. Dairy Sci. 55:232–237.

Eicher, S. D., J. L. Morrill, F. Blecha, C. G. Chitko-McKown, N. V. Anderson, and J. J. Higgins. 1994. Leukocyte functions of young dairy calves fed milk replacers supplemented with vitamins A and E. J. Dairy Sci. 77:1399–1407.

Eicher-Pruiett, S. D., J. L. Morrill, T. G. Nagaraja, J. J. Higgins, N. V. Anderson, and P. G. Reddy. 1992. Response of young dairy calves with lasalocid delivery varied in feed sources. J. Dairy Sci. 75:857–862.

Flatt, W. G., R. G. Warner, and J. K. Loosli. 1958. Influence of purified materials on the development of the ruminant stomach. J. Dairy Sci. 41:1593–1600.

Foley, J. A., and D. E. Otterby. 1978. Availability, storage, treatment, composition, and feeding value of surplus colostrum: a review. J. Dairy Sci. 61:1033–1060.

Garrett, W. N. 1980. Energy utilization by growing cattle as determined in 72 comparative slaughter experiments. In Energy Metabolism edited by L.E. Mount, EAAP Publ. No 26, 3–7. London: Butterworths.

Garry, F. B., R. Adams, M. B. Cattell, and R. P. Dinsmore. 1996. Comparison of passive immunoglobulin transfer to dairy calves fed colostrum or commercially available colostral supplement products. J. Am. Vet. Med. Assoc. 1:107–110.
Garthwaite, B. D., J. K. Drackley, G. C. McCoy, and E.H. Jaster. 1994. Whole milk and oral rehydration solution for calves with diarrhea of spontaneous origin. J. Dairy Sci. 77:835–843.
Gerrits, W. J. J., G. H. Tolman, J. W. Schrama, S. Tamminga, M. W. Bosch, and M.W.A. Verstegen. 1996. Effect of protein and protein-free energy intake on protein and fat deposition rates in preruminant calves of 80 to 240 kg live weight. J. Anim. Sci. 74:2129–2139.
Gonzalez-Jimenez, E., and K. L. Blaxter. 1962. The metabolism and thermal regulation of calves in the first month of life. Br. J. Nutr. 16:199–212.
Greenwood, R. H., J. L. Morrill, E. C. Titgemeyer, and G. A. Kennedy. 1997. A new method of measuring diet abrasion and its effect on the development of the forestomach. J. Dairy Sci. 80:2534–2541.
Griebel, P. J., M. Schoonderwoerd, and L. A. Babiuk. 1987. Ontogeny of the immune response: effect of protein energy malnutrition in neonatal calves. Can. J. Vet. Res. 51:428–435.
Hammon, H. M., and J. W. Blum. 1998. Metabolic and endocrine traits of neonatal calves are influenced by feeding colostrum for different durations or only milk replacer. J. Nutr. 128:624–632.
Heinrichs, A. J. 1993. Raising dairy replacements to meet the needs of the 21st century J. Dairy Sci. 76:3179–3187.
Heinrichs, A. J. 1994. Milk replacers for dairy calves—part I. Compend. Contin. Educ. Prac. Vet. 16:1605–1612.
Heinrichs, A. J. 1995. Milk replacers for dairy calves—part II. Compend. Contin. Educ. Prac. Vet. 17:433–438.
Heinrichs, A. J., and G. J. Bush. 1991. Evaluation of decoquinate or lasalocid against coccidiosis from natural exposure in neonatal dairy calves. J. Dairy Sci. 74:3223–3227.
Heinrichs, A. J., L. A. Swartz, T. R. Drake, and P. A. Travis. 1990. Influence of decoquinate fed to neonatal dairy calves on early and conventional weaning systems. J. Dairy Sci. 73:1851–1856.
Heinrichs, A. J., S. J. Wells, and W. C. Losinger. 1995. A study of the use of milk replacers for dairy calves in the United States. J. Dairy Sci. 78:2831–2837.
Hidiroglou, M., and J. E. Knipfel. 1981. Maternal-fetal relationships of copper, manganese, and sulfur in ruminants: a review. J. Dairy Sci. 64:1637–1647.
Higginbotham, G. E., and D. L. Bath. 1993. Evaluation of Lactobacillus fermentation cultures in calf feeding systems. J. Dairy Sci. 76:615–620.
Hoblet, K. H., T. P. Charles, and R. P. Howard. 1989. Evaluation of lasalocid and decoquinate against coccidiosis resulting from natural exposure in weaned dairy calves. Am. J. Vet. Res. 50:1060–1064.
Hodgson, J. 1971. The development of solid food intake in calves. 5. The relationship between liquid and solid food intake. Anim. Prod. 13:593–597.
Holmes, C. W., and A. W. F. Davey. 1976. The energy metabolism of young Jersey and Friesian calves fed fresh milk. Anim. Prod. 23:43–53.
Hopkins, B. A., and J. D. Quigley, III. 1997. Effects of method of colostrum feeding and colostrum supplementation on concentrations of immunoglobulin G in the serum of neonatal calves. J. Dairy Sci. 80:979–983.
Huber, J. T., A. G. Silva, O. F. Campos, and C. M. Mathieu. 1984. Influence of feeding different amounts of milk on performance, health, and absorption capability of baby calves. J. Dairy Sci. 67:2957–2963.
Huisman, J. 1989. Antinutritional factors (ANFs) in the nutrition of monogastric farm animals. In Nutrition and Digestive Physiology in Monogastric Farm Animals, 17–35. Wageningen, Netherlands: Pudoc.
Jackson, J. A., and R. W. Hemken. 1994. Calcium and cation-anion effects on feed intake, body weight gain, and humoral response of dairy calves. J. Dairy Sci. 77:1430–1436.
Jaster, E. H., G. C. McCoy, and R. L. Fernando. 1990. Dietary fat in milk or milk replacers for young calves raised in hutches during winter. J. Dairy Sci. 73: 1843–1850.
Jaster, E. H., G. C. McCoy, N. Spanski, and T. Tomkins. 1992. Effect of extra energy as fat or milk replacer solids in diets of young dairy calves on growth during cold weather. J. Dairy Sci. 75:2524–2531.
Jenkins, K. J., J. K. G. Kramer, F. D. Sauer, and D. B. Emmons. 1985. Influence of triglycerides and free fatty acids in milk replacers on calf performance, blood plasma, and adipose lipids. J. Dairy Sci. 68:669–680.
Jenny, B. F., S. E. Mills, W. E. Johnston, and G. D. O'Dell. 1978. Effect of fluid intake and dry matter concentration on scours and water intake in calves fed once daily. J. Dairy Sci. 61:765–770.
Jenny, B. F., H. J. Vandijk, and J. A. Collins. 1991. Performance and fecal flora of calves fed a Bacillus subtilis concentrate. J. Dairy Sci. 74:1968–1973.
Johnson, P. T. C., and R. C. Elliott. 1972a. Dietary energy intake and utilization by young Friesland calves. 2. Digestibility and metabolizable energy contents of whole milk and spray-dried skimmilk powder, and energy retentions of calves given these foods. Rhod. J. Agric. Res. 10:125–133.
Johnson, P. T. C., and R. C. Elliott. 1972b. Dietary energy intake and utilization by young Friesland calves. 3. The utilization by calves of energy in whole milk. Rhod. J. Agric. Res. 10:135–142.
Kertz, A. F., L. R. Prewitt, and J. P. Everett, Jr. 1979. An early weaning calf program: summarization and review. J. Dairy Sci. 62:1835–1843.
Kertz, A. F., L. F. Reutzel, and J.H. Mahoney. 1984. Ad libitum water intake by neonatal calves and its relationship to calf starter intake, weight gain, fecal score, and season. J. Dairy Sci. 76: 2964–2969.
Khouri, R. H., and F. S. Pickering. 1968. Nutrition of the milk-fed calf. I. Performance of calves fed on different levels of whole milk relative to body weight. N.Z. J. Agric. Res. 11:227–236.
Kincaid, R. L., B. P. Chew, and J. D. Cronrath. 1997. Zinc oxide and amino acids as sources of dietary zinc for calves: effects on uptake and immunity. J. Dairy Sci. 80:1381–1388.
Kuehn, C. S., D. E. Otterby, J. G. Linn, W. G. Olson, H. Chester-Jones, G. D. Marx, and J. A. Barmore. 1994. The effect of dietary energy concentration on calf performance. J. Dairy Sci. 77:2621–2629.
Lallès, J. P. 1993. Nutritional and antinutritional aspects of soyabean and field pea proteins used in veal calf production: a review. Livestock Prod. Sci. 34:181–202.
Lammers, B. P., A. J. Heinrichs, and A. Aydin. 1998. The effect of whey protein concentrate or dried skim milk in milk replacer on calf performance and blood metabolites. J. Dairy Sci. 81:1940–1945.
Leaver, J. D., and N. H. Yarrow. 1972. Rearing of dairy cattle. 2. Weaning calves according to their concentrate intake. Anim. Prod. 14:161–165.
Lewis, L. D., and R. W. Phillips. 1978. Pathophysiologic changes due to coronavirus-induced diarrhea in the calf. J. Am. Vet. Med. Assoc. 173:636–642.
Maiga, H. A., D. J. Schingoethe, F. C. Ludens, W. L. Tucker, and D. P. Casper. 1994. Response of calves to diets that varied in amounts of ruminally degradable carbohydrate and protein. J. Dairy Sci. 77:278–283.
McCoy, G. C., J. K. Reneau, A. G. Hunter, and J. B. Williams. 1970. Effects of diet and time on blood serum proteins in the newborn calf. J. Dairy Sci. 53:358–362.
McDowell, L. R. 1992. Minerals in Animal and Human Nutrition. San Diego, CA: Academic Press, Inc.
McGavin, M. D., and J. L. Morrill. 1976. Scanning electron microscopy of ruminal papillae in calves fed various amounts and forms of roughage. Am. J. Vet Res. 37:497–508.
McGuirk, S. M. 1992. New approach to electrolyte therapy. Proc. 17th World Buiatrics Congress and 25th American Association Bovine Prac-

titioners Conference, vol. 2, 182–186, West Lafayette, IN: American Association of Bovine Practitioners.

Morin, D. E., G. C. McCoy, and W. L. Hurley. 1997. Effects of quality, quantity, and timing of colostrum feeding and addition of a colostrum supplement on immunoglobulin G1 absorption in Holstein bull calves. J. Dairy Sci. 80:747–753.

Morrill, J. L., A. D. Dayton, and R. Mickelsen. 1977. Cultured milk and antibiotics for young calves. J. Dairy Sci. 60:1105–1109.

Morrill, J. L., J. M. Morrill, A. M. Feyerherm, and J. F. Laster. 1995. Plasma proteins and a probiotic as ingredients in milk replacer. J. Dairy Sci. 78:902–907.

National Research Council. 1968. Prenatal and Postnatal Mortality in Cattle, Publication 1685. Washington, DC: Natl. Acad. Sci.

National Research Council. 1978. Nutrient Requirements of Dairy Cattle, 5th rev. ed. Washington, DC: Natl. Acad. Sci.

National Research Council. 1981. Nutritional Energetics of Domestic Animals. Washington, DC: National Academy Press.

National Research Council. 1987. Vitamin Tolerance of Animals. Washington, DC: National Academy Press.

National Research Council, 1989. Nutrient Requirements of Dairy Cattle, 6th rev. ed. Washington, DC: National Academy Press.

National Research Council, 1996. Nutrient Requirements of Beef Cattle, 7th ed. Washington, DC: National Academy Press.

Neergard, L. 1976. A comparative study of nitrogen and energy metabolism in young calves fed three liquid diets. In Energy Metabolism of Farm Animals, edited by M. Vermorel, 205–208. European Association of Animal Production, Claremont-Ferrand, France.

Nocek, J. E., and D. G. Braund. 1986. Performance, health, and postweaning growth on calves fed cold, acidified milk replacer ad libitum. J. Dairy Sci. 69:1871–1883.

Nonnecke, B. J., R. L. Horst, W. R. Waters, P. Dubeski, and J. A. Harp. 1999. Modulation of fat-soluble vitamin concentrations and blood mononuclear leukocyte populations in milk replacer-fed calves by dietary vitamin A and β-carotene. J. Dairy Sci. 82:2632–2641.

Okamoto, M., J. B. Robinson, R. J. Christopherson, and B. A. Young. 1986. Summit metabolism of newborn calves with and without colostrum feeding. Can. J. Anim. Sci. 66: 937–944.

Orskov, E. R. 1972. Reflex closure of the oesophageal groove and its potential application in ruminant nutrition. S. Afr. J. Anim. Sci. 2: 169–176.

Ortigues, I., C. Martin, M. Vermorel, and Y. Anglaret. 1994. Energy cost of standing and circadian changes in energy expenditure in the preruminant calf. J. Anim. Sci. 72:2131–2140.

Phillips, R. W. 1985. Fluid therapy for diarrheic calves. What, how, and how much? Vet. Clin. North Am. Food Anim. Pract. 1:541–562.

Pollock, J. M., T. G. Rowan, J. B. Dixon, S. D. Carter, D. Spiller, and H. Warenius. 1993. Alteration of cellular immune responses by nutrition and weaning in calves. Res. Vet. Sci. 55:298–306.

Pollock, J. M., T. G. Rowan, J. B. Dixon, and S. D. Carter. 1994. Level of nutrition and age at weaning: effects on humoral immunity in young calves. Br. J. Nutr. 71:239–248.

Pritchett, L. C., C. C. Gay, T. E. Besser, and D. D. Hancock. 1991. Management and production factors influencing immunoglobulin $G_1$ concentration in colostrum from Holstein cows. J. Dairy Sci. 74:2336–2341.

Quigley, III, J. D. 1996a. Feeding prior to weaning. In Calves, Heifers, and Dairy Profitability. Facilties, Nutrition, and Health, 245–255, Northeast Regional Agricultural Engineering Service, Ithaca, NY.

Quigley, III, J. D. 1996b. Influence of weaning method on growth, intake, and selected blood metabolites in Jersey calves. J. Dairy Sci. 79:2255–2260.

Quigley, III, J. D., and J. K. Bernard. 1996. Milk replacers with or without animal plasma for dairy calves. J. Dairy Sci. 79:1881–1884.

Quigley, III, J. D., and M. G. Welborn. 1996. Influence of injectable immunoglobulin on serum immunoglobulin concentrations in dairy calves. J. Dairy Sci. 79:2032–2037.

Quigley, III, J. D., and J. J. Drewry. 1998. Nutrient and immunity transfer from cow to calf pre- and postcalving. J. Dairy Sci. 81:2779–2790.

Quigley, III, J. D., C. G. Schwab, and W. E. Hylton. 1985. Development of rumen function in calves: nature of protein reaching the abomasum. J. Dairy Sci. 68:694–702.

Quigley, III, J. D., L. A. Caldwell, G. D. Sinks, and R. N. Heitmann. 1991. Changes in blood glucose, nonesterified fatty acids, and ketones in response to weaning and feed intake in young calves. J. Dairy Sci. 74:250–257.

Quigley, III, J. D., L. B. Wallis, H. H. Dowlen, and R. N. Heitmann. 1992. Sodium bicarbonate and yeast culture effects on ruminal fermentation, growth, and intake in dairy calves. J. Dairy Sci. 75:3531–3538.

Quigley, III, J. D., J. K. Bernard, T. L Tyberendt, and K. R. Martin. 1994a. Intake, growth, and selected blood parameters in calves fed calf starter via bucket or bottle. J. Dairy Sci. 77:354–357.

Quigley, III, J. D., J. J. Rejman, and K. R. Martin. 1994b. Response of peripheral blood mononuclear cells to mitogenic stimulation in young calves. J. Dairy Sci. 77:259–263.

Quigley, III, J. D., K. R. Martin, D. A. Bemis, L.N.D. Potgieter, C. R. Reinemeyer, B. W. Rohrbach, H. H. Dowlen, and K. C. Lamar. 1995. Effects of housing and colostrum feeding on serum immunoglobulins, growth, and fecal score of Jersey calves. J. Dairy Sci. 78:893–901.

Quigley, III, J. D., J. J. Drewry, L. M. Murray, and S. J. Ivey. 1997a. Body weight gain, feed efficiency, and fecal scores of dairy calves in response to galactosyl-lactose or antibiotics in milk replacers. J. Dairy Sci. 80:1751–1754.

Quigley, III, J. D., J. J. Drewry, L. M. Murray, and S. J. Ivey. 1997b. Effects of lasalocid in milk replacer or calf starter on health and performance of calves challenged with Eimeria species. J. Dairy Sci. 80:2972–2976.

Raven, A. M. 1970. Fat in milk replacers for calves. J. Sci. Food Agric. 21:352–359.

Reddy, P. G., J. L. Morrill, H. C. Minocha, M. B. Morrill, A. D. Dayton, and R. A. Frey. 1986. Effect of supplemental vitamin E on the immune system of calves. J. Dairy Sci. 69:164–171.

Reddy, P. G., J. L. Morrill, and R. A. Frey. 1987a. Vitamin E requirements of dairy calves. J. Dairy Sci. 70:123–129.

Reddy, P. G., J. L. Morrill, H. C. Minocha, and J. S. Stevenson. 1987b. Vitamin E is immunostimulatory in calves. J. Dairy Sci. 70:993–999.

Reddy, P. V., J. L. Morrill, and L. S. Bates. 1993. Effect of roasting temperatures on soybean utilization by young dairy calves. J. Dairy Sci. 76:1387–1393.

Richard, A. L., L. D. Muller, and A. J. Heinrichs. 1988. Ad libitum or twice daily feeding of acidified milk replacer to calves housed individually in warm and cold environments. J. Dairy Sci. 71:2193–2202.

Ridder, T. A., J. W. Young, K. A. Anderson, D. W. Lodman, K. G. Odde, and D. E. Johnson. 1991. Effects of prepartum energy nutrition and body condition on birthweight and basal metabolism in bovine neonates. J. Anim. Sci. 69(Suppl. 1):450. (Abstr.).

Roy, J. H. B. 1970. Protein in milk replacers for calves. J. Sci. Food Agric. 21:346–351.

Roy, J. H. B. 1980. The Calf, 4th ed. Boston: Butterworths.

Roy, J. H. B., C. F. Huffman, and E. P. Reineke. 1957. The basal metabolism of the newborn calf. Br. J. Nutr. 11:373–381.

Rowan, T. G. 1992. Thermoregulation in neonatal ruminants. In Neonatal Survival and Growth, edited by M.A. Varley, P. E. V. Williams, and T. L. J. Lawrence, Occasional Pulb. No. 15, 13–24; Edinburgh, UK: Br. Soc. Anim. Prod.

Sander, E. G., R. G. Warner, H. N. Harrison, and J. K. Loosli. 1959. The stimulatory effect of sodium butyrate and sodium propionate on the development of rumen mucosa in the young calf. J. Dairy Sci. 42:1600–1605.

Schingoethe, D. J., D. P. Casper, J. K. Drackley, and F. C. Ludens. 1986. Increased solids intake and feeding frequency for calves in hutches during cold weather. J. Dairy Sci. 69:1063–1069.

Schrama, J. W. 1993. Energy Metabolism of Young Unadapted Calves. Ph.D. diss., Department of Animal Husbandry and Department of Animal Nutrition, Wageningen, The Netherlands: Wageningen Agricultural University.

Schrama, J. W., W. van der Hel, A. Arieli, and M. W. A. Verstegen. 1992. Alteration of energy metabolism of calves fed below maintenance during 6 to 14 days of age. J. Anim. Sci. 70:2527–2532.

Scibilia, L. S., L. D. Muller, R. S. Kensinger, T. F. Sweeney, and P. R. Shellenberger. 1987. Effect of environmental temperature and dietary fat on growth and physiological responses of newborn calves. J. Dairy Sci. 70:1426–1433.

Spanski, N. A., J. K. Drackley, C. L. Davis, and E. H. Jaster. 1997. Utilization of supplemental triglycerides or free fatty acids by calves from 4 to 10 weeks of age. J. Dairy Sci. 80:573–585.

Stewart, G. D., and D. J. Schingoethe. 1984. Evaluation of high starch and high fat rations for dairy calves. J. Dairy Sci. 67:598–605.

Stobo, I. J. F. 1983. Milk replacers for calves. In Recent Advances in Animal Nutrition, 113–140. London: Butterworths.

Stobo, I. J. F., J. H. B. Roy, and H. J. Gaston. 1966. Rumen development in the calf. I. The effect of diets containing different proportions of concentrates to hay on rumen development. Br. J. Nutr. 20:171–188.

Swanson, K. S., N. R. Merchen, J. W. Erdman, Jr., J. K. Drackley, F. Orias, D. E. Morin, and M. F. Haddad. 2000. Influence of vitamin A content on serum and liver vitamin A concentrations and health in preruminant Holstein calves fed milk replacer. J. Dairy Sci. 83:2027–2036.

Ternouth, J. H., I. J. F. Stobo, J. H. B. Roy, and A. W. Beattie. 1985. The effect of milk substitute concentration upon the intake, digestion and growth of calves. Anim. Prod. 41:151–159.

Terosky, T. L., A. J. Heinrichs, and L. L. Wilson. 1997. A comparison of milk protein sources in diets of calves up to eight weeks of age. J. Dairy Sci. 80:2977–2983.

Terui, H., J. L. Morrill, and J. J. Higgins. 1996. Evaluation of wheat gluten in milk replacers and calf starters. J. Dairy Sci. 79:1261–1266.

Tomkins, T., and E. H. Jaster. 1991. Preruminant calf nutrition. Vet. Clin. North Am. Food Anim. Pract. 7:557–576.

Toullec, R. 1989. Veal calves. In Ruminant Nutrition- Recommended Allowances and Feed Tables, edited by R. Jarrige. London; INRA, John Libby.

Toullec, R., and P. Guilloteau. 1989. Research into the digestive physiology of the milk-fed calf. In: Nutrition and Digestive Physiology in Monogastric Farm Animals, edited by E. J. Van Weerdon and J. Huisman, 37–55. Wageningen, The Netherlands: Pudoc.

Toullec, R., M. Theriez, and P. Thivend. 1980. Milk replacers for calves and lambs. World Anim. Rev. 33:32–42.

Van Es, A. J. H., H. J. Nijkamp, E. J. Vanweerden, and K. K. Hellemond. 1969. Energy, carbon, and nitrogen balance experiments with veal calves. In Energy Metabolism of Farm Animals, edited by K. L. Blaxter, J. Kielowski, and G. Thorbeck, 197–202, Oriel Press, Newcastle-upon-Tyne, UK.

Van Saun, R. J., T. H. Herdt, and H. D. Stowe. 1989a. Maternal and fetal selenium concentrations and their interrelationships in dairy cattle. J. Nutr. 119:1128–1137.

Van Saun, R. J., T. H. Herdt, and H. D. Stowe. 1989b. Maternal and fetal vitamin E concentrations and selenium-vitamin E interrelationships in dairy cattle. J. Nutr. 119:1156–1164.

Vermorel, M., J. C. Bouvier, P. Thivend, and R. Toullec. 1974. Utilisation energetique des aliments d'allaitement par le veau preruminant a l'engrais de differents poids. In Energy Metabolism of Farm Animals, edited by K. H. Menke, H. J. Lantzch, and J. R. Reichl, 143–146, Universitat Hohenheim Dokumentationsstelle, Hohenheim, BRD.

Vermorel, M., C. Dardillat, J. Vernat, Saido, and C. Demigne. 1983. Energy metabolism and thermoregulation in the newborn calf. Ann. Rech. Vet. 14:382–389.

Walker, P. G., P. D. Constable, D. E. Morin, J. K. Drackley, J. H. Foreman, and J. C. Thurmon. 1998. A reliable, practical, and economical protocol for inducing diarrhea and severe dehydration in the neonatal calf. Can. J. Vet. Res. 62:205–213.

Warner, R. G. 1991. Nutritional factors affecting the development of a functional ruminant—A historical perspective. Proc. Cornell Nutr. Conf., 1–12. Ithaca, NY: Cornell University.

Webster, A. J. F., H. Donnelly, J. M. Brockway, and J. S. Smith. 1975. Energy exchanges of veal calves fed high-fat milk replacer diet containing different amounts of iron. Anim. Prod. 20:69–75.

Webster, A. J. F., J. G. Gordon, and R. McGregor. 1978. The cold tolerance of beef and dairy type calves in the first weeks of life. Anim. Prod. 26:85–92.

Weil, A. B., W. B. Tucker, and R. W. Hemken. 1988. Potassium requirement of dairy calves. J. Dairy Sci. 71:1868–1872.

Williams, P. E. V., and A. J. Frost. 1992. Feeding the young ruminant. In Neonatal Survival and Growth, edited by M. Varley, P. E. V. Williams, and T. L. J. Lawrence, Occasional Publ. No. 15, 109–118. Edinburgh, UK: Br. Soc. Anim. Prod.

Williams, P. E. V., D. Day, A. M. Raven, and J. A. McLean. 1981. The effect of climatic housing and level of nutrition on the performance of calves. Anim. Prod. 32:133–141.

Wilson, G. A., and J. V. Wheelock. 1972. Factors affecting the action of rennin in heated milk. J. Dairy Res. 39:413–419.

# 11 Growth

## ENERGY AND PROTEIN REQUIREMENTS FOR GROWING DAIRY HEIFERS

Since the publication of the last National Research Council review of nutrient requirements of dairy cattle (National Research Council, 1989), several articles on use of accelerated growth programs for heifers and their effects on milk production have been published (Lammers et al., 1999; Radcliff et al., 1997; Van Amburgh et al., 1998a, 1998b). In addition, there have been several reports of studies on protein requirements of heifers (Pirlo et al., 1997; Tomlinson et al., 1997). This renewed interest in rearing heifers is largely due to the costs of raising replacement animals and the impact of the growing period on lifetime milk production. These economic imperatives underscore the importance of accurate prediction of heifer nutrient requirements. Energy and protein requirements for growth are estimated from the energy and protein content of the tissue deposited during growth (National Research Council, 1996). The amount of energy required for growth is calculated from the net energy deposited. The amount of protein that must be consumed daily to achieve the target growth rate is the sum of 1) rumen degradable protein (RDP) required for microbial growth that can be achieved given the level of ruminally available carbohydrates, and 2) rumen undegradable protein (RUP) required to supplement the microbial protein produced to support the energy allowable average daily gain (ADG). Preston (1982) indicated that protein requirements for growth could be expressed as a ratio of dietary crude protein (CP) to dietary total digestible nutrients (TDN). However, this approach does not account for differences in RDP and RUP requirements, and in mature body size.

Tomlinson et al. (1997) reported a growth response when RUP was added to heifer diets. A growth response also was evident when RUP was added to low energy, but not high energy, diets fed to heifers less than 385 days old (Bethard et al., 1997). Heifers responded to both supplemental TDN and CP when the basal diet contained 90 percent of National Research Council-predicted requirements (Pirlo et al., 1997). Accurate estimation of dietary requirements for protein should be based on ruminal and tissue requirements in varied production environments (National Research Council, 1996; Van Amburgh et al., 1998a).

### *Terminology*

In this section on growth, several terms are used which are less familiar to those in the dairy industry than to those who work primarily with growing animals. In the 1989 publication on requirements of dairy cattle (National Research Council, 1989), all calculations were done on a full body weight (BW or FBW) basis. In this publication, the terms shrunk body weight (SBW) and empty body weight (EBW) also are used. These terms permit better description of biologic functions than reliance on live weight alone. For example, SBW, which is defined as 96 percent of FBW, is equivalent to an animal's weight after an overnight fast without feed or water. It is used to compute $NE_M$ requirements, which are measured as fasting heat production (National Research Council, 1984). Shrunk body weight also is used in calculations to determine the amount of net energy available for growth in the diet (NEFG) and target shrunk weight gain (SWG). Empty body weight (weight without ingesta), which is 89.1 percent of SBW or 85.5 percent of BW, was used to develop the equation to predict the energy required for SWG because net energy requirements are a function of the proportion of fat and protein in the empty body tissue gain (EBG) (Garrett et al., 1959). Empty body gain is 96 percent of SWG.

### *Growth Requirements and Composition of Gain*

The strong relationship between weight and height (Heinrichs and Losinger, 1998) makes it possible to use linear measurements to describe dimensional changes as an animal matures (Hoffman, 1997; Kertz et al., 1998; Lammers et al., 1999). Although these measurements have several useful field applications, skeletal growth cannot be directly used to compute energy and protein requirements for growth for two reasons: 1) net energy for gain ($NE_G$) is defined as the energy content of the tissue deposited during growth, and 2) most of the data relating stature and weight are from Holsteins so that the system would be unworkable for other breeds. It is a function of the proportion of fat and protein in EBG (Garrett et al., 1959). Simpfendorfer (1974) summarized data on the body composition of growing cattle from birth to maturity and found that 95.6–98.9 percent of the variation in chemical composition was associated with differences in the weights of cattle of similar mature sizes. If an animal is fed a diet containing adequate energy, the percentage of protein diminishes and the percentage of fat increases in the empty body as the animal matures (National Research Council, 1996). Chemical maturity is achieved when weight gain contains little additional protein (National Research Council, 1996). Previous subcommittees on beef and dairy nutrition (National Research Council, 1984, 1989, 1996) adopted the equation developed by Garrett (1980) to predict the energy content of weight gain. Garrett's data set included 72 comparative slaughter experiments conducted at the University of California between 1960 and 1980 with approximately 3,500 cattle (predominantly British breed beef steers) fed a variety of diets. The Garrett equation describes the relationship between retained energy (RE) and EBG for a given EBW. The same data were used to derive the relationships between FBW, SBW, and EBW and to describe the composition of ingesta-free BW gain at a particular stage of growth of cattle (National Research Council, 1996).

Because the weight at which cattle reach a given chemical composition varies depending on mature size and gender, body composition may differ among animals of similar weights (National Research Council, 1996). Following the approach adopted in the 1984 *Nutrient Requirements of Beef Cattle* (National Research Council, 1984) and in the 1989 *Nutrient Requirements of Dairy Cattle* (National Research Council, 1989), recently developed systems to predict animal requirements have used a size scaling approach to account for these effects (National Research Council, 1996). The size-scaling approach adopted in the Australian system (Commonwealth Scientific and Industrial Research Organization [CSIRO], 1990) involves calculation of the relationship between an animal's current weight and a standard reference weight. The standard reference weight is defined as the weight at which skeletal development is complete and the empty body contains 25 percent fat corresponding to a body condition score (BCS) of 3 on a 0 to 5 scale. To facilitate ration balancing, standard reference weights for different breeds are provided in a table in the CSIRO system (1990).

Oltjen et al. (1986) developed a simulation model of growth and body composition based on differential equations describing whole body DNA accretion and protein synthesis and degradation. He assumed that the difference between net energy available for gain and that required for protein synthesis deposited as fat. By using the ratio between the animal's current weight and its mature weight, it was possible to adjust for differences in mature size.

In the model developed by the Institut National de la Recherche Agronomique (INRA) system (Institut National de la Recherche Agronomique, 1989), the amounts of protein and lipid retained daily are predicted considering the type, live weight, and daily live weight gain of the animal. The INRA approach to prediction of energy and protein requirements involves use of allometric relationships between EBW and live weight, between lipid content (kg) and EBW, and between protein content and fat-free body mass. The coefficients in the INRA equations are the parameters obtained by fitting data on live weight and age to the Gompertz equation (Taylor, 1968). The French system includes initial and final weights and growth curve coefficients for six classes of bulls, two classes of steers, and two classes of heifers for finishing cattle, and two classes each for male and female growing cattle. The amount of lipid deposited daily is proportional to the daily live weight gain raised to the power 1.8 ($BW^{1.8}$). Daily protein accretion is calculated from the gain in the fat-free body mass because protein content of fat-free gain varies little with type of animal, growth rate, or feeding level (Garrett, 1987).

The mature weights of dairy cattle vary from 400 kg for small breeds to more than 680 kg for large breeds. Because of the considerable variation in mature size within and among breeds, this committee decided that it was necessary to consider mature size in estimating growth requirements. In the previous publication on the nutrient requirements of dairy cattle (National Research Council, 1989), size effects were taken into account by including requirements for small, medium, and large breeds in the nutrient requirement tables. However, the equations used to compute the net energy and protein content of gain were not adjusted to account for the effect of mature weight.

The National Research Council *Nutrient Requirements of Beef Cattle* (1996) adopted the size scaling system developed by Fox et al. (1992) with refinements published by Tylutki et al. (1994). This system is used to account for differences in mature size of cattle (Equations 11-1 and 11-2) with further modifications made to adapt it for use with dairy heifers (except for pre-ruminant calves) (Fox et al., 1999). As in the CSIRO (1990) and INRA (1989) systems, it is assumed in this model that the chemical composition of gain is similar among animals at the same proportion of mature BW. The size scaling equation in the beef growth model (National Research Council, 1996) is similar to the approach adopted by CSIRO (1990).

The equations of Garrett (1980), with the adjustments for mature size shown in Equations 11-2 and 11-5, are used to compute the energy content of gain at various stages of growth and rates of gain. These equations were chosen because: a) they were developed from a large, robust data set (Garrett, 1980), b) they have been used with success in previous National Research Council publications (National Research Council, 1984, 1989, 1996), and c) they accurately described the net energy and protein content of Holstein heifers (Fox et al., 1999) using the adjustments for mature body size in Equations 11-2 and 11-5.

$$\text{EQSBW} = \text{SBW} \times (478/\text{MSBW}) \qquad (11\text{-}1)$$

$$\text{RE, Mcal} = 0.0635 \times \text{EQEBW}^{0.75} \times \text{EQEBG}^{1.097} \qquad (11\text{-}2)$$

where EQEBW is 0.891 × EQSBW and EQEBG is 0.956 × SWG.

In this growth model, EQSBW is the weight at which the standard reference animal has the same energy content of gain as the dairy heifer being evaluated. An analysis of the California data set indicated that the mature SBW for the animals in the serial slaughter studies averaged 478 kg. Equation 11-2, which describes the energy content of gain at a particular weight for the California data base (National Research Council, 1996), is used in the current model to describe the growth curve of dairy heifers. As a result, the standard reference animal is assumed to have a mature weight of 478 kg (National Research Council, 1996). In Equation 11-2, energy content of gain increases with weight and rate of growth. If we assume that the average Holstein has a full BW (FBW) of 677 kg or SBW of 650 kg, the relationship between this animal and the standard reference animal can be determined using Equation 11-1. The ratio of the reference SBW to the mature SBW (478/650) is used to determine that the standard reference animal weighs 73.5 percent as much as the Holstein at chemical maturity. Assuming an average SBW of 650 kg, Equation 11-1 indicates the standard reference animal weighs 478/650 = 73.5 percent as much at maturity, and therefore weighs 73.5 percent as much as this Holstein at the same stage of chemical maturity. For example, the "size-scaled" weight of a Holstein heifer with an SBW of 300 kg (313 FBW) and a mature SBW of 650 kg (677 FBW) is 300 × (478/650) = 221 kg. This value is then adjusted to an empty body basis (221 × 0.891 = 197 kg) and used in Equation 11-2 to compute her net energy requirement. For a 300 kg SBW Holstein heifer with a mature weight of 800 kg, the size-scaled weight is 300 × (478/800) = 179 kg, with an EBW of 159 kg. The size-scaled weight of a Jersey heifer weighing 300 kg SBW with a mature weight of 400 kg is 300 × 478/400 = 359 kg with an EBW of 320 kg, which is used in Equation 11-2 to compute her net energy requirement. Although these three heifers weigh the same amount (300 kg SBW), the Jersey heifer is at 75 percent of her mature weight, while the average and large Holstein heifers are at 46 percent and 38 percent of their respective mature weights. When these size-scaled weights are used in Equation 11-2 with a rate of gain of 0.7 kg (EBG = 0.7 × 0.956 = 0.669), the Jersey heifer will have the highest net energy content of gain, followed by the average and large mature size Holstein heifers (3.09, 2.15, and 1.83 Mcal, respectively). The validation by Fox et al. (1999) showed that this size scaling approach can be used for dairy heifers.

Given the relationship between energy retained and protein content of gain, protein content of SWG (net protein for gain, $NP_g$) is computed from the following equation (National Research Council, 1984, 1996):

$$NP_g\text{, g/d} = \text{SWG} \times (268 - (29.4 \times (\text{RE/SWG}))) \qquad (11\text{-}3)$$

The retained protein predicted in Equation 11-3 is adjusted for mature size because the RE used in that equation is based on EQEBW. The absorbed protein requirement is:

$$\text{MPGrowth} = NP_g / (0.834 - (\text{EQSBW} \times 0.00114))$$
$$\text{If EQSBW is} > 478 \text{ kg, then EQSBW} = 478 \text{ kg.} \qquad (11\text{-}4)$$

To develop feeding programs and evaluate heifer performance, daily gain must be predicted from the diet being fed. This is accomplished by substituting EQSBW for SBW and the net energy available for growth (NEFG) for RE in the Garrett (1980) equation (Equation 11-5) to predict SWG:

$$\text{SWG} = 13.91 \times \text{NEGrowthDiet}^{0.9116} \times \text{EQSBW}^{-0.6837} \qquad (11\text{-}5)$$

Actual SWG and NEGrowthDiet can be substituted into Equation 11-3 to compute the protein required for the observed SWG and NEFG. Equation 11-4 can then be used to compute the MP required for the observed SWG to evaluate whether protein requirements have been met.

### *Evaluation of Model Predictions of Energy and Protein Requirements for Growth of Dairy Heifers*

Table 11-1 shows the net energy requirements of heifers of different mature sizes (650, 800, and 400 kg) growing at different rates (0.6, 0.8, and 1.0 kg/day). Several important relationships are shown in this table. First, as BW increases, the energy content of the gain increases and protein content of the gain decreases, because more energy is deposited as fat. Second, as SWG increases, energy content of the gain increases and protein content of the gain decreases because the gain contains a higher proportion of fat as

TABLE 11-1 Relationship Between Mature Size and Growth Requirements[a]

| Mature weight | Live Body Weight During Growth (kg) | | | | | | |
|---|---|---|---|---|---|---|---|
| 650 kg Holstein | 200 | 250 | 300 | 350 | 400 | 450 | 500 |
| 800 kg Holstein | 246 | 308 | 369 | 431 | 493 | 554 | 616 |
| 400 kg Jersey | 139 | 173 | 208 | 242 | 277 | 312 | 346 |
| SWG (kg/day) | $NE_G$ required, Mcal/d[b] | | | | | | |
| 0.6 | 1.34 | 1.58 | 1.81 | 2.03 | 2.25 | 2.46 | 2.66 |
| 0.8 | 1.83 | 2.17 | 2.48 | 2.79 | 3.08 | 3.37 | 3.64 |
| 1.0 | 2.34 | 2.77 | 3.17 | 3.56 | 3.94 | 4.30 | 4.65 |
| | Net protein required for growth, g/d[c] | | | | | | |
| 0.6 | 122 | 114 | 108 | 101 | 95 | 89 | 83 |
| 0.8 | 161 | 151 | 141 | 132 | 124 | 115 | 107 |
| 1.0 | 199 | 187 | 175 | 163 | 152 | 142 | 131 |
| | Metabolizable protein required for growth, g/d[d] | | | | | | |
| 0.6 | 182 | 183 | 185 | 187 | 190 | 194 | 199 |
| 0.8 | 241 | 241 | 243 | 245 | 248 | 253 | 259 |
| 1.0 | 299 | 299 | 300 | 302 | 305 | 310 | 316 |

[a]The body weights are full, not shrunk, body weights. The weights within the same column are at the same stage of growth.

[b]$NE_G$ requirement is computed from Equation 11-2: Retained energy (RE), Mcal $= 0.0635\ EQEBW^{0.75}\ EQEBG^{1.097}$, where EQEBW is equivalent empty body weight and EQEBG is $0.956 \times$ SWG.

[c]Net protein in the gain is computed from Equation 11-3: $NP_g$ (g/d) $=$ SWG $\times (268 - (29.4 \times (RE/SWG)))$

[d]Metabolizable protein required is computed from Equation 11-4: MPGrowth $= NP_g / (0.834 - (EQSBW \times 0.00114))$; If EQSBW is $> 478$ kg, then EQSBW $= 478$ kg.

growth rate increases. Third, as animals increase in weight, metabolizable protein required does not decrease as rapidly as net protein required, because the efficiency of protein absorption declines. As energy intake above maintenance increases, it is assumed that the rate of protein deposition becomes limiting, and excess energy is deposited as fat. The fat dilutes the body content of protein, ash, and water, which are deposited at nearly constant ratios to each other at a given age (Garrett, 1987). The carcasses of Holstein heifers growing from 344 to 388 kg SBW that gained either 0.8 or 1.2 kg/d contained 12.1 or 18.5 percent body fat in the SBW (Radcliff et al., 1997). Holstein heifers grown to 321 kg SBW (334 kg FBW) deposited 1.93 Mcal/d (2.58 Mcal/kg SBG) when grown at 0.75 kg/d compared to 2.75 Mcal/d (3.67 Mcal/kg SBG) when the heifers grew at 0.95 kg/d (Waldo et al., 1997).

The equations used to predict energy and protein retained during growth were validated using data from experiments with Holstein heifers that were serially slaughtered (Fortin et al., 1980; Anrique et al., 1990, as described by Fox et al., 1999). Although these animals were fed diets that were pelleted and contained less fiber than usually is fed to growing animals, the energy retained for the observed daily gain can be used to validate this model. Plots of observed and predicted values and plots of residuals of data on composition of gain of Angus and Holstein heifers showed that the composition of gain for beef and dairy breeds was similar when the size scaling approach was used. The slope and intercept of the regression describing the composition of gain of the Holstein heifers was similar to the regression for the combined data set. The $r^2$ was 0.86 when observed and predicted data on RE of Holstein heifers were regressed using the equations from *Nutrient Requirements of Dairy Cattle* (National Research Council, 1989) with a bias of $-11$ percent. The $r^2$ was 0.96 for the model presented here, with a bias of $-4$ percent. When similar regressions were performed to evaluate prediction of RP in Holstein heifers, the $r^2$ was 0.91 for the 1989 equations and 0.71 for the model presented here, with biases of $-13$ and $-10$ percent, respectively. The bias for the 1989 National Research Council equations was nonuniform, with under prediction of RP at lower BW. These results indicate the present model can be used to predict RE and RP for dairy heifers. We suggest, however that more research is needed to account for factors influencing RP, as indicated by the lower $r^2$ and higher bias in predicting RP compared to RE.

Information from 32 Holstein heifers fed alfalfa or corn silage diets at two rates of ADG (0.78 and 0.99 kg/d) from 181 to 334 kg of FBW (Waldo et al., 1997) was used to evaluate the prediction of EBW and EBG. The EBW averaged 89 percent of SBW compared to 89.1 percent in the Garrett (1980) data-base, which was used to develop this model. The EBG averaged 87.4 percent of SWG compared to 95.6 percent in the Garrett (1980) data-base. In Holstein steers at the same stage of growth as the heifers in the trials conducted by Waldo et al. (1997) ($< 400$ kg SBW), EBW was 89 percent of SBW and EBG averaged 95.7 percent of SWG (Abdalla et al., 1988). These values are nearly identical to those used in this model.

Based on these evaluations of the model, errors in predicting net energy and protein requirements and SWG may occur due to one or more of the following factors:

- Using an incorrect MSBW.
- Short-term, transitory effects of previous nutrition.
- Variation in the $NE_M$ requirement.
- Variation in the ME value assigned to the feed because of variations in feed composition and extent of ruminal or intestinal digestion.
- Variation in $NE_M$ and $NE_G$ derived from the ME because of variation in end products of digestion and their metabolizability.
- Variations in gut fill.

Although ionophores are commonly fed to replacement heifers, the computer model accompanying this publication includes no adjustments for ionophores for several reasons. The relative importance of the various effects of ionophores such as changes in intake, protein sparing, influence on ruminal pH, increased energetic efficiency of the ruminal microbes and reduced problems with protozoal pathogens has not been fully elucidated. The effects of ionophores vary with diet, animal condition, environmental conditions, and the types of ionophore used. The model may not predict accurately when ionophores are fed unless the user adjusts either intake or the digestibility of nutrients in the ration.

## SETTING TARGET GROWTH RATES

Growth rates of replacement heifers affect economic returns on dairy farms (Cady and Smith, 1996). Inadequate size at first parturition may limit milk production and conception rate during first lactation (Hoffman et al., 1996). Excess energy intake, however, can have negative effects on mammary development by affecting the mammary parenchyma (ductular epithelial tissue) (Harrison et al., 1983; Foldager and Serjsen, 1987). There was an interaction between protein and energy because, when adequate amounts of metabolizable protein were supplied to animals receiving high-energy diets, fewer effects on mammary development were evident (Radcliff et al., 1997). Follow-up research showed that heifers fed diets high in energy and protein decreased age at first parturition and milk production at first lactation (Radcliff et al., 2000) but milk production was not reduced in the first lactation in other heifers raised on an accelerated (0.9 kg ADG/day) growth program (Abeni et al., 2000). Because puberty is associated with BW and weight is not linearly related to growth, parenchyma tissue growth may be truncated before full ductal development occurs if excess energy is consumed before puberty (Van Amburgh et al., 1991). Excessive energy intake, indicated by over-conditioning from 2 to 3 months of age until after conception, can reduce first lactation milk production (Van Amburgh et al., 1998b). Numerous data are available to support the concept of a genetically determined threshold age and weight at which heifers attain puberty (National Research Council, 1996). Joubert (1963) proposed that heifers would not attain puberty until they reached a given degree of physiologic maturity, which is similar to the "target weight" concept proposed by Lamond (1970). Simply stated, the concept is to feed heifers to attain a pre-selected or target weight at a given age to achieve optimum first lactation performance while controlling the costs of rearing replacements. Heifers of beef breeds usually attain puberty at about 60 percent of mature weight, while dual purpose and dairy heifers reach puberty at a younger age at about 55 percent of mature weight (National Research Council, 1996).

Optimum growth rates for heifers to minimize replacement costs while maximizing first lactation milk production have been described recently (Ferguson and Otto, 1989; Hoffman, 1997; Van Amburgh et al., 1998b). The *Nutrient Requirements of Beef Cattle* (National Research Council, 1996) equations to predict target weights, modified and evaluated by Fox et al. (1999), are used to predict target weights for dairy heifers. Further modifications included in this version of *Nutrient Requirements of Dairy Cattle*, compared to those outlined by Fox et al. (1999), are that the target weights after first and third calving were set to 82 and 100 percent of mature weight respectively, instead of 85 percent and 96 percent. In the following equations, calving weights are weights after parturition. The equations to predict target weights and rates of gain are as follows:

$$\text{Target weight first bred} = \text{Mature SBW} \times 0.55 \qquad (11\text{-}6)$$

$$\text{Target age for 1st pregnancy} = \text{Target first calving age} - 280 \qquad (11\text{-}7)$$

$$\text{Target SWG before 1st pregnancy} = (\text{Target weight first bred} - \text{current SBW})/(\text{Target age for 1st pregnancy} - \text{current age}) \qquad (11\text{-}8)$$

$$\text{Target 1st calving weight} = \text{Mature SBW} \times 0.82 \qquad (11\text{-}9)$$

$$\text{Target 2nd calving weight} = \text{Mature SBW} \times 0.92 \qquad (11\text{-}10)$$

$$\text{Target 3rd calving weight} = \text{Mature SBW} \times 1.00 \qquad (11\text{-}11)$$

$$\text{First pregnant SWG} = (\text{Target 1st calving weight} - \text{Target weight first bred})/280 \qquad (11\text{-}12)$$

$$\text{1st lactation SWG} = (\text{Target 2nd calving weight} - \text{Target 1st calving weight})/\text{Calving interval} \qquad (11\text{-}13)$$

$$\text{2nd lactation SWG} = (\text{Target 3rd calving weight} - \text{Target 2nd calving weight})/\text{Calving interval} \qquad (11\text{-}14)$$

Where calving interval (CI) is in days.

For all target rates of gain, Equation 11-2 is used to compute the $NE_G$ requirement and Equations 11-3 and 11-4 are used to compute the protein requirement for growth. Observed weights can be substituted for the previous target weight and divided by days left to reach the next target weight to determine SWG required to achieve the next target weight. The $NE_G$ required to reach the target weight can then be calculated. The target ADG will be small when the actual weight is close to the target weight. For pregnant animals, weight gain due to growth of the gravid uterus should be added to predicted daily shrunk weight gain (SWG) as follows:

$$ADG_{preg} = 665 \times (CBW/45) \text{ if DaysPreg} > 190 \qquad (11\text{-}15)$$

Where CBW = expected calf birth weight (kg).

For pregnant heifers, weight of fetal and associated uterine tissue and fluids should be subtracted from SBW to compute growth requirements. The conceptus weight (CW) can be calculated as follows:

$$CW = (18 + ((\text{DaysPreg} - 190) \times 0.665)) \times (CBW/45) \quad (11\text{-}16)$$

When evaluating requirements and rations with the accompanying computer model, the user must choose whether to use the target gains predicted by the model using the system described above or to enter desired rates of gain (for example, 500g/day) to determine nutrient requirements. The only difference between these two systems is the rate of gain used to calculate the requirements; all the other computations are similar.

### *Evaluation of Target Weight Equations*

The $NE_G$ required for growth of replacement heifers can be calculated from published data (Van Amburgh et al., 1998a). This study involved 273 Holstein heifers fed from an average of 77 d of age through the first lactation. Average mature weight of the herd determined at all stages of lactation was 641 kg. The weight after weaning (calves were weaned at 6–8 wk and there was a 3-wk transition period) was 84 kg, average age at first calving was 687 d, and calving interval was 431 d. Targets computed with the model presented are shown in Table 11-2. Average BW and SWG observed in this experiment compared well with model predicted values. The SWG before first calving averaged 0.82 kg/d compared to a target of 0.87 kg/d; weight at first pregnancy was 370 kg vs. the target of 352 kg; the SWG during first pregnancy averaged 0.63 kg/d vs. a target of 0.62 kg/d; weight post first calving averaged 533 kg vs. a target of 526 kg; first lactation SWG averaged 0.136 kg/d vs. a target of 0.148 kg/d; and the weight after the second calving was 592 kg (projected from 40 wk of lactation SBW and SWG) compared to a target of 590 kg.

Using the data from Table 11-2, the target growth rates and energy and protein requirements are calculated using the data from Van Amburgh et al. (1998a). This example outlines the calculations performed by the model.

Recent studies have provided target weights and growth rates for Holstein heifers (Hoffman, 1997; Kertz et al., 1998). The target postpartum weight for the Van Amburgh study (1998a) (526 kg) agrees with the actual weight of 533 kg, and both of these weights are within the ranges suggested by Hoffman (1997) (515–558 kg). The data of Kertz et al. (1997, 1998) indicated that postpartum weight of replacement heifers should be 77 percent of mature BW, compared to 83 percent in the study of Van Amburgh et al. (1998a) and the target of 82 percent in this model. The target weight at conception of 352 kg is within the range proposed by Hoffman (1997). The target daily gain before conception in this study (0.87 kg/d), which was set for animals calving at 22.5 months of age, agrees with the upper range of 0.84 kg/d suggested by Hoffman (1997) for animals calving at 24 months of age. The target ADG in the study by Van Amburgh et al. (1998a) (0.87 kg/d) was between the standard and accelerated ADG reported by Lammers et al. (1999) (0.70 and 1.01 kg/d, respectively), and is within the range suggested by Kertz et al. (1998) (0.82–0.93 kg/d). Thus, this model appears to give target weights and growth rates within the ranges suggested by recent research with Holstein cattle (Table 11-3).

TABLE 11-2 Calculation of Target Weights and Daily Gain Using the Data Set of Van Amburgh et al. (1998a)

| Target | Input variables and calculations of target |
|---|---|
| Target first pregnant weight, kg | 641 × 0.55 = 352 kg |
| Target first calving age, days | = 687 d |
| Target age at first pregnancy, days | 687 − 280 = 407 d |
| Target SWG before conception, kg | (352 − 84) / (407 − 77) = 0.87 kg/d |
| Target weight post-first calving, kg | 641 × 0.82 = 526 kg |
| Target SWG after first conception, kg | (526 − 352) / 280 = 0.62 kg/d |
| Target weight post-second calving, kg | 641 × 0.92 = 590 kg |
| Calving interval, days | = 431 d |
| Target SWG after first calving, kg | (590 − 526) / 431 = 0.148 kg/d |
| Target weight post-third calving, kg | 641 × 1 = 641 kg |
| Target SWG after second calving, kg | (641 − 590) / 431 = 0.118 kg/d |

## MAINTENANCE REQUIREMENT EFFECTS ON GROWTH

The growth rate of heifers depends on the net energy available after maintenance requirements have been met. Data collected on growth of dairy heifers on farms in Wisconsin indicated that environment had a substantial effect on heifer growth (Hoffman et al., 1994). The National Research Council (1996) provided a summary of the effects of environment on maintenance requirements of cattle. The maintenance model published by the National Research Council (1996) was adapted by this committee, with modifications for dairy heifers based on Fox and Tylutki (1998).

The maintenance requirement for energy was defined in *Nutrient Requirements of Beef Cattle* (National Research Council, 1996) as the intake of feed energy that results in no net loss or gain of energy from the tissues of the animal's body. This energy is required for essential metabolic processes, body temperature regulation and physical activity. To predict the amount of feed intake required for these purposes in diverse situations, the maintenance require-

TABLE 11-3 Application of Equations to Predict Energy and Protein Requirements, Using Target Weights and Daily Gains from Table 11-2 (Van Amburgh et al., 1998a)

| Variable | Calculation of requirement |
|---|---|
| *$NE_G$ required for target SWG for growth before first conception:* | |
| Mean target SBW | (352 + 84) / 2 = 218 kg |
| EQSBW | (478/641) × 218 = 163 kg |
| EQEBW | 163 × 0.891 = 145 kg |
| EQEBG | 0.87 × 0.956 = 0.83 kg/d |
| $NE_G$ required | $0.0635 \times 145^{0.75} \times 0.83^{1.097}$ = 2.16 Mcal/d |
| *$NE_G$ required for target SWG for heifer growth during first pregnancy:* | |
| Mean target SBW | (352 + 526) / 2 = 439 kg |
| EQSBW | (478/641) × 439 = 327 kg |
| EQEBW | 327 × 0.891 = 292 kg |
| EQEBG | 0.956 × 0.62 = 0.59 kg/d |
| RE (or $NE_G$ required) during pregnancy | $0.0635 \times 292^{0.75} \times 0.59^{1.097}$ = 2.51 Mcal/d |
| *$NE_G$ required for target SWG during first lactation:* | |
| Mean target SBW | (526 + 590) / 2 = 558 kg |
| EQSBW | (478/641) × 558 = 416 kg |
| EQEBW | 416 × 0.891 = 371 kg |
| EQEBG | 0.956 × 0.148 = 0.141 kg/d |
| $NE_G$ required | $0.0635 \times 371^{0.75} \times 0.141^{1.097}$ = 0.63 Mcal/d |
| *$NE_G$ required for target SWG during second lactation:* | |
| Mean target SBW | (590 + 641) / 2 = 616 kg |
| EQSBW | (478/641) × 616 = 459 kg |
| EQEBW | 459 × 0.891 = 409 kg |
| EQEBG | 0.956 × 0.118 = 0.113 kg/d |
| $NE_G$ required | $0.0635 \times 409^{0.75} \times 0.113^{1.097}$ = 0.53 Mcal/d |

ment must be partitioned into the energy required for basal metabolism, physical activity, and temperature regulation.

### *Basal Maintenance Requirement*

Fox and Tylutki (1998) defined the maintenance requirement for dairy heifers in a thermoneutral environment with minimal activity as follows:

$$NE_M = (0.086 \times SBW^{0.75} \times COMP) + a2 \qquad (11\text{-}17)$$

Where COMP = compensatory effect for previous plane of nutrition, and a2 = maintenance adjustment for previous temperature effect (Mcal/d/kg $SBW^{0.75}$).

The coefficient of 0.086 for dairy heifers is based on calorimetric data (Haaland et al., 1980; 1981) and comparative slaughter studies (Fox and Black, 1984). Approximately 10 percent of this requirement is for activity (Fox and Tylutki, 1998). Fox and Tyltuki (1998) presented a more complicated model to account for variation in heat stress.

### *Adjustment for Previous Temperature*

The a2 value is used to adjust for the effect of the previous temperature on metabolic rate. The National Research Council (1981) concluded that the temperature to which the animal had been exposed previously (PrevTemp) has an effect on the animal's current basal metabolic rate. A temperature of 20°C is thermoneutral because it has no effect on basal metabolic rate. The studies of Young (1975a,b) were used to describe how the $NE_M$ requirement of cattle adapted to a given thermal environment is related to the previous ambient air temperature.

$$a2 = 0.0007 \times (20 - \text{PrevTemp}) \qquad (11\text{-}18)$$

The current temperature (Temp) affects how much energy is required to respond to the current effects of cold or heat stress. On average, temperatures move slowly from one season to the next, but can fluctuate widely from day to day. To avoid a model that is too sensitive to temperature effects, we recommend using the average mean daily temperature over the previous month to which the animals have been exposed as the value for PrevTemp. The recommended input for current temperature is the average daily temperature for the previous week. To account for local environmental effects, it is best to measure these temperatures in the animal's environment (barn, outside lot, etc.).

### *Adjustment for Previous Plane of Nutrition*

Recent summaries of the literature (CSIRO, 1990; National Research Council, 1996) documented the effect of restricted feeding on fasting heat production. Sheep and cattle kept in drought conditions averaged 16 percent lower fasting metabolism than those with access to adequate feed supplies (CSIRO, 1990). These changes in basal metabolic requirement are due to changes in the activity of ionic pumps, metabolite cycling, and, most importantly, alterations in the size and metabolic activity of visceral organs (National Research Council, 1996). The National Research Council (1996) concluded that the requirement for metabolism of fasted animals was reduced by an average of 20 percent in published studies. Clearly, the extent and duration of undernutrition, as well as the plane of nutrition during the period of repletion, affect this average. An assumption made in the current model is that the BCS reflects the previous plane of nutrition. A change of 10 percent in the energy requirement for fasting metabolism is predicted for each increase or decrease in condition score from the average of 3. For example, animals with a BCS of 2 and 4 would have a basal metabolic requirements equal to 90 and 110 percent of the requirements of an animal with a BCS of 3.

$$COMP = 0.8 + ((BCS - 1) \times 0.05) \quad (11\text{-}19)$$

*Adjustment for the Direct Effects of Cold Stress*

The following series of equations are used to compute the energy required to maintain a normal body temperature during cold stress.

$$SA = 0.09 \times SBW^{0.67} \quad (11\text{-}20)$$

$$HP = (MEI - NEFP) / SA \quad (11\text{-}21)$$

$$EI = ((7.36 - (0.296 \times WINDSPEED) + (2.55 \times HAIRDEPTH)) \times COAT) \times 0.8 \quad (11\text{-}22)$$

Where SA = surface area ($m^2$), HP = heat production ($Mcal/m^2/d$), MEI = metabolizable energy intake (Mcal/d), NEFP = net energy available for production, Mcal/d, EI = external insulation value ($°C/Mcal/m^2/d$), WINDSPEED = wind speed (kph), HAIRDEPTH = hair depth (cm), and COAT = adjustment factor for external insulation. COAT is a discrete variable that is used to describe the insulation value of the coat with a choice of 4 codes; 1 = clean and dry, 2 = some mud on lower body, 3 = wet and matted, and 4 = covered with wet snow or mud. When the COAT variable equals 1, no change is made in the effectiveness of the insulation provided by the coat, but, when the COAT variable is equal to 2, 3, or 4, the coat insulation is 0.8, 0.5 or 0.2 times that of the clean, dry coat.

$$INS = TI + EI \quad (11\text{-}23)$$

Where I = insulation value ($°C/Mcal/m^2/d$), and TI = tissue (internal) insulation value ($°C/Mcal/m^2/d$) and is

2.5 for newborn calf,
6.5 for 1-mo old calf,
5.1875 + (0.3125 × BCS) for yearlings, and
5.25 + (0.75 × BCS) for adult cattle.

$$LCT = 39 - (INS \times HP \times 0.85) \quad (11\text{-}24)$$

$$ME_{cs} = SA \times (LCT - Tc) / INS \quad (11\text{-}25)$$

$$NE_{Mcs} = k_m \times ME_{cs} \quad (11\text{-}26)$$

$$\text{DMI for maintenance} = NE_M / NE_{Ma} \quad (11\text{-}27)$$

Where LCT = animal's lower critical temperature (°C), $ME_{cs}$ = metabolizable energy required for cold stress (Mcal/d), $NE_{Mcs}$ = net energy required for cold stress (Mcal/d), $k_m$ = diet $NE_M$/diet ME, $NE_M$ = net energy required for maintenance adjusted for acclimatization and cold stress, and $NE_{Ma}$ = net energy value of diet for maintenance (Mcal/kg).

*Adjustment for the Direct Effects of Heat Stress*

The $NE_M$ requirement increases when temperature increases above thermoneutral because of the energy cost of dissipating excess heat (National Research Council, 1996). Because of the difficulty in accounting for the complex interactions involved in predicting the upper critical temperature, a panting index ($NE_M$ multiplier of 1.07 if an animal has rapid, shallow breathing or 1.18 if open mouth panting is evident) is used to adjust for the energy cost to dissipate excess heat. A more complex model was developed Fox and Tylutki (1998) to account for the effects of humidity and temperatures above thermoneutral on the maintenance requirement.

*Model Evaluation*

The effects of temperature, relative humidity, wind, and hair coat condition on maintenance energy requirements are shown in Table 11-4. The effects of acclimatization are

TABLE 11-4 Multipliers Used to Adjust the Maintenance Energy Requirement to Reflect Various Environmental Conditions[a,b]

| | −1.1°C | | −12°C | | −23°C | |
|---|---|---|---|---|---|---|
| Hair Coat Code | 1[c] | 3[c] | 1[c] | 3[c] | 1[c] | 3[c] |
| Wind velocity (kph) | | | | | | |
| 1.6 | 1.17 | 1.41 | 1.37 | 1.90 | 1.74 | 2.39 |
| 16 | 1.33 | 1.70 | 1.80 | 2.27 | 2.26 | 2.84 |

[a]Temperature values reflect current temperature (Temp).
[b]Values given are net energy maintenance requirement ($NE_M$) required for these conditions divided by the maintenance requirement without stress.
[c]Hair coat code: 1 = dry and clean, 2 = mud on lower body (values not shown), and 3 = wet and matted.

accounted for by using the average temperature for the previous month for PrevTemp. Current environmental effects on energy requirements are computed by determining heat loss relative to heat production, based on current temperature, internal and external insulation, wind, and hair coat depth and condition. This calculation becomes important when the animal is in an environment below the model's lower critical temperature. No effect is evident at 20°C, but when the hide is dirty and it is −12°C with a 16 kph wind, the maintenance requirement is nearly three times as high as the requirement of a clean animal in a thermoneutral environment without wind. The maintenance requirement multiplier of 1.17 at −1.1°C with a clean and dry hair coat reflects the adjustment for acclimatization, because in this environment the animals are above their lower critical temperature. Energy intake also affects cold stress because increased ME intake results in a larger heat increment that can be used to alleviate cold stress.

Table 11-5 shows the predicted impact of the environment on the performance of heifers from 8 weeks to calving (Fox and Tylutki, 1998). At a thermoneutral temperature (20°C), the revised model yields the same maintenance requirement as the National Research Council (1989) requirements. In Table 11-5, the "northern" environment category has mean monthly temperatures similar to the those in the north central and northeastern United States, while "southwest" reflects mean monthly temperatures found in the southwestern United States. In situation 1, the animal's coat is clean and dry, while in situation 2 the coat is moderately matted. In situation 3, the hair coat is moderately matted from April through November and the animal is housed in a lot with 10 cm of mud from November through March. Situation 4 is the same as situation 1 except that there is a 16 kph wind. The specific effects of temperature and hair coat insulation are shown in Table 11-4. The energy available for growth depended on interactions among DMI, heat increment, and animal insulation, variables that were influenced by environmental temperature, wind, and animal heat production and loss. When environmental stress delayed puberty, age at first calving was increased. Weight at first calving was decreased if environmental stress occurred after conception.

## REFERENCES


Abdalla, H. O., D. G. Fox, and M. L. Thonney. 1988. Compensatory gain by Holstein calves after underfeeding protein. J. Anim. Sci. 66:2687–2695.

Abeni, F., L. Calamari, L. Stefanini, and G. Pirlo. 2000. Effects of daily gain in pre- and postpubertal replacement dairy heifers on body condition score, body size, metabolic profile, and future milk production. J. Dairy Sci. 83:1468–1478.

Anrique, R. G., M. L. Thonney, and H. J. Ayala. 1990. Dietary energy losses of cattle influenced by body type, size, sex and intake. Anim. Prod. 50:467–474.

Berthard, G. L., R. E. James, and M. L. McGilliard. 1997. Effect of rumen-undegradable protein and energy on growth and feed efficiency of growing Holstein heifers. J. Dairy Sci. 80:2149–2155.

Cady, R. A., and T. R. Smith. 1996. Economics of heifer raising programs. Proc. Calves, Heifers and Dairy Profitability National Conference. Northeast Regional Agricultural Engineering Service Pub. No. 74 pp. 7–24. Cornell University, Ithaca, NY 14853.

Commonwealth Scientific and Industrial Research Organization. 1990. Feeding standards for Australian livestock: Ruminants. East Melbourne, Victoria, Australia:CSIRO Publications.

Ferguson, J. D., and K. A. Otto. 1989. Managing body condition in cows. Proc. Cornell Nutr. Conf. Feed Manuf. Conf. pp. 75–87.

Foldager, J., and K. Serjsen. 1987. Research in Cattle Production: Danish Status and Perspectives. Tryk Denmark: Landhusholdningsselskabets Forlag.

Fortin, A., S. Simpfendorfer, J. T. Reid, H. J. Ayala, R. Anrique, and A. F. Kertz. 1980. Effect of level of energy intake and influence of breed and sex on the chemical composition of cattle. J. Anim. Sci. 51:604–614.

Fox, D. G., and J. R. Black. 1984. A system for predicting body composition and performance of growing cattle. J. Anim. Sci. 58:725–739.

Fox, D. G., C. J. Sniffen, J. D. O'Connor, J. B. Russell, and P. J. Van Soest. 1992. A net carbohydrate and protein system for evaluating cattle diets. III. Cattle requirements and diet adequacy. J. Anim. Sci. 70:3578–3596.

Fox, D. G. and T. P. Tylutki. 1998. Accounting for the effects of environment on the nutrient requirements of dairy cattle. J. Dairy Sci. 81:3085–3095.

Fox, D. G., M. E. Van Amburgh, and T. P. Tylutki. 1999. Predicting requirements for growth, maturity, and body reserves in dairy cattle. J. Dairy Sci. 82:1968–1977.


TABLE 11-5 Predicted Effects of Four Environments on Heifer Performance (Fox and Tylutki, 1998)

| | Neutral[a] | Northern[b] | | | | Southwest[c] | | | |
|---|---|---|---|---|---|---|---|---|---|
| | 1 | 1 | 2 | 3 | 4 | 1 | 2 | 3 | 4 |
| ADG[d], kg/d | 0.94 | 0.88 | 0.60 | 0.53 | 0.68 | 0.88 | 0.88 | 0.78 | 0.88 |
| Calving age, mo | 20.3 | 21.1 | 28.5 | 28.5 | 25.9 | 20.7 | 20.7 | 22.4 | 20.7 |
| Calving BW, kg | 603 | 588 | 560 | 501 | 574 | 580 | 580 | 561 | 580 |

[a]Same maintenance requirement as the National Research Council (1989).

[b]Mean monthly temperatures similar to the northcentral and northeastern United States. Situation 1 = clean and dry, situation 2 = moderately matted hair coat, situation 3 = situation 2 plus 10 cm mud from November through March, and situation 4 = situation 1 plus 16 kph wind velocity.

[c]Mean monthly temperatures similar to the southwestern region of the United States.

[d]Average daily gain.

Garrett, W. N. 1980. Energy utilization by growing cattle as determined in 72 comparative slaughter experiments. Energy Metab. Proc. Symp. 26:3–7.

Garrett, W. N. 1987. Relationship between energy metabolism and the amounts of protein and fat deposited in growing cattle. Energy Metab. Proc. Symp. 32 98–101.

Garrett, W. N., J. H. Meyer, and G. P. Lofgreen. 1959. The comparative energy requirements of sheep and cattle for maintenance and gain. J. Anim. Sci. 18:528–547.

Haaland, G. L., H. F. Tyrrell, and P. W. Moe. 1980. The effect of dietary protein and cattle breed on energy utilization for growth. J. Anim. Sci. 51(Suppl. 1):365.(Abstr.).

Haaland, G. L., H. F. Tyrrell, and P. W. Moe. 1981. The effect of dietary protein level and cattle breed on energy utilization of corn-corn silage diets for growth assessed by respiration calorimetry. J. Anim. Sci. 52(Suppl. 1):403.(Abstr.).

Harrison, R. D., I. P. Reynolds, and W. Little. 1983. A quantitative analysis of mammary glands of dairy heifers reared at different rates of live weight gain. J. Dairy Res. 50:405–412.

Heinrichs, A.J., and W.C. Losinger. 1998. Growth of Holstein heifers in the United States. J. Anim. Sci. 76:1254–1260.

Hoffman, P. C., N. M. Brehm, W. T. Howard, and D. A. Funk. 1994. The influence of nutrition and environment on growth of Holstein replacement heifers in commercial dairy herds. Professional Anim. Sci. 10:59–65.

Hoffman, P. C., N. M. Brehm, S. G. Price, and A. Prill-Adams. 1996. Effect of accelerated post-pubertal growth and early calving on lactation performance of primiparous Holstein heifers. J. Dairy Sci. 79:2024–2031.

Hoffman, P. C. 1997. Optimum body size of Holstein replacement heifers. J. Anim. Sci. 75:836–845.

Institut National de la Recherche Agronomique. 1989. Ruminant Nutrition. Montrouge, France: John Libbey Eurotext.

Joubert, D. M. 1963. Puberty in female farm animals. Anim. Breed. Abstr. 31:295–306.

Kertz, A. F., B. A. Barton, L. F. Reutzel and R. L. Ely. 1997. Body weight, body condition score, and wither height of prepartum Holstein cows and birth weight and sex of calves by parity: a data base and summary. J. Dairy Sci. 80:525–529.

Kertz, A. F., B. A. Barton, and L. F. Reutzel. 1998. Relative efficiencies of wither height and body weight increase from birth until first calving in Holstein cattle. J. Dairy Sci. 81:1479–1482.

Lammers, B. P., A. J. Heinrichs, and R. S. Kensinger. 1999. The effects of accelerated growth rates and estrogen implants in prepubertal Holstein heifers on growth, feed efficiency, and blood parameters. J. Dairy Sci. 82:1746–1752.

Lamond, D. R. 1970. The influence of undernutrition on reproduction in the cow. Anim. Breed. Abstr. 38:359–372.

National Research Council. 1981. Effect of Environment on Nutrient Requirements of Domestic Animals. Washington, DC: National Academy Press.

National Research Council. 1984. Nutrient Requirements of Beef Cattle, Sixth Revised Ed. Washington, DC: National Academy Press.

National Research Council. 1989. Nutrient Requirements of Dairy Cattle, Seventh Revised Ed. Washington, DC: National Academy Press.

National Research Council. 1996. Nutrient Requirements of Beef Cattle, Seventh Revised Ed. Washington, D.C.: National Academy Press.

Oltjen, J. W., A. C. Bywater, R. L. Baldwin, and W. N. Garrett. 1986. Development of a dynamic model of beef cattle growth and composition. J. Anim. Sci. 62:86–97.

Pirlo, G., M. Capelletti, and G. Marchetto. 1997. Effects of energy and protein allowances in the diets of prepubertal heifers on growth and milk production. J. Dairy Sci. 80:730–739.

Preston, R. L. 1982. Emperical value of crude protein systems for feedlot cattle. Proceedings Protein Requirements for cattle Symposium. Oklahoma State Univ. publication MP 109:201–217.

Radcliff, R. P., M. J. Vandehaar, L. T. Chapin, T. E. Pilbeam, D. K. Beede, E. P. Staniseiewski, and H. A. Tucker. 2000. Effects of diet and injection of bovine somatotropin on prepubertal growth and first-lactation milk yields of Holstein cows. J. Dairy Sci. 83:23–29.

Radcliff, R. P., M. J. Vandehaar, A. L. Skidmore, L. T. Chapin, B. R. Radke, J. W. Lloyd, E. P. Stanisiewski, and H. A. Tucker. 1997. Effects of diet and bovine somatotropin on heifer growth and mammary development. J. Dairy Sci. 80:1996–2003.

Simpfendorfer, S. 1974. Relationship of Body Type, Size, Sex, and Energy Intake to the Body Composition of Cattle. Ph.D. dissertation. Cornell University, Ithaca, N.Y.

Taylor, C. S. 1968. Time taken to mature in relation to mature weight for sexes, strains, and species for domesticated mammals and birds. Anim. Prod. 10:157–169.

Tomlinson, D. L., R. E. James, G. L. Bethard, and M. L. McGilliard. 1997. Influence of undegradability of protein in the diet on intake, daily gain, feed efficiency, and body composition of Holstein heifers. J. Dairy Sci. 80:943–948.

Tylutki, T. P., D. G. Fox, and R. G. Anrique. 1994. Predicting net energy and protein requirements for growth of implanted and nonimplanted heifers and steers and nonimplanted bulls varying in body size. J. Anim. Sci. 72:1806–1813.

Van Amburgh, M. E., D. G. Fox, D. M Galton, D. E. Bauman, and L. E. Chase. 1998a. Evaluation of National Research Council and Cornell Net Carbohydrate and Protein Systems for predicting requirements of Holstein heifers. J. Dairy Sci. 81:509–526.

Van Amburgh, M. E., D. M Galton, D. E. Bauman, R. W. Everett, D. G. Fox, L. E. Chase, and H. N. Erb. 1998b. Effects of three pre pubertal body growth rates in Holstein heifers during first lactation performance. J. Dairy Sci. 81:527–538.

Van Amburgh, M. E., D. M. Galton, D. G. Fox, and D. E. Bauman. 1991. Optimizing heifer growth. Proc. Cornell Nutr. Conf. Feed Manuf. Conf. pp. 85–93.

Waldo, D. R., H. F. Tyrrell, A. V. Capuco, and C. E. Rexroad, Jr. 1997. Components of growth in Holstein heifers fed either alfalfa or corn silage diets to produce two daily gains. J. Dairy Sci. 80:1674–1684.

Young, B. A. 1975a. Effects of winter acclimatization on resting metabolism of beef cows. Can. J. Anim. Sci. 55:619–625.

Young, B. A. 1975b. Temperature-induced changes in metabolism and body weight of cattle. Can. J. Physiol. Pharmacol. 53:947–953.

# 12 Dairy Cattle Nutrition and the Environment

The dairy industry is developing intensive management systems in which cows are fed and housed in large groups. Consolidation of large numbers of dairy cattle into small land areas to improve the efficiency of milk production may contribute to environmental problems unless animals are fed and managed properly. However, any size dairy herd that does not have proper nutrition, feeding, management, and waste-disposal programs has the potential to pollute the environment. If cows are fed excessive amounts of dietary nutrients that are not used efficiently for milk production, large amounts of the nutrients will be excreted in feces and urine, resulting in pollution of the environment and increased cost of milk production (Chandler, 1996).

Developments in dairy cattle nutrition will be important in determining the ability of the dairy industry to produce a nutritious, wholesome product at an economic cost without polluting the environment (Clark and Overton, 1995). Dairy cattle should continue to be fed and managed to increase the production and the efficiency of production of milk and milk components because this will require fewer cows to produce the same quantity of milk and milk components; this will increase the efficiency of nutrient use and decrease the excretion of waste products. Although high-producing dairy cows are the ruminants most efficient at converting nutrients in feed to food for human consumption, not all nutrients consumed by dairy cows are secreted in milk. Dairy cattle must be fed to meet their requirements with minimal excesses of nutrients in the diet if the efficiency of nutrient use and milk production by dairy cows are to be maximized and nutrient losses to the environment reduced. The most successful feeding regimens will be the ones that supply nutrients in amounts required to optimize synthesis of milk and milk components, maximize ruminal fermentation and growth of ruminal microbes, and minimize nutrient losses to the environment. Development and adoption of improved dairy cattle feeding systems driven by the concept of nutrient management to meet nutrient requirements and to prevent environmental pollution will result in increased efficiency of nutrient use.

The U.S. Environmental Protection Agency has issued its definition of the term "concentrated animal feeding operation" for purposes of permit requirements and specifying limits on pollutant discharges from feedlots (Meyer and Mullinax, 1999; Meyer, 2000). The U.S. Environmental Protection Agency and the U.S. Department of Agriculture have drafted national guidelines that suggest comprehensive nutrient management plans for concentrated animal feeding operations. Users should become informed to be sure they are in compliance with all federal and state regulations. These activities have taken place because of the quantity and odor of the solid, liquid, and gaseous waste products produced when waste from large numbers of animals concentrated in a small area is not well managed (Lanyon, 1994; Miner, 1997; Van Horn et al., 1994). Large amounts of waste can create disposal problems and odors and result in more strict actions for waste disposal unless the cows are fed to meet but not exceed the required amount of nutrients and waste is properly managed to prevent environmental pollution. Components of voluntary guidelines and future plans, if implemented by the government, are concerned with feed management to reduce excreted nutrients, manure handling and storage, the application of manure and other wastes to crops and land, and recordkeeping.

From an environmental standpoint, nitrogen and phosphorus are the nutrients of primary concern, and ammonia, carbon dioxide, hydrogen sulfide, and methane are the gases of primary concern (Tamminga, 1992; Chase, 1994; Van Horn et al., 1994; Chandler, 1996; Johnson et al., 1996; Koelsch and Lesoing, 1999; Kuipers et al., 1999; Nelson, 1999). The loss of other mineral nutrients in animal waste might become important in the future. Successfully defining nutrient requirements of dairy cattle will minimize nutrient losses in feces, urine, and gases. Reducing nutrient losses in waste from cattle and developing good waste management practices will decrease the concerns about the effects of waste disposal on the environment.

## NITROGEN

Nitrogen is of primary environmental concern because of losses of ammonia in the air and because of nitrate contamination of surface water and groundwater (Tamminga, 1992; Van Horn et al., 1994). Large amounts of nitrogen are brought onto dairy farms in purchased feeds. Much of this nitrogen remains on the farm rather than being incorporated into milk, animal tissue, and crops that are sold from the farm (Korevaar, 1992; Aarts et al., 1992; Klausner, 1993). Klausner (1993) indicated that purchased feeds supplied 62–87 percent of the total nitrogen on farms and that the percentage of total nitrogen taken to farms in feeds increased as herd size increased because a larger percentage of the feeds was purchased rather than grown on the farms. The percentage of the total nitrogen inputs that remained on the farm ranged between 64 and 76 percent but was not related to herd size (Klausner, 1993). The fraction of total nitrogen that remained on Dutch farms was 85 percent (Korevaar, 1992). To prevent environmental pollution and ensure efficient nutrient use, a nutrient management plan should be developed for the farm that will determine the movement and quantity of nutrients entering, leaving, and remaining on the farm; a nutrient application schedule that ensures that the rate and timing of manure and fertilizer applications are in concert with crop requirements while minimizing loss; and a crop selection and rotational sequence that provides quality feed, improves nutrient recycling, and reduces runoff and erosion (Klausner, 1993).

Dairy cows on average secrete in milk 25–35 percent of the nitrogen that they consume (Chase, 1994; Chandler, 1996), and almost all the remaining nitrogen is excreted in feces and urine. Van Horn et al. (1994) indicated that total excretion of nitrogen in waste products can be determined by subtracting the amount secreted in milk from the amount consumed. Feeding nitrogen in excess of requirements, feeding excessive amounts of ruminally degradable protein, or feeding diets not properly balanced for ruminally degradable and undegradable protein, amino acids, or energy may increase nitrogen excretion in feces or urine (Pell, 1992; St-Pierre and Thraen, 1999). As milk production increases, nitrogen excretion in feces and urine per unit of milk produced decreases (Chandler, 1996; St-Pierre and Thraen, 1999).

Ammonia and organic nitrogen are the major forms of nitrogen in manure (Van Horn et al., 1994). This nitrogen is from undigested feed, microbial protein, endogenous nitrogen, and urea and ammonia nitrogen excreted in urine. Some 40–50 percent of the total nitrogen excreted in manure is from urea and ammonia nitrogen excreted in urine (Van Horn et al., 1994). Urea is rapidly converted to ammonia in the presence of urease. In an acidic environment ammonia ($NH_3$) reacts with $H^+$ to form the nongaseous ammonium ion ($NH_4^+$); this reaction prevents the loss of $NH_3$ to the atmosphere. However, most dairy cow manure provides little acid for converting $NH_3$ to $NH_4^+$, and it releases large amounts of $NH_3$ into the atmosphere. In fact, 50–75 percent of the nitrogen can be lost from manure mostly as $NH_3$ before nitrification to nitrate ($NO_3^-$) (Van Horn et al., 1994). Excessive concentrations of $NH_3$ in closed buildings can lower animal performance and pose a potential health hazard for cows and people. In addition, $NH_3$ emitted into the air can cause acid rain. If excessive nitrogen is applied to land in manure, $NO_3^-$ can contaminate surface water and leach into the groundwater.

Many aspects of dairy cattle nutrition will probably contribute to improving the efficiency of nitrogen use in the future, including optimizing the intake of nitrogen, ruminal fermentation, the synthesis of microbial protein, and the passage of ruminally protected amino acids to the small intestine; absorption and postabsorption metabolism of nitrogen; and the further development of integrated computer models, feeding systems, and waste-management systems based on new scientific information generated from research to determine nutrient requirements, increase efficiency of nutrient use, and decrease excretion of nutrients into the environment (Clark and Overton, 1995).

It will be difficult to determine an exact amount of crude protein to include in the diet that will provide optimal performance in all situations. The amount of crude protein needed in the diet will be influenced by milk yield, milk protein percentage, growth rate, body size, amount and type of energy in the diet, and amino acid composition and degradability of dietary protein. Feeding diets that do not meet requirements of ruminal microbes and dairy cows decrease nutrient digestibility and production of milk and milk components. An adequate supply of nitrogen is essential for maximizing carbohydrate digestibility in the rumen (Oldham, 1984). Carbohydrate makes up the largest percentage of diets fed to dairy cattle, and anything that increases carbohydrate digestibility increases energy availability to cows, decreases the volume of manure produced, and reduces concerns about waste disposal. In contrast, feeding a diet that contains too much crude protein is wasteful, detrimental to the environment, inefficient for dairy cattle because energy must be used to synthesize urea that is excreted in urine, and costly to dairy farmers because the protein is not used for productive functions by dairy cows.

Feeding high-quality forages that are produced on the farm will improve nutrient management and increase dry matter (DM) intake. Maximizing DM intake will allow dairy producers to feed diets that contain a lower percentage of crude protein and that will improve the efficiency of nitrogen use by dairy cows and decrease the amount of protein supplement that must be purchased (Chase, 1994). A 5 percent increase in DM intake decreases the percentage of crude protein required in diets by about 1 percentage point (Chase, 1994). Feeding total mixed rations formulated from feeds analyzed to supply the exact amount of nutrients required by dairy cows on the basis of milk production, milk composition, body size, and pregnancy status will be essential for maximizing efficiency of nitrogen use and minimizing environmental pollution.

Optimizing ruminal fermentation, microbial protein synthesis, and passage of selected nutrients to the small intestine of dairy cattle offers potential for improving nutrient management (Clark and Davis, 1983). During ruminal fermentation, dietary protein is degraded to a mixture of peptides, amino acids, and ammonia, and this supplies precursors for synthesis of microbial protein. Excess ammonia is absorbed through the ruminal wall and transported to the liver to be detoxified by synthesizing urea. Any urea that is not recycled to the gastrointestinal tract is excreted in urine; this represents a nitrogen loss from cows to the environment. Both nitrogen and carbohydrates are required for microbial growth; synchronization of carbohydrate and protein degradation should increase incorporation of nitrogen into microbial protein (Hoover and Stokes, 1991; Clark et al., 1992). Digestibility of dry matter, efficiency of microbial protein synthesis, and synthesis of microbial protein in the rumen were maximized when diets contained 10–13 percent of the dietary DM as ruminally degradable protein and 56 percent of the total carbohydrate as nonstructural carbohydrate (Hoover and Stokes, 1991); however, further refinement of these estimates is needed. Increasing feed intake and the amount of organic matter digested in the rumen will supply additional energy to fuel microbial growth if both protein and carbohydrates are in adequate supply and their degradation is synchronized (Clark et al., 1992). Faster growth of microorganisms coupled with faster passage of microorganisms to the small intestine resulting from increased feed intake should decrease recycling of energy and nitrogen in the rumen because of decreased cell lysis; this will decrease maintenance requirements and trap more nutrients for growth of the microorganisms (Clark et al., 1992; Russell et al., 1992).

Microbial protein supplies a large quantity of the total amino acids passing to the small intestine; therefore, differences in passage of individual amino acids to the small intestine when different diets are fed often are small (Clark et al., 1992). From a nutrient-management perspective, it is essential that use of amino acids be optimized for production of milk and milk protein if dairy cows are to use crude protein from the diet most efficiently. Schwab (1994) reported that methionine and lysine were limiting for production of milk and milk protein when they made up less than 5 and 15 percent respectively of the total essential amino acids passing to the small intestine. Feeding protein supplements of low ruminal degradability to cows has not consistently increased the passage of methionine and lysine to the small intestine, probably because synthesis of microbial protein often is decreased (Clark et al., 1992). Even though passage of methionine and lysine to the small intestine can increase in some situations, passage of other amino acids to the small intestine probably will increase also, and the desired ratio of amino acids will not be correctly balanced; the imbalance will result in inefficient use. Feeding diets that contain lower concentrations of crude protein supplemented with balanced quantities of rumen-protected amino acids should minimize excretion of nitrogen in the urine.

The contributions of small peptides to microbial growth in the rumen have not been quantified in dairy cattle. Ruminal bacteria might transport peptides more rapidly and efficiently than single amino acids (Chen et al., 1987), and growth and efficiency of growth of ruminal bacteria are improved when amino acids or peptides are supplied, as opposed to ammonia (Maeng and Baldwin, 1976a, b; Maeng et al., 1976). Therefore, the potential exists to improve the efficiency of microbial protein synthesis by manipulating the quantity and composition of peptides supplied to the ruminal microorganisms.

Few data are available to quantify the absorption and metabolism of amino acids by splanchnic tissues of lactating dairy cows, but the use of many amino acids by the portal-drained viscera is substantial (Reynolds et al., 1994). Furthermore, the contribution of peptides to amino acid absorption and transport is relatively unknown (Reynolds et al., 1994). Substantial quantities of amino acids are probably absorbed from the gut as short peptides (Webb et al., 1992, 1993), but research is needed to provide a better understanding of absorption and metabolism of amino acids and peptides by tissues of lactating dairy cows. Data on the effects of amount and composition of peptides on ruminal microorganisms and tissues of dairy cattle could unlock mechanisms that will improve the efficiency of nitrogen use and decrease nitrogen output in urine and feces.

## PHOSPHORUS

In some parts of the United States and in many other countries, the amount of waste that can be generated by a farm operation is regulated and limited by law. For instance, in the Netherlands in 1987, laws were enacted that limited the amount of phosphorus that could be applied to the land to 55 kg/hectare. That corresponded to limiting agriculture to about three cows or 17 pigs per hectare (Korevaar and den Boer, 1990). Regulatory agencies usually give special attention to the role of phosphate as an environmental pollutant, because it is relatively easy to measure and does not volatilize or leach away, as does much of the nitrogen excreted into manure and applied to the land. Phosphate in manure that is applied to the land is usually adsorbed onto soil particles, so it does not leach into water tables or into waterways; therefore, it builds up in the soil (Pierzynski et al., 1994). It will erode into waterways with soil and causes environmental concern because it is considered to be the nutrient that limits growth of most aquatic plants (Sharpley et al., 1994). From a regulatory standpoint, it is also felt probable that if an excessive amount of phosphate is being excreted and applied to the land, an excessive amount of nitrogen is also being lost to the environment.

Nearly two-thirds of the phosphorus found in common feedstuffs is unavailable to nonruminant animals because it is bound to the organic acid phytate. In contrast, ruminal microorganisms effectively break down phytate, making a greater proportion of dietary phosphorus available to ruminant animals. In the subcommittee's model the coefficients of absorption of phosphorus from the diet are 64 percent for forages, 70 percent for concentrates, and > 70 percent for most of the inorganic sources of phosphorus.

Once the phosphorus needs of cows have been met by the diet, most of the extra phosphorus will be excreted in the feces and urine. Morse et al. (1992) fed lactating Holstein cows diets that contained phosphorus at 0.30, 0.41, and 0.56 percent, which supplied 60, 82, and 112 g of phosphorus/day, respectively. On the basis of the 1989 National Research Council requirements, the cows were fed 79, 108, and 147 percent of their phosphorus requirement. According to the current model in this publication, the cows required a diet that provided 58–62 g of phosphorus/day. Cows fed 60 g/day of phosphorus in the diet, which provided less than required, excreted 42.1 g of phosphorus in feces and urine. Cows fed 82 g/day of phosphorus excreted 50.6 g/day of phosphorus in feces and urine, or 5 g for each 22 g of phosphorus fed in excess of requirements. Cows fed 112 g/day of phosphorus excreted 79.9 in feces and urine. Increasing dietary phosphorus intake from 82 g/d to 112 g/d (a 30 g/d increase) increased phosphorus excretion in feces and urine by 29.3 g/d. Wu et al. (1998) and Satter and Wu (1999) showed that the loss of fecal phosphorus increased greatly once the needs of the animal were met, which occurred at about 0.35 percent dietary P in their experiment. They also showed that the dietary requirement for phosphorus can be met with diets that are below the requirement suggested in the 1989 National Research Council publication which was 0.48 percent in diets for cows in early lactation and 0.41 percent in diets for cows in later lactation. Many dairy rations contain phosphorus in excess of the needs of cows. A survey of nutritionists indicated that the average concentration of phosphorus in diets fed to commercial herds was about 0.52 percent for high-producing dairy cows (Sansinena et al., 1999).

## SUMMARY

Dairy cattle should be fed to meet but not to exceed their nutrient requirements. Feeding diets that are deficient in any nutrient will decrease production of milk and milk components; however, feeding excessive amounts of a nutrient will decrease the efficiency of nutrient utilization, which results in increased nutrient excretion into the environment, increased cost of milk production, decreased profits for dairy producers, and increased costs for the consumers of dairy products. Production of milk by dairy cows causes losses of nutrients in feces and urine that can not be prevented. Because nutrients accumulate on dairy farms, nutrients should be managed to ensure efficient nutrient cycling with a minimum impact on the environment.

## REFERENCES

Aarts, H. F. M., E. E. Biewinga, and H. Van Keulen. 1992. Dairy farming systems based on efficient nutrient management. Neth. J. Agric. Sci. 40:285–299.

Chandler, P. T. 1996. Environmental challenges as related to animal agriculture—dairy. pp. 7–19 *in* Nutrient Management of Food Animals to Enhance and Protect the Environment. E. T. Kornegay ed. CRC Press, Inc., Boca Raton, FL.

Chase, L. E. 1994. Environmental considerations in developing dairy rations. pp. 56–62 *in* Proc. Cornell Nutr. Conf. Feed Manuf., Rochester, NY. Cornell Univ., Ithaca, NY.

Chen, G., J. B. Russell, and C. J. Sniffen. 1987. A procedure for measuring peptides in rumen fluid and evidence that peptide uptake can be a rate-limiting step in ruminal protein degradation. J. Dairy Sci. 70:1211–1219.

Clark, J. H., and C. L. Davis. 1983. Future improvement of milk production: Potential for nutritional improvement. J. Animal Sci. 57:750–764.

Clark, J. H., T. H. Klusmeyer, and M. R. Cameron. 1992. Microbial protein synthesis and flows of nitrogen fractions to the duodenum of dairy cows. J. Dairy Sci. 75:2304–2323.

Clark, J. H., and T. R. Overton. 1995. The dairy industry and dairy cattle nutrition in the 21st century. pp. 4–59 *in* Proc. California Anim. Nutr. Conf., Fresno, CA. California State Polytechnic University, Pomona, CA.

Hoover, W. H., and S. R. Stokes. 1991. Balancing carbohydrates and proteins for optimum rumen microbial yield. J. Dairy Sci. 74:3630–3644.

Johnson, D. E., G. M. Ward, and J. J. Ramsey. 1996. Livestock methane: Current emissions and mitigation potential. pp. 219–233 *in* Nutrient Management of Food Animals to Enhance and Protect the Environment. E. T. Kornegay ed. CRC Press, Inc., Boca Raton, FL.

Klausner, S. D. 1993. Mass nutrient balances on dairy farms. pp. 126–129 *in* Proc. Cornell Nutr. Conf. Feed Manuf., Rochester, NY. Cornell Univ., Ithaca, NY.

Koelsch, R., and G. Lesoing. 1999. Nutrient balance on Nebraska livestock confinement systems. J. Dairy Sci. 82(Suppl. 2):63–71.

Korevaar, H. 1992. The nitrogen balance on intensive Dutch dairy farms: A review. Livestock Prod. Sci. 31:17–27.

Korevaar, H., and D. J. den Boer. 1990. Practical measures to reduce nutrient losses from grassland systems. The Fertilizer Soc., London. p. 33.

Kuipers, A., F. Mandersloot, and R. L. G. Zom. 1999. An approach to nutrient management on dairy farms. J. Dairy Sci. 82(Suppl. 2):84–89.

Lanyon, L. E. 1994. Dairy manure and plant nutrient management issues affecting water quality and the dairy industry. J. Dairy Sci. 77:1999–2007.

Maeng, W. J., and R. L. Baldwin. 1976a. Factors influencing rumen microbial growth rates and yields: Effects of urea and amino acids over time. J. Dairy Sci. 59:643–647.

Maeng, W. J., and R. L. Baldwin. 1976b. Factors influencing rumen microbial growth rates and yields: Effects of amino acid additions to a purified diet with nitrogen from urea. J. Dairy Sci. 59:648–655.

Maeng, W. J., C. J. Van Nevel, R. L. Baldwin, and J. G. Morris. 1976. Rumen microbial growth rates and yields: Effects of amino acids and protein. J. Dairy Sci. 59:68–79.

Meyer, D. 2000. Dairying and the environment. J. Dairy Sci. 83:1419–1427.

Meyer, D., and D. D. Mullinax. 1999. Livestock nutrient management concerns: Regulatory and legislative overview. J. Dairy Sci. 82(Suppl. 2):51–62.

Miner, J. R. 1997. Nuisance concerns and odor control. J. Dairy Sci. 80:2667–2672.

Morse, D., H. H. Head, C. J. Wilcox, H. H. van Horn, C. D. Hissem, and B. Harris, Jr. 1992. Effects of concentration of dietary phosphorus on amount and route of excretion. J. Dairy Sci. 75:3039–3049.

National Research Council. 1989. Nutrient Requirements of Dairy Cattle, 6th Rev. ed. Natl. Acad. Sci., Washington, DC.

Nelson, C. J. 1999. Managing nutrients across regions of the United States. J. Dairy Sci. 82(Suppl. 2):90–100.

Oldham, J. D. 1984. Protein-energy interrelationships in dairy cows. J. Dairy Sci. 67:1090–1114.

Pell, A. N. 1992. Does ration balancing affect nutrient management? pp. 23–31 *in* Proc. Cornell Nutr. Conf. Feed Manuf., Rochester, NY. Cornell Univ., Ithaca, NY.

Pierzynski, G. M., J. T. Sims, and G. F. Vance. 1994. Soils and Environmental Quality. Boca Raton, FL: Lewis Publishers, CRC Press. 313 p.

Reynolds, C. K., D. L. Harmon, and M. J. Cecava. 1994. Absorption and delivery of nutrients for milk protein synthesis by portal-drained viscera. J. Dairy Sci. 77:2787–2808.

Russell, J. B., J. D. O'Connor, D. G. Fox, P. J. Van Soest, and C. J. Sniffen. 1992. A net carbohydrate and protein system for evaluating cattle diets: I. Ruminal fermentation. J. Animal Sci. 70:3551–3561.

Sansinena, M., L. D. Bunting, S. R. Stokes, and E. R. Jordan. 1999. A survey of trends and rationales for dietary phosphorus recommendations among mid-south dairy nutritionists. Proceedings of the 1999 Mid-South Ruminant Nutrition Conference. Texas Agricultural Extension Service, May 6–7, Dallas, TX. p. 51–54.

Satter, L. D., and Z. Wu. 1999. New strategies in ruminant nutrition. Getting ready for the next millenium. pp. 1–24 *in* Southwest Nutr. and Mgt. Conf. Proc. Phoenix, AZ. Univ. of Arizona, Tucson.

Schwab, C. G. 1994. Optimizing amino acid nutrition for optimum yields of milk and milk protein. pp. 114–129 *in* Proc. Southwest Nutr. and Mgt. Conf., Phoenix, AZ. Univ. of Arizona, Tucson.

Sharpley, A. N., S. C. Chapra, R. Wedepohl, J. T. Sims, T. C. Daniel, and K. R. Reddy. 1994. Managing agricultural phosphorus for protection of surface waters: Issues and options. J. Environ. Qual. 23:437–451.

St-Pierre, N. R., and C. S. Thraen. 1999. Animal grouping strategies, sources of variation, and economic factors affecting nutrient balance on dairy farms. J. Dairy Sci. 82(Suppl. 2):72–83.

Tamminga, S. 1992. Nutrition management of dairy cows as a contribution to pollution control. J. Dairy Sci. 75:345–357.

Van Horn, H. H., A. C. Wilkie, W. J. Powers, and R. A. Nordstedt. 1994. Components of dairy manure management systems. J. Dairy Sci. 77:2008–2030.

Webb, K. E., Jr., D. B. DiRienzo, and J. C. Matthews. 1993. Recent developments in gastrointestinal absorption and tissue utilization of peptides: A review. J. Dairy Sci. 76:351–361.

Webb, K. E., Jr., J. C. Matthews, and D. B. DiRienzo. 1992. Peptide absorption: A review of current concepts and future perspectives. J. Animal Sci. 70:3248–3257.

Wu, Z., L.D. Satter, R. Sojo, and A. Blohowiak. 1998. Phosphorus balance of dairy cows in early lactation at three levels of dietary phosphorus. J. Dairy Sci. 81(Suppl.1):358.

# 13 Carbohydrate Chemistry and Feed Processing

## NONSTRUCTURAL CARBOHYDRATES

The more readily digestible carbohydrates in animal feeds lack a satisfactory system of classification, even though they represent the major energy yielding components of feedstuffs. The lack of an adequate definition is partly a function of the diversity of the chemical fraction as well as lack of basic research into their specific nutritive characteristics. The nonstructural carbohydrates are those carbohydrates not included in the cell wall matrix and they are not recovered in NDF. By this definition, the nonstructural carbohydrates are comprised of sugars, starches, organic acids, and other reserve carbohydrates such as fructans.

Nonstructural carbohydrates can be classified as water-soluble (including monosaccharides, disaccharides, oligosaccharides, and some polysaccharides) and larger polysaccharides that are insoluble in water. Water soluble nonstructural carbohydrates, such as sugars (glucose and fructose) and disaccharides (sucrose and lactose) are rapidly fermented in the rumen and comprise a significant fraction of certain feeds (molasses, sugar beets, high sugar corn grain, and whey). Sugar content of fresh grasses and legumes is variable and may exceed 10 percent of the dry matter (DM), but hay and silage have lower concentrations because of losses from fermentation and respiration. Temperate grasses store fructans in leaves and stems as water-soluble levan. Fructosan is increased by cool weather and may increase to as much as 30 percent of the DM for cool season perennial ryegrass (Van Soest, 1983). Although water-soluble carbohydrates may be high in individual feeds, concentrations are generally low in ruminant diets. Galactans are the storage carbohydrate of leguminous plants, and the B-glucan gums are found in the bran of barley, oats, and rye, and the cell wall of grasses (Aman and Hesselman, 1985). Pectins are associated with the cell wall but are not covalently linked to the lignified portions and are almost completely digested (90 to 100 percent) in the rumen. Pectin concentrations on a DM basis are high in citrus and beet pulps, soybean hulls, and dicotyledonous legume forages but are low in grasses (Allen and Knowlton, 1995). Starch is the major storage carbohydrate in most cereal grains. It is composed of two major molecules: amylose and amylopectin. Amylose is a linear polymer of α 1-4, D-glucose units while amylopectin is a branched polymer with linear chains of α D-glucose that has a branch point every 20 to 25 glucose units (French, 1973). Most forages contain little starch with the exception of small grain silage (10 to 20 percent of DM), grain sorghum silage (25 to 35 percent), and corn silage (25 to 35 percent of DM). The ruminal degradation of starch is variable ranging from 40 to over 90 percent depending on source, processing, and other factors.

## ANALYTIC PROCEDURES

### *Neutral Detergent Fiber*

The accuracy of feed composition data and requirements for NDF and NSC is compromised by the lack of standard methods. The neutral detergent fraction includes cellulose, hemicellulose, and lignin as the major components. There are three major modifications of the NDF method, each of which generates different values depending upon the feed that is analyzed. The original NDF method (Van Soest and Wine, 1967, Goering and Van Soest, 1970) used sodium sulfite to remove contaminating proteins from NDF by cleaving disulfide bonds and dissolving many crosslinked proteins. It was discovered that the original method did not adequately remove starch from grains and corn silage. The neutral detergent residue modification was developed that included a heat-stable amylase in the procedure to remove starch, however, sulfite was removed from the procedure because of concerns about the possible loss of lignin and phenolic compounds (Van Soest et al., 1991). The amylase-treated NDF modification (aNDF) was developed to measure NDF in all types of feeds and uses both heat-stable amylase and sodium sulfite to obtain NDF with minimum contamination by either starch or protein. It has been adopted as the reference method for NDF by the National Forage Testing Association (Undersander et al., 1993), and is being evaluated in a collaborative study for AOAC approval as an official method. The use of sodium sulfite is crucial for the removal of nitrogenous contamination from heated feeds (Hintz et al., 1996). If the objective is to accurately measure total fiber in feeds with minimum contamination by digestible protein or starch the aNDF method is preferred. Sodium sulfite improves the filtration of fiber residues during the NDF procedure and allows the method to be used on all types of feeds and feed mixtures, including heated feeds and protein supplements. The aNDF method cannot be used to measure the slowly degraded protein (B3) fraction in feeds in the Net Protein and Carbohydrate Model which is defined as the difference between neutral detergent insoluble crude protein (measured without the use of sulfite) and acid detergent insoluble crude protein. When NDF is measured without the use of sodium sulfite it probably should be corrected for protein contamination. However, for routine analysis the aNDF procedure will provide an accurate estimate of NDF with minimum contamination by protein or starch. The NDF concentrations shown in Table 15-1 were determined using amylase and sulfite.

*Neutral Detergent Insoluble Nitrogen*

The nitrogen associated with NDF is mostly cell wall-bound protein plus other nitrogen compounds and includes indigestible nitrogen found in the acid-detergent residue. A major cell-wall associated protein is extensin that is covalently linked to hemicellulosic carbohydrate (Fry, 1988). The nitrogen insoluble in neutral detergent solution (NDIN), but soluble in acid detergent, is digestible and consists of slowly degraded protein (Licitra et al., 1996). Pichard (1977) reported a positive correlation between the slowly solubilized pool of nitrogen and NDIN in forage samples. Krishnamoorthy et al. (1982) demonstrated that over 30 percent of total nitrogen in forages and fermented grains was NDIN (sulfite was not used).

Protein contamination of NDF for unheated forages is not a major problem, but neutral detergent insoluble CP (NDICP) is still in the range of 8 to 12 percent of the NDF with sulfite. For certain concentrate feeds such as distillers' and brewers' grains, CP contamination can greatly inflate NDF values. The concentration of NDICP (as a percentage of NDF) for brewers' and distillers' grains can be as high as 40 percent (Weiss et al., 1989). Adding sulfite to the NDF solution reduces CP contamination but does not quantitatively remove all the contamination (Dong and Rasco, 1987). Standardization of procedures for nitrogen fractionation of ruminant feeds has been reviewed by Licitra et al. (1996).

*Acid Detergent Fiber*

The acid detergent fiber (ADF) fraction of feedstuffs includes cellulose and lignin as primary components and should be analyzed according to AOAC (1973). The residue also contains variable amounts of ash and nitrogen compounds.

*Acid Detergent Insoluble Nitrogen*

The concentration of acid detergent insoluble nitrogen (ADIN) is used to determine protein availability in heated feeds. Tannins, if present, are one possibility for increased insoluble protein associated with the plant cell wall. Another is the Maillard or nonenzymatic browning reaction caused by heating and drying. The nitrogen in these fractions has low biologic availability and tends to be recovered in ADF (Van Soest, 1965b; Van Soest and Mason, 1991). Heat drying of forages at temperatures above 60° C results in significant increases in yields of lignin and fiber. The increased yield of ADF can be accounted for largely by the production of artifact lignin via nonezymatic Browning Reaction (Van Soest, 1965b). The ADIN can be a sensitive assay for nonenzymatic Browning Reaction due to overheating of certain feeds (Van Soest and Mason, 1991). The ADIN concentration in forages has a strong negative correlation to apparent protein digestibility (Thomas et al., 1982). Nakamura et al. (1994), however, demonstrated a weak correlation between ADIN concentrations in eight different nonforage fiber sources and nitrogen digestibility. Their results indicated that ADIN values in nonforage sources of protein predicted more protein damage than that measured by in vivo nitrogen digestibility. The chemical composition of ADIN (Weiss et al., 1986) and the relationship between ADIN concentrations and digestibility are different between concentrates and forages, therefore the use of a single equation to relate ADIN to nitrogen digestibility for all feeds is not correct.

*Lignin*

Lignin is a noncarbohydrate, high molecular weight compound that constitutes a diverse class of phenolic compounds (Van Soest, 1983). The acid detergent lignin (ADL) procedure of Van Soest (1965a) includes both hydrolytic (sulfuric acid) and oxidative (potassium permanganate) methods; the sulfuric acid variant of ADL is the most popular (Jung et al., 1997). The Klason lignin is the residue remaining after a two stage sulfuric acid hydrolysis that is commonly used to determine the neutral sugar components of cell wall polysaccharides (Theander and Westerlund, 1986). Differences in the ADL and Klason lignin methods ( i.e., order of acid strength use, detergent in the ADF step, and addition of the filtration step to the ADL procedure) account for the difference in lignin values as measured by these two methods (Lowry et al., 1994). Klason lignin values are typically two to four times greater for grasses than the sulfuric ADL estimates and 30 percent higher for legumes (Jung et al., 1997). Hatfield et al. (1994) concluded that the Klason lignin is a more accurate estimate of plant cell wall lignin content than is ADL. Other evidence suggests that an acid soluble lignin fraction is lost in the ADF step of the ADL procedure, thereby resulting in underestimates of lignin content by the ADL method (Lowry et al., 1994).

The Klason lignin procedure was approved by the AOAC (1973) at the same time as ADF. Klason lignin is a better marker for digestibility than permanganate lignin; however, Klason lignin followed by treatment with permanganate yields lignin by difference that is more recoverable in feces (Van Soest et al., 1991). The fraction resistant to both 72 percent sulfuric acid detergent lignin and permanganate is cutin, which is in many seed hulls. The correlation between forage digestibility and concentrations of 72 percent sulfuric acid detergent lignin and Klason lignin were compared by Jung et al. (1997). Thirty-six forages, including C3 legumes and C3 and C4 grasses, were analyzed for sulfuric acid detergent lignin, Klason lignin, and in vitro digestibilities of DM and NDF. Twenty of these forages were also fed to lambs at restricted intake for measurement of DM and NDF digestibilities. Lignin concentrations determined by the two lignin methods were positively correlated, and the Klason lignin value was always greater than the acid detergent lignin concentration. The largest differences were observed for grass forages. In vivo and in vitro digestibilities of DM and NDF in forages were negatively correlated with both lignin measurements. The degree of correlation for the two lignin methods with digestibility was generally similar across all forages and within forage classes. Slopes of linear regressions of digestibility on lignin concentration did not differ between legumes and grasses. Although the sulfuric acid detergent lignin and Klason lignin procedures gave very different estimates of the lignin concentration in forage, they were similarly correlated with digestibility.

### *Total Nonstructural Carbohydrates*

Total nonstructural carbohydrates (NSC) include starch, sugar, and fructan measured using the procedure of Smith (1981) when modified to use ferriccyanide as the colorimetric indicator. The method of Salomonsson et al. (1984) as modified by Herrera-Saldana et al. (1990) measures only starch by an enzymatic method. Crude enzyme preparations such as taka-diastase (derived from Aspergillis oryzae) represents more than 30 different enzymatic functions, including amylolytic, proteolytic, and lipolytic (Nocek, 1991). Considerable variation may be associated with the specificity and/or lack of specificity of enzymes used in the starch and NSC analysis. In most cases the starch and modified Smith (1981) procedure are synonymous. The difference calculation usually accounts for more carbohydrate types (mainly pectin), especially for forages and byproduct feeds. Table 4-1 provides a summary of several common feed sources with measured values for NSC and calculated NFC values as a percentage of DM.

Generally, wheat has the highest content of starch for the grains (77 percent of the DM; ranging from 66 to 82 percent), followed by corn and sorghum (72 percent of the DM; ranging from 65 to 80 percent) and then by barley (57 percent of the DM; ranging from 55 to 75 percent), and oats (58 percent of the DM; ranging from 45 to 69 percent); (Nocek and Tamminga, 1991; Huntington, 1994). Starch content of corn silage (35 percent of the DM) is a function of plant maturity and proportion of grain in the whole plant. Corn silage with 32 percent grain should contain about 22 percent starch. Alfalfa hay or silage contains from 2.7 to 20 percent starch and protein supplements such as soybean meal and cottonseed meal contain from 2.5 to 27 percent starch (Nocek and Tamminga, 1991).

## EFFECTS OF PROCESSING ON ENERGY IN FEED

### *Sources of Starch*

#### BARLEY GRAIN

Cows digest whole barley poorly because of the cutinous nature of the seed husk (Nordin and Campling, 1976). Less than 10 percent of DM from whole barley is digested after 48 hours of in situ incubation in the rumen (McAllister et al., 1990). When grains were broken into halves or quarters, in situ DM digestibility was about 60 percent after 24 hour of incubation. Treatment of barley with an aqueous solution of NaOH (30 to 40 g of NaOH/kg of barley) can substitute for mechanical processing (Ørskov and Greenhalgh, 1977). Barley treated with NaOH has higher concentrations of ash (corresponding to the Na added); the concentrations of the other nutrients are reduced because of ash dilution (McNiven et al., 1995). Dry matter digestibility of NaOH-treated barley in the total tract was similar, digestibility of NDF was higher, and digestibility of starch was lower than for rolled barley. Ruminal digestibility of CP and DM was reduced about 30 percent by NaOH treatment (McNiven et al., 1995). Cows fed NaOH-treated barley or rolled barley produced similar amounts of milk in a 10-week study (Bettenay, 1980), but fat and protein concentrations in milk were reduced when NaOH-treated barley was fed in a short-term study (McNiven et al., 1995).

Milk production and digestibility of DM were similar when cows are fed rolled high-moisture barley or dry rolled barley (Kennelly et al., 1988; Christen et al., 1996). Heat-treatment of dry barley (exit temperatures of 135 or 175° C) has little effect on its gross nutrient composition, energy value, or milk production compared with dry rolled barley (Robinson and McNiven, 1994; McNiven et al., 1995). High producing cows fed twice daily produced more milk when fed heat-treated barley than when fed rolled barley but when cows were fed seven times per day no differences were observed (Robinson and McNiven, 1994).

### CORN GRAIN

Mechanical processing (grinding) significantly increases the digestibility of dry corn. The digestibility of whole corn was increased approximately 25 percent by either rolling (Clark et al., 1975) or cracking (Moe et al., 1973). Ground dry corn has 4 to 6 percent more digestible energy than either rolled or coarsely cracked corn (Moe et al., 1973; Knowlton et al., 1996; Wilkerson et al., 1997). Most of the difference in digestibility between cracked and ground corn is caused by a 7 to 10 percent improvement in digestibility of starch (or nonfiber carbohydrate), but part of the increase is offset by a reduction in digestibility of NDF (Knowlton et al., 1996; Wilkerson et al., 1997). The site of digestion of starch is affected more by grinding than is the digestibility of starch in the total tract. Based on in situ studies, approximately 44 percent of the starch in coarsely cracked corn is digested in the rumen compared with 60 to 65 percent for finely ground corn (Cerneau and Michalet-Doreau, 1991; Lykos et al., 1997).

Because of changes in the site of digestion, the difference in measured $NE_L$ concentrations between cracked and ground corn should be less than the differences in digestibility. The difference in measured $NE_L$ concentrations between cracked and ground dry corn is between 0 and 4 percent (Moe et al., 1973; Wilkerson et al., 1997). Milk production increased 3.5 to 6 percent when high producing (35 kg/d) cows were fed ground dry corn compared with dry cracked corn (Mitzner et al., 1994; Knowlton et al., 1996; Wilkerson et al., 1997). Milk composition was not consistently affected by the fineness of the grind of dry corn. Based on production and calorimetry data, average dry ground corn should have about 6 percent more $NE_L$ than average cracked corn when fed at 3 X maintenance (Table 15-1).

Dry matter digestibility of steam-flaked corn is not consistently higher than that of rolled or ground dry corn when fed to cows (Joy et al., 1997; Crocker et al., 1998; Yu et al., 1998). Plascencia and Zinn (1996) however, reported a 10 percentage unit increase (15 percent) in digestibility of OM between steam-flaked and dry-rolled corn when fed to lactating cows. In that study, digestibility of the dry-rolled corn diet was much lower than would be expected. Generally steam-flaking increases digestibility of starch by 10 to 20 percent but digestibility of NDF decreases by a similar amount (Plascencia and Zinn, 1996; Joy et al., 1997; Crocker et al., 1998; Yu et al., 1998; Dann et al., 1999). Digestibility of starch in the total tract was consistently increased as the density of the corn following steam-flaking was reduced (Chen et al., 1994; Plascencia and Zinn, 1996; Joy et al., 1997; Yu et al., 1998). However, variable responses of flake density have been found for digestibility of OM because digestibility of NDF usually decreases as flake density is reduced. Steam-flaking generally increased the proportion of starch digestion occurring in the rumen. The optimal flake density based on milk production is about 0.36 kg/L (28 lbs/bushel).

The average response in yield of fat-corrected milk was 4.5 percent when steam-flaked corn replaced dry ground corn (Chen et al., 1994; Plascencia and Zinn, 1996; Joy et al., 1997; Yu et al., 1998; Dann et al., 1999). Milk fat percentage was either not affected or tended to decrease and milk protein percentage was either not affected or tended to increase when steam-flaked corn replaced dry rolled corn. Based on milk production and changes in digestibility, the $NE_L$ value for average steam-flaked corn is about 11 percent higher than that for average dry cracked corn and about 4 percent higher than that for average dry finely ground corn when fed at 3 X maintenance (Table 15-1). Theurer et al. (1999) calculated that steam-flaked corn had 18 percent more $NE_L$ than cracked corn. These differences are highly related to DMI and differences between cracked corn and other forms of corn should increase as DMI increases.

The chemical composition of high-moisture corn is similar to that of dry corn except that high moisture corn contains two to three times more soluble CP (Prigge et al., 1976). The concentration of NDF tends to be higher in high moisture corn probably because of contamination by the cob. On average, high-moisture corn was about 9 percent more digestible than dry corn when fed to lactating cows (Tyrrell and Varga, 1987; Wilkerson et al., 1997). When similar diets were fed to nonlactating cows (at approximately maintenance) the difference in digestibility was $<1$ percent (McCaffree and Merrill, 1968; Tyrrell and Varga, 1987). Grinding high-moisture corn increased the digestibility of energy or organic matter of diets about 5 percent compared with diets with rolled high moisture corn (Ekinci and Broderick, 1997; Wilkerson et al., 1997).

Measured $NE_L$ of diets containing rolled high-moisture corn is about 5 percent higher than that of diets containing rolled dry corn when fed to lactating cows (Tyrrell and Varga, 1987; Wilkerson et al., 1997). If no associative effects are assumed, the $NE_L$ value of rolled high-moisture corn was 12 to 13 percent higher than that for rolled dry corn. When the corn was ground, diets with high-moisture corn had 13 percent more $NE_L$ than did diets with dry corn. Assuming no associative effects, the $NE_L$ of the ground high-moisture corn was 32 percent higher than that for the ground dry corn (Wilkerson et al., 1997). The difference in $NE_L$ values between high-moisture and dry corn was about twice as large as the difference in digestibility. Ruminal digestibility of starch is 15 to 25 percent higher when rolled high-moisture corn is fed to high producing cows than when rolled dry corn is fed (Aldrich et al., 1993; Knowlton et al., 1998). Energetic losses should be higher when starch is digested in the rumen rather than the small intestine; $NE_L$ values should differ less than digestibility.

Clark (1975) reviewed the early literature and found no difference in dry matter intake (DMI) (ca. 17 kg/d) or FCM production (ca. 20 kg/d) between cows fed high-moisture or dry corn. In short term studies (Lykos et al., 1997; Wilkerson et al., 1997), DMI was not affected, but milk production increased about 5 percent when dry corn was replaced with high-moisture corn in diets of high producing cows. In a longer term study (Dhiman and Satter, 1995), with diets based on alfalfa and corn silage, cows fed high-moisture corn (either rolled or finely ground) produced 6 percent more 3.5 percent fat-corrected milk (34.2 vs. 32.2 kg/d) than cows fed dry-rolled corn. Conversely, Knowlton et al. (1998) reported that DMI (23.5 kg/d), milk production (35 kg/d), and milk composition were not different between cows fed high-moisture or dry corn. Diets in that study were the same as those used in the calorimetry study conducted by Wilkerson et al. (1997).

Based on digestibility, measured $NE_L$ values, and milk production data, rolled high-moisture corn averages about 7 percent higher in $NE_L$ than dry cracked corn at 3X maintenance. Based on similar criteria, ground high-moisture corn has about 11 percent more $NE_L$ than cracked dry corn at 3X maintenance (Table 15-1).

### CORN SILAGE

Based on limited data, digestibility of starch from normal corn silage (ca. 35 percent DM) is similar to that of cracked corn but digestibility of starch from mature corn silage is about 10 percent less when fed to cows at approximately 3X maintenance (Harrison et al., 1996; Bal et al., 1997). Mechanical rolling of corn silage (i.e., kernel processing) increased digestibility of starch in the total diet by about 6 percent (Bal et al., 1998; Weiss and Wyatt, 2000; Bal et al., 2000). Digestibility of energy in a diet with processed mature corn silage (27 percent of DM) was about 7 percent higher than for a diet with mature unprocessed corn silage, but processing did not affect digestibility of energy in diets with less mature corn silage (Johnson et al., 1998). In another study, processing increased the TDN of one hybrid of corn silage by about 8 percent but had essentially no effect on another hybrid (Weiss and Wyatt, 2000). Milk yield of high producing cows has not been consistently affected by processing corn silage (Bal et al., 1998; Bal et al., 2000; Weiss and Wyatt, 2000). Because of the paucity of published data with lactating cows, an appropriate factor to adjust the energy value of processed corn silage cannot be developed at this time.

### OAT GRAIN

More than 90 percent of the starch in oats is soluble and almost 100 percent of the starch in ground oats disappeared in situ within 4 hour of incubation (Herrera-Saldana et al., 1990). The DM digestibility of diets containing 25 percent whole or rolled oats was not different when fed to lactating cows and milk production was similar (Moran, 1986). Current data do not support extensive processing of oat grain for feeding to moderately producing dairy cows or changing the $NE_L$ value of processed oats.

### SORGHUM GRAIN

Whole sorghum is poorly digested (Nordin and Campling, 1976). The digestibility of starch from dry rolled sorghum is 7 to 18 percent less than that of ground or steam-rolled corn (Oliveira et al., 1993), and barley (Herrera-Saldana and Huber, 1989) when fed to lactating cows. In those studies, yield of solid or fat-corrected milk was slightly (ca. 2 percent) lower when cows were fed dry-rolled sorghum rather than when fed steam-flaked corn, finely ground corn, or barley. Milk production was similar for cows fed dry-rolled sorghum and rolled corn (Mitzner et al., 1994).

Steam-flaked sorghum has consistently higher digestibility of starch than dry rolled sorghum when fed to lactating cows. In three studies, digestibility of starch from diets based on steam-flaked sorghum was 8 percent higher than that for starch from diets based on dry-rolled sorghum (Chen et al., 1994; Santos et al., 1997a; Simas et al., 1998). Another study indicated a 27 percent increase in digestibility of starch when sorghum was steam-flaked (Moore et al., 1992), but the digestibility of the starch in the dry-rolled sorghum diet was very low. On average, digestibility of starch for diets based on stream-flaked sorghum was 98 percent. The digestibility of DM or OM for diets with steam-flaked sorghum was about 8 percent higher than for diets based on dry rolled sorghum (Moore et al., 1992; Chen et al., 1994; Santos et al., 1997a; Simas et al., 1998). The degree to which steam flaking increases the feeding value of sorghum is primarily a function of flake density. The optimal density of steam-flaked sorghum is about 0.36 kg/L (Chen et al., 1994; Plascencia and Zinn, 1996; Santos et al., 1997a; Santos et al., 1997b). Extremely thin flakes (density $< 0.3$ kg/L) often result in reduced DMI and lower production (Moore et al., 1992; Santos et al., 1997a).

Milk production and gross efficiency of feed utilization (FCM yield/DMI) when steam-flaked sorghum was fed was about 10 percent higher than when dry-rolled sorghum was fed (Moore et al., 1992; Chen et al., 1994; Santos et al., 1997a; Simas et al., 1998). Based on milk production and DM digestibility data, the $NE_L$ value of steam-flaked sorghum is about 13 percent higher than for dry-rolled sorghum. Compared with cracked corn, dry rolled sorghum contains about 4 percent less $NE_L$ at 3X maintenance (a function of less fat and lower starch digestibility). Steam-flaked sorghum (mainly because of improved digestibility of starch) has about 9 percent more $NE_L$ than cracked corn at 3X maintenance (Table 15-1). This difference is less than the difference (16 percent) calculated by Theurer et al. (1999).

#### WHEAT GRAIN

Data on the effects of processing wheat fed to dairy cows are lacking. In situ DM disappearance of intact wheat is low but once the kernel is broken, particle size does not greatly affect extent or rate of DM disappearance (McAllister et al., 1990). In a study with nonlactating cows fed a diet with 33 percent wheat, OM digestibility of the diet was increased by 30 percent when the wheat was rolled rather than when fed whole (Nordin and Campling, 1976). The digestibility of OM was 88 percent for rolled wheat and 41 percent for whole wheat grain. Based on that study, wheat should undergo some mechanical processing prior to feeding to dairy cows. Ground wheat to supply up to 33 percent of dietary DM has been fed to moderately producing cows (ca. 30 kg/d) without negative effects (Faldet et al., 1989). The benefits, if any, of feeding ground wheat rather than rolled wheat to dairy cows are not known.

### *Oilseeds*

#### COTTONSEED

The majority of cottonseed fed in the United States is not processed; however, the effects of mechanical processing and heat-treatment of cottonseeds have been investigated (Arieli, 1998). The DM digestibility of diets with 15 percent intact, cracked, or ground Pima cottonseed (naturally delinted) was not different when fed to lactating cows although approximately 12 percent of the intact seeds (weight basis) were excreted in the feces (Sullivan et al., 1993a,b). Digestibility of fiber tended to be reduced and digestibility of crude fat was increased by cracking or grinding. Based on the digestibility data in those experiments, the TDN of cracked and ground Pima seeds would be about 7 percentage units higher (ca. 10 percent ) than that of intact Pima seeds. Milk production and gross efficiency of feed utilization were not different when cows were fed intact or cracked Pima cottonseed but gross efficiency was 9 percent higher for the diet with ground Pima seeds compared with the diet that contained intact cottonseed (Sullivan et al., 1993a,b). Similar to the data with Pima cottonseed, 11 percent of the acid delinted cottonseeds consumed by lactating cows were voided in the feces compared with $<1$ percent of whole linted cottonseed (Coppock et al., 1985). Because of lack of dilution by lint, delinted seeds generally have higher ether extract concentrations than linted seeds; therefore differences in TDN are less than differences in digestibiilty. However, based on the data of Coppock et al. (1985) whole delinted cottonseeds have about 10 percent less TDN than whole linted seeds. When the delinted seeds were cracked TDN values were slightly higher than those for whole linted seeds (Coppock et al., 1985). Grinding linted cottonseeds had little effect on extent and site of digestibility of most nutrients or on milk production when fed to low producing cows (Pires et al., 1997).

The effect of heat-treatment of whole linted cottonseed on OM digestibility has been inconsistent. Heat-treatment of cottonseeds has either not affected OM digestibility (Pena et al., 1986) or decreased it (Pires et al., 1997). In the Pires et al. (1997) study, digestibility of NDF and CP was reduced but digestibility of fatty acids was not affected by heat-treatment. When heat-treated cottonseeds were ground, digestibility of OM was similar to that for raw cottonseeds (Pires et al., 1997). Feed intake and milk production were not different when low to moderate producing cows were fed raw or heat-treated cottonseed (Smith and Vosloo, 1994; Pires et al., 1997). Pires et al. (1997) reported increased milk protein when heat-treated cottonseed was fed.

Currently available data do not support adjusting the $NE_L$ value of linted cottonseeds when they are ground or cracked. Grinding significantly increases the energy value of delinted cottonseeds. Even though chemical data suggest that delinted cottonseeds would have more energy than linted seeds, based on digestibility, linted seeds have approximately 10 percent more available energy than delinted seeds when intact seeds are fed.

#### SOYBEANS

Heat-treatment of soybeans generally consists of heating the whole seed to 120 to 140° C and steeping for 30 to

120 minutes. Digestibility of diets with 10 to 18 percent soybeans were not different when roasted or raw soybeans were fed to dairy cows or steers (Bernard, 1990; Tice et al., 1993; Aldrich et al., 1995), but one study (Scott et al., 1991) found that OM digestibility of a diet that contained 16 percent soybeans was reduced (69 vs. 60 percent ) when roasted soybeans were fed compared with raw soybeans. Roasting soybeans has not consistently altered crude fat or fatty acid digestibility (Aldrich et al., 1995; Bernard, 1990; Scott et al., 1991; Tice et al., 1993).

Milk production was generally, but not always, increased when cows were fed roasted soybeans compared with cows fed raw soybeans. Two studies (Bernard, 1990; Scott et al., 1991) with cows producing approximately 30 kg/d of milk indicated no difference between raw and roasted soybeans. Four other studies (Faldet and Satter, 1991; Tice et al., 1993; Chouinard et al., 1997; Dhiman et al., 1997) indicated that cows fed roasted soybeans produced 10 to 16 percent more milk than did cows fed raw soybeans. Source of forage did not seem to influence the results. Some of the inconsistency could be caused by different heat-treatments.

Digestibility of OM from diets that contained whole, cracked, or ground roasted soybeans was not different (Tice et al., 1993). Milk production (38.5 vs. 37.2 kg/d) was higher for cows fed coarsely cracked roasted soybeans than for cows fed ground roasted soybeans (Dhiman et al., 1997). With low-producing cows (19 kg/d) mechanical processing of roasted soybeans did not affect milk production (Tice et al., 1993).

Data comparing the digestibility of diets that contained extruded soybeans with diets that contained raw or roasted soybeans are limited. Scott et al. (1991) reported similar digestibility of diets that contained either 16 percent extruded or roasted soybeans and both were lower than the digestibility of the diet that contained raw soybeans. Milk production by cows fed extruded soybeans was similar or higher than that of cows fed raw or roasted soybeans (Guillaume et al., 1991; Scott et al., 1991; Chouinard et al., 1997). Digestibility data do not support adjusting $NE_L$ concentrations when soybeans are roasted, or extruded, or when roasted soybeans are mechanically processed.

## REFERENCES


Aldrich, C. G., N. R. Merchen, and J. K. Drackley. 1995. The effect of roasting temperature applied to whole soybeans on site of digestion by steers: 1. Organic matter, energy, fiber and fatty acid digestion. J. Anim. Sci. 73 2120–2130.

Aldrich, J. M., L. D. Muller, G. A. Varga, and J. L. C. Griel. 1993. Nonstructural carbohydrate and protein effects on rumen fermentation, nutrient flow and performance of dairy cows. J. Dairy Sci. 76:1091–1105.

Allen, M. S., and K. F. Knowlton. 1995. Non-structural carbohydrates important for ruminants. Feedstuffs, April 17, 1995, pp. 13–15.

Aman, P. and K. Hesselman. 1985. An enzyme method for analysis of total mixed linkage beta glucans in cereal grains. J. Cereal Sci. 3:231–237.

Association of Official Analytical Chemists. 1973. Official Methods of Analysis. Washington, D.C.

Arieli, A. 1998. Whole cottonseed in dairy cattle feeding: a review. Anim. Feed Sci. Tech. 72:97–110.

Bal, M. A., J. G. Coors, and R. D. Shaver. 1997. Impact of the maturity of corn for use as silage in the diets of dairy cows on intake, digestion, and milk production. J. Dairy Sci. 80:2497–2503.

Bal, M. A., R. D. Shaver, K. J. Shinners, and L. D. Satter. 1998. Effect of mechanical processing on the utilization of whole-plant corn silage by lactating dairy cows. J. Dairy Sci. 81(Suppl. 1):334 (abstr.).

Bal, M. A., R. D. Shaver, A. G. Jirovec, K. J. Shinners, and J. G. Coors. 2000. Crop processing and chop length of corn silage: effects on intake, digestion, and milk production by dairy cows. J. Dairy Sci. 83:1264–1273.

Bernard, J. K. 1990. Effect of raw or roasted whole soybeans on digestibility of dietary nutrients and milk production of lactating dairy cows. J. Dairy Sci. 73:3231–3236.

Bettenay, R. A. 1980. Comparison of caustic soda-treated barley and rolled barley in the ration of dairy cows. Austral. J. Exp. Ag. Anim. Husb. 20:394–397.

Cerneau, P., and B. Michalet-Doreau. 1991. In situ starch degradation of different feeds in the rumen. Reprod. Nutr. Dev. 1:65–72.

Chen, K. H., J. T. Huber, C. B. Theurer, R. S. Swingle, J. Simas, S. C. Chan, Z. Wu, and J. L. Sullivan. 1994. Effect of steam flaking of corn and sorghum grains on performance of lactating cows. J. Dairy Sci. 77:1038–1043.

Chouinard, P. Y., V. Girard, and G. J. Brisson. 1997. Performance and profiles of milk fatty acids of cows fed full fat, heat-treated soybeans using various processing methods. J. Dairy Sci. 80:334–342.

Christen, S. D., T. M. Hill, and M. S. Williams. 1996. Effects of tempered barley on milk yield, intake, and digestion kinetics of lactating Holstein cows. J. Dairy Sci. 79:1394–1399.

Clark. 1975. Utilization of high moisture grains by dairy and beef cattle. Proc 2nd Int'l Silage Res. Conf. 2:205–238.

Clark, J. H., W. J. Croom, and K. E. Harshbarger. 1975. Feeding value of dry, ensiled, and acid treated high moisture corn fed whole or rolled to lactating cows. J. Dairy Sci. 58:907–921.

Coppock, C. E., J. R. Moya, J. W. West, D. H. Nave, J. M. Labore, and C. E. Gates. 1985. Effect of lint on whole cottonseed passage and digestibility and diet choice on intake of whole cottonseed by Holstein cows. J. Dairy Sci. 68:1198–1206.

Crocker, L. M., E. J. DePeters, J. G. Fadel, H. Perez-Monti, S. J. Taylor, J. A. Wyckoff, and R. A. Zinn. 1998. Influence of processed corn grain in diets of dairy cows on digestion of nutrients and milk composition. J. Dairy Sci. 81:2394–2407.

Dann, H. M., G. A. Varga, D. E. Putnam, and J. L. C. Griel. 1999. Improving energy supply to late gestation and early postpartum dairy cows. J. Dairy Sci. 82:1765–1778.

Dhiman, T. R., and L. D. Satter. 1995. Particle size and moisture content of corn grain and their effect on dairy cow performance. J. Dairy Sci. 78(Suppl. 1):210(abstr.).

Dhiman, T. R., A. C. Korevaar, and L. D. Satter. 1997. Particle size of roasted soybeans and the effect on milk production of dairy cows. J. Dairy Sci. 80:1722–1727.

Dong, F. M., and B. A. Rasco. 1987. The neutral detergent fiber, acid detergent fiber, crude fiber, and lignin contents of distiller's grains with solubles. J. Food Sci. 52:403–410.

Ekinci, C., and G. A. Broderick. 1997. Effects of processing high moisture ear corn on ruminal fermentation and milk yield. J. Dairy Sci. 80:3298–3307.

Faldet, M. A., T. Nalsen, L. J. Bush, and G. D. Adams. 1989. Utilization of wheat in complete rations for lactating cows. J. Dairy Sci. 72:1243–1251.

Faldet, M. A., and L. D. Satter. 1991. Feeding heat-treated full fat soybeans to cows in early lactation. J. Dairy Sci. 74:3047–3054.

French, D. 1973. Chemical and physical properties of starch. J. Anim. Sci. 37:1048–1061.

Fry, S. C. 1988. The Growing Plant Cell Wall: Chemical and Metabolic Analysis, Wiley, p. 352. Longman Scientific & Technical:New York, Wiley.

Goering, H. K., and P. J. Van Soest. 1970. Forage fiber analysis. U.S. Department of Agriculture Handbook, No. 379, Washington, D.C.

Guillaume, B., D. E. Otterby, M. D. Stern, J. G. Linn, and D. G. Johnson. 1991. Raw or extruded soybeans and rumen-protected methionine and lysine in alfalfa-based diets for dairy cows. J. Dairy Sci. 74:1912–1922.

Harrison, J. H., L. Johnson, R. Riley, S. Xu, K. Loney, C. W. Hunt, and D. Sapienza. 1996. Effect of harvest maturity of whole plant corn silage on milk production and component yield and passage of corn grain and starch into feces. J. Dairy Sci. 79(Suppl. 1):149(Abstr.).

Hatfield, R. D., H. G. Jung, J. Ralph, D. R. Buxton, and P.J. Weimer. 1994. Comparison of the insoluble residues produced by the Klason lignin and acid detergent lignin procedure. J. Sci. Food Ag. 65:51–58.

Herrera-Saldana, R., and J. T. Huber. 1989. Influence of varying protein and starch digestibilities on performance of lactating cows. J. Dairy Sci. 72:1477–1483.

Herrera-Saldana, R. E., J. T. Huber, and M. H. Poore. 1990. Dry matter, crude protein, and starch degradability of five cereal grains. J. Dairy Sci. 73:2386–2393.

Hintz, R.W., D. R. Mertens, and K. A. Albrecht. 1996. Effects of sodium sulfite on recovery and composition of detergent fiber and lignin. J. AOAC Int. 1996 79:16–22.

Huntington, G. B. 1994. Ruminant starch utilization progress has been extensive. Feedstuffs 66:16–18, 38–43.

Johnson, L. M., J. H. Harrison, R. E. Riley, and A. Tintzman. 1998. Effect of maturity and mechanical processing of corn silage on energy content of corn silage based total mixed rations. J. Dairy Sci. 81(Suppl. 1): 199(abstr.).

Joy, M. T., E. J. DePeters, J. G. Fadel, and R. A. Zinn. 1997. Effects of corn processing on the site and extent of digestion in lactating cows. J. Dairy Sci. 80:2087–2097.

Jung, H. G., D. R. Mertens, and A. J. Payne. 1997. Correlation of acid detergent and Klason lignin with digestibility of forage dry matter and neutral detergent fiber. J. Dairy Sci. 80:1622–1628.

Kennelly, J. J., D. L. Dalton, and J. K. Ha. 1988. Digestion and utilization of high moisture barley by lactating dairy cows. J. Dairy Sci. 71:1259–1266.

Knowlton, K. F., M. S. Allen, and P. S. Erickson. 1996. Lasalocid and particle size of corn grain for dairy cows in early lactation. 1. Effect on performance, serum metabolites and nutrient digestibility. J. Dairy Sci. 79:557–564.

Knowlton, K. F., B. P. Glenn, and R. A. Erdman. 1998. Performance, ruminal fermentation, and site of starch digestion in early lactation Holstein cows fed corn grain harvested and processed differently. J. Dairy Sci. 81:1972–1985.

Krishnamoorthy, U., T. V. Muscato, C. J. Sniffen, and P. J. Van Soest. 1982. Nitrogen fractions in selected feedstuffs. J. Dairy Sci. 65:217–225.

Licitra, G., T. M. Hernandez, and P. J. Van Soest. 1996. Standardization of procedures for nitrogen fractionation of ruminant feeds. Anim. Sci. Feed Tech. 57:347–358.

Lowry, J. B., L. L. Conlan, A. C. Schlink, and C. S. McSweeney. 1994. Acid detergent dispersible lignin in tropical grasses. J. Sci. Food Ag. 65:41–49.

Lykos, T., G. A. Varga, and D. Casper. 1997. Varying degradation rates of total nonstructural carbohydrates: effects on ruminal fermentation, blood metabolites, and milk production and composition in high producing Holstein cows. J. Dairy Sci. 80:3341–3355.

McAllister, T. A., L. M. Rode, D. J. Major, K.-J. Cheng, and J. G. Buchanan-Smith. 1990. Effect of ruminal microbial colonization on cereal grain digestion. Can. J. Anim. Sci. 70:571–579.

McCaffree, J. D., and W. G. Merrill. 1968. High moisture corn for dairy cows in early lactation. J. Dairy Sci. 51:553–560.

McNiven, M. A., M. R. Weisbjerg, and T. Hvelplund. 1995. Influence of roasting or sodium hydroxide treatment of barley on digestion in lactating cows. J. Dairy Sci. 78:1106–1115.

Mitzner, K. C., F. G. Owen, and R. J. Grant. 1994. Comparison of sorghum and corn grains in early and midlactation diets for dairy cows. J. Dairy Sci. 77:1044–1051.

Moe, P. W., H. F. Tyrrell, and J. N. W. Hooven. 1973. Physical form and energy value of corn grain. J. Dairy Sci. 56:1298–1304.

Moore, J. A., M. H. Poore, T. P. Eck, R. S. Swingle, J. T. Huber, and M. J. Arana. 1992. Sorghum grain processing and buffer addition for early lactation cows. J. Dairy Sci. 75:3465–3472.

Moran, J. B. 1986. Cereal grains in complete diets for dairy cows: a comparison of rolled barley, wheat and oats and of three methods of processing oats. Anim. Prod. 43:27–36.

Nakamura, T., T. J. Klopfenstein, and R. A. Britton. 1994. Evaluation of acid detergent insoluble nitrogen as an indicator of protein quality in nonforage proteins. J. Anim. Sci. 72:1043–1048.

Nocek, J. E. 1991. New concepts in carbohydrate nutrition for high producing cows. Prof. Anim. Sci. 8:5–16.

Nocek, J. E., and S. Tamminga. 1991. Site of digestion of starch in the gastrointestinal tract of dairy cows and its effect on milk production. J. Dairy Sci. 74:3598–3629.

Nordin, M., and R. C. Campling. 1976. Digestibility studies with cows given whole and rolled cereal grains. Anim. Prod. 23:305–315.

Oliveira, J. S., J. T. Huber, D. Ben-Ghedalia, R. S. Swingle, C. B. Theurer, and M. Pessarakli. 1993. Influence of sorghum grain processing on performance of lactating dairy cows. J. Dairy Sci. 76:575–581.

Ørskov, E. R., and J. F. D. Greenhalgh. 1977. Alkali treatment as a method of processing whole grain for cattle. J. Ag. Sci. (Camb.) 89:253–255.

Pena, F., H. Tagari, and L. D. Satter. 1986. The effect of heat treatment of whole cottonseed on site and extent of protein digestion in dairy cows. J. Anim. Sci. 62:1423–1433.

Pichard, D.G. R. 1977. Forage nutritive value. Continuous and batch in vitro rumen fermentations and nitrogen solubility. Ph.D. dissertation. Cornell Univ., Ithaca, NY.

Pires, A. V., M. L. Eastridge, J. L. Firkins, and Y. C. Lin. 1997. Effects of heat treatment and physical processing of cottonseed on nutrient digestibility and production performance by lactating cows. J. Dairy Sci. 80:1685–1694.

Plascencia, A., and R. A. Zinn. 1996. Influence of flake density on the feeding value of steam-processed corn in diets for lactating cows. J. Anim. Sci. 74:310–316.

Prigge, E. C., R. R. Johnson, F. N. Owens, and D. Williams. 1976. Soluble nitrogen and acid production of high moisture corn. J. Anim. Sci. 42:490–496.

Robinson, P. H., and M. A. McNiven. 1994. Influence of flame roasting and feeding frequency of barley on performance of dairy cows. J. Dairy Sci. 77:3631–3643.

Salomonsson, A,-C., O. Theander, and E. Westerlund. 1984. Chemical characterization of some Swedish cereal whole meal and bran fractions. Swed. J. Ag. Res. 14:111–118.

Santos, F. A., J. T. Huber, C. B. Theurer, R. S. Swingle, and J. M. Simas. 1997a. Response of lactating dairy cows to various densities of sorghum grain. J. Anim. Sci. 75:1681–1685.

Santos, F. A. P., J. T. Huber, C. B. Theurer, R. S. Swingle, K. H. Chen, S. C. Chan, J. Santos, and E. J. DePeters. 1997b. Comparison of barley and sorghum grain processed at different densities for lactating dairy cows. J. Dairy Sci. 80:2098–2103.

Scott, T. A., D. K. Combs, and R. R. Grummer. 1991. Effects of roasting, extrusion, and particle size on the feeding value of soybeans for dairy cattle. J. Dairy Sci. 74:2555–2562.

Simas, J. M., J. T. Huber, C. B. Theurer, K. H. Chen, F. A. P. Santos, and Z. Wu. 1998. Influence of sorghum grain processing on performance and nutrient digestibilities in dairy cows fed varying concentrations of fat. J. Dairy Sci. 81:1966–1971.

Smith, D. 1981. Removing and analyzing total non-structural carbohydrates from plant tissues. Wisconsin Ag., Exp. Stn. Rep. No. R2107, Madison.

Smith, W. A., and L. P. Vosloo. 1994. Effect of whole cottonseed, heat-treated whole cottonseed and whole cottonseed plus lanolin on milk production and composition. S. African J. Anim. Sci. 24:45–48.

Sullivan, J. L., J. T. Huber, and J. M. Harper. 1993a. Performance of dairy cows fed short staple, pima, and cracked pima cottonseed and feed characteristics. J. Dairy Sci. 76:3555–3561.

Sullivan, J. L., J. T. Huber, R. L. Price, and J. M. Harper. 1993b. Comparison of digestibility, nutritive value, and storage characteristics of different forms of cottonseed in diets fed to lactating dairy cows. J. Anim. Sci. 71:2837–2842.

Theander, O., and E. A. Westerlund. 1986. Studies on dietary fiber. 3. Improved procedures for analysis of dietary fiber. J. Ag. Food Chem. 34:330–336.

Theurer, C. B., J. T. Huber, A. DelgadoElorduy, and R. Wanderley. 1999. Invited review: Summary of steam-flaking corn or sorghum grain for lactating dairy cows. J. Dairy Sci. 82:1950–1959.

Thomas, J. W., Y. Yu, T. Middleton, and C. Stallings. 1982. Estimations of protein damage. pp. 81–98 *in* Protein Requirements for Cattle: Symposium. F. N. Owens, ed. Oklahoma State Univ. MP-109, Stillwater, OK.

Tice, E. M., M. L. Eastridge, and J. L. Firkins. 1993. Raw soybeans and roasted soybeans of different particle sizes. 1. Digestibility and utilization by lactating cows. J. Dairy Sci. 76:224–235.

Tyrrell, H. F., and G. A. Varga. 1987. Energy value for lactation of rations containing ground whole ear maize or maize meal both conserved dry or ensiled at high moisture. Eur. Assoc. Anim. Prod. 32:308–309.

Undersander, D., D. R. Mertens, and N. Thiex. 1993. Forage Analyses Procedures. National Forage Testing Association Proceedings, Omaha, NE, pp. 95–103.

Van Soest, P. J. 1965a. Use of detergents in analyses of fibrous feeds. II. A rapid method for the determination of fiber and lignin. J. Assoc. Offic. Agric. Chem. 46:829–835.

Van Soest, P. J. 1965b. Use of detergents in analysis of fibrous feeds. III. Study of effects of heating and drying on yields of fiber and lignin in feeds. J. Assoc. Offic. Agric. Chem. 48:785–791.

Van Soest, P. J. 1983. Nutritional ecology of the ruminant. Comstock, Cornell Univ. Press, Ithaca, NY.

Van Soest, P. J., and R. H. Wine. 1967. Use of detergents in the analysis of fibrous feeds. IV. J. Assoc. Offic. Agric. Chem. 50:50–55.

Van Soest, P. J., and V. C. Mason. 1991. The influence of the Maillard reaction upon the nutritive value of fibrous feeds. Anim. Feed Sci. Tech. 32:45–53.

Van Soest, P. J., J. B. Robertson, and B. A. Lewis. 1991. Methods for dietary fiber, neutral detergent fiber, and nonstarch polysaccharides in relation to animal nutrition. J. Dairy Sci. 74:3583–3587.

Weiss, W. P., H. R. Conrad, and W. L. Shockey. 1986. Digestibility of nitrogen in heat-damaged alfalfa. J. Dairy Sci. 69:2658–2670.

Weiss, W. P., D. O. Erickson, G. M. Erickson, and G. R. Fisher. 1989. Barley distillers grains as a protein supplement for dairy cows. J. Dairy Sci. 72:980–987.

Weiss, W. P., and D. J. Wyatt. 2000. Effect of oil content and kernel processing of corn silage on digestibility and milk production by dairy cows. J. Dairy Sci. 83:351–358.

Wilkerson, V. A., B. P. Glenn, and K. R. McLeod. 1997. Energy and nitrogen balance in lactating cows fed diets containing dry or high moisture corn in either rolled or ground form. J. Dairy Sci. 80:2487–2496.

Yu, P., J. T. Huber, F. A. P. Santos, J. M. Simas, and C. B. Theurer. 1998. Effects of ground, steam-flaked, and steam-rolled corn grains on performance of lactating cows. J. Dairy Sci. 81:777–783.

# 14 Nutrient Requirement Tables

Requirements for rumen degradable protein (RDP), rumen undegradable protein (RUP), and total protein are dependent on animal factors, the concentration of available energy in the diet, and dry matter intake. The dietary requirement for minerals depends on animal factors and the bioavailability of the minerals which differs among feedstuffs and diets. Tables of nutrient requirements are included to provide users with general guidelines and to illustrate how dietary factors influence requirements of some nutrients. The computer model uses animal and dietary factors to estimate requirements and will produce the most accurate estimates of requirements for specific situations and specific diet formulations. Users are strongly encouraged to use model-generated requirements.

## LACTATING COWS

Tables 14-1 through 14-6 show RDP, RUP, and total crude protein (CP) requirements for small and large breed lactating cows at different production levels as generated by the computer model. These tables also illustrate the effect of dietary energy concentration (Tables 14-2 vs. 14-3 and 14-5 vs. 14-6) and the effect of intake (Tables 14-1 vs. 14-2 and 14-4 vs. 14-5) on protein requirements. Tables 14-7 through 14-9 provide estimates of nutrient requirements of lactating (early and mid) and dry cows. These tables were also generated using the computer model, but the subcommittee has included its recommendations for certain nutrients that require special consideration, when using the model. Dietary requirements for minerals shown in Tables 14-7 through 14-9 are applicable only to the diets included in the tables. Different diets, because of differences in bioavailability of minerals may yield different dietary requirements for minerals.

The values in the tables are the subcommittee's best estimates of requirements when cattle are fed specific dietary formulations under nonstressful environmental conditions. These tables (Tables 14-1 through 14-16) are intended as guides, and readers are encouraged to pay careful attention to footnotes in the tables. The computer model allows great flexibility in accounting for many dietary, environmental, and management factors that affect animal performance in contrast to the static numbers presented in tables.

## HEIFERS

The equations outlined in Chapter 16 were used to develop tables containing guidelines for the nutrient requirements of dairy replacement heifers (Tables 14-12 through 14-16). At a predicted DMI, the TDN concentration needed to meet the requirements for maintenance and gain were determined. The requirements obtained with the computer program may differ slightly from those in Tables 14-12 through 14-15 because the model-predicted supply of nutrients affects the calculation of some dietary requirements. These differences are due to variation in RUP intestinal digestibility, predicted diet TDN, and mineral bioavailabilities as described below. These tables are guidelines only and the NRC computer program should be used to evaluate the nutritional adequacy of specific diets. These requirement tables were calculated to approximate the requirements obtained with the computer program when heifers are fed a typical diet at the model-predicted dry matter intake, using the following assumptions.

1. The TDN used is the TDN discounted to account for depression in digestibility at intakes above maintenance.
2. DE (Mcal) was assumed to equal 4.409 x TDN (kg). In the model, this value varies slightly among diets.
3. An RUP intestinal digestibility of 67 percent was assumed. This value ranges from 60 percent for diets based entirely on very mature forages fed to heifers with low requirements to approximately 75 percent for diets typi-

cally fed to animals with high requirements in which much of the supplemental protein comes from concentrates. Thus, the dietary RUP needed to meet the requirement for metabolizable protein should be increased approximately 10 percent if most of the diet consists of mature forages and can be decreased 10 percent if the diet is based on combinations of forages and concentrates typically fed to animals with high requirements.

4. Body weights and daily gains in the table are expressed on a full body weight basis although, in the model, they are converted to shrunk (96 percent of BW) and empty body (89.1 percent of SBW) weights to compute requirements.

5. It is assumed that there is no stress due to weather and that the body condition score of the animal is 3.

6. Net requirements were converted to dietary requirements by assuming an average bioavailability of 40 percent for calcium and 67 percent for phosphorus. These values were obtained by formulating diets for target ADG across a range of body weights. Across these diets, the bioavailability of phosphorus was relatively constant (near 67 percent), but calcium bioavailability ranged from 32 percent for diets with no supplemental calcium to 41 percent for diets supplemented with calcium carbonate.

7. For pregnant heifers, body weight (BW) includes the conceptus weight (kg) shown, which is computed using the equation in the model assuming that birth weight equals 6.275 percent of mature weight.

8. For pregnant heifers, reported daily gains are heifer ADG with and without conceptus (ADG in parentheses include the conceptus gain (kg/d), which is computed with the model equation). The requirements for pregnancy are included in the total requirements.

The body weights and daily gains in the tables were selected to reflect likely values for heifers in both typical and accelerated heifer rearing programs. Some of the trends that are apparent in the tables include:

1. The effects of mature weight and current body weight on net energy and protein requirements are evident in the tables. Animals that have higher rates of gain have higher energy and protein requirements for growth and, as the animal matures, the amount of energy required for a particular daily gain increases. However, RUP and RDP requirements are more complicated. The factors affecting these calculations are: If two heifers have similar current body weights, but different mature weights, the required TDN concentration of the diet is higher for animals with the smaller mature weight because the $NE_G$ requirement is higher. The higher TDN permits the growth of more microbes provided that adequate RDP is available. Thus, the RDP requirements are higher in the animals with the smaller mature size.

2. Stage of growth of the heifer also affects CP and RUP requirements. When mature size increases, the physiological age at which an animal reaches a specific weight is reduced. The result is that the efficiency with which protein is used for growth increases. The increase in the amount of net protein required for growth by animals with larger mature sizes at a set body weight and ADG may be offset by the higher efficiency of use of the absorbed protein.

3. As a result of these two factors, RUP and CP required may actually be lower for animals with a larger mature weight at a given body weight and ADG than for animals with smaller mature weights. These interactions are illustrated below for a body weight of 300 kg and an ADG of 0.8 kg/day for both mature sizes.

| | | |
|---|---|---|
| Mature weight, kg | 450 | 650 |
| % of mature weight | 67 | 41 |
| $NE_G$ required, Mcal/day | 3.13 | 2.38 |
| DMI, kg/d | 7.1 | 7.1 |
| Diet TDN, % | 67.7 | 63.4 |
| Net protein required, g/d | 114 | 136 |
| Equivalent body weight, kg | 319 | 221 |
| Efficiency of MP use for NP, % | 47.1 | 58.2 |
| MP required, g/d | 524 | 525 |
| MP from microbial protein, g/d | 443 | 409 |
| RDP required/ g/d | 736 | 685 |
| RUP required, g/d | 151 | 183 |
| CP required, g/d | 887 | 868 |

TABLE 14-1 Daily Nutrient Requirements of Small Breed Cows (live weight = 454 kg) in Early Lactation (intake estimated at 11 days in milk). Values are Appropriate for the Diet Below With 78% TDN[a]

| Milk (kg) | Fat (%) | True Protein (%) | DMI (kg) | LW change (kg) | $NE_L$ (Mcal) | RDP (g) | RUP (g) | RDP (%) | RUP (%) | CP (%) |
|---|---|---|---|---|---|---|---|---|---|---|
| 15 | 4.0 | 3.0 | 9.4 | −0.3 | 19.0 | 1060 | 500 | 11.3 | 5.3 | 16.6 |
| 15 | 4.0 | 3.5 | 9.4 | −0.3 | 19.4 | 1060 | 630 | 11.3 | 6.7 | 18.0 |
| 15 | 4.0 | 4.0 | 9.4 | −0.4 | 19.8 | 1060 | 760 | 11.3 | 8.1 | 19.4 |
| 15 | 4.5 | 3.0 | 9.7 | −0.3 | 19.7 | 1090 | 490 | 11.2 | 5.1 | 16.3 |
| 15 | 4.5 | 3.5 | 9.7 | −0.4 | 20.1 | 1090 | 620 | 11.2 | 6.4 | 17.6 |
| 15 | 4.5 | 4.0 | 9.7 | −0.5 | 20.5 | 1090 | 750 | 11.2 | 7.7 | 18.9 |
| 15 | 5.0 | 3.0 | 9.9 | −0.4 | 20.4 | 1110 | 480 | 11.2 | 4.8 | 16.0 |
| 15 | 5.0 | 3.5 | 9.9 | −0.5 | 20.8 | 1110 | 610 | 11.2 | 6.2 | 17.4 |
| 15 | 5.0 | 4.0 | 9.9 | −0.5 | 21.2 | 1110 | 740 | 11.2 | 7.5 | 18.7 |
| 30 | 4.0 | 3.0 | 12.9 | −1.4 | 30.1 | 1410 | 1170 | 10.9 | 9.1 | 20.0 |
| 30 | 4.0 | 3.5 | 12.9 | −1.6 | 30.9 | 1410 | 1430 | 10.9 | 11.1 | 22.0 |
| 30 | 4.0 | 4.0 | 12.9 | −1.7 | 31.8 | 1410 | 1690 | 10.9 | 13.1 | 24.0 |
| 30 | 4.5 | 3.0 | 13.5 | −1.5 | 31.5 | 1460 | 1150 | 10.8 | 8.5 | 19.3 |
| 30 | 4.5 | 3.5 | 13.5 | −1.7 | 32.3 | 1460 | 1410 | 10.8 | 10.4 | 21.2 |
| 30 | 4.5 | 4.0 | 13.5 | −1.9 | 33.2 | 1460 | 1670 | 10.8 | 12.4 | 23.2 |
| 30 | 5.0 | 3.0 | 14.0 | −1.6 | 32.8 | 1510 | 1140 | 10.8 | 8.1 | 18.9 |
| 30 | 5.0 | 3.5 | 14.0 | −1.8 | 33.7 | 1510 | 1400 | 10.8 | 10.0 | 20.8 |
| 30 | 5.0 | 4.0 | 14.0 | −2.0 | 34.6 | 1510 | 1660 | 10.8 | 11.9 | 22.7 |

[a]Diet used for this table consisted of 15% immature legume silage, 33% normal corn silage, 34% ground high moisture shelled corn, 12% soybean meal (48% crude protein), 2.5% tallow, 1.5% menhaden fish meal, and 2% mineral and vitamin mix. Requirements are dependent upon the diet fed. Requirements shown do not include nutrients needed for live weight change. Live weight change is based on assumed $NE_L$ intake minus requirements. Requirements for RUP do not include protein provided by loss in body reserves or required for gain in body reserves. Requirement for total CP assumes RDP and RUP are met. Requirement for total CP will increase if RDP requirement is not met.

TABLE 14-2 Daily Nutrient Requirements of Small Breed Cows (live weight = 454 kg) in Midlactation (intake estimated at 90 days in milk). Values Are Appropriate for the Diet Below with 78% TDN[a]

| Milk (kg) | Fat (%) | True Protein (%) | DMI (kg) | LW change (kg) | $NE_L$ (Mcal) | RDP (g) | RUP (g) | RDP (%) | RUP (%) | CP (%) |
|---|---|---|---|---|---|---|---|---|---|---|
| 20 | 4.0 | 3.0 | 16.0 | 1.0 | 22.7 | 1680 | 560 | 10.5 | 3.5 | 14.0 |
| 20 | 4.0 | 3.5 | 16.0 | 0.8 | 23.2 | 1680 | 740 | 10.5 | 4.6 | 15.1 |
| 20 | 4.0 | 4.0 | 16.0 | 0.7 | 23.8 | 1680 | 910 | 10.5 | 5.7 | 16.2 |
| 20 | 4.5 | 3.0 | 16.5 | 0.9 | 23.6 | 1730 | 550 | 10.5 | 3.3 | 13.8 |
| 20 | 4.5 | 3.5 | 16.5 | 0.8 | 24.2 | 1730 | 720 | 10.5 | 4.4 | 14.9 |
| 20 | 4.5 | 4.0 | 16.5 | 0.7 | 24.8 | 1730 | 900 | 10.5 | 5.5 | 16.0 |
| 20 | 5.0 | 3.0 | 17.0 | 0.9 | 24.5 | 1770 | 540 | 10.4 | 3.2 | 13.6 |
| 20 | 5.0 | 3.5 | 17.0 | 0.8 | 25.1 | 1770 | 710 | 10.4 | 4.2 | 14.6 |
| 20 | 5.0 | 4.0 | 17.0 | 0.6 | 25.7 | 1770 | 880 | 10.4 | 5.2 | 15.6 |
| 30 | 4.0 | 3.0 | 19.5 | 0.4 | 30.1 | 1980 | 1010 | 10.2 | 5.2 | 15.4 |
| 30 | 4.0 | 3.5 | 19.5 | 0.2 | 30.9 | 1980 | 1270 | 10.2 | 6.5 | 16.7 |
| 30 | 4.0 | 4.0 | 19.5 | 0 | 31.8 | 1980 | 1530 | 10.2 | 7.8 | 18.0 |
| 30 | 4.5 | 3.0 | 20.3 | 0.3 | 31.5 | 2040 | 990 | 10.0 | 4.9 | 14.9 |
| 30 | 4.5 | 3.5 | 20.3 | 0.1 | 32.3 | 2040 | 1250 | 10.0 | 6.2 | 16.2 |
| 30 | 4.5 | 4.0 | 20.3 | −0.1 | 33.2 | 2040 | 1510 | 10.0 | 7.4 | 17.4 |
| 30 | 5.0 | 3.0 | 21.1 | 0.2 | 32.8 | 2100 | 980 | 10.0 | 4.6 | 14.6 |
| 30 | 5.0 | 3.5 | 21.1 | 0 | 33.7 | 2100 | 1240 | 10.0 | 5.9 | 15.9 |
| 30 | 5.0 | 4.0 | 21.1 | −0.2 | 34.6 | 2100 | 1500 | 10.0 | 7.1 | 17.1 |
| 40 | 4.0 | 3.0 | 23.1 | −0.3 | 37.5 | 2240 | 1470 | 9.7 | 6.4 | 16.1 |
| 40 | 4.0 | 3.5 | 23.1 | −0.6 | 38.6 | 2240 | 1820 | 9.7 | 7.9 | 17.6 |
| 40 | 4.0 | 4.0 | 23.1 | −0.8 | 39.8 | 2240 | 2160 | 9.7 | 9.4 | 19.1 |
| 40 | 4.5 | 3.0 | 24.2 | −0.5 | 39.3 | 2310 | 1460 | 9.5 | 6.0 | 15.5 |
| 40 | 4.5 | 3.5 | 24.2 | −0.7 | 40.5 | 2310 | 1800 | 9.5 | 7.4 | 16.9 |
| 40 | 4.5 | 4.0 | 24.2 | −1.0 | 41.7 | 2310 | 2150 | 9.5 | 8.9 | 18.4 |
| 40 | 5.0 | 3.0 | 25.2 | −0.7 | 41.2 | 2390 | 1450 | 9.5 | 5.8 | 15.3 |
| 40 | 5.0 | 3.5 | 25.2 | −0.9 | 42.3 | 2390 | 1790 | 9.5 | 7.1 | 16.6 |
| 40 | 5.0 | 4.0 | 25.2 | −1.1 | 43.5 | 2390 | 2140 | 9.5 | 8.5 | 18.0 |

[a]Diet used for this table consisted of 15% immature legume silage, 33% normal corn silage, 34% ground high moisture shelled corn, 12% soybean meal (48% crude protein), 2.5% tallow, 1.5% menhaden fish meal, and 2% mineral and vitamin mix. Requirements are dependent upon the diet fed. Requirements shown do not include nutrients needed for live weight change. Live weight change is based on assumed $NE_L$ intake minus requirements. Requirements for RUP do not include protein provided by loss in body reserves or required for gain in body reserves. Requirement for total CP assumes RDP and RUP are met. Requirement for total CP will increase if RDP requirement is not met.

TABLE 14-3 Daily Nutrient Requirements of Small Breed Cows (live weight = 454 kg) in Midlactation (intake estimated at 90 days in milk). Values are Appropriate for the Diet Below with 68% TDN[a]

| Milk (kg) | Fat (%) | True Protein (%) | DMI (kg) | LW change (kg) | $NE_L$ (Mcal) | RDP (g) | RUP (g) | RDP (%) | RUP (%) | CP (%) |
|---|---|---|---|---|---|---|---|---|---|---|
| 10 | 4.0 | 3.0 | 12.4 | 0.9 | 15.3 | 1240 | 230 | 10.0 | 1.9 | 11.9 |
| 10 | 4.0 | 3.5 | 12.4 | 0.8 | 15.6 | 1240 | 320 | 10.0 | 2.6 | 12.6 |
| 10 | 4.0 | 4.0 | 12.4 | 0.8 | 15.9 | 1240 | 420 | 10.0 | 3.4 | 13.4 |
| 10 | 4.5 | 3.0 | 12.7 | 0.9 | 15.7 | 1270 | 230 | 10.0 | 1.8 | 11.8 |
| 10 | 4.5 | 3.5 | 12.7 | 0.8 | 16.0 | 1270 | 320 | 10.0 | 2.5 | 12.5 |
| 10 | 4.5 | 4.0 | 12.7 | 0.8 | 16.3 | 1270 | 410 | 10.0 | 3.2 | 13.2 |
| 10 | 5.0 | 3.0 | 12.9 | 0.9 | 16.2 | 1290 | 220 | 10.0 | 1.7 | 11.7 |
| 10 | 5.0 | 3.5 | 12.9 | 0.8 | 16.5 | 1290 | 310 | 10.0 | 2.4 | 12.4 |
| 10 | 5.0 | 4.0 | 12.9 | 0.8 | 16.8 | 1290 | 400 | 10.0 | 3.1 | 13.1 |
| 20 | 4.0 | 3.0 | 16.0 | 0.4 | 22.7 | 1560 | 680 | 9.8 | 4.3 | 14.1 |
| 20 | 4.0 | 3.5 | 16.0 | 0.3 | 23.2 | 1560 | 860 | 9.8 | 5.4 | 15.2 |
| 20 | 4.0 | 4.0 | 16.0 | 0.2 | 23.8 | 1560 | 1040 | 9.8 | 6.5 | 16.3 |
| 20 | 4.5 | 3.0 | 16.5 | 0.4 | 23.6 | 1610 | 660 | 9.8 | 4.0 | 13.8 |
| 20 | 4.5 | 3.5 | 16.5 | 0.3 | 24.2 | 1610 | 840 | 9.8 | 5.1 | 14.9 |
| 20 | 4.5 | 4.0 | 16.5 | 0.2 | 24.8 | 1610 | 1030 | 9.8 | 6.2 | 16.0 |
| 20 | 5.0 | 3.0 | 17.0 | 0.4 | 24.5 | 1660 | 650 | 9.8 | 3.8 | 13.6 |
| 20 | 5.0 | 3.5 | 17.0 | 0.2 | 25.1 | 1660 | 830 | 9.8 | 4.9 | 14.7 |
| 20 | 5.0 | 4.0 | 17.0 | 0.1 | 25.7 | 1660 | 1010 | 9.8 | 5.9 | 15.7 |
| 30 | 4.0 | 3.0 | 19.5 | −0.1 | 30.1 | 1870 | 1130 | 9.6 | 5.8 | 15.4 |
| 30 | 4.0 | 3.5 | 19.5 | −0.3 | 30.9 | 1870 | 1400 | 9.6 | 7.2 | 16.8 |
| 30 | 4.0 | 4.0 | 19.5 | −0.4 | 31.8 | 1870 | 1670 | 9.6 | 8.6 | 18.2 |
| 30 | 4.5 | 3.0 | 20.3 | −0.2 | 31.5 | 1940 | 1110 | 9.6 | 5.5 | 15.1 |
| 30 | 4.5 | 3.5 | 20.3 | −0.3 | 32.3 | 1940 | 1380 | 9.6 | 6.8 | 16.4 |
| 30 | 4.5 | 4.0 | 20.3 | −0.5 | 33.2 | 1940 | 1650 | 9.6 | 8.1 | 17.7 |
| 30 | 5.0 | 3.0 | 21.1 | −0.2 | 32.8 | 2000 | 1090 | 9.5 | 5.2 | 14.7 |
| 30 | 5.0 | 3.5 | 21.1 | −0.4 | 33.7 | 2000 | 1360 | 9.5 | 6.4 | 15.9 |
| 30 | 5.0 | 4.0 | 21.1 | −0.6 | 34.6 | 2000 | 1630 | 9.5 | 7.7 | 17.2 |

[a]Diet used for this table consisted of 40% mid-maturity legume hay, 27% normal corn silage, 23% cracked dry shelled corn, 8% soybean meal (48% crude protein), and 2% mineral and vitamin mix. Requirements are dependent upon the diet fed. Requirements shown do not include nutrients needed for live weight change. Live weight change is based on assumed $NE_L$ intake minus requirements. Requirements for RUP do not include protein provided by loss in body reserves or required for gain in body reserves. Requirement for total CP assumes RDP and RUP are met. Requirement for total CP will increase if RDP requirement is not met.

TABLE 14-4 Daily Nutrient Requirements Of Large Breed Cows (Live Weight = 680 kg) In Early Lactation (intake estimated at 11 days in milk). Values Are Appropriate For The Diet Below With 78% TDN[a]

| Milk (kg) | Fat (%) | True Protein (%) | DMI (kg) | LW change (kg) | $NE_L$ (Mcal) | RDP (g) | RUP (g) | RDP (%) | RUP (%) | CP (%) |
|---|---|---|---|---|---|---|---|---|---|---|
| 20 | 3.0 | 2.5 | 12.0 | 0 | 23.0 | 1360 | 500 | 11.3 | 4.2 | 15.5 |
| 20 | 3.0 | 3.0 | 12.0 | −0.2 | 23.6 | 1360 | 670 | 11.3 | 5.6 | 16.9 |
| 20 | 3.0 | 3.5 | 12.0 | −0.3 | 24.2 | 1360 | 850 | 11.3 | 7.1 | 18.4 |
| 20 | 3.5 | 2.5 | 12.4 | −0.1 | 23.9 | 1400 | 480 | 11.3 | 3.9 | 15.2 |
| 20 | 3.5 | 3.0 | 12.4 | −0.2 | 24.5 | 1400 | 660 | 11.3 | 5.3 | 16.6 |
| 20 | 3.5 | 3.5 | 12.4 | −0.4 | 25.1 | 1400 | 840 | 11.3 | 6.8 | 18.1 |
| 20 | 4.0 | 2.5 | 12.7 | −0.2 | 24.9 | 1440 | 470 | 11.3 | 3.7 | 15.0 |
| 20 | 4.0 | 3.0 | 12.7 | −0.3 | 25.4 | 1440 | 650 | 11.3 | 5.1 | 16.5 |
| 20 | 4.0 | 3.5 | 12.7 | −0.4 | 26.0 | 1440 | 820 | 11.3 | 6.5 | 17.8 |
| 30 | 3.0 | 2.5 | 14.0 | −0.6 | 29.2 | 1570 | 860 | 11.2 | 6.1 | 17.4 |
| 30 | 3.0 | 3.0 | 14.0 | −0.8 | 30.1 | 1570 | 1130 | 11.2 | 8.1 | 19.3 |
| 30 | 3.0 | 3.5 | 14.0 | −1.0 | 30.9 | 1570 | 1390 | 11.2 | 9.9 | 21.1 |
| 30 | 3.5 | 2.5 | 14.5 | −0.7 | 30.6 | 1620 | 850 | 11.2 | 5.9 | 17.0 |
| 30 | 3.5 | 3.0 | 14.5 | −0.9 | 31.4 | 1620 | 1110 | 11.2 | 7.7 | 18.8 |
| 30 | 3.5 | 3.5 | 14.5 | −1.1 | 32.3 | 1620 | 1370 | 11.2 | 9.4 | 20.6 |
| 30 | 4.0 | 2.5 | 15.1 | −0.9 | 32.0 | 1670 | 830 | 11.1 | 5.5 | 16.6 |
| 30 | 4.0 | 3.0 | 15.1 | −1.0 | 32.8 | 1670 | 1090 | 11.1 | 7.2 | 18.3 |
| 30 | 4.0 | 3.5 | 15.1 | −1.2 | 33.7 | 1670 | 1350 | 11.1 | 8.9 | 20.0 |
| 40 | 3.0 | 2.5 | 16.0 | −1.2 | 35.3 | 1760 | 1230 | 11.0 | 7.7 | 18.7 |
| 40 | 3.0 | 3.0 | 16.0 | −1.5 | 36.5 | 1760 | 1580 | 11.0 | 9.9 | 20.9 |
| 40 | 3.0 | 3.5 | 16.0 | −1.7 | 37.7 | 1760 | 1930 | 11.0 | 12.1 | 23.1 |
| 40 | 3.5 | 2.5 | 16.7 | −1.4 | 37.2 | 1830 | 1210 | 11.0 | 7.2 | 18.2 |
| 40 | 3.5 | 3.0 | 16.7 | −1.6 | 38.4 | 1830 | 1560 | 11.0 | 9.3 | 20.3 |
| 40 | 3.5 | 3.5 | 16.7 | −1.9 | 39.6 | 1830 | 1910 | 11.0 | 11.4 | 22.4 |
| 40 | 4.0 | 2.5 | 17.4 | −1.6 | 39.1 | 1900 | 1190 | 10.9 | 6.8 | 17.8 |
| 40 | 4.0 | 3.0 | 17.4 | −1.8 | 40.2 | 1900 | 1540 | 10.9 | 8.9 | 19.8 |
| 40 | 4.0 | 3.5 | 17.4 | −2.0 | 41.4 | 1900 | 1890 | 10.9 | 10.9 | 21.8 |

[a]Diet used for this table consisted of 15% immature legume silage, 33% normal corn silage, 34% ground high moisture shelled corn, 12% soybean meal (48% crude protein), 2.5% tallow, 1.5% Menhaden fish meal, and 2% mineral and vitamin mix. Requirements are dependent upon the diet fed. Requirements shown do not include nutrients needed for live weight change. Live weight change is based on assumed $NE_L$ intake minus requirements. Requirements for RUP do not include protein provided by loss in body reserves or required for gain in body reserves. Requirement for total CP assumes RDP and RUP are met. Requirement for total CP will increase if RDP requirement is not met.

TABLE 14-5 Daily Nutrient Requirements Of Large Breed Cows (Live Weight = 680 kg) In Midlactation (intake estimated at 90 days in milk). Values Are Appropriate For The Diet Below With 78% TDN[a]

| Milk (kg) | Fat (%) | True Protein (%) | DMI (kg) | LW change (kg) | $NE_L$ (Mcal) | RDP (g) | RUP (g) | RDP (%) | RUP (%) | CP (%) |
|---|---|---|---|---|---|---|---|---|---|---|
| 35 | 3.0 | 2.5 | 22.7 | 1.3 | 32.2 | 2370 | 820 | 10.4 | 3.6 | 14.1 |
| 35 | 3.0 | 3.0 | 22.7 | 1.1 | 33.2 | 2370 | 1130 | 10.4 | 5.0 | 15.4 |
| 35 | 3.0 | 3.5 | 22.7 | 0.9 | 34.2 | 2370 | 1430 | 10.4 | 6.3 | 16.7 |
| 35 | 3.5 | 2.5 | 23.6 | 1.2 | 33.8 | 2450 | 800 | 10.4 | 3.4 | 13.8 |
| 35 | 3.5 | 3.0 | 23.6 | 1.0 | 34.8 | 2450 | 1110 | 10.4 | 4.7 | 15.1 |
| 35 | 3.5 | 3.5 | 23.6 | 0.8 | 35.9 | 2450 | 1410 | 10.4 | 6.0 | 16.4 |
| 35 | 4.0 | 2.5 | 24.5 | 1.1 | 35.4 | 2520 | 780 | 10.3 | 3.2 | 13.5 |
| 35 | 4.0 | 3.0 | 24.5 | 0.9 | 36.5 | 2520 | 1090 | 10.3 | 4.4 | 14.7 |
| 35 | 4.0 | 3.5 | 24.5 | 0.7 | 37.5 | 2520 | 1390 | 10.3 | 5.7 | 16.0 |
| 45 | 3.0 | 2.5 | 25.7 | 0.8 | 38.3 | 2620 | 1190 | 10.2 | 4.6 | 14.8 |
| 45 | 3.0 | 3.0 | 25.7 | 0.5 | 39.7 | 2620 | 1580 | 10.2 | 6.1 | 16.3 |
| 45 | 3.0 | 3.5 | 25.7 | 0.3 | 41.0 | 2620 | 1970 | 10.2 | 7.7 | 17.9 |
| 45 | 3.5 | 2.5 | 26.9 | 0.7 | 40.4 | 2710 | 1170 | 10.1 | 4.3 | 14.4 |
| 45 | 3.5 | 3.0 | 26.9 | 0.4 | 41.8 | 2710 | 1560 | 10.1 | 5.8 | 15.9 |
| 45 | 3.5 | 3.5 | 26.9 | 0.2 | 43.1 | 2710 | 1950 | 10.1 | 7.2 | 17.3 |
| 45 | 4.0 | 2.5 | 28.1 | 0.5 | 42.5 | 2800 | 1150 | 10.0 | 4.1 | 14.1 |
| 45 | 4.0 | 3.0 | 28.1 | 0.3 | 43.8 | 2800 | 1540 | 10.0 | 5.5 | 15.4 |
| 45 | 4.0 | 3.5 | 28.1 | 0 | 45.2 | 2800 | 1930 | 10.0 | 6.9 | 16.8 |
| 55 | 3.0 | 2.5 | 28.7 | 0.3 | 44.5 | 2850 | 1570 | 9.9 | 5.5 | 15.4 |
| 55 | 3.0 | 3.0 | 28.7 | 0 | 46.1 | 2850 | 2060 | 9.9 | 7.2 | 17.1 |
| 55 | 3.0 | 3.5 | 28.7 | −0.4 | 47.7 | 2850 | 2540 | 9.9 | 8.9 | 18.8 |
| 55 | 3.5 | 2.5 | 30.2 | 0.1 | 47.1 | 2960 | 1560 | 9.8 | 5.2 | 15.0 |
| 55 | 3.5 | 3.0 | 30.2 | −0.2 | 48.7 | 2960 | 2040 | 9.8 | 6.8 | 16.6 |
| 55 | 3.5 | 3.5 | 30.2 | −0.6 | 50.7 | 2960 | 2510 | 9.8 | 8.3 | 18.1 |
| 55 | 4.0 | 2.5 | 31.7 | −0.1 | 49.6 | 3060 | 1540 | 9.7 | 4.9 | 14.5 |
| 55 | 4.0 | 3.0 | 31.7 | −0.5 | 51.2 | 3060 | 2020 | 9.7 | 6.4 | 16.0 |
| 55 | 4.0 | 3.5 | 31.7 | −0.8 | 52.8 | 3060 | 2490 | 9.7 | 7.9 | 17.5 |

[a]Diet used for this table consisted of 15% immature legume silage, 33% normal corn silage, 34% ground high moisture shelled corn, 12% soybean meal (48% crude protein), 2.5% tallow, 1.5% menhaden fish meal, and 2% mineral and vitamin mix. Requirements are dependent upon the diet fed. Requirements shown do not include nutrients needed for live weight change. Live weight change is based on assumed $NE_L$ intake minus requirements. Requirements for RUP do not include protein provided by loss in body reserves or required for gain in body reserves. Requirement for total CP assumes RDP and RUP are met. Requirement for total CP will increase if RDP requirement is not met.

TABLE 14-6 Daily Nutrient Requirements Of Large Breed Cows (Live Weight = 680 kg) In Midlactation (intake estimated at 90 days in milk). Values Are Appropriate For The Diet Below With 68% TDN[a]

| Milk (kg) | Fat (%) | True Protein (%) | DMI (kg) | LW change (kg) | $NE_L$ (Mcal) | RDP (g) | RUP (g) | RDP (%) | RUP (%) | CP (%) |
|---|---|---|---|---|---|---|---|---|---|---|
| 25 | 3.0 | 2.5 | 19.6 | 1.0 | 26.0 | 1940 | 620 | 9.9 | 3.2 | 13.1 |
| 25 | 3.0 | 3.0 | 19.6 | 0.8 | 26.8 | 1940 | 840 | 9.9 | 4.3 | 14.2 |
| 25 | 3.0 | 3.5 | 19.6 | 0.7 | 27.5 | 1940 | 1070 | 9.9 | 5.5 | 15.4 |
| 25 | 3.5 | 2.5 | 20.3 | 0.9 | 27.2 | 2000 | 600 | 9.9 | 3.0 | 12.9 |
| 25 | 3.5 | 3.0 | 20.3 | 0.8 | 27.9 | 2000 | 820 | 9.9 | 4.0 | 13.9 |
| 25 | 3.5 | 3.5 | 20.3 | 0.6 | 28.7 | 2000 | 1050 | 9.9 | 5.2 | 15.1 |
| 25 | 4.0 | 2.5 | 21.0 | 0.9 | 28.4 | 2060 | 580 | 9.8 | 2.8 | 12.6 |
| 25 | 4.0 | 3.0 | 21.0 | 0.7 | 29.1 | 2060 | 810 | 9.8 | 3.9 | 13.7 |
| 25 | 4.0 | 3.5 | 21.0 | 0.6 | 29.8 | 2060 | 1030 | 9.8 | 4.9 | 14.7 |
| 35 | 3.0 | 2.5 | 22.7 | 0.6 | 32.2 | 2210 | 990 | 9.7 | 4.4 | 14.1 |
| 35 | 3.0 | 3.0 | 22.7 | 0.4 | 33.2 | 2210 | 1300 | 9.7 | 5.7 | 15.4 |
| 35 | 3.0 | 3.5 | 22.7 | 0.2 | 34.2 | 2210 | 1620 | 9.7 | 7.1 | 16.8 |
| 35 | 3.5 | 2.5 | 23.6 | 0.5 | 33.8 | 2290 | 960 | 9.7 | 4.1 | 13.8 |
| 35 | 3.5 | 3.0 | 23.6 | 0.3 | 34.8 | 2290 | 1280 | 9.7 | 5.4 | 15.1 |
| 35 | 3.5 | 3.5 | 23.6 | 0.1 | 35.9 | 2290 | 1600 | 9.7 | 6.7 | 16.4 |
| 35 | 4.0 | 2.5 | 24.5 | 0.4 | 35.4 | 2370 | 940 | 9.7 | 3.8 | 13.5 |
| 35 | 4.0 | 3.0 | 24.5 | 0.2 | 36.5 | 2370 | 1260 | 9.7 | 5.1 | 14.8 |
| 35 | 4.0 | 3.5 | 24.5 | 0 | 37.5 | 2370 | 1570 | 9.7 | 6.4 | 16.1 |
| 45 | 3.0 | 2.5 | 25.7 | 0.1 | 28.3 | 2470 | 1370 | 9.6 | 5.3 | 14.9 |
| 45 | 3.0 | 3.0 | 25.7 | −0.1 | 39.7 | 2470 | 1780 | 9.6 | 6.9 | 16.5 |
| 45 | 3.0 | 3.5 | 25.7 | −0.4 | 41.0 | 2470 | 2180 | 9.6 | 8.5 | 18.1 |
| 45 | 3.5 | 2.5 | 26.9 | 0 | 40.4 | 2570 | 1340 | 9.6 | 5.0 | 14.6 |
| 45 | 3.5 | 3.0 | 26.9 | −0.2 | 41.8 | 2570 | 1750 | 9.6 | 6.5 | 16.1 |
| 45 | 3.5 | 3.5 | 26.9 | −0.5 | 43.1 | 2570 | 2160 | 9.6 | 8.0 | 17.6 |
| 45 | 4.0 | 2.5 | 28.1 | −0.1 | 42.5 | 2670 | 1310 | 9.5 | 4.7 | 14.2 |
| 45 | 4.0 | 3.0 | 28.1 | −0.3 | 43.8 | 2670 | 1720 | 9.5 | 6.1 | 15.6 |
| 45 | 4.0 | 3.5 | 28.1 | −0.6 | 45.2 | 2670 | 2130 | 9.5 | 7.6 | 17.1 |

[a] Diet used for this table consisted of 40% mid-maturity legume hay, 27% normal corn silage, 23% cracked dry shelled corn, 8% soybean meal (48% crude protein), and 2% mineral and vitamin mix. Requirements are dependent upon the diet fed. Requirements shown do not include nutrients needed for live weight change. Live weight change is based on assumed $NE_L$ intake minus $NE_L$ requirements. Requirements for RUP do not include protein provided by loss in body reserves or required for gain in body reserves. Requirement for total CP assumes RDP and RUP are met. Requirement for total CP will increase if RDP requirement is not met.

TABLE 14-7 Nutrient Requirements of Lactating Dairy Cows as Determined Using Sample Diets

| | Holstein = 680 kg Bwt, Mature Bwt = 680 kg, BCS = 3.0, 65 mos age, Milk fat = 3.5%, milk true protein = 3.0%, lactose = 4.8%, Default environmental conditions | | | | Jersey = 454 kg Bwt, mature Bwt = 454 kg, BCS = 3.0, 65 mos age milk fat = 4.2%, milk true protein = 3.6%, lactose = 4.8% Default environmental conditions | | | | | |
|---|---|---|---|---|---|---|---|---|---|---|
| Days in milk | 90 | 90 | 90 | 90 | 90 | 90 | 90 | 50 | 120 | 90 |
| Dry matter intake input | Model predicted | Model predicted | Model predicted | Model predicted | Model predicted | Model predicted[h] | Model predicted | Model predicted[h] | Model predicted[h] | Model predicted + 5%[h] |
| Milk production (kg) | 25 | 35 | 45 | 54.4 | 25 | 35 | 40 | 35 | 35 | 35 |
| Milk production (lbs) | 55 | 77 | 99 | 120 | 55 | 77 | 88 | 77 | 77 | 77 |
| Dry matter intake (kg) | 20.3 | 23.6 | 26.9 | 30 | 18 | 21.7 | 23.5 | 19.8 | 22.2 | 22.7 |
| Dry matter intake (lbs) | 44.7 | 51.9 | 59.2 | 66 | 39.6 | 47.7 | 51.7 | 43.6 | 48.8 | 49.9 |
| Daily wt change (kg) | 0.5 | 0.3 | 0.1 | −0.2 | 0 | −0.2 | −0.5 | −0.7 | −0.1 | 0 |
| Days to gain one condition score | 221 | 316 | 1166 | | 3777 | | | | | 4247 |
| Days to lose one condition score | | | | 544 | | 241 | 110 | 80 | 532 | |
| Energy[a] | | | | | | | | | | |
| $NE_L$ (Mcal /day) | 27.9 | 34.8 | 41.8 | 48.3 | 27.7 | 35.6 | 39.5 | 35.6 | 35.6 | 35.6 |
| $NE_L$ ( Mcal/ kg) | 1.37 | 1.47 | 1.55 | 1.61 | 1.54 | 1.64 | 1.68 | 1.8 a | 1.6 | 1.57 |
| $NE_L$ (Mcal/ lb) | 0.62 | 0.67 | 0.7 | 0.73 | 0.7 | 0.74 | 0.76 | 0.82 | 0.73 | 0.71 |
| Protein | | | | | | | | | | |
| Metabolizable protein (g/d) | 1862 | 2407 | 2954 | 3476 | 1991 | 2639 | 2965 | 2579 | 2656 | 2672 |
| Diet % MP | 9.2 | 10.2 | 11 | 11.6 | 11.1 | 12.2 | 12.6 | 13 | 12 | 11.8 |
| Rumen degradable protein (g/d) | 1937 | 2298 | 2636 | 2947 | 1747 | 2125 | 2288 | 1971 | 2167 | 2206 |
| Diet % RDP | 9.5 | 9.7 | 9.8 | 9.8 | 9.7 | 9.8 | 9.7 | 10 | 9.8 | 9.7 |
| Rumen undegradable protein (g/d) | 933 | 1291 | 1677 | 2089 | 1151 | 1632 | 1865 | 1670 | 1619 | 1611 |
| Diet % RUP | 4.6 | 5.5 | 6.2 | 6.9 | 6.4 | 7.5 | 7.9 | 8.4 | 7.3 | 7.1 |
| % RDP + % RUP (crude protein)[b] | 14.1 | 15.2 | 16.0 | 16.7 | 16.1 | 17.3 | 17.6 | 18.4 | 17.1 | 16.8 |
| Fiber and carbohydrate[c] | | | | | | | | | | |
| NDF, min % | 25–33 | 25–33 | 25–33 | 25–33 | 25–33 | 25–33 | 25–33 | 25–33 | 25–33 | 25–33 |
| ADF, min % | 17–21 | 17–21 | 17–21 | 17–21 | 17–21 | 17–21 | 17–21 | 17–21 | 17–21 | 17–21 |
| NFC, max % | 36–44 | 36–44 | 36–44 | 36–44 | 36–44 | 36–44 | 36–44 | 36–44 | 36–44 | 36–44 |
| Minerals | | | | | | | | | | |
| Absorbable calcium (g/day) | 52.1 | 65 | 76.5 | 88 | 50.7 | 65.2 | 72.4 | 65.2 | 65.2 | 65.2 |
| Dietary Ca % | 0.62 | 0.61 | 0.67 | 0.6 | 0.57 | 0.57 | 0.63 | 0.66 | 0.54 | 0.53 |
| Absorbable phosphorus (g/day) | 44.2 | 56.5 | 68.8 | 80.3 | 41.4 | 54.1 | 60.4 | 52.2 | 54.6 | 55.1 |
| Dietary P % | 0.32 | 0.35 | 0.36 | 0.38 | 0.33 | 0.37 | 0.36 | 0.44 | 0.35 | 0.34 |
| Mg[d] % | 0.18 | 0.19 | 0.2 | 0.21 | 0.18 | 0.19 | 0.2 | 0.21 | 0.19 | 0.19 |
| Cl % | 0.24 | 0.26 | 0.28 | 0.29 | 0.24 | 0.26 | 0.27 | 0.28 | 0.25 | 0.25 |
| K[e] % | 1 | 1.04 | 1.06 | 1.07 | 1.02 | 1.03 | 1.04 | 1.07 | 1.03 | 1.02 |
| Na % | 0.22 | 0.23 | 0.22 | 0.22 | 0.2 | 0.2 | 0.2 | 0.22 | 0.2 | 0.19 |
| S % | 0.2 | 0.2 | 0.2 | 0.2 | 0.2 | 0.2 | 0.2 | 0.2 | 0.2 | 0.2 |
| Co mg/kg | 0.11 | 0.11 | 0.11 | 0.11 | 0.11 | 0.11 | 0.11 | 0.11 | 0.11 | 0.11 |
| Cu mg/kg[f] | 11 | 11 | 11 | 11 | 10 | 10 | 10 | 11 | 10 | 9 |
| I mg/kg[g] | 0.6 | 0.5 | 0.44 | 0.4 | 0.44 | 0.4 | 0.34 | 0.4 | 0.36 | 0.35 |
| Fe mg/kg | 12.3 | 15 | 17 | 18 | 14 | 16 | 17 | 18 | 16 | 15 |
| Mn mg/kg | 14 | 14 | 13 | 13 | 12 | 12 | 12 | 13 | 12 | 12 |
| Se mg/kg | 0.3 | 0.3 | 0.3 | 0.3 | 0.3 | 0.3 | 0.3 | 0.3 | 0.3 | 0.3 |
| Zn mg/kg | 43 | 48 | 52 | 55 | 45 | 49 | 51 | 54 | 48 | 47 |
| Vitamin A (IU/day) | 75000 | 75000 | 75000 | 75000 | 49500 | 49500 | 49500 | 49500 | 49500 | 49500 |
| Vitamin D (IU/day) | 21000 | 21000 | 21000 | 21000 | 13500 | 13500 | 13500 | 13500 | 13500 | 13500 |
| Vitamin E (IU/day) | 545 | 545 | 545 | 545 | 360 | 360 | 360 | 360 | 360 | 360 |
| Vitamin A (IU/kg) | 3685 | 3169 | 2780 | 2500 | 2772 | 2300 | 2123 | 2520 | 2247 | 2198 |
| Vitamin D (IU/kg) | 1004 | 864 | 758 | 680 | 755 | 627 | 579 | 687 | 613 | 600 |
| Vitamin E (IU/kg) | 27 | 23 | 20 | 18 | 20 | 17 | 16 | 18 | 16 | 16 |
| Sample diets used in model to generate tables. Ingredients listed as kg /day DM. | | | | | | | | | | |
| Corn silage, normal | 8.48 | 8.21 | 5.61 | 12.02 | 8.96 | 7.77 | 7.39 | 7.1 | 7.96 | 8.15 |
| Soybean meal, solv. 48% CP | 1.01 | 1.62 | 1.41 | 2.39 | 2.16 | 2.78 | 1.67 | 2.54 | 2.85 | 2.91 |
| Legume forage silage, mid-maturity | 3.85 | 4.57 | | | 2.67 | 3.1 | | 2.83 | 3.18 | 3.25 |
| Corn grain, steam flaked | 1.8 | 4.33 | 7.08 | 6.35 | 2.6 | 4.91 | 5.88 | 4.48 | 5.03 | 5.15 |
| Calcium carbonate | 0.04 | 0.07 | 0.09 | 0.02 | 0.06 | 0.04 | 0.03 | 0.04 | 0.04 | 0.04 |
| Monosodium phosphate (1 H2O) | 0.02 | 0.02 | 0.04 | 0.06 | 0.01 | 0.01 | 0.03 | 0.01 | 0.01 | 0.01 |
| Soybean meal, expellers | | | | | | | 1.16 | | | |
| Legume forage hay, immature | | | 6.16 | 5.42 | | | 4.59 | | | |
| Sodium chloride | 0.12 | 0.011 | 0.12 | 0.14 | 0.1 | 0.1 | 0.12 | 0.09 | 0.1 | 0.1 |
| Grass hay, c-3, mid-mat | 4.47 | 3.21 | 0.98 | 0.93 | 0.85 | 0.95 | 0.97 | | | |
| Vitamin and mineral premix | 0.54 | 0.49 | 0.51 | 0.49 | 0.5 | 0.5 | 0.5 | 0.45 | 0.51 | 0.52 |
| Bermudagrass hay, coastal | | | 0.87 | | | | | | | |

*Continues*

TABLE 14-7 *(continued)*

| | Holstein = 680 kg Bwt, Mature Bwt = 680 kg, BCS = 3.0, 65 mos age, Milk fat = 3.5%, milk true protein = 3.0%, lactose = 4.8%, Default environmental conditions | | | | Jersey = 454 kg Bwt, mature Bwt = 454 kg, BCS = 3.0, 65 mos age milk fat = 4.2%, milk true protein = 3.6%, lactose = 4.8% Default environmental conditions | | | | | |
|---|---|---|---|---|---|---|---|---|---|---|
| Days in milk | 90 | 90 | 90 | 90 | 90 | 90 | 90 | 50 | 120 | 90 |
| Dry matter intake input | Model predicted | Model predicted | Model predicted | Model predicted | Model predicted | Model predicted[h] | Model predicted | Model predicted[h] | Model predicted[h] | Model predicted + 5%[h] |
| Cottonseed, whole with lint | | | 2.53 | 2.24 | | 1.02 | 1.64 | 0.94 | 1.05 | 1.07 |
| Tallow | | | | 0.29 | | 0.24 | 0.21 | 0.22 | 0.24 | 0.25 |
| Calcium soaps of fatty acids | | | | 0.29 | | 0.18 | 0.21 | 0.17 | 0.19 | 0.19 |
| Blood meal, ring dried | | | 0.23 | 0.31 | | 0.11 | 0.1 | 0.1 | 0.11 | 0.12 |
| Sorghum, sudan type, silage | | | 2.26 | | | | | | | |
| Sample diet evaluation | | | | | | | | | | |
| $NE_L$ (Mcal/kg) | 1.49 | 1.55 | 1.57 | 1.58 | 1.54 | 1.59 | 1.57 | 1.62 | 1.58 | 1.57 |
| Undiscounted TDN % | 65 | 69 | 71 | 74 | 69 | 73 | 75 | 73 | 73 | 73 |

[a] Recommended energy content of early lactation rations must be limited to prevent rumen acidosis. Cow must therefore be expected to utilize body reserves to meet energy needs at highest levels of milk production. See fiber and NFC restrictions.

[b] Equivalent to crude protein requirement only if RDP and RUP are perfectly balanced.

[c] These are the minimum fiber (or maximum NFC) concentrations needed to maintain rumen health and milk fat test (see Chapter 4).

[d] Assumes that active transport of magnesium across the rumen wall is intact. High dietary potassium and excess non-protein nitrogen often interfere with Mg absorption. Under these conditions dietary Mg should be increased to 0.3%–0.35% (see Chapter 6).

[e] Heat stress may increase the need for potassium (see Chapter 6).

[f] High dietary molybdenum, sulfur, and iron can interfere with copper absorption increasing the requirement (see Chapter 6).

[g] Diets high in goitrogenic substances increase the iodine requirement (see Chapter 6).

[h] Diet composition is the same in all four cases of the Jersey cow producing 35 kg milk. Amount of dry matter consumed varies with days in milk and the use of predicted vs. actual dry matter intake in the model.

TABLE 14-8 Nutrient Requirements and Required Diet Nutrient Concentrations for Fresh Cows Fed an Example Fresh-Cow Ration

| | Holstein = 680 kg Bwt, Mature Bwt = 680 kg, BCS = 3.3, 58 mos age; milk fat = 3.5%, milk true protein = 3.0%, milk lactose = 4.8%; Default environmental conditions | | | | Jersey = 454 kg Bwt, Mature Bwt = 454 kg, BCS = 3.3, 58 mos. Age; milk fat = 4.2%, milk true protein = 3.6%, milk lactose = 4.8%; Default environmental conditions | |
|---|---|---|---|---|---|---|
| Days in milk | 11 | 11 | 11 | 11 | 11 | 11 |
| Dry matter intake input | Model predicted | Model predicted + 20% | Model predicted | Model predicted + 20% | Model predicted | Model predicted + 20% |
| Milk production (kg) | 25 | 25 | 35 | 35 | 25 | 25 |
| Milk production (lbs) | 55 | 55 | 77 | 77 | 55 | 55 |
| Dry matter intake (kg) | 13.5 | 16.1 | 15.6 | 18.8 | 11.9 | 14.3 |
| Dry matter intake (lbs) | 29.7 | 35.4 | 34.3 | 41.4 | 26.2 | 31.5 |
| Daily wt change (kg) | −0.9 | 0 | −1.6 | −0.6 | −1.4 | −0.7 |
| Days to gain one condition score | | | | | | |
| Days to lose one condition score | 99 | 4886 | 55 | 143 | 41 | 83 |
| Energy[a] | | | | | | |
| $NE_L$ (Mcal/day) | 27.9 | 27.9 | 34.8 | 34.8 | 27.7 | 27.7 |
| $NE_L$ (Mcal/kg) | 2.06 | 1.73 | 2.23 | 1.85 | 2.33 | 1.93 |
| $NE_L$ (Mcal/lb) | 0.94 | 0.79 | 1.01 | 0.84 | 1.06 | 0.88 |
| Protein[b] | | | | | | |
| Metabolizable protein (g/d) | 1643 | 1725 | 2157 | 2254 | 1801 | 1875 |
| Diet % MP | 12.2 | 10.7 | 13.8 | 12.0 | 15.1 | 13.1 |
| Rumen degradable protein (g/d) | 1421 | 1683 | 1634 | 1931 | 1244 | 1469 |
| Diet % RDP | 10.5 | 10.5 | 10.5 | 10.3 | 10.5 | 10.3 |
| Rumen undegradable protein (g/d) | 949 | 863 | 1405 | 1045 | 1265 | 1202 |
| Diet % RUP | 7.0 | 5.4 | 9.0 | 5.6 | 10.6 | 8.4 |
| % RDP + % RUP (crude protein)[c] | 17.5 | 15.9 | 19.5 | 15.9 | 21.1 | 18.7 |
| Fiber and carbohydrate[d] | | | | | | |
| NDF, min % | 25–33 | 25–33 | 25–33 | 25–33 | 25–33 | 25–33 |
| ADF, min % | 17–21 | 17–21 | 17–21 | 17–21 | 17–21 | 17–21 |
| NFC, max % | 36–44 | 36–44 | 36–44 | 36–44 | 36–44 | 36–44 |
| Minerals | | | | | | |
| Absorbable calcium (g/day) | 52.1 | 52.1 | 64 | 64 | 51 | 51 |
| Dietary Ca % | 0.74 | 0.65 | 0.79 | 0.68 | 0.80 | 0.70 |
| Absorbable phosphorus (g/ day) | 37.3 | 40.0 | 49.0 | 52.0 | 35.0 | 37.7 |
| Dietary P % | 0.38 | 0.34 | 0.42 | 0.37 | 0.40 | 0.36 |
| Mg[e] % | 0.27 | 0.23 | 0.29 | 0.24 | 0.27 | 0.22 |
| Cl % | 0.36 | 0.30 | 0.40 | 0.33 | 0.36 | 0.30 |
| K[f] % | 1.19 | 1.11 | 1.24 | 1.14 | 1.19 | 1.10 |
| Na % | 0.34 | 0.29 | 0.34 | 0.28 | 0.31 | 0.26 |
| S % | 0.2 | 0.2 | 0.2 | 0.2 | 0.2 | 0.2 |
| Co mg/kg | 0.11 | 0.11 | 0.11 | 0.11 | 0.11 | 0.11 |
| Cu mg/kg[g] | 16 | 13 | 16 | 13 | 15 | 12 |
| I mg/kg[h] | 0.88 | 0.74 | 0.77 | 0.64 | 0.67 | 0.56 |
| Fe mg/kg | 19 | 16 | 22 | 19 | 21 | 17 |
| Mn mg/kg | 21 | 17 | 21 | 17 | 19 | 15 |
| Se mg/kg | 0.3 | 0.3 | 0.3 | 0.3 | 0.3 | 0.3 |
| Zn mg/kg | 65 | 54 | 73 | 60 | 67 | 56 |
| Vitamin A (IU/day) | 75000 | 75000 | 75000 | 75000 | 49900 | 49900 |
| Vitamin D (IU/day) | 21000 | 21000 | 21000 | 21000 | 13600 | 13600 |
| Vitamin E (IU/day) | 545 | 545 | 545 | 545 | 363 | 363 |
| Vitamin A (IU/kg) | 5540 | 4646 | 4795 | 3978 | 4193 | 3490 |
| Vitamin D (IU/kg) | 1511 | 1267 | 1308 | 1085 | 1143 | 951 |
| Vitamin E (IU/kg) | 40 | 34 | 35 | 29 | 31 | 25 |

*Continues*

TABLE 14-8 *(continued)*

| | | | | | | |
|---|---|---|---|---|---|---|
| Sample diet used in model to generate tables. Ingredients listed as % DM. | | | | | | |
| Corn silage, normal | 36.44 | | | | | |
| Corn grain, steam flaked | 18.29 | | | | | |
| Soybean meal, expellers | 7.65 | | | | | |
| Soybean meal, solv. 48% CP | 2.53 | | | | | |
| Legume forage hay, immature | 20.17 | | | | | |
| Cottonseed, whole with lint | 8.41 | | | | | |
| Calcium soaps of fatty acids | 0.65 | | | | | |
| Blood meal, ring dried | 1.02 | | | | | |
| Calcium carbonate | 0.56 | | | | | |
| Monosodium phosphate (1 H2O) | 0.4 | | | | | |
| Sodium chloride | 0.7 | | | | | |
| Vitamin and mineral premix | 3.18 | | | | | |
| Sample "fresh cow" diet evaluation | | | | | | |
| NDF % | 31.6 | | | | | |
| Forage NDF % | 23.7 | | | | | |
| ADF % | 21 | | | | | |
| NFC % | 41.4 | | | | | |
| Undiscounted TDN | 71 | | | | | |
| Diet $NE_L$ (Mcal/kg), dependent on DMI | 1.75 | 1.73 | 1.73 | 1.70 | 1.72 | 1.69 |
| Crude protein % | 17.4 | | | | | |

[a] Recommended energy content of early lactation rations must be limited to prevent rumen acidosis. Cow must therefore be expected to utilize body reserves to meet energy and protein requirements of early lactation. See fiber and NFC restrictions.

[b] It will be nearly impossible to meet the metabolizable protein needs of the high producing fresh cow due to low dry matter intake and the difficulty formulating rations with such high RUP.

[c] Equivalent to crude protein requirement only if RDP and RUP are perfectly balanced.

[d] These are the minimum fiber (or maximum NFC) concentrations needed to maintain rumen health and milk fat test (see Chapter 4).

[e] Assumes that active transport of magnesium across the rumen wall is intact. High dietary potassium and excess non-protein nitrogen often interfere with Mg absorption. Under these conditions dietary Mg should be increased to 0.3%–0.35% (see Chapter 6).

[f] Heat stress may increase the need for potassium (see Chapter 6).

[g] High dietary molybdenum, sulfur, and iron can interfere with copper absorption increasing the requirement (see Chapter 6).

[h] Diets high in goitrogenic substances increase the iodine requirement (see Chapter 6).

TABLE 14-9 Nutrient Requirements and Diet Concentrations Needed to Meet Requirements for Dry Cows as Determined Using Example Diets

| | REQUIREMENTS OF A DIET TO MEET TISSUE DEMANDS<br>Holstein Cow, mature body weight without conceptus = 680 kg, BCS = 3.3, Calf wt = 45 kg<br>Gaining 0.67 kg/day with conceptus | | |
|---|---|---|---|
| Days pregnant | 240 | 270 | 279 |
| Current body wt (with conceptus) kg | 730 | 751 | 757 |
| Age (months) | 57 | 58 | 58 |
| Dry matter intake (kg) | 14.4 | 13.7 | 10.1 |
| Dry matter intake (lbs) | 31.7 | 30.1 | 22.2 |
| Energy | | | |
| $NE_L$ (Mcal/day required) | 14.0 | 14.4 | 14.5 |
| $NE_L$ (Mcal/kg required) | 0.97 | 1.05 | 1.44 |
| Protein | | | |
| Metabolizable protein (g/d) | 871 | 901 | 810 |
| Diet % MP | 6.0 | 6.6 | 8.0 |
| Rumen degradable protein (g/day) | 1114 | 1197 | 965 |
| Diet % RDP | 7.7 | 8.7 | 9.6 |
| Rumen undegradable protein (g/day) | 317 | 292 | 286[a] |
| Diet % RUP | 2.2 | 2.1 | 2.8[a] |
| % RDP + % RUP (crude protein)[b] | 9.9 | 10.8 | 12.4 |
| Fiber and carbohydrate[c] | | | |
| Minimum % NDF | 33 | 33 | 33 |
| Minimum % ADF | 21 | 21 | 21 |
| Maximum % NFC | 42 | 42 | 42 |
| Minerals | | | |
| Absorbable calcium (g) | 18.1 | 21.5 | 22.5 |
| Dietary Ca % | 0.44 | 0.45 | 0.48 |
| Absorbable phosphorus (g) | 19.9 | 20.3 | 16.9 |
| Dietary P % | 0.22 | 0.23 | 0.26 |
| Mg[d] % | 0.11 | 0.12 | 0.16 |
| Cl % | 0.13 | 0.15 | 0.20 |
| K % | 0.51 | 0.52 | 0.62 |
| Na % | 0.10 | 0.10 | 0.14 |
| S % | 0.2 | 0.2 | 0.2 |
| Co mg/kg | 0.11 | 0.11 | 0.11 |
| Cu mg/kg[e] | 12 | 13 | 18 |
| I mg/kg[f] | 0.4 | 0.4 | 0.5 |
| Fe mg/kg | 13 | 13 | 18 |
| Mn mg/kg | 16 | 18 | 24 |
| Se mg/kg | 0.3 | 0.3 | 0.3 |
| Zn mg/kg | 21 | 22 | 30 |
| Vitamin A (IU/day) | 80300 | 82610 | 83270 |
| Vitamin D (IU/day) | 21900 | 21530 | 22710 |
| Vitamin E (IU/day) | 1168 | 1202 | 1211 |
| Vitamin A (IU/kg) | 5576 | 6030 | 8244 |
| Vitamin D (IU/kg) | 1520 | 1645 | 2249 |
| Vitamin E (IU/kg) | 81 | 88 | 120 |
| Sample diets used in model to generate tables | | | |
| Ingredient (kg DM) | | | |
| Corn silage, normal | | 4.32 | 4.03 |
| Soybean meal, solv. 48% CP | | | 0.27 |
| Grass silage, C-3, mid-mat | 8.1 | 7.35 | 3.73 |
| Corn grain, ground hi moist | | | 0.31 |
| Beet sugar pulp, dried | | | 1.42 |
| Wheat straw | 5.79 | 1.56 | |
| Sodium chloride | 0.02 | 0.02 | 0.02 |
| Vitamin and mineral premix | 0.46 | 0.41 | 0.31 |
| Calcium carbonate | | | |
| Monosodium phosphate (1 H2O) | | | |
| Magnesium oxide | | | |
| Calcium phosphate (Di-) | | | |

*Continues*

TABLE 14-9 *(continued)*

| | REQUIREMENTS OF A DIET TO MEET TISSUE DEMANDS Holstein Cow, mature body weight without conceptus = 680 kg, BCS = 3.3, Calf wt = 45 kg Gaining 0.67 kg/day with conceptus | | |
|---|---|---|---|
| Sample dry cow diet evaluation | | | |
| NDF % | 62.2 | 53.9 | 46.5 |
| Forage NDF % | 62.2 | 53.9 | 39.5 |
| ADF % | 39.7 | 33.5 | 27.8 |
| NFC % | 19.6 | 27.2 | 34.7 |
| Undiscounted TDN | 51 | 57 | 63 |
| Diet $NE_L$ (Mcal/kg), dependent on DMI | 1.12 | 1.33 | 1.49 |
| $NE_L$ (Mcal/day supplied by example diet) | 16.1 | 18.1 | 15 |

[a] RUP corrected from model prediction to provide actual RUP requirement if diet had been formulated to meet RDP requirement. Protein in many cases will not be balanced for RDP before the metabolizable protein requirement of the dry cow is met. When this occurs the RUP requirement determined by the model increases to compensate for the lost microbial protein. When RDP is inadequate the energy derived from the diet may be less than predicted by model due to incomplete digestion as a result of reduced bacterial activity in the rumen.

[b] % RUP + % RDP = Crude protein required only if ration is perfectly balanced for RDP and RUP. Rumen function may require that the crude protein content of the dry cow ration be 12%, despite the needs of the cow being met at lower CP levels.

[c] These are the minimum fiber (or maximum NFC) concentrations needed to maintain rumen health and milk fat test (see Chapter 4). Actual concentrations may need to be higher (or lower for NFC) depending on energy requirements of the cow. For transition and early lactation cows, diets should meet these minimum and maximum constraints and be formulated to contain 1.60 Mcal/kg of $NE_L$ (see Chapter 9).

[d] High dietary potassium and excess non-protein nitrogen can interfere with Mg absorption.

[e] High dietary molybdenum, sulfur, and iron can interfere with copper absorption increasing the requirement (see text).

[f] Diets high in goitrogenic substances increase the iodine requirement (see text).

TABLE 14-10 Example Diet Incorporating Dietary Guidelines Suggested in Chapter 9 for Transitioning a Heifer (entering first lactation) During the Later Dry Period to Acclimate Her To the Lactating Ration and To Reduce Metabolic Disease

This animal must be entered into the model as a replacement heifer to accommodate growth requirements. Tissue requirements for a heifer (270 d pregnant, weighing 625 kg with conceptus, mature body weight of 680 kg, consuming 10.6 kg dry matter / day, gaining 300 g body weight plus 660 g conceptus weight each day, and a current body condition score of 3.3) and nutrient densities of an example ration that follows the recommendation guidelines.

| | Guidelines for close-up heifer diet | Nutrients required by tissues (as assessed with the example diet) | Example close-up heifer ration |
|---|---|---|---|
| | Recommendations that differ from requirement | | Nutrients supplied |
| Energy | | | |
| $NE_L$ (Mcal/day) | | 14.8 | 16.9 |
| $NE_L$ (Mcal/kg) | 1.54–1.62[a] | 1.40 | 1.59 |
| Protein | | | |
| Metabolizable protein (g/d) | | 888 | 1027 |
| Diet % MP | | 8.4 | 9.7 |
| Rumen degradable protein (g/day) | | 1052 | 1067 |
| Diet % RDP | | 9.9 | 10.2 |
| Rumen undegradable protein (g/day) | | 336 | 511 |
| Diet % RUP | | 3.2 | 4.9 |
| % RDP+ % RUP (crude protein[b]) | 13.5–15.0[c] | 13.1 | 15.0 |
| Fiber and carbohydrate[d] | | | |
| Minimum % NDF | 33[c] | 25–33 | 39.1 |
| Minimum % ADF | 21[c] | 17–21 | 23.4 |
| Maximum % NFC | 43[c] | 36–43 | 39.4 |
| Minerals | | | |
| Absorbable calcium (g) | | 22.4 | 24.5 |
| Dietary Ca % | | 0.40 | 0.44 |
| Absorbable phosphorus (g) | | 16.6 | 25.4 |
| Dietary P % | 0.3–0.4[e] | 0.23 | 0.37 |
| Mg % | 0.35–0.40[f] | 0.14 | 0.40 |
| Cl % | | 0.16 | 0.44 |
| K % | 0.55[g] | 0.55 | 1.54 |
| Na % | | 0.12 | 0.13 |
| S % | | 0.20 | 0.19 |
| Co mg/kg | | 0.11 | 0.11 |
| Cu mg/kg | | 16 | 16 |
| I mg/kg | | 0.4 | 0.4 |
| Fe mg/kg | | 26 | 26 |
| Mn mg/kg | | 22 | 22 |
| Se mg/kg | | 0.3 | 0.3 |
| Zn mg/kg | | 30 | 30 |
| Vitamin A (IU/day) | 75000[h] | 68750 | 75000 |
| Vitamin D (IU/day) | 20000[h] | 18750 | 20000 |
| Vitamin E (IU/day) | 1200[h] | 848 | 1200 |
| Vitamin A (IU/kg) | | 6486 | 7075 |
| Vitamin D (IU/kg) | | 1769 | 1887 |
| Vitamin E (IU/kg) | | 80 | 113 |
| Dietary cation-anion difference (Na + K) − (Cl + S), meq/kg | | 24 | 203 |

*Continues*

TABLE 14-10 *(continued)*

| Sample diet used in model to generate tables | Ingredient (kg DM/day) | Example Close-up heifer diet |
|---|---|---|
| | Corn silage, normal | 4.58 |
| | Soybean meal, solv. 48% CP | 1.07 |
| | Grass silage, C-3, mid-mat | 2.44 |
| | Corn grain, ground high moist | 1.04 |
| | Beet sugar pulp, dried | 0.95 |
| | Sodium chloride | 0.02 |
| | Vitamin and mineral premix | 0.39 |
| | Magnesium oxide | 0.04 |
| | Calcium phosphate (Di-) | 0.02 |

[a]Energy increased to prepare rumen for lactation ration, promote feed intake, and reduce displaced abomasum after calving.

[b]% RUP + % RDP = Crude protein required only if ration is perfectly balanced for RDP and RUP.

[c]Protein may not be balanced for RDP before the metabolizable protein requirement of the animals is met. When this occurs the RUP requirement is increased to compensate for the lost microbial protein. In addition energy derived from the diet may be diminished due to incomplete digestion as a result of reduced bacterial activity in the rumen.

[d]Suggested carbohydrate profile to reduce displacement of the abomasum.

[e]A level which will provide adequate phosphorus even on the day of calving when DMI is low.

[f]A level which will allow passive absorption of magnesium across the rumen wall to maintain adequate blood magnesium concentration.

[g]Goal would be to limit potassium to the requirement of the heifer to reduce udder edema. Very difficult to achieve.

[h]A level which will provide adequate vitamins even on the day of calving when DMI is low, utilizing requirements of cows, not replacement heifers.

TABLE 14-11 Example Diet Incorporating Dietary Guidelines Suggested in Chapter 9 for Transitioning a Cow (entering 2nd lactation or greater) During the Last Weeks of Gestation to Acclimate Her To a Lactating Ration and To Reduce Metabolic Disease

Tissue requirements for a cow (270 d pregnant, weighing 751 kg with conceptus, mature body weight of 680 kg, consuming 13.7 kg dry matter/day, and a current body condition score of 3.3) with the nutrients supplied by the example rations that follow the recommendation guidelines.

| | Nutrients needed to meet requirement of tissues as determined with example diet | Guidelines for standard close-up diet | Guidelines for "anionic" close-up diet | Example standard close-up diet | Example "anionic" close-up diet |
|---|---|---|---|---|---|
| | | Recommendations that differ from simply meeting tissue requirement | Recommendations that differ from simply meeting tissue requirement | Nutrients supplied | Nutrients supplied |
| Energy | | | | | |
| $NE_L$ (Mcal/day) | 14.4 | | | 22.0 | 21.5 |
| $NE_L$ (Mcal/kg diet) | 1.05 | 1.54–1.62[a] | 1.54–1.62[a] | 1.61 | 1.58 |
| Protein | | | | | |
| Metabolizable protein (g/d) | 910 | | | 164 | 1133 |
| Diet % MP | 6.6 | | | 8.5 | 8.3 |
| Rumen degradable protein (g/day) | 1358 | | | 1104 | 1075 |
| Diet % RDP | 9.9 | | | 8.1 | 7.8 |
| Rumen undegradable protein (g/day) | 172[b] | | | 640 | 621 |
| Diet % RUP | 1.3[b] | | | 4.7 | 4.5 |
| % RDP + % RUP (crude protein)[c] | 10.2 | 12.0[d] | 12.0[d] | 12.8 | 12.3 |
| Fiber and carbohydrate[e] | | | | | |
| Minimum % NDF | 25–33 | 33 | 33 | 38.2 | 37.2 |
| Minimum % ADF | 17–21 | 21 | 21 | 22.4 | 21.8 |
| Maximum % NFC | 36–44 | 43 | 43 | 42.8 | 41.6 |
| Minerals | | | | | |
| Absorbable calcium (g) | 21.5 | | | 32.0 | 95.0 |
| Dietary Ca % | 0.45 | | 0.6–1.5[f] | 0.43 | 0.98 |
| Absorbable phosphorus (g) | 20.3 | | | 28 | 36 |
| Dietary P % | 0.23 | 0.3–0.4[g] | 0.3–0.4 | 0.3 | 0.37 |
| Mg % | 0.12 | 0.35–0.40[h] | 0.35–0.40[h] | 0.39 | 0.38 |
| Cl % | 0.15 | | 0.8–1.2[i] | 0.42 | 0.89 |
| K[j] % | 0.52 | | | 1.35 | 1.32 |
| Na % | 0.1 | | | 0.16 | 0.15 |
| S % | 0.2 | | 0.3–0.4[i] | 0.18 | 0.31 |
| Co mg/kg | 0.11 | | | 0.11 | 0.11 |
| Cu mg/kg | 13 | | | 13 | 13 |
| I mg/kg | 0.4 | | | 0.4 | 0.4 |
| Fe mg/kg | 13 | | | 13 | 13 |
| Mn mg/kg | 18 | | | 18 | 18 |
| Se mg/kg | 0.3 | | | 0.3 | 0.3 |
| Zn mg/kg | 22 | | | 22 | 22 |
| Vitamin A (IU/day) | 82610 | 100000[k] | 100000[k] | 100000 | 100000 |
| Vitamin D (IU/day) | 22530 | 25000[k] | 25000[k] | 25000 | 25000 |
| Vitamin E (IU/day) | 1202 | 1200[k] | 1200[k] | 1803 | 1803 |
| Vitamin A (IU/kg) | 6030 | | | 7300 | 7300 |
| Vitamin D (IU/kg) | 1644 | | | 1824 | 1824 |
| Vitamin E (IU/kg) | 88 | | | 132 | 132 |
| Dietary cation-anion difference (Na + K) − (Cl + S), meq/kg | 10 | 10 | −75 to 0[l] | 185 | −41 |

*Continues*

TABLE 14-11 *(continued)*

Tissue requirements for a cow (270 d pregnant, weighing 751 kg with conceptus, mature body weight of 680 kg, consuming 13.7 kg dry matter/day, and a current body condition score of 3.3) with the nutrients supplied by the example rations that follow the recommendation guidelines.

| | Nutrients needed to meet requirement of tissues as determined with example diet | Guidelines for standard close-up diet | Guidelines for "anionic" close-up diet | Example standard close-up diet | Example "anionic" close-up diet |
|---|---|---|---|---|---|
| | | Recommendations that differ from simply meeting tissue requirement | Recommendations that differ from simply meeting tissue requirement | Nutrients supplied | Nutrients supplied |
| Sample diets used in model to generate tables | | | | | |
| Ingredient (kg DM/day) | | | | No added anion diet | Anionic diet |
| Corn silage, normal | | | | 5.55 | 5.40 |
| Soybean meal, solv. 48% CP | | | | 0.79 | 0.77 |
| Grass silage, C-3, mid-mat | | | | 2.48 | 2.42 |
| Corn grain, ground hi moist | | | | 2.16 | 2.10 |
| Beet sugar pulp, dried | | | | 2.15 | 2.09 |
| Sodium chloride | | | | 0.03 | 0.03 |
| Vitamin and mineral premix | | | | 0.43 | 0.42 |
| Calcium carbonate | | | | | 0.07 |
| Magnesium oxide | | | | 0.05 | 0.03 |
| Calcium phosphate (Di−) | | | | 0.02 | 0.07 |
| Magnesium sulfate (7 H2O, Epsom salts)[m] | | | | | 0.14 |
| Calcium chloride (2 H2O, 77–80% CaCl2)[m] | | | | | 0.14 |

[a] Energy increased to prepare rumen for lactation ration, promote feed intake, and reduce displaced abomasum after calving.

[b] RUP corrected from model prediction to provide RUP requirement if diet can be formulated to meet RDP requirement.

[c] % RUP + % RDP = Crude Protein Required only if ration is perfectly balanced for RDP and RUP.

[d] Protein in most cases will not be balanced for RDP before the metabolizable protein requirement of the dry cow is met. When this occurs the RUP requirement determined by the model increases to compensate for the lost microbial protein. When RDP is inadequate the energy derived from the diet may be less than predicted by model due to incomplete digestion as a result of reduced bacterial activity in the rumen. In order to improve rumen digestion the recommendation is to exceed the cow's requirement for metabolizable protein to meet the RDP requirement of the rumen.

[e] Suggested carbohydrate profile to reduce displacement of the abomasum.

[f] Utilizing the DCAD concept to prevent milk fever, diet calcium does not have to be limited.

[g] A level which will provide adequate phosphorus even on the day of calving when DMI is low.

[h] A level which will allow passive absorption of magnesium across the rumen wall to maintain adequate blood magnesium concentration.

[i] Adding anions to the ration to reduce hypocalcemia.

[j] Goal would be to limit potassium to the requirement of the cow. Very difficult to achieve.

[k] A level which will provide adequate vitamins even on the day of calving when DMI is low.

[l] Monitoring urine pH can help titrate the correct DCAD of the ration.

[m] More palatable sources of anions than used in this example are available and would likely impair DMI less.

TABLE 14-12 Daily Nutrient Requirements (DM basis) of Small Breed (mature weight = 450 kg) Non-Bred Heifers

| BW kg | ADG kg/d | DMI kg/d | TDN % | NEm Mcal/d | $NE_G$ Mcal/d | ME Mcal/d | RDP g/d | RUP g/d | RDP % | RUP % | CP[a] % | Ca g/d | P g/d |
|---|---|---|---|---|---|---|---|---|---|---|---|---|---|
| 100 | 0.3 | 3.0 | 56.5 | 2.64 | 0.47 | 6.0 | 255 | 110 | 8.6 | 3.7 | 12.4 | 14 | 7 |
| | 0.4 | 3.0 | 58.6 | 2.64 | 0.64 | 6.4 | 270 | 143 | 9.0 | 4.7 | 13.7 | 18 | 8 |
| | 0.5 | 3.1 | 60.7 | 2.64 | 0.82 | 6.7 | 284 | 175 | 9.3 | 5.7 | 15.0 | 21 | 10 |
| | 0.6 | 3.1 | 62.9 | 2.64 | 1.00 | 7.0 | 298 | 207 | 9.6 | 6.7 | 16.3 | 25 | 11 |
| | 0.7 | 3.1 | 65.2 | 2.64 | 1.19 | 7.3 | 310 | 239 | 10.0 | 7.7 | 17.7 | 28 | 12 |
| | 0.8 | 3.1 | 67.7 | 2.64 | 1.37 | 7.6 | 323 | 270 | 10.4 | 8.7 | 19.0 | 31 | 13 |
| 150 | 0.3 | 4.0 | 56.5 | 3.57 | 0.63 | 8.2 | 346 | 95 | 8.6 | 2.4 | 11.0 | 15 | 8 |
| | 0.4 | 4.1 | 58.6 | 3.57 | 0.87 | 8.7 | 366 | 124 | 9.0 | 3.0 | 12.0 | 19 | 10 |
| | 0.5 | 4.1 | 60.7 | 3.57 | 1.11 | 9.1 | 385 | 152 | 9.3 | 3.7 | 12.9 | 22 | 11 |
| | 0.6 | 4.2 | 62.9 | 3.57 | 1.36 | 9.5 | 403 | 180 | 9.6 | 4.3 | 13.9 | 25 | 12 |
| | 0.7 | 4.2 | 65.3 | 3.57 | 1.61 | 9.9 | 421 | 207 | 10.0 | 4.9 | 14.9 | 28 | 13 |
| | 0.8 | 4.2 | 67.7 | 3.57 | 1.86 | 10.3 | 437 | 234 | 10.4 | 5.5 | 15.9 | 31 | 14 |
| 200 | 0.3 | 5.0 | 56.5 | 4.44 | 0.79 | 10.2 | 429 | 81 | 8.6 | 1.6 | 10.3 | 17 | 10 |
| | 0.4 | 5.1 | 58.6 | 4.44 | 1.08 | 10.7 | 454 | 106 | 9.0 | 2.1 | 11.1 | 20 | 11 |
| | 0.5 | 5.1 | 60.7 | 4.44 | 1.38 | 11.3 | 478 | 131 | 9.3 | 2.6 | 11.8 | 23 | 12 |
| | 0.6 | 5.2 | 62.9 | 4.44 | 1.68 | 11.8 | 500 | 156 | 9.6 | 3.0 | 12.6 | 26 | 13 |
| | 0.7 | 5.2 | 65.3 | 4.44 | 1.99 | 12.3 | 522 | 179 | 10.0 | 3.4 | 13.4 | 29 | 14 |
| | 0.8 | 5.2 | 67.7 | 4.44 | 2.31 | 12.8 | 543 | 202 | 10.4 | 3.9 | 14.2 | 32 | 15 |
| 250 | 0.3 | 5.9 | 56.5 | 5.24 | 0.93 | 12.0 | 508 | 69 | 8.6 | 1.2 | 9.8 | 19 | 11 |
| | 0.4 | 6.0 | 58.6 | 5.24 | 1.28 | 12.7 | 537 | 91 | 9.0 | 1.5 | 10.5 | 21 | 12 |
| | 0.5 | 6.1 | 60.7 | 5.24 | 1.63 | 13.4 | 565 | 113 | 9.3 | 1.9 | 11.1 | 24 | 13 |
| | 0.6 | 6.1 | 62.9 | 5.24 | 1.99 | 14.0 | 592 | 135 | 9.6 | 2.2 | 11.8 | 27 | 14 |
| | 0.7 | 6.2 | 65.3 | 5.24 | 2.36 | 14.6 | 617 | 155 | 10.0 | 2.5 | 12.5 | 30 | 15 |
| | 0.8 | 6.2 | 67.7 | 5.24 | 2.73 | 15.2 | 642 | 175 | 10.4 | 2.8 | 13.2 | 32 | 16 |
| 300 | 0.3 | 6.7 | 56.5 | 6.01 | 1.07 | 13.8 | 582 | 58 | 8.6 | 0.9 | 9.5 | 20 | 12 |
| | 0.4 | 6.9 | 58.6 | 6.01 | 1.46 | 14.6 | 616 | 79 | 9.0 | 1.1 | 10.1 | 23 | 13 |
| | 0.5 | 7.0 | 60.7 | 6.01 | 1.87 | 15.3 | 648 | 98 | 9.3 | 1.4 | 10.7 | 26 | 14 |
| | 0.6 | 7.0 | 62.9 | 6.01 | 2.28 | 16.0 | 678 | 117 | 9.6 | 1.7 | 11.3 | 28 | 15 |
| | 0.7 | 7.1 | 65.3 | 6.01 | 2.70 | 16.7 | 707 | 135 | 10.0 | 1.9 | 11.9 | 31 | 16 |
| | 0.8 | 7.1 | 67.7 | 6.01 | 3.13 | 17.4 | 736 | 151 | 10.4 | 2.1 | 12.5 | 34 | 17 |

[a]Crude protein required only if ration is perfectly balanced for RDP and RUP.

TABLE 14-13 Daily Nutrient Requirements (DM basis) of Large Breed (mature weight = 650 kg) Non-Bred Heifers

| BW kg | ADG kg/d | DMI kg/d | TDN % | NEm Mcal/d | $NE_G$ Mcal/d | ME Mcal/d | RDP g/d | RUP g/d | RDP % | RUP % | CP[a] % | Ca g/d | P g/d |
|---|---|---|---|---|---|---|---|---|---|---|---|---|---|
| 150 | 0.5 | 4.1 | 58.4 | 3.57 | 0.84 | 8.6 | 364 | 167 | 8.9 | 4.1 | 13.0 | 23 | 11 |
| | 0.6 | 4.1 | 60.0 | 3.57 | 1.03 | 9.0 | 379 | 199 | 9.2 | 4.8 | 14.0 | 26 | 12 |
| | 0.7 | 4.2 | 61.7 | 3.57 | 1.22 | 9.3 | 393 | 230 | 9.4 | 5.5 | 14.9 | 30 | 13 |
| | 0.8 | 4.2 | 63.4 | 3.57 | 1.41 | 9.6 | 407 | 261 | 9.7 | 6.2 | 15.9 | 33 | 15 |
| | 0.9 | 4.2 | 65.3 | 3.57 | 1.61 | 9.9 | 421 | 292 | 10.0 | 6.9 | 16.9 | 37 | 16 |
| | 1.0 | 4.2 | 67.2 | 3.57 | 1.80 | 10.3 | 434 | 322 | 10.3 | 7.6 | 17.9 | 40 | 17 |
| | 1.1 | 4.2 | 69.2 | 3.57 | 2.00 | 10.6 | 446 | 352 | 10.6 | 8.3 | 18.9 | 43 | 18 |
| 200 | 0.5 | 5.1 | 58.4 | 4.44 | 1.05 | 10.7 | 452 | 148 | 8.9 | 2.9 | 11.9 | 24 | 12 |
| | 0.6 | 5.1 | 60.0 | 4.44 | 1.28 | 11.1 | 470 | 177 | 9.2 | 3.4 | 12.6 | 27 | 13 |
| | 0.7 | 5.2 | 61.7 | 4.44 | 1.51 | 11.5 | 488 | 205 | 9.4 | 4.0 | 13.4 | 30 | 14 |
| | 0.8 | 5.2 | 63.4 | 4.44 | 1.75 | 11.9 | 505 | 233 | 9.7 | 4.5 | 14.2 | 34 | 15 |
| | 0.9 | 5.2 | 65.3 | 4.44 | 1.99 | 12.3 | 522 | 260 | 10.0 | 5.0 | 15.0 | 37 | 17 |
| | 1.0 | 5.2 | 67.2 | 4.44 | 2.24 | 12.7 | 538 | 287 | 10.3 | 5.5 | 15.8 | 40 | 18 |
| | 1.1 | 5.2 | 69.2 | 4.44 | 2.49 | 13.1 | 554 | 314 | 10.6 | 6.0 | 16.6 | 43 | 19 |
| 250 | 0.5 | 6.0 | 58.4 | 5.24 | 1.24 | 12.6 | 534 | 131 | 8.9 | 2.2 | 11.1 | 25 | 13 |
| | 0.6 | 6.1 | 60.0 | 5.24 | 1.51 | 13.1 | 556 | 156 | 9.2 | 2.6 | 11.8 | 28 | 14 |
| | 0.7 | 6.1 | 61.7 | 5.24 | 1.79 | 13.6 | 577 | 182 | 9.4 | 3.0 | 12.4 | 31 | 15 |
| | 0.8 | 6.2 | 63.4 | 5.24 | 2.07 | 14.1 | 597 | 207 | 9.7 | 3.4 | 13.1 | 34 | 16 |
| | 0.9 | 6.2 | 65.3 | 5.24 | 2.36 | 14.6 | 617 | 232 | 10.0 | 3.7 | 13.7 | 37 | 17 |
| | 1.0 | 6.2 | 67.2 | 5.24 | 2.65 | 15.0 | 636 | 256 | 10.3 | 4.1 | 14.4 | 40 | 18 |
| | 1.1 | 6.2 | 69.2 | 5.24 | 2.94 | 15.5 | 655 | 280 | 10.6 | 4.5 | 15.1 | 43 | 19 |
| 300 | 0.5 | 6.9 | 58.4 | 6.01 | 1.42 | 14.5 | 612 | 114 | 8.9 | 1.7 | 10.6 | 27 | 14 |
| | 0.6 | 6.9 | 60.0 | 6.01 | 1.73 | 15.1 | 637 | 138 | 9.2 | 2.0 | 11.2 | 30 | 15 |
| | 0.7 | 7.0 | 61.7 | 6.01 | 2.05 | 15.6 | 661 | 161 | 9.4 | 2.3 | 11.7 | 33 | 16 |
| | 0.8 | 7.1 | 63.4 | 6.01 | 2.38 | 16.2 | 685 | 183 | 9.7 | 2.6 | 12.3 | 35 | 17 |
| | 0.9 | 7.1 | 65.3 | 6.01 | 2.70 | 16.7 | 707 | 205 | 10.0 | 2.9 | 12.9 | 38 | 18 |
| | 1.0 | 7.1 | 67.2 | 6.01 | 3.03 | 17.2 | 729 | 227 | 10.3 | 3.2 | 13.5 | 41 | 19 |
| | 1.1 | 7.1 | 69.2 | 6.01 | 3.37 | 17.7 | 751 | 248 | 10.6 | 3.5 | 14.1 | 44 | 20 |
| 350 | 0.5 | 7.7 | 58.4 | 6.75 | 1.59 | 16.2 | 687 | 99 | 8.9 | 1.3 | 10.2 | 28 | 15 |
| | 0.6 | 7.8 | 60.0 | 6.75 | 1.94 | 16.9 | 715 | 121 | 9.2 | 1.5 | 10.7 | 31 | 16 |
| | 0.7 | 7.9 | 61.7 | 6.75 | 2.30 | 17.6 | 742 | 141 | 9.4 | 1.8 | 11.2 | 34 | 17 |
| | 0.8 | 7.9 | 63.4 | 6.75 | 2.67 | 18.2 | 769 | 162 | 9.7 | 2.0 | 11.7 | 37 | 18 |
| | 0.9 | 8.0 | 65.3 | 6.75 | 3.03 | 18.8 | 794 | 181 | 10.0 | 2.3 | 12.3 | 40 | 19 |
| | 1.0 | 8.0 | 67.2 | 6.75 | 3.41 | 19.4 | 819 | 200 | 10.3 | 2.5 | 12.8 | 42 | 20 |
| | 1.1 | 8.0 | 69.2 | 6.75 | 3.78 | 19.9 | 843 | 218 | 10.6 | 2.7 | 13.3 | 45 | 21 |
| 400 | 0.5 | 8.5 | 58.4 | 7.46 | 1.76 | 18.0 | 760 | 86 | 8.9 | 1.0 | 9.9 | 30 | 16 |
| | 0.6 | 8.6 | 60.0 | 7.46 | 2.15 | 18.7 | 791 | 105 | 9.2 | 1.2 | 10.4 | 33 | 17 |
| | 0.7 | 8.7 | 61.7 | 7.46 | 2.55 | 19.4 | 821 | 124 | 9.4 | 1.4 | 10.9 | 35 | 18 |
| | 0.8 | 8.8 | 63.4 | 7.46 | 2.95 | 20.1 | 850 | 142 | 9.7 | 1.6 | 11.3 | 38 | 19 |
| | 0.9 | 8.8 | 65.3 | 7.46 | 3.35 | 20.7 | 878 | 159 | 10.0 | 1.8 | 11.8 | 41 | 20 |
| | 1.0 | 8.8 | 67.2 | 7.46 | 3.76 | 21.4 | 905 | 176 | 10.3 | 2.0 | 12.3 | 44 | 21 |
| | 1.1 | 8.8 | 69.2 | 7.46 | 4.18 | 22.0 | 931 | 192 | 10.6 | 2.2 | 12.8 | 46 | 22 |

[a]Crude protein required only if ration is perfectly balanced for RDP and RUP.

TABLE 14-14 Daily Nutrient Requirements (DM basis) of Small Breed (mature weight = 450 kg) Bred Heifers

| BW kg | ADG kg/d | DMI kg/d | TDN % | NEm Mcal/d | $NE_G$ Mcal/d | ME Mcal/d | RDP g/d | RUP g/d | RDP % | RUP % | CP[a] % | Ca g/d | P g/d |
|---|---|---|---|---|---|---|---|---|---|---|---|---|---|
| | | | | 240 days pregnant (Conceptus weight of 39 kg and ADG of 0.4 kg/day) | | | | | | | | | |
| 300 | 0.3 (0.7)[b] | 7.7 | 56.5 | 5.42 | 0.96 | 15.7 | 663 | 291 | 8.6 | 3.8 | 12.4 | 36 | 19 |
| | 0.4 (0.8) | 7.7 | 58.6 | 5.42 | 1.32 | 16.4 | 693 | 310 | 9.0 | 4.0 | 13.0 | 39 | 20 |
| | 0.5 (0.9) | 7.7 | 60.8 | 5.42 | 1.68 | 17.0 | 721 | 329 | 9.3 | 4.2 | 13.5 | 41 | 21 |
| | 0.6 (1.0) | 7.7 | 63.1 | 5.42 | 2.06 | 17.7 | 748 | 346 | 9.7 | 4.5 | 14.1 | 44 | 22 |
| | 0.7 (1.1) | 7.7 | 65.5 | 5.42 | 2.44 | 18.3 | 774 | 364 | 10.0 | 4.7 | 14.7 | 47 | 23 |
| | 0.8 (1.2) | 7.7 | 68.1 | 5.42 | 2.82 | 18.9 | 798 | 380 | 10.4 | 5.0 | 15.4 | 49 | 24 |
| | 0.9 (1.3) | 7.6 | 70.9 | 5.42 | 3.21 | 19.4 | 822 | 395 | 10.8 | 5.2 | 16.1 | 52 | 24 |
| 350 | 0.3 (0.7) | 8.6 | 56.2 | 6.18 | 1.10 | 17.5 | 739 | 282 | 8.6 | 3.3 | 11.9 | 38 | 20 |
| | 0.4 (0.8) | 8.7 | 58.3 | 6.18 | 1.50 | 18.3 | 773 | 299 | 8.9 | 3.4 | 12.4 | 40 | 21 |
| | 0.5 (0.9) | 8.7 | 60.5 | 6.18 | 1.92 | 19.0 | 805 | 315 | 9.3 | 3.6 | 12.9 | 43 | 22 |
| | 0.6 (1.0) | 8.7 | 62.8 | 6.18 | 2.35 | 19.8 | 836 | 330 | 9.6 | 3.8 | 13.4 | 46 | 23 |
| | 0.7 (1.1) | 8.7 | 65.3 | 6.18 | 2.78 | 20.4 | 865 | 345 | 10.0 | 4.0 | 14.0 | 48 | 24 |
| | 0.8 (1.2) | 8.6 | 67.8 | 6.18 | 3.22 | 21.1 | 893 | 358 | 10.4 | 4.2 | 14.5 | 51 | 25 |
| | 0.9 (1.3) | 8.5 | 70.6 | 6.18 | 3.66 | 21.8 | 921 | 371 | 10.8 | 4.3 | 15.1 | 53 | 25 |
| 400 | 0.3 (0.7) | 9.5 | 56.0 | 6.91 | 1.23 | 19.2 | 813 | 275 | 8.6 | 2.9 | 11.5 | 40 | 21 |
| | 0.4 (0.8) | 9.6 | 58.1 | 6.91 | 1.68 | 20.1 | 851 | 291 | 8.9 | 3.0 | 11.9 | 42 | 22 |
| | 0.5 (0.9) | 9.6 | 60.3 | 6.91 | 2.15 | 21.0 | 887 | 305 | 9.2 | 3.2 | 12.4 | 45 | 23 |
| | 0.6 (1.0) | 9.6 | 62.6 | 6.91 | 2.62 | 21.8 | 921 | 319 | 9.6 | 3.3 | 12.9 | 47 | 24 |
| | 0.7 (1.1) | 9.6 | 65.0 | 6.91 | 3.11 | 22.5 | 953 | 331 | 9.9 | 3.5 | 13.4 | 50 | 25 |
| | 0.8 (1.2) | 9.5 | 67.6 | 6.91 | 3.60 | 23.3 | 985 | 342 | 10.3 | 3.6 | 13.9 | 52 | 26 |
| | 0.9 (1.3) | 9.4 | 70.3 | 6.91 | 4.09 | 24.0 | 1015 | 352 | 10.8 | 3.7 | 14.5 | 55 | 26 |
| 450 | 0.3 (0.7) | 10.4 | 55.8 | 7.62 | 1.35 | 20.9 | 884 | 273 | 8.5 | 2.6 | 11.2 | 41 | 22 |
| | 0.4 (0.8) | 10.5 | 57.9 | 7.62 | 1.85 | 21.9 | 926 | 288 | 8.9 | 2.8 | 11.6 | 44 | 23 |
| | 0.5 (0.9) | 10.5 | 60.1 | 7.62 | 2.37 | 22.8 | 965 | 301 | 9.2 | 2.9 | 12.1 | 46 | 24 |
| | 0.6 (1.0) | 10.5 | 62.4 | 7.62 | 2.89 | 23.7 | 1003 | 313 | 9.5 | 3.0 | 12.5 | 49 | 25 |
| | 0.7 (1.1) | 10.5 | 64.8 | 7.62 | 3.42 | 24.5 | 1038 | 324 | 9.9 | 3.1 | 13.0 | 51 | 26 |
| | 0.8 (1.2) | 10.4 | 67.4 | 7.62 | 3.96 | 25.4 | 1073 | 333 | 10.3 | 3.2 | 13.5 | 54 | 27 |
| | 0.9 (1.3) | 10.3 | 70.1 | 7.62 | 4.51 | 26.1 | 1106 | 341 | 10.7 | 3.3 | 14.0 | 56 | 28 |

[a] Crude protein required only if ration is perfectly balanced for RDP and RUP.
[b] Values in parentheses are ADG (lbs/d).

TABLE 14-15 Daily Nutrient Requirements (DM basis) of Large Breed (mature weight = 650 kg) Bred Heifers

| BW kg | ADG kg/d | DMI kg/d | TDN % | NEm Mcal/d | $NE_G$ Mcal/d | ME Mcal/d | RDP g/d | RUP g/d | RDP % | RUP % | CP[a] % | Ca g/d | P g/d |
|---|---|---|---|---|---|---|---|---|---|---|---|---|---|
| | | | 240 days pregnant (Conceptus weight of 48 kg and ADG of 0.6 kg/day) | | | | | | | | | | |
| 450 | 0.5 (1.1)[b] | 10.5 | 59.3 | 7.49 | 1.77 | 22.5 | 951 | 402 | 9.1 | 3.8 | 12.9 | 47 | 25 |
| | 0.6 (1.2) | 10.5 | 61.1 | 7.49 | 2.16 | 23.2 | 981 | 418 | 9.3 | 4.0 | 13.3 | 50 | 25 |
| | 0.7 (1.3) | 10.5 | 62.9 | 7.49 | 2.55 | 23.9 | 1010 | 433 | 9.6 | 4.1 | 13.7 | 53 | 26 |
| | 0.8 (1.4) | 10.5 | 64.8 | 7.49 | 2.96 | 24.5 | 1038 | 448 | 9.9 | 4.3 | 14.2 | 55 | 27 |
| | 0.9 (1.5) | 10.4 | 66.8 | 7.49 | 3.37 | 25.2 | 1066 | 462 | 10.2 | 4.4 | 14.7 | 58 | 28 |
| | 1.0 (1.6) | 10.4 | 68.9 | 7.49 | 3.78 | 25.8 | 1092 | 475 | 10.5 | 4.6 | 15.1 | 61 | 29 |
| | 1.1 (1.7) | 10.3 | 71.2 | 7.49 | 4.19 | 26.4 | 1118 | 488 | 10.9 | 4.8 | 15.6 | 63 | 30 |
| 500 | 0.5 (1.1) | 11.3 | 59.0 | 8.17 | 1.93 | 24.2 | 1024 | 391 | 9.0 | 3.4 | 12.5 | 49 | 26 |
| | 0.6 (1.2) | 11.4 | 60.8 | 8.17 | 2.36 | 25.0 | 1057 | 405 | 9.3 | 3.6 | 12.9 | 52 | 27 |
| | 0.7 (1.3) | 11.4 | 62.6 | 8.17 | 2.79 | 25.7 | 1088 | 419 | 9.6 | 3.7 | 13.3 | 54 | 27 |
| | 0.8 (1.4) | 11.3 | 64.5 | 8.17 | 3.23 | 26.4 | 1119 | 432 | 9.9 | 3.8 | 13.7 | 57 | 28 |
| | 0.9 (1.5) | 11.3 | 66.5 | 8.17 | 3.67 | 27.2 | 1149 | 444 | 10.2 | 3.9 | 14.1 | 59 | 29 |
| | 1.0 (1.6) | 11.2 | 68.6 | 8.17 | 4.13 | 27.8 | 1177 | 455 | 10.5 | 4.1 | 14.5 | 62 | 30 |
| | 1.1 (1.7) | 11.1 | 70.8 | 8.17 | 4.58 | 28.5 | 1206 | 465 | 10.8 | 4.2 | 15.0 | 65 | 31 |
| 550 | 0.5 (1.1) | 12.2 | 58.8 | 8.84 | 2.09 | 25.9 | 1094 | 382 | 9.0 | 3.1 | 12.1 | 51 | 27 |
| | 0.6 (1.2) | 12.2 | 60.5 | 8.84 | 2.55 | 26.7 | 1130 | 395 | 9.3 | 3.2 | 12.5 | 53 | 28 |
| | 0.7 (1.3) | 12.2 | 62.3 | 8.84 | 3.02 | 27.5 | 1164 | 407 | 9.5 | 3.3 | 12.9 | 56 | 29 |
| | 0.8 (1.4) | 12.2 | 64.2 | 8.84 | 3.49 | 28.3 | 1197 | 418 | 9.8 | 3.4 | 13.3 | 58 | 29 |
| | 0.9 (1.5) | 12.1 | 66.2 | 8.84 | 3.98 | 29.1 | 1229 | 428 | 10.1 | 3.5 | 13.7 | 61 | 30 |
| | 1.0 (1.6) | 12.1 | 68.3 | 8.84 | 4.46 | 29.8 | 1260 | 437 | 10.4 | 3.6 | 14.1 | 64 | 31 |
| | 1.1 (1.7) | 12.0 | 70.5 | 8.84 | 4.95 | 30.5 | 1291 | 445 | 10.8 | 3.7 | 14.5 | 66 | 32 |
| 600 | 0.5 (1.1) | 13.0 | 58.6 | 9.50 | 2.24 | 27.5 | 1163 | 375 | 9.0 | 2.9 | 11.8 | 53 | 28 |
| | 0.6 (1.2) | 13.0 | 60.3 | 9.50 | 2.74 | 28.4 | 1202 | 387 | 9.2 | 3.0 | 12.2 | 55 | 29 |
| | 0.7 (1.3) | 13.0 | 62.1 | 9.50 | 3.24 | 29.3 | 1238 | 397 | 9.5 | 3.0 | 12.5 | 58 | 30 |
| | 0.8 (1.4) | 13.0 | 64.0 | 9.50 | 3.75 | 30.1 | 1274 | 407 | 9.8 | 3.1 | 12.9 | 60 | 30 |
| | 0.9 (1.5) | 13.0 | 66.0 | 9.50 | 4.27 | 30.9 | 1308 | 416 | 10.1 | 3.2 | 13.3 | 63 | 31 |
| | 1.0 (1.6) | 12.9 | 68.0 | 9.50 | 4.79 | 31.7 | 1342 | 423 | 10.4 | 3.3 | 13.7 | 65 | 32 |
| | 1.1 (1.7) | 12.8 | 70.2 | 9.50 | 5.32 | 32.5 | 1374 | 430 | 10.7 | 3.4 | 14.1 | 68 | 33 |
| 650 | 0.5 (1.1) | 13.8 | 58.4 | 10.14 | 2.39 | 29.1 | 1231 | 371 | 8.9 | 2.7 | 11.6 | 54 | 29 |
| | 0.6 (1.2) | 13.8 | 60.1 | 10.14 | 2.92 | 30.1 | 1272 | 382 | 9.2 | 2.8 | 12.0 | 57 | 30 |
| | 0.7 (1.3) | 13.8 | 61.9 | 10.14 | 3.46 | 31.0 | 1311 | 392 | 9.5 | 2.8 | 12.3 | 59 | 31 |
| | 0.8 (1.4) | 13.8 | 63.8 | 10.14 | 4.00 | 31.9 | 1349 | 400 | 9.8 | 2.9 | 12.7 | 62 | 31 |
| | 0.9 (1.5) | 13.8 | 65.8 | 10.14 | 4.56 | 32.7 | 1385 | 408 | 10.1 | 3.0 | 13.0 | 64 | 32 |
| | 1.0 (1.6) | 13.7 | 67.8 | 10.14 | 5.11 | 33.6 | 1421 | 414 | 10.4 | 3.0 | 13.4 | 67 | 33 |
| | 1.1 (1.7) | 13.6 | 70.0 | 10.14 | 5.68 | 34.4 | 1456 | 418 | 10.7 | 3.1 | 13.8 | 69 | 34 |

[a]Crude protein required only if ration is perfectly balanced for RDP and RUP.
[b]Values in parentheses are ADG (lbs/d).

TABLE 14-16 Nutrient Requirements of Growing Holstein Heifers Using Model to Predict Target Average Daily Gain Needed to Attain a Mature Body Weight of 680 Kg

| | 6 mos. (200 kg) BCS = 3.0 to calve at 24 mos age | 12 mos. (300 kg) BCS = 3.0 to calve at 24 mos age | 18 mos. (450 kg) BCS = 3.0 90 days gestation to calve at 24 mos age |
|---|---|---|---|
| Dry matter intake predicted by model (kg) | 5.2 | 7.1 | 11.3 |
| Dry matter intake predicted by model (lbs) | 11.4 | 15.62 | 24.9 |
| Energy | | | |
| ME (Mcal/day) | 10.6 | 16.2 | 20.3 |
| ME (Mcal/kg) | 2.04 | 2.28 | 1.79 |
| ME (Mcal/lb) | 0.93 | 1.03 | 0.82 |
| Protein | | | |
| Metabolizable protein (g/d) | 415 | 550 | 635 |
| Diet % MP | 8.0 | 7.7 | 5.6 |
| Rumen degradable protein | 481 | 667 | 970 |
| Diet % RDP | 9.3 | 9.4 | 8.6 |
| Rumen undegradable protein | 176 | 209 | 88 |
| Diet % RUP | 3.4 | 2.9 | 0.8 |
| % RDP + % RUP (crude protein)[a] | 12.7 | 12.3 | 9.4 |
| Fiber and carbohydrate[b] | | | |
| NDF, min % | 30–33 | 30–33 | 30–33 |
| ADF, min % | 20–21 | 20–21 | 20–21 |
| NFC, max % | 34–38 | 34–38 | 34–38 |
| Minerals | | | |
| Absorbable calcium (g) | 11.3 | 15.0 | 13.0 |
| Dietary Ca % | 0.41 | 0.41 | 0.37 |
| Absorbable phosphorus (g) | 9.1 | 10.6 | 13 |
| Dietary P % | 0.28 | 0.23 | 0.18 |
| Mg[c] % | 0.11 | 0.11 | 0.08 |
| Cl % | 0.11 | 0.12 | 0.10 |
| K % | 0.47 | 0.48 | 0.46 |
| Na % | 0.08 | 0.08 | 0.07 |
| S % | 0.2 | 0.2 | 0.2 |
| Co mg/kg | 0.11 | 0.11 | 0.11 |
| Cu mg/kg[d] | 10 | 10 | 9 |
| I mg/kg[e] | 0.27 | 0.30 | 0.30 |
| Fe mg/kg | 43 | 31 | 13 |
| Mn mg/kg | 22 | 20 | 14 |
| Se mg/kg | 0.3 | 0.3 | 0.3 |
| Zn mg/kg | 32 | 27 | 18 |
| Vitamin A (IU/ day) | 16000 | 24000 | 36000 |
| Vitamin D (IU/ day) | 6000 | 9000 | 13500 |
| Vitamin E (IU /day) | 160 | 240 | 360 |
| Vitamin A (IU/kg) | 3076 | 3380 | 3185 |
| Vitamin D (IU/kg) | 1154 | 1268 | 1195 |
| Vitamin E (IU /kg) | 31 | 34 | 32 |
| Sample Diets used in model to generate tables | | | |
| Ingredient (kg/d) | | | |
| Corn silage, normal | 2.90 | 4.08 | 1.51 |
| Soybean meal, solv. 48% CP | 0.30 | 0.41 | 0 |
| Grass silage, C-3, mid-mat | 1.68 | 2.29 | 9.52 |
| Limestone | 0.03 | 0.02 | 0 |
| Vitamin premix | 0.30 | 0.27 | 0.30 |
| Diet ME (Mcal/kg) | 2.24 | 2.29 | 2.08 |
| Diet undiscounted TDN % | 61 | 62 | 56 |
| Target ADG without conceptus (kg) | 0.65 | 0.87 | 0.59 |
| Target ADG with conceptus (kg) | 0.65 | 0.87 | 0.59 |
| ME allowable ADG without conceptus of diet | 0.82 | 0.87 | 0.86 |
| ME allowable ADG with conceptus of diet | 0.82 | 0.87 | 0.86 |
| MP allowable ADG without conceptus of diet | 0.76 | 1.09 | 1.30 |
| MP allowable ADG with conceptus of diet | 0.76 | 1.09 | 1.30 |

[a]Equivalent to crude protein requirement only if RDP and RUP are perfectly balanced.
[b]These are the minimum fiber (or maximum NFC) concentrations needed to maintain rumen health (see Chapter 4). Actual concentrations may need to be higher (or lower for NFC) depending on energy requirements of the heifer.
[c]Assumes that active transport of magnesium across the rumen wall is intact. High dietary potassium and excess non-protein nitrogen often interfere with Mg absorption. Under these conditions dietary Mg should be increased. (see Chapter 6).
[d]High dietary Mo, sulfur, and Fe can interfere with Cu absorption increasing the requirement (see Chapter 6).
[e]Diets high in goitrogenic substances increase the iodine requirement (see Chapter 6).

# 15 Nutrient Composition of Feeds

Data in Table 15-1 were compiled from commercial laboratories, literature data, *Nutrient Requirements of Beef Cattle* (National Research Council, 1996), and unpublished data provided by university researchers. When commercial laboratory data disagreed greatly with published data (>1.5 SD from the mean), the published data were used. The table includes means, standard deviations, and the number of samples (N) used to generate those statistics. Users should examine the standard deviation and N before using the mean value as an estimate of the nutritional content of a specific feed sample. Means derived from a large N will better reflect the total population. Means with a large standard deviation may represent the total population but may be a poor estimate for a specific sample.

All energy values in Table 15-1 were calculated from the mean nutrient data for each entry. Values for ME and $NE_L$ assume the diet has 74 percent TDN. Neutral detergent insoluble crude protein (NDICP) and acid detergent insoluble crude protein (ADICP) are not used directly to formulate diets but are used to calculate energy. Ether extract values represent the total lipid content of a feed but is a poor index of the true fat content of many feeds. The concentration of fatty acids in a feed is a measure of the true fat content and should replace the ether extract assay (Sukhija and Palmquist, 1988). Ether extract values were retained in this edition because of the limited availability of fatty acid data for most feedstuffs. In some cases, data were used that were derived with different analytic techniques, especially neutral detergent fiber (NDF) because other data were not available (see section on Analytic Procedures in chapter 13). Lignin and ash concentrations are used only to estimate energy values and the majority of lignin values were determined using sulfuric acid acid detergent lignin (ADL). Fiber concentrations are not presented for animal-based feedstuffs because the values have little meaning. Concentrations of macro and trace minerals are included in the table; however, before using these values, examine the standard deviations. Soil concentrations of minerals are highly variable; geographic differences exist for the mineral concentrations of many feeds. For most trace minerals, the standard deviation is high. The use of mean values for copper, iron, manganese, selenium, and zinc is discouraged. Concentrations of molybdenum are provided only in reference to copper availability.

For a very limited number of entries, the concentrations of certain nutrients (NDICP, ADICP, and some minerals) were estimated. Values in the table with no N were estimated. Generally the estimates were from a larger population (e.g., the sulfur concentration for normal corn silage also was used for immature corn silage). For some hay crop forages, values for a specific maturity class were estimated from the *all samples* entries. For some forage classifications, estimates of NDICP and ADICP were calculated from the mean value as a percent of crude protein (CP) for the *all sample* entries and multiplying that value by the mean CP for the specific entry. Data for ground corn (dry and high moisture) was used for cracked dry and high moisture corn. Data for dry rolled sorghum was used for steam-flaked sorghum.

Common names were used to designate feeds. In contrast with previous editions, data for different species of cool season grasses (C-3) were combined into a single classification (Grasses, Cool Season). The classification was simplified because nutrient composition does not vary greatly among different species (Cherney et al., 1993). Similarly, common legumes (alfalfa, clover, trefoil) were combined into a single classification (Legumes, Forage). The standard maturity classifications were eliminated because data from commercial labs and published data often do not include specific maturity designations. Within the cool season grasses and forage legume categories entries were broken into low NDF, medium NDF, and high NDF. Typically less mature forages contain lower NDF concentrations, but growing conditions can alter that relationship. The NDF concentrations, included in each entry are in the table. Because of the widespread use of mixed legume and grass forages, entries were included for this type of forage. The difference in hemicellulose concentrations between legumes and grasses was used to partition feeds into mostly (>70 percent) grass mixtures, mixtures with approximately equal amount grass and legume, and mostly (>70 percent) legume mixtures. Maturity classification for mixed forages was also based on NDF concentrations. Maturity of corn silage was estimated from dry matter content. Generally, as corn plants mature, dry matter increases (Wiersma et al., 1993).

## REFERENCES

Cherney, D. J., J. H. Cherney, and R. F. Lucey. 1993. In vitro digestion kinetics and quality of perennial grasses as influenced by forage maturity. J. Dairy Sci. 76:790–797.

National Research Council. 1996. Nutrient Requirements of Beef Cattle. 7th rev. ed. National Academy Press, Washington, D.C.

Sukhija, P. S., and D. L. Palmquist. 1988. Rapid method for determination of total fatty acid content and composition of feedstuffs and feces. J. Agric. Food Chem. 36:1202–1206.

Wiersma, D. W., P. R. Carter, K. A. Albrecht, and J. G. Coors. 1993. Kernel milkline stage and corn forage yield, quality, and dry matter content. J. Prod. Agr. 6:94–99.

TABLE 15-1 Nutrient Composition and Variability of Some Feedstuffs Commonly Fed to Dairy Cattle (all values on a dry basis)

| Entry No. | Feed Name/Description | International Feed No. | TDN-1X % | TDN Equation Class | PAF | DE-1X Mcal/kg | ME-3X Mcal/kg | NEL-3X Mcal/kg | NEL-4X Mcal/kg | NEM-3X Mcal/kg | NEG-3X Mcal/kg | DM % | CP % | NDICP % | ADICP % | Ether Extract % | NDF % | ADF % | Lignin % | Ash % |
|---|---|---|---|---|---|---|---|---|---|---|---|---|---|---|---|---|---|---|---|---|
| | ALFALFA *Medicago sativa* | Also see LEGUMES, FORAGE | | | | | | | | | | | | | | | | | | |
| 1 | Meal, 17% CP | 1-00-023 | 56.4 | Forage | 1.00 | 2.60 | 1.96 | 1.19 | 1.11 | 1.27 | 0.70 | 90.3 | 19.2 | 3.1 | 2.4 | 2.5 | 41.6 | 32.8 | 7.6 | 11.0 |
| | | N | | | | | | | | | | 222 | 221 | 3 | 70 | 54 | 221 | 220 | 70 | 84 |
| | | SD | | | | | | | | | | 1.4 | 3.3 | 0.3 | 0.1 | 0.6 | 7.1 | 5.1 | 1.2 | 2.3 |
| | ALMOND | | | | | | | | | | | | | | | | | | | |
| 2 | Hulls | 4-00-359 | 58.4 | Conc | 1.00 | 2.53 | 1.89 | 1.14 | 1.07 | 1.22 | 0.65 | 86.9 | 6.5 | 2.3 | 1.8 | 2.9 | 36.8 | 28.7 | 14.9 | 6.1 |
| | | N | | | | | | | | | | 23 | 32 | 4 | 3 | 23 | 30 | 30 | 11 | 16 |
| | | SD | | | | | | | | | | 5.6 | 2.5 | 0.3 | 0.4 | 2.0 | 11.2 | 8.5 | 3.0 | 0.5 |
| | APPLE | | | | | | | | | | | | | | | | | | | |
| 3 | Pomace, wet | 4-25-450 | 57.1 | Conc | 1.00 | 2.48 | 1.86 | 1.12 | 1.06 | 1.18 | 0.62 | 35.9 | 7.7 | 3.7 | 3.1 | 5.0 | 52.5 | 43.2 | 15.4 | 2.6 |
| | | N | | | | | | | | | | 65 | 65 | 3 | 4 | 22 | 65 | 65 | 5 | 16 |
| | | SD | | | | | | | | | | 29.4 | 3.8 | 0.9 | 0.7 | 1.9 | 9.5 | 6.6 | 2.6 | 1.1 |
| | BAKERY BYPRODUCT | | | | | | | | | | | | | | | | | | | |
| 4 | Byproduct meal | 4-00-466 | 93.5 | Conc | 1.04 | 4.09 | 3.37 | 2.21 | 2.09 | 2.32 | 1.61 | 84.7 | 12.5 | 2.3 | 1.1 | 9.5 | 13.9 | 6.5 | 1.6 | 3.8 |
| | | N | | | | | | | | | | 192 | 188 | 5 | 3 | 136 | 133 | 132 | 6 | 71 |
| | | SD | | | | | | | | | | 10.7 | 3.6 | 1.1 | 0.6 | 6.2 | 10.7 | 6.5 | 0.4 | 1.6 |
| 5 | Bread, waste | 4-00-466 | 89.3 | Conc | 1.04 | 3.99 | 3.25 | 2.09 | 1.98 | 2.21 | 1.52 | 68.3 | 15.0 | 0.6 | 0.5 | 2.2 | 8.9 | 3.1 | 0.1 | 2.8 |
| | | N | | | | | | | | | | 72 | 70 | 1 | 2 | 2 | 66 | 66 | 1 | 10 |
| | | SD | | | | | | | | | | 10.7 | 2.7 | | | | 10.5 | 4.3 | | 1.4 |
| 6 | Cereal byproduct | 4-00-466 | 87.6 | Conc | 1.04 | 3.79 | 3.07 | 1.97 | 1.88 | 2.12 | 1.45 | 88.5 | 9.1 | 3.2 | 1.2 | 3.5 | 10.0 | 3.9 | 2.6 | 3.2 |
| | | N | | | | | | | | | | 61 | 61 | 5 | 6 | 36 | 53 | 56 | 5 | 21 |
| | | SD | | | | | | | | | | 10.2 | 2.1 | 1.4 | 0.7 | 2.9 | 6.5 | 3.1 | 2.1 | 1.3 |
| 7 | Cookie byproduct | 4-24-852 | 95.0 | Conc | 1.04 | 4.11 | 3.40 | 2.24 | 2.12 | 2.33 | 1.63 | 90.1 | 9.7 | 1.9 | 0.5 | 10.6 | 12.7 | 6.5 | 2.6 | 3.0 |
| | | N | | | | | | | | | | 37 | 36 | 4 | 4 | 25 | 33 | 33 | 4 | 5 |
| | | SD | | | | | | | | | | 4.3 | 3.1 | 1.0 | 0.3 | 4.5 | 8.9 | 5.3 | 2.1 | 1.1 |
| | BARLEY | | | | | | | | | | | | | | | | | | | |
| 8 | Grain, rolled | 4-00-528 | 82.7 | Conc | 1.04 | 3.64 | 2.92 | 1.86 | 1.76 | 2.02 | 1.36 | 91.0 | 12.4 | 1.8 | 0.5 | 2.2 | 20.8 | 7.2 | 1.9 | 2.9 |
| | | N | | | | | | | | | | 823 | 795 | 60 | 61 | 247 | 331 | 727 | 69 | 257 |
| | | SD | | | | | | | | | | 3.5 | 2.1 | 1.1 | 0.4 | 0.6 | 8.6 | 2.8 | 1.1 | 0.8 |
| 9 | Malt sprouts | 5-00-545 | 66.4 | Conc | 1.00 | 3.06 | 2.38 | 1.49 | 1.40 | 1.61 | 1.01 | 90.5 | 20.1 | 3.7 | 1.1 | 2.3 | 47.0 | 21.8 | 3.4 | 7.4 |
| | | N | | | | | | | | | | 42 | 40 | 2 | 2 | 21 | 37 | 37 | 2 | 9 |
| | | SD | | | | | | | | | | 5.5 | 3.5 | | | 0.4 | 7.6 | 4.9 | | 1.3 |
| 10 | Silage, headed | 3-00-512 | 60.2 | Forage | 1.00 | 2.68 | 2.03 | 1.24 | 1.17 | 1.33 | 0.76 | 35.5 | 12.0 | 1.6 | 0.9 | 3.5 | 56.3 | 34.5 | 5.6 | 7.5 |
| | | N | | | | | | | | | | 504 | 528 | 25 | 265 | 68 | 387 | 528 | 84 | 166 |
| | | SD | | | | | | | | | | 9.6 | 2.6 | 0.6 | 0.4 | 0.7 | 7.0 | 4.9 | 1.5 | 2.1 |
| | BEET, SUGAR | | | | | | | | | | | | | | | | | | | |
| 11 | Pulp, dried | 4-00-669 | 69.1 | Conc | 1.00 | 3.03 | 2.36 | 1.47 | 1.38 | 1.60 | 0.99 | 88.3 | 10.0 | 5.5 | 0.6 | 1.1 | 45.8 | 23.1 | 1.6 | 7.3 |
| | | N | | | | | | | | | | 198 | 181 | 18 | 5 | 122 | 151 | 161 | 11 | 54 |
| | | SD | | | | | | | | | | 9.4 | 1.1 | 1.3 | 0.3 | 0.4 | 6.6 | 3.6 | 0.9 | 1.9 |
| | BERMUDAGRASS *Cynodon dactlyon* | | | | | | | | | | | | | | | | | | | |
| 12 | Coastal, hay, early head | 1-20-900 | 52.9 | Forage | 1.00 | 2.35 | 1.73 | 1.02 | 0.96 | 1.08 | 0.52 | 87.1 | 10.4 | 4.0 | 0.9 | 2.7 | 73.3 | 36.8 | 6.5 | 8.1 |
| | | N | | | | | | | | | | 326 | 325 | 7 | 12 | 2 | 41 | 41 | 10 | 34 |
| | | SD | | | | | | | | | | 0.9 | 2.3 | 0.7 | 0.2 | | 5.1 | 4.6 | 1.5 | 1.9 |
| 13 | Tifton-85, hay, 3-4 wk growth | IFN | 55.3 | Forage | 1.00 | 2.49 | 1.86 | 1.12 | 1.05 | 1.19 | 0.63 | 87.3 | 13.7 | 5.3 | 1.2 | 2.7 | 76.9 | 36.2 | 5.4 | 6.5 |
| | | N | | | | | | | | | | 5 | 5 | | | | 5 | 5 | 2 | 2 |
| | | SD | | | | | | | | | | 2.3 | 1.9 | | | | 1.5 | 1.5 | | |
| | BLOOD | | | | | | | | | | | | | | | | | | | |
| 14 | Meal, ring dried | 5-00-380 | 76.4 | Animal | 1.00 | 4.35 | 3.58 | 2.33 | 2.21 | 2.49 | 1.76 | 90.2 | 95.5 | NA | NA | 1.2 | NA | NA | NA | 2.5 |
| | | N | | | | | | | | | | 97 | 84 | | | 47 | | | | 31 |
| | | SD | | | | | | | | | | 4.0 | 8.3 | | | 2.0 | | | | 1.4 |
| 15 | Meal, batch dried (composition data from ring-dried) | | 65.9 | Animal | 1.00 | 3.76 | 3.04 | 1.95 | 1.84 | 2.11 | 1.41 | 90.2 | 95.5 | NA | NA | 1.2 | NA | NA | NA | 2.5 |
| | BLUEGRASS *Poa pratensis* | See GRASSES, COOL SEASON | | | | | | | | | | | | | | | | | | |
| | BREWERS GRAINS | | | | | | | | | | | | | | | | | | | |
| 16 | Dried | 5-12-024 | 71.3 | Conc | 1.00 | 3.38 | 2.69 | 1.71 | 1.62 | 1.84 | 1.21 | 90.7 | 29.2 | 9.1 | 3.5 | 5.2 | 47.4 | 22.2 | 5.0 | 4.3 |
| | | N | | | | | | | | | | 698 | 688 | 32 | 30 | 88 | 221 | 88 | 34 | 138 |
| | | SD | | | | | | | | | | 3.5 | 4.0 | 3.7 | 0.9 | 1.6 | 6.6 | 3.9 | 2.7 | 0.9 |
| 17 | Wet | 5-00-517 | 71.6 | Conc | 1.00 | 3.38 | 2.69 | 1.71 | 1.62 | 1.84 | 1.21 | 21.8 | 28.4 | 9.3 | 2.9 | 5.2 | 47.1 | 23.1 | 4.7 | 4.9 |
| | | N | | | | | | | | | | 1309 | 1127 | 23 | 29 | | 685 | 686 | 35 | 110 |
| | | SD | | | | | | | | | | 5.0 | 4.0 | 3.9 | 0.9 | | 6.8 | 3.8 | 0.9 | 1.1 |
| | BROME, SMOOTH *Bromus inermis* | See GRASSES, COOL SEASON | | | | | | | | | | | | | | | | | | |
| | CANARYGRASS, REED *Phalaris arundianacea* | See GRASSES, COOL SEASON | | | | | | | | | | | | | | | | | | |
| | CANOLA | | | | | | | | | | | | | | | | | | | |
| 18 | Seed | 5-08-109 | 127.4 | Conc | 1.00 | 5.60 | 4.92 | 3.52 | 3.36 | 3.28 | 2.38 | 89.9 | 20.5 | 3.4 | 1.3 | 40.5 | 17.8 | 11.6 | 2.7 | 4.6 |
| | | N | | | | | | | | | | 1 | 1 | | | 1 | 1 | 1 | 1 | 1 |
| | | SD | | | | | | | | | | | | | | | | | | |

*(continues)*

TABLE 15-1 *(continued)*

| Entry No. | Feed Name/Description | International Feed No. | TDN-1X % | TDN Equation Class | PAF | DE-1X Mcal/kg | ME-3X Mcal/kg | NEL-3X Mcal/kg | NEL-4X Mcal/kg | NEM-3X Mcal/kg | NEG-3X Mcal/kg | DM % | CP % | NDICP % | ADICP % | Ether Extract % | NDF % | ADF % | Lignin % | Ash % |
|---|---|---|---|---|---|---|---|---|---|---|---|---|---|---|---|---|---|---|---|---|
| 19 | Meal, mech. extracted | 5-03-870 | 69.9 | Conc | 1.00 | 3.44 | 2.75 | 1.76 | 1.66 | 1.88 | 1.25 | 90.3 | 37.8 | 6.3 | 2.4 | 5.4 | 29.8 | 20.5 | 9.5 | 7.4 |
| | | N | | | | | | | | | | 230 | 230 | 16 | 19 | 71 | 81 | 82 | 18 | 27 |
| | | SD | | | | | | | | | | 1.1 | 1.1 | 2.5 | 0.7 | 5.5 | 6.6 | 5.1 | 4.3 | 1.2 |
| | CHOCOLATE | | | | | | | | | | | | | | | | | | | |
| 20 | Byproduct | | 102.7 | Conc | 1.04 | 4.46 | 3.77 | 2.56 | 2.43 | 2.56 | 1.81 | 95.2 | 11.9 | 0 | 0 | 20.5 | 23.8 | 15.7 | 3.2 | 2.1 |
| | | N | | | | | | | | | | 21 | 21 | 1 | | 16 | 19 | 19 | 1 | 15 |
| | | SD | | | | | | | | | | 3.1 | 7.2 | | | 8.8 | 15.8 | 12.6 | | 2.0 |
| | CITRUS | | | | | | | | | | | | | | | | | | | |
| 21 | Pulp dried | 4-01-237 | 79.8 | Conc | 1.00 | 3.44 | 2.76 | 1.76 | 1.66 | 1.89 | 1.25 | 85.8 | 6.9 | 0.4 | 0.3 | 4.9 | 24.2 | 22.2 | 0.9 | 7.2 |
| | | N | | | | | | | | | | 380 | 469 | 3 | 3 | 39 | 99 | 99 | 7 | 35 |
| | | SD | | | | | | | | | | 8.5 | 0.6 | 0.3 | 0.1 | 1.3 | 3.5 | 4.5 | 0.1 | 4.2 |
| | CLOVER, LADINO *Trifolium pratense* | See LEGUMES, FORAGE | | | | | | | | | | | | | | | | | | |
| | CLOVER, RED *Trifolium repens* | See LEGUMES, FORAGE | | | | | | | | | | | | | | | | | | |
| | CORN, YELLOW | | | | | | | | | | | | | | | | | | | |
| 22 | Cobs | 1-28-234 | 54.2 | Conc | 1.00 | 2.31 | 1.68 | 0.99 | 0.93 | 1.04 | 0.48 | 90.8 | 3.0 | 1.7 | 0.8 | 0.6 | 86.2 | 42.2 | 5.9 | 2.2 |
| | | N | | | | | | | | | | 5 | 7 | 1 | 1 | 4 | 6 | 4 | 3 | 2 |
| | | SD | | | | | | | | | | 0.3 | 0.3 | | | 0.1 | 7.3 | 3.5 | | |
| 23 | Distillers grains with solubles, dried | 5-28-236 | 79.5 | Conc | 1.00 | 3.72 | 3.03 | 1.97 | 1.87 | 2.07 | 1.41 | 90.2 | 29.7 | 8.6 | 5.0 | 10.0 | 38.8 | 19.7 | 4.3 | 5.2 |
| | | N | | | | | | | | | | 892 | 879 | 37 | 392 | 464 | 493 | 710 | 46 | 134 |
| | | SD | | | | | | | | | | 1.8 | 3.3 | 3.4 | 2.6 | 3.4 | 7.8 | 4.6 | 2.8 | 1.1 |
| 24 | Gluten feed, dried | 5-28-243 | 74.1 | Conc | 1.00 | 3.43 | 2.73 | 1.73 | 1.64 | 1.87 | 1.24 | 89.4 | 23.8 | 3.6 | 1.4 | 3.5 | 35.5 | 12.1 | 2.0 | 6.8 |
| | | N | | | | | | | | | | 131 | 186 | 9 | 22 | 68 | 122 | 142 | 10 | 25 |
| | | SD | | | | | | | | | | 1.2 | 5.7 | 1.5 | 2.0 | 1.1 | 6.8 | 3.0 | 1.1 | 1.5 |
| 25 | Gluten meal, dried | 5-28-242 | 84.4 | Conc | 1.00 | 4.43 | 3.66 | 2.38 | 2.25 | 2.54 | 1.79 | 86.4 | 65.0 | 3.6 | 3.0 | 2.5 | 11.1 | 8.2 | 1.5 | 3.3 |
| | | N | | | | | | | | | | 66 | 57 | 11 | 13 | 42 | 39 | 52 | 10 | 20 |
| | | SD | | | | | | | | | | 10.1 | 7.8 | 2.7 | 2.0 | 1.1 | 10.1 | 4.7 | 0.8 | 1.2 |
| 26 | Grain, cracked, dry | 4-02-854 | 85.0 | Conc | 0.95 | 3.69 | 2.98 | 1.91 | 1.80 | 2.05 | 1.39 | 88.1 | 9.4 | 0.7 | 0.3 | 4.2 | 9.5 | 3.4 | 0.9 | 1.5 |
| | | N | | | | | | | | | | | | | | | | | | |
| | | SD | | | | | | | | | | | | | | | | | | |
| 27 | Grain, ground, dry | 4-02-854 | 88.7 | Conc | 1.00 | 3.85 | 3.12 | 2.01 | 1.90 | 2.16 | 1.48 | 88.1 | 9.4 | 0.7 | 0.3 | 4.2 | 9.5 | 3.4 | 0.9 | 1.5 |
| | | | | | | | | | | | | 1448 | 4457 | 66 | 50 | 659 | 1239 | 1204 | 157 | 567 |
| | | | | | | | | | | | | 3.1 | 1.3 | 0.3 | 0.2 | 1.0 | 2.3 | 1.0 | 0.4 | 0.5 |
| 28 | Grain, steam-flaked | 4-02-854 | 91.7 | Conc | 1.04 | 3.97 | 3.24 | 2.09 | 1.98 | 2.24 | 1.55 | 88.1 | 9.4 | 0.7 | 0.3 | 4.2 | 9.5 | 3.4 | 0.9 | 1.5 |
| 29 | Grain, rolled, high moisture | 4-28-265 | 88.5 | Conc | 1.00 | 3.84 | 3.11 | 2.01 | 1.90 | 2.15 | 1.48 | 71.8 | 9.2 | 0.6 | 0.3 | 4.3 | 10.3 | 3.6 | 0.9 | 1.5 |
| | | N | | | | | | | | | | | | | | | | | | |
| | | SD | | | | | | | | | | | | | | | | | | |
| 30 | Grain, ground, high moisture | 4-28-265 | 91.5 | Conc | 1.04 | 3.96 | 3.23 | 2.09 | 1.97 | 2.23 | 1.55 | 71.8 | 9.2 | 0.6 | 0.3 | 4.3 | 10.3 | 3.6 | 0.9 | 1.5 |
| | | | | | | | | | | | | 4845 | 4761 | 61 | 38 | 1357 | 4729 | 4728 | 1123 | 2544 |
| | | | | | | | | | | | | 5.1 | 0.9 | 0.3 | 0.3 | 0.7 | 2.7 | 1.6 | 0.2 | 0.6 |
| 31 | Grain and cob, dry, ground | 4-02-849 | 83.5 | Conc | 1.00 | 3.62 | 2.91 | 1.86 | 1.76 | 2.00 | 1.35 | 89.2 | 8.6 | 0.9 | 0.4 | 3.9 | 21.5 | 8.0 | 1.6 | 1.7 |
| | | N | | | | | | | | | | 198 | 190 | 4 | 6 | 68 | 183 | 167 | 37 | 83 |
| | | SD | | | | | | | | | | 3.0 | 1.6 | 0.1 | 0.3 | 1.4 | 12.5 | 4.3 | 0.5 | 0.5 |
| 32 | Grain and cob, high moisture, ground | 4-26-240 | 86.6 | Conc | 1.04 | 3.74 | 3.03 | 1.94 | 1.83 | 2.09 | 1.42 | 67.1 | 8.4 | 0.7 | 0.3 | 3.9 | 21.0 | 9.4 | 1.4 | 1.7 |
| | | N | | | | | | | | | | 2708 | 2684 | 49 | 33 | 622 | 2675 | 2673 | 802 | 1381 |
| | | SD | | | | | | | | | | 6.8 | 1.0 | 0.3 | 0.1 | 1.8 | 6.9 | 3.7 | 0.4 | 0.3 |
| 33 | Hominy | 4-02-887 | 83.1 | Conc | 1.00 | 3.64 | 2.94 | 1.88 | 1.78 | 2.02 | 1.37 | 88.5 | 11.9 | 1.5 | 0.5 | 4.2 | 21.1 | 6.2 | 1.7 | 2.7 |
| | | N | | | | | | | | | | 364 | 358 | 15 | 20 | 228 | 315 | 309 | 15 | 118 |
| | | SD | | | | | | | | | | 1.5 | 2.4 | 0.5 | 0.2 | 2.0 | 5.5 | 1.8 | 0.5 | 1.1 |
| 34 | Silage, immature <25% DM | 3-28-247 | 65.6 | Forage | 1.00 | 2.87 | 2.21 | 1.36 | 1.28 | 1.48 | 0.89 | 23.5 | 9.7 | 1.4 | 0.9 | 2.5 | 54.1 | 34.1 | 3.5 | 4.8 |
| | | N | | | | | | | | | | 70 | 70 | | 9 | 37 | 70 | 70 | 8 | 69 |
| | | SD | | | | | | | | | | 2.0 | 2.2 | | 0.1 | 1.1 | 4.6 | 4.1 | 0.3 | 2.1 |
| 35 | Silage, normal 32-38% DM | 3-28-248 | 68.8 | Forage | 0.94 | 2.99 | 2.33 | 1.45 | 1.38 | 1.57 | 0.97 | 35.1 | 8.8 | 1.3 | 0.8 | 3.2 | 45 | 28.1 | 2.6 | 4.3 |
| | | N | | | | | | | | | | 1033 | 1033 | 667 | 77 | 75 | 1033 | 1033 | 79 | 1027 |
| | | SD | | | | | | | | | | 1.7 | 1.2 | 0.5 | 0.2 | 0.5 | 5.3 | 3.3 | 0.8 | 1.0 |
| 36 | Silage, mature >40% DM | 3-28-249 | 65.4 | Forage | 0.87 | 2.84 | 2.19 | 1.35 | 1.28 | 1.46 | 0.87 | 44.2 | 8.5 | 1.3 | 0.9 | 3.2 | 44.5 | 27.5 | 3.1 | 4.0 |
| | | N | | | | | | | | | | 705 | 705 | | 41 | 41 | 705 | 705 | 33 | 704 |
| | | SD | | | | | | | | | | 3.9 | 3.9 | | 0.2 | 0.7 | 5.9 | 3.9 | 0.7 | 1.3 |
| | COTTON SEED | | | | | | | | | | | | | | | | | | | |
| 37 | Whole seeds with lint | 5-01-614 | 77.2 | Conc | 1.00 | 3.55 | 2.91 | 1.94 | 1.83 | 1.96 | 1.31 | 90.1 | 23.5 | 2.4 | 1.9 | 19.3 | 50.3 | 40.1 | 12.9 | 4.2 |
| | | N | | | | | | | | | | 1059 | 1124 | 71 | 4 | 27 | 953 | 1024 | 76 | 193 |
| | | SD | | | | | | | | | | 4.6 | 2.6 | 1.2 | 0.1 | 1.4 | 5.8 | 4.4 | 3.2 | 2.1 |

*(continues)*

TABLE 15-1 *(continued)*

| Entry No. | Feed Name/Description | International Feed No. | TDN-1X % | TDN Equation Class | PAF | DE-1X Mcal/kg | ME-3X Mcal/kg | NEL-3X Mcal/kg | NEL-4X Mcal/kg | NEM-3X Mcal/kg | NEG-3X Mcal/kg | DM % | CP % | NDICP % | ADICP % | Ether Extract % | NDF % | ADF % | Lignin % | Ash % |
|---|---|---|---|---|---|---|---|---|---|---|---|---|---|---|---|---|---|---|---|---|
| 38 | Hulls | 1-01-599 | 34.3 | Conc | 1.00 | 1.51 | 0.95 | 0.48 | 0.44 | 0.39 | -0.13 | 89.0 | 6.2 | 3.0 | 1.1 | 2.5 | 85.0 | 64.9 | 22.5 | 2.8 |
| | | N | | | | | | | | | | 135 | 134 | 10 | 1 | 84 | 106 | 108 | 10 | 75 |
| | | SD | | | | | | | | | | 3.5 | 3.6 | 0.3 | | 1.3 | 5.9 | 5.0 | 3.0 | 0.5 |
| 39 | Meal, solvent, 41% CP | 5-01-630 | 66.4 | Conc | 1.00 | 3.40 | 2.70 | 1.71 | 1.61 | 1.84 | 1.23 | 90.5 | 44.9 | 3.3 | 1.8 | 1.9 | 30.8 | 19.9 | 7.6 | 6.7 |
| | | N | | | | | | | | | | 180 | 158 | 7 | 8 | 113 | 47 | 58 | 3 | 44 |
| | | SD | | | | | | | | | | 1.9 | 4.1 | 0.9 | 0.5 | 2.2 | 9.0 | 5.4 | | 0.7 |
| | FATS AND OILS | | | | | | | | | | | | | | | | | | | |
| 40 | Calcium soaps | IFN | 163.5 | Fat | 1.00 | 6.83 | 6.27 | 5.02 | 4.80 | 5.02 | 3.45 | 95.3 | 0 | 0 | 0 | 84.5 | 0 | 0 | 0 | 15.5 |
| | | N | | | | | | | | | | | | | | | | | | |
| | | SD | | | | | | | | | | | | | | | | | | |
| 41 | Hydrolyzed tallow fatty acids | IFN | 176.3 | Fat | 1.00 | 7.37 | 6.76 | 5.41 | 5.17 | 5.41 | 3.72 | 99.8 | 0 | 0 | 0 | 99.2 | NA | NA | NA | 0 |
| | | N | | | | | | | | | | | | | | | | | | |
| | | SD | | | | | | | | | | | | | | | | | | |
| 42 | Partially hydrogenated tallow | IFN | 96.6 | Fat+G | 1.00 | 4.05 | 3.72 | 2.97 | 2.84 | 2.97 | 2.04 | 100.0 | 0 | 0 | 0 | 99.5 | NA | NA | NA | 0 |
| | | N | | | | | | | | | | | | | | | | | | |
| | | SD | | | | | | | | | | | | | | | | | | |
| 43 | Tallow | IFN | 147.4 | Fat+G | 1.00 | 6.17 | 5.66 | 4.53 | 4.33 | 4.53 | 3.12 | 99.8 | 0 | 0 | 0 | 99.8 | NA | NA | NA | 0 |
| | | N | | | | | | | | | | | | | | | | | | |
| | | SD | | | | | | | | | | | | | | | | | | |
| 44 | Vegetable oil | 4-05-077 | 184.0 | Fat+G | 1.00 | 7.70 | 7.07 | 5.65 | 5.41 | 5.65 | 3.89 | 100.0 | 0 | 0 | 0 | 99.9 | 0 | 0 | 0 | 0 |
| | | N | | | | | | | | | | | | | | | | | | |
| | | SD | | | | | | | | | | | | | | | | | | |
| | FEATHERS | | | | | | | | | | | | | | | | | | | |
| 45 | Hydrolyzed meal | | 72.8 | Animal | 1.00 | 4.05 | 3.32 | 2.15 | 2.03 | 2.29 | 1.60 | 93.3 | 92 | NA | NA | 4.6 | NA | NA | NA | 3.5 |
| | | N | | | | | | | | | | 19 | | | | | | | | |
| | | SD | | | | | | | | | | 2.2 | | | | | | | | |
| 46 | Hydrolyzed meal with some viscera | 5-13-540 | 80.1 | Animal | 1.00 | 4.32 | 3.58 | 2.36 | 2.24 | 2.47 | 1.73 | 91.5 | 85.0 | NA | NA | 8.8 | NA | NA | NA | 5.5 |
| | | N | | | | | | | | | | 38 | 39 | | | 24 | | | | 12 |
| | | SD | | | | | | | | | | 6.1 | 9.8 | | | 5.6 | | | | 2.1 |
| | FESCUE *Festuca sp.* | See GRASSES, COOL SEASON | | | | | | | | | | | | | | | | | | |
| | FISH BYPRODUCTS | | | | | | | | | | | | | | | | | | | |
| 47 | Anchovy, meal, mech. | 5-01-985 | 76.1 | Animal | 1.00 | 4.16 | 3.42 | 2.22 | 2.10 | 2.34 | 1.65 | 92.0 | 71.2 | NA | NA | 4.6 | NA | NA | NA | 16.0 |
| | | N | | | | | | | | | | 67 | 58 | | | 36 | | | | 47 |
| | | SD | | | | | | | | | | 1.2 | 2.2 | | | 1.6 | | | | 1.5 |
| 48 | Menhaden, meal, mech. | 5-02-009 | 79.9 | Animal | 1.00 | 4.25 | 3.52 | 2.33 | 2.20 | 2.44 | 1.70 | 91.2 | 68.5 | NA | NA | 10.4 | NA | NA | NA | 19.7 |
| | | N | | | | | | | | | | 135 | 147 | | | 143 | | | | 113 |
| | | SD | | | | | | | | | | 3.3 | 4.4 | | | 2.0 | | | | 2.4 |
| | GRASSES, COOL SEASON | | | | | | | | | | | | | | | | | | | |
| 49 | Pasture, intensively managed | 2-02-260 | 66.6 | Forage | 1.00 | 3.14 | 2.46 | 1.54 | 1.45 | 1.67 | 1.06 | 20.1 | 26.5 | 3.9 | 1.1 | 2.7 | 45.8 | 25.0 | 2.1 | 9.8 |
| | | N | | | | | | | | | | 13 | 13 | | 11 | 1 | 13 | 13 | 1 | 13 |
| | | SD | | | | | | | | | | 1.7 | 5.6 | | 0.4 | | 7.5 | 5.8 | | 1.2 |
| 50 | Hay, all samples | 1-02-250 | 56.3 | Forage | 1.00 | 2.49 | 1.86 | 1.12 | 1.05 | 1.19 | 0.63 | 88.1 | 10.6 | 3.8 | 1.1 | 2.6 | 64.4 | 39.5 | 6.4 | 7.0 |
| | | N | | | | | | | | | | 4767 | 4702 | 53 | 182 | 542 | 4695 | 4695 | 1010 | 1791 |
| | | SD | | | | | | | | | | 1.1 | 3.1 | 1.3 | 0.5 | 0.7 | 6.2 | 4.0 | 1.1 | 1.5 |
| 51 | Hay, immature <55% NDF | 1-02-212 | 63.1 | Forage | 1.00 | 2.88 | 2.22 | 1.37 | 1.29 | 1.48 | 0.89 | 84.0 | 18.0 | 3.4 | 1.3 | 3.3 | 49.6 | 31.4 | 3.9 | 9.2 |
| | | N | | | | | | | | | | 31 | 44 | 1 | 38 | 26 | 44 | 44 | 16 | 34 |
| | | SD | | | | | | | | | | 4.9 | 3.3 | | 0.3 | 2.0 | 5.0 | 4.1 | 1.6 | 1.1 |
| 52 | Hay, mid maturity 55-60% NDF | 1-02-243 | 59.7 | Forage | 1.00 | 2.67 | 2.02 | 1.23 | 1.16 | 1.33 | 0.75 | 83.8 | 13.3 | 3.9 | 1.2 | 2.5 | 57.7 | 36.9 | 4.3 | 8.8 |
| | | N | | | | | | | | | | 51 | 55 | 2 | 35 | 30 | 55 | 55 | 14 | 50 |
| | | SD | | | | | | | | | | 3.7 | 3.4 | 0.2 | 0.3 | 0.6 | 1.6 | 3.3 | 1.2 | 1.6 |
| 53 | Hay, mature <60% NDF | 1-02-244 | 56.0 | Forage | 1.00 | 2.48 | 1.85 | 1.11 | 1.04 | 1.18 | 0.62 | 84.4 | 10.8 | 7.4 | 1.1 | 2.0 | 69.1 | 41.6 | 5.9 | 7.0 |
| | | N | | | | | | | | | | 402 | 413 | 1 | 61 | 51 | 413 | 413 | 19 | 399 |
| | | SD | | | | | | | | | | 3.9 | 2.8 | | 0.3 | 0.6 | 5.1 | 4.0 | 1.6 | 1.7 |
| 54 | Silage, all samples | 3-02-222 | 55.7 | Forage | 1.00 | 2.49 | 1.86 | 1.12 | 1.05 | 1.19 | 0.63 | 36.5 | 12.8 | 3.3 | 1.5 | 3.1 | 60.7 | 40.3 | 6.9 | 8.1 |
| | | N | | | | | | | | | | 4377 | 4401 | 68 | 4388 | 456 | 4390 | 4390 | 1079 | 988 |
| | | SD | | | | | | | | | | 11 | 3.7 | 1.3 | 0.8 | 0.9 | 7.5 | 5.4 | 1.8 | 2.1 |
| 55 | Silage, immature <55% NDF | 3-02-217 | 60.4 | Forage | 1.00 | 2.75 | 2.10 | 1.29 | 1.21 | 1.39 | 0.81 | 36.2 | 16.8 | 4.3 | 1.1 | 2.8 | 51.0 | 32.9 | 4.8 | 9.9 |
| | | N | | | | | | | | | | 35 | 35 | | 5 | 23 | 35 | 35 | 17 | 34 |
| | | SD | | | | | | | | | | 10.5 | 3.0 | | 0.4 | 0.3 | 3.4 | 3.5 | 1.2 | 1.8 |
| 56 | Silage, mid maturity 55-60% NDF | 3-02-218 | 56.0 | Forage | 1.00 | 2.56 | 1.92 | 1.16 | 1.09 | 1.25 | 0.68 | 42.0 | 16.8 | 4.3 | 1.1 | 2.4 | 58.2 | 35.2 | 6.8 | 8.7 |
| | | N | | | | | | | | | | 41 | 41 | | 26 | 6 | 41 | 41 | 5 | 41 |
| | | SD | | | | | | | | | | 13.5 | 3.8 | | 0.4 | 0.3 | 1.3 | 3 | 1.8 | 1.5 |
| 57 | Silage, mature >60% NDF | 3-02-219 | 53.2 | Forage | 1.00 | 2.39 | 1.76 | 1.05 | 0.98 | 1.11 | 0.55 | 38.7 | 12.7 | 3.2 | 1.4 | 3.0 | 66.6 | 41.1 | 7.4 | 8.0 |
| | | N | | | | | | | | | | 135 | 135 | | 110 | 6 | 135 | 135 | 5 | 135 |
| | | SD | | | | | | | | | | 10.6 | 2.9 | | 0.5 | 1.3 | 3.9 | 3.7 | 1.5 | 1.8 |

*(continues)*

TABLE 15-1 *(continued)*

| Entry No. | Feed Name/Description | International Feed No. | TDN-1X % | TDN Equation Class | PAF | DE-1X Mcal/kg | ME-3X Mcal/kg | NEL-3X Mcal/kg | NEL-4X Mcal/kg | NEM-3X Mcal/kg | NEG-3X Mcal/kg | DM % | CP % | NDICP % | ADICP % | Ether Extract % | NDF % | ADF % | Lignin % | Ash % |
|---|---|---|---|---|---|---|---|---|---|---|---|---|---|---|---|---|---|---|---|---|
| | GRASS-LEGUME MIXTURES Predominantly grass (17-22% Hemicellulose) | | | | | | | | | | | | | | | | | | | |
| 58 | Hay, immature <51% NDF | 1-02-275 | 62.1 | Forage | 1.00 | 2.84 | 2.18 | 1.34 | 1.26 | 1.45 | 0.87 | 84.3 | 18.4 | 4.2 | 1.3 | 2.4 | 49.6 | 31.5 | 4.0 | 9.2 |
| | | N | | | | | | | | | | 21 | 21 | | 7 | 7 | 21 | 21 | 7 | 21 |
| | | SD | | | | | | | | | | 2.3 | 3.1 | | 0.3 | 0.5 | 1.8 | 2.0 | 1.0 | 1.2 |
| 59 | Hay, mid maturity 51-57% NDF | 1-02-277 | 59.5 | Forage | 1.00 | 2.71 | 2.07 | 1.26 | 1.19 | 1.36 | 0.78 | 87.3 | 17.4 | 4.2 | 1.4 | 2.6 | 55.1 | 36.4 | 4.5 | 9.5 |
| | | N | | | | | | | | | | 155 | 155 | 52 | 81 | 25 | 155 | 155 | 27 | 155 |
| | | SD | | | | | | | | | | 5.3 | 2.9 | 0.7 | 0.3 | 0.6 | 1.5 | 2.1 | 1.1 | 1.7 |
| 60 | Hay, mature >57% NDF | 1-02-280 | 57.0 | Forage | 1.00 | 2.55 | 1.92 | 1.16 | 1.09 | 1.24 | 0.67 | 84.7 | 13.3 | 4.4 | 1.3 | 2.3 | 62.5 | 42.1 | 5.5 | 7.9 |
| | | N | | | | | | | | | | 149 | 149 | 3 | 68 | 52 | 149 | 149 | 51 | 149 |
| | | SD | | | | | | | | | | 3.5 | 3.3 | 0.1 | 0.8 | 0.4 | 3.6 | 3.5 | 1.0 | 1.4 |
| 61 | Silage, immature <51% NDF | 3-02-302 | 60.9 | Forage | 1.00 | 2.78 | 2.13 | 1.31 | 1.23 | 1.42 | 0.79 | 47.1 | 18.0 | 3.1 | 1.2 | 2.9 | 49.9 | 31.8 | 5.0 | 9.1 |
| | | N | | | | | | | | | | 18 | 18 | | 16 | 1 | 18 | 18 | 1 | 18 |
| | | SD | | | | | | | | | | 14.7 | 2.5 | | 0.4 | | 1.0 | 1.3 | | 1.3 |
| 62 | Silage, mid maturity 51-57% NDF | 3-02-265 | 56.7 | Forage | 1.00 | 2.60 | 1.96 | 1.19 | 1.11 | 1.29 | 0.73 | 44.5 | 17.6 | 3.1 | 1.4 | 2.9 | 54.5 | 35.7 | 6.5 | 9.5 |
| | | N | | | | | | | | | | 95 | 95 | | 88 | 6 | 95 | 95 | 6 | 95 |
| | | SD | | | | | | | | | | 12.6 | 3.0 | | 0.5 | 0.6 | 1.6 | 1.9 | 0.8 | 1.6 |
| 63 | Silage, mature >57% NDF | 3-02-266 | 53.6 | Forage | 1.00 | 2.43 | 1.80 | 1.08 | 1.01 | 1.15 | 0.59 | 38.5 | 15.4 | 3.1 | 1.8 | 2.6 | 61.7 | 42.2 | 6.9 | 9.0 |
| | | N | | | | | | | | | | 166 | 166 | | 159 | 9 | 166 | 166 | 9 | 166 |
| | | SD | | | | | | | | | | 12.6 | 2.4 | | 0.7 | 0.4 | 3.7 | 3.5 | 1.0 | 1.5 |
| | Mixed Grass and Legume (12-15% Hemicellulose) | | | | | | | | | | | | | | | | | | | |
| 64 | Hay, immature <47% NDF | 1-02-275 | 62.1 | Forage | 1.00 | 2.86 | 2.20 | 1.35 | 1.27 | 1.47 | 0.88 | 83.1 | 19.7 | 3.9 | 1.3 | 2.5 | 45.4 | 30.8 | 5.1 | 8.8 |
| | | N | | | | | | | | | | 42 | 42 | | 19 | 16 | 42 | 42 | 16 | 42 |
| | | SD | | | | | | | | | | 4.0 | 1.9 | | 0.3 | 0.3 | 1.5 | 1.6 | 0.8 | 0.9 |
| 65 | Hay, mid maturity 47-53% NDF | 1-02-277 | 58.8 | Forage | 1.00 | 2.70 | 2.05 | 1.25 | 1.17 | 1.35 | 0.77 | 85.3 | 18.4 | 4.6 | 1.5 | 2.3 | 50.8 | 35.8 | 5.7 | 9.3 |
| | | N | | | | | | | | | | 184 | 184 | 5 | 90 | 61 | 184 | 184 | 61 | 184 |
| | | SD | | | | | | | | | | 3.6 | 2.2 | 0.5 | 0.3 | 0.4 | 1.8 | 1.9 | 0.8 | 1.4 |
| 66 | Hay, mature >53% NDF | 1-02-280 | 54.1 | Forage | 1.00 | 2.49 | 1.86 | 1.12 | 1.05 | 1.19 | 0.63 | 89.7 | 18.2 | 4.4 | 1.7 | 2.0 | 56.0 | 40.1 | 7.0 | 9.9 |
| | | N | | | | | | | | | | 233 | 233 | 121 | 179 | 35 | 233 | 233 | 42 | 233 |
| | | SD | | | | | | | | | | 4.9 | 2.2 | 0.7 | 0.6 | 0.4 | 2.4 | 2.6 | 1.1 | 1.6 |
| 67 | Silage, immature <47% NDF | 3-02-302 | 59.5 | Forage | 1.00 | 2.76 | 2.10 | 1.29 | 1.21 | 1.39 | 0.81 | 45.9 | 20.3 | 3.1 | 1.4 | 2.3 | 45.3 | 30.8 | 5.8 | 9.8 |
| | | N | | | | | | | | | | 45 | 45 | | 41 | 8 | 45 | 45 | 8 | 45 |
| | | SD | | | | | | | | | | 10.3 | 3.7 | | 0.4 | 0.3 | 1.3 | 1.5 | 1.4 | 1.7 |
| 68 | Silage, mid maturity 47-53% NDF | 3-02-265 | 57.7 | Forage | 1.00 | 2.66 | 2.01 | 1.23 | 1.15 | 1.32 | 0.74 | 44.1 | 19.1 | 3.5 | 1.6 | 2.5 | 50.4 | 35.4 | 5.9 | 10.1 |
| | | N | | | | | | | | | | 171 | 171 | 1 | 164 | 29 | 171 | 171 | 30 | 171 |
| | | SD | | | | | | | | | | 12.3 | 2.3 | | 0.5 | 0.5 | 1.8 | 2.1 | 1.6 | 1.5 |
| 69 | Silage, mature <47% NDF | 3-02-266 | 53.6 | Forage | 1.00 | 2.46 | 1.83 | 1.09 | 1.02 | 1.16 | 0.60 | 42.8 | 17.4 | 3.5 | 2.0 | 2.3 | 57.4 | 42.1 | 7.1 | 9.6 |
| | | N | | | | | | | | | | 255 | 255 | | 255 | 33 | 255 | 255 | 33 | 255 |
| | | SD | | | | | | | | | | 13.5 | 2.3 | | 0.8 | 0.3 | 2.9 | 2.9 | 1.0 | 1.3 |
| | Predominantly Legume (10-13% Hemicellulose) | | | | | | | | | | | | | | | | | | | |
| 70 | Hay, immature <44% NDF | 1-02-275 | 60.7 | Forage | 1.00 | 2.81 | 2.15 | 1.32 | 1.24 | 1.43 | 0.85 | 83.8 | 20.5 | 2.9 | 1.5 | 2.0 | 41.7 | 30.5 | 5.8 | 9.2 |
| | | N | | | | | | | | | | 157 | 157 | | 120 | 119 | 157 | 157 | 119 | 157 |
| | | SD | | | | | | | | | | 2.4 | 2.4 | | 1.2 | 0.4 | 1.9 | 1.8 | 0.8 | 1.4 |
| 71 | Hay, mid maturity 44-50% NDF | 1-02-277 | 57.8 | Forage | 1.00 | 2.66 | 2.02 | 1.23 | 1.15 | 1.32 | 0.75 | 84.2 | 19.1 | 3.1 | 1.6 | 2.0 | 47.2 | 35.4 | 6.7 | 9.1 |
| | | N | | | | | | | | | | 296 | 296 | | 210 | 195 | 296 | 296 | 195 | 296 |
| | | SD | | | | | | | | | | 2.3 | 2.0 | | 0.3 | 0.4 | 1.7 | 1.8 | 1.0 | 1.2 |
| 72 | Hay, mature >50% NDF | 1-02-280 | 53.9 | Forage | 1.00 | 2.47 | 1.84 | 1.10 | 1.03 | 1.18 | 0.61 | 84.3 | 17.2 | 3.6 | 1.7 | 1.7 | 53.6 | 41.5 | 8.1 | 8.7 |
| | | N | | | | | | | | | | 134 | 134 | 1 | 85 | 72 | 134 | 134 | 71 | 134 |
| | | SD | | | | | | | | | | 2.5 | 2.4 | | 0.5 | 0.3 | 3.3 | 3.5 | 1.3 | 1.4 |
| 73 | Silage, immature <44% NDF | 3-02-302 | 57.1 | Forage | 1.00 | 2.65 | 2.00 | 1.22 | 1.14 | 1.31 | 0.74 | 43.2 | 20.0 | 2.8 | 1.7 | 2.2 | 42.2 | 31.1 | 6.7 | 11.5 |
| | | N | | | | | | | | | | 193 | 193 | | 191 | 165 | 193 | 193 | 165 | 193 |
| | | SD | | | | | | | | | | 9.9 | 2.2 | | 0.4 | 0.1 | 1.9 | 2.0 | 1.2 | 2.1 |
| 74 | Silage, mid maturity 44-50% NDF | 3-02-265 | 55.3 | Forage | 1.00 | 2.55 | 1.92 | 1.16 | 1.09 | 1.24 | 0.67 | 43.3 | 19.0 | 2.7 | 1.7 | 2.1 | 47.0 | 35.4 | 7.3 | 10.8 |
| | | N | | | | | | | | | | 505 | 505 | | 496 | 314 | 505 | 505 | 314 | 504 |
| | | SD | | | | | | | | | | 9.9 | 2.3 | | 0.5 | 0.4 | 1.7 | 1.6 | 1.2 | 1.6 |

*(continues)*

TABLE 15-1 (continued)

| Entry No. | Feed Name/Description | International Feed No. | TDN-1X % | TDN Equation Class | PAF | DE-1X Mcal/kg | ME-3X Mcal/kg | NEL-3X Mcal/kg | NEL-4X Mcal/kg | NEM-3X Mcal/kg | NEG-3X Mcal/kg | DM % | CP % | NDICP % | ADICP % | Ether Extract % | NDF % | ADF % | Lignin % | Ash % |
|---|---|---|---|---|---|---|---|---|---|---|---|---|---|---|---|---|---|---|---|---|
| 75 | Silage, mature >50% NDF | 3-02-266 | 51.8 | Forage | 1.00 | 2.39 | 1.77 | 1.05 | 0.99 | 1.12 | 0.56 | 42.9 | 18.3 | 2.7 | 2.0 | 2.0 | 53.7 | 41.6 | 8.4 | 10.2 |
| | | N | | | | | | | | | | 339 | 339 | 2 | 337 | 87 | 339 | 339 | 92 | 339 |
| | | SD | | | | | | | | | | 11.6 | 2.4 | 0.5 | 0.8 | 0.4 | 3.0 | 3.1 | 1.8 | 1.8 |
| | LEGUMES, FORAGE | | | | | | | | | | | | | | | | | | | |
| 76 | Pasture, intensively managed | 2-29-431 | 66.3 | Forage | 1.00 | 3.13 | 2.46 | 1.54 | 1.45 | 1.66 | 1.05 | 21.4 | 26.5 | 3.8 | 1.1 | 3.7 | 33.1 | 23.9 | 5.4 | 10.0 |
| | | N | | | | | | | | | | 17 | 24 | 2 | 2 | 2 | 24 | 24 | 4 | 11 |
| | | SD | | | | | | | | | | 6.5 | 5.6 | | | | 7.8 | 6.4 | 0.9 | 1.4 |
| 77 | Hay, all samples | 1-20-648 | 58.9 | Forage | 1.00 | 2.73 | 2.08 | 1.27 | 1.19 | 1.37 | 0.79 | 87.8 | 20.2 | 2.4 | 1.6 | 2.1 | 39.6 | 31.2 | 7.0 | 10.0 |
| | | N | | | | | | | | | | 12292 | 12218 | 237 | 825 | 1434 | 12178 | 12195 | 3692 | 4527 |
| | | SD | | | | | | | | | | 1.4 | 2.6 | 0.9 | 0.4 | 0.5 | 6.3 | 4.6 | 0.9 | 1.2 |
| 78 | Hay, immature <40% NDF | 1-07-792 | 62.1 | Forage | 1.00 | 2.89 | 2.23 | 1.38 | 1.30 | 1.49 | 0.90 | 84.2 | 22.8 | 2.7 | 1.6 | 2.1 | 36.3 | 28.6 | 5.9 | 9.5 |
| | | N | | | | | | | | | | 181 | 210 | | 210 | 125 | 210 | 210 | 50 | 159 |
| | | SD | | | | | | | | | | 3.3 | 2.1 | | 0.3 | 0.5 | 2.4 | 2.6 | 2.2 | 1.3 |
| 79 | Hay, mid maturity 40-46% NDF | 1-07-788 | 59.1 | Forage | 1.00 | 2.74 | 2.09 | 1.28 | 1.20 | 1.38 | 0.80 | 83.9 | 20.8 | 2.5 | 1.6 | 2.0 | 42.9 | 33.4 | 6.4 | 9.4 |
| | | N | | | | | | | | | | 268 | 296 | | 296 | 214 | 296 | 296 | 107 | 262 |
| | | SD | | | | | | | | | | 3.2 | 2.3 | | 0.3 | 0.4 | 1.2 | 2.0 | 1.0 | 1.1 |
| 80 | Hay, mature >46% NDF | 1-07-789 | 54.7 | Forage | 1.00 | 2.51 | 1.88 | 1.13 | 1.06 | 1.21 | 0.65 | 83.8 | 17.8 | 2.1 | 1.7 | 1.6 | 50.9 | 39.5 | 7.3 | 9.2 |
| | | N | | | | | | | | | | 218 | 237 | | 237 | 155 | 237 | 237 | 56 | 205 |
| | | SD | | | | | | | | | | 2.9 | 2.6 | | 0.4 | 0.4 | 3.7 | 3.6 | 1.1 | 1.6 |
| 81 | Silage, all samples | 3-07-796 | 56.6 | Forage | 1.00 | 2.62 | 1.98 | 1.20 | 1.13 | 1.29 | 0.72 | 39.1 | 20.0 | 2.9 | 1.6 | 3.1 | 45.7 | 37.0 | 8.1 | 10.4 |
| | | N | | | | | | | | | | 8555 | 8576 | 255 | 8567 | 1325 | 8567 | 8562 | 2770 | 5183 |
| | | SD | | | | | | | | | | 10.5 | 3.0 | 1.1 | 0.6 | 0.7 | 6.5 | 4.8 | 1.8 | 1.7 |
| 82 | Silage, immature <40% NDF | 3-07-795 | 60.5 | Forage | 1.00 | 2.83 | 2.18 | 1.34 | 1.26 | 1.45 | 0.86 | 41.2 | 23.2 | 3.4 | 1.6 | 2.3 | 36.7 | 30.2 | 6.2 | 11.1 |
| | | N | | | | | | | | | | 361 | 322 | | 189 | 148 | 322 | 322 | 93 | 322 |
| | | SD | | | | | | | | | | 8.6 | 2.1 | | 0.3 | 0.4 | 2.5 | 2.7 | 0.9 | 1.5 |
| 83 | Silage, mid maturity 40-46% NDF | 3-07-797 | 56.7 | Forage | 1.00 | 2.65 | 2.01 | 1.22 | 1.15 | 1.32 | 0.74 | 42.9 | 21.9 | 3.1 | 1.8 | 2.2 | 43.2 | 35.2 | 7.3 | 10.8 |
| | | N | | | | | | | | | | 884 | 750 | 2 | 250 | 188 | 750 | 750 | 129 | 749 |
| | | SD | | | | | | | | | | 10.0 | 1.8 | | 0.5 | 0.3 | 1.5 | 2.1 | 1.2 | 1.5 |
| 84 | Silage, mature >46% NDF | 3-07-798 | 53.0 | Forage | 1.00 | 2.47 | 1.84 | 1.10 | 1.03 | 1.18 | 0.62 | 42.6 | 20.3 | 2.9 | 2.1 | 2.1 | 50.0 | 40.9 | 8.4 | 10.3 |
| | | N | | | | | | | | | | 754 | 731 | | 121 | 99 | 731 | 731 | 74 | 731 |
| | | SD | | | | | | | | | | 10.2 | 1.8 | | 0.6 | 0.4 | 3.0 | 3.1 | 1.3 | 1.6 |
| 85 | LINSEED (Flax) meal, solvent | 5-30-288 | 65.4 | Conc | 1.00 | 3.19 | 2.51 | 1.57 | 1.48 | 1.48 | 1.10 | 90.3 | 32.6 | 7.9 | 1.1 | 1.7 | 36.1 | 22.1 | 8.3 | 6.5 |
| | | N | | | | | | | | | | 6 | 6 | 1 | 2 | 2 | 6 | 6 | 1 | 1 |
| | | SD | | | | | | | | | | 1.5 | 4.9 | | | | 5.7 | 3.1 | | |
| | MEAT | | | | | | | | | | | | | | | | | | | |
| 86 | Meal, rendered | 5-09-323 | 79.6 | Animal | 1.00 | 4.05 | 3.35 | 2.21 | 2.10 | 2.29 | 1.59 | 93.9 | 57.6 | NA | NA | 12.7 | NA | NA | NA | 22.9 |
| | | N | | | | | | | | | | 78 | 66 | | | 32 | | | | 12 |
| | | SD | | | | | | | | | | 4.0 | 7.6 | | | 3.8 | | | | 5.6 |
| 87 | Meat and bone, rendered | 5-00-388 | 61.9 | Animal | 1.00 | 3.19 | 2.54 | 1.63 | 1.54 | 1.71 | 1.09 | 94.0 | 54.2 | NA | NA | 10.4 | NA | NA | NA | 30.4 |
| | | N | | | | | | | | | | 62 | 62 | | | 54 | | | | 13 |
| | | SD | | | | | | | | | | 4.9 | 5.6 | | | 2.8 | | | | 7.5 |
| | MOLASSES | | | | | | | | | | | | | | | | | | | |
| 88 | Beet sugar | 4-00-668 | 82.9 | Conc | 1.04 | 3.60 | 2.88 | 1.84 | 1.73 | 1.99 | 1.33 | 77.9 | 8.5 | 0.0 | 0.0 | 0.2 | 0.1 | 0.1 | 0.0 | 11.4 |
| | | N | | | | | | | | | | 21 | 12 | | | 3 | 3 | 3 | | 9 |
| | | SD | | | | | | | | | | 1.7 | 1.1 | | | 0.1 | | | | 1.3 |
| 89 | Sugarcane | 4-04-696 | 81.0 | Conc | 1.04 | 3.48 | 2.78 | 1.76 | 1.66 | 1.91 | 1.28 | 74.3 | 5.8 | 0.0 | 0.0 | 0.2 | 0.4 | 0.2 | 0.0 | 13.3 |
| | | N | | | | | | | | | | 84 | 64 | | | 6 | 1 | 1 | | 52 |
| | | SD | | | | | | | | | | 3.3 | 2.1 | | | 0.2 | | | | 2.3 |
| | OATS | | | | | | | | | | | | | | | | | | | |
| 90 | Grain, rolled | 4-03-309 | 78.5 | Conc | 1.04 | 3.47 | 2.78 | 1.77 | 1.67 | 1.90 | 1.26 | 90.0 | 13.2 | 1.8 | 0.3 | 5.1 | 30.0 | 14.6 | 4.9 | 3.3 |
| | | N | | | | | | | | | | 176 | 308 | | 2 | 145 | 120 | 173 | 6 | 104 |
| | | SD | | | | | | | | | | 2.0 | 1.8 | | | 0.9 | 10.5 | 5.6 | 2.5 | 0.5 |
| 91 | Hay, headed | 1-09-099 | 55.9 | Forage | 1.00 | 2.46 | 1.83 | 1.10 | 1.03 | 1.17 | 0.61 | 91.9 | 9.1 | 1.3 | 0.6 | 2.2 | 58.0 | 36.4 | 6.5 | 8.5 |
| | | N | | | | | | | | | | 433 | 422 | 7 | 8 | 54 | 419 | 419 | 9 | 22 |
| | | SD | | | | | | | | | | 1.2 | 2.9 | 0.3 | 0.4 | 0.6 | 6.3 | 4.5 | 1.4 | 4.0 |
| 92 | Silage, headed | 3-21-843 | 56.8 | Forage | 1.00 | 2.54 | 1.91 | 1.15 | 1.08 | 1.23 | 0.66 | 34.6 | 12.9 | 2.1 | 1.0 | 3.4 | 60.6 | 38.9 | 5.5 | 9.8 |
| | | N | | | | | | | | | | 626 | 634 | 5 | 630 | 53 | 632 | 631 | 135 | 182 |
| | | SD | | | | | | | | | | 10.6 | 1.6 | 0.4 | 0.5 | 0.8 | 5.7 | 4.2 | 1.4 | 2.3 |
| | ORCHARDGRASS *Dactylis glomerata* | see GRASSES, COOL SEASON | | | | | | | | | | | | | | | | | | |
| | PEANUT | | | | | | | | | | | | | | | | | | | |
| 93 | Meal, solvent | 5-08-605 | 74.8 | Conc | 1.00 | 3.85 | 3.12 | 2.00 | 1.90 | 2.14 | 1.48 | 92.3 | 51.8 | 5.8 | 1.1 | 1.4 | 21.4 | 13.5 | 4.6 | 5.8 |
| | | N | | | | | | | | | | 55 | 51 | 2 | 2 | 25 | 15 | 15 | 1 | 11 |
| | | SD | | | | | | | | | | 1.7 | 4.4 | | | 2.6 | 5.7 | 4.4 | | 1.5 |

*(continues)*

TABLE 15-1 *(continued)*

| Entry No. | Feed Name/Description | International Feed No. | TDN-1X % | TDN Equation Class | PAF | DE-1X Mcal/kg | ME-3X Mcal/kg | NEL-3X Mcal/kg | NEL-4X Mcal/kg | NEM-3X Mcal/kg | NEG-3X Mcal/kg | DM % | CP % | NDICP % | ADICP % | Ether Extract % | NDF % | ADF % | Lignin % | Ash % |
|---|---|---|---|---|---|---|---|---|---|---|---|---|---|---|---|---|---|---|---|---|
| | POTATO | | | | | | | | | | | | | | | | | | | |
| 94 | Byproduct meal | 4-03-775 | 80.7 | Conc | 1.00 | 3.51 | 2.84 | 1.85 | 1.75 | 1.94 | 1.30 | 35.4 | 10.5 | 5.2 | 2.3 | 10.8 | 22.1 | 16.5 | 2.3 | 12.8 |
| | | N | | | | | | | | | | 79 | 79 | 2 | 2 | 28 | 79 | 79 | 2 | 22 |
| | | SD | | | | | | | | | | 23.1 | 8.4 | | | 7.8 | 14.3 | 11.0 | | 7.4 |
| | RICE | | | | | | | | | | | | | | | | | | | |
| 95 | Bran | 4-03-928 | 84.8 | Conc | 1.00 | 3.76 | 3.09 | 2.05 | 1.94 | 2.10 | 1.43 | 90.6 | 15.5 | 3.7 | 0.4 | 15.2 | 26.1 | 13.1 | 4.6 | 10.4 |
| | | N | | | | | | | | | | 72 | 86 | 11 | 3 | 77 | 59 | 51 | 30 | 69 |
| | | SD | | | | | | | | | | 1.3 | 2.2 | 1.7 | 0.1 | 4.2 | 6.8 | 4.3 | 1.4 | 1.9 |
| | RYE, ANNUAL | | | | | | | | | | | | | | | | | | | |
| 96 | Silage, vegetative | 3-21-853 | 60.0 | Forage | 1.00 | 2.72 | 2.08 | 1.28 | 1.20 | 1.37 | 0.79 | 29.7 | 16.1 | 1.9 | 0.9 | 3.8 | 57.8 | 34.9 | 4.5 | 9.6 |
| | | N | | | | | | | | | | 787 | 1175 | 31 | 504 | 63 | 1174 | 1173 | 169 | 844 |
| | | SD | | | | | | | | | | 8.8 | 3.1 | 1.4 | 0.4 | 1.2 | 6.3 | 4.9 | 1.6 | 3.9 |
| | RYEGRASS *Lolium sp.* | see GRASSES, COOL SEASON | | | | | | | | | | | | | | | | | | |
| | SAFFLOWER | | | | | | | | | | | | | | | | | | | |
| 97 | Meal, solvent | 5-04-110 | 52.5 | Conc | 1.00 | 2.60 | 1.96 | 1.19 | 1.11 | 1.27 | 0.70 | 93.5 | 29.0 | 2.0 | 1.2 | 2.4 | 53.8 | 39.1 | 14.5 | 4.7 |
| | | N | | | | | | | | | | 5 | 5 | 1 | 1 | 3 | 5 | 5 | 1 | 1 |
| | | SD | | | | | | | | | | 0.3 | 0.2 | | | | 2.9 | 1.6 | | |
| | SORGHUM, GRAIN TYPE | | | | | | | | | | | | | | | | | | | |
| 98 | Grain, dry rolled | 4-04-380 | 80.6 | Conc | 0.92 | 3.53 | 2.83 | 1.80 | 1.70 | 1.95 | 1.30 | 88.6 | 11.6 | 2.8 | 1.0 | 3.1 | 10.9 | 5.9 | 1.1 | 2.0 |
| | | N | | | | | | | | | | 438 | 437 | 2 | 2 | 90 | 61 | 62 | 2 | 74 |
| | | SD | | | | | | | | | | 3.4 | 1.8 | | | 0.8 | 5.0 | 2.7 | | 0.6 |
| 99 | Grain, steam-flaked | 4-04-380 | 89.4 | Conc | 1.04 | 3.91 | 3.17 | 2.04 | 1.93 | 2.20 | 1.51 | 88.6 | 11.6 | 2.8 | 1.0 | 3.1 | 10.9 | 5.9 | 1.1 | 2.0 |
| 100 | Silage | 3-22-371 | 56.7 | Forage | 1.00 | 2.48 | 1.85 | 1.11 | 1.04 | 1.18 | 0.62 | 28.8 | 9.1 | 2.4 | 1.2 | 2.9 | 60.7 | 38.7 | 6.5 | 7.5 |
| | | N | | | | | | | | | | 1160 | 1168 | 18 | 581 | 78 | 864 | 1162 | 144 | 181 |
| | | SD | | | | | | | | | | 10.7 | 2.6 | 1.0 | 0.6 | 0.7 | 8.2 | 5.9 | 1.4 | 2.9 |
| | SORGHUM, SUDAN TYPE | | | | | | | | | | | | | | | | | | | |
| 101 | Hay | 1-04-480 | 54.4 | Forage | 1.00 | 2.39 | 1.77 | 1.05 | 0.98 | 1.11 | 0.56 | 86.5 | 9.4 | 2.8 | 1.2 | 2.3 | 64.8 | 40.0 | 6.0 | 8.7 |
| | | N | | | | | | | | | | 487 | 726 | 7 | | 48 | 717 | 717 | 130 | 172 |
| | | SD | | | | | | | | | | 1.2 | 2.2 | 0.5 | | 0.6 | 5.2 | 4.1 | 1.3 | 2.2 |
| 102 | Silage | 3-04-499 | 54.4 | Forage | 1.00 | 2.41 | 1.79 | 1.07 | 1.00 | 1.13 | 0.57 | 28.8 | 10.8 | 2.4 | 1.2 | 3.6 | 63.3 | 40.7 | 5.9 | 10.9 |
| | | N | | | | | | | | | | 438 | 140 | 1 | 138 | 14 | 139 | 139 | 32 | 37 |
| | | SD | | | | | | | | | | 9.2 | 3.2 | | 0.4 | 1.0 | 7.2 | 5.1 | 1.5 | 3.2 |
| | SOYBEAN | | | | | | | | | | | | | | | | | | | |
| 103 | Hulls | 1-04-560 | 67.3 | Conc | 1.00 | 3.01 | 2.34 | 1.46 | 1.37 | 1.58 | 0.98 | 90.9 | 13.9 | 3.5 | 1.0 | 2.7 | 60.3 | 44.6 | 2.5 | 4.8 |
| | | N | | | | | | | | | | 130 | 138 | 18 | 16 | 77 | 88 | 87 | 24 | 45 |
| | | SD | | | | | | | | | | 1.9 | 4.6 | 0.5 | 0.3 | 1.4 | 7.4 | 5.1 | 2.5 | 0.7 |
| 104 | Meal, expellers, 45% CP | 5-12-820 | 88.5 | Conc | 1.00 | 4.35 | 3.61 | 2.38 | 2.25 | 2.49 | 1.76 | 89.6 | 46.3 | 9.6 | 0.4 | 8.1 | 21.7 | 10.4 | 1.5 | 5.5 |
| | | N | | | | | | | | | | 546 | 546 | 16 | 3 | 473 | 70 | 70 | 16 | 20 |
| | | SD | | | | | | | | | | 2.5 | 3.2 | 5.9 | 0.1 | 3.2 | 8.0 | 2.8 | 0.8 | 0.9 |
| 105 | Meal, nonenzymatically browned | | 82.9 | Conc | 1.00 | 4.17 | 3.41 | 2.21 | 2.09 | 2.37 | 1.66 | 89.0 | 50.0 | 27.0 | 1.6 | 2.3 | 29.7 | 9.5 | 3.7 | 6.8 |
| | | N | | | | | | | | | | 2 | 14 | 2 | 2 | 8 | 14 | 14 | 2 | 8 |
| | | SD | | | | | | | | | | 0.1 | 1.6 | 4.9 | 0.8 | 0.3 | 6.2 | 1.9 | 0.6 | 0.6 |
| 106 | Meal, solvent, 44% CP | 5-20-637 | 80.0 | Conc | 1.00 | 4.05 | 3.31 | 2.13 | 2.02 | 2.29 | 1.59 | 89.1 | 49.9 | 0.7 | 0.4 | 1.6 | 14.9 | 10.0 | 0.7 | 6.6 |
| | | N | | | | | | | | | | 11 | 111 | | 44 | 87 | 2 | 3 | | 66 |
| | | SD | | | | | | | | | | 1.2 | 1.2 | | 0.2 | 0.7 | 1.3 | 0.1 | | 0.6 |
| 107 | Meal, solvent, 48% CP | 5-20-638 | 81.4 | Conc | 1.00 | 4.16 | 3.41 | 2.21 | 2.09 | 2.37 | 1.66 | 89.5 | 53.8 | 0.7 | 0.4 | 1.1 | 9.8 | 6.2 | 0.5 | 6.4 |
| | | N | | | | | | | | | | 561 | 549 | 21 | | 41 | 248 | 248 | 8 | 119 |
| | | SD | | | | | | | | | | 1.9 | 2.1 | 0.2 | | 0.4 | 5.6 | 3.0 | 0.5 | 0.7 |
| 108 | Seeds, whole | 5-04-610 | 101.0 | Conc | 1.00 | 4.77 | 4.05 | 2.75 | 2.62 | 2.76 | 1.97 | 90.0 | 39.2 | 2.3 | 0.6 | 19.2 | 19.5 | 13.1 | 1.2 | 5.9 |
| | | N | | | | | | | | | | 51 | 48 | 2 | 3 | 12 | 27 | 27 | 1 | 7 |
| | | SD | | | | | | | | | | 6.7 | 5.4 | | 0.3 | 4.5 | 9.2 | 7.0 | | 0.4 |
| 109 | Seeds, whole roasted | 5-04-597 | 98.8 | Conc | 1.00 | 4.72 | 4.00 | 2.72 | 2.58 | 2.73 | 1.95 | 91.0 | 43.0 | 6.1 | 2.0 | 19.0 | 22.1 | 14.7 | 3.1 | 5.0 |
| | | N | | | | | | | | | | 413 | 410 | 18 | 4 | 52 | 128 | 128 | 22 | 32 |
| | | SD | | | | | | | | | | 2.8 | 3.8 | 4.8 | 0.9 | 4.4 | 6.0 | 3.3 | 1.5 | 0.5 |
| 110 | Silage, early maturity | 3-04-579 | 59.9 | Forage | 1.00 | 2.73 | 2.09 | 1.29 | 1.21 | 1.37 | 0.79 | 40.4 | 17.4 | 2.5 | 1.4 | 5.7 | 46.6 | 36.9 | 6.5 | 12.2 |
| | | N | | | | | | | | | | 18 | 20 | | 17 | 2 | 20 | 20 | 3 | 3 |
| | | SD | | | | | | | | | | 17.6 | 5.1 | | 0.7 | | 6.0 | 4.0 | 0.5 | |
| | SUNFLOWER | | | | | | | | | | | | | | | | | | | |
| 111 | Meal, solvent | 5-30-032 | 59.9 | Conc | 1.00 | 2.90 | 2.24 | 1.38 | 1.30 | 1.49 | 0.92 | 92.2 | 28.4 | 5.5 | 1.4 | 1.4 | 40.3 | 30.0 | 9.5 | 7.7 |
| | | N | | | | | | | | | | 47 | 48 | 3 | 3 | 36 | 16 | 16 | 3 | 20 |
| | | SD | | | | | | | | | | 1.4 | 5.0 | | 0.4 | 2.3 | 6.6 | 6.4 | | 0.4 |
| 112 | Oil seeds, whole | 5-08-530 | 122.3 | Conc | 1.00 | 5.37 | 4.71 | 3.38 | 3.22 | 3.13 | 2.27 | 91.8 | 19.2 | 2.9 | 1.9 | 41.9 | 24.0 | 16.7 | 6.0 | 5.1 |
| | | N | | | | | | | | | | 13 | 15 | 1 | 1 | 4 | 1 | 2 | 1 | 5 |
| | | SD | | | | | | | | | | 2.5 | 4.2 | | | 3.5 | | | | 1.5 |
| | TIMOTHY *Phleum pratense* | See GRASSES, COOL SEASON | | | | | | | | | | | | | | | | | | |
| | TREFOIL, BIRDSFOOT *Lotus corniculatus* | See LEGUMES, FORAGE | | | | | | | | | | | | | | | | | | |

*(continues)*

TABLE 15-1 (*continued*)

| Entry No. | Feed Name/Description | International Feed No. | TDN-1X % | TDN Equation Class | PAF | DE-1X Mcal/kg | ME-3X Mcal/kg | NEL-3X Mcal/kg | NEL-4X Mcal/kg | NEM-3X Mcal/kg | NEG-3X Mcal/kg | DM % | CP % | NDICP % | ADICP % | Ether Extract % | NDF % | ADF % | Lignin % | Ash % |
|---|---|---|---|---|---|---|---|---|---|---|---|---|---|---|---|---|---|---|---|---|
| | TOMATO | | | | | | | | | | | | | | | | | | | |
| 113 | Pomace | 5-05-042 | 65.5 | Conc | 1.00 | 2.99 | 2.37 | 1.52 | 1.43 | 1.56 | 0.96 | 24.7 | 19.3 | 8.0 | 3.8 | 13.3 | 60.0 | 47.6 | 13.3 | 5.5 |
| | | N | | | | | | | | | | 4 | 22 | 1 | 2 | 4 | 4 | 4 | 3 | 3 |
| | | SD | | | | | | | | | | 20.1 | 4.8 | | 0.1 | 4.9 | 5.8 | 2.8 | 10.8 | 1.9 |
| | TRITICALE | | | | | | | | | | | | | | | | | | | |
| 114 | Silage, headed | 3-26-208 | 57.2 | Forage | 1.00 | 2.57 | 1.94 | 1.18 | 1.10 | 1.25 | 0.69 | 32.0 | 13.8 | 2.2 | 1.0 | 3.8 | 59.7 | 39.6 | 5.8 | 9.7 |
| | | N | | | | | | | | | | 107 | 107 | 2 | 86 | 16 | 107 | 107 | 18 | 41 |
| | | SD | | | | | | | | | | 10.9 | 4.0 | | 0.8 | 0.6 | 8.3 | 5.7 | 3.4 | 3.8 |
| | WHEAT | | | | | | | | | | | | | | | | | | | |
| 115 | Bran | 4-05-190 | 71.5 | Conc | 1.00 | 3.23 | 2.55 | 1.61 | 1.52 | 1.74 | 1.12 | 89.1 | 17.3 | 2.8 | 1.4 | 4.3 | 42.5 | 15.5 | 3.0 | 6.3 |
| | | N | | | | | | | | | | 103 | 81 | | 8 | 64 | 22 | 22 | 1 | 43 |
| | | SD | | | | | | | | | | 1.3 | 1.1 | | 0.3 | 0.8 | 8.4 | 5.5 | | 1.6 |
| 116 | Grain, rolled | 4-13-245 | 86.6 | Conc | 1.04 | 3.83 | 3.10 | 1.99 | 1.88 | 2.15 | 1.47 | 89.4 | 14.2 | 1.7 | 0.2 | 2.3 | 13.4 | 4.4 | 1.7 | 2.0 |
| | | N | | | | | | | | | | 215 | 165 | 5 | 5 | 55 | 61 | 91 | 2 | 39 |
| | | SD | | | | | | | | | | 2.6 | 2.3 | 0.7 | 0.1 | 1.1 | 6.2 | 3.6 | | 0.3 |
| 117 | Hay, headed | 1-05-170 | 52.7 | Forage | 1.00 | 2.33 | 1.71 | 1.01 | 0.94 | 1.06 | 0.51 | 86.8 | 9.4 | 1.1 | 0.8 | 1.7 | 61.1 | 38.1 | 8.7 | 6.7 |
| | | N | | | | | | | | | | 121 | 120 | 7 | 17 | 9 | 116 | 116 | 5 | 10 |
| | | SD | | | | | | | | | | 1.5 | 3.8 | 0.2 | 0.1 | 0.4 | 9.7 | 7.3 | 2.6 | 1.5 |
| 118 | Middlings | 4-05-205 | 73.3 | Conc | 1.00 | 3.33 | 2.64 | 1.67 | 1.58 | 1.80 | 1.18 | 89.5 | 18.5 | 2.8 | 0.5 | 4.5 | 36.7 | 12.1 | 4.2 | 5.0 |
| | | N | | | | | | | | | | 293 | 245 | 26 | 30 | 211 | 146 | 158 | 34 | 87 |
| | | SD | | | | | | | | | | 1.4 | 2.1 | 0.4 | 0.1 | 1.3 | 7.5 | 2.7 | 0.6 | 0.8 |
| 119 | Silage, early head | 3-21-865 | 57.2 | Forage | 1.00 | 2.55 | 1.91 | 1.16 | 1.08 | 1.24 | 0.67 | 33.3 | 12.0 | 1.5 | 1.0 | 3.2 | 59.9 | 37.6 | 5.8 | 8.6 |
| | | N | | | | | | | | | | 459 | 471 | 30 | 397 | 46 | 471 | 470 | 121 | 211 |
| | | SD | | | | | | | | | | 8.9 | 3.0 | 0.8 | 0.4 | 1.1 | 7.4 | 4.9 | 1.5 | 2.6 |
| 120 | Straw | 1-05-175 | 47.5 | Forage | 1.00 | 2.04 | 1.44 | 0.82 | 0.76 | 0.83 | 0.29 | 92.7 | 4.8 | 2.1 | 1.4 | 1.6 | 73.0 | 49.4 | 8.8 | 7.6 |
| | | N | | | | | | | | | | 131 | 161 | 8 | 8 | 37 | 107 | 109 | 9 | 64 |
| | | SD | | | | | | | | | | 1.9 | 1.9 | 0.2 | 0.3 | 0.6 | 7.1 | 6.4 | 0.9 | 2.8 |
| | WHEY | | | | | | | | | | | | | | | | | | | |
| 121 | Wet, cattle | 4-08-134 | 80.3 | Animal | 1.00 | 3.63 | 2.92 | 1.86 | 1.76 | 1.96 | 1.41 | 20.8 | 14.6 | NA | NA | 0.7 | NA | NA | NA | 9.8 |
| | | N | | | | | | | | | | 73 | 68 | | | 62 | | | | 16 |
| | | SD | | | | | | | | | | 26.2 | 14.1 | | | 0.9 | | | | 2.7 |

TABLE 15-2a. Nitrogen Fractions, RUP Digestibility, and Amino Acids of Feedstuffs

| Entry No. | Feed Name/ Description | International Feed No. | Feed Type | CP % | NDICP % | ADICP % | N Fractions (% CP) A | B | C | Kd (%/h) of B | Example RUP (%CP) DMI = 2.0% BW Forage = 25% DMI | DMI = 4.0% BW Forage = 50% DMI | RUP Digest % | Arg %CP | His %CP | Ile %CP | Leu %CP | Lys %CP | Met %CP | Cys %CP | Phe %CP | Thr %CP | Trp %CP | Val %CP | TEAA %CP | Lys %EAA | Met %EAA |
|---|---|---|---|---|---|---|---|---|---|---|---|---|---|---|---|---|---|---|---|---|---|---|---|---|---|---|---|
| | ALFALFA | | | | | | | | | | | | | | | | | | | | | | | | | | |
| 1 | Meal, 17% CP | 1-00-023 | Conc | 19.2 | 3.1 | 2.4 | 27.8 | 66.0 | 6.2 | 6.7 | 31.6 | 40.9 | 75 | 4.14 | 2.16 | 3.98 | 7.11 | 4.34 | 1.46 | 1.08 | 4.89 | 4.10 | 1.39 | 5.03 | 38.60 | 11.24 | 3.78 |
| | | N | | 221 | 3 | 70 | 4 | 4 | 3 | 4 | | | | 15 | 15 | 15 | 15 | 15 | 15 | 15 | 15 | 15 | 15 | 15 | | | |
| | | SD | | 3.3 | 0.3 | 0.1 | 7.2 | 9.2 | 3.9 | 4.0 | | | | 0.39 | 0.11 | 0.21 | 0.37 | 0.31 | 0.08 | 0.07 | 0.33 | 0.14 | 0.07 | 0.22 | | | |
| | ALMOND | | | | | | | | | | | | | | | | | | | | | | | | | | |
| 2 | Hulls (N fractions and Kd from canola hulls) | 4-00-359 | Conc | 6.5 | 2.3 | 1.8 | 29.6 | 35.4 | 35.0 | 5.3 | 50.6 | 55.7 | 50 | 2.23 | 0.86 | 2.35 | 4.05 | 2.74 | 0.90 | 0.71 | 2.80 | 2.70 | 1.00 | 3.53 | 23.16 | 11.83 | 3.89 |
| | | N | | 32 | 4 | 3 | | | | | | | | 7 | 7 | 7 | 7 | 7 | 7 | 7 | 7 | 7 | | 7 | | | |
| | | SD | | 2.5 | 0.3 | 0.4 | | | | | | | | 0.28 | 0.06 | 0.29 | 0.32 | 0.32 | 0.26 | 0.08 | 0.33 | 0.34 | | 0.38 | | | |
| | APPLE | | | | | | | | | | | | | | | | | | | | | | | | | | |
| 3 | Pomace, wet (N fractions and Kd from citrus pulp, dried) | 4-25-450 | Conc | 7.7 | 3.7 | 3.1 | 41.7 | 53.3 | 5.0 | 7.4 | 24.2 | 31.7 | 80 | 4.52 | 1.86 | 3.13 | 5.58 | 3.93 | 1.38 | 1.18 | 3.31 | 3.04 | 0.88 | 4.11 | 31.74 | 12.38 | 4.35 |
| | | N | | 65 | 3 | 4 | | | | | | | | 3 | 3 | 3 | 3 | 3 | 3 | 3 | 3 | 3 | 3 | 3 | | | |
| | | SD | | 3.8 | 0.9 | 0.7 | | | | | | | | 0.03 | 0.10 | 0.03 | 0.05 | 0.01 | 0.04 | 0.04 | 0.06 | 0.06 | 0.04 | 0.04 | | | |
| | BAKERY BYPRODUCT | | | | | | | | | | | | | | | | | | | | | | | | | | |
| 4 | Byproduct meal (N fractions and Kd from wheat middlings) | 4-00-466 | Conc | 12.5 | 2.3 | 1.1 | 40.3 | 53.6 | 6.1 | 15.2 | 17.7 | 23.7 | 90 | 4.74 | 2.61 | 4.00 | 7.77 | 2.91 | 1.73 | 2.14 | 5.44 | 3.36 | 1.15 | 4.42 | 38.12 | 7.63 | 4.54 |
| | | N | | 188 | 5 | 3 | | | | | | | | 104 | 104 | 104 | 104 | 104 | 104 | 104 | 104 | 104 | 104 | 104 | | | |
| | | SD | | 3.6 | 1.1 | 0.6 | | | | | | | | 0.52 | 0.24 | 0.25 | 0.38 | 0.38 | 0.16 | 0.22 | 0.11 | 0.19 | 0.06 | 0.28 | | | |
| 5 | Bread, waste (N fractions and Kd from wheat middlings; amino acids from bakery byproduct meal) | 4-00-466 | Conc | 15.0 | 0.6 | 0.5 | 40.3 | 53.6 | 6.1 | 15.2 | 17.7 | 23.7 | 90 | 4.74 | 2.61 | 4.00 | 7.77 | 2.91 | 1.73 | 2.14 | 5.44 | 3.36 | 1.15 | 4.42 | 38.12 | 7.63 | 4.54 |
| | | N | | 70 | 1 | 2 | | | | | | | | | | | | | | | | | | | | | |
| | | SD | | 2.7 | | | | | | | | | | | | | | | | | | | | | | | |
| 6 | Cereal byproduct (N fractions, Kd, and amino acids from wheat bran) | 4-00-466 | Conc | 9.1 | 3.2 | 1.2 | 33.7 | 62.5 | 3.8 | 20 | 14.6 | 20.7 | 75 | 6.84 | 2.82 | 3.15 | 6.16 | 4.05 | 1.57 | 2.10 | 3.97 | 3.26 | 1.37 | 4.50 | 37.88 | 10.75 | 4.17 |
| | | N | | 61 | 5 | 6 | | | | | | | | | | | | | | | | | | | | | |
| | | SD | | 2.1 | 1.4 | 0.7 | | | | | | | | | | | | | | | | | | | | | |
| 7 | Cookie byproduct (N fractions and Kd from wheat middlings) | 4-24-852 | Conc | 9.7 | 1.9 | 0.5 | 40.3 | 53.6 | 6.1 | 15.2 | 17.7 | 23.7 | 90 | 4.19 | 1.77 | 3.12 | 7.12 | 1.71 | 1.83 | 1.94 | 4.78 | 3.14 | 0.88 | 4.58 | 33.12 | 5.16 | 5.53 |
| | | N | | 36 | 4 | 4 | | | | | | | | 2 | 2 | 2 | 2 | 2 | 2 | 2 | 2 | 2 | 2 | 2 | | | |
| | | SD | | 3.1 | 1.0 | 0.3 | | | | | | | | 0.74 | 0.24 | 0.16 | 0.93 | 0.28 | 0.45 | 0.30 | 0.37 | 0.32 | 0.32 | 0.23 | | | |
| | BARLEY | | | | | | | | | | | | | | | | | | | | | | | | | | |
| 8 | Grain, rolled | 4-00-528 | Conc | 12.4 | 1.8 | 0.5 | 30.2 | 61.2 | 8.6 | 22.7 | 18.1 | 23.7 | 85 | 5.07 | 2.30 | 3.47 | 6.97 | 3.63 | 1.70 | 2.28 | 5.11 | 3.42 | 1.17 | 4.90 | 37.74 | 9.62 | 4.50 |
| | | N | | 795 | 60 | 61 | 37 | 37 | 37 | 37 | | | | 116 | 116 | 116 | 116 | 116 | 116 | 116 | 116 | 116 | 116 | 116 | | | |
| | | SD | | 2.1 | 1.1 | 0.4 | 13.5 | 13.9 | 4.6 | 8.9 | | | | 0.27 | 0.21 | 0.14 | 0.25 | 0.25 | 0.09 | 0.17 | 0.23 | 0.13 | 0.07 | 0.24 | | | |
| 9 | Malt sprouts | 5-00-545 | Conc | 20.1 | 3.7 | 1.1 | 56.0 | 44.0 | 0.0 | 4.5 | 21.2 | 27.4 | 80 | 4.25 | 1.84 | 4.00 | 6.00 | 4.38 | 1.33 | 1.10 | 3.20 | 3.61 | 0.90 | 5.38 | 34.89 | 12.55 | 3.81 |
| | | N | | 40 | 2 | 2 | 1 | 1 | 1 | 1 | | | | 4 | 4 | 4 | 4 | 4 | 4 | 4 | 4 | 4 | 4 | 4 | | | |
| | | SD | | 3.5 | | | | | | | | | | 0.85 | 0.44 | 0.31 | 0.36 | 0.94 | 0.13 | 0.23 | 0.64 | 0.32 | 0.28 | 0.55 | | | |
| 10 | Silage, headed (Amino acids from rye silage) | 3-00-512 | Wet | 12.0 | 1.6 | 0.9 | 56.6 | 32.9 | 10.5 | 5.9 | 24.3 | 26.4 | 65 | 1.04 | 1.21 | 3.45 | 4.88 | 2.35 | 1.16 | 0.66 | 3.42 | 2.51 | 1.42 | 4.80 | 26.42 | 8.96 | 4.39 |
| | | N | | 528 | 25 | 265 | 6 | 6 | 6 | 6 | | | | | | | | | | | | | | | | | |
| | | SD | | 2.6 | 0.6 | 0.4 | 29.7 | 29.9 | 3.3 | 2.0 | | | | | | | | | | | | | | | | | |

| | | | | | | | | | | | | | | | | | | | | | | | | | | | |
|---|---|---|---|---|---|---|---|---|---|---|---|---|---|---|---|---|---|---|---|---|---|---|---|---|---|---|---|
| | BEET, SUGAR | | | | | | | | | | | | | | | | | | | | | | | | | | |
| 11 | Pulp, dried | 4-00-669 | Conc | 10.0 | 5.5 | 0.6 | 4.5 | 90.5 | 5.0 | 2.0 | 66.2 | 76.3 | 80 | 3.23 | 2.54 | 3.18 | 5.10 | 4.35 | 1.24 | 1.10 | 2.93 | 3.38 | 0.81 | 4.70 | 31.46 | 13.83 | 3.94 |
| | | N | | 181 | 18 | 5 | 2 | 2 | 1 | 2 | | | | 11 | 11 | 11 | 11 | 11 | 11 | 11 | 11 | 11 | 11 | 11 | | | |
| | | SD | | 1.1 | 1.3 | 0.3 | 4.6 | 4.6 | | 1.8 | | | | 0.96 | 0.36 | 0.24 | 0.46 | 0.59 | 0.19 | 0.19 | 0.20 | 0.39 | 0.09 | 0.50 | | | |
| | BERMUDAGRASS (*Cynodon dactylon*) | | | | | | | | | | | | | | | | | | | | | | | | | | |
| 12 | Coastal, hay, early head | 1-20-900 | Dry | 10.4 | 4.0 | 0.9 | 36.7 | 51.7 | 11.6 | 8.1 | 27.6 | 29.8 | 65 | 3.88 | 1.63 | 3.32 | 6.22 | 3.49 | 1.30 | 1.16 | 3.92 | 3.60 | 1.24 | 4.51 | 33.05 | 10.53 | 3.93 |
| | | N | | 325 | 7 | 12 | | | | | | | | | | | | | | | | | | | | | |
| | | SD | | 2.3 | 0.7 | 0.2 | | | | | | | | | | | | | | | | | | | | | |
| 13 | Tifton-85, hay, 3-4 wk growth | IFN | Dry | 13.7 | 5.3 | 1.2 | 36.7 | 51.7 | 11.6 | 8.1 | 27.4 | 29.6 | 65 | 3.88 | 1.63 | 3.32 | 6.22 | 3.49 | 1.30 | 1.16 | 3.92 | 3.60 | 1.24 | 4.51 | 33.05 | 10.53 | 3.93 |
| | | N | | 5 | | | | | | | | | | | | | | | | | | | | | | | |
| | | SD | | 1.9 | | | | | | | | | | | | | | | | | | | | | | | |
| | BLOOD | | | | | | | | | | | | | | | | | | | | | | | | | | |
| 14 | Meal, ring dried | 5-00-380 | Conc | 95.5 | NA | NA | 10.1 | 60.9 | 29.0 | 1.9 | 70.9 | 77.5 | 80 | 4.38 | 6.36 | 1.26 | 12.82 | 8.98 | 1.17 | 1.28 | 6.85 | 4.34 | 1.59 | 8.68 | 56.43 | 15.91 | 2.07 |
| | | N | | 84 | | | 8 | 8 | 5 | 8 | | | | 53 | 53 | 53 | 53 | 53 | 53 | 53 | 53 | 53 | 53 | 53 | | | |
| | | SD | | 8.3 | | | 8.5 | 39.7 | 33.3 | 2.3 | | | | 0.23 | 0.35 | 0.20 | 0.38 | 0.34 | 0.15 | 0.16 | 0.31 | 0.36 | 0.13 | 0.33 | | | |
| 15 | Meal, batch dried (CP and amino acids from blood meal, ring dried) | | Conc | 95.5 | NA | NA | 10.1 | 60.9 | 29.0 | 1.9 | 70.9 | 77.5 | 65 | 4.38 | 6.36 | 1.26 | 12.82 | 8.98 | 1.17 | 1.28 | 6.85 | 4.34 | 1.59 | 8.68 | 56.43 | 15.91 | 2.07 |
| | | N | | | | | | | | | | | | | | | | | | | | | | | | | |
| | | SD | | | | | | | | | | | | | | | | | | | | | | | | | |
| | BREWERS GRAINS | | | | | | | | | | | | | | | | | | | | | | | | | | |
| 16 | Dried | 5-12-024 | Conc | 29.2 | 9.1 | 3.5 | 18.3 | 64.6 | 17.1 | 4.7 | 47.5 | 56.6 | 80 | 5.77 | 2.00 | 3.85 | 7.85 | 4.08 | 1.70 | 1.85 | 4.60 | 3.58 | 0.98 | 4.75 | 39.16 | 10.42 | 4.34 |
| | | N | | 688 | 32 | 30 | 14 | 14 | 14 | 14 | | | | | | | | | | | | | | | | | |
| | | SD | | 4.0 | 3.7 | 0.9 | 7.9 | 13.8 | 10.3 | 1.4 | | | | | | | | | | | | | | | | | |
| 17 | Wet (Trp from brewers grains, dried) | 5-00-517 | Conc | 28.4 | 9.3 | 2.9 | 48.3 | 42.5 | 9.2 | 4.6 | 29.4 | 35.4 | 85 | 4.47 | 2.25 | 3.85 | 9.61 | 3.40 | 1.93 | 1.96 | 5.57 | 3.61 | 0.98 | 5.14 | 40.81 | 8.33 | 4.66 |
| | | N | | 1127 | 23 | 29 | 4 | 4 | 4 | 4 | | | | 4 | 4 | 4 | 4 | 4 | 4 | 4 | 4 | 4 | | 4 | | | |
| | | SD | | 4.0 | 3.9 | 0.9 | 3.3 | 5.2 | 3.8 | 2.3 | | | | 0.31 | 0.04 | 0.21 | 1.03 | 0.03 | 0.06 | 0.24 | 0.37 | 0.08 | | 0.41 | | | |
| | CANOLA | | | | | | | | | | | | | | | | | | | | | | | | | | |
| 18 | Seeds, ground (Amino acids from canola meal) | 5-08-109 | Conc | 20.5 | 3.4 | 1.3 | 35.2 | 59.5 | 5.3 | 20.1 | 15.5 | 21.3 | 50 | 7.01 | 2.80 | 3.83 | 6.77 | 5.62 | 1.87 | 2.54 | 4.06 | 4.42 | 1.46 | 4.73 | 42.56 | 13.20 | 4.39 |
| | | N | | 1 | | | 2 | 2 | 1 | 2 | | | | | | | | | | | | | | | | | |
| | | SD | | | | | 4.4 | 0.6 | | 1.7 | | | | | | | | | | | | | | | | | |
| 19 | Meal, mech. extracted | 5-03-870 | Conc | 37.8 | 6.3 | 2.4 | 23.2 | 70.4 | 6.4 | 10.4 | 26.6 | 35.7 | 75 | 7.01 | 2.80 | 3.83 | 6.77 | 5.62 | 1.87 | 2.54 | 4.06 | 4.42 | 1.46 | 4.73 | 42.56 | 13.20 | 4.39 |
| | | N | | 230 | 16 | 19 | 22 | 22 | 22 | 22 | | | | 58 | 58 | 58 | 58 | 58 | 58 | 58 | 58 | 58 | 58 | 58 | | | |
| | | SD | | 1.1 | 2.5 | 0.7 | 5.8 | 7.0 | 5.4 | 3.7 | | | | 0.46 | 0.25 | 0.12 | 0.32 | 0.28 | 0.10 | 0.19 | 0.33 | 0.18 | 0.12 | 0.18 | | | |
| | CHOCOLATE | | | | | | | | | | | | | | | | | | | | | | | | | | |
| 20 | Byproduct (N fractions and Kd from molasses, beet sugar) | | Conc | 11.9 | 0 | 0 | 74.1 | 25.9 | 0.0 | 3.2 | 14.7 | 18.1 | 90 | 2.25 | 1.57 | 3.60 | 6.52 | 2.25 | 1.57 | 0.90 | 3.82 | 3.82 | 0.67 | 5.84 | 31.91 | 7.05 | 4.92 |
| | | N | | 21 | 1 | | | | | | | | | 1 | 1 | 1 | 1 | 1 | 1 | 1 | 1 | 1 | 1 | 1 | | | |
| | | SD | | 7.2 | | | | | | | | | | | | | | | | | | | | | | | |
| | CITRUS | | | | | | | | | | | | | | | | | | | | | | | | | | |
| 21 | Pulp dried | 4-01-237 | Conc | 6.9 | 0.4 | 0.3 | 41.7 | 53.3 | 5.0 | 7.4 | 24.2 | 31.7 | 80 | 3.39 | 1.88 | 2.79 | 5.01 | 2.56 | 1.03 | 1.38 | 3.63 | 2.91 | 0.76 | 3.78 | 27.74 | 9.23 | 3.71 |
| | | N | | 469 | 3 | 3 | 1 | 1 | 1 | 1 | | | | 15 | 15 | 15 | 15 | 15 | 15 | 15 | 15 | 15 | 15 | 15 | | | |
| | | SD | | 0.6 | 0.3 | 0.1 | | | | | | | | 0.29 | 0.41 | 0.18 | 0.22 | 0.28 | 0.09 | 0.27 | 0.38 | 0.11 | 0.10 | 0.37 | | | |
| | CORN, YELLOW | | | | | | | | | | | | | | | | | | | | | | | | | | |
| 22 | Cobs | 1-28-234 | Conc | 3.0 | 1.7 | 0.8 | 45.0 | 49.4 | 5.6 | 2.8 | 35.2 | 41.5 | 60 | 4.00 | 2.94 | 3.50 | 12.66 | 2.78 | 2.50 | 2.12 | 4.72 | 3.59 | 0.69 | 4.78 | 42.16 | 6.59 | 5.93 |
| | | N | | 7 | 1 | 1 | 2 | 2 | 2 | 2 | | | | 1 | 1 | 1 | 1 | 1 | 1 | 1 | 1 | 1 | 1 | 1 | | | |
| | | SD | | 0.3 | | | 12.9 | 7.9 | 0.6 | 2.9 | | | | | | | | | | | | | | | | | |
| 23 | Distillers grains with solubles, dried | 5-28-236 | Conc | 29.7 | 8.6 | 5.0 | 28.5 | 63.3 | 8.2 | 3.6 | 42.2 | 50.8 | 80 | 4.06 | 2.50 | 3.71 | 9.59 | 2.24 | 1.82 | 1.86 | 4.87 | 3.44 | 0.87 | 4.70 | 37.80 | 5.93 | 4.81 |
| | | N | | 879 | 37 | 392 | 3 | 3 | 3 | 3 | | | | 12 | 12 | 12 | 12 | 12 | 12 | 12 | 12 | 12 | 12 | 12 | | | |
| | | SD | | 3.3 | 3.4 | 2.6 | 2.6 | 5.0 | 6.8 | 0.7 | | | | 0.28 | 0.21 | 0.13 | 2.80 | 0.39 | 0.21 | 0.13 | 0.37 | 0.34 | 0.16 | 0.27 | | | |
| 24 | Gluten feed, dried | 5-28-243 | Conc | 23.8 | 3.6 | 1.4 | 48.0 | 43.2 | 8.8 | 7.7 | 24.0 | 30.0 | 85 | 3.85 | 2.93 | 3.10 | 8.98 | 2.74 | 1.61 | 2.13 | 3.68 | 3.48 | 0.56 | 4.46 | 35.39 | 7.74 | 4.55 |
| | | N | | 186 | 9 | 22 | 7 | 7 | 7 | 7 | | | | 11 | 11 | 11 | 11 | 11 | 11 | 11 | 11 | 11 | 11 | 11 | | | |
| | | SD | | 5.7 | 1.5 | 2.0 | 8.5 | 9.8 | 3.5 | 2.9 | | | | 0.7 | 0.23 | 0.17 | 0.57 | 0.27 | 0.1 | 0.21 | 0.26 | 0.15 | 0.07 | 0.13 | | | |

*(continues)*

TABLE 15-2a. *(continued)*

| Entry No. | Feed Name/ Description | International Feed No. | Feed Type | CP % | NDICP % | ADICP % | N Fractions (% CP) A | B | C | Kd (%/h) of B | Example RUP (%CP) DMI = 2.0% BW Forage = 25% DMI | DMI = 4.0% BW Forage = 50% DMI | RUP Digest % | Arg %CP | His %CP | Ile %CP | Leu %CP | Lys %CP | Met %CP | Cys %CP | Phe %CP | Thr %CP | Trp %CP | Val %CP | TEAA %CP | Lys %EAA | Met %EAA |
|---|---|---|---|---|---|---|---|---|---|---|---|---|---|---|---|---|---|---|---|---|---|---|---|---|---|---|---|
| 25 | Gluten meal, dried | 5-28-242 | Conc | 65.0 | 3.6 | 3.0 | 3.9 | 90.9 | 5.2 | 2.3 | 63.8 | 74.6 | 92 | 3.20 | 2.13 | 4.11 | 16.79 | 1.69 | 2.37 | 1.80 | 6.35 | 3.38 | 0.53 | 4.64 | 45.20 | 3.74 | 5.24 |
| | | N | | 57 | 11 | 13 | 3 | 3 | 3 | 3 | | | | 118 | 118 | 118 | 118 | 118 | 118 | 118 | 118 | 118 | 118 | 118 | | | |
| | | SD | | 7.8 | 2.7 | 2.0 | 5.8 | 5.3 | 2.9 | 0.5 | | | | 0.21 | 0.13 | 0.10 | 0.52 | 0.15 | 0.16 | 0.14 | 0.13 | 0.11 | 0.04 | 0.16 | | | |
| 26 | Grain, cracked, dry (Amino acids from ground dry corn) | 4-02-854 | Conc | 9.4 | 0.7 | 0.3 | 23.9 | 72.5 | 3.6 | 4.9 | 37.0 | 47.3 | 90 | 4.61 | 3.13 | 3.31 | 11.20 | 2.84 | 2.13 | 2.13 | 4.62 | 3.55 | 0.72 | 4.02 | 40.13 | 7.08 | 5.31 |
| | | N | | 1388 | 66 | 50 | | | | | | | | | | | | | | | | | | | | | |
| | | SD | | 1.3 | 0.3 | 0.2 | | | | | | | | | | | | | | | | | | | | | |
| 27 | Grain, ground, dry (CP, NDICP, and ADICP from cracked corn) | 4-02-854 | Conc | 9.4 | 0.7 | 0.3 | 23.9 | 72.5 | 3.6 | 4.9 | 37.0 | 47.3 | 90 | 4.61 | 3.13 | 3.31 | 11.20 | 2.84 | 2.13 | 2.13 | 4.62 | 3.55 | 0.72 | 4.02 | 40.13 | 7.08 | 5.31 |
| | | N | | | | | 27 | 27 | 27 | 27 | | | | 599 | 599 | 599 | 599 | 599 | 599 | 599 | 599 | 599 | 599 | 599 | | | |
| | | SD | | | | | 12.5 | 14.7 | 8.3 | 2.0 | | | | 0.05 | 0.05 | 0.04 | 0.14 | 0.03 | 0.02 | 0.02 | 0.05 | 0.03 | 0.04 | 0.04 | | | |
| 28 | Grain, steam-flaked | 4-02-854 | Conc | 9.4 | 0.7 | 0.3 | 1.7 | 82.8 | 15.5 | 3.0 | 63.7 | 74.5 | 90 | 4.73 | 3.13 | 3.34 | 10.87 | 3.05 | 2.04 | 2.22 | 4.62 | 3.66 | 0.72 | 4.75 | 40.19 | 7.45 | 4.99 |
| | | N | | | | | 1 | 1 | 1 | 1 | | | | 6 | | 6 | 6 | 6 | 6 | 6 | | 6 | | 6 | | | |
| | | SD | | | | | | | | | | | | 0.51 | | 0.26 | 1.60 | 0.47 | 0.20 | 0.08 | | 0.10 | | 0.27 | | | |
| 29 | Grain, rolled, high moisture (N fractions, Kd, and amino acids from ground grain, high moisture) | 4-28-265 | Conc | 9.2 | 0.6 | 0.3 | 27.9 | 71.4 | 0.7 | 5.1 | 32.9 | 43.0 | 90 | 3.85 | 2.54 | 3.38 | 11.60 | 2.64 | 2.11 | 2.08 | 4.56 | 3.68 | 0.98 | 4.90 | 40.24 | 6.56 | 5.24 |
| | | N | | 4761 | 61 | 38 | | | | | | | | | | | | | | | | | | | | | |
| | | SD | | 0.9 | 0.3 | 0.3 | | | | | | | | | | | | | | | | | | | | | |
| 30 | Grain, ground, high moisture | 4-28-265 | Conc | 9.2 | 0.6 | 0.3 | 27.9 | 71.4 | 0.7 | 5.1 | 32.9 | 43.0 | 90 | 3.85 | 2.54 | 3.38 | 11.60 | 2.64 | 2.11 | 2.08 | 4.56 | 3.68 | 0.98 | 4.90 | 40.24 | 6.56 | 5.24 |
| | | N | | | | | 3 | 3 | 3 | 3 | | | | 37 | 37 | 37 | 37 | 37 | 37 | 37 | 37 | 37 | 37 | 37 | | | |
| | | SD | | | | | 2.9 | 2.0 | 0.9 | 2.5 | | | | 0.74 | 0.22 | 0.25 | 0.93 | 0.41 | 0.28 | 0.21 | 0.33 | 0.30 | 0.10 | 0.38 | | | |
| 31 | Grain and cob, dry, ground | 4-02-849 | Conc | 8.6 | 0.9 | 0.4 | 30.0 | 68.3 | 1.7 | 5.0 | 32.8 | 42.5 | 90 | 3.30 | 2.79 | 3.54 | 12.97 | 2.60 | 2.00 | 1.96 | 4.50 | 3.56 | 0.68 | 4.74 | 40.68 | 6.39 | 4.92 |
| | | N | | 190 | 4 | 6 | 1 | 1 | 1 | 1 | | | | 56 | 56 | 56 | 56 | 56 | 56 | 56 | 56 | 56 | 56 | 56 | | | |
| | | SD | | 1.6 | 0.1 | 0.3 | | | | | | | | 0.61 | 0.32 | 0.15 | 0.66 | 0.17 | 0.15 | 0.11 | 0.30 | 0.09 | 0.07 | 0.16 | | | |
| 32 | Grain and cob, high moisture, ground (N fractions and Kd calculated from dry and high moisture grains) | 4-26-240 | Conc | 8.4 | 0.7 | 0.3 | 34.0 | 65.7 | 0.3 | 5.2 | 29.6 | 38.9 | 90 | 3.30 | 2.79 | 3.56 | 14.56 | 2.28 | 1.70 | 1.96 | 4.50 | 3.32 | 0.66 | 4.51 | 41.17 | 5..54 | 4.13 |
| | | N | | 2684 | 49 | 33 | | | | | | | | 12 | 12 | 12 | 12 | 12 | 12 | 12 | 12 | 12 | 12 | 12 | | | |
| | | SD | | 1.0 | 0.29 | 0.1 | | | | | | | | 0.34 | 0.28 | 0.21 | 0.83 | 0.31 | 0.14 | 0.23 | 0.34 | 0.18 | 0.07 | 0.28 | | | |
| 33 | Hominy | 4-02-887 | Conc | 11.9 | 1.5 | 0.5 | 45.0 | 49.0 | 6.0 | 7.0 | 24.3 | 31.2 | 90 | 5.44 | 2.72 | 3.50 | 9.51 | 3.69 | 1.75 | 1.75 | 4.17 | 3.88 | 0.97 | 5.05 | 40.68 | 9.07 | 4.30 |
| | | N | | 358 | 15 | 20 | 1 | 1 | 1 | 1 | | | | | | | | | | | | | | | | | |
| | | SD | | 2.4 | 0.49 | 0.2 | | | | | | | | | | | | | | | | | | | | | |
| 34 | Silage, immature <25% DM (Amino acids from normal corn silage) | 3-28-247 | Wet | 9.7 | 1.4 | 0.9 | 57.8 | 23.7 | 18.5 | 4.0 | 30.8 | 32.2 | 70 | 1.97 | 1.79 | 3.34 | 8.59 | 2.51 | 1.53 | 1.34 | 3.83 | 3.19 | 0.44 | 4.47 | 31.64 | 7.93 | 4.84 |
| | | N | | 70 | | 9 | 7 | 7 | 7 | 7 | | | | | | | | | | | | | | | | | |
| | | SD | | 2.2 | | 0.1 | 8 | 5.7 | 4.6 | 1.3 | | | | | | | | | | | | | | | | | |
| 35 | Silage, normal 32–38% DM | 3-28-248 | Wet | 8.8 | 1.3 | 0.8 | 51.3 | 30.2 | 18.5 | 4.4 | 33.3 | 35.3 | 70 | 1.97 | 1.79 | 3.34 | 8.59 | 2.51 | 1.53 | 1.34 | 3.83 | 3.19 | 0.44 | 4.47 | 31.64 | 7.93 | 4.84 |
| | | N | | 1033 | 667 | 77 | 11 | 11 | 11 | 11 | | | | 122 | 122 | 122 | 122 | 122 | 122 | 122 | 122 | 122 | 122 | 122 | | | |
| | | SD | | 1.2 | 0.5 | 0.2 | 16.9 | 14.8 | 5.3 | 1.5 | | | | 0.41 | 0.30 | 0.23 | 0.91 | 0.35 | 0.12 | 0.23 | | 0.30 | 0.08 | 0.28 | | | |

| | | | | | | | | | | | | | | | | | | | | | | | | | | | |
|---|---|---|---|---|---|---|---|---|---|---|---|---|---|---|---|---|---|---|---|---|---|---|---|---|---|---|---|
| 36 | Silage, mature >40% DM (Amino acids from normal corn silage) | 3-28-249 | Wet | 8.5 | 1.3 | 0.9 | 48.8 | 27.6 | 23.6 | 3.2 | 39.3 | 41.1 | 70 | 1.97 | 1.79 | 3.34 | 8.59 | 2.51 | 1.53 | 1.34 | 3.83 | 3.19 | 0.44 | 4.47 | 31.64 | 7.93 | 4.84 |
| | | N | | 705 | | 41 | 5 | 5 | 5 | 5 | | | | | | | | | | | | | | | | | |
| | | SD | | 3.9 | | 0.2 | 11.5 | 6.2 | 5.9 | 1.2 | | | | | | | | | | | | | | | | | |
| | COTTON SEED | | | | | | | | | | | | | | | | | | | | | | | | | | |
| 37 | Whole seeds with lint | 5-01-614 | Conc | 23.5 | 2.4 | 1.9 | 45.4 | 46.7 | 7.9 | 15.7 | 17.7 | 22.9 | 80 | 11.52 | 3.11 | 3.20 | 5.88 | 4.35 | 1.71 | 1.76 | 5.30 | 3.46 | 1.27 | 4.70 | 44.51 | 9.77 | 3.84 |
| | | N | | 1124 | 71 | 4 | 4 | 4 | 4 | 4 | | | | 79 | 79 | 79 | 79 | 79 | 79 | 79 | 79 | 79 | 79 | 79 | | | |
| | | SD | | 2.6 | 1.2 | 0.1 | 5 | 7.9 | 4.0 | 6.9 | | | | 2.21 | 0.70 | 0.34 | 0.90 | 0.48 | 0.26 | 0.23 | 0.63 | 0.91 | 0.53 | 0.52 | | | |
| 38 | Hulls (N fractions and Kd from canola hulls) | 1-01-599 | Conc | 6.2 | 3.0 | 1.1 | 29.6 | 35.4 | 35.0 | 5.3 | 50.6 | 55.7 | 50 | 11.42 | 3.32 | 3.39 | 7.22 | 4.66 | 1.83 | 1.62 | 5.63 | 3.81 | 1.42 | 5.00 | 47.68 | 9.77 | 3.84 |
| | | N | | 134 | 10 | 1 | | | | | | | | 3 | 3 | 3 | 3 | 3 | 3 | 3 | 3 | 3 | 3 | 3 | | | |
| | | SD | | 3.6 | 0.3 | | | | | | | | | 1.57 | 0.21 | 0.14 | 0.56 | 0.61 | 0.10 | 0.17 | 0.29 | 0.20 | 0.15 | 0.21 | | | |
| 39 | Meal, solvent, 41% CP | 5-01-630 | Conc | 44.9 | 3.3 | 1.8 | 25.6 | 55.5 | 18.9 | 6.8 | 40.0 | 47.9 | 92 | 11.05 | 2.82 | 3.09 | 5.89 | 4.13 | 1.59 | 1.68 | 5.31 | 3.23 | 1.21 | 4.24 | 42.55 | 9.71 | 3.74 |
| | | N | | 158 | 7 | 8 | 14 | 14 | 14 | 14 | | | | 50 | 50 | 50 | 50 | 50 | 50 | 50 | 50 | 50 | 50 | 50 | | | |
| | | SD | | 4.1 | 0.9 | 0.5 | 6.1 | 16.5 | 15.9 | 2.8 | | | | 0.73 | 0.20 | 0.20 | 0.25 | 0.29 | 0.10 | 0.23 | 0.14 | 0.15 | 0.06 | 0.31 | | | |
| | FATS AND OILS | | | | | | | | | | | | | | | | | | | | | | | | | | |
| 40 | Calcium soaps | IFN | Conc | 0 | 0 | 0 | 0 | 0 | 0 | 0 | | | 0 | | | | | | | | | | | | | | |
| | | N | | | | | | | | | | | | | | | | | | | | | | | | | |
| | | SD | | | | | | | | | | | | | | | | | | | | | | | | | |
| 41 | Hydrolyzed Tallow | IFN | Conc | 0 | 0 | 0 | 0 | 0 | 0 | 0 | | | 0 | | | | | | | | | | | | | | |
| | | N | | | | | | | | | | | | | | | | | | | | | | | | | |
| | | SD | | | | | | | | | | | | | | | | | | | | | | | | | |
| 42 | Partially hydrogenated tallow | IFN | Conc | 0 | 0 | 0 | 0 | 0 | 0 | 0 | | | 0 | | | | | | | | | | | | | | |
| | | N | | | | | | | | | | | | | | | | | | | | | | | | | |
| | | SD | | | | | | | | | | | | | | | | | | | | | | | | | |
| 43 | Tallow | IFN | Conc | 0 | 0 | 0 | 0 | 0 | 0 | 0 | | | 0 | | | | | | | | | | | | | | |
| | | N | | | | | | | | | | | | | | | | | | | | | | | | | |
| | | SD | | | | | | | | | | | | | | | | | | | | | | | | | |
| 44 | Vegetable oil | 4-05-077 | Conc | 0 | 0 | 0 | 0 | 0 | 0 | 0 | | | 0 | | | | | | | | | | | | | | |
| | | N | | | | | | | | | | | | | | | | | | | | | | | | | |
| | | SD | | | | | | | | | | | | | | | | | | | | | | | | | |
| | FEATHERS | | | | | | | | | | | | | | | | | | | | | | | | | | |
| 45 | Hydrolyzed meal | . | Conc | 92.0 | NA | NA | 23.4 | 23.7 | 52.9 | 6.6 | 62.1 | 65.4 | 65 | 6.93 | 1.15 | 4.85 | 8.51 | 2.57 | 0.75 | 5.09 | 4.93 | 4.73 | 0.73 | 7.52 | 42.68 | 6.02 | 1.76 |
| | | N | | | | | 3 | 3 | 3 | 3 | | | | 156 | 156 | 156 | 156 | 156 | 156 | 156 | 156 | 156 | 156 | 156 | | | |
| | | SD | | | | | 2.4 | 17.6 | 19.9 | 10.0 | | | | 0.62 | 0.02 | 0.27 | 0.39 | 0.35 | 0.07 | 0.71 | 0.19 | 0.25 | 0.14 | 0.40 | | | |
| 46 | Hydrolyzed meal with some viscera (N fractions and Kd from feather meal) | 5-13-540 | Conc | 85.0 | NA | NA | 23.4 | 23.7 | 52.9 | 6.6 | 62.1 | 65.4 | 70 | 6.27 | 1.33 | 4.34 | 8.44 | 2.90 | 0.84 | 4.34 | 4.83 | 4.70 | 0.73 | 6.76 | 41.14 | 7.05 | 2.04 |
| | | N | | 39 | | | | | | | | | | | | | | | | | | | | | | | |
| | | SD | | 9.8 | | | | | | | | | | | | | | | | | | | | | | | |
| | FISH BYPRODUCTS | | | | | | | | | | | | | | | | | | | | | | | | | | |
| 47 | Anchovy, meal, mech. | 5-01-985 | Conc | 71.2 | NA | NA | 32.4 | 37.9 | 29.7 | 3.2 | 51.2 | 56.2 | 90 | 5.70 | 2.41 | 4.74 | 7.74 | 7.91 | 3.02 | 0.94 | 4.12 | 4.37 | 1.18 | 5.43 | 46.62 | 16.97 | 6.48 |
| | | N | | 58 | | | 7 | 7 | 7 | 7 | | | | | | | | | | | | | | | | | |
| | | SD | | 2.2 | | | 11.3 | 19.8 | 17.5 | 2.0 | | | | | | | | | | | | | | | | | |
| 48 | Menhaden, meal, mech. | 5-02-009 | Conc | 68.5 | NA | NA | 22.8 | 72.0 | 5.2 | 1.4 | 59.1 | 65.8 | 90 | 5.82 | 2.83 | 4.09 | 7.22 | 7.65 | 2.81 | 0.91 | 3.99 | 4.20 | 1.05 | 4.82 | 44.48 | 17.20 | 6.32 |
| | | N | | 147 | | | 10 | 10 | 10 | 10 | | | | | | | | | | | | | | | | | |
| | | SD | | 4.4 | | | 8.0 | 19.1 | 11.8 | 0.4 | | | | | | | | | | | | | | | | | |
| | GRASSES, COOL SEASON | | | | | | | | | | | | | | | | | | | | | | | | | | |
| 49 | Pasture, intensively managed | 2-02-260 | Wet | 26.5 | 3.9 | 1.1 | 30.7 | 63.5 | 5.8 | 12.3 | 22.2 | 25.5 | 75 | 4.28 | 1.88 | 3.38 | 6.22 | 3.46 | 1.37 | 0.93 | 4.60 | 3.56 | 1.33 | 4.41 | 34.49 | 10.03 | 3.97 |
| | | N | | 13 | | 11 | 14 | 14 | 14 | 14 | | | | | | | | | | | | | | | | | |
| | | SD | | 5.6 | | 0.4 | 18.3 | 17.8 | 3.4 | 4.5 | | | | | | | | | | | | | | | | | |
| 50 | Hay, all samples | 1-02-250 | Dry | 10.6 | 3.8 | 1.1 | 36.7 | 50.4 | 12.9 | 8.5 | 28.4 | 30.5 | 65 | 3.83 | 1.63 | 3.32 | 6.22 | 3.48 | 1.30 | 1.17 | 3.92 | 3.60 | 1.24 | 4.51 | 33.05 | 10.53 | 3.93 |
| | | N | | 4702 | 53 | 182 | | | | | | | | | | | | | | | | | | | | | |
| | | SD | | 3.1 | 1.3 | 0.5 | | | | | | | | | | | | | | | | | | | | | |

*(continues)*

TABLE 15-2a. *(continued)*

| Entry No. | Feed Name/ Description | International Feed No. | Feed Type | CP % | NDICP % | ADICP % | N Fractions (% CP) A | B | C | Kd (%/h) of B | Example RUP (%CP) DMI = 2.0% BW Forage = 25% DMI | DMI = 4.0% BW Forage = 50% DMI | RUP Digest % | Arg %CP | His %CP | Ile %CP | Leu %CP | Lys %CP | Met %CP | Cys %CP | Phe %CP | Thr %CP | Trp %CP | Val %CP | TEAA %CP | Lys %EAA | Met %EAA |
|---|---|---|---|---|---|---|---|---|---|---|---|---|---|---|---|---|---|---|---|---|---|---|---|---|---|---|---|
| 51 | Hay, immature <55% NDF | 1-02-212 | Dry | 18.0 | 3.4 | 1.3 | 45.0 | 46.7 | 8.3 | 12.4 | 19.7 | 21.3 | 70 | 3.83 | 1.63 | 3.32 | 6.22 | 3.48 | 1.30 | 1.17 | 3.92 | 3.60 | 1.24 | 4.51 | 33.05 | 10.53 | 3.93 |
| | | N | | 44 | 1 | 38 | 18 | 18 | 18 | 18 | | | | | | | | | | | | | | | | | |
| | | SD | | 3.3 | | 0.3 | 13.4 | 11.8 | 4.6 | 5.9 | | | | | | | | | | | | | | | | | |
| 52 | Hay, mid maturity 55-60% NDF | 1-02-243 | Dry | 13.3 | 3.9 | 1.2 | 36.7 | 51.7 | 11.6 | 8.1 | 28.4 | 30.5 | 65 | 3.88 | 1.63 | 3.32 | 6.22 | 3.49 | 1.30 | 1.16 | 3.92 | 3.60 | 1.24 | 4.51 | 33.05 | 10.53 | 3.93 |
| | | N | | 55 | 2 | 35 | 27 | 27 | 27 | 27 | | | | | | | | | | | | | | | | | |
| | | SD | | 3.4 | 0.2 | 0.3 | 8.7 | 10.7 | 5.4 | 3.9 | | | | | | | | | | | | | | | | | |
| 53 | Hay, mature >60% NDF | 1-02-244 | Dry | 10.8 | 7.4 | 1.1 | 28.4 | 52.9 | 18.7 | 5.0 | 41.2 | 43.7 | 60 | 3.83 | 1.63 | 3.32 | 6.22 | 3.48 | 1.30 | 1.17 | 3.92 | 3.60 | 1.24 | 4.51 | 33.05 | 10.53 | 3.93 |
| | | N | | 413 | 1 | 61 | 68 | 68 | 68 | 68 | | | | | | | | | | | | | | | | | |
| | | SD | | 2.8 | | 0.3 | 13.9 | 18.8 | 12.0 | 3.3 | | | | | | | | | | | | | | | | | |
| 54 | Silage, all samples | 3-02-222 | Wet | 12.8 | 3.3 | 1.5 | 56.1 | 33.2 | 10.7 | 5.8 | 24.8 | 26.9 | 60 | 3.06 | 1.66 | 3.58 | 6.16 | 3.30 | 1.22 | 0.78 | 4.37 | 3.37 | 1.07 | 4.89 | 32.68 | 10.10 | 3.73 |
| | | N | | 4401 | 68 | 4388 | | | | | | | | | | | | | | | | | | | | | |
| | | SD | | 3.7 | 1.3 | 0.8 | | | | | | | | | | | | | | | | | | | | | |
| 55 | Silage, immature <55% NDF | 3-02-217 | Wet | 16.8 | 4.3 | 1.1 | 60.1 | 31.8 | 8.1 | 8.1 | 19.1 | 21.0 | 65 | 3.06 | 1.66 | 3.57 | 6.12 | 3.28 | 1.21 | 0.78 | 4.37 | 3.34 | 1.07 | 4.89 | 32.57 | 10.07 | 3.72 |
| | | N | | 35 | | 5 | 57 | 57 | 57 | 57 | | | | | | | | | | | | | | | | | |
| | | SD | | 3.0 | | 0.4 | 9.9 | 8.8 | 3.6 | 4.6 | | | | | | | | | | | | | | | | | |
| 56 | Silage, mid-maturity 55-60% NDF | 3-02-218 | Wet | 16.8 | 4.3 | 1.1 | 60.4 | 31.0 | 8.6 | 4.8 | 23.2 | 25.2 | 60 | 3.06 | 1.66 | 3.57 | 6.12 | 3.28 | 1.21 | 0.78 | 4.37 | 3.34 | 1.07 | 4.89 | 32.57 | 10.07 | 3.72 |
| | | N | | 41 | | 26 | 16 | 16 | 16 | 16 | | | | | | | | | | | | | | | | | |
| | | SD | | 3.8 | | 0.4 | 11.4 | 8.0 | 7.3 | 1.8 | | | | | | | | | | | | | | | | | |
| 57 | Silage, mature >60% NDF | 3-02-219 | Wet | 12.7 | 3.2 | 1.4 | 47.9 | 37.1 | 15.0 | 4.6 | 32.9 | 35.2 | 55 | 3.06 | 1.66 | 3.60 | 6.23 | 3.35 | 1.23 | 0.77 | 4.37 | 3.42 | 1.07 | 4.91 | 32.90 | 10.18 | 3.74 |
| | | N | | 135 | | 110 | 15 | 15 | 15 | 15 | | | | | | | | | | | | | | | | | |
| | | SD | | 2.9 | | 0.5 | 13.9 | 12.0 | 10.3 | 1.9 | | | | | | | | | | | | | | | | | |
| | GRASS-LEGUME MIXTURES Predominantly grass (17-22% Hemicellulose) | | | | | | | | | | | | | | | | | | | | | | | | | | |
| 58 | Hay, immature <51% NDF | 1-02-275 | Dry | 18.4 | 4.2 | 1.3 | 44.4 | 47.7 | 7.9 | 13.8 | 18.7 | 20.3 | 70 | 4.16 | 1.71 | 3.56 | 6.51 | 3.89 | 1.37 | 1.23 | 4.13 | 3.80 | 1.31 | 4.70 | 35.14 | 11.07 | 3.90 |
| | | N | | 21 | | 7 | | | | | | | | | | | | | | | | | | | | | |
| | | SD | | 3.1 | | 0.3 | | | | | | | | | | | | | | | | | | | | | |
| 59 | Hay, mid-maturity 51-57% NDF | 1-02-277 | Dry | 17.4 | 4.2 | 1.4 | 38.6 | 50.5 | 10.9 | 10.6 | 24.6 | 26.5 | 65 | 4.20 | 1.71 | 3.55 | 6.51 | 3.89 | 1.37 | 1.23 | 4.13 | 3.80 | 1.31 | 4.69 | 35.16 | 11.06 | 3.90 |
| | | N | | 155 | 52 | 81 | | | | | | | | | | | | | | | | | | | | | |
| | | SD | | 2.9 | 0.7 | 0.3 | | | | | | | | | | | | | | | | | | | | | |
| 60 | Hay, mature >57% NDF | 1-02-280 | Dry | 13.3 | 4.4 | 1.3 | 31.0 | 52.1 | 16.9 | 7.25 | 34.8 | 37.1 | 60 | 4.15 | 1.71 | 3.54 | 6.49 | 3.86 | 1.36 | 1.24 | 4.13 | 3.79 | 1.30 | 4.68 | 35.01 | 11.03 | 3.88 |
| | | N | | 149 | 3 | 68 | | | | | | | | | | | | | | | | | | | | | |
| | | SD | | 3.3 | 0.1 | 0.8 | | | | | | | | | | | | | | | | | | | | | |
| 61 | Silage, immature <51% NDF | 3-02-302 | Wet | 18.0 | 3.1 | 1.2 | 60.5 | 31.1 | 8.4 | 9.4 | 18.2 | 20.0 | 65 | 3.26 | 1.67 | 3.61 | 6.09 | 3.58 | 1.25 | 0.78 | 4.32 | 3.46 | 1.04 | 4.92 | 33.20 | 10.78 | 3.77 |
| | | N | | 18 | | 16 | | | | | | | | | | | | | | | | | | | | | |
| | | SD | | 2.5 | | 0.4 | | | | | | | | | | | | | | | | | | | | | |
| 62 | Silage, mid-maturity 51-57% NDF | 3-02-265 | Wet | 17.6 | 3.1 | 1.4 | 59.6 | 32.1 | 8.3 | 6.7 | 20.9 | 22.8 | 60 | 3.26 | 1.67 | 3.67 | 6.18 | 3.56 | 1.25 | 0.78 | 4.32 | 3.46 | 1.04 | 4.92 | 33.33 | 10.68 | 3.75 |
| | | N | | 95 | | 88 | | | | | | | | | | | | | | | | | | | | | |
| | | SD | | 3.0 | | 0.5 | | | | | | | | | | | | | | | | | | | | | |

| | | | | | | | | | | | | | | | | | | | | | | | | | | | |
|---|---|---|---|---|---|---|---|---|---|---|---|---|---|---|---|---|---|---|---|---|---|---|---|---|---|---|---|
| 63 | Silage, mature >57% NDF | 3-02-266 | Wet | 15.4 | 3.1 | 1.8 | 49.2 | 36.4 | 14.4 | 5.5 | 30.5 | 32.7 | 55 | 3.26 | 1.67 | 3.68 | 6.27 | 3.59 | 1.27 | 0.77 | 4.32 | 3.52 | 1.04 | 4.94 | 33.56 | 10.70 | 3.78 |
| | | N | | 166 | | 159 | | | | | | | | | | | | | | | | | | | | | |
| | | SD | | 2.4 | | 0.7 | | | | | | | | | | | | | | | | | | | | | |
| | Mixed grass and legume (12-15% Hemicellulose) | | | | | | | | | | | | | | | | | | | | | | | | | | |
| 64 | Hay, immature <47% NDF | 1-02-275 | Dry | 19.7 | 3.9 | 1.3 | 43.0 | 40.6 | 7.4 | 15.1 | 17.9 | 19.4 | 75 | 4.50 | 1.79 | 3.79 | 6.81 | 4.31 | 1.43 | 1.30 | 4.34 | 4.00 | 1.38 | 4.89 | 37.24 | 11.57 | 3.84 |
| | | N | | 42 | | 19 | | | | | | | | | | | | | | | | | | | | | |
| | | SD | | 1.9 | | 0.3 | | | | | | | | | | | | | | | | | | | | | |
| 65 | Hay, mid-maturity 47-53% NDF | 1-02-277 | Dry | 18.4 | 4.6 | 1.5 | 40.5 | 49.3 | 10.2 | 13.0 | 21.8 | 23.5 | 70 | 4.51 | 1.79 | 3.78 | 6.79 | 4.29 | 1.43 | 1.29 | 4.34 | 3.99 | 1.37 | 4.88 | 37.17 | 11.54 | 3.85 |
| | | N | | 184 | 5 | 90 | | | | | | | | | | | | | | | | | | | | | |
| | | SD | | 2.2 | 0.5 | 0.3 | | | | | | | | | | | | | | | | | | | | | |
| 66 | Hay, mature >53% NDF | 1-02-280 | Dry | 18.2 | 4.4 | 1.7 | 33.6 | 51.3 | 15.1 | 9.5 | 30.1 | 32.0 | 65 | 4.47 | 1.79 | 3.75 | 6.76 | 4.25 | 1.43 | 1.30 | 4.34 | 3.98 | 1.36 | 4.86 | 36.99 | 11.49 | 3.87 |
| | | N | | 233 | 121 | 179 | | | | | | | | | | | | | | | | | | | | | |
| | | SD | | 2.2 | 0.7 | 0.6 | | | | | | | | | | | | | | | | | | | | | |
| 67 | Silage, immature <47% NDF | 3-02-302 | Wet | 20.3 | 3.1 | 1.4 | 60.9 | 30.4 | 8.7 | 10.6 | 17.5 | 19.2 | 70 | 3.47 | 1.68 | 3.76 | 6.24 | 3.85 | 1.29 | 0.79 | 4.28 | 3.59 | 1.01 | 4.95 | 34.12 | 11.28 | 3.78 |
| | | N | | 45 | | 41 | | | | | | | | | | | | | | | | | | | | | |
| | | SD | | 3.7 | | 0.4 | | | | | | | | | | | | | | | | | | | | | |
| 68 | Silage, mid-maturity 47-53% NDF | 3-02-265 | Wet | 19.1 | 3.5 | 1.6 | 58.9 | 33.2 | 8.0 | 8.5 | 19.1 | 21.0 | 65 | 3.47 | 1.68 | 3.76 | 6.24 | 3.85 | 1.29 | 0.79 | 4.28 | 3.59 | 1.01 | 4.95 | 34.12 | 11.28 | 3.78 |
| | | N | | 171 | 1 | 164 | | | | | | | | | | | | | | | | | | | | | |
| | | SD | | 2.3 | | 0.5 | | | | | | | | | | | | | | | | | | | | | |
| 69 | Silage, mature >53% NDF | 3-02-266 | Wet | 17.4 | 3.5 | 2.0 | 50.4 | 35.7 | 13.9 | 6.3 | 28.3 | 30.6 | 60 | 3.47 | 1.68 | 3.76 | 6.30 | 3.83 | 1.30 | 0.78 | 4.28 | 3.62 | 1.02 | 4.97 | 34.23 | 11.19 | 3.80 |
| | | N | | 255 | | 255 | | | | | | | | | | | | | | | | | | | | | |
| | | SD | | 2.3 | | 0.8 | | | | | | | | | | | | | | | | | | | | | |
| | Predominantly Legume (10-13.5% Hemicellulose) | | | | | | | | | | | | | | | | | | | | | | | | | | |
| 70 | Hay, immature <44% NDF | 1-02-275 | Dry | 20.5 | 2.9 | 1.5 | 43.1 | 49.9 | 7.0 | 16.5 | 17.0 | 18.5 | 75 | 4.83 | 1.87 | 4.03 | 7.10 | 4.72 | 1.50 | 1.36 | 4.55 | 4.19 | 1.45 | 5.07 | 39.31 | 12.01 | 3.82 |
| | | N | | 157 | | 120 | | | | | | | | | | | | | | | | | | | | | |
| | | SD | | 2.4 | | 1.2 | | | | | | | | | | | | | | | | | | | | | |
| 71 | Hay, mid-maturity 44-50% NDF | 1-02-277 | Dry | 19.1 | 3.1 | 1.6 | 42.4 | 48.1 | 9.5 | 15.5 | 19.5 | 21.0 | 70 | 4.83 | 1.87 | 4.00 | 7.08 | 4.69 | 1.50 | 1.36 | 4.55 | 4.19 | 1.44 | 5.06 | 39.21 | 11.96 | 3.83 |
| | | N | | 296 | | 210 | | | | | | | | | | | | | | | | | | | | | |
| | | SD | | 2.0 | | 0.3 | | | | | | | | | | | | | | | | | | | | | |
| 72 | Hay, mature >50% NDF | 1-02-280 | Dry | 17.2 | 3.6 | 1.7 | 36.3 | 50.4 | 13.3 | 11.8 | 26.0 | 27.8 | 65 | 4.79 | 1.87 | 3.97 | 7.03 | 4.63 | 1.49 | 1.37 | 4.55 | 4.16 | 1.41 | 5.03 | 38.93 | 11.89 | 3.83 |
| | | N | | 134 | 1 | 85 | | | | | | | | | | | | | | | | | | | | | |
| | | SD | | 2.4 | | 0.5 | | | | | | | | | | | | | | | | | | | | | |
| 73 | Silage, immature <44% NDF | 3-02-302 | Wet | 20.0 | 2.8 | 1.7 | 61.2 | 29.8 | 9.0 | 11.9 | 16.9 | 18.4 | 70 | 3.67 | 1.68 | 3.69 | 6.03 | 4.18 | 1.33 | 0.78 | 4.23 | 3.71 | 0.97 | 4.97 | 34.46 | 12.13 | 3.86 |
| | | N | | 193 | | 191 | | | | | | | | | | | | | | | | | | | | | |
| | | SD | | 2.2 | | 0.4 | | | | | | | | | | | | | | | | | | | | | |
| 74 | Silage, mid-maturity 44-50% NDF | 3-02-265 | Wet | 19.0 | 2.7 | 1.7 | 58.1 | 34.2 | 7.7 | 10.4 | 17.7 | 19.6 | 65 | 3.67 | 1.68 | 3.86 | 6.30 | 4.13 | 1.33 | 0.79 | 4.23 | 3.71 | 0.97 | 4.97 | 34.85 | 11.85 | 3.82 |
| | | N | | 505 | | 496 | | | | | | | | | | | | | | | | | | | | | |
| | | SD | | 2.3 | | 0.5 | | | | | | | | | | | | | | | | | | | | | |
| 75 | Silage, mature >50% NDF | 3-02-266 | Wet | 18.3 | 2.7 | 2.0 | 51.6 | 35.1 | 13.3 | 7.2 | 26.4 | 28.6 | 60 | 3.67 | 1.68 | 3.84 | 6.34 | 4.06 | 1.34 | 0.78 | 4.23 | 3.72 | 0.99 | 4.99 | 34.86 | 11.65 | 3.84 |
| | | N | | 339 | 2 | 337 | | | | | | | | | | | | | | | | | | | | | |
| | | SD | | 2.4 | 0.5 | 0.8 | | | | | | | | | | | | | | | | | | | | | |
| | LEGUMES, FORAGE | | | | | | | | | | | | | | | | | | | | | | | | | | |
| 76 | Pasture, intensively managed | 2-29-431 | Wet | 26.5 | 3.8 | 1.1 | 31.1 | 61.6 | 7.3 | 12.3 | 23.2 | 26.4 | 75 | 5.21 | 1.97 | 4.30 | 7.46 | 5.18 | 1.58 | 1.44 | 4.81 | 4.44 | 1.54 | 5.31 | 41.80 | 12.39 | 3.78 |
| | | N | | 24 | 2 | 2 | 8 | 8 | 8 | 8 | | | | | | | | | | | | | | | | | |
| | | SD | | 5.6 | | | 16.5 | 15.5 | 2.1 | 4.9 | | | | | | | | | | | | | | | | | |
| 77 | Hay, all samples | 1-20-648 | Dry | 20.2 | 2.4 | 1.6 | 41.9 | 49.2 | 8.9 | 16.6 | 18.8 | 20.2 | 70 | 5.14 | 1.95 | 4.22 | 7.35 | 5.08 | 1.56 | 1.42 | 4.78 | 4.37 | 1.50 | 5.23 | 41.18 | 12.34 | 3.79 |
| | | N | | 12218 | 237 | 825 | | | | | | | | | | | | | | | | | | | | | |
| | | SD | | 2.6 | 0.9 | 0.4 | | | | | | | | | | | | | | | | | | | | | |

*(continues)*

TABLE 15-2a. *(continued)*

| Entry No. | Feed Name/ Description | International Feed No. | Feed Type | CP % | NDICP % | ADICP % | N Fractions (% CP) A | B | C | Kd (%/h) of B | Example RUP (%CP) DMI = 2.0% BW Forage = 25% DMI | DMI = 4.0% BW Forage = 50% DMI | RUP Digest % | Arg %CP | His %CP | Ile %CP | Leu %CP | Lys %CP | Met %CP | Cys %CP | Phe %CP | Thr %CP | Trp %CP | Val %CP | TEAA %CP | Lys %EAA | Met %EAA |
|---|---|---|---|---|---|---|---|---|---|---|---|---|---|---|---|---|---|---|---|---|---|---|---|---|---|---|---|
| 78 | Hay, immature <40% NDF | 1-07-792 | Dry | 22.8 | 2.7 | 1.6 | 42.5 | 51.0 | 6.5 | 17.8 | 16.3 | 17.7 | 75 | 5.16 | 1.95 | 4.26 | 7.39 | 5.13 | 1.56 | 1.42 | 4.76 | 4.39 | 1.52 | 5.26 | 41.38 | 12.40 | 3.77 |
| | | N | | 210 | | 210 | 27 | 27 | 27 | 27 | | | | | | | | | | | | | | | | | |
| | | SD | | 2.1 | | 0.3 | 10.4 | 10.6 | 3.6 | 7.8 | | | | | | | | | | | | | | | | | |
| 79 | Hay, mid-maturity 40- 46% NDF | 1-07-788 | Dry | 20.8 | 2.5 | 1.6 | 44.3 | 46.9 | 8.8 | 17.9 | 17.6 | 18.9 | 70 | 5.14 | 1.95 | 4.23 | 7.36 | 5.09 | 1.56 | 1.42 | 4.76 | 4.38 | 1.50 | 5.24 | 41.21 | 12.35 | 3.79 |
| | | N | | 296 | | 296 | 25 | 25 | 25 | 25 | | | | | | | | | | | | | | | | | |
| | | SD | | 2.3 | | 0.3 | 10.3 | 9.6 | 3.7 | 5.4 | | | | | | | | | | | | | | | | | |
| 80 | Hay, mature >46% NDF | 1-07-789 | Dry | 17.8 | 2.1 | 1.7 | 38.9 | 49.6 | 11.5 | 14.0 | 22.5 | 24.1 | 65 | 5.11 | 1.95 | 4.18 | 7.30 | 5.01 | 1.55 | 1.43 | 4.76 | 4.35 | 1.47 | 5.20 | 40.88 | 12.26 | 3.79 |
| | | N | | 237 | | 237 | 31 | 31 | 31 | 31 | | | | | | | | | | | | | | | | | |
| | | SD | | 2.6 | | 0.4 | 12.4 | 14.1 | 6.9 | 7.0 | | | | | | | | | | | | | | | | | |
| 81 | Silage, all samples | 3-07-796 | Wet | 20.0 | 2.9 | 1.6 | 57.3 | 33.0 | 9.9 | 11.1 | 18.9 | 20.6 | 65 | 3.87 | 1.69 | 3.87 | 6.24 | 4.40 | 1.37 | 0.78 | 4.18 | 3.83 | 0.94 | 5.00 | 35.39 | 12.43 | 3.87 |
| | | N | | 8576 | 255 | 8567 | | | | | | | | | | | | | | | | | | | | | |
| | | SD | | 3.0 | 1.1 | 0.6 | | | | | | | | | | | | | | | | | | | | | |
| 82 | Silage, immature <40% NDF | 3-07-795 | Wet | 23.2 | 3.4 | 1.6 | 61.6 | 29.1 | 9.3 | 13.1 | 16.5 | 17.9 | 70 | 3.87 | 1.69 | 3.73 | 6.00 | 4.48 | 1.37 | 0.78 | 4.18 | 3.83 | 0.93 | 5.00 | 35.08 | 12.77 | 3.91 |
| | | N | | 322 | | 189 | 21 | 21 | 21 | 21 | | | | | | | | | | | | | | | | | |
| | | SD | | 2.1 | | 0.3 | 16.8 | 13.8 | 6.5 | 7.6 | | | | | | | | | | | | | | | | | |
| 83 | Silage, mid-maturity 40-46% NDF | 3-07-797 | Wet | 21.9 | 3.1 | 1.8 | 57.3 | 35.3 | 7.4 | 12.2 | 16.6 | 18.4 | 65 | 3.87 | 1.69 | 3.95 | 6.36 | 4.41 | 1.37 | 0.79 | 4.18 | 3.83 | 0.94 | 5.00 | 35.60 | 12.39 | 3.85 |
| | | N | | 750 | 2 | 250 | 10 | 10 | 10 | 10 | | | | | | | | | | | | | | | | | |
| | | SD | | 1.8 | | 0.5 | 10.2 | 9.2 | 2.3 | 7.1 | | | | | | | | | | | | | | | | | |
| 84 | Silage, mature >47% NDF | 3-07-798 | Wet | 20.3 | 2.9 | 2.1 | 52.9 | 34.4 | 12.7 | 8.0 | 24.7 | 26.7 | 60 | 3.87 | 1.69 | 3.92 | 6.37 | 4.30 | 1.37 | 0.78 | 4.18 | 3.82 | 0.96 | 5.02 | 35.50 | 12.11 | 3.86 |
| | | N | | 731 | | 121 | 18 | 18 | 18 | 18 | | | | | | | | | | | | | | | | | |
| | | SD | | 1.8 | | 0.6 | 14.1 | 12.7 | 6.3 | 3.6 | | | | | | | | | | | | | | | | | |
| 85 | LINSEED (Flax) meal, solvent | 5-30-288 | Conc | 32.6 | 7.9 | 1.1 | 17.6 | 69.9 | 12.5 | 5.4 | 43.0 | 53.0 | 85 | 8.84 | 2.02 | 4.64 | 6.13 | 3.69 | 1.76 | 1.76 | 4.67 | 3.75 | 1.55 | 5.18 | 42.23 | 8.74 | 4.17 |
| | | N | | 6 | 1 | 2 | 2 | 2 | 2 | 2 | | | | | | | | | | | | | | | | | |
| | | SD | | | | | 17.5 | 35.1 | 17.6 | 2.3 | | | | | | | | | | | | | | | | | |
| | MEAT | | | | | | | | | | | | | | | | | | | | | | | | | | |
| 86 | Meal, rendered | 5-09-323 | Conc | 57.6 | NA | NA | 34.9 | 40.1 | 25.0 | 6.0 | 41.5 | 47.2 | 80 | 7.06 | 2.06 | 2.96 | 6.31 | 5.38 | 1.43 | 1.12 | 3.57 | 3.38 | 0.67 | 4.44 | 37.26 | 14.44 | 3.84 |
| | | N | | 66 | | | 1 | 1 | 1 | 1 | | | | 435 | 435 | 435 | 435 | 435 | 435 | 435 | 435 | 435 | 435 | 435 | | | |
| | | SD | | 7.6 | | | | | | | | | | 0.75 | 0.26 | 0.40 | 0.54 | 0.57 | 0.21 | 0.42 | 0.29 | 0.29 | 0.07 | 0.49 | | | |
| 87 | Meat and bone, rendered | 5-00-388 | Conc | 54.2 | NA | NA | 18.1 | 48.2 | 33.7 | 7.2 | 51.4 | 58.2 | 60 | 6.98 | 1.89 | 2.76 | 6.13 | 5.18 | 1.40 | 1.01 | 3.36 | 3.27 | 0.58 | 4.20 | 35.74 | 14.49 | 3.92 |
| | | N | | 62 | | | 8 | 8 | 4 | 8 | | | | 227 | 227 | 227 | 227 | 227 | 227 | 227 | 227 | 227 | 227 | 227 | | | |
| | | SD | | 5.6 | | | 8.2 | 19.1 | 11.7 | 6.5 | | | | 0.53 | 0.33 | 0.32 | 0.59 | 0.42 | 0.18 | 0.27 | 0.29 | 0.26 | 0.14 | 0.45 | | | |
| | MOLASSES | | | | | | | | | | | | | | | | | | | | | | | | | | |
| 88 | Beet sugar (Amino acids from molasses, sugarcane) | 4-00-668 | Conc | 8.5 | 0 | 0 | 74.1 | 25.9 | 0.0 | 3.2 | 14.7 | 18.1 | 100 | 4.91 | 1.59 | 4.44 | 3.59 | 1.00 | 0.22 | 0.83 | 2.71 | 1.57 | 0.45 | 3.36 | 23.84 | 4.19 | 0.92 |
| | | N | | 12 | | | 2 | 2 | 2 | 2 | | | | | | | | | | | | | | | | | |
| | | SD | | 1.1 | | | 20.4 | 20.3 | | 3.2 | | | | | | | | | | | | | | | | | |
| 89 | Sugarcane (N fractions and Kd from molasses, beet sugar) | 4-04-696 | Conc | 5.8 | 0 | 0 | 74.1 | 25.9 | 0.0 | 3.2 | 14.7 | 18.1 | 100 | 4.91 | 1.59 | 4.44 | 3.59 | 1.00 | 0.22 | 0.83 | 2.71 | 1.57 | 0.45 | 3.36 | 23.84 | 4.19 | 0.92 |
| | | N | | 64 | | | | | | | | | | 10 | 10 | 10 | 10 | 10 | 10 | 10 | 10 | 10 | 10 | 10 | | | |
| | | SD | | 2.0 | | | | | | | | | | 2.91 | 0.51 | 0.08 | 1.21 | 0.40 | 0.05 | 0.18 | 1.25 | 0.33 | 0.07 | 0.83 | | | |

| | | | | | | | | | | | | | | | | | | | | | | | | | | | |
|---|---|---|---|---|---|---|---|---|---|---|---|---|---|---|---|---|---|---|---|---|---|---|---|---|---|---|---|
| 90 | OATS<br>Grain, rolled | 4-03-309 | Conc | 13.2 | 1.8 | 0.3 | 65.2 | 28.8 | 6.0 | 17.4 | 11.6 | 14.6 | 75 | 6.82 | 2.44 | 3.75 | 7.30 | 4.18 | 1.71 | 2.85 | 5.16 | 3.46 | 1.19 | 5.19 | 41.20 | 10.15 | 4.15 |
| | | N | | 308 | | 2 | 4 | 4 | 2 | 4 | | | | 18 | 18 | 18 | 18 | 18 | 18 | 18 | 18 | 18 | 18 | 18 | | | |
| | | SD | | 1.8 | | | 27.3 | 28.3 | 2.4 | 14.8 | | | | 0.44 | 0.25 | 0.22 | 0.34 | 0.25 | 0.09 | 0.18 | 0.22 | 0.13 | 0.09 | 0.41 | | | |
| 91 | Hay, headed<br>(Amino acids from oat silage, headed) | 1-09-099 | Dry | 9.1 | 1.3 | 0.6 | 35.0 | 53.1 | 11.9 | 4.3 | 37.1 | 39.5 | 70 | 2.18 | 1.94 | 5.50 | 6.65 | 3.56 | 1.87 | 0.74 | 4.70 | 4.13 | 1.42 | 4.13 | 36.09 | 9.86 | 5.18 |
| | | N | | 422 | 7 | 8 | | | | | | | | | | | | | | | | | | | | | |
| | | SD | | 2.9 | 0.3 | 0.4 | | | | | | | | | | | | | | | | | | | | | |
| 92 | Silage, headed | 3-21-843 | Wet | 12.9 | 2.1 | 1.0 | 45.6 | 30.9 | 23.5 | 5.4 | 37.2 | 39.1 | 65 | 2.18 | 1.94 | 5.50 | 6.65 | 3.56 | 1.87 | 0.74 | 4.70 | 4.13 | 1.42 | 4.13 | 36.09 | 9.86 | 5.18 |
| | | N | | 634 | 5 | 630 | 2 | 2 | 2 | 2 | | | | 3 | 3 | 3 | 3 | 3 | 3 | 3 | 3 | 3 | 3 | 3 | | | |
| | | SD | | 1.6 | 0.4 | 0.5 | 0.8 | 11.6 | 12.2 | 3.4 | | | | 0.28 | 0.21 | 0.30 | 0.43 | 0.34 | 0.25 | 0.06 | 0.46 | 0.24 | 0.15 | 0.26 | | | |
| 93 | PEANUT<br>Meal, solvent | 5-08-605 | Conc | 51.8 | 5.8 | 1.1 | 61.7 | 36.6 | 1.7 | 16.1 | 9.2 | 13.2 | 90 | 11.07 | 2.42 | 3.27 | 6.40 | 3.34 | 1.17 | 1.38 | 4.85 | 2.69 | 0.98 | 3.94 | 40.13 | 8.32 | 2.92 |
| | | N | | 51 | 2 | 2 | 2 | 2 | 2 | 2 | | | | 22 | 22 | 22 | 22 | 22 | 22 | 22 | 22 | 22 | 22 | 22 | | | |
| | | SD | | 4.4 | | | 26.4 | 29.2 | 2.4 | 4.4 | | | | 0.44 | 0.15 | 0.11 | 0.14 | 0.25 | 0.10 | 0.10 | 0.22 | 0.10 | 0.08 | 0.18 | | | |
| 94 | POTATO<br>Byproduct meal<br>(N fractions and Kd from beet pulp) | 4-03-775 | Conc | 10.5 | 5.2 | 2.3 | 4.5 | 90.5 | 5.0 | 2.0 | 66.2 | 76.3 | 90 | 2.47 | 1.84 | 3.14 | 5.34 | 4.21 | 0.95 | 1.34 | 3.62 | 3.11 | 0.67 | 4.40 | 29.75 | 14.15 | 3.19 |
| | | N | | 79 | 2 | 2 | | | | | | | | 3 | 3 | 3 | 3 | 3 | 3 | 3 | 3 | 3 | 3 | 3 | | | |
| | | SD | | 8.4 | | | | | | | | | | 0.30 | 0.20 | 0.13 | 0.25 | 0.73 | 0.08 | 0.19 | 0.14 | 0.26 | 0.04 | 0.19 | | | |
| 95 | RICE<br>Bran | 4-03-928 | Conc | 15.5 | 3.7 | 0.4 | 32.6 | 49.0 | 18.4 | 5.0 | 40.7 | 47.7 | 65 | 7.80 | 2.78 | 3.42 | 7.10 | 4.65 | 2.05 | 2.23 | 4.76 | 3.87 | 1.17 | 5.24 | 42.84 | 10.85 | 4.79 |
| | | N | | 86 | 11 | 3 | 1 | 1 | 1 | 1 | | | | 14 | 14 | 14 | 14 | 14 | 14 | 14 | 14 | 14 | 14 | 14 | | | |
| | | SD | | 2.2 | 1.7 | 0.1 | | | | | | | | 0.33 | 0.07 | 0.19 | 0.32 | 0.18 | 0.12 | 0.11 | 0.39 | 0.15 | 0.03 | 0.24 | | | |
| 96 | RYE, ANNUAL<br>Silage, vegetative<br>(N fractions and Kd from barley silage) | 3-21-853 | Wet | 16.1 | 1.9 | 0.9 | 56.6 | 33.0 | 10.4 | 5.9 | 24.3 | 26.3 | 65 | 1.04 | 1.21 | 3.45 | 4.88 | 2.35 | 1.16 | 0.66 | 3.42 | 2.51 | 0.60 | 4.80 | 25.42 | 9.24 | 4.56 |
| | | N | | 1175 | 31 | 504 | | | | | | | | 10 | 10 | 10 | 10 | 10 | 10 | 10 | 10 | 10 | | 10 | | | |
| | | SD | | 3.1 | 1.4 | 0.4 | | | | | | | | 0.13 | 0.23 | 0.78 | 2.53 | 1.23 | 0.15 | 0.01 | 0.80 | 0.37 | | 1.21 | | | |
| 97 | SAFFLOWER<br>Meal, solvent<br>(N fractions and Kd from canola meal) | 5-04-110 | Conc | 29.0 | 2.0 | 1.2 | 23.2 | 70.4 | 6.4 | 10.4 | 26.6 | 35.7 | 75 | 8.72 | 2.52 | 2.86 | 6.50 | 3.16 | 1.45 | 1.62 | 4.57 | 2.78 | 1.41 | 5.04 | 39.01 | 8.10 | 3.72 |
| | | N | | 5 | 1 | 1 | | | | | | | | | | | | | | | | | | | | | |
| | | SD | | 0.2 | | | | | | | | | | | | | | | | | | | | | | | |
| 98 | SORGHUM, GRAIN TYPE<br>Grain, dry rolled | 4-04-380 | Conc | 11.6 | 2.8 | 1.0 | 18.9 | 79.4 | 1.7 | 5.5 | 36.0 | 47.3 | 85 | 4.09 | 2.44 | 3.94 | 13.06 | 2.38 | 1.81 | 1.88 | 5.25 | 3.37 | 1.09 | 4.95 | 42.38 | 5.62 | 4.27 |
| | | N | | 437 | 2 | 2 | 2 | 2 | 1 | 2 | | | | 115 | 115 | 115 | 115 | 115 | 115 | 115 | 115 | 115 | 115 | 115 | | | |
| | | SD | | 1.8 | | | 6.4 | 7.6 | | 0.7 | | | | 0.32 | 0.17 | 0.19 | 0.69 | 0.24 | 0.15 | 0.18 | 0.32 | 0.12 | 0.06 | 0.27 | | | |
| 99 | Grain, steam-flaked<br>(Amino acid data from sorghum grain) | 4-04-380 | Conc | 11.6 | 2.8 | 1.0 | 33.2 | 21.9 | 44.9 | 2.5 | 58.6 | 61.3 | 85 | 4.09 | 2.44 | 3.94 | 13.06 | 2.38 | 1.81 | 1.88 | 5.25 | 3.37 | 1.09 | 4.95 | 42.38 | 5.62 | 4.27 |
| 100 | Silage<br>(N fractions and Kd from corn silage, normal) | 3-22-371 | Wet | 9.1 | 2.4 | 1.2 | 42.4 | 37.3 | 20.3 | 4.1 | 39.4 | 41.7 | 70 | 4.07 | 2.47 | 3.91 | 13.04 | 2.64 | 1.93 | 0.64 | 5.24 | 3.59 | 1.16 | 5.00 | 43.04 | 6.13 | 4.48 |
| | | N | | 1168 | 18 | 581 | | | | | | | | 4 | 4 | 4 | 4 | 4 | 4 | 4 | 4 | 4 | 4 | 4 | | | |
| | | SD | | 2.6 | 1.0 | 0.6 | | | | | | | | 0.80 | 0.43 | 0.25 | 0.94 | 0.36 | 0.01 | 0.09 | 0.49 | 0.30 | 0.11 | 0.38 | | | |
| 101 | SORGHUM, SUDAN TYPE<br>Hay<br>(Data from grass hay, mature) | 1-04-480 | Dry | 9.4 | 2.8 | 1.2 | 28.4 | 52.9 | 18.7 | 5.0 | 41.4 | 43.9 | 60 | 3.83 | 1.63 | 3.32 | 6.22 | 3.48 | 1.30 | 1.17 | 3.92 | 3.60 | 1.24 | 4.51 | 33.05 | 10.53 | 3.93 |
| | | N | | 726 | 7 | | | | | | | | | | | | | | | | | | | | | | |
| | | SD | | 2.2 | 0.5 | | | | | | | | | | | | | | | | | | | | | | |
| 102 | Silage<br>(Amino acids from grass silage, mature) | 3-04-499 | Wet | 10.8 | 2.4 | 1.2 | 37.6 | 29.7 | 32.7 | 3.7 | 48.6 | 50.5 | 55 | 3.06 | 1.66 | 3.60 | 6.23 | 3.35 | 1.23 | 0.77 | 4.37 | 3.42 | 1.07 | 4.91 | 32.90 | 10.18 | 3.74 |
| | | N | | 140 | 1 | 138 | 1 | 1 | 1 | 1 | | | | | | | | | | | | | | | | | |
| | | SD | | 3.2 | | 0.4 | | | | | | | | | | | | | | | | | | | | | |

(continues)

TABLE 15-2a. *(continued)*

| Entry No. | Feed Name/ Description | International Feed No. | Feed Type | CP % | NDICP % | ADICP % | N Fractions (% CP) A | B | C | Kd (%/h) of B | Example RUP (%CP) DMI = 2.0% BW Forage = 25% DMI | DMI = 4.0% BW Forage = 50% DMI | RUP Digest % | Arg %CP | His %CP | Ile %CP | Leu %CP | Lys %CP | Met %CP | Cys %CP | Phe %CP | Thr %CP | Trp %CP | Val %CP | TEAA %CP | Lys %EAA | Met %EAA |
|---|---|---|---|---|---|---|---|---|---|---|---|---|---|---|---|---|---|---|---|---|---|---|---|---|---|---|---|
| | SOYBEAN | | | | | | | | | | | | | | | | | | | | | | | | | | |
| 103 | Hulls | 1-04-560 | Conc | 13.9 | 3.5 | 1.0 | 22.5 | 72.2 | 5.3 | 6.2 | 34.4 | 44.6 | 70 | 5.18 | 2.88 | 3.86 | 6.50 | 6.27 | 1.16 | 1.76 | 4.33 | 3.60 | 1.08 | 4.56 | 39.43 | 15.90 | 2.94 |
| | | N | | 138 | 18 | 16 | 2 | 2 | 2 | 2 | | | | 8 | 8 | 8 | 8 | 8 | 8 | 8 | 8 | 8 | 8 | 8 | | | |
| | | SD | | 4.6 | 0.5 | 0.3 | 5.5 | 6.9 | 1.4 | 0.1 | | | | 0.33 | 0.12 | 0.01 | 0.22 | 0.36 | 0.07 | 0.13 | 0.20 | 0.12 | 0.10 | 0.16 | | | |
| 104 | Meal, expellers, 45% CP | 5-12-820 | Conc | 46.3 | 9.6 | 0.4 | 8.7 | 91.3 | 0.0 | 2.4 | 58.0 | 69.0 | 93 | 7.40 | 2.77 | 4.56 | 7.81 | 6.27 | 1.45 | 1.48 | 5.26 | 3.98 | 1.27 | 4.71 | 45.47 | 13.79 | 3.19 |
| | | N | | 546 | 16 | 3 | 3 | 3 | 1 | 3 | | | | 9 | 9 | 9 | 9 | 9 | 9 | 9 | 9 | 9 | 9 | 9 | | | |
| | | SD | | 3.2 | 5.9 | 0.1 | 9.7 | 9.7 | | 0.8 | | | | 0.28 | 0.05 | 0.21 | 0.16 | 0.07 | 0.01 | 0.01 | 0.27 | 0.09 | 0.04 | 0.16 | | | |
| 105 | Meal, nonenzymatically browned | | Conc | 50.0 | 27.0 | 1.6 | 2.4 | 97.6 | 0.0 | 1.7 | 69.4 | 79.4 | 93 | 6.78 | 2.40 | 4.56 | 8.92 | 5.78 | 1.32 | 1.46 | 5.60 | 4.31 | 1.27 | 5.46 | 46.40 | 12.46 | 2.84 |
| | | N | | 14 | 2 | 2 | 7 | 7 | 1 | 7 | | | | 4 | 4 | | 4 | 4 | 4 | 4 | 4 | 4 | | 4 | | | |
| | | SD | | 1.6 | 4.9 | 0.8 | 1.8 | 1.8 | | 0.2 | | | | 0.17 | 0.06 | | 0.18 | 0.25 | 0.09 | 0.04 | 0.09 | 0.08 | | 0.11 | | | |
| 106 | Meal, solvent, 44% CP | 5-20-637 | Conc | 49.9 | 0.7 | 0.4 | 22.5 | 76.8 | 0.7 | 9.4 | 24.3 | 34.6 | 93 | 7.38 | 2.77 | 4.56 | 7.81 | 6.28 | 1.45 | 1.52 | 5.26 | 3.98 | 1.27 | 4.69 | 45.43 | 13.82 | 3.19 |
| | | N | | 111 | | 44 | 14 | 14 | 10 | 14 | | | | 345 | 345 | 345 | 345 | 345 | 345 | 345 | 345 | 345 | 345 | 345 | | | |
| | | SD | | 1.2 | | 0.2 | 13.4 | 14.0 | 0.8 | 2.6 | | | | 0.35 | 0.20 | 0.19 | 0.19 | 0.22 | 0.07 | 0.13 | 0.20 | 0.13 | 0.07 | 0.22 | | | |
| 107 | Meal, solvent, 48% CP | 5-20-638 | Conc | 53.8 | 0.7 | 0.4 | 15 | 84.4 | 0.6 | 7.5 | 30.8 | 42.6 | 93 | 7.32 | 2.77 | 4.56 | 7.81 | 6.29 | 1.44 | 1.50 | 5.26 | 3.96 | 1.26 | 4.64 | 45.30 | 13.89 | 3.18 |
| | | N | | 549 | 21 | | 14 | 14 | 11 | 14 | | | | 295 | 295 | 295 | 295 | 295 | 295 | 295 | 295 | 295 | 295 | 295 | | | |
| | | SD | | 2.1 | 0.2 | | 6.2 | 5.6 | 1.9 | 2.4 | | | | 0.36 | 0.17 | 0.22 | 0.24 | 0.27 | 0.09 | 0.15 | 0.21 | 0.14 | 0.07 | 0.26 | | | |
| 108 | Seeds, whole | 5-04-610 | Conc | 39.2 | 2.3 | 0.6 | 27.8 | 70.2 | 2.0 | 10.9 | 21.5 | 30.4 | 85 | 7.52 | 2.76 | 4.42 | 7.41 | 5.98 | 1.47 | 1.46 | 4.99 | 3.96 | 1.30 | 4.70 | 44.51 | 13.44 | 3.30 |
| | | N | | 48 | 2 | 3 | 5 | 5 | 1 | 5 | | | | 17 | 17 | 17 | 17 | 17 | 17 | 17 | 17 | 17 | 17 | 17 | | | |
| | | SD | | 5.4 | | 0.3 | 16.1 | 16.2 | | 4.1 | | | | 0.47 | 0.01 | 0.19 | 0.21 | 0.09 | 0.03 | 0.00 | 0.35 | 0.08 | 0.06 | 0.00 | | | |
| 109 | Seeds, whole roasted | 5-04-597 | Conc | 43.0 | 6.1 | 2.04 | 17.8 | 77.0 | 5.2 | 9.3 | 29.1 | 39.4 | 85 | 6.79 | 2.61 | 4.22 | 7.13 | 5.98 | 1.40 | 1.44 | 4.32 | 3.80 | 1.13 | 4.59 | 41.98 | 14.24 | 3.33 |
| | | N | | 410 | 18 | 4 | 11 | 11 | 1 | 11 | | | | 13 | 13 | 13 | 13 | 13 | 13 | 13 | 13 | 13 | 13 | 13 | | | |
| | | SD | | 3.8 | 4.8 | 0.9 | 8.5 | 12.8 | | 3.5 | | | | 0.38 | 0.10 | 0.03 | 0.12 | 0.08 | 0.00 | 0.00 | 0.24 | 0.03 | 0.00 | 0.05 | | | |
| 110 | Silage, early maturity (N fractions, Kd, and amino acids from legume silage, mid maturity) | 3-04-579 | Wet | 17.4 | 2.5 | 1.4 | 57.3 | 35.3 | 7.4 | 12.2 | 16.6 | 18.4 | 65 | 3.87 | 1.69 | 3.73 | 6.00 | 4.48 | 1.37 | 0.78 | 4.18 | 3.83 | 0.93 | 5.00 | 35.08 | 12.77 | 3.91 |
| | | N | | 20 | | 17 | | | | | | | | | | | | | | | | | | | | | |
| | | SD | | 5.1 | | 0.7 | | | | | | | | | | | | | | | | | | | | | |
| | SUNFLOWER | | | | | | | | | | | | | | | | | | | | | | | | | | |
| 111 | Meal, solvent | 5-30-032 | Conc | 28.4 | 5.5 | 1.4 | 42.0 | 52.8 | 5.2 | 29.2 | 11.8 | 15.9 | 90 | 8.18 | 2.60 | 4.09 | 6.41 | 3.56 | 2.29 | 1.77 | 4.62 | 3.72 | 1.19 | 4.95 | 41.61 | 8.56 | 5.50 |
| | | N | | 48 | 3 | 3 | 5 | 5 | 5 | 5 | | | | 109 | 109 | 109 | 109 | 109 | 109 | 109 | 109 | 109 | 109 | 109 | | | |
| | | SD | | 5.0 | | 0.4 | 17.7 | 17.3 | 4.4 | 15.2 | | | | 0.45 | 0.18 | 0.15 | 0.21 | 0.19 | 0.12 | 0.12 | 0.22 | 0.13 | 0.06 | 0.20 | | | |
| 112 | Oil seeds, whole (Amino acids from sunflower meal, solvent) | 5-08-530 | Conc | 19.2 | 2.9 | 1.9 | 66.7 | 31.7 | 1.6 | 17.0 | 7.9 | 11.2 | 80 | 8.18 | 2.60 | 4.09 | 6.41 | 3.56 | 2.29 | 1.77 | 4.62 | 3.72 | 1.19 | 4.95 | 41.61 | 8.56 | 5.50 |
| | | N | | 15 | 1 | 1 | 1 | 1 | 1 | 1 | | | | | | | | | | | | | | | | | |
| | | SD | | 4.2 | | | | | | | | | | | | | | | | | | | | | | | |
| | TOMATO | | | | | | | | | | | | | | | | | | | | | | | | | | |
| 113 | Pomace (N fractions and Kd from citrus pulp, dried) | 5-05-042 | Conc | 19.3 | 8.0 | 3.8 | 41.7 | 53.3 | 5.0 | 7.4 | 24.2 | 31.7 | 80 | 5.53 | 1.83 | 3.23 | 7.87 | 7.40 | 0.47 | 0.47 | 4.17 | 3.23 | 0.94 | 4.64 | 39.31 | 18.80 | 1.20 |
| | | N | | 22 | 1 | 2 | | | | | | | | | | | | | | | | | | | | | |
| | | SD | | 4.8 | | 0.1 | | | | | | | | | | | | | | | | | | | | | |

| | | | | | | | | | | | | | | | | | | | | | | | | | | | |
|---|---|---|---|---|---|---|---|---|---|---|---|---|---|---|---|---|---|---|---|---|---|---|---|---|---|---|---|
| | TRITICALE | | | | | | | | | | | | | | | | | | | | | | | | | | |
| 114 | Silage, headed (N fractions and Kd from barley silage) | 3-26-208 | Wet | 13.8 | 2.2 | 1.0 | 56.6 | 32.9 | 10.5 | 5.9 | 24.3 | 26.4 | 65 | 3.84 | 2.53 | 3.04 | 5.86 | 1.83 | 1.31 | 1.43 | 4.78 | 2.14 | 1.03 | 3.68 | 31.47 | 5.82 | 4.16 |
| | | N | | 107 | 2 | 86 | | | | | | | | 3 | 3 | 3 | 3 | 3 | 3 | 3 | 3 | 3 | | 3 | | | |
| | | SD | | 4.0 | | 0.8 | | | | | | | | 0.45 | 0.33 | 0.22 | 0.08 | 0.19 | 0.11 | 0.11 | 0.47 | 0.16 | | 0.36 | | | |
| | WHEAT | | | | | | | | | | | | | | | | | | | | | | | | | | |
| 115 | Bran | 4-05-190 | Conc | 17.3 | 2.8 | 1.4 | 33.7 | 62.5 | 3.8 | 20.0 | 14.6 | 20.7 | 75 | 6.84 | 2.82 | 3.15 | 6.16 | 4.05 | 1.57 | 2.10 | 3.97 | 3.26 | 1.37 | 4.50 | 37.68 | 10.75 | 4.17 |
| | | N | | 81 | | 8 | 4 | 4 | 3 | 4 | | | | 75 | 75 | 75 | 75 | 75 | 75 | 75 | 75 | 75 | 75 | 75 | | | |
| | | SD | | 1.1 | | 0.3 | 13.1 | 15.3 | 2.3 | 8.1 | | | | 0.34 | 0.19 | 0.13 | 0.19 | 0.24 | 0.09 | 0.15 | 0.21 | 0.13 | 0.15 | 0.24 | | | |
| 116 | Grain, rolled | 4-13-245 | Conc | 14.2 | 1.7 | 0.2 | 27.1 | 65.1 | 7.8 | 18.8 | 19.6 | 26.2 | 95 | 4.69 | 2.43 | 3.32 | 6.64 | 2.81 | 1.60 | 2.20 | 4.59 | 2.90 | 1.19 | 4.24 | 34.42 | 8.16 | 4.65 |
| | | N | | 165 | 5 | 5 | 6 | 6 | 6 | 6 | | | | 278 | 278 | 278 | 278 | 278 | 278 | 278 | 278 | 278 | 278 | 278 | | | |
| | | SD | | 2.3 | 0.7 | 0.1 | 18.6 | 28.2 | 16.2 | 8.5 | | | | 0.47 | 0.18 | 0.15 | 0.27 | 0.30 | 0.10 | 0.15 | 0.23 | 0.13 | 0.10 | 0.27 | | | |
| 117 | Hay, headed (N fractions and Kd from oat hay; amino acids from wheat silage) | 1-05-170 | Dry | 9.4 | 1.1 | 0.8 | 35 | 53.1 | 11.9 | 4.3 | 36.9 | 39.4 | 70 | 2.02 | 3.60 | 4.01 | 6.64 | 4.21 | 1.77 | 0.61 | 4.24 | 4.21 | 1.03 | 5.80 | 37.51 | 11.22 | 4.72 |
| | | N | | 120 | 7 | 17 | | | | | | | | | | | | | | | | | | | | | |
| | | SD | | 3.8 | 0.2 | 0.1 | | | | | | | | | | | | | | | | | | | | | |
| 118 | Middlings | 4-05-205 | Conc | 18.5 | 2.8 | 0.5 | 40.3 | 53.6 | 6.1 | 15.2 | 17.7 | 23.7 | 90 | 5.86 | 2.75 | 3.44 | 6.65 | 3.63 | 1.60 | 2.04 | 4.43 | 3.11 | 1.28 | 4.63 | 37.38 | 9.71 | 4.28 |
| | | N | | 245 | 26 | 30 | 4 | 4 | 3 | 4 | | | | 120 | 120 | 120 | 120 | 120 | 120 | 120 | 120 | 120 | 120 | 120 | | | |
| | | SD | | 2.1 | 0.4 | 0.1 | 23 | 25.3 | 3.1 | 3.4 | | | | 0.44 | 0.10 | 0.14 | 0.23 | 0.31 | 0.09 | 0.11 | 0.23 | 0.09 | 0.12 | 0.16 | | | |
| 119 | Silage, early head | 3-21-865 | Wet | 12.0 | 1.5 | 1.0 | 69.5 | 8.7 | 21.8 | 29.0 | 22.9 | 23.2 | 70 | 2.02 | 3.60 | 4.01 | 6.64 | 4.21 | 1.77 | 0.61 | 4.24 | 4.21 | 1.03 | 5.80 | 37.51 | 11.22 | 4.72 |
| | | N | | 471 | 30 | 397 | 2 | 2 | 2 | 2 | | | | 5 | 5 | 5 | 5 | 5 | 5 | 5 | 5 | 5 | 5 | 5 | | | |
| | | SD | | 3.0 | 0.8 | 0.4 | 0.4 | 1.6 | 1.2 | 11.7 | | | | 0.26 | 0.50 | 0.25 | 0.43 | 0.41 | 0.04 | 0.10 | 0.00 | 0.28 | 0.09 | 0.31 | | | |
| 120 | Straw (Amino acids estimated) | 1-05-175 | Dry | 4.8 | 2.1 | 1.4 | 9.3 | 51.4 | 39.3 | 1.4 | 76.4 | 78.3 | 65 | 1.08 | 1.64 | 1.78 | 3.25 | 3.25 | 1.19 | 1.07 | 2.08 | 3.25 | 1.42 | 2.67 | 21.61 | 15.04 | 5.51 |
| | | N | | 161 | 8 | 8 | 2 | 2 | 2 | 2 | | | | | | | | | | | | | | | | | |
| | | SD | | 1.9 | 0.2 | 0.3 | 3.7 | 47.2 | 50.6 | 0.8 | | | | | | | | | | | | | | | | | |
| | WHEY | | | | | | | | | | | | | | | | | | | | | | | | | | |
| 121 | Wet, cattle (N fractions and Kd estimated) | 4-08-134 | Conc | 14.6 | NA | NA | 90.0 | 10.0 | 0.0 | 5.0 | 4.6 | 6.0 | 95 | 2.09 | 1.89 | 5.12 | 8.95 | 7.42 | 1.41 | 2.04 | 2.94 | 5.94 | 1.48 | 4.92 | 42.16 | 17.60 | 3.34 |
| | | N | | 68 | | | | | | | | | | 13 | 13 | 13 | 13 | 13 | 13 | 13 | 13 | 13 | 13 | 13 | | | |
| | | SD | | 14.1 | | | | | | | | | | 0.12 | 0.17 | 0.24 | 0.39 | 0.45 | 0.10 | 0.21 | 0.47 | 0.28 | 0.13 | 0.30 | | | |

NOTE: Values for CP, NDICP, and ADICP are the same as those presented in Table 15-1. The N fraction and Kd data are a summary of published values. The example RUP values were calculated using the equations in the text and in the case of dry forages the N fractions (A,B, and C), the Kd of the B fraction, and the NDF values reported in the feed tables. Most of the amino acid values are courtesy of Degussa Corporation with a majority of the values obtained from the book, "The Amino Acid Composition of Feedstuffs" (Fickler et al., 1996). Exceptions are values for extruded soybean meal, whole sunflower seeds, safflower meal, and some of the data for nonenzymatically browned soybean meal (courtesy of Rhone-Poulenc Animal Nutrition), values for feather meal with some viscera (Cunningham et al, 1994), values for tomato pomace (US-Canadian Table of Feed Composition, 1982), and values for dried brewers grains, hominy, fish byproducts, linseed meal, and safflower meal (NRC, 1998). The amino acid values for the grass-legume mixtures of hays and silages were calculated from the values for all grass and all legume forages assuming 75% grass and 25% legume for predominantly grass, 50% grass and 50% legume for mixed grass and legume, and 25% grass and 75% legume for predominantly legume.

Table 15-2b. Nitrogen Fractions and Amino Acid Composition of Less Commonly Used Feedstuffs, Which Are Cited in the Literature, But Were Not Included as Commonly Used Feedstuffs in Table 15-2a

| Entry No. | Feed Name/Description | N and SD | Feed Type | CP % | N Fractions (% CP) A | B | C | Kd (%/h) of B | RUP Digest % | Arg %CP | His %CP | Ile %CP | Leu %CP | Lys %CP | Met %CP | Cys %CP | Phe %CP | Thr %CP | Trp %CP | Val %CP | TEAA %CP | Lys %EAA | Met %EAA |
|---|---|---|---|---|---|---|---|---|---|---|---|---|---|---|---|---|---|---|---|---|---|---|---|
| | ALFALFA | | | | | | | | | | | | | | | | | | | | | | |
| 1 | Cubes, dry (Amino acids from mid-maturity legume hay) | | Dry | 19.5 | 37.9 | 52.7 | 9.4 | 10.8 | 75 | 5.14 | 1.95 | 4.23 | 7.36 | 5.09 | 1.56 | 1.42 | 4.76 | 4.38 | 1.50 | 5.24 | 41.21 | 12.35 | 3.79 |
| | | N | | 4 | 4 | 4 | 4 | 4 | | | | | | | | | | | | | | | |
| | | SD | | 0.3 | 4.8 | 7.3 | 2.5 | 3.6 | | | | | | | | | | | | | | | |
| 2 | Cubes, ensiled (Amino acids from mid-maturity legume silage) | | Wet | 18.7 | 68.6 | 20.7 | 10.7 | 14.5 | 65 | 3.87 | 1.69 | 3.95 | 6.36 | 4.41 | 1.37 | 0.79 | 4.18 | 3.83 | 0.94 | 5.00 | 35.60 | 12.39 | 3.85 |
| | | N | | 1 | 1 | 1 | 1 | 1 | | | | | | | | | | | | | | | |
| | | SD | | | | | | | | | | | | | | | | | | | | | |
| | BARLEY | | | | | | | | | | | | | | | | | | | | | | |
| 3 | Grain, dry, hulless (His and Phe from barley grain, rolled) | | Conc | 12.8 | 31.8 | 62.6 | 5.6 | 24.6 | 90 | 4.26 | 2.30 | 3.04 | 5.99 | 3.07 | 1.53 | 2.04 | 5.11 | 2.94 | 1.18 | 4.55 | 36.00 | 8.53 | 4.25 |
| | | N | | 2 | 8 | 8 | 8 | 8 | | 42 | | 42 | 42 | 42 | 42 | 42 | | 42 | 14 | 42 | 42 | 42 | 42 |
| | | SD | | 0.4 | 7.6 | 8 | 0.9 | 5.8 | | 0.21 | | 0.12 | 0.70 | 0.26 | 0.12 | 0.20 | | 0.16 | 0.10 | 0.49 | | | |
| 4 | Grain, heat treated (Amino acids from barley grain, rolled) | | Conc | 12.1 | 27 | 60.7 | 12.3 | 7 | 85 | 4.82 | 2.30 | 3.44 | 6.96 | 3.33 | 1.66 | 2.28 | 5.11 | 3.32 | 1.12 | 4.73 | 36.80 | 9.05 | 4.51 |
| | | N | | 3 | 3 | 3 | 3 | 3 | | | | | | | | | | | | | | | |
| | | SD | | 1.3 | 15.5 | 31.3 | 15.8 | 3.4 | | | | | | | | | | | | | | | |
| 5 | Grain, high moisture (Amino acids from barley grain, rolled) | | Conc | 13.1 | 25.6 | 65.6 | 8.8 | 15 | 85 | 4.82 | 2.30 | 3.44 | 6.96 | 3.33 | 1.66 | 2.28 | 5.11 | 3.32 | 1.12 | 4.73 | 36.80 | 9.05 | 4.51 |
| | | N | | 2 | 4 | 4 | 4 | 4 | | | | | | | | | | | | | | | |
| | | SD | | 0.6 | 21.9 | 22.6 | 9.1 | 10.2 | | | | | | | | | | | | | | | |
| 6 | Grain, high moisture, ammoniated (Amino acids from barley grain, rolled) | | Conc | 15.4 | 33.8 | 52.4 | 13.8 | 20.7 | 85 | 4.82 | 2.30 | 3.44 | 6.96 | 3.33 | 1.66 | 2.28 | 5.11 | 3.32 | 1.12 | 4.73 | 36.80 | 9.05 | 4.51 |
| | | N | | 5 | 5 | 5 | 5 | 5 | | | | | | | | | | | | | | | |
| | | SD | | 1.6 | 18.2 | 13 | 5.3 | 11.9 | | | | | | | | | | | | | | | |
| 7 | Mill run, 80% NDF | | Conc | 6.6 | 38.2 | 29.7 | 32.1 | 11.2 | 70 | | | | | | | | | | | | | | |
| | | N | | 2 | 2 | 2 | 2 | 2 | | | | | | | | | | | | | | | |
| | | SD | | 0.4 | 2 | 0.8 | 2.8 | 2.2 | | | | | | | | | | | | | | | |
| 8 | Mill run, 60% NDF | | Conc | 12.6 | 35.6 | 50.4 | 14 | 12.8 | 70 | | | | | | | | | | | | | | |
| | | N | | 1 | 1 | 1 | 1 | 1 | | | | | | | | | | | | | | | |
| 9 | Grain, temper-rolled, hulless (Amino acids from barley grain, hulless) | | Conc | 12.5 | 11.8 | 81.2 | 7 | 14.5 | 85 | 4.26 | 2.30 | 3.04 | 5.99 | 3.07 | 1.53 | 2.04 | 5.11 | 2.94 | 1.18 | 4.55 | 36.00 | 8.53 | 4.25 |
| | | N | | 5 | 5 | 5 | 5 | 5 | | | | | | | | | | | | | | | |
| | | SD | | 0.4 | 3.2 | 3.6 | 1.2 | 2.1 | | | | | | | | | | | | | | | |
| 10 | Silage, vegetative (Amino acids from rye silage) | | Wet | 16.6 | 77.4 | 16.8 | 5.8 | 12.3 | 65 | 1.04 | 1.21 | 3.45 | 4.88 | 2.35 | 1.16 | 0.66 | 3.42 | 2.51 | 1.42 | 4.80 | 26.42 | 8.96 | 4.39 |
| | | N | | 1 | 1 | 1 | 1 | 1 | | | | | | | | | | | | | | | |
| | | SD | | | | | | | | | | | | | | | | | | | | | |

| | | | | | | | | | | | | | | | | | | | | | | | |
|---|---|---|---|---|---|---|---|---|---|---|---|---|---|---|---|---|---|---|---|---|---|---|---|
| 11 | Straw (CP and amino acids estimated) | | Dry | 4.3 | 46.9 | 27.4 | 25.7 | 1.3 | 65 | 1.08 | 1.64 | 1.78 | 3.25 | 3.25 | 1.19 | | 2.08 | 3.25 | 1.42 | 2.67 | 21.61 | 15.04 | 5.51 |
| | | N | | | 1 | 1 | 1 | 1 | | | | | | | | | | | | | | | |
| | | SD | | | | | | | | | | | | | | | | | | | | | |
| | BORAGE (*Borago officinalis*) | | | | | | | | | | | | | | | | | | | | | | |
| 12 | Meal, dry | | Conc | 32.5 | 31.8 | 48.6 | 19.6 | 7.9 | | | | | | | | | | | | | | | |
| | | N | | 2 | 2 | 2 | 2 | 2 | | | | | | | | | | | | | | | |
| | | SD | | 1.3 | 0.1 | 4.5 | 4.4 | 2.7 | | | | | | | | | | | | | | | |
| | CANOLA | | | | | | | | | | | | | | | | | | | | | | |
| 13 | Hulls | | Conc | 16.1 | 29.5 | 35.5 | 35 | 5.3 | 70 | | | | | | | | | | | | | | |
| | | N | | 2 | 2 | 2 | 2 | 2 | | | | | | | | | | | | | | | |
| | | SD | | 1 | 5.7 | 5.3 | 0.4 | 0.8 | | | | | | | | | | | | | | | |
| 14 | Seeds, coarse grind (AA from canola meal, mech. extracted) | | Conc | 25 | 3.6 | 84.6 | 11.8 | 7.4 | 50 | 7.01 | 2.80 | 3.83 | 6.77 | 5.62 | 1.87 | 2.54 | 4.06 | 4.42 | 1.46 | 4.73 | 42.56 | 13.20 | 4.39 |
| | | N | | 1 | 1 | 1 | 1 | 1 | | | | | | | | | | | | | | | |
| | | SD | | | | | | | | | | | | | | | | | | | | | |
| 15 | Meal, mech. extracted, heated (Amino acids from canola meal, mech. extracted) | | Conc | 39.3 | 18.3 | 80.7 | 1.0 | 4.4 | 70 | 7.01 | 2.8 | 3.83 | 6.77 | 5.62 | 1.87 | 2.54 | 4.06 | 4.42 | 1.46 | 4.73 | 42.56 | 13.2 | 4.39 |
| | | N | | | | | | | | | | | | | | | | | | | | | |
| | | SD | | | | | | | | | | | | | | | | | | | | | |
| | COCONUT | | | | | | | | | | | | | | | | | | | | | | |
| 16 | Meal (Amino acids from NRC, 1998) | | Conc | 21.3 | 28.0 | 65.1 | 6.9 | 8.7 | 90 | 10.87 | 1.78 | 3.42 | 6.21 | 2.65 | 1.60 | 1.32 | 3.84 | 3.06 | 0.87 | 4.89 | 39.19 | 6.76 | 4.08 |
| | | N | | 2 | 2 | 2 | 2 | 2 | | | | | | | | | | | | | | | |
| | | SD | | 3.5 | 1.3 | 5.9 | 7.2 | 1.8 | | | | | | | | | | | | | | | |
| | CORN, YELLOW | | | | | | | | | | | | | | | | | | | | | | |
| 17 | Distillers grains, dried (Amino acids from 1998 Swine NRC) | | Conc | 22.2 | 39.5 | 41.6 | 18.9 | 7.9 | 75 | 3.63 | 2.54 | 3.83 | 10.6 | 2.98 | 1.73 | 1.13 | 3.99 | 2.50 | 0.81 | 5.00 | 37.61 | 7.92 | 4.60 |
| | | N | | 4 | 5 | 5 | 5 | 5 | | | | | | | | | | | | | | | |
| | | SD | | 6.2 | 13.1 | 12.8 | 12.2 | 4.3 | | | | | | | | | | | | | | | |
| 18 | Grain, dry, extruded (Amino acids from corn grain, dry) | | Conc | 8.1 | 42.3 | 23.0 | 34.7 | 3.9 | 90 | 4.47 | 3.07 | 3.51 | 12.80 | 2.65 | 2.03 | 1.93 | 4.92 | 3.56 | 0.68 | 4.77 | 42.46 | 6.24 | 4.78 |
| | | N | | 1 | 1 | 1 | 1 | 1 | | | | | | | | | | | | | | | |
| | | SD | | | | | | | | | | | | | | | | | | | | | |
| 19 | Silage <45% NDF (Amino acids from corn silage, mature) | | Wet | 8.1 | 65.7 | 15.3 | 19.0 | 2.1 | 70 | 1.96 | 1.79 | 3.33 | 8.59 | 2.43 | 1.52 | 1.28 | 3.83 | 3.19 | 0.44 | 4.49 | 31.59 | 7.69 | 4.81 |
| | | N | | 3 | 4 | 4 | 4 | 4 | | | | | | | | | | | | | | | |
| | | SD | | 0.6 | 10.5 | 4.2 | 7.4 | 0.9 | | | | | | | | | | | | | | | |
| 20 | Silage 45 to 50% NDF (Amino acids from corn silage, normal) | | Wet | 8.4 | 54.8 | 28.8 | 16.4 | 4.5 | 70 | 1.97 | 1.79 | 3.34 | 8.59 | 2.51 | 1.53 | 1.34 | 3.83 | 3.19 | 0.44 | 4.47 | 31.64 | 7.93 | 4.84 |
| | | N | | 7 | 7 | 7 | 7 | 7 | | | | | | | | | | | | | | | |
| | | SD | | 0.6 | 18.2 | 14 | 5.7 | 1.6 | | | | | | | | | | | | | | | |
| 21 | Silage 45 to 50% NDF (Amino acids from corn silage, normal) | | Wet | 9.5 | 51.2 | 29.0 | 19.8 | 3.9 | 70 | 1.97 | 1.79 | 3.34 | 8.59 | 2.51 | 1.53 | 1.34 | 3.83 | 3.19 | 0.44 | 4.47 | 31.64 | 7.93 | 4.84 |
| | | N | | 8 | 8 | 8 | 8 | 8 | | | | | | | | | | | | | | | |
| | | SD | | 1.5 | 17.3 | 14.0 | 5.3 | 1.2 | | | | | | | | | | | | | | | |

*(continues)*

Table 15-2b. *(continued)*

| Entry No. | Feed Name/Description | N and SD | Feed Type | CP % | N Fractions (% CP) A | B | C | Kd (%/h) of B | RUP Digest % | Arg %CP | His %CP | Ile %CP | Leu %CP | Lys %CP | Met %CP | Cys %CP | Phe %CP | Thr %CP | Trp %CP | Val %CP | TEAA %CP | Lys %EAA | Met %EAA |
|---|---|---|---|---|---|---|---|---|---|---|---|---|---|---|---|---|---|---|---|---|---|---|---|
| 22 | Silage >50% NDF (Amino acids from corn silage, immature) | | Wet | 9.5 | 50.9 | 26.4 | 22.7 | 4.6 | 70 | 1.96 | 1.79 | 3.36 | 8.58 | 2.58 | 1.54 | 1.42 | 3.83 | 3.19 | 0.44 | 4.46 | 31.72 | 8.13 | 4.85 |
| | | N | | 5 | 5 | 5 | 5 | 5 | | | | | | | | | | | | | | | |
| | | SD | | 1.3 | 6.7 | 5.8 | 3.6 | 1.6 | | | | | | | | | | | | | | | |
| | COTTON SEED | | | | | | | | | | | | | | | | | | | | | | |
| 23 | Whole seeds with lint, heated (Amino acids from whole seeds with lint) | | Conc | 23 | 24.4 | 64.5 | 11.1 | 8.2 | 80 | 11.52 | 3.11 | 3.2 | 5.88 | 4.35 | 1.71 | 1.76 | 5.3 | 3.46 | 1.27 | 4.70 | 44.51 | 9.77 | 3.84 |
| | | N | | 5 | 6 | 6 | 6 | 6 | | | | | | | | | | | | | | | |
| | | SD | | 0 | 11 | 13.1 | 5.8 | 5.2 | | | | | | | | | | | | | | | |
| | CRAMBE (*Crabme abyssinica*) | | | | | | | | | | | | | | | | | | | | | | |
| 24 | Meal, solvent, dehulled | | Conc | 49.4 | 56.0 | 42.0 | 2.0 | 18.4 | 90 | | | | | | | | | | | | | | |
| | | N | | 1 | 1 | 1 | 1 | 1 | | | | | | | | | | | | | | | |
| | | SD | | | | | | | | | | | | | | | | | | | | | |
| 25 | Meal, solvent, partly hulled | | Conc | 29.2 | 78.0 | 13.0 | 9.0 | 11.4 | 90 | | | | | | | | | | | | | | |
| | | N | | 1 | 1 | 1 | 1 | 1 | | | | | | | | | | | | | | | |
| | | SD | | | | | | | | | | | | | | | | | | | | | |
| | FABA BEANS | | | | | | | | | | | | | | | | | | | | | | |
| 26 | Seed, raw, cracked (Amino acids from 1998 Swine NRC) | | Conc | 31.4 | 67.0 | 33.0 | 0.0 | 3.9 | 90 | 8.98 | 2.64 | 4.06 | 7.44 | 6.38 | 0.79 | 1.26 | 4.06 | 3.5 | 0.87 | 4.49 | 43.21 | 14.77 | 1.83 |
| | | N | | 1 | 1 | 1 | 1 | 1 | | | | | | | | | | | | | | | |
| | | SD | | | | | | | | | | | | | | | | | | | | | |
| | HEMP (*Cannabis sativa* L.) | | | | | | | | | | | | | | | | | | | | | | |
| 27 | Meal | | Conc | 32.1 | 6.5 | 90.1 | 3.4 | 2.9 | 85 | | | | | | | | | | | | | | |
| | | N | | 1 | 1 | 1 | 1 | 1 | 1 | | | | | | | | | | | | | | |
| | | SD | | | | | | | | | | | | | | | | | | | | | |
| | LINSEED (Flax) | | | | | | | | | | | | | | | | | | | | | | |
| 28 | Meal, expellers (Amino acids from meal, solvent) | | Conc | 37.8 | 19.3 | 59.7 | 21 | 5.3 | 85 | 8.84 | 2.02 | 4.64 | 6.13 | 3.69 | 1.76 | 1.76 | 4.67 | 3.75 | 1.55 | 5.18 | 42.23 | 8.74 | 4.17 |
| | | N | | 1 | 1 | 1 | 1 | 1 | | | | | | | | | | | | | | | |
| | | SD | | | | | | | | | | | | | | | | | | | | | |
| | LUPIN | | | | | | | | | | | | | | | | | | | | | | |
| 29 | Seed, cracked, raw | | Conc | 34.5 | 30.1 | 66.5 | 3.4 | 26.1 | 75 | 10.08 | 2.38 | 4.13 | 7.23 | 4.49 | 0.81 | 1.51 | 3.80 | 3.50 | 0.76 | 3.80 | 40.99 | 10.95 | 1.98 |
| | | N | | 7 | 7 | 7 | 7 | 7 | | 9 | 9 | 9 | 9 | 9 | 9 | 9 | 9 | 9 | 9 | 9 | 9 | 9 | 9 |
| | | SD | | 2.4 | 27.3 | 24.9 | 4.6 | 21.3 | | 1.1 | 0.35 | 0.13 | 0.24 | 0.25 | 0.09 | 0.38 | 0.18 | 0.15 | 0.04 | 0.15 | | | |
| 30 | Seed, extruded (Amino acids from seed, cracked, raw) | | Conc | 37.9 | 41.3 | 57.9 | 0.8 | 4.6 | 95 | 10.08 | 2.38 | 4.13 | 7.23 | 4.49 | 0.81 | 1.51 | 3.80 | 3.50 | 0.76 | 3.80 | 40.99 | 10.95 | 1.98 |
| | | N | | 7 | 7 | 7 | 7 | 7 | | | | | | | | | | | | | | | |
| | | SD | | 2.7 | 23.7 | 24.2 | 0.6 | 2.2 | | | | | | | | | | | | | | | |
| 31 | Silage, 45% NDF | | Wet | 16.0 | 39.8 | 47.2 | 13.0 | 24.0 | 75 | | | | | | | | | | | | | | |
| | | N | | 1 | 1 | 1 | 1 | 1 | | | | | | | | | | | | | | | |
| | | SD | | | | | | | | | | | | | | | | | | | | | |

| | | | | | | | | | | | | | | | | | | | | | |
|---|---|---|---|---|---|---|---|---|---|---|---|---|---|---|---|---|---|---|---|---|---|
| 32 | MILK<br>Skim, dry powder | Conc | 38.5 | | | | | 95 | 3.37 | 2.84 | 5.13 | 9.84 | 7.71 | 2.49 | 0.79 | 4.88 | 4.41 | 1.37 | 6.32 | 48.36 | 15.94 | 5.15 |
| | | N | 15 | | | | | | 15 | 15 | 15 | 15 | 15 | 15 | 15 | 15 | 15 | 15 | 15 | 15 | 15 | 15 |
| | | SD | 1.5 | | | | | | 0.2 | 0.14 | 0.24 | 0.39 | 0.48 | 0.14 | 0.05 | 0.18 | 0.22 | 0.02 | 0.17 | | | |
| 33 | PALM KERNEL<br>Byproduct meal | Conc | 18.9 | 9.6 | 80.8 | 9.6 | 1.6 | 75 | | | | | | | | | | | | | | |
| | | N | 7 | 7 | 7 | 7 | 7 | | | | | | | | | | | | | | | |
| | | SD | 1.9 | 6.1 | 7.6 | 2.2 | 0.4 | | | | | | | | | | | | | | | |
| 34 | PEAS<br>Field, raw | Conc | 25.6 | 55.5 | 44.4 | 0.1 | 16.7 | 80 | 8.93 | 2.59 | 4.09 | 7.24 | 7.17 | 1.00 | 1.47 | 4.70 | 3.75 | 0.90 | 4.67 | 46.51 | 15.42 | 2.15 |
| | | N | 2 | 5 | 5 | 5 | 5 | | 77 | 77 | 77 | 77 | 77 | 77 | 77 | 77 | 77 | 77 | 77 | 77 | 77 | 77 |
| | | SD | 1.7 | 11.5 | 11.5 | 0.1 | 8.1 | | 0.98 | 0.15 | 0.15 | 0.19 | 0.25 | 0.08 | 0.12 | 0.22 | 0.13 | 0.04 | 0.18 | | | |
| 35 | Field, extruded (Amino acids from field, raw) | Conc | 24.5 | 15.7 | 75.4 | 8.9 | 13.1 | 90 | 8.93 | 2.59 | 4.09 | 7.24 | 7.17 | 1.00 | 1.47 | 4.70 | 3.75 | 0.90 | 4.67 | 46.51 | 15.42 | 2.15 |
| | | N | 4 | 4 | 4 | 4 | 4 | | | | | | | | | | | | | | | |
| | | SD | 0.8 | 3.5 | 3.9 | 7 | 6.6 | | | | | | | | | | | | | | | |
| | POULTRY LITTER | Conc | 21.8 | 70.9 | 18.6 | 10.6 | 11.8 | 80 | | | | | | | | | | | | | | |
| | | N | 1 | 2 | 2 | 2 | 2 | | | | | | | | | | | | | | | |
| | | SD | | 0 | 0.4 | 0.4 | 8.8 | | | | | | | | | | | | | | | |
| 36 | RAPESEED<br>Meal, solvent | Conc | 38.4 | 23.4 | 69.2 | 7.4 | 13.1 | 70 | 6.17 | 2.80 | 3.93 | 7.09 | 5.62 | 2.04 | 2.54 | 4.06 | 4.42 | 1.30 | 5.09 | 42.52 | 13.22 | 4.80 |
| | | N | 6 | 6 | 6 | 6 | 6 | | 268 | 268 | 268 | 268 | 268 | 268 | 268 | 268 | 268 | 268 | 268 | 268 | 268 | 268 |
| | | SD | 2.5 | 6.6 | 6.6 | 2.6 | 4.3 | | 0.52 | 0.21 | 0.15 | 0.18 | 0.41 | 0.10 | 0.18 | 0.16 | 0.18 | 0.08 | 0.23 | | | |
| 37 | Meal, solvent, heated (Amino acids from meal, solvent) | Conc | 38.4 | 18.3 | 74.8 | 6.9 | 10.4 | 75 | 6.17 | 2.80 | 3.93 | 7.09 | 5.62 | 2.04 | 2.54 | 4.06 | 4.42 | 1.30 | 5.09 | 42.52 | 13.22 | 4.80 |
| | | N | 6 | 6 | 6 | 6 | 6 | | | | | | | | | | | | | | | |
| | | SD | 2.5 | 8 | 7.5 | 3.3 | 2.6 | | | | | | | | | | | | | | | |
| 38 | RYE<br>Grain | Conc | 10.9 | | | | | 80 | 5.4 | 2.59 | 3.57 | 6.54 | 4.05 | 1.81 | 2.55 | 4.89 | 3.58 | 0.99 | 5.08 | 38.50 | 10.52 | 4.70 |
| | | N | 14 | | | | | | 14 | 14 | 14 | 14 | 14 | 14 | 14 | 14 | 14 | 14 | 14 | | | |
| | | SD | 1.5 | | | | | | 0.38 | 0.21 | 0.28 | 0.37 | 0.36 | 0.13 | 0.19 | 0.31 | 0.24 | 0.06 | 0.36 | | | |
| 39 | SORGHUM, GRAIN TYPE<br>Grain, extruded (Amino acids from grain, dry rolled) | Conc | 8.3 | 33.2 | 21.9 | 44.9 | 2.5 | 85 | 4.09 | 2.44 | 3.94 | 13.06 | 2.38 | 1.81 | 1.88 | 5.25 | 3.37 | 1.09 | 4.95 | 42.38 | 5.62 | 4.27 |
| | | N | 1 | 1 | 1 | 1 | 1 | | | | | | | | | | | | | | | |
| | | SD | | | | | | | | | | | | | | | | | | | | |
| 40 | SUNFLOWER<br>Meal, solvent, roasted (CP and amino acids from meal, solvent) | Conc | 28.4 | 33.4 | 32.3 | 34.3 | 4.4 | 90 | 8.77 | 2.60 | 4.16 | 6.42 | 3.38 | 2.36 | 1.77 | 4.62 | 3.68 | 1.24 | 4.95 | 42.19 | 8.01 | 5.59 |
| | | N | | 6 | 6 | 6 | 6 | | | | | | | | | | | | | | | |
| | | SD | | 2.9 | 11 | 11.9 | 0.8 | | | | | | | | | | | | | | | |
| 41 | Silage (Trp estimated) | Wet | 12.5 | | | | | 70 | 6.67 | 2.18 | 3.44 | 5.38 | 2.99 | 1.92 | 1.74 | 3.88 | 3.12 | 1.24 | 4.16 | 35.02 | 8.54 | 5.48 |
| | | N | | | | | | | 5 | 5 | 5 | 5 | 5 | 5 | 5 | 5 | 5 | | 5 | 5 | 5 | 5 |
| | | SD | | | | | | | 0.87 | 0.38 | 0.18 | 0.34 | 0.16 | 0.09 | 0.20 | 0.18 | 0.11 | | 0.31 | | | |
| 42 | TRITICALE<br>Grain, ground | Conc | 14.5 | 51.3 | 45.9 | 2.8 | 43 | 90 | 5.29 | 2.53 | 3.59 | 6.82 | 3.62 | 1.79 | 2.45 | 4.78 | 3.35 | 1.04 | 4.78 | 37.59 | 9.63 | 4.76 |
| | | N | 1 | | | | | | 31 | 31 | 31 | 31 | 31 | 31 | 31 | 31 | 31 | 31 | 31 | 31 | 31 | 31 |
| | | SD | | | | | | | 0.28 | 0.51 | 0.66 | 0.74 | 0.46 | 0.20 | 0.35 | 0.80 | 0.40 | 0.12 | 0.65 | | | |
| 43 | WHEAT<br>Distillers grains, dried | Conc | 42.3 | 21.1 | 76.9 | 2 | 26.1 | 80 | 2.59 | 3.16 | 3.53 | 6.12 | 1.55 | 1.41 | | 4.43 | 3.05 | 1.09 | 4.54 | 31.47 | 4.93 | 4.48 |
| | | N | 2 | 2 | 2 | 2 | 2 | | 1 | 1 | 1 | 1 | 1 | 1 | | 1 | 1 | 1 | 1 | 1 | 1 | 1 |
| | | SD | 1.8 | 2.1 | 2.5 | 0.4 | 0.8 | | | | | | | | | | | | | | | |

NOTE: Amino acid values are courtesy of Degussa Corporation; exceptions are values for wheat distillers grains (Rhone-Poulenc Animal Nutrition).

TABLE 15-3 Mineral Composition of Some Feedstuffs Commonly Fed to Dairy Cattle (all values on a dry basis)

| Entry No. | Feed Name/Description | International Feed No. | Ash % | Ca % | P % | Mg % | K % | Na % | Cl % | S % | Co mg/kg | Cu mg/kg | I mg/kg | Fe mg/kg | Mn mg/kg | Se mg/kg | Zn mg/kg | Mo mg/kg |
|---|---|---|---|---|---|---|---|---|---|---|---|---|---|---|---|---|---|---|
| | ALFALFA *Medicago sativa* | Also see LEGUMES, FORAGE | | | | | | | | | | | | | | | | |
| 1 | Meal, 17% CP | 1-00-023 | 11.0 | 1.47 | 0.28 | 0.29 | 2.37 | 0.10 | 0.65 | 0.26 | 0.31 | 9 | 0.16 | 619 | 44 | 0.36 | 28 | 2.8 |
| | | N | 84 | 206 | 206 | 206 | 206 | 110 | 17 | 72 | | 110 | 1 | 110 | 110 | 2 | 110 | 110 |
| | | SD | 2.3 | 0.36 | 0.07 | 0.06 | 0.42 | 0.08 | 0.27 | 0.04 | | 4 | | 617 | 20 | 0.04 | 19 | 1.2 |
| | ALMOND | | | | | | | | | | | | | | | | | |
| 2 | Hulls | 4-00-359 | 6.1 | 0.28 | 0.13 | 0.13 | 2.62 | 0.02 | 0.03 | 0.04 | | 7 | | 247 | 22 | 0.07 | 22 | 1.0 |
| | | N | 16 | 30 | 30 | 30 | 30 | 30 | 9 | 14 | | 30 | | 16 | 30 | 7 | 30 | 23 |
| | | SD | 0.5 | 0.11 | 0.08 | 0.05 | 0.52 | 0.01 | 0.03 | 0.01 | | 4 | | 11 | 18 | 0.02 | 15 | 0.6 |
| | APPLE | | | | | | | | | | | | | | | | | |
| 3 | Pomace, wet | 4-25-450 | 2.6 | 0.20 | 0.14 | 0.09 | 0.73 | 0.04 | 0.03 | 0.07 | | 11 | | 185 | 17 | | 14 | 0.7 |
| | | N | 16 | 54 | 54 | 54 | 54 | 54 | 3 | 18 | | 54 | | 54 | 54 | | 54 | 54 |
| | | SD | 1.1 | 0.11 | 0.03 | 0.03 | 0.25 | 0.04 | | 0.01 | | 5 | | 190 | 18 | | 10 | 0.5 |
| | BAKERY BYPRODUCT | | | | | | | | | | | | | | | | | |
| 4 | Byproduct meal | 4-00-466 | 3.8 | 0.20 | 0.36 | 0.13 | 0.42 | 0.72 | 1.20 | 0.14 | 1.05 | 5 | | 273 | 30 | 0.29 | 46 | 1.1 |
| | | N | 71 | 168 | 168 | 168 | 168 | 168 | 13 | 41 | 1 | 168 | | 168 | 168 | 5 | 168 | 168 |
| | | SD | 1.6 | 0.20 | 0.24 | 0.10 | 0.26 | 0.50 | 0.73 | 0.05 | | 4 | | 330 | 27 | 0.21 | 50 | 0.7 |
| 5 | Bread, waste | 4-00-466 | 2.8 | 0.14 | 0.20 | 0.05 | 0.23 | 0.85 | 0.94 | 0.17 | | 4 | | 140 | 10 | | 16 | 0.6 |
| | | N | 10 | 57 | 57 | 57 | 57 | 57 | 5 | 21 | | 57 | | 57 | 57 | | 57 | 57 |
| | | SD | 1.4 | 0.10 | 0.06 | 0.06 | 0.06 | 0.33 | 0.41 | 0.03 | | 8 | | 170 | 3 | | 6 | 0.6 |
| 6 | Cereal byproduct | 4-00-466 | 3.2 | 0.17 | 0.29 | 0.10 | 0.33 | 0.59 | 0.69 | 0.10 | | 4 | | 252 | 26 | | 80 | 1 |
| | | N | 21 | 48 | 48 | 48 | 48 | 48 | 5 | 24 | | 48 | | 48 | 48 | | 48 | 48 |
| | | SD | 1.3 | 0.27 | 0.16 | 0.05 | 0.16 | 0.27 | 0.39 | 0.03 | | 1 | | 164 | 16 | | 47 | 0.5 |
| 7 | Cookie byproduct | 4-24-852 | 3.0 | 0.23 | 0.29 | 0.13 | 0.46 | 0.68 | 1.20 | 0.13 | | 5 | | 235 | 27 | | 38 | 1.0 |
| | | N | 5 | 29 | 29 | 29 | 29 | 29 | 1 | 20 | | 29 | | 29 | 29 | | 29 | 29 |
| | | SD | | 0.28 | 0.16 | 0.13 | 0.17 | 0.46 | | 0.08 | | 5 | | 288 | 20 | | 31 | 0.7 |
| | BARLEY | | | | | | | | | | | | | | | | | |
| 8 | Grain, rolled | 4-00-528 | 2.9 | 0.06 | 0.39 | 0.14 | 0.56 | 0.02 | 0.13 | 0.12 | 0.35 | 6 | | 70 | 22 | 0.11 | 38 | 1.1 |
| | | N | 257 | 319 | 321 | 287 | 287 | 229 | 31 | 139 | 16 | 241 | | 253 | 241 | 519 | 241 | 237 |
| | | SD | 0.8 | 0.02 | 0.96 | 0.02 | 0.12 | 0.02 | 0.07 | 0.01 | 0.28 | 3 | | 60 | 12 | 0.09 | 30 | 0.6 |
| 9 | Malt sprouts | 5-00-545 | 7.4 | 0.24 | 0.51 | 0.18 | 1.19 | 0.04 | | 0.29 | | 9 | | 353 | 49 | 0.67 | 65 | 2.0 |
| | | N | 9 | 31 | 31 | 31 | 31 | 31 | | 10 | | 31 | | 31 | 31 | 6 | 31 | 31 |
| | | SD | 1.3 | 0.16 | 0.11 | 0.04 | 0.18 | 0.00 | | 0.05 | | 2 | | 207 | 14 | 0.55 | 13 | 0.6 |
| 10 | Silage, headed | 3-00-512 | 7.5 | 0.48 | 0.30 | 0.18 | 2.43 | 0.13 | 0.72 | 0.17 | 0.72 | 7 | | 343 | 43 | 0.12 | 30 | 1.6 |
| | | N | 166 | 525 | 525 | 420 | 420 | 214 | 11 | 97 | 6 | 291 | | 291 | 291 | 197 | 291 | 214 |
| | | SD | 2.1 | 0.19 | 0.06 | 0.05 | 0.78 | 0.23 | 0.54 | 0.04 | 0.41 | 3 | | 458 | 25 | 0.09 | 13 | 0.8 |
| | BEET, SUGAR | | | | | | | | | | | | | | | | | |
| 11 | Pulp, dried | 4-00-669 | 7.3 | 0.91 | 0.09 | 0.23 | 0.96 | 0.31 | 0.18 | 0.30 | | 11 | | 642 | 62 | 0.14 | 22 | 1.5 |
| | | N | 54 | 170 | 152 | 152 | 152 | 152 | 16 | 55 | | 152 | | 152 | 152 | 10 | 152 | 143 |
| | | SD | 1.9 | 0.27 | 0.03 | 0.05 | 0.50 | 0.28 | 0.25 | 0.11 | | 6 | | 269 | 30 | 0.09 | 9 | 0.7 |
| | BERMUDAGRASS *Cynodon dactylon* | | | | | | | | | | | | | | | | | |
| 12 | Coastal, hay, early head | 1-20-900 | 8.1 | 0.49 | 0.27 | 0.19 | 1.80 | 0.17 | 0.67 | 0.48 | | 8 | | 224 | 62 | | 32 | |
| | | N | 34 | 8 | 8 | 7 | 7 | 7 | 7 | 7 | | 7 | | 7 | 7 | | 7 | |
| | | SD | 1.9 | 0.07 | 0.03 | 0.05 | 0.34 | 0.10 | 0.22 | 0.10 | | 10 | | 126 | 25 | | 15 | |
| 13 | Tifton-85, hay, 3-4 wk growth (Data from Coastal hay, adj. for ash) | IFN | 6.5 | 0.39 | 0.22 | 0.15 | 1.40 | 0.14 | 0.54 | 0.38 | | 8 | | 224 | 62 | | 32 | |
| | | N | 2 | | | | | | | | | | | | | | | |
| | | SD | | | | | | | | | | | | | | | | |
| | BLOOD | | | | | | | | | | | | | | | | | |
| 14 | Meal, ring dried | 5-00-380 | 2.5 | 0.30 | 0.30 | 0.03 | 0.33 | 0.40 | 0.33 | 0.77 | | 10 | | 2453 | 9 | 0.77 | 33 | 0.6 |
| | | N | 31 | 75 | 75 | 75 | 75 | 75 | 7 | 46 | | 75 | | 75 | 75 | 13 | 75 | 75 |
| | | SD | 1.4 | 0.40 | 0.26 | 0.02 | 0.22 | 0.28 | 0.16 | 0.34 | | 4 | | 420 | 6 | 0.84 | 14 | 0.8 |
| 15 | Meal, batch dried (Composition data from ring-dried) | | 2.5 | 0.30 | 0.30 | 0.03 | 0.33 | 0.40 | 0.33 | 0.77 | | 10 | | 2453 | 9 | 0.77 | 33 | 0.6 |
| | BLUEGRASS *Poa pratensis* | See GRASSES, COOL SEASON | | | | | | | | | | | | | | | | |
| | BREWERS GRAINS | | | | | | | | | | | | | | | | | |
| 16 | Dried | 5-12-024 | 4.3 | 0.30 | 0.67 | 0.26 | 0.50 | 0.04 | 0.07 | 0.38 | | 11 | | 224 | 45 | 1.06 | 85 | 3.2 |
| | | N | 138 | 344 | 344 | 344 | 344 | 77 | 22 | 138 | | 344 | | 344 | 344 | 4 | 344 | 340 |
| | | SD | 0.9 | 0.11 | 0.06 | 0.35 | 0.26 | 0.06 | 0.02 | 0.08 | | 6 | | 119 | 12 | 0.28 | 15 | 0.8 |
| 17 | Wet | 5-00-517 | 4.9 | 0.35 | 0.59 | 0.21 | 0.47 | 0.01 | 0.12 | 0.33 | | 9 | | 247 | 49 | 1.06 | 91 | 3.4 |
| | | N | 110 | 427 | 427 | 427 | 427 | 13 | 1 | 190 | | 389 | | 389 | 389 | | 389 | 389.0 |
| | | SD | 1.1 | 0.22 | 0.10 | 0.26 | 0.26 | 0.01 | | 0.06 | | 7 | | 270 | 13 | | 17 | 1 |
| | BROME, SMOOTH *Bromus inermis* | See GRASSES, COOL SEASON | | | | | | | | | | | | | | | | |
| | CANARYGRASS, REED *Phalaris arundianacea* | See GRASSES, COOL SEASON | | | | | | | | | | | | | | | | |
| | CANOLA | | | | | | | | | | | | | | | | | |
| 18 | Seed | 5-08-109 | 4.6 | 0.44 | 0.68 | 0.21 | 0.91 | 0.03 | | 0.42 | | 12 | | 253 | 48 | | 88 | |
| | | N | 1 | 1 | 1 | 1 | 1 | 1 | | 1 | | 1 | | 1 | 1 | | 1 | |
| | | SD | | | | | | | | | | | | | | | | |

*(continues)*

TABLE 15-3 *(continued)*

| Entry No. | Feed Name/Description | International Feed No. | Ash % | Ca % | P % | Mg % | K % | Na % | Cl % | S % | Co mg/kg | Cu mg/kg | I mg/kg | Fe mg/kg | Mn mg/kg | Se mg/kg | Zn mg/kg | Mo mg/kg |
|---|---|---|---|---|---|---|---|---|---|---|---|---|---|---|---|---|---|---|
| 19 | Meal, mech. extracted | 5-03-870 | 7.4 | 0.75 | 1.10 | 0.53 | 1.41 | 0.07 | 0.04 | 0.73 | | 5 | | 296 | 62 | 1.09 | 61 | 2.7 |
| | | N | 27 | 79 | 79 | 79 | 79 | 79 | 9 | 32 | | 29 | | 79 | 79 | 19 | 79 | 79 |
| | | SD | 1.2 | 0.11 | 0.20 | 0.07 | 0.13 | 0.10 | 0.01 | 0.19 | | 3 | | 251 | 12 | 0.99 | 7 | 0.6 |
| | CHOCOLATE | | | | | | | | | | | | | | | | | |
| 20 | Byproduct | | 2.1 | 0.22 | 0.30 | 0.22 | 1.18 | 0.07 | | 0.11 | | 15 | | 461 | 31 | | 40 | 1.6 |
| | | N | 15 | 14 | 14 | 14 | 14 | 14 | | 5 | | 14 | | 14 | 14 | | 14 | 14 |
| | | SD | 2.0 | 0.12 | 0.20 | 0.22 | 1.20 | 0.03 | | 0.02 | | 19 | | 800 | 32 | | 28 | 1.6 |
| | CITRUS | | | | | | | | | | | | | | | | | |
| 21 | Pulp dried | 4-01-237 | 7.2 | 1.92 | 0.12 | 0.12 | 1.10 | 0.06 | 0.08 | 0.10 | | 8 | | 151 | 9 | | 11 | 0.9 |
| | | N | 35 | 90 | 90 | 90 | 90 | 90 | 18 | 47 | | 90 | | 90 | 90 | | 57 | 90 |
| | | SD | 4.2 | 0.53 | 0.03 | 0.01 | 0.16 | 0.06 | 0.05 | 0.03 | | 3 | | 145 | 3 | | 3 | 0.5 |
| | CLOVER, LADINO *Trifolium pratense* | See LEGUMES, FORAGE | | | | | | | | | | | | | | | | |
| | CLOVER, RED *Trifolium pratense* | See LEGUMES, FORAGE | | | | | | | | | | | | | | | | |
| | CORN, YELLOW | | | | | | | | | | | | | | | | | |
| 22 | Cobs | 1-28-234 | 2.2 | 0.10 | 0.06 | 0.06 | 0.90 | 0.04 | | 0.07 | | 6 | | 254 | 5 | 0.08 | 11 | 0.13 |
| | | N | 2 | 3 | 3 | 3 | 3 | 2 | | 2 | | 2 | | 2 | 2 | 1 | 2 | 1 |
| | | SD | | | | | | | | | | | | | | | | |
| 23 | Distillers grains with solubles, dried | 5-28-236 | 5.2 | 0.22 | 0.83 | 0.33 | 1.10 | 0.30 | 0.26 | 0.44 | | 8 | | 178 | 27 | 0.39 | 65 | 1.9 |
| | | N | 134 | 649 | 649 | 648 | 648 | 647 | 90 | 278 | | 648 | | 265 | 648 | 12 | 648 | 556 |
| | | SD | 1.15 | 0.10 | 0.14 | 0.07 | 0.23 | 0.27 | 0.10 | 0.15 | | 7 | | 82 | 15 | 0.44 | 19 | 0.5 |
| 24 | Gluten feed, dried | 5-28-243 | 6.8 | 0.07 | 1.00 | 0.42 | 1.46 | 0.13 | 0.20 | 0.44 | | 6 | | 196 | 23 | 0.19 | 75 | 2.2 |
| | | N | 25 | 144 | 144 | 144 | 144 | 83 | 2 | 65 | | 144 | | 144 | 144 | 12 | 144 | 131 |
| | | SD | 1.5 | 0.08 | 0.23 | 0.11 | 0.33 | 0.12 | | 0.09 | | 3 | | 103 | 9 | 0.11 | 16 | 0.7 |
| 25 | Gluten meal, dried | 5-28-242 | 3.3 | 0.06 | 0.60 | 0.14 | 0.46 | 0.05 | 0.11 | 0.86 | | 4 | | 138 | 15 | 0.34 | 49 | 1.1 |
| | | N | 20 | 57 | 57 | 57 | 57 | 57 | 1 | 23 | | 57 | | 57 | 57 | 11 | 57 | 57 |
| | | SD | 1.2 | 0.06 | 0.28 | 0.16 | 0.29 | 0.09 | | 0.17 | | 5 | | 73 | 24 | 0.3 | 59 | 0.8 |
| 26 | Grain, cracked, dry (Data from dry ground corn) | 4-02-854 | 1.5 | 0.04 | 0.30 | 0.12 | 0.42 | 0.02 | 0.08 | 0.10 | | 3 | | 54 | 11 | 0.07 | 27 | 0.8 |
| | | N | | | | | | | | | | | | | | | | |
| | | SD | | | | | | | | | | | | | | | | |
| 27 | Grain, ground, dry | 4-02-854 | 1.5 | 0.04 | 0.30 | 0.12 | 0.42 | 0.02 | 0.08 | 0.10 | | 3 | | 54 | 11 | 0.07 | 27 | 0.8 |
| | | | 567 | 1185 | 1185 | 1185 | 1185 | 554 | 143 | 322 | | 572 | | 572 | 327 | 45.00 | 327 | 542.0 |
| | | | 0.5 | 0.07 | 0.05 | 0.03 | 0.06 | 0.08 | 0.07 | 0.01 | | 4 | | 53 | 24 | 0.05 | 20 | 0.5 |
| 28 | Grain, steam-flaked (Data from dry ground corn) | 4-02-854 | 1.5 | 0.04 | 0.30 | 0.12 | 0.42 | 0.02 | 0.08 | 0.10 | | 3 | | 54 | 11 | 0.07 | 27 | 0.8 |
| 29 | Grain, rolled, high moisture (Data from ground high moisture corn) | 4-28-265 | 1.5 | 0.03 | 0.30 | 0.12 | 0.43 | 0.01 | 0 05 | 0.10 | | 1 | | 59 | 7 | 0.07 | 21 | 0.7 |
| | | N | | | | | | | | | | | | | | | | |
| | | SD | | | | | | | | | | | | | | | | |
| 30 | Grain, ground, high moisture | 4-28-265 | 1.5 | 0.03 | 0.30 | 0.12 | 0.43 | 0.01 | 0.05 | 0.10 | | 1 | | 59 | 7 | 0.07 | 21 | 0.7 |
| | | | 2544 | 4633 | 4633 | 4633 | 4633 | 439 | 107 | 1317 | | 853 | | 853 | 853 | | 853 | 694 |
| | | | 0.6 | 0.03 | 0.03 | 0.03 | 0.06 | 0.01 | 0.01 | 0.01 | | 1 | | 87 | 3 | | 5 | 0.4 |
| 31 | Grain and cob, dry, ground | 4-02-849 | 1.7 | 0.06 | 0.29 | 0.13 | 0.49 | 0.03 | 0.07 | 0.10 | | 3 | | 91 | 10 | 0.07 | 27 | 0.8 |
| | | N | 83 | 158 | 158 | 158 | 158 | 55 | 2 | 48 | | 54 | | 54 | 54 | | 54 | 52.0 |
| | | SD | 0.5 | 0.09 | 0.07 | 0.04 | 0.14 | 0.16 | | 0.01 | | 1 | | 71 | 6 | | 9 | 0.5 |
| 32 | Grain and cob, high moisture | 4-26-240 | 1.7 | 0.05 | 0.28 | 0.12 | 0.48 | 0.01 | 0.07 | 0.09 | | 3 | | 68 | 9 | 0.07 | 22 | 0.7 |
| | | N | 1381 | 2608 | 2608 | 2608 | 2608 | 470 | 54 | 907 | | 599 | | 599 | 599 | | 599 | 470 |
| | | SD | 0.28 | 0.03 | 0.03 | 0.01 | 0.07 | 0.03 | 0.03 | 0.01 | | 2 | | 60 | 4 | | 5 | 0.4 |
| 33 | Hominy | 4-02-887 | 2.7 | 0.03 | 0.65 | 0.26 | 0.82 | 0.01 | 0.10 | 0.12 | | 3 | | 87 | 14 | | 49 | 1.2 |
| | | N | 118 | 287 | 287 | 287 | 287 | 287 | 58 | 141 | | 287 | | 287 | 287 | | 287 | 287 |
| | | SD | 1.1 | 0.03 | 0.29 | 0.12 | 0.34 | 0.01 | 0.08 | 0.02 | | 1 | | 77 | 9 | | 21 | 0.6 |
| 34 | Silage, immature <25% DM | 3-28-247 | 4.8 | 0.29 | 0.24 | 0.19 | 1.30 | 0.01 | 0.30 | 0.14 | | 6 | | 157 | 46 | 0.04 | 29 | |
| | | N | 69 | 70 | 70 | 70 | 70 | 20 | 20 | | | 56 | | 55 | 56 | | 56 | |
| | | SD | 2.1 | 0.10 | 0.10 | 0.10 | 0.50 | 0.01 | 0.15 | | | 2 | | 130 | 18 | | 10 | |
| 35 | Silage, normal 32-38% DM | 3-28-248 | 4.3 | 0.28 | 0.26 | 0.17 | 1.20 | 0.01 | 0.29 | 0.14 | | 6 | | 104 | 36 | 0.04 | 24 | |
| | | N | 1027 | 1033 | 1033 | 1033 | 1033 | 6991 | 468 | 27 | | 912 | | 909 | 914 | 11 | 915 | |
| | | SD | 1 | 0.10 | 0.04 | 0.04 | 0.30 | 0.01 | 0.10 | 0.02 | | 7 | | 109 | 19 | 0.02 | 8 | |
| 36 | Silage, mature >40% DM | 3-28-249 | 4.0 | 0.26 | 0.25 | 0.16 | 1.10 | 0.01 | 0.17 | 0.10 | | 6 | | 92 | 36 | 0.04 | 23 | |
| | | N | 704 | 705 | 705 | 705 | 705 | 11 | 11 | 10 | | 622 | | 622 | 622 | | 624 | |
| | | SD | 1.3 | 0.10 | 0.04 | 0.04 | 0.30 | 0.00 | 0.06 | 0.01 | | 2 | | 79 | 17 | | 7 | |
| | COTTON SEED | | | | | | | | | | | | | | | | | |
| 37 | Whole seeds with lint | 5-01-614 | 4.2 | 0.17 | 0.60 | 0.37 | 1.13 | 0.02 | 0.06 | 0.23 | | 7 | | 94 | 18 | 0.14 | 37 | 1.3 |
| | | N | 193 | 928 | 928 | 928 | 928 | 928 | 148 | 424 | | 928 | | 928 | 928 | 9 | 928 | 919 |
| | | SD | 2.1 | 0.08 | 0.08 | 0.04 | 0.07 | 0.02 | 0.03 | 0.04 | | 3 | | 185 | 13 | 0.11 | 18 | 0.6 |

*(continues)*

TABLE 15-3 *(continued)*

| Entry No. | Feed Name/Description | International Feed No. | Ash % | Ca % | P % | Mg % | K % | Na % | Cl % | S % | Co mg/kg | Cu mg/kg | I mg/kg | Fe mg/kg | Mn mg/kg | Se mg/kg | Zn mg/kg | Mo mg/kg |
|---|---|---|---|---|---|---|---|---|---|---|---|---|---|---|---|---|---|---|
| 38 | Hulls | 1-01-599 | 2.8 | 0.18 | 0.12 | 0.17 | 1.16 | 0.02 | 0.06 | 0.07 | | 5 | | 68 | 22 | | 17 | 0.8 |
| | | N | 75 | 118 | 118 | 112 | 113 | 109 | 11 | 68 | | 106 | | 107 | 102 | | 105 | 102 |
| | | SD | 0.5 | 0.10 | 0.06 | 0.04 | 0.07 | 0.03 | 0.03 | 0.03 | | 3 | | 61 | 8 | | 11 | 0.5 |
| 39 | Meal, solvent, 41% CP | 5-01-630 | 6.7 | 0.20 | 1.15 | 0.61 | 1.64 | 0.07 | 0.07 | 0.40 | | 14 | | 149 | 24 | 0.30 | 67 | 3 |
| | | N | 44 | 185 | 185 | 65 | 185 | 97 | 3 | 30 | | 59 | | 60 | 61 | 2 | 55 | 18.0 |
| | | SD | 0.7 | 0.10 | 0.10 | 0.11 | 0.38 | 0.06 | | 0.11 | | 3 | | 47 | 11 | | 15 | 0.8 |
| | FATS AND OILS | | | | | | | | | | | | | | | | | |
| 40 | Calcium soaps | IFN | 15.5 | 12.00 | 0 | 0 | 0 | 0 | 0 | 0 | 0 | 0 | 0 | 0 | 0 | 0 | 0 | 0 |
| | | N | | | | | | | | | | | | | | | | |
| | | SD | | | | | | | | | | | | | | | | |
| 41 | Hydrolyzed tallow fatty acids | IFN | 0 | 0 | 0 | 0 | 0 | 0 | 0 | 0 | 0 | 0 | 0 | 0 | 0 | 0 | 0 | 0 |
| | | N | | | | | | | | | | | | | | | | |
| | | SD | | | | | | | | | | | | | | | | |
| 42 | Partially hydrogenated tallow | IFN | 0 | 0 | 0 | 0 | 0 | 0 | 0 | 0 | 0 | 0 | 0 | 0 | 0 | 0 | 0 | 0 |
| | | N | | | | | | | | | | | | | | | | |
| | | SD | | | | | | | | | | | | | | | | |
| 43 | Tallow | IFN | 0 | 0 | 0 | 0 | 0 | 0 | 0 | 0 | 0 | 0 | 0 | 0 | 0 | 0 | 0 | 0 |
| | | N | | | | | | | | | | | | | | | | |
| | | SD | | | | | | | | | | | | | | | | |
| 44 | Vegetable oil | 4-05-077 | 0 | 0 | 0 | 0 | 0 | 0 | 0 | 0 | 0 | 0 | 0 | 0 | 0 | 0 | 0 | 0 |
| | | N | | | | | | | | | | | | | | | | |
| | | SD | | | | | | | | | | | | | | | | |
| | FEATHERS | | | | | | | | | | | | | | | | | |
| 45 | Meal | | 3.5 | 0.33 | 0.50 | 0.22 | 0.33 | 0.34 | 0.26 | 1.39 | 0.04 | 10 | 0.04 | 76 | 10 | 0.69 | 111 | |
| | | N | | | | | | | | | | | | | | | | |
| | | SD | | | | | | | | | | | | | | | | |
| 46 | Meal with some viscera | 5-13-540 | 5.5 | 1.36 | 0.77 | 0.06 | 0.24 | 0.27 | 0.47 | 1.75 | | 12 | | 625 | 12 | 0.69 | 100 | 0.8 |
| | | N | 12 | 29 | 29 | 29 | 29 | 29 | 1 | 24 | | 29 | | 29 | 29 | 1 | 29 | 29 |
| | | SD | 2.1 | 1.75 | 0.90 | 0.05 | 0.13 | 0.14 | | 0.50 | | 6 | | 372 | 36 | | 9 | 0.5 |
| | FESCUE *Festuca sp.* | See GRASSES, COOL SEASON | | | | | | | | | | | | | | | | |
| | FISH BYPRODUCTS | | | | | | | | | | | | | | | | | |
| 47 | Anchovy, meal, mech. | 5-01-985 | 16.0 | 4.06 | 2.69 | 0.27 | 0.79 | 0.96 | 0.80 | 0.78 | | 10 | 3.41 | 234 | 12 | 1.47 | 114 | 0.2 |
| | | N | 47 | 51 | 52 | 32 | 35 | 32 | | 4 | | 27 | 2 | 28 | 31 | 27 | 31 | 1 |
| | | SD | 1.5 | 0.54 | 0.45 | 0.05 | 0.27 | 0.33 | | 0.23 | | 2 | | 63 | 6 | 0.25 | 17 | |
| 48 | Menhaden, meal, mech. | 5-02-009 | 19.7 | 5.34 | 3.05 | 0.20 | 0.74 | 0.68 | 0.80 | 1.16 | | 7 | 1.19 | 562 | 32 | 2.26 | 112 | 1.8 |
| | | N | 113 | 112 | 111 | 63 | 65 | 66 | 2 | 34 | | 64 | 2 | 65 | 65 | 30 | 62 | 46 |
| | | SD | 2.4 | 1.15 | 0.53 | 0.05 | 0.25 | 0.27 | | 1.01 | | 4 | | 354 | 23 | 1.5 | 24 | 0.9 |
| | GRASSES, COOL SEASON | | | | | | | | | | | | | | | | | |
| 49 | Pasture, intensively managed | 2-02-260 | 9.8 | 0.56 | 0.44 | 0.20 | 3.36 | 0.02 | 0.56 | 0.20 | | 10 | | 275 | 75 | | 36 | |
| | | N | 13 | 13 | 13 | 13 | 13 | 1 | | | | 13 | | 13 | 13 | | 13 | |
| | | SD | 1.2 | 0.15 | 0.06 | 0.03 | 0.49 | | | | | 3 | | 209 | 36 | | 6 | |
| 50 | Hay, all samples | 1-02-250 | 7 | 0.58 | 0.23 | 0.20 | 2.01 | 0.04 | 0.50 | 0.21 | | 9 | | 156 | 72 | 0.06 | 31 | 1.5 |
| | | N | 1791 | 4653 | 4653 | 4653 | 4653 | 1321 | 161 | 1448 | | 1321 | | 1321 | 1321 | 5 | 1321 | 1321 |
| | | SD | 1.5 | 0.23 | 0.06 | 0.05 | 0.53 | 0.08 | 0.32 | 0.06 | | 6 | | 157 | 52 | 0.06 | 30 | 1 |
| 51 | Hay, immature <55% NDF | 1-02-212 | 9.2 | 0.72 | 0.34 | 0.23 | 2.57 | 0.03 | 0.42 | 0.24 | | 9 | | 199 | 84 | 0.06 | 27 | |
| | | N | 34 | 42 | 42 | 42 | 42 | 4 | 3 | 5 | | 8 | | 8 | 8 | | 8 | |
| | | SD | 1.1 | 0.23 | 0.07 | 0.06 | 0.56 | 0.03 | 0.49 | 0.03 | | 3 | | 93 | 20 | | 8 | |
| 52 | Hay, mid-maturity 55-60% NDF | 1-02-243 | 8.8 | 0.66 | 0.29 | 0.23 | 2.13 | 0.08 | 0.92 | 0.24 | | 9 | | 194 | 72 | 0.06 | 25 | |
| | | N | 50 | 54 | 54 | 54 | 54 | 8 | 1 | 7 | | 23 | | 23 | 23 | | 23 | |
| | | SD | 1.6 | 0.23 | 0.13 | 0.11 | 0.72 | 0.06 | | 0.15 | | 4 | | 146 | 26 | | 7 | |
| 53 | Hay, mature >60% NDF | 1-02-244 | 7.0 | 0.47 | 0.26 | 0.18 | 1.97 | 0.02 | 0.66 | 0.17 | | 8 | | 180 | 90 | 0.06 | 25 | |
| | | N | 399 | 413 | 413 | 413 | 413 | 51 | 49 | 56 | | 342 | | 342 | 342 | | 342 | |
| | | SD | 1.7 | 0.18 | 0.07 | 0.08 | 0.59 | 0.06 | 0.67 | 0.04 | | 3 | | 233 | 51 | | 8 | |
| 54 | Silage, all samples | 3-02-222 | 8.1 | 0.55 | 0.29 | 0.23 | 2.54 | 0.05 | 0.67 | 0.21 | | 9 | | 331 | 74 | 0.09 | 30 | 2.2 |
| | | N | 988 | 4365 | 4365 | 4365 | 4365 | 839 | 118 | 1388 | | 879 | | 879 | 879 | 3 | 879 | 879 |
| | | SD | 2.1 | 0.28 | 0.08 | 0.05 | 0.73 | 0.07 | 0.38 | 0.05 | | 3 | | 324 | 47 | | 12 | 1.4 |
| 55 | Silage, immature <55% NDF | 3-02-217 | 9.9 | 0.57 | 0.36 | 0.22 | 3.11 | 0.05 | 0.67 | 0.21 | | 9 | | 280 | 56 | 0.09 | 31 | |
| | | N | 34 | 35 | 35 | 35 | 35 | | | | | 11 | | 11 | 11 | | 11 | |
| | | SD | 1.8 | 0.19 | 0.07 | 0.05 | 0.62 | | | | | 3 | | 159 | 20 | | 10 | |
| 56 | Silage, mid-maturity 55-60% NDF | 3-02-218 | 8.7 | 0.60 | 0.36 | 0.21 | 2.78 | 0.05 | 0.67 | 0.21 | | 9 | | 275 | 79 | 0.09 | 31 | |
| | | N | 41 | 41 | 41 | 41 | 41 | | | | | 35 | | 35 | 35 | | 35 | |
| | | SD | 1.5 | 0.21 | 0.07 | 0.04 | 0.71 | | | | | 2 | | 181 | 35 | | 9 | |

*(continues)*

TABLE 15-3 *(continued)*

| Entry No. | Feed Name/Description | International Feed No. | Ash % | Ca % | P % | Mg % | K % | Na % | Cl % | S % | Co mg/kg | Cu mg/kg | I mg/kg | Fe mg/kg | Mn mg/kg | Se mg/kg | Zn mg/kg | Mo mg/kg |
|---|---|---|---|---|---|---|---|---|---|---|---|---|---|---|---|---|---|---|
| 57 | Silage, mature >60% NDF | 3-02-219 | 8.0 | 0.56 | 0.31 | 0.20 | 2.42 | 0.05 | 0.89 | 0.20 | | 9 | | 327 | 90 | 0.09 | 30 | |
| | | N | 135 | 135 | 135 | 135 | 135 | | 5 | 7 | | 128 | | 127 | 128 | | 128 | |
| | | SD | 1.8 | 0.20 | 0.07 | 0.06 | 0.72 | | 0.32 | 0.04 | | 3 | | 396 | 45 | | 8 | |
| | GRASS-LEGUME MIXTURES Predominantly Grass (17-22% Hemicellulose) | | | | | | | | | | | | | | | | | |
| 58 | Hay, immature <51% NDF | 1-02-275 | 9.2 | 1.01 | 0.31 | 0.26 | 2.83 | 0.03 | 0.74 | 0.28 | | 9 | | 117 | 53 | 0.09 | 25 | |
| | | N | 21 | 21 | 21 | 21 | 21 | | | | | 14 | | 14 | 14 | | 14 | |
| | | SD | 1.2 | 0.32 | 0.06 | 0.08 | 0.65 | | | | | 3 | | 110 | 17 | | 3 | |
| 59 | Hay, mid maturity 51-57% NDF | 1-02-277 | 9.5 | 0.88 | 0.36 | 0.25 | 2.45 | 0.01 | 0.77 | 0.27 | | 9 | | 358 | 75 | 0.09 | 26 | |
| | | N | 155 | 155 | 155 | 155 | 155 | 52 | 9 | 3 | | 124 | | 124 | 124 | | 124 | |
| | | SD | 1.7 | 0.22 | 0.07 | 0.05 | 0.74 | 0.01 | 0.41 | 0.02 | | 2 | | 302 | 20 | | 5 | |
| 60 | Hay, mature >57% NDF | 1-02-280 | 7.9 | 0.73 | 0.27 | 0.21 | 2.09 | 0.10 | 0.71 | 0.29 | | 8 | | 124 | 74 | 0.09 | 24 | |
| | | N | 149 | 149 | 149 | 149 | 149 | 14 | 8 | 9 | | 98 | | 98 | 98 | | 98 | |
| | | SD | 1.4 | 0.73 | 0.06 | 0.06 | 0.66 | 0.21 | 0.50 | 0.04 | | 3 | | 271 | 46 | | 5 | |
| 61 | Silage, immature <51% NDF | 3-02-302 | 9.1 | 1.02 | 0.34 | 0.25 | 2.88 | 0.03 | 0.74 | 0.27 | | 9 | | 234 | 74 | 0.11 | 27 | |
| | | N | 18 | 18 | 18 | 18 | 18 | | | | | 17 | | 17 | 17 | | 17 | |
| | | SD | 1.3 | 0.31 | 0.05 | 0.05 | 0.44 | | | | | 2 | | 217 | 31 | | 5 | |
| 62 | Silage, mid-maturity 51-57% NDF | 3-02-265 | 9.5 | 0.89 | 0.36 | 0.26 | 2.64 | 0.01 | 0.45 | 0.25 | | 9 | | 264 | 78 | 0.11 | 30 | |
| | | N | 95 | 95 | 95 | 95 | 95 | | 2 | 3 | | 85 | | 85 | 85 | | 85 | |
| | | SD | 1.6 | 0.26 | 0.06 | 0.07 | 0.73 | | | 0.02 | | 2 | | 325 | 30 | | 8 | |
| 63 | Silage, mature >57% NDF | 3-02-266 | 9.0 | 0.85 | 0.33 | 0.23 | 2.51 | 0.10 | 0.90 | 0.34 | | 9 | | 241 | 73 | 0.11 | 28 | |
| | | N | 166 | 166 | 166 | 166 | 166 | | 4 | | | 151 | | 151 | 151 | | 151 | |
| | | SD | 1.5 | 0.22 | 0.06 | 0.06 | 0.61 | | 0.33 | | | 2 | | 321 | 35 | | 6 | |
| | Mixed Grass and Legume (12-15% Hemicellulose) | | | | | | | | | | | | | | | | | |
| 64 | Hay, immature <47% NDF | 1-02-275 | 8.8 | 1.20 | 0.31 | 0.29 | 3.06 | 0.07 | 0.50 | 0.27 | | 10 | | 160 | 59 | 0.12 | 24 | |
| | | N | 42 | 42 | 42 | 42 | 42 | 3 | 1 | 6.00 | | 27 | | 27 | 27 | | 27 | |
| | | SD | 0.9 | 0.26 | 0.04 | 0.06 | 0.62 | 0.06 | | 0.10 | | 3 | | 452 | 18 | | 8 | |
| 65 | Hay, mid-maturity 47-53% NDF | 1-02-277 | 9.3 | 1.04 | 0.32 | 0.25 | 2.59 | 0.03 | 0.80 | 0.24 | | 9 | | 197 | 59 | 0.12 | 25 | |
| | | N | 184 | 184 | 184 | 184 | 184 | 23 | 3 | 11 | | 115 | | 115 | 115 | | 115 | |
| | | SD | 1.4 | 0.18 | 0.06 | 0.05 | 0.64 | 0.06 | 0.24 | 0.03 | | 2 | | 247 | 20 | | 5 | |
| 66 | Hay, mature >53% NDF | 1-02-280 | 9.9 | 0.97 | 0.37 | 0.26 | 2.24 | 0.01 | 0.93 | 0.28 | | 9 | | 403 | 75 | 0.12 | 27 | |
| | | N | 233 | 233 | 233 | 233 | 233 | 128 | 16 | 6 | | 195 | | 195 | 195 | | 195 | |
| | | SD | 1.6 | 0.17 | 0.08 | 0.04 | 0.85 | 0.01 | 0.14 | 0.04 | | 2 | | 249 | 19 | | 5 | |
| 67 | Silage, immature <47% NDF | 3-02-302 | 9.8 | 1.08 | 0.35 | 0.28 | 2.89 | 0.01 | 1.77 | 0.16 | | 9 | | 328 | 71 | 0.14 | 29 | |
| | | N | 45 | 45 | 45 | 45 | 45 | 1 | 1 | 3 | | 2 | | 36 | 36 | | 36 | |
| | | SD | 1.7 | 0.30 | 0.06 | 0.07 | 0.72 | | | 0.05 | | 36 | | 202 | 25 | | 7 | |
| 68 | Silage, mid-maturity 47-53% NDF | 3-02-265 | 10.1 | 1.09 | 0.35 | 0.27 | 2.80 | 0.01 | 1.10 | 0.26 | | 9 | | 252 | 71 | 0.14 | 31 | |
| | | N | 171 | 171 | 171 | 171 | 171 | 1 | 2 | 9 | | 139 | | 139 | 139 | | 139 | |
| | | SD | 1.5 | 0.26 | 0.05 | 0.06 | 0.63 | | | 0.10 | | 3 | | 219 | 26 | | 9 | |
| 69 | Silage, mature <47% NDF | 3-02-266 | 9.6 | 1.06 | 0.33 | 0.24 | 2.70 | 0.02 | 0.52 | 0.31 | | 9 | | 262 | 72 | 0.14 | 30 | |
| | | N | 255 | 255 | 255 | 255 | 255 | 2 | 3 | 5 | | 210 | | 210 | 210 | | 210 | |
| | | SD | 1.3 | 0.27 | 0.05 | 0.06 | 0.59 | | 0.30 | 0.07 | | 2 | | 317 | 26 | | 13 | |
| | Predominantly Legume (10-13.5% Hemicellulose) | | | | | | | | | | | | | | | | | |
| 70 | Hay, immature <44% NDF | 1-02-275 | 9.2 | 1.30 | 0.30 | 0.30 | 2.41 | 0.03 | 0.60 | 0.20 | | 10 | | 167 | 58 | 0.15 | 24 | |
| | | N | 157 | 157 | 157 | 157 | 157 | | | 4.00 | | 40 | | 40 | 40 | | 40 | |
| | | SD | 1.4 | 0.18 | 0.04 | 0.06 | 0.49 | | | 0.06 | | 6 | | 165 | 18 | | 6 | |
| 71 | Hay, mid-maturity 44-50% NDF | 1-02-277 | 9.1 | 1.17 | 0.30 | 0.27 | 2.34 | 0.08 | 0.43 | 0.26 | | 9 | | 141 | 49 | 0.15 | 24 | |
| | | N | 296 | 296 | 296 | 296 | 296 | 8 | 1 | 13 | | 103 | | 103 | 103 | | 103 | |
| | | SD | 1.2 | 0.15 | 0.04 | 0.06 | 0.46 | 0.03 | | 0.02 | | 3 | | 131 | 16 | | 6 | |
| 72 | Hay, mature >50% NDF | 1-02-280 | 8.7 | 1.09 | 0.28 | 0.25 | 2.23 | 0.01 | 0.21 | 0.26 | | 8 | | 141 | 43 | 0.15 | 24 | |
| | | N | 134 | 134 | 134 | 134 | 134 | 2 | 2 | 15 | | 60 | | 60 | 60 | | 60 | |
| | | SD | 1.4 | 0.17 | 0.04 | 0.04 | 0.51 | 0.01 | | 0.04 | | 2 | | 299 | 15 | | 6 | |
| 73 | Silage, immature <44% NDF | 3-02-302 | 11.5 | 1.16 | 0.36 | 0.30 | 2.95 | 0.01 | 0.60 | 0.32 | | 11 | | 279 | 70 | 0.17 | 36 | |
| | | N | 193 | 193 | 193 | 193 | 193 | 4 | | 4 | | 31 | | 31 | 31 | | 31 | |
| | | SD | 2.1 | 0.20 | 0.05 | 0.06 | 0.61 | 0.07 | | 0.09 | | 4 | | 206 | 20 | | 15 | |

*(continues)*

TABLE 15-3 *(continued)*

| Entry No. | Feed Name/Description | International Feed No. | Ash % | Ca % | P % | Mg % | K % | Na % | Cl % | S % | Co mg/kg | Cu mg/kg | I mg/kg | Fe mg/kg | Mn mg/kg | Se mg/kg | Zn mg/kg | Mo mg/kg |
|---|---|---|---|---|---|---|---|---|---|---|---|---|---|---|---|---|---|---|
| 74 | Silage, mid-maturity 44-50% NDF | 3-02-265 | 10.8 | 1.14 | 0.34 | 0.28 | 2.88 | 0.01 | 0.60 | 0.25 | | 9 | | 244 | 64 | 0.17 | 28 | |
| | | N | 504 | 505 | 505 | 505 | 505 | 5 | | 17 | | 185 | | 185 | 185 | | 185 | |
| | | SD | 1.6 | 0.21 | 0.04 | 0.06 | 0.52 | 0.08 | | 0.06 | | 2 | | 231 | 21 | | 6 | |
| 75 | Silage, mature >50% NDF | 3-02-266 | 10.2 | 1.17 | 0.33 | 0.26 | 2.77 | 0.03 | 0.60 | 0.26 | | 9 | | 339 | 66 | 0.17 | 29 | |
| | | N | 339 | 339 | 339 | 339 | 339 | 4 | | 13 | | 240 | | 240 | 240 | | 240 | |
| | | SD | 1.8 | 0.24 | 0.06 | 0.06 | 0.60 | 0.03 | | 0.04 | | 3 | | 379 | 23 | | 8 | |
| | LEGUMES, FORAGE | | | | | | | | | | | | | | | | | |
| 76 | Pasture, intensively managed | 2-29-431 | 10 | 1.31 | 0.37 | 0.28 | 3.21 | 0.01 | 0.60 | 0.31 | 0.44 | 10 | | 215 | 54 | 0.20 | 33 | 2.3 |
| | | N | 11 | 24 | 24 | 24 | 24 | 11 | 1 | 7 | 6 | 20 | | 20 | 20 | | 20 | 11 |
| | | SD | 1.4 | 0.36 | 0.08 | 0.09 | 0.94 | 0.11 | | 0.06 | 0.05 | 5 | | 120 | 27 | | 8 | 1.7 |
| 77 | Hay, all samples | 1-20-648 | 10.0 | 1.52 | 0.26 | 0.30 | 2.53 | 0.01 | 0.74 | 0.25 | 0.65 | 9 | | 286 | 35 | 0.20 | 24 | 2.9 |
| | | N | 4527 | 11212 | 11272 | 11212 | 11212 | 4242 | 565 | 4250 | 38 | 4242 | | 4242 | 4242 | 902 | 4242 | 4242 |
| | | SD | 1.2 | 0.27 | 0.05 | 0.06 | 0.49 | 0.12 | 0.39 | 0.05 | 0.34 | 4 | | 270 | 13 | 0.18 | 19 | 1.6 |
| 78 | Hay, immature <40% NDF | 1-07-792 | 9.5 | 1.56 | 0.31 | 0.33 | 2.56 | 0.03 | 0.55 | 0.33 | 0.65 | 10 | | 213 | 49 | 0.20 | 26 | |
| | | N | 159 | 210 | 210 | 210 | 210 | | | 41 | | 42 | | 42 | 42 | | 42 | |
| | | SD | 1.3 | 0.27 | 0.04 | 0.06 | 0.47 | | | 0.06 | | 2 | | 135 | 17 | | 6 | |
| 79 | Hay, mid-maturity 40- 46% NDF | 1-07-788 | 9.4 | 1.37 | 0.30 | 0.30 | 2.45 | 0.02 | 0.61 | 0.31 | 0.65 | 9 | | 207 | 46 | 0.20 | 24 | |
| | | N | 262 | 296 | 296 | 296 | 296 | | | 26 | | 56 | | 56 | 56 | | 56 | |
| | | SD | 1.1 | 0.20 | 0.04 | 0.06 | 0.41 | | | 0.07 | | 2 | | 113 | 14 | | 5 | |
| 80 | Hay, mature >46% NDF | 1-07-789 | 9.2 | 1.22 | 0.28 | 0.27 | 2.38 | 0.02 | 0.48 | 0.23 | 0.65 | 9 | | 250 | 44 | 0.2 | 24 | |
| | | N | 205 | 237 | 237 | 237 | 237 | | | 21 | | 53 | | 53 | 53 | | 53 | |
| | | SD | 1.6 | 0.21 | 0.04 | 0.05 | 0.49 | | | 0.08 | | 2 | | 299 | 17 | | 6 | |
| 81 | Silage, all samples | 3-07-796 | 10.4 | 1.34 | 0.32 | 0.27 | 2.87 | 0.06 | 0.62 | 0.24 | 0.65 | 10 | | 367 | 50 | 0.18 | 29 | 2.4 |
| | | N | 5183 | 8479 | 8479 | 8479 | 8479 | 2729 | 374 | 3255 | 2 | 2729 | | 2729 | 2729 | 199 | 2729 | 2729 |
| | | SD | 1.7 | 0.26 | 0.06 | 0.05 | 0.59 | 0.09 | 0.33 | 0.04 | 0.15 | 3 | | 490 | 22 | 0.17 | 8 | 1.3 |
| 82 | Silage, immature <40% NDF | 3-07-795 | 11.1 | 1.39 | 0.36 | 0.30 | 3.03 | 0.03 | 0.55 | 0.30 | 0.65 | 9 | | 401 | 67 | 0.18 | 31 | |
| | | N | 322 | 322 | 322 | 322 | 322 | 36 | 36 | 16 | | 171 | | 171 | 171 | | 171 | |
| | | SD | 1.5 | 0.21 | 0.05 | 0.06 | 0.57 | 0.02 | 0.30 | 0.06 | | 3 | | 353 | 24 | | 7 | |
| 83 | Silage, mid-maturity 40-46% NDF | 3-07-797 | 10.8 | 1.36 | 0.35 | 0.28 | 3.00 | 0.02 | 0.61 | 0.28 | 0.65 | 9 | | 395 | 64 | 0.18 | 30 | |
| | | N | 749 | 750 | 750 | 750 | 750 | 48 | 48 | 20 | | 607 | | 610 | 610 | | 610 | |
| | | SD | 1.5 | 0.23 | 0.05 | 0.05 | 0.56 | 0.01 | 0.41 | 0.05 | | 3 | | 311 | 26 | | 8 | |
| 84 | Silage, mature >46% NDF | 3-07-798 | 10.3 | 1.3 | 0.33 | 0.26 | 2.87 | 0.02 | 0.48 | 0.28 | 0.65 | 9 | | 403 | 63 | 0.18 | 29 | |
| | | N | 731 | 731 | 731 | 731 | 731 | 81 | 81 | 9 | | 607 | | 610 | 610 | | 610 | |
| | | SD | 1.6 | 0.23 | 0.05 | 0.05 | 0.58 | 0.01 | 0.3 | 0.05 | | 2 | | 311 | 26 | | 8 | |
| 85 | LINSEED (Flax) Meal, solvent | 5-30-288 | 6.5 | 0.40 | 0.83 | 0.55 | 1.22 | 0.09 | | 0.37 | | 19 | | 369 | 39 | 1.05 | 69 | 2.0 |
| | | N | 1 | 5 | 5 | 5 | 5 | 5 | | 2 | | 5 | | 5 | 5 | 10 | 5 | 5 |
| | | SD | | | | | | | | | | | | | | 0.63 | | 0.6 |
| | MEAT | | | | | | | | | | | | | | | | | |
| 86 | Meal, rendered | 5-09-323 | 22.9 | 8.86 | 4.20 | 0.26 | 0.49 | 0.78 | 0.44 | 0.51 | | 21 | | 701 | 26 | 0.45 | 114 | 2.4 |
| | | N | 12 | 62 | 62 | 62 | 62 | 62 | | 29 | | 62 | | 62 | 10 | 34 | 10 | 62 |
| | | SD | 5.6 | 2.58 | 1.14 | 0.27 | 0.16 | 0.31 | | 0.13 | | 8 | | 560 | 33 | 0.68 | 82 | 1.9 |
| 87 | Meat and bone, rendered | 5-00-388 | 30.4 | 10.60 | 4.73 | 0.24 | 1.02 | 0.71 | 0.44 | 0.39 | | 10 | | 602 | 22 | | 94 | 2.7 |
| | | N | 13 | 51 | 51 | 51 | 51 | 51 | 2 | 13 | | 51 | | 51 | 51 | | 51 | 51 |
| | | SD | 7.5 | 2.35 | 1.06 | 0.05 | 0.12 | 0.16 | | 0.08 | | 4 | | 322 | 8 | | 17 | 2.3 |
| | MOLASSES | | | | | | | | | | | | | | | | | |
| 88 | Beet sugar | 4-00-668 | 11.4 | 0.15 | 0.03 | 0.29 | 6.06 | 1.48 | | 0.60 | | 22 | | 87 | 66 | | 18 | 0.5 |
| | | N | 9 | 13 | 11 | 10 | 10 | 8 | | 9 | | 7 | | 8 | 7 | | 5 | 1 |
| | | SD | 1.3 | 0.05 | 0.01 | 0.01 | 0.29 | 0.08 | | 0.05 | | 1 | | 25 | 12 | | 0 | |
| 89 | Sugarcane | 4-04-696 | 13.3 | 1.00 | 0.10 | 0.42 | 4.01 | 0.22 | | 0.47 | | 66 | | 263 | 59 | | 21 | 1.6 |
| | | N | 52 | 32 | 31 | 12 | 16 | 9 | | 9 | | 8 | | 11 | 11 | | 5 | 4 |
| | | SD | 2.3 | 0.18 | 0.02 | 0.10 | 0.88 | 0.02 | | 0.02 | | 26 | | 34 | 6 | | 6 | 0.7 |
| | OATS | | | | | | | | | | | | | | | | | |
| 90 | Grain, rolled | 4-03-309 | 3.3 | 0.11 | 0.40 | 0.16 | 0.52 | 0.03 | | 0.19 | 0.06 | 8 | | 106 | 43 | 0.48 | 41 | 1.7 |
| | | N | 104 | 221 | 228 | 205 | 204 | 101 | | 30 | 8 | 183 | | 184 | 193 | 68 | 196 | 156 |
| | | SD | 0.5 | 0.05 | 0.06 | 0.02 | 0.09 | 0.07 | | 0.02 | 0.02 | 4 | | 62 | 16 | 0.30 | 10 | 0.7 |
| 91 | Hay, headed | 1-09-099 | 8.5 | 0.37 | 0.22 | 0.17 | 2.01 | 0.33 | 1.08 | 0.14 | | 8 | | 250 | 59 | | 23 | 1.6 |
| | | N | 22 | 403 | 403 | 403 | 403 | 403 | 51 | 180 | | 403 | | 403 | 403 | | 403 | 403 |
| | | SD | 4.0 | 0.22 | 0.07 | 0.06 | 0.71 | 0.28 | 0.51 | 0.06 | | 3 | | 370 | 28 | | 27 | 1.0 |
| 92 | Silage, headed | 3-21-843 | 9.8 | 0.52 | 0.31 | 0.20 | 2.89 | 0.24 | 1.34 | 0.19 | | 9 | | 500 | 66 | | 29 | 2.2 |
| | | N | 182 | 615 | 615 | 615 | 615 | 207 | 28 | 194 | | 212 | | 212 | 212 | | 212 | 212 |
| | | SD | 2.3 | 0.21 | 0.07 | 0.05 | 0.77 | 0.30 | 0.91 | 0.05 | | 4 | | 595 | 30 | | 9 | 1.3 |
| | ORCHARDGRASS *Dactylis glomerata* | see GRASSES, COOL SEASON | | | | | | | | | | | | | | | | |

*(continues)*

TABLE 15-3 *(continued)*

| Entry No. | Feed Name/Description | International Feed No. | Ash % | Ca % | P % | Mg % | K % | Na % | Cl % | S % | Co mg/kg | Cu mg/kg | I mg/kg | Fe mg/kg | Mn mg/kg | Se mg/kg | Zn mg/kg | Mo mg/kg |
|---|---|---|---|---|---|---|---|---|---|---|---|---|---|---|---|---|---|---|
| | PEANUT | | | | | | | | | | | | | | | | | |
| 93 | Meal, solvent | 5-08-605 | 5.8 | 0.20 | 0.64 | 0.32 | 1.32 | 0.03 | 0.10 | 0.32 | | 13 | 0.07 | 302 | 33 | 0.21 | 54 | 3.8 |
| | | N | 11 | 15 | 16 | 14 | 15 | 14 | 1 | 8 | | 14 | 1 | 14 | 14 | 1 | 14 | 14 |
| | | SD | 1.5 | 0.15 | 0.06 | 0.03 | 0.08 | 0.04 | | 0.02 | | 3 | | 115 | 5 | | 11 | 2 |
| | POTATO | | | | | | | | | | | | | | | | | |
| 94 | Byproduct meal | 4-03-775 | 12.8 | 0.49 | 0.29 | 0.11 | 1.04 | 0.26 | 0.19 | 0.11 | | 11 | | 1006 | 26 | | 25 | 1.6 |
| | | N | 22 | 72 | 72 | 72 | 64 | 64 | 5 | 33 | | 72 | | 72 | 72 | | 72 | 64 |
| | | SD | 7.4 | 0.77 | 0.32 | 0.05 | 0.84 | 0.34 | 0.21 | 0.08 | | 10 | | 608 | 20 | | 10 | 1.2 |
| | RICE | | | | | | | | | | | | | | | | | |
| 95 | Bran | 4-03-928 | 10.4 | 0.07 | 1.78 | 0.81 | 1.57 | 0.03 | 0.09 | 0.19 | | 10 | | 239 | 186 | 0.17 | 71 | 2.8 |
| | | N | 69 | 69 | 69 | 61 | 66 | 54 | 2 | 26 | | 57 | | 57 | 23 | 8 | 55 | 32 |
| | | SD | 1.9 | 0.06 | 0.36 | 0.17 | 0.24 | 0.02 | | 0.02 | | 6 | | 266 | 62 | 0.09 | 20 | 0.7 |
| | RYE, ANNUAL | | | | | | | | | | | | | | | | | |
| 96 | Silage, vegetative | 3-21-853 | 9.6 | 0.43 | 0.42 | 0.16 | 3.34 | 0.05 | 0.90 | 0.20 | | 9 | | 373 | 63 | | 32 | 2.0 |
| | | N | 844 | 1155 | 1155 | 1155 | 1155 | 563 | 24 | 240 | | 859 | | 859 | 859 | | 859 | 722 |
| | | SD | 3.9 | 0.16 | 0.08 | 0.10 | 0.66 | 0.08 | 0.51 | 0.05 | | 5 | | 446 | 34 | | 8 | 1.2 |
| | RYEGRASS *Lolium sp.* | see GRASSES, COOL SEASON | | | | | | | | | | | | | | | | |
| | SAFFLOWER | | | | | | | | | | | | | | | | | |
| 97 | Meal, solvent | 5-04-110 | 4.7 | 0.38 | 0.72 | 0.39 | 1.21 | 0.04 | | 0.32 | | 22 | | 319 | 30 | | 77 | 2.3 |
| | | N | 1 | 5 | 5 | 5 | 5 | 5 | | 2 | | 5 | | 5 | 5 | | 5 | 5 |
| | | SD | | 0.04 | 0.08 | 0.04 | 0.06 | 0.04 | | | | 4 | | 53 | 4 | | 5 | 0.8 |
| | SORGHUM, GRAIN TYPE | | | | | | | | | | | | | | | | | |
| 98 | Grain, dry rolled | 4-04-380 | 2 | 0.07 | 0.35 | 0.17 | 0.47 | 0.01 | 0.06 | 0.11 | | 6 | | 89 | 21 | 0.46 | 25 | 1.0 |
| | | N | 74 | 78 | 77 | 75 | 66 | 38 | 7 | 20 | | 64 | | 74 | 72 | 3 | 51 | 38 |
| | | SD | 0.6 | 0.04 | 0.07 | 0.05 | 0.16 | 0.01 | 0.02 | 0.03 | | 2 | | 61 | 4 | 0.58 | 4 | 0.7 |
| 99 | Grain, steam-flaked (Data from dry-rolled sorghum) | 4-04-380 | 2 | 0.07 | 0.35 | 0.17 | 0.47 | 0.01 | 0.06 | 0.11 | | 6 | | 89 | 21 | 0.46 | 25 | 1.0 |
| 100 | Silage | 3-22-371 | 7.5 | 0.50 | 0.21 | 0.27 | 1.75 | 0.02 | 0.60 | 0.12 | | 9 | | 392 | 65 | 0.03 | 31 | 1.9 |
| | | N | 181 | 1097 | 1097 | 1097 | 1097 | 865 | 26 | 317 | | 865 | | 805 | 865 | 2 | 298 | 298 |
| | | SD | 2.9 | 0.26 | 0.08 | 0.09 | 0.70 | 0.04 | 0.19 | 0.03 | | 6 | | 309 | 56 | 0.01 | 18 | 1.4 |
| | SORGHUM, SUDAN TYPE | | | | | | | | | | | | | | | | | |
| 101 | Hay | 1-04-480 | 8.7 | 0.54 | 0.20 | 0.32 | 2.36 | 0.03 | 1.16 | 0.13 | | 10 | | 284 | 44 | | 34 | 2.3 |
| | | N | 172 | 681 | 681 | 681 | 681 | 528 | 102 | 329 | | 528 | | 528 | 528 | | 528 | 528 |
| | | SD | 2.2 | 0.21 | 0.06 | 0.09 | 0.71 | 0.06 | 0.42 | 0.03 | | 5 | | 307 | 11 | | 12 | 0.9 |
| 102 | Silage | 3-04-499 | 10.9 | 0.64 | 0.24 | 0.31 | 2.57 | 0.03 | 0.56 | 0.15 | | 11 | | 990 | 79 | | 33 | 2.7 |
| | | N | 37 | 131 | 131 | 131 | 131 | 63 | 5 | 53 | | 63 | | 63 | 63 | | 63 | 63 |
| | | SD | 3.2 | 0.41 | 0.07 | 0.08 | 0.97 | 0.05 | 0.22 | 0.05 | | 6 | | 796 | 72 | | 15 | 2.2 |
| | SOYBEAN | | | | | | | | | | | | | | | | | |
| 103 | Hulls | 1-04-560 | 4.8 | 0.63 | 0.17 | 0.25 | 1.51 | 0.01 | 0.05 | 0.12 | 0.12 | 10 | | 604 | 26 | 0.21 | 35 | 1.6 |
| | | N | 45 | 81 | 79 | 73 | 71 | 75 | 5 | 37 | 1 | 72 | | 73 | 74 | 4 | 73 | 67 |
| | | SD | 0.7 | 0.07 | 0.07 | 0.03 | 0.14 | 0.02 | 0.03 | 0.04 | | 2 | | 249 | 8 | 0.10 | 6 | 0.7 |
| 104 | Meal, expellers, 45% CP | 5-12-820 | 5.5 | 0.36 | 0.66 | 0.30 | 2.12 | 0.04 | 0.10 | 0.34 | | 17 | 0.12 | 169 | 39 | | 72 | 3.8 |
| | | N | 20 | 64 | 64 | 64 | 64 | 64 | 9 | 15 | | 64 | 1 | 64 | 64 | | 64 | 64 |
| | | SD | 0.9 | 0.23 | 0.08 | 0.17 | 0.39 | 0.04 | 0.09 | 0.06 | | 4 | | 115 | 7 | | 30 | 2 |
| 105 | Meal, nonenzymatically browned | | 6.8 | 0.39 | 0.75 | 0.30 | 2.32 | 0.10 | | 0.40 | | 15 | | 111 | 38 | | 54 | 3.0 |
| | | N | 8 | 14 | 14 | 14 | 14 | 14 | | 14 | | 14 | | 14 | 14 | | 14 | 14 |
| | | SD | 0.6 | 0.08 | 0.05 | 0.01 | 0.08 | 0.03 | | 0.03 | | 1 | | 9 | 6 | | 6 | 0.5 |
| 106 | Meal, solvent, 44% CP | 5-20-637 | 6.6 | 0.40 | 0.71 | 0.31 | 2.22 | 0.04 | 0.13 | 0.46 | | 22 | | 185 | 35 | 0.21 | 57 | 0.1 |
| | | N | 66 | 26 | 29 | 19 | 21 | 12 | | 6 | | 15 | | 15 | 15 | 42 | 13 | 1 |
| | | SD | 0.6 | 0.11 | 0.04 | 0.03 | 0.24 | 0.03 | | 0.04 | | 8 | | 39 | 3 | 0.16 | 7 | |
| 107 | Meal, solvent, 48% CP | 5-20-638 | 6.4 | 0.35 | 0.70 | 0.29 | 2.41 | 0.03 | 0.13 | 0.39 | | 16 | | 206 | 40 | 0.13 | 58 | 5.9 |
| | | N | 119 | 256 | 256 | 243 | 246 | 237 | 96 | 142 | | 243 | | 237 | 237 | 34 | 237 | 237 |
| | | SD | 0.7 | 0.10 | 0.08 | 0.03 | 0.25 | 0.25 | 0.65 | 0.05 | | 4 | | 124 | 12 | 0.19 | 17 | 2.5 |
| 108 | Seeds, whole | 5-04-610 | 5.9 | 0.32 | 0.60 | 0.25 | 1.99 | 0.01 | 0.04 | 0.31 | | 13 | | 148 | 29 | 0.28 | 49 | 3.8 |
| | | N | 7 | 27 | 27 | 27 | 27 | 27 | 2 | 12 | | 27 | | 27 | 27 | 6 | 27 | 27 |
| | | SD | 0.4 | 0.19 | 0.12 | 0.04 | 0.29 | 0.02 | | 0.06 | | 3 | | 85 | 6 | 0.15 | 7 | 2.8 |
| 109 | Seeds, whole roasted | 5-04-597 | 5.0 | 0.26 | 0.64 | 0.25 | 1.99 | 0.01 | 0.06 | 0.32 | | 15 | | 142 | 29 | 0.28 | 48 | 5.3 |
| | | N | 32 | 106 | 106 | 106 | 106 | 106 | 15 | 70 | | 106 | | 106 | 106 | | 50 | 106 |
| | | SD | 0.5 | 0.07 | 0.08 | 0.03 | 0.18 | 0.02 | 0.03 | 0.05 | | 3 | | 98 | 8 | | 9 | 4.0 |
| 110 | Silage, early maturity | 3-04-579 | 12.2 | 1.07 | 0.37 | 0.35 | 2.25 | 0.01 | | 0.22 | | 14 | | 656 | 75 | | 42 | 3.1 |
| | | N | 3 | 18 | 18 | 18 | 18 | 18 | | 3 | | 9 | | 9 | 9 | | 9 | 9 |
| | | SD | | 0.29 | 0.13 | 0.07 | 0.80 | 0.01 | | | | 4 | | 263 | 30 | | 11 | 1.4 |
| | SUNFLOWER | | | | | | | | | | | | | | | | | |
| 111 | Meal, solvent | 5-30-032 | 7.7 | 0.48 | 1.00 | 0.63 | 1.50 | 0.04 | 0.12 | 0.39 | | 32 | | 298 | 45 | 0.50 | 88 | 2.7 |
| | | N | 20 | 23 | 23 | 19 | 19 | 14 | 1 | 9 | | 12 | | 12 | 12 | 1 | 12 | 12 |
| | | SD | 0.4 | 0.17 | 0.25 | 0.10 | 0.24 | 0.03 | | 0.10 | | 20 | | 70 | 5 | | 8 | 0.8 |
| 112 | Oil seeds, whole | 5-08-530 | 5.1 | 0.71 | 0.51 | 0.34 | 1.06 | 0.01 | | 0.21 | | 20 | | 144 | 35 | | 53 | 1.8 |
| | | N | 5 | 6 | 6 | 6 | 6 | 6 | | 4 | | 6 | | 6 | 6 | | 6 | 6 |
| | | SD | 1.5 | 0.47 | 0.18 | 0.06 | 0.69 | 0.01 | | 0.03 | | 7 | | 46 | 10 | | 21 | 0.8 |
| | TIMOTHY *Phleum pratense* | See GRASSES, COOL SEASON | | | | | | | | | | | | | | | | |

*(continues)*

TABLE 15-3 *(continued)*

| Entry No. | Feed Name/Description | International Feed No. | Ash % | Ca % | P % | Mg % | K % | Na % | Cl % | S % | Co mg/kg | Cu mg/kg | I mg/kg | Fe mg/kg | Mn mg/kg | Se mg/kg | Zn mg/kg | Mo mg/kg |
|---|---|---|---|---|---|---|---|---|---|---|---|---|---|---|---|---|---|---|
| | TREFOIL, BIRDSFOOT *Lotus corniculatus* | See LEGUMES, FORAGE | | | | | | | | | | | | | | | | |
| | TOMATO | | | | | | | | | | | | | | | | | |
| 113 | Pomace | 5-05-042 | 5.5 | 0.22 | 0.47 | 0.28 | 0.98 | 0.12 | | 0.15 | | 11 | | 541 | 11 | | 54 | 1.8 |
| | | N | 3 | 10 | 10 | 9 | 9 | 9 | | 6 | | 9 | | 9 | 9 | | 9 | 9 |
| | | SD | 1.9 | 0.11 | 0.20 | 0.07 | 0.26 | 0.23 | | 0.06 | | 3 | | 574 | 3 | | 10 | 0.3 |
| | TRITICALE | | | | | | | | | | | | | | | | | |
| 114 | Silage, headed | 3-26-208 | 9.7 | 0.57 | 0.33 | 0.19 | 3.01 | 0.05 | | 0.21 | | 7 | | 404 | 66 | | 37 | 1.8 |
| | | N | 41 | 107 | 107 | 107 | 107 | 40 | | 25 | | 60 | | 60 | 60 | | 47 | 40 |
| | | SD | 3.8 | 0.30 | 0.07 | 0.06 | 0.88 | 0.08 | | 0.06 | | 2 | | 323 | 34 | | 12 | 1 |
| | WHEAT | | | | | | | | | | | | | | | | | |
| 115 | Bran | 4-05-190 | 6.3 | 0.13 | 1.18 | 0.53 | 1.32 | 0.04 | 0.16 | 0.21 | | 11 | | 157 | 122 | 0.50 | 85 | 2.5 |
| | | N | 43 | 44 | 43 | 31 | 31 | 27 | 4 | 16 | | 22 | | 24 | 22 | 7 | 20 | 14 |
| | | SD | 1.6 | 0.03 | 0.23 | 0.09 | 0.16 | 0.01 | 0.03 | 0.03 | | 2 | | 51 | 29 | 0.37 | 27 | 0.9 |
| 116 | Grain, rolled | 4-13-245 | 2.0 | 0.05 | 0.43 | 0.15 | 0.50 | 0.01 | 0.11 | 0.15 | | 5 | | 72 | 42 | 0.28 | 40 | 1.3 |
| | | N | 39 | 135 | 136 | 61 | 61 | 22 | 3 | 35 | | 56 | | 56 | 56 | 35 | 55 | 40 |
| | | SD | 0.3 | 0.03 | 0.14 | 0.03 | 0.14 | 0.01 | 0.03 | 0.03 | | 3 | | 55 | 17 | 0.37 | 13 | 0.8 |
| 117 | Hay, headed | 1-05-170 | 6.7 | 0.31 | 0.20 | 0.13 | 1.71 | 0.06 | 0.38 | 0.13 | | 8 | | 319 | 62 | | 25 | 1.4 |
| | | N | 10 | 110 | 110 | 110 | 110 | 110 | 20 | 44 | | 110 | | 110 | 110 | | 110 | 110 |
| | | SD | 1.5 | 0.18 | 0.07 | 0.04 | 0.72 | 0.12 | 0.24 | 0.05 | | 4 | | 419 | 36 | | 13 | 1.5 |
| 118 | Middlings | 4-05-205 | 5 | 0.16 | 1.02 | 0.42 | 1.38 | 0.03 | 0.10 | 0.18 | | 10 | | 158 | 125 | 0.46 | 91 | 2.5 |
| | | N | 87 | 195 | 196 | 181 | 182 | 170 | 16 | 58 | | 176 | | 177 | 175 | 9 | 171 | 165 |
| | | SD | 0.8 | 0.15 | 0.20 | 0.11 | 0.18 | 0.03 | 0.02 | 0.05 | | 4 | | 80 | 27 | 0.42 | 24 | 0.8 |
| 119 | Silage, early head | 3-21-865 | 8.6 | 0.38 | 0.29 | 0.16 | 2.28 | 0.07 | 0.83 | 0.17 | | 7 | | 391 | 72 | | 27 | 1.7 |
| | | N | 211 | 223 | 459 | 459 | 459 | 249 | 36 | 179 | | 322 | | 322 | 322 | | 322 | 249 |
| | | SD | 2.6 | 0.16 | 0.08 | 0.05 | 0.69 | 0.13 | 0.49 | 0.05 | | 4 | | 399 | 36 | | 10 | 1.0 |
| 120 | Straw | 1-05-175 | 7.6 | 0.31 | 0.10 | 0.14 | 1.55 | 0.12 | 0.60 | 0.11 | | 6 | | 172 | 67 | | 16 | 1.3 |
| | | N | 64 | 137 | 134 | 123 | 125 | 91 | 8 | 41 | | 120 | | 121 | 69 | | 116 | 88 |
| | | SD | 2.8 | 0.22 | 0.05 | 0.08 | 0.62 | 0.23 | 0.35 | 0.04 | | 4 | | 113 | 81 | | 7 | 1.5 |
| | WHEY | | | | | | | | | | | | | | | | | |
| 121 | Wet, cattle | 4-08-134 | 3.1 | 1.37 | 1.04 | 0.22 | 3.32 | 1.40 | 2.41 | 1.15 | | 2 | | 131 | 4 | 0.06 | 16 | 1.3 |
| | | N | 16 | 58 | 58 | 58 | 58 | 58 | 16 | 18 | | 58 | | 58 | 58 | 11 | 33 | 9 |
| | | SD | 2.7 | 1.20 | 0.70 | 0.13 | 0.84 | 2.55 | 3.70 | 1.42 | | 7 | | 195 | 5 | 0.06 | 24 | 2.7 |

TABLE 15-4 Compositions of Inorganic Mineral Sources and Element Absorption Coefficients for Dairy Cattle on a 100% Dry Matter Basis

| Mineral Element Source | International Feed No.[a] | Dry Matter[b] | Crude Protein Equivalent (CPE) = N% x 6.25 | Primary Mineral Element Content | Absorption Coefficient (AC) of Primary Element |
|---|---|---|---|---|---|
| Calcium Sources | | (DM%) | (CPE%) | Ca (%) | AC of Ca |
| Bone meal, steamed, fg[c] | 6-00-400 | 97 | 13.2 | 30.71 | 0.95 |
| Calcium carbonate, $CaCO_3$, fg | 6-01-069 | 100 | —[d] | 39.39 | 0.75 |
| Calcium chloride anhydrous, $CaCl_2$, cp[e,g] | NA[f] | 100 | — | 36.11 | 0.95 |
| Calcium chloride dihydrate, $CaCl_2 \cdot 2H_2O$, cp[g] | NA | 100 | — | 27.53 | 0.95 |
| Calcium hydroxide, $Ca(OH)_2$, cp | NA | 100 | — | 54.09 | 0.55 |
| Calcium oxide, CaO, cp[g] | NA | 100 | — | 71.47 | 0.50 |
| Calcium phosphate (monobasic), $Ca(H_2PO_4)_2$, from defluorinated phosphoric acid fg | 6-01-082 | 97 | — | 16.40 | 0.95 |
| Calcium sulfate dihydrate, $CaSO_4 \cdot 2H_2O$, cp | 6-01-089 | 97 | — | 23.28 | 0.70 |
| Curacao, phosphate, fg | 6-05-586 | 99 | — | 34.34 | 0.70 |
| Dicalcium phosphate (dibasic), $CaHPO_4$, from defluorinated phosphoric acid, fg | 6-01-080 | 97 | — | 22.00 | 0.94 |
| Dolomitic limestone (magnesium), fg | 6-02-633 | 99 | — | 22.30 | 0.60 |
| Limestone, ground, fg | 6-02-632 | 100 | — | 34.00 | 0.70 |
| Magnesium oxide, MgO, fg | 6-02-756 | 98 | — | 3.07 | 0.70 |
| Oystershell, flour (ground), fg | 6-03-481 | 99 | — | 38.00 | 0.75 |
| Phosphate, defluorinated, fg | 6-01-780 | 100 | — | 32.00 | 0.70 |
| Phosphate rock, fg | 6-03-945 | 100 | — | 35.00 | 0.30 |
| Phosphate rock, low-fluorine, fg | 6-03-946 | 100 | — | 36.00 | 0.30 |
| Soft rock phosphate colloidal clay, fg | 6-03-947 | 100 | — | 17.00 | 0.30 |
| Phosphorus Sources | | (DM%) | (CPE%) | P (%) | AC of P |
| Ammonium phosphate (dibasic), $(NH_4)_2HPO_4$, fg | 6-00-370 | 97 | 115.9 | 20.60 | 0.80 |
| Ammonium phosphate (monobasic), $(NH_4)H_2PO_4$, fg | 6-09-338 | 97 | 70.9 | 24.74 | 0.80 |
| Bone meal, steamed, fg | 6-00-400 | 97 | 13.2 | 12.86 | 0.80 |
| Calcium phosphate (monobasic), $Ca(H_2PO_4)_2$, from defluorinated phosphoric acid, fg | 6-01-082 | 97 | — | 21.60 | 0.80 |
| Curacao, phosphate, fg | 6-05-586 | 99 | — | 14.14 | 0.85 |
| Dicalcium phosphate (dibasic), $CaHPO_4$, from defluorinated phosphoric acid, fg | 6-01-080 | 97 | — | 19.30 | 0.75 |
| Phosphate, defluorinated, fg | 6-01-780 | 100 | — | 18.00 | 0.65 |
| Phosphate rock, fg | 6-03-945 | 100 | — | 13.00 | 0.30 |
| Phosphate rock, low-fluorine, fg | 6-03-946 | 100 | — | 14.00 | 0.30 |
| Phosphoric acid, $-H_3PO_4$, fg[g-l] | 6-03-707 | 75 | — | 31.60 | 0.90 |
| Sodium phosphate (monobasic) monohydrate, $NaH_2PO_4 \cdot H_2O$, fg | 6-04-288 | 97 | — | 22.50 | 0.90 |
| Sodium tripolyphosphate (meta- and pyro-phosphate) $Na_5P_3O_{10}$, fg | 6-08-076 | 96 | — | 25.00 | 0.75 |
| Soft rock phosphate, colloidal clay, fg | 6-03-947 | 100 | — | 9.00 | 0.30 |
| Sodium Sources | | (DM%) | (CPE%) | Na (%) | AC of Na |
| Bone meal, steamed, fg | 6-00-400 | 97 | 13.2 | 5.69 | 0.90 |
| Phosphate, defluorinated, fg | 6-01-780 | 100 | — | 4.90 | 0.90 |
| Potassium chloride, KCl, fg | 6-03-755 | 100 | — | 1.00 | 0.90 |
| Sodium bicarbonate, $NaHCO_3$, fg | 6-04-272 | 100 | — | 27.00 | 0.90 |
| Sodium carbonate monohydrate, $Na_2CO_3 \cdot H_2O$, cp | NA | 100 | — | 37.08 | 0.90 |
| Sodium chloride, NaCl, fg | 6-04-152 | 100 | — | 39.34 | 0.90 |
| Sodium phosphate (monobasic) monohydrate, $NaH_2PO_4 \cdot H_2O$, fg | 6-04-288 | 97 | — | 16.68 | 0.90 |
| Sodium selenate decahydrate, $Na_2SeO_4 \cdot 10H_2O$, cp | NA | 100 | — | 12.46 | 0.90 |
| Sodium selenite, $Na_2SeO_3$, fg | 6-26-013 | 98 | — | 26.60 | 0.90 |
| Sodium sesquicarbonate dihydrate, $Na_2CO_3 + NaHCO_3 \cdot 2H_2O$, fg | NA | 100 | — | 30.50 | 0.90 |
| Sodium sulfate decahydrate, $Na_2SO_4 \cdot 10H_2O$, cp | 6-04-292 | 97 | — | 14.27 | 0.90 |

*(continues)*

TABLE 15-4 *(continued)*

| Mineral Element Source | International Feed No.[a] | Dry Matter[b] | Crude Protein Equivalent (CPE) = N% x 6.25 | Primary Mineral Element Content | Absorption Coefficient (AC) of Primary Element |
|---|---|---|---|---|---|
| Sodium Sources *(continued)* | | *(DM%)* | *(CPE%)* | *Na (%)* | *AC of Na* |
| Sodium tripolyphosphate(meta- and pyro-phosphate, $Na_5P_3O_{10}$, fg | 6-08-076 | 96 | — | 31.00 | 0.90 |
| Chloride Sources | | *(DM%)* | *(CPE%)* | *Cl (%)* | *AC of Cl* |
| Ammonium chloride, cp | NA | 100 | 163.63 | 66.28 | 0.90 |
| Calcium chloride anhydrous, $CaCl_2$, cp[g] | NA | 100 | — | 63.89 | 0.90 |
| Calcium chloride dihydrate, $CaCl_2 \cdot 2H_2O$, cp[g] | NA | 100 | — | 48.23 | 0.90 |
| Cobalt dichloride hexahydrate, $CoCl_2 \cdot 6H_2O$, cp | NA | 100 | — | 29.80 | 0.90 |
| Cupric chloride dihydrate, $CuCl_2 \cdot 2H_2O$, cp | NA | 100 | — | 41.65 | 0.90 |
| Magnesium chloride hexahydrate, $MgCl_2 \cdot 6H_2O$, cp | NA | 100 | — | 34.88 | 0.90 |
| Manganese dichloride, $MnCl_2$, cp | NA | 100 | — | 56.34 | 0.90 |
| Manganese chloride tetrahydrate, $MnCl_2 \cdot 4H_2O$, cp | NA | 100 | — | 35.80 | 0.90 |
| Potassium chloride, KCl, fg | 6-03-755 | 100 | — | 47.30 | 0.90 |
| Sodium chloride, NaCl, fg | 6-04-152 | 100 | — | 60.66 | 0.90 |
| Zinc chloride, $ZnCl_2$, cp | NA | 100 | — | 52.03 | 0.90 |
| Potassium Sources | | *(DM%)* | *(CPE%)* | *K (%)* | *AC of K* |
| Potassium bicarbonate, $KHCO_3$, cp | 6-29-493 | 99 | — | 39.05 | 0.90 |
| Potassium carbonate, $K_2CO_3$, cp | NA | 100 | — | 56.58 | 0.90 |
| Potassium chloride, KCl, fg | 6-03-755 | 100 | — | 50.00 | 0.90 |
| Potassium iodide, KI, fg | 6-03-759 | 100 | — | 21.00 | 0.90 |
| Potassium sulfate, $K_2SO_4$, fg | 6-06-098 | 98 | — | 41.84 | 0.90 |
| Magnesium Sources | | *(DM%)* | *(CPE%)* | *Mg (%)* | *AC of Mg* |
| Dolomitic limestone (magnesium), fg | 6-02-633 | 99 | — | 9.99 | 0.30 |
| Limestone, ground, fg | 6-02-632 | 100 | — | 2.06 | 0.30 |
| Magnesium carbonate, $MgCO_3 + Mg(OH)_2$ fg | 6-02-754 | 98 | | 30.81 | 0.35 |
| Magnesium chloride hexahydrate, $MgCl_2 \cdot 6H_2O$, cp | NA | 100 | — | 11.96 | 0.90 |
| Magnesium hydroxide, $Mg(OH)_2$, cp | NA | 100 | — | 41.69 | 0.70 |
| Magnesium oxide, MgO, fg | 6-02-756 | 98 | — | 56.20 | 0.70 |
| Magnesium sulfate heptahydrate, $MgSO_4 \cdot 7H_2O$, fg | 6-02-758 | 98 | — | 9.80 | 0.90 |
| Sulfur Sources | | *(DM%)* | *(CPE%)* | *S (%)* | *AC of S* |
| Ammonium phosphate (dibasic), $(NH_4)_2HPO_4$, fg | 6-00-370 | 97 | 115.9 | 2.16 | |
| Ammonium phosphate (monobasic), $(NH_4)H_2PO_4$, fg | 6-09-338 | 97 | 70.9 | 1.46 | |
| Ammonium sulfate, $(NH_4)_2SO_4$, fg | 6-09-339 | 100 | 134.1 | 24.10 | |
| Bone meal, steamed, fg | 6-00-400 | 97 | 13.2 | 2.51 | |
| Calcium phosphate (monobasic), $Ca(H_2PO_4)_2$, from defluorinated phosphoric acid, fg | 6-01-082 | 97 | — | 1.22 | |
| Calcium sulfate, dihydrate $CaSO_4 \cdot 2H_2O$, fg | 6-01-089 | 97 | — | 18.62 | |
| Cupric sulfate pentahydrate, $CuSO_4 \cdot 5H_2O$ | 6-01-720 | 100 | — | 12.84 | |
| Dicalcium phosphate (dibasic), $CaHPO_4$, from defluorinated phosphoric acid, fg | 6-01-080 | 97 | — | 1.14 | |
| Ferrous sulfate heptahydrate, $FeSO_4 \cdot 7H_2O$, fg | 6-20-734 | 98 | — | 12.35 | |
| Magnesium sulfate heptahydrate, $MgSO_4 \cdot 7H_2O$, fg | NA | 98 | — | 13.31 | |
| Manganese sulfate monohydrate, $MnSO_4 \cdot H_2O$, cp | NA | 100 | — | 18.97 | |
| Manganese sulfate pentahydrate, $MnSO_4 \cdot 5H_2O$, cp | NA | 100 | — | 13.30 | |

*(continues)*

TABLE 15-4 *(continued)*

| Mineral Element Source | International Feed No.[a] | Dry Matter[b] | Crude Protein Equivalent (CPE) = N% x 6.25 | Primary Mineral Element Content | Absorption Coefficient (AC) of Primary Element |
|---|---|---|---|---|---|
| *Sulfur Sources (continued)* | | *(DM%)* | *(CPE%)* | *S (%)* | *AC of S* |
| Phosphoric acid, -$H_3PO_4$, fg[g] | 6-03-707 | 75 | — | 1.55 | |
| Potassium sulfate, $K_2SO_4$, fg | 6-06-098 | 98 | — | 17.35 | |
| Sodium sulfate decahydrate, $Na_2SO_4 \cdot 10H_2O$, cp | 6-04-292 | 97 | — | 9.95 | |
| Zinc sulfate monohydrate, $ZnSO_4 \cdot H_2O$, fg | 6-05-555 | 99 | — | 17.68 | |
| Cobalt Sources | | *(DM%)* | *(CPE%)* | *Co (mg/kg)* | *AC of CO* |
| Cobalt carbonate, $CoCO_3$, fg | 6-01-566 | 99 | — | 460,000 | |
| Cobalt carbonate hexahydrate, $CoCO_3 \cdot 6H_2O$, cp | NA | 100 | — | 259,000 | |
| Cobalt dichloride hexahydrate, $CoCl_2 \cdot 6H_2O$, cp | NA | 100 | — | 247,800 | |
| Copper (Cupric) Sources | | *(DM%)* | *(CPE%)* | *Cu (mg/kg)* | *AC of Cu* |
| Cupric chloride dihydrate, $CuCl_2 \cdot 2H_2O$, cp | NA | 100 | — | 372,000 | 0.05 |
| Cupric oxide, CuO, cp | NA | 100 | — | 798,800 | 0.01 |
| Cupric sulfate pentahydrate, $CuSO_4 \cdot 5H_2O$, cp | 6-01-720 | 100 | — | 254,500 | 0.05 |
| Iodine Sources | | *(DM%)* | *(CPE%)* | *I (mg/kg)* | *AC of I* |
| Ethylenediaminodihydroiodide (EDDI), fg | 6-01-842 | 98 | — | 803,400 | 0.90 |
| Potassium iodide, KI, fg | 6-03-759 | 100 | — | 681,700 | 0.90 |
| Iron Sources | | *(DM%)* | *(CPE%)* | *Fe (mg/kg)* | *AC of Fe* |
| Ammonium phosphate (dibasic), $(NH_4)_2HPO_4$, fg | 6-00-370 | 97 | 115.9 | 12,400 | 0.40 |
| Ammonium phosphate (monobasic), $(NH_4)H_2PO_4$, fg | 6-09-338 | 97 | 70.9 | 17,400 | 0.40 |
| Bone meal, steamed, fg | 6-00-400 | 97 | 13.2 | 26,700 | 0.40 |
| Calcium phosphate (monobasic), $Ca(H_2PO_4)_2$, from defluorinated phosphoric acid, fg | 6-01-082 | 97 | — | 15,800 | 0.40 |
| Dicalcium phosphate (dibasic), $CaHPO_4$, from defluorinated phosphoric acid, fg | 6-01-080 | 97 | — | 14,400 | 0.40 |
| Ferrous sulfate heptahydrate, $FeSO_4 \cdot 7H_2O$, fg | 6-20-734 | 98 | — | 218,400 | 0.60 |
| Phosphate rock, fg | 6-03-945 | 100 | — | 16,800 | 0.40 |
| Phosphoric acid, -$H_3PO_4$, fg[g] | 6-03-707 | 75 | — | 17,500 | 0.40 |
| Soft rock phosphate, colloidal clay, fg | 6-03-947 | 100 | — | 19,000 | 0.40 |
| Manganese (Manganous) Sources | | *(DM%)* | *(CPE%)* | *Mn (mg/kg)* | *AC of Mn* |
| Manganese carbonate, $MnCO_3$, cp | 6-03-036 | 97 | — | 478,000 | 0.0015 |
| Manganese chloride, $MnCl_2$, cp | NA | 100 | — | 430,000 | 0.0120 |
| Manganese chloride tetrahydrate, $MnCl_2 \cdot 4H_2O$, cp | NA | 100 | — | 277,000 | 0.0120 |
| Manganese oxide, MnO, cp | 6-03-056 | 99 | — | 774,500 | 0.0025 |
| Manganese sulfate monohydrate, $MnSO_4 \cdot H_2O$, cp | NA | 100 | — | 325,069 | 0.0120 |
| Manganese sulfate pentahydrate, $MnSO_4 \cdot 5H_2O$, cp | NA | 100 | — | 227,891 | 0.0100 |
| Selenium Sources | | *(DM%)* | *(CPE%)* | *Se(mg/kg)* | |
| Sodium selenate decahydrate, $Na_2SeO_4 \cdot 10H_2O$, cp | NA | 100 | — | 213,920 | |
| Sodium selenite, $Na_2SeO_3$, cp | 6-26-013 | 98 | — | 456,000 | |
| Zinc Sources | | *(DM%)* | *(CPE%)* | *Zn (mg/kg)* | *AC of Zn* |
| Zinc carbonate, $ZnCO_3$, cp | NA | 100 | — | 521,400 | 0.10 |
| Zinc chloride, $ZnCl_2$, cp | NA | 100 | — | 479,700 | 0.20 |
| Zinc oxide, ZnO, cp | 6-05-533 | 100 | — | 780,000 | 0.12 |
| Zinc sulfate monohydrate, $ZnSO_4 \cdot H_2O$, fg | 6-05-555 | 99 | — | 363,600 | 0.20 |

*(continues)*

TABLE 15-4 *(continued)*

| Mineral Element Source | International Feed No.[a] | Dry Matter[b] | Crude Protein Equivalent (CPE) = N% x 6.25 | Primary Mineral Element Content | Absorption Coefficient (AC) of Primary Element |
|---|---|---|---|---|---|
| **Fluorine Sources** | | *(DM%)* | *(CPE%)* | *Fl (mg/kg)* | |
| Ammonium phosphate (dibasic), $(NH_4)_2HPO_4$, fg | 6-00-370 | 97 | 115.9 | 2,100 | |
| Ammonium phosphate (monobasic), $(NH_4)H_2PO_4$, fg | 6-09-338 | 97 | 70.9 | 2,500 | |
| Calcium phosphate (monobasic), $Ca(H_2PO_4)_2$, from defluorinated phosphoric acid, fg | 6-01-082 | 97 | — | 2,100 | |
| Curacao, phosphate, fg | 6-05-586 | 99 | — | 5,550 | |
| Dicalcium phosphate (dibasic), $CaHPO_4$, from defluorinated phosphoric acid, fg | 6-01-080 | 97 | — | 1,800 | |
| Phosphate, defluorinated, fg | 6-01-780 | 100 | — | 1,800 | |
| Phosphate rock, fg | 6-03-945 | 100 | — | 35,000 | |
| Phosphoric acid, $H_3PO_4$, fg[g] | 6-03-707 | 75 | — | 3,100 | |
| Soft rock phosphate, colloidal clay, fg | 6-03-947 | 100 | — | 15,000 | |

NOTE: The compositions of hydrated mineral sources (e.g., $CaSO_4 \cdot 2H_2O$) are shown including the waters of hydration. Mineral element compositions of feed-grade sources vary by source, processing method, site of mining, and manufacturer. Sources should be analyzed or manufacturer's analyses should be used when available. Element composition of a source is listed if specific element concentration is $\geq$*1.0% for macromineral elements, or* $\geq$*10,000 mg/kg for micromineral elements, except for fluorine concentrations which are listed because of potential toxicity.*

[a]First digit denotes the class of feed: 1, dry forages and roughages; 2, pastured, range plants, and forages fed green; 3, silages; 4, energy feeds; 5, protein supplement; 6, minerals; 7, vitamins; 8, additives. The other five digits identify the individual feed.

[b]Dry matter contents have been estimated for the sources; actual analysis will be more accurate.

[c]fg = Feed-grade source.

[d]None present.

[e]cp = Chemically pure form.

[f]NA = Not available.

[g]Use caution when handling and mixing; can be extremely hazardous.

# 16 Model Evaluation and Prediction Equations

The evaluation of specific components of the model can be found in the relevant chapters. This chapter concerns the evaluation of the overall model relative to energy, protein, and intake. The model equations are also presented in this chapter for reference.

## METHODOLOGY

Data from experiments published in the *Journal of Dairy Science* from 1992 through February 2000 were used to evaluate the model. Only data from continuous lactation experiments that lasted at least 6 weeks were used (data from cross-over type experiments were not used). Twenty-five papers representing 100 different diets were selected. The papers were selected so that a wide variety of ingredients and production levels of cows could be evaluated. The selection was made prior to diet evaluation; all selected diets are shown in the plots. Diets varied in:

1. Forage source (corn silage and alfalfa were used in most experiments)
2. Forage:concentrate ratio
3. Fat supplementation (without and with a wide variety of fat sources)
4. Nonforage fiber sources (without and with a wide variety of nonforage fiber sources)
5. Source of starch (mostly corn grain but sorghum and barley was also fed in some experiments)
6. Corn grain processing (dry and high moisture, grind size, steam-treatment)

Cows varied with respect to days in milk, milk yield, and milk composition. Twenty-three papers used Holstein cows, two papers used Jersey cows.

Diet composition (ingredients) was entered into the model. Published nutrient composition of the individual ingredients was used when available. When nutrient composition data were missing, values from the feed composition table (Table 15-1) were used. When nutrient composition of ingredients was not published but nutrient composition of the total diet was included, nutrient composition of individual ingredients (usually only the forages) were changed by no more than one standard deviation so that composition (NDF and CP) of the diet was the same as the published composition. Most studies did not include measured lignin, ash, and neutral and acid detergent insoluble crude protein. The protein fraction and digestion rate data in the composition tables (Tables 15-2a and b) were used in all evaluations. Few papers published data on mineral composition of the ingredients or diets, and because mean composition data on minerals (Table 15-3) has a large variance, provision of minerals was not evaluated. However, the concentration of mineral supplements was included in the diets.

Mean production data (days in milk, lactation number, body weight, and milk yield and composition) were entered into the model. Day of gestation usually was not published so a reasonable estimate was entered based on days in milk. Most papers did not include data on the age of the cows. Therefore, growth requirements were set to zero for all cows except those that were exclusively primiparous (for those cows, model generated growth requirements were used).

## EVALUATION

After diet and cow data were entered into the model, predicted dry matter intake, net energy allowable milk, and metabolizable protein allowable milk were compared with actual intake and milk production. Predicted net energy balance was compared with actual net energy balance by including net energy provided by or needed for the measured body weight change. Sources of data used in the evaluation are shown in Table 16-1.

### *Dry Matter Intake*

Mean observed dry matter intake was 22.3 kg/d and mean predicted intake was 22.1 kg/d. No evidence of a linear bias was found (Figure 16-1). Root mean square error (predicted minus observed) was 2.0 kg/d. Predicted intake was within ± 5 percent of observed intake in 41 percent of the observations and 73 percent of the predicted intakes were within ± 10 percent of observed intake.

### *Energy*

To evaluate the energy portion of the model, intake of $NE_L$ (based on actual DMI and model predicted $NE_L$ concentration) was compared with $NE_L$ utilization (model predicted $NE_L$ for maintenance, based on actual body weight, model predicted $NE_L$ for actual milk produced, and $NE_L$ used for measured body weight change). The data set was as described above except two studies (4 treatment means) could not be used because body weight change was not reported. If the model is accurate, $NE_L$ intake and $NE_L$ use should be equal with no apparent bias. Overall, the accuracy of the model was acceptable (Figure 16-2). Intake of $NE_L$ and $NE_L$ use were highly correlated ($r^2 = 0.61$; $P<0.01$). Energy use was within ± 5 percent of $NE_L$ intake for 46 percent of the observations and within 10 percent for 76 percent of the observations. Mean $NE_L$ intake was 35.4 Mcal/d compared with mean $NE_L$ use of 34.5, therefore, a small mean bias (0.9 Mcal of $NE_L$ intake or 2.5 percent) was present. A linear bias is apparent ($NE_L$ intake $= 7.8 + 0.8 \times NE_L$ Use); however, within the range of $NE_L$ used for most lactating cows in the United States the bias will be small (at 20 Mcal of $NE_L$ use, estimated mean $NE_L$ intake is 23.8 Mcal/day; at 30 Mcal/d $NE_L$ use, estimated mean $NE_L$ intake is 31.8 Mcal/day; and at 45 Mcal of $NE_L$ use, estimated mean $NE_L$ intake is 43.8 Mcal/day).

TABLE 16-1 Sources of Data Used in the Model Evaluation (see also Figures 16-1 to 16-5)

| | | |
|---|---|---|
| Aydin et al. (1999) | Knowlton et al. (1998) | Soder and Holden (1999) |
| Bertrand et al. (1998) | Kuehn et al. (1999) | Stegeman et al. (1992) |
| Coomer et al. (1993) | Messman et al. (1992) | Tackett et al. (1996) |
| Dann et al. (2000) | Mowrey et al. (1999) | Wattiaux et al. (1994) |
| Dhiman and Satter (1993) | Overton et al. (1998) | Weiss (1995) |
| Kalscheur et al. (1999) | Pereira et al. (1999) | Weiss and Shockey (1991) |
| Khorasani et al. (1993) | Santos et al. (1998) | Weiss and Wyatt (2000) |
| Khorasani et al. (1996) | Santos et al. (1999) | Wilkerson et al. (1997) |
| Kim et al. (1993) | | |

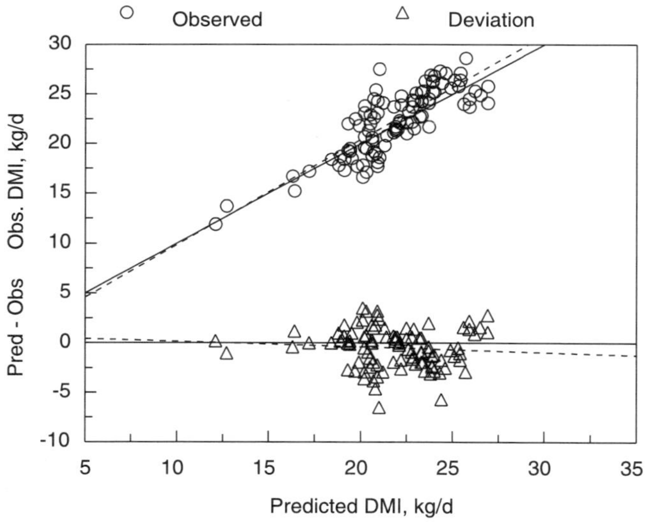


FIGURE 16-1 Model predicted vs. actual dry matter intake. Values from 100 published treatments means from 25 studies.

### *Protein*

Evaluation of the protein portion of the model by comparing MP allowable milk with actual milk is equivocal. When MP allowable milk is greater than actual milk, milk production could be limited by the physiologic state or genetic potential of the cow or by a nutrient other than MP. Higher MP allowable milk than actual milk could also mean that the model underpredicted MP requirements of the cow. When MP allowable milk was compared with actual milk, MP allowable milk was less than actual milk in only 18 (18 percent) observations (Figure 16-3). Of those 18 observations, MP allowable milk for 5, 8, and 5 observations were within 10 to 17 percent, 5 to 10 percent, or less than 5 percent of actual milk. Eighty-two percent of all treatment groups in this data set produced less milk than the model predicted could be produced from the amount of MP available. In 67 percent of the observations, MP allowable milk was more than 10 percent greater than actual milk. Other than energy, the most likely nutrients

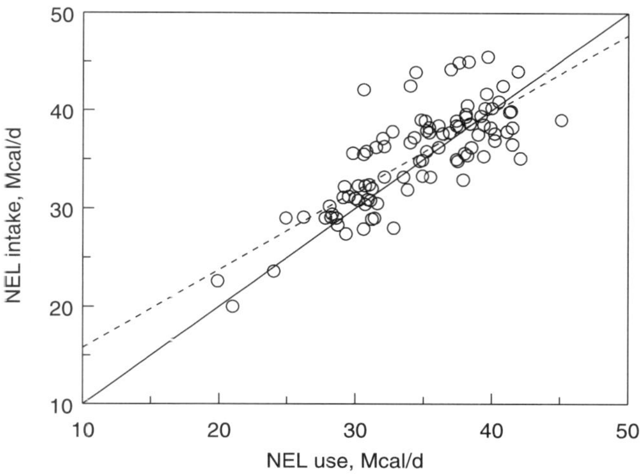


FIGURE 16-2 NEL intake (estimated from observed dry matter intake and model estimated NEL concentration) versus NEL use (estimated from model predicted maintenance and lactation requirement plus NEL needed to meet observed body weight change). Values from a data base of 96 published treatment means from 23 studies. The solid line represents y=x, the dashed line represents y=7.8 + 0.8X.

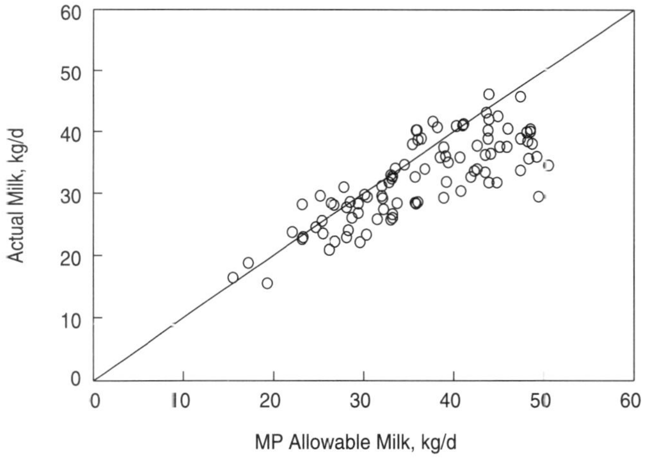


FIGURE 16-3 Actual milk production versus model predicted MP allowable milk production. Values from 100 published treatment means from 25 studies.

limiting milk production and causing MP allowable milk to be greater than actual milk are specific amino acids. The difference between MP allowable milk and actual milk increased as the concentration of lysine decreased from 6.5 percent of MP (Figure 16-4) and as the concentration of methionine decreased from 1.9 percent of MP (Figure 16-5). This suggests that although supply of total MP was adequate in many of these experiments, the balance of absorbable amino acids may have been incorrect and limited milk production. Experiments specifically designed to test the MP requirements predicted by the model are needed.

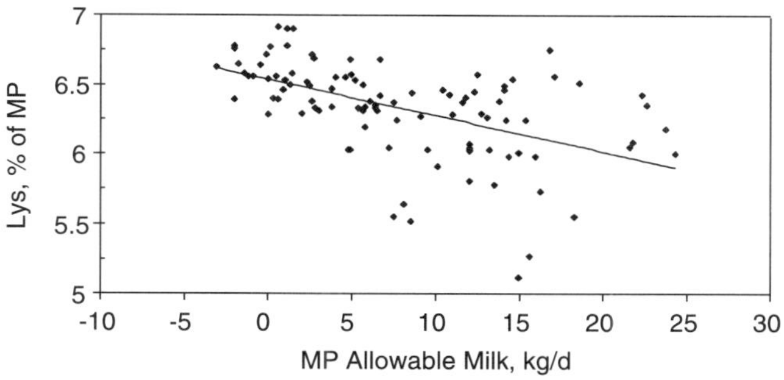


FIGURE 16-4 Difference between MP allowable milk and actual milk versus model predicted lysine concentration of MP. Values from 100 published treatment means from 25 studies. Regression line: y = 6.54 − 0.026x.

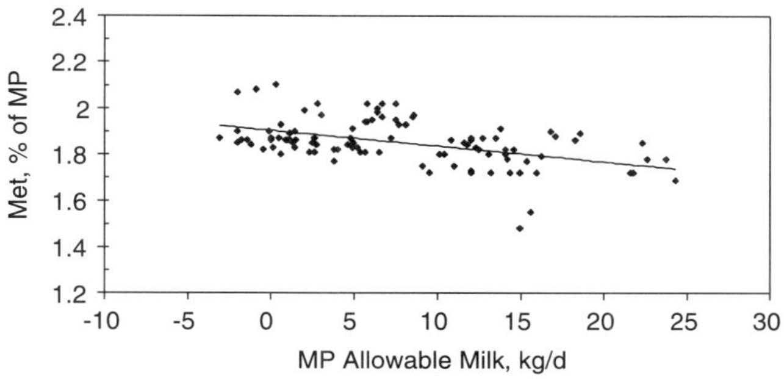


FIGURE 16-5 Difference between MP allowable milk and actual milk versus model predicted methionine concentration of MP. Values from 100 published treatment means from 25 studies. Regression line: y = 1.90 − 0.0067x.

## MODEL PREDICTION EQUATIONS

### *Model Structure*

The model is divided into two major components: prediction of requirements and supply of nutrients. Within this structure, there are submodels for young calves, maintenance, pregnancy, growth, lactation, dry matter intake, minerals, reserves, energy and protein supply, amino acids, and diet evaluation. A glossary of the terms used in the equations is included at the end of the chapter. Background information explaining the committee's rationale in choosing the approach and coefficients used in the model is presented in the appropriate chapters. A complete listing of all of the equations in the model is included in a file on the compact disk that contains the model itself. Note, MEng is used to denote metabolizable energy (ME) in the computer program and in the equations below because ME can not be used as a variable in the programming language that we used.

### *Animal Requirements*

The requirements section is divided into four main sections based on physiological function: maintenance, growth, lactation, and pregnancy. Adjustments made for grazing activity are included in the maintenance section. There are four classes of animals in this model, lactating cow, dry cow, replacement heifer, and young calf. If different equations are used for heifers, lactating cows, or dry cows, they will be presented under the appropriate physiologic function. The equations used to predict the requirements and nutrient supply of the young calves are in a separate section.

*Maintenance*

MAINTENANCE ENERGY REQUIREMENTS

Maintenance requirements are computed by adjusting the NEm requirement for fasting metabolism for the effects of physiologic state, activity, and, in the case of heifers, heat and cold stress.

*Lactating and Dry Cows* The maintenance requirement for lactating cows is calculated using metabolic body size ($BW^{0.75}$), and calculated with the following equation which includes an adjustment for activity:

$$\text{NEmaint (Mcal/d)} = ((\text{BW} - \text{CW})^{0.75} \times \text{a1}) + \text{NEmact}$$

Where a1 = 0.08 for mature cows based on the requirement for NEm (80 kcal/kg $BW^{0.75}$) (NRC, 1989), CW is conceptus weight and NEmact is the variable to calculate the requirement for activity.

$$\text{NEmact} = ((((\text{Distance}/1000) \times \text{Trips}) \times (0.00045 \times \text{BW})) + (0.0012 \times (\text{BW}))$$

Where Distance is the distance from the pasture to the milking parlor (km), Trips is the number of times that animals go to and from the milking parlor daily, and Pasture is an adjustment for percent of the predicted dry matter intake supplied by grazing.

NEmact is adjusted for differences in topography for grazing animals. Topography may be either flat or hilly. No adjustment is made if the topography is flat.

If Topography = 'Hilly' Then NEmact = NEmact + (0.006 × BW)

The following equations are used to calculate the net energy concentration of the diet and the amount of feed that is required to meet the maintenance requirement.

$$\text{NEFP} = (\text{TotalDMFed} - \text{FeedMaint}) \times (\text{NEl\_Total} / \text{TotalDMFed}) \times 0.65$$

Where NEFP = Net energy for production, TotalDMFed = Total dry matter consumed, NEl_Total = total NE (in Mcals) and 0.65 is the assumed efficiency of conversion of metabolizable protein to net protein

*Heifers* The maintenance requirements for heifers without stress (NEmaintNS) are calculated with the following equation:

$$\text{NEmaintNS (Mcal/d)} = (((\text{SBW} - \text{CW})^{0.75}) \times ((\text{a1} \times \text{COMP}) + \text{a2})) + \text{NEmact}$$

Where:
SBW = shrunk body weight = 0.96 × BW, CW = conceptus weight (kg),
a1 = 0.086 (thermoneutral maintenance requirement (Mcal/day)),
a2 = 0.0007 × (20 − PrevTemp) (Adjustment for previous temperature effect),
COMP = 0.8 + ((CS9 − 1) × 0.05) (Adjustment for previous plane of nutrition) NEmact = energy required for activity

In the model, a 1–9 system for body condition scoring is used so the following equation is used to convert from the 1–5 system more commonly used in the dairy industry to the 1–9 system. The conversion to the 9-point condition score from the 5-point system is:

$$\text{CS9} = ((\text{CS} - 1) \times 2) + 1$$

The following equation is used to calculate the activity requirement for grazing heifers:

NEmact = ((0.0009 BW) + (0.0016 BW)) if the heifer is grazing, otherwise it is 0.
If Topography = 'Hilly' then NEmact = NEmact + (0.006 × BW)

For heifers, these requirements then are adjusted for the effects of temperature that are based on surface area, heat production, tissue and coat insulation, coat condition, and temperature. First surface area (SA) and heat production (HP) ($Mcal/m^2/day$) are calculated:

$$\text{SA} = 0.09 \times (\text{SBW}^{0.67})$$
$$\text{HP} = (\text{MEI} - \text{NEFP})/\text{SA}$$

Where NEFP = Net energy for production which equals NEGrowthDietNS (Net energy for growth available in the diet with no stress, Mcal/day), HP = Heat production ($Mcal/m^2/day$), MEI = Metabolizable energy intake (Mcal), and NEGrowthDietNS = (TotalDMFed − FeedMaint) × (NEg_Total / TotalDMFed)

The next step is to calculate tissue insulation (TI, $Mcal/m^2/°C/day$). For younger animals, these factors are based on age alone but, for older animals, body condition score is also considered. These factors are:

| *Age (days)* | *TI Factor* |
|---|---|
| ≤ 30 | 2.5 |
| 31 to 183 | 6.5 |
| 184 to 362 | 5.1875 × (0.3125 × CS9) |
| ≥ 363 | 5.25 × (0.75 × CS9) |

The insulation is further affected by coat condition (Coat):

| *Coat condition* | *Factor* |
|---|---|
| Clean/dry | 1.0 |
| Some mud | 0.8 |
| Wet/matted | 0.5 |
| Coated with snow/mud | 0.2 |

The external insulation value, EI (°C/Mcal/m²/day) is:

$$EI = ((7.36 - (0.296 \times WindSpeed) + (2.55 \times HairDepth)) \times Coat) \times 0.8$$

Where WindSpeed (kph) is the average wind speed and typical HairDepth values for animals in summer are 0.63 cm (0.25 inches) and for winter 1.27 cm (0.5 inches) and Coat is the coat condition factor.

The total insulation (INS, Mcal/m²/°C/day) is INS = TI + EI

The effects of heat and cold stress are based on lower and upper critical temperatures.
The animal's lower critical temperature (LCT, °C) is:

$$LCT = 39 - (INS \times HP \times 0.85)$$

If the LCT > ambient temperature (Temp), then

$$MEcs = SA \times (LCT - Temp)/INS$$

Where MEcs is Metabolizable energy required for cold stress (Mcal/day).
Otherwise, there is no cold stress.

$$ColdStr = (((NEDietConc/MEng\_Total/TotalDMFed)) \times MEcs)$$

Where NEDietConc is the concentration of net energy in the diet (kg DM/day), MEng_Total is Total ME intake (Mcal/day), and TotalDMFed is total dry matter fed (kg).
To calculate the effects of heat, the HeatStress variable is used. An index based on visible changes in breathing in response to heat based on breathing is used:

If HeatStress = 'None' or Temp < 30 then HeatStr = 1
If HeatStress = 'Rapid/Shallow' then HeatStr = 1.07
If HeatStress = 'Open Mouth' then HeatStr = 1.18

The final equation to calculate the maintenance requirement for replacement heifers is:

$$NEMaint = ((NEMaintNS + ColdStr) \times HeatStr) + NEmact$$

*Maintenance Protein Requirement*

LACTATING AND DRY COWS AND REPLACEMENT HEIFERS

The protein requirements for maintenance for all classes of cattle except for the young calves are calculated with the following equation:

$$MPMaint = (0.3 \times (BW - CW)^{0.6}) + (4.1 \times (BW - CW)^{0.5}) + (TotalDMFed \times 1000 \times 0.03 - 0.5 \times ((MPBact / 0.8) - MPBact) + MPEndoReq$$

Where MPMaint = Metabolizable protein required for maintenance (g/day)
CW = conceptus weight
Scurf Requirement = $(0.3 \times (BW - CW)^{0.6})$;
Urinary Requirement = $(4.1 \times (BW - CW)^{0.5})$;
Metabolic Fecal Protein Requirement = (TotalDMFed × 1000 × 0.03 − 0.5 × ((MPBact / 0.8) − MPBact));
MP required for Endogenous Protein (MPEndoReq) = MPEndo/0.67;
MPBact = Metabolizable protein supplied by microbial protein (g/day);
MPEndo = Endogenous metabolizable protein (g/day) = 0.4 × EndCP and
EndCP = Endogenous crude protein (g/day) = 11.8 × TotalDMFed.

*Growth*

ENERGY REQUIREMENTS FOR GROWTH

Replacement Heifers, Lactating and Dry Cows (1st and 2nd Lactation only)

In this section of the model, requirements for growth are calculated from shrunk body weight, SBW (0.96 × BW) and empty body weight (EBW) (see Chapter 11 for rationale). The user may choose to enter a desired rate of gain or may use the model-generated target gains. For both options, a size-scaling approach is used which requires information on mature body weight (MBW) and mature shrunk body weight (MSBW). The user may use data on mature weights from his/her herd or may rely on default values generated in the program. Accurate estimates of mature weight are needed for accurate predictions of requirements. Representative weights of mature culls cows with average body condition scores may be used to estimate mature weights (MW).

MSBW = Mature shrunk body weight = 0.96 × MW
SBW = Shrunk body weight = 0.96 × BW
EBW = Empty body weight = 0.891 × SBW
EBG = Empty body weight gain = 0.956 × SWG

The following calculation is used to calculate the ratio of the standard reference weight to mature shrunk body weight (SRW_to_MSBW).

$$SRW\_to\_MSBW = 478 / MSBW$$

$$EQSBW = (SBW - CW) \times SRW\_to\_MSBW$$

Where EQSBW = Equivalent shrunk body weight (kg) and CW = Conceptus weight (kg).

The equation is used to compute shrunk weight gain (SWG):

$SWG = 13.91 \times (NEGrowthDiet^{0.9116}) \times (EQSBW^{-0.6837})$

Where SWG = shrunk weight gain (kg), NEGrowthDiet = NEg in the diet (Mcal)

If the animal is a replacement heifer, then WG (weight gain) = SWG (shrunk weight gain),
Otherwise, WG = ADG (Average daily gain)

The following equations are conversions to equivalent (size-scaled) weights:

EQEBW = Size-scaled empty body weight = 0.891 × EQSBW
EQEBG = Size-scaled empty body weight gain = 0.956 × WG

Retained energy (RE) is calculated with the following equation:

$RE = 0.0635 \times (EQEBW^{0.75}) \times (EQEBG^{1.097})$

*Protein Requirements for Growth*

REPLACEMENT HEIFERS, LACTATING AND DRY COWS (1ST AND 2ND LACTATION ONLY)

Net protein for growth (NPg) is calculated as follows:

NPg = WG × (268 − (29.4 × (RE / WG)))

Where WG = weight gain (kg) (always positive) and RE = retained energy (Mcal).

The efficiency with which net protein is used for gain (EffMP_NPg) is then computed:

If EQSBW ≤ 478 then EffMP_NPg = (83.4 − (0.114 × EQSBW)) / 100
Otherwise EffMP_NPg = 0.28908

The next step is to calculate the metabolizable protein required for growth (MPGrowth) by dividing NPg by the efficiency with which MP is converted to NP:

MPGrowth = NPg / EffMP_NPg

If the animal is a replacement heifer,
DMIAvailGrowth = TotalDMFed − DMIMaint − DMIPreg
Otherwise
DMIAvailGrowth = TotalDMFed − DMIMaint − DMIPreg − DMILact

Where DMIAvailGrowth is the dry matter intake for growth.

If Age < FirstCalf, then ADGwPreg = SWG + (ADGPreg / 1000)
Otherwise, ADGwPreg = (EQEBG / 0.956) + (ADGPreg/ 1000)

For replacement heifers only,
If NEfOverMEng > 0, then MEGrowth = NEGrowth / NEgOverMEng

Calculation of Target Weights and Average Daily Gain for Replacement Heifers and Animals in 1st and 2nd Lactations

The following set of calculations is used to compute the gain required to achieve specified target weights at first breeding, calving, and maturity which is assumed to occur at the beginning of the third lactation. It is important to ensure that appropriate mature weights, age at first calving, and calving interval data are entered or the predictions for target gain will be unrealistic.

The following equations are used to calculate age at different calvings:

Age1st = FirstCalf
Age2nd = Age1st + CalfInt
Age3rd = Age2nd + CalfInt
Age1stBred = Age1st − (280 / 30.4)

It is assumed that heifers will achieve 0.55 of their mature shrunk body weight at first breeding, 0.82 at first calving, and 0.92 at 2nd calving. At the onset of their third lactation, they are assumed to have reached their mature weight.

Wt1stBred = MSBW × 0.55
Wt1st = MSBW × 0.82
Wt2nd = MSBW × 0.92
Wt3rd = MSBW

ADG1stBred = (Wt1st − Wt1stBred) / ((Age1st − Age1stBred) × 30.4)
ADG1st = (Wt2nd − Wt1st) / (CI × 30.4)
ADG2nd = (Wt3rd − Wt2nd) / (CI × 30.4)

If AnimalType = “Replacement Heifer” and Age < Age1stBred Then ADGNonBred = (Wt1stBred − SBW) / ((Age1stBred − Age) × 30.4)
Otherwise, ADGNonBred = 0

If AnimalType ≠ “Replacement Heifer”, then ADGNonBred = 0

If AnimalType = “Replacement Heifer” and is pregnant then
ADG = ADG1stBred
Otherwise, ADG = ADGNonBred

*Pregnancy*

PREGNANT REPLACEMENT HEIFERS AND MATURE COWS

Constants used in pregnancy calculations are:

Km = conversion of ME to NE = 0.64
EffMEPreg = The efficiency with which ME is used for pregnancy = 0.14
EffMPPreg = The efficiency with which MP is used for pregnancy = 0.33

Until day 190 of pregnancy, no requirements for pregnancy are computed in the model. The maximum number of days that a cow can be pregnant is assumed to be 279.

CBW (calf birth weight) = MW × 0.06275
CW (conceptus weight) = (18 + ((DaysPreg − 190) × 0.665)) × (CBW / 45)
ADGPreg (ADG of the conceptus) = 665 × (CBW / 45)
MEPreg (ME required for pregnancy) = ((2 × 0.00159 × DaysPreg − 0.0352) × (CBW / 45)) / EffMEPreg
MPPreg (MP required for pregnancy) = ((0.69 × DaysPreg − 69.2) × (CBW / 45)) / EffMPPreg
NEPreg = Net energy required for pregnancy = MEPreg × Km

*Lactation*

If lactose content of milk is not available,

MilkEn (energy content of milk) = (0.0929 × MilkFat) + (0.0547 × MilkTrueProtein / 0.93) + 0.192

If lactose content is known,

MilkEn = (0.0929 × MilkFat) + (0.0547 × MilkTrueProtein / 0.93) + (0.0395 × Lactose)

The amounts of energy, protein, and fat in milk then are computed:

YEn = NELact (energy in milk daily, Mcal/day) = MilkEn × MilkProd
YProtn (daily protein yield in milk, kg/day) = MilkProd × (MilkTrueProtein / 100)
Yfatn (daily fat yield in milk, kg/day) = MilkProd × (MilkFat / 100)

MPLact (Metabolizable protein required for lactation) = (Yprotn / 0.67) × 1000

The following equation is used to convert to fat-corrected milk (FCM):

FCM = 0.4 × MilkProd + 15 × (MilkFat / 100) × MilkProd

*Reserves*

The factors used to adjust weight at the current CS to expected weight at CS3.

| | |
|---|---|
| $CS\_F_1$ = 0.726 | $CS\_F_6$ = 1.069 |
| $CS\_F_2$ = 0.794 | $CS\_F_7$ = 1.137 |
| $CS\_F_3$ = 0.863 | $CS\_F_8$ = 1.206 |
| $CS\_F_4$ = 0.931 | $CS\_F_9$ = 1.274 |
| $CS\_F_5$ = 1.000 | |

CS5EBW = (SBW × 0.851) / ( $CS\_F_X$)

Where CS5EBW = Empty body weight at CS5 using the 1 to 9 scale and CS_F = factor to calculate reserves at CS1 to 9.

$EBW_X$ (Empty body weight at $CS_X$) = $CS\_F_X$ × CS5EBW
$AF_X$ (Proportion of fat at $CS_X$) = 0.037683 × X
$TF_X$ (Weight of fat at $CS_X$) = $AF_X$ × $EBW_X$
$AP_X$ (Proportion of protein at $CS_X$) = 0.200886 − (0.0066762 × X)
$TP_X$ (Weight of protein at $CS_X$) = $AP_X$ × $EBW_X$
$ER_X$ (Energy reserves at $CS_X$) = (9.4 × $TF_X$) + (5.55 × $TP_X$)

Where X varies from 1 to 9.

If CS9 ≥ 3, then Lose1CS = $ER_{CS9}$ − $ER_{CS9-2}$,
Otherwise, Lose1CS = 1000000

If CS9 ≥ 3, then NElSub = 0.82 × Lose1CS
Otherwise, NElSub = 0.82 × ($ER_{CS9}$ − $ER_1$)

If CS9 ≤ 7, then Gain1CS = $ER_{CS9+2}$ − $ER_{CS9}$
Otherwise, Gain1CS = 1000000

If CS9 ≤ 7, then NElReq = (0.644 / 0.75) × Gain1CS
Otherwise, NElReq = (0.644 / 0.75) × ($ER_9$ − $ER_{CS9}$)

If EnergyBal > 0, then deltaER = NElReq
Otherwise, deltaER = NElSub

Days to change condition score is calculated only for cows:

If AnimalType = "Replacement Heifer", then DaysToChange = 0.
Otherwise, DaysToChange = deltaER / EnergyBal

Energy balance is calculated in the following equations.

For Dry Cows and Lactating Cows:
NEBalance = NEl_Total − (NEMaint + NEPreg + NELact + NEGrowth)
(These groups of animals use an NE-based system.)

For Replacement Heifers:
MEBalance = (MEng_Total − (MEMaint + MEPreg + MEGrowth))
(Heifers use an ME-based system).

Weight change in cows due to energy balance is computed in the following equations:

For Lactating Cows:

If NEBalance < 0, Then kg weight change = NEBalance / 4.92
If NEBalance > 0, Then kg weight change = NEBalance / 5.12

For Dry Cows:
If NEBalance < 0, Then kg weight change = NEBalance / 4.92
If NEBalance > 0, Then kg weight change = NEBalance / 6.40

If the animal is gaining weight, the protein requirement for this gain must be computed.

If NEBalance > 0 Then
MPReqReserves = (Reserves_WG × ProteinInGain) / 0.492
MPProvReserves = 0
RUPReqReserves = MPReqReserves / DietRUPDigest

If NEBalance < 0 Then
MPReqReserves = 0

If the animal is losing weight, the protein provided by catabolism is computed.

MPProvReserves = (−1 × Reserves_WG) × ProteinInGain × 0.67
RUPReqReserves = MPProvReserves /DietRUPDigest

Where MPReqReserves = metabolizable protein required for reserves, MPProvReserves = metabolizable protein provided by mobilization of reserves, RUPReqReserves = RUP required for repletion of reserves and RUPProvReserves = RUP provided by mobilization of reserves.

### *Mineral Requirements*

In most cases, the requirements for minerals are determined for each physiologic function, maintenance, growth, lactation, and pregnancy, but for some minerals this approach has not been followed. The maintenance component of the mineral requirement includes fecal, urinary, sweat, and miscellaneous losses. Because the bioavailability of minerals from various sources differs, the amount of the total mineral in the diet that is absorbable is determined. Growth requirements for minerals are calculated for heifers during their first lactation, but not during their first dry period or during the second lactation.

All calculations for milk mineral requirements are done on a 4 percent fat corrected milk basis (FCM). The equation to convert to FCM is:

FCM = (0.4 × MilkProd) + (15 × ( MilkFat / 100) × MilkProd)

CALCIUM (g/d)

*Fecal*
If DaysInMilk > 0, then Fecal = 3.1 × (BW / 100)
If DaysInMilk = 0, then Fecal = 1.54 × (BW / 100)

*Urinary*
Urine = 0.08 × (BW / 100)

*Miscellaneous*
Misc = 0

*Sweat*
Sweat = 0

*Pregnancy*
If DaysPreg > 190, then
Fetal = 0.02456 × Exp((0.05581 − (0.00007 × DaysPreg)) × DaysPreg) − 0.02456 × Exp((0.05581 − (0.00007 × (DaysPreg − 1))) × (DaysPreg − 1))

If DaysPreg ≤ 190, then Fetal = 0

*Lactation*
If DaysInMilk > 0, then
If breed = Holstein or Milking Shorthorn, then
Milk = 1.22 × Milk Prod
If breed = Jersey, then
Milk = 1.45 × Milk Prod
Otherwise, Milk = 1.37 × Milk Prod

*Growth*
If BW > 0 and WG > 0, Then
Growth = (9.83 × ($MW^{0.22}$) × ($BW^{-0.22}$)) × (WG / 0.96)

PHOSPHORUS (g/d)

*Fecal*
If AnimalType = Cow, then Fecal = 1 × TotalDMFed
Otherwise, Fecal = 0.8 × TotalDMFed

*Urine*
Urine = 0.002 × BW

*Miscellaneous*
Misc = 0

*Sweat*
Sweat = 0

*Pregnancy*
If DaysPreg ≥ 190 Then
Fetal = 0.02743 × Exp(((0.05527 − (0.000075 × DaysPreg)) × DaysPreg)) − 0.02743 ×

Exp(((0.05527 − (0.000075 × (DaysPreg − 1))) × (DaysPreg − 1)))
Otherwise, Fetal = 0

*Lactation*
If DaysInMilk > 0, then Milk phosphorus = 0.9 × MilkProd

*Growth*
If BW > 0 and WG > 0, then
Growth = $(1.2 + (4.635 \times (MW^{0.22}) \times (BW^{-0.22}))) \times (WG / 0.96)$

MAGNESIUM (g/day)

*Fecal*
Fecal = 0.003 × BW

*Urine*
Urine = 0

*Miscellaneous*
Misc = 0

*Sweat*
Sweat = 0

*Pregnancy*
If DaysPreg > 190 Then Fetal = 0.33 g/day
Otherwise, Fetal = 0

*Lactation*
If DaysInMilk > 0, Then Milk = 0.15 × MilkProd

*Growth*
Growth = 0.45 × (WG / 0.96)

CHLORINE (g/day)

*Fecal*
Fecal = 2.25 × (BW / 100)

*Urine*
Urine = 0

*Miscellaneous*
Misc = 0

*Sweat*
Sweat = 0

*Pregnancy*
If DaysPreg > 190 Then Fetal = 1
Otherwise, Fetal = 0

*Lactation*
Milk = 1.15 × MilkProd

*Growth*
Growth = 1 × (WG / 0.96)

POTASSIUM (g/day)

*Fecal*
If AnimalType = Lactating cow
Fecal = 6.1 × TotalDMFed
Otherwise Fecal = 2.6 × TotalDMFed

*Urine*
Urine = 0.038 × BW

*Sweat*
If Temp < 25, then Sweat = 0
If Temp 25 to 30, then Sweat = 0.04 × (BW / 100)
If Temp > 30, then Sweat = 0.4 × (BW / 100)

*Miscellaneous*
Misc = 0

*Pregnancy*
If DaysPreg > 190 Then Fetal = 1.027
Otherwise, Fetal = 0

*Lactation*
Milk = 1.5 × MilkProd

*Growth*
Growth = 1.6 × (WG / 0.96)

SODIUM (g/day)

*Fecal*
For lactating cows, Fecal = 0.038 × BW
Otherwise, Fecal = 0.015 × BW

*Urine*
Urine = 0

*Miscellaneous*
Misc = 0

*Sweat*
If Temp < 25, then Sweat = 0
If Temp 25 to 30, then Sweat = 0.1 × (BW / 100)
If Temp > 30, then Sweat = 0.5 × (BW / 100)

*Pregnancy*
If DaysPreg > 190, then Fetal = 1.39
If DaysPreg ≤ 190, then Fetal = 0

*Lactation*
Milk = 0.63 × MilkProd

*Growth*
Growth = 1.4 × (WG / 0.96)

SULFUR (g/day)

A non-factorial approach is used to determine the sulfur requirement.

Total = 2 × TotalDMFed

COBALT (mg/day)

A non-factorial approach is used to determine the cobalt requirement.

Total = 0.11 × TotalDMFed

COPPER (mg/day)

*Fecal*
Fecal = (0.0071 × BW)

*Urine*
Urine = 0

*Sweat*
Sweat = 0

*Miscellaneous*
Misc = 0

*Pregnancy*
If DaysPreg $<$ 100, then Fetal = 0.5 mg/day
If 100 $\leq$ DaysPreg $\leq$ 225, then Fetal = 1.5 mg/day
If DaysPreg $>$ 225, then Fetal = 2 mg/day

*Lactation*
Milk = 0.15 × MilkProd

*Growth*
Growth = 1.15 × (WG / 0.96)

IODINE (mg/day)

*Fecal*
Fecal = 0

*Urine*
Urine = 0

*Sweat*
Sweat = 0

*Miscellaneous*
Misc = 0

*Fetal*
Fetal = 0

*Lactation*
If DaysInMilk $>$ 0, then Milk = 1.5 × (BW / 100)
If DaysInMilk = 0, then Misc = 0.6 × (BW / 100)

*Growth*
Growth = 0

IRON (mg/day)

*Fecal*
Fecal = 0

*Urine*
Urine = 0

*Sweat*
Sweat = 0

*Miscellaneous*
Misc = 0

*Pregnancy*
If DaysPreg $>$ 190, then Fetal = 18
Otherwise, Fetal = 0

*Lactation*
Milk = 1 × MilkProd

*Growth*
Growth = 34 × (WG / 0.96)

MANGANESE (mg/day)

*Fecal*
Fecal = 0.002 × BW

*Urine*
Urine = 0

*Sweat*
Sweat = 0

*Miscellaneous*
Misc = 0

*Pregnancy*
If DaysPreg $>$ 190, then Fetal = 0.3
Otherwise, Fetal = 0

*Lactation*
If DaysInMilk $>$ 0, then Milk = 0.03 × MilkProd

*Growth*
Growth = 0.7 × (WG / 0.96)

SELENIUM (mg/d)

A non-factorial approach is used to determine the selenium requirement.

Total = 0.3 × TotalDMFed

ZINC (mg/day)

*Fecal*
Fecal = 0.033 × BW

*Urine*
Urine = 0.012 × BW

*Sweat*
Sweat = 0

*Miscellaneous*
Misc = 0

*Pregnancy*
If DaysPreg > 190, then Fetal = 12
Otherwise, Fetal = 0

*Lactation*
Milk = 4 × MilkProd

*Growth*
Growth = 24 × (WG / 0.96)

VITAMIN A (1000 IU/kg)

A non-factorial approach is used to determine the Vitamin A requirement.

If AnimalType = Lactating Cow, Dry Cow, or Replacement Heifer with DaysPreg > 259, then Total = 0.11 × BW
If AnimalType = Replacement Heifer with DaysPreg ≤ 259, then Total = 0.08 × BW

VITAMIN D (1000 IU/kg)

A non-factorial approach is used to determine the Vitamin D requirement.

The requirement is 0.03 × BW.

VITAMIN E (IU/kg)

A non-factorial approach is used to determine the Vitamin E requirement.

If the animal is grazing and the AnimalType = Dry Cow, then Vit E required = 0.5 × BW
If the animal is grazing and the AnimalType = Lactating Cow or Replacement Heifer,
Then Vit E required = 0.26 × BW
If the animal is not grazing and the AnimalType = Dry Cow, then Total = 1.6 × BW
If the animal is not grazing and the AnimalType = Lactating Cow or Replacement Heifer, then Vit E required = 0.8 × BW

## *Dry Matter Intake Predictions*

LACTATING AND DRY COWS

The equation to predict intake for lactating cows (DMILact) is:

$$DMILact = (((BW^{0.75}) \times 0.0968) + (0.372 \times FCM) - 0.293) \times Lag$$

Low intake in early lactation is adjusted using the Lag variable for lactating cows:

$$Lag = 1 - e^{(-1 \times 0.192 \times (WOL + 3.67))}$$

The equation for predicting the dry matter intake of dry cows (DMIDry) in the last 21 days of pregnancy is:

$$DMIDry = ((1.97 - (0.75 \times e^{(0.16 \times (DaysPreg - 280))})) / 100) \times BW$$

REPLACEMENT HEIFERS

Heifer intakes are adjusted for environmental temperature and conditions using the coat condition (CoatCond) variable to calculate CCFact, the adjustment factor. In the following section, we describe how the environmental adjustments are made and then provide the equation for heifer intake (DMI_RH).

If CoatCond = Clean/Dry, then CCFact = 1
If CoatCond = Some Mud, then CCFact = 1
If CoatCond = Wet/Matted, then CCFact = 0.85
If CoatCond = Covered with Snow/Mud, then CCFact = 0.7

Heifer intake also is adjusted for temperature effects (TempFact). At temperatures > 35, night cooling also affects intake:

If Temp < -15, then TempFact = 1.16
If -15 ≤ Temp ≤ -5, then TempFact = 1.07
If -5 ≤ Temp ≤ 5 , then TempFact = 1.05
If 5 ≤ Temp ≤ 15, then TempFact = 1.03
If 15 ≤ Temp ≤ 25, then TempFact = 1.00
If 25 ≤ Temp ≤ 35, then TempFact = 0.9
If Temp > 35 without night cooling, then TempFact = 0.65
If Temp > 35 with night cooling, then TempFact = 0.9

Predicted intake also is adjusted for the effects of age with the SubFact variable:

If Age ≤ 12, Then SubFact = 0.1128
If Age > 12, Then SubFact = 0.0869

The energy concentration of the diet affects intake using the DivFact variable. For lactating and dry cows, net energy diet concentration is calculated as follows:

NEDietConc = NEl_Total / Total DMFed

For replacement heifers, the equation is: NEDietConc = NEm_Total / Total DMFed

If NEDietConc < 1, then DivFact = 0.95
Otherwise DivFact = NEDietConc

Because intake decreases immediately prior to calving, an adjustment to intake is made in this period as well.

If DaysPreg < 210 and if DivFact > 0, then

$$DMI\_RH = ((BW^{0.75}) \times (((0.2435 \times NEDietConc) - (0.0466 \times (NEDietConc^{2})) - SubFact) / DivFact)) \times TempFact \times CCFact$$

If DaysPreg > 210 and < 259, then an intake adjustment factor (DMIRH_Factor) is used to adjust the intake of heifers. This DMIRH_Factor is multipled by DMI_RH to obtain the predicted DMI for heifers. The DMIRH-_Factor is calculated as follows:

$$DMIRH\_Factor = (1 + ((210 - DaysPreg) \times 0.0025))$$
if DaysPreg > 210 and < 259
Otherwise DMIRH_Factor = 1

If DaysPreg > 259, then $DMI\_RH = ((1.71 - (0.69e^{(0.35 \times DaysPreg - 280)}))) / 100 \times BW$

SUPPLY CALCULATIONS

*Energy*

The percent concentrate in the ration is calculated based on the amounts of feeds designated as "Concentrate" that are fed.

$$PercentConc = (ConcSum / TotalDMFed) \times 100$$

For feeds that are not classified as Vitamin/Mineral supplements, TDN at 1X maintenance ($TDN_{1x}$) and at the actual increment above maintenance is calculated.

$$TDN_{X} = (Feed_{X}.TDN / 100) \times (DMFed \times 1000)$$
$$TDN\_Act_{X} = (Feed_{X}.TDN\_Act_{X} / 100) \times (DMFed \times 1000)$$

The following calculations are used to determine the energy value of all feeds that are not classified as Calf Feeds or as Vitamins/Minerals. A different set of calculations is used to calculate the energy value of the milk-based calf feeds, and vitamin and mineral supplements are assumed not to contain energy.

*Non-fiber Carbohydrate (NFC) amounts and digestibility*

It is assumed that non-fiber carbohydrate digestibility, NFCDigest = 0.98
The total digestible NFC = tdNFC = NFCDigest × (100 − NDF − CP − Fat − Ash + NDFIP) × PAF

Where NFCDigestibility = non-fiber carbohydrate digestibility, NDF = neutral detergent fiber, CP = crude protein, Fat = Fat, NDFIP = neutral detergent insoluble protein, and PAF = processing adjustment factor.

The tdNFC is calculated for each feed and the amounts from the individual ration components are added together.

*Crude Protein Contribution to Energy*

The contribution of protein to the energy supply is computed in the next set of calculations. Different routines are used to calculate protein digestibility depending on how the feed is classified using the energy equation class (EnergyEqClass) that divides feeds into forages, concentrates, or feeds of animal origin also is used.

Protein digestibility of forages is calculated with the following equation:

$$tdCP = Exp((-1.2 \times (ADFIP / CP))) \times CP$$

Where tdCP = total digestible Crude Protein, ADFIP = Acid detergent insoluble protein, and CP = crude protein.

Below is the equation to calculate protein digestibility of feeds (tdCP) containing proteins from animal sources:

$$tdCP = (CPDigest \times CP)$$

For all other classes of feeds, $tdCP = (1 - (0.4 \times (ADFIP / CP))) \times CP$

*Contribution of Fat to the Energy Supply*

If Fat < 1, then tdFat = 0
Otherwise, tdFat = (Fat − 1) × 2.25
If Category = Fat and EnergyEqClass = Fatty Acid,
TDN = Fat × FatDigest × 2.25
DE = 0.094 × FatDigest × Fat
If Category = Fat and EnergyEqClass = Fat,
TDN = 10 + ((Fat − 10) × FatDigest × 2.25)
DE = (FatDigest × (Fat − 10) × 0.094) + 0.43

*TDN Calculations*

Adjustments are made based on feed type in the calculations of TDN. TDN and DE are computed with the following equations if the feed is an Animal Protein:

$$TDN = (CPDigest \times CP) + ((Fat - 1) \times 2.25) + ((NFCDigest \times (100 - CP - Ash - Fat)) - 7)$$
$$DE = (tdNFC \times 0.042) + (tdCP \times 0.056) + (0.094 \times (tdFat / 2.25)) - 0.3$$

For feeds that are not Animal Proteins or Fats and that do contain some NDF (forages, many by-products, concentrates), the following equations are used:

$$TDN = tdNFC + tdCP + tdFat + dNDF - 7$$
$$DE = (tdNFC \times 0.042) + (dNDF \times 0.042) + (tdCP \times 0.056) + (0.094 \times (tdFat / 2.25)) - 0.3$$

The equation below is used for feeds that do not contain NDF, that are not primarily fat and that are not derived from animals (molasses, for example):

$TDN = ((0.98 \times PAF) \times (100 - CP - Fat - Ash)) + (CP \times (1 - (0.4 \times (ADFIP / CP)))) + ((2.25 \times (Fat - 1) - 7))$

$DE = (0.98 \times PAF) \times (0.042 \times (100 - CP - Fat - Ash)) + (CP \times (0.056 \times (1 - (0.4 \times (ADFIP / CP))))) + (0.094 \times (Fat - 1)) - 0.3$

The equations for feeds with fat and ash are:

$TDN = ((0.98 \times PAF) \times (100 - Fat - Ash)) + ((2.25 \times (Fat - 1) - 7))$

$DE = (0.98 \times PAF) \times (0.042 \times (100 - Fat - Ash)) + (0.094 \times (Fat - 1)) - 0.3$

No energy values are calculated for Vitamins or Minerals.

*Energy Calculations and Conversions*

For animals other than young calves, the ratio of total dry matter intake to intake used to meet the maintenance requirement (DMI_to_DMIMaint) is calculated with the following equations.

For replacement heifers

$DMI\_to\_DMIMaint = TotalTDN / (0.035 \times (SBW^{0.75}))$
Where DMI_to_DMIMaint is the amount of intake needed to meet the maintenance requirement, TotalTDN = Total dietary TDN, and SBW = shrunk body weight.

For lactating and mature cows

$DMI\_to\_DMIMaint = TotalTDN / (0.035 \times (BW^{0.75}))$

For young calves

$DMI\_to\_DMIMaint = TotalTDN / (0.035 \times (CalfBW^{0.75}))$

*Fat Adjustment*

After the total amount of fat in the diet has been determined (code not shown), it is necessary to make an adjustment to the TDN value if the diet contains more than 3 percent fat. Fat digestibility is calculated differently for feeds classified as fatty acids than for other fats. The equations below show how fat digestibility is calculated for 1) fat supplements classified as fats, 2) fat supplements classified as fatty acids, and 3) for other feeds:

1). $DigestibleFat = 10 + ((Fat - 10) \times FatDigest)$
2). $DigestibleFat = Fat \times FatDigest$
3). $DigestibleFat = Fat - 1$

If $(Fat\_Total / TotalRegDMFed) > 0.03$ Then
$Adj\_TDN = TDNConc - (((TotalFat) - 3) \times (TotalDigestibleFat / TotalFat) \times 2.25)$
$TDNConc = Adj\_TDN / ((100 - (TotalFat - 3)) / 100)$

*Discount Variable*

This variable is used to discount TDN to account for depressed digestibility of feeds above maintenance levels. It used to calculate energy availability for all classes of animals except young calves.

If a feed is not a milk-based calf feed and contains energy, then
$DiscountVariable = ((0.18 \times TDNConc) - 10.3) \times (DMI\_to\_DMIMaint - 1)$
Where DiscountVariable = Factor used to discount TDN, TDNConc = TDN concentration in the ration, and DMI_to_DMIMaint is the amount of the specified ration needed to meet the maintenance requirement.

The discount variable cannot be $< 0$ and, if the TDN of a feed is $< 60$, then the DiscountVariable = 1. Otherwise $Discount = (TDNConc - DiscountVariable) / TDNConc$

For feeds other than milk-based calf feeds and if $TDNConc > 0$, then
$TDN\_ActX = TDN \times Discount$

Different discounts are applied depending on the fat content of the ration. These discounts apply to all classes of animals except young calves.

If $Fat \geq 3$ and if the animal is a dry cow or a lactating cow, then
$MEng = (1.01 \times DiscDE) - 0.45 + (0.0046 \times (Fat - 3))$

If $Fat \geq 3$ and the animal is a heifer, then
$MEng = 0.82 \times DE$

Net energy for lactation for feeds having more than 3% fat is computed.
$NEl = (0.703 \times MEng) - 0.19 + ((((0.097 \times MEng) + 0.19) / 97) \times (Fat - 3))$

If the feeds have < 3% fat, the equation to compute ME for lactating and dry cows is
$MEng = (1.01 \times DiscDE) - 0.45$

The equation for heifers is
$MEng = 0.82 \times DE$

The equation to compute the NEl of low fat feeds is:

$NEl = (0.703 \times MEng) - 0.19$

For feeds that are not classified as fats

$MEforNEg = 0.82 \times DE$
$NEg = 1.42 \times MEforNEg - 0.174 \times MEforNEg^2 + 0.0122 \times MEforNEg^3 - 1.65$
$NEm = 1.37 \times MEforNEg - 0.138 \times MEforNEg^2 + 0.0105 \times MEforNEg^3 - 1.12$

Otherwise,
MEng = DiscDE
NEl = 0.8 × DiscDE
NEm = 0.8 × MEng
NEg = 0.55 × MEng

Computation of the total energy values for the diet.

MEng_Total = TotalMEConc × TotalRegDMFed
NEl_Total = TotalNElConc × TotalRegDMFed
NEg_Total = TotalNEgConc × TotalRegDMFed
NEm_Total = TotalNEmConc × TotalRegDMFed

If AnimalType is not "Replacement Heifer", then
NEDietConc = NE_Total / TotalRegDMFed
If AnimalType is "Replacement Heifer", then
NEDietConc = NEm_ Total / TotalRegDMFed

### *Protein Supply and Requirements*

Microbial yield (MCP_Total) is calculated as a percentage of discounted TDN (TDN_Act_Total):

MCP_Total = 0.13 × TDN_Act_Total

The following equation is used to calculate the amount of crude protein from each feed.

$CP_X$ = ($Feed_X$CP / 100) × (DMFed × 1000)

To calculate the site of digestion of protein, both passage (kp) and digestion (kd) rates are needed. Separate passage equations are used for concentrates, dry forages, and wet forages.

*Concentrate*

Kp = 2.904 + (1.375 × BW_DMI) − (0.02 × PercentConc)

*Dry Forage*

Kp = 3.362 + (0.479 × BW_DMI) − (0.017 × $Feed_X$NDF) − (0.007 × PercentConc)

*Wet Forage*

Kp = 3.054 + (0.614 × BW_DMI)

The amount of RDP in a specific feed is calculated using the following equation. It is assumed that all of Protein A is ruminally available and that none of Protein C is degraded in the rumen. Thus, only Protein B is affected by digestion and passage rates.

If ($Feed_X$.Kd + Kp) > 0 Then
$RDP_X$ = (($Feed_X$.Kd / ($Feed_X$.Kd + Kp)) × (((($Feed_X$.PrtB / 100) × ($Feed_X$CP /100)) × $Feed_X$DMFed))) + ((($Feed_X$PrtA / 100) × ($Feed_X$CP / 100)) × $Feed_X$DMFed)
Otherwise, $RDP_X$ = 0

The amount of ruminally-undegraded protein is obtained by subtraction:

$RUP_X$ = ($CP_X$ − ($RDP_X$ × 1000)) / 1000

If RUP_Total > 0, then DietRUPDigest = TotalDigestedRUP / RUP_Total
Otherwise, DietRUPDigest = 0.

The requirement for RDP is calculated in the following equation.

RDPReq = 0.15294 × TDN_Act_Total

RDPSup = TotalDMFed × 1000 × DietCP × CP_RDP

RDPBal = RDPSup − RDPReq

RUPSup = CP_Total − RDPSup

RUPReq = TotalCPReq − (MPBact + MPEndo))/ DietRUPDigest

The efficiency of microbial crude protein synthesis cannot exceed 0.85.

If MCP_Total > (0.85 × (RDP_Total × 1000)), then

MCP_Total = (0.85 × (RDP_Total × 1000))

CP required = RUPreq + RDPReq

MPBalance = (((MPFeed × 1000) + MPBact + MPEndo) − (MPMaint + MPPreg + MPLact + MPGrowth))

### *Amino Acids*

The amino acid supply is calculated using the following equation with arginine (Arg) as an example. The structure of this equation is similar for all of the amino acids that are considered in the model.

TArg = TArg + (((DMFed / TotalDMFed) × (CP / 100) × (($RUP_X$ × 1000) / $CP_X$) × (Arg / 100) × TotalDMFed) × 1000)

Where TArg = Total arginine, DMFed = quantity of feed X fed, TotalDMFed = Total dry matter fed, CP = % Crude Protein, $RUP_X$ = RUP in feed X, $CP_X$ = crude protein in feed X.

The next step is to calculate the total digestible supply of each amino acid. Below is the equation for Dig_TArg. The equations for the other amino acids have the same format.

Dig_TArg = Dig_TArg + (((DMFed / TotalDMFed) × (CP / 100) × (($RUP_X$ × 1000) / $CP_X$) × ($Feed_X$RUPDigest / 100) × (Arg / 100) × TotalDMFed) × 1000)

Where Dig_TArg = Total digestible arginine,
RUPDigest = RUP digestibility of feed X

The total essential amino acid supply before the contribution of the microbial protein has been added (EAATotalBeforeMP) is calculated.

$$EAATotalBeforeMP = (TArg + THis + TIle + TLeu + TLys + TMet + TPhe + TThr + TTrp + TVal)$$

The variables x1 and x2 are used in the following sets of calculations of the total amount of each amino acid supplied. The equations to calculate the total amounts of each amino acid follow. In all equations, it is assumed that:

If EAATotalBeforeMP > 0 then
x1 = ((TArg (or other amino acid) / EAATotalBeforeMPP × 100)
Otherwise x1 = 0

If ((RUP_Total × 1000) + EndCP + MCP_Total) > 0 then
x2 = ((RUP_Total × 1000) / ((RUP_Total × 1000) + EndCP + MCP_Total)) × 100
Otherwise, x2 = 0

$$TotalArg = 7.31 + (0.251 \times x1)$$
$$TotalHis = 2.07 + (0.393 \times x1) + (0.0122 \times x2)$$
$$TotalIle = 7.59 + (0.391 \times x1) - (0.0123 \times x2)$$
$$TotalLeu = 8.53 + (0.41 \times x1) + (0.0746 \times x2)$$
$$TotalLys = 13.66 + (0.3276 \times x1) - (0.07497 \times x2)$$
$$TotalMet = 2.9 + (0.391 \times x1) - (0.00742 \times x2)$$
$$TotalPhe = 7.32 + (0.244 \times x1) + (0.029 \times x2)$$
$$TotalThr = 7.55 + (0.45 \times x1) - (0.0212 \times x2)$$
$$TotalVal = 8.68 + (0.314 \times x1)$$

The total essential amino acid supply is calculated below:

$$TotalEAA = 30.9 + (0.863 \times EAATotalBeforeMP) + (0.433 \times MCP\_Total)$$

Total flows of RUP of specific amino acids are calculated below:

$$TotalRUPArgFlow = 0.863 \times TArg$$
$$TotalRUPHisFlow = 0.863 \times THis$$
$$TotalRUPIleFlow = 0.863 \times TIle$$
$$TotalRUPLeuFlow = 0.863 \times TLeu$$
$$TotalRUPLysFlow = 0.863 \times TLys$$
$$TotalRUPMetFlow = 0.863 \times TMet$$
$$TotalRUPPheFlow = 0.863 \times TPhe$$
$$TotalRUPThrFlow = 0.863 \times TThr$$
$$TotalRUPTrpFlow = 0.863 \times TTrp$$
$$TotalRUPValFlow = 0.863 \times TVal$$

Duodenal flow (g/day) is calculated using an equation of the form below for each amino acid. Arginine is given as an example.

$$Arg\_Flow = (TotalArg / 100) \times TotalEAA$$

The contribution of microbial crude protein and endogenous protein to the amino acid supply is calculated as follows. The form of this equation is similar for all amino acids.

$$TotalMCPEndArgFlow = Arg\_Flow - TotalRUPArgFlow$$

The next step is to calculate the supply of each amino acid in RUP that is digestible. The form of the equation for each amino acid is similar to that given for arginine below:

If TArg > 0, then dTotalRUPArg = TotalRUPArgFlow × (Dig_TArg / TArg)
Otherwise, dTotalRUPArg = 0

The amount of a specific amino acid that is digestible and is of microbial or endogenous origin then is calculated. Arginine is used as the example but similar calculations are made for all amino acids.

$$dTotalMCPEndArg = 0.8 \times TotalMCPEndArgFlow$$

The flow of digestible arginine, or other amino acids) then is calculated.

$$Dig\_Arg\_Flow = dTotalRUPArg + dTotalMCPEndArg$$

The protein in the duodenum must be converted from crude protein to a metabolizable protein basis. Microbial crude protein is converted to metabolizable protein with an efficiency of 0.64:

$$MPBact = 0.64 \times MCP\_Total$$
$$MPFeed = TotalDigestedRUP$$
$$MPEndo = 0.4 \times EndCP$$

The next computation is to determine the percent of a specific amino acid of metabolizable protein. The arginine equation is similar to those of the other amino acids.

If (MPBact + (MPFeed × 1000) + MPEndo) > 0, then
ArgPctMP = 100 × (Dig_Arg_Flow / (MPBact + (MPFeed × 1000) + MPEndo))
Otherwise, ArgPctMP = 0

*Minerals*

Two sets of equations for the calculation of the supply of minerals are presented here for all classes of animals except for young calves. Both the amount of mineral supplied and the amount of the mineral that is absorbable are calculated. The first equations are for the macrominerals using calcium as an example. In the mineral equations, d is used for mineral supplements instead of x to denote the feed.

$\text{Supplied} = \text{Supplied} + ((\text{Feed}_d\text{Ca} / 100) \times \text{Feed}_d\text{DMFed})$
$\text{Absorbable} = \text{Absorbable} + (((\text{Feed}_d\text{Ca} / 100) \times \text{Feed}_d\text{DMFed}) \times (\text{Feed}_d\text{CaBio}))$

The second set of equations represents those used for trace minerals using zinc as an example.

$\text{Supplied} = \text{Supplied} + (\text{Feed}_d\text{Zn} \times \text{Feed}_d\text{DMFed})$
$\text{Absorbable} = \text{Absorbable} + ((\text{Feed}_d\text{Zn} \times \text{Feed}_d\text{DMFed}) \times (\text{Feed}_d\text{ZnBio}))$

Ration density (RD) = Supplied / TotalDMFed

## YOUNG CALF SUB-MODEL

Both the requirements and supply portions of the young calf sub-model are in this section.

### *Requirements*

#### ENERGY REQUIREMENTS

For young calves, the efficiencies with which feeds are used for maintenance and gain, Km and Kg, for milk-based and other feeds are fixed.

*Milk-fed*
CalfKm = 0.8 for milk-based feeds
CalfKg = 0.69 for milk-based feeds

*Fed Milk and Starter*
CalfKm = 0.75 if the feed is not milk-based
CalfKg = 0.57 if the feed is not milk-based

The equation to calculate the basal maintenance requirement of a calf without stress is:

$\text{NEmCalf} = 0.086 \times (\text{CalfBW}^{0.75})$

The next step is to calculate the CalfKm and CalfKg for the proposed ration using the fixed efficiencies of conversion of ME to NEm and NEg.

If the feed is classified as a calf feed (milk-based) and if cMEng ≠ 0, Then
$\text{CalfKm} = \text{CalfKm} + (0.86 \times (\text{Feed}_X\text{DMFed} \times \text{Feed}_X\text{cMEng}))$
$\text{CalfKg} = \text{CalfKg} + (0.69 \times (\text{Feed}_X\text{DMFed} \times \text{Feed}_X\text{cMEng}))$

An adjustment is made to ensure that no energy values are computed from mineral supplements:

$\text{NonMineralFeeds} = \text{NonMineralFeeds} + (\text{Feed}_X\text{DMFed} \times \text{Feed}_X\text{cMEng})$

For all other classes of feeds if MEng ≠ 0
$\text{CalfKm} = \text{CalfKm} + (0.75 \times (\text{Feed}_X\text{DMFed} \times \text{Feed}_X\text{MEng}))$
$\text{CalfKg} = \text{CalfKg} + (0.57 \times (\text{Feed}_X\text{DMFed} \times \text{Feed}_X\text{MEng}))$
$\text{NonMineralFeeds} = \text{NonMineralFeeds} + (\text{Feed}_X\text{DMFed} \times \text{Feed}_X\text{MEng})$

If NonMineralFeeds > 0 Then
CalfKm = CalfKm / NonMineralFeeds
CalfKg = CalfKg / NonMineralFeeds

#### LOWER TEMPERATURE ADJUSTMENTS TO CALF MAINTENANCE REQUIREMENT

The maintenance requirement for young calves is adjusted to account for cold stress as follows:

| *Temperature (° C)* | *Calves > 2 months* | *Temperature (° C)* | *Calves < 2 months* |
|---|---|---|---|
| > 5 | 0 | > 15 | 0 |
| 0 to 5 | 0.13 | 10 to 15 | 0.13 |
| −5 to 0 | 0.27 | 5 to 10 | 0.27 |
| −10 to −5 | 0.40 | 0 to 5 | 0.40 |
| −15 to −10 | 0.54 | −5 to 0 | 0.54 |
| −20 to −15 | 0.68 | −10 to −5 | 0.68 |
| −25 to −20 | 0.81 | −15 to −10 | 0.86 |
| −30 to −25 | 0.94 | −20 to −15 | 0.94 |
| <−30 | 1.07 | −25 to −20 | 1.08 |
| | | −25 to −30 | 1.21 |
| | | <−30 | 1.34 |

The resulting equation for the maintenance requirement of young calves with the temperature adjustment is:

$\text{NEmCalf} = (\text{NEmCalf} \times (1 + \text{TempFactor}))$

The next step is to recalculate ME required for maintenance with the NEm that has been adjusted for temperature effects.

If CalfKm ≠ 0 Then
MEMaint = NEmCalf / CalfKm
Otherwise MEMaint = 0

The following equation is used to calculate the amount of intake devoted to meeting the maintenance requirement:

If DietNEmCalf ≠ 0 Then
DMIForNEmCalf = NEmCalf / DietNEmCalf
Else DMIForNEmCalf = 0

A similar calculation is used to calculate the dry matter intake available for growth and the net energy available for growth:

DMIForGrowth = (TotalDMFed − DMIForNEmCalf)

NEFGCalf = DMIForGrowth × DietNEmCalf

If CalfKg ≠ 0 Then MEFGCalf = NEFGCalf / CalfKg
Else MEFGCalf = 0

If NEFGCalf > 0 Then
EnergyADGCalf = Exp((0.8333 × (Log((1.19 × NEFGCalf) / (0.69 × (CalfBW$^{0.355}$))))))

CALF PROTEIN REQUIREMENTS

Calf protein requirements are computed with the following equation:

ProteinReqCalf = CalfADG × 0.188 (30 g N/kg gain = 187.5 g Net Protein / kg gain)

Total apparently digested protein (TotalADP) is calculated as follows where 0.93 and 0.75 are the assumed digestibilities of milk-based feeds and starter feeds respectively:

TotalADP + ((TotalMilkCP × 0.93) + (TotalStarterCP× 0.75)) × 1000

The ratio of ADP to CP is calculated as follows:

ADP_to_CP = TotalADP / ((TotalMilkCP + TotalStarterCP) × 1000)

*Calf Protein Maintenance Requirements*

EUN = Endogenous urinary N losses = 0.2 × (CalfBW$^{0.75}$)
MFN = Metabolic fecal N = (MilkDMI × 1.9) + (StarterDMI × 3.3))
BV = Biological value = (0.8 × (TotalMilkCP / TotalCP)) + (0.7 × (TotalStarterCP / TotalCP))

ADPmaint = 6.25 × (((1 / BV) × (EUN + MFN)) − MFN)

CPmCalf = ADPMaint / ADP_to_CP if ADP_to_CP>0

ADPgrowth = (ProteinReqCalf × 1000) / BV

ADPAllowGain = ((TotalADP − ADPmaint) × BV) / 0.188

CALF MINERAL REQUIREMENTS

A factorial approach is not used to estimate mineral requirements for young calves. The requirements for calves are based on the amounts of milk-based feed, starter, and grower that are offered. It is assumed that the values presented in Table 10 = 6 for milk replacers, calf starter, and grower meet the mineral requirements of the young calf. Table 16-2 indicates the desired ration densities for each of the three categories of feeds (milk-based calf feeds, calf starter, and calf grower). The densities for calf grower are used as the standard for all feeds in the Feed Library except milk-based feeds and calf starter.

To calculate the desired concentrations of each mineral, the following equation is used:

TABLE 16-2 Ration Densities of Required Minerals for Three Categories of Feeds for Calves

| Mineral | Milk-Replacer | Starter | Grower |
|---|---|---|---|
| Calcium | 1.0 | 0.7 | 0.6 |
| Phosphorus | 0.7 | 0.45 | 0.4 |
| Magnesium | 0.07 | 0.1 | 0.1 |
| Sodium | 0.4 | 0.15 | 0.14 |
| Potassium | 0.65 | 0.65 | 0.65 |
| Chlorine | 0.25 | 0.2 | 0.2 |
| Sulfur | 0.29 | 0.2 | 0.2 |
| Iron | 100 | 50 | 50 |
| Manganese | 40 | 40 | 40 |
| Zinc | 40 | 40 | 40 |
| Copper | 10 | 10 | 10 |
| Iodine | 0.5 | 0.25 | 0.25 |
| Cobalt | 0.11 | 0.1 | 0.1 |
| Selenium | 0.3 | 0.3 | 0.3 |
| Vitamin A | 9 | 4 | 4 |
| Vitamin D | 0.6 | 0.6 | 0.6 |
| Vitamin E | 50 | 25 | 25 |

If TotalDMFed>0 Then
RDReq = ((MilkFeeds × m) + (CalfStarter × n) + (RegFeeds × o)) / TotalDMFed
Where m = concentration of mineral X in MilkFeeds,
n = concentration of mineral X in calf starter, and
o = concentration of mineral X in regular feeds.

*Calf Supply and Diet Evaluation*

In the calf submodel, milk-based feeds are in a separate category in the feed library because the energy values for these feeds are calculated differently from feeds that may be used as starter feeds. Any feed in the library except for the milk-based calf feeds may be used as a starter feed. The information for the starter feeds is taken from the appropriate category of the main feed library.

*Calf Energy and Protein*

The energy calculations to obtain TDN, DE, and ME are included in the main energy computation section. To get the appropriate energy and protein values, the totals from the calf feeds are calculated and then the totals from the other feeds are obtained. Finally, the contributions from the two groups of feeds are added together.

In the following sets of calculations, it is assumed that the initial value of the variable is 0.

TotalNEm = TotalNEm + (DMFed × cNEm)
TotalNEg = TotalNEg + (DMFed × cNEg)
TotalME = TotalME + (DMFed × cMEng)
TotalCP = TotalCP + (DMFed × (cCP / 100))
TotalDCP = TotalDCP + (DMFed × (cDCP / 100))

If Category = "Calf Feed − Milk" Then
MilkDMI = MilkDMI + DMFed
MilkME = MilkME + (DMFed × cMEng)

TotalMilkADP = TotalMilkADP + (DMFed × (cDCP / 100))
TotalMilkCP = TotalMilkCP + (DMFed × (cCP / 100))

Otherwise
StarterDMI = StarterDMI + DMFed
StarterME = StarterME + (DMFed × cMEng)
TotalStarterADP = TotalStarterADP + (DMFed × (cDCP / 100))
TotalStarterCP = TotalStarterCP + (DMFed × (cCP / 100))

To convert starter/regular feeds from CP to cDCP:

$$cDCP = 0.75 \times CP$$

Here are the equations to obtain the total values:

TotalNEm = TotalNEm + NEm_Total
TotalNEg = TotalNEg + NEg_Total
TotalME = TotalME + MEng_Total

DietNEmCalf = TotalNEm / TotalDMFed
DietNEgCalf = TotalNEg / TotalDMFed
DietMECalf = TotalME / TotalDMFed

Mature Weights

Mature weight is used both to estimate the target growth rates of replacement heifers and to predict calf birth weights. The user has the option of entering the mature weight based on herd observations or of using default values.

The default weights for various breeds are:

| | |
|---|---|
| Aryshire | 545 kg |
| Brown Swiss | 682 kg |
| Guernsey | 500 kg |
| Holstein | 682 kg |
| Jersey | 454 kg |
| Milking Shorthorn | 568 kg |

Calf birth weight is calculated from mature weight using the following equation:

$$CBW\_From\_MW = 0.06275 \times MW$$

## REFERENCES


Aydin, G., R. J. Grant, and O. R. J. 1999. Brown midrib sorghum in diets for lactating dairy cows. J. Dairy Sci. 82:2127–2135.

Bertrand, J. A., F. E. Pardue, and T. C. Jenkins. 1998. Effect of ruminally protected amino acids on milk yield and composition of Jersey cows fed whole cottonseed. J. Dairy Sci. 81:2215–2220.

Coomer, J. C., H. E. Amos, C. C. Williams, and J. G. Wheeler. 1993. Response of early lactation cows to fat supplementation in diets with different nonstructural carbohydrate concentrations. J. Dairy Sci. 76:3747–3754.

Dann, H. M., J. K. Drackley, G. C. McCoy, M. F. Hutjens, and J. E. Garrett. 2000. Effects of yeast culture (*Saccharomyces cerevisiae*) on prepartum intake and postpartum intake and milk production of Jersey cows. J. Dairy Sci. 83:123–127.

Dhiman, T. R., and L. D. Satter. 1993. Protein as the first-limiting nutrient for lactating dairy cows fed high proportions of good quality alfalfa silage. J. Dairy Sci. 76:1960–1971.

Kalscheur, K. F., J. H. Vandersall, R. A. Erdman, R. A. Kohn, and E. Russek Cohen. 1999. Effects of dietary crude protein concentration and degradability on milk production responses of early, mid, and late lactation dairy cows. J. Dairy Sci. 82:545–554.

Khorasani, G. R., G. D. Boer, and J. J. Kennelly. 1996. Response of early lactation cows to ruminally undegradable protein in the diet. J. Dairy Sci. 79:446–453.

Khorasani, G. R., E. K. Okine, J. J. Kennelly, and J. H. Helm. 1993. Effect of whole crop cereal grain silage substituted for alfalfa silage on performance of lactating dairy cows. J. Dairy Sci. 76: 3536–3546.

Kim, Y. K., D. J. Schingoethe, D. P. Casper, and F. C. Ludens. 1993. Supplemental dietary fat from extruded soybeans and calcium soaps of fatty acids for lactating dairy cows. J. Dairy Sci. 76:197–204.

Knowlton, K. F., B. P. Glenn, and R. A. Erdman. 1998. Performance, ruminal fermentation, and site of starch digestion in early lactation Holstein cows fed corn grain harvested and processed differently. J. Dairy Sci. 81:1972–1985.

Kuehn, C. S., J. G. Linn, D. G. Johnson, H. G. Jung, and M. I. Endres. 1999. Effect of feeding silages from corn hybrids selected for leafiness or grain to lactating dairy cattle. J. Dairy Sci. 82:2746–2755.

Messman, M. A., W. P. Weiss, P. R. Henderlong, and W. L. Shockey. 1992. Evaluation of pearl millet and field peas plus triticale silages for midlactation dairy cows. J. Dairy Sci. 75:2769–2775.

Mowrey, A., M. R. Ellersieck, and J. N. Spain. 1999. Effect of fibrous by-products on production and ruminal fermentation in lactating dairy cows. J. Dairy Sci. 82:2709–2715.

National Research Council. 1989. Nutrient Requirements of Dairy Cattle, 6th rev. ed., Washington, DC: National Academy Press.

Overton, T. R., L. S. Emmert, and J. H. Clark. 1998. Effects of source of carbohydrate and protein and rumen-protected methionine on performance of cows. J. Dairy Sci. 81:221–228.

Pereira, M. N., E. F. Garrett, G. R. Oetzel, and L. E. Armentano. 1999. Partial replacement of forage with nonforage fiber sources in lactating cow diets. I. Performance and health. J. Dairy Sci. 82:2716–2730.

Santos, F. A. P., J. T. Huber, C. B. Theurer, R. S. Swingle, J. M. Simas, K. H. Chen, and P. Yu. 1998. Milk yield and composition of lactating cows fed steam-flaked sorghum and graded concentrations of ruminally degradable protein. J. Dairy Sci. 81:215–220.

Santos, J. E. P., J. T. Huber, C. B. Theurer, L. G. Nussio, M. Tarazon, and F. A. P. Santos. 1999. Response of lactating dairy cows to steam-flaked sorghum, steam-flaked corn, or steam-rolled corn and protein sources of differing degradability. J. Dairy Sci. 82:728–737.

Soder, K. J., and L. A. Holden. 1999. Dry matter intake and milk yield and composition of cows fed yeast prepartum and postpartum. J. Dairy Sci. 82:605–610.

Stegeman, G. A., D. P. Casper, D. J. Schingoethe, and R. J. Baer. 1992. Lactational responses of dairy cows fed unsaturated dietary fat and receiving bovine somatotropin. J. Dairy Sci. 75:1936–1945.

Tackett, V. L., J. A. Bertrand, T. C. Jenkins, F. E. Pardue, and L. W. Grimes. 1996. Interaction of dietary fat and acid detergent fiber diets of lactating dairy cows. J. Dairy Sci. 79:270–275.

Wattiaux, M. A., D. K. Combs, and R. D. Shaver. 1994. Lactational responses to ruminally undegradable protein by dairy cows fed diets based on alfalfa silage. J. Dairy Sci. 77:1604–1617.

Weiss, W. P. 1995. Full lactation response of cows fed diets with different sources and amounts of fiber and ruminal degradable protein. J. Dairy Sci. 78:1802–1814.

Weiss, W. P., and W. L. Shockey. 1991. Value of orchardgrass and alfalfa silages fed with varying amounts of concentrates to dairy cows. J. Dairy Sci. 74:1933–1943.

Weiss, W. P., and D. J. Wyatt. 2000. Effect of oil content and kernel processing of corn silage on digestibility and milk production by dairy cows. J. Dairy Sci. 83:351–358.

Wilkerson, V. A., B. P. Glenn, and K. R. McLeod. 1997. Energy and nitrogen balance in lactating cows fed diets containing dry or high moisture corn in either rolled or ground form. J. Dairy Sci. 80:2487–2496.

# Glossary

A glossary of terms used in the computer model and text description is provided here. This glossary provides definitions for terms, abbreviations, and acronyms used throughout the model and text revision. The user should note that the metric system is used internally for all calculations in the model, even if the user has chosen to use English units. No units are specified for variables used to calculate mineral requirements or supply because different units are used for different minerals.

**a1:** The thermoneutral maintenance requirement (Mcal/day/kg $BW^{0.75}$).

**a2:** Adjustment for previous temperature effect on maintenance requirement for heifers. (Mcal/day/kg $SBW^{0.75}$).

**Absorbable:** Total quantity of absorbable mineral supplied by the diet.

**ADF():** Acid detergent fiber (% DM).

**ADF_Total:** Total ADF intake (g/day).

**ADFIP:** Acid detergent insoluble protein (% DM).

**ADG:** Average daily gain for animal given current age and weight status (kg/day).

**ADG1st:** Average daily gain at first calving (kg/day).

**ADG1stBred:** Average daily gain at first breeding (kg/day).

**ADGNonBred:** Average daily gain of non-pregnant replacement heifers (kg/day).

**ADG2nd:** Average daily gain at second calving (kg/day).

**ADG3rd:** Average daily gain at third calving (kg/day).

**ADGPreg:** Average daily gain due to conceptus growth (g/day).

**ADGwoPreg:** Average daily gain without pregnancy (kg/day).

**ADGwPreg:** Average daily gain with pregnancy (kg/day).

**ADP:** Apparently digestible protein (g/day).

**ADPAllowGain:** ADP allowable gain for young calves (g/day).

**ADPGrowth:** Apparently digested crude protein available for growth for young calves (g/day).

**ADPMaint:** Apparently digested crude protein for maintenance for young calves (g/day).

**AF(1 To 9):** Proportion of fat in the animal at specified condition score.

**Age:** Current age (months).

**Age1st:** Age at first calving (months).

**Age1stBred:** Age at first breeding (months).

**Age2nd:** Age at second calving (months).

**Age3rd:** Age at third calving (months).

**AnimalType:** Lactating cow, dry cow, replacement heifer, or young calf are the choices.

**AP(1 To 9):** Proportion of protein in animal at specified condition score.

**Arg:** Arginine (% CP).

**Arg_Flow:** Flow of arginine to the small intestine (g/day).

**ArgPctMP:** Arginine as a percent of metabolizable protein (%).

**Ash:** Dietary ash (% DM).

**Balance:** Difference between the quantity of the mineral required and supplied.

**Breed:** Breed of animal. The choices are Ayrshire, Brown Swiss, Guernsey, Holstein, and Jersey.

**BV:** Biological value used in apparently digested protein (ADP) calculation for young calves.

**BW:** Body weight (kg).

**Ca:** Calcium (% DM).

**CaBio:** Bioavailability of calcium in a feed (%).

**CalfADG:** Average daily gain of young calves (g/day).

**CalfADPBal:** Digestible apparently digested protein balance for young calves (g/day).
**CalfAge:** Calf age (weeks).
**CalfBW:** Calf body weight (kg).
**CalfCPBal:** Digestible crude protein balance for young calves (g/day).
**CalfFat:** Dietary fat in calf rations (kg/day).
**CalfInt:** Calving interval (months).
**CalfKg:** Efficiency of use of ME for NEg.
**CalfKm:** Efficiency of use of ME for NEm.
**CBWFromMW:** Used to compute calf birth weight from mature weight of cow if CalfBW is not available (kg).
**CalfTemp:** Environmental temperature for calves (° C).
**cAsh:** Calf ash (% DM).
**Ca_TargetDietConc:** Ration density for calcium required to meet animal's requirements.
**CBW:** Calf birth weight (kg).
**CCFact:** Coat condition factor used to adjust dry matter intake predictions for replacement heifers.
**cCP:** Calf crude protein (% DM).
**cDCP:** Calf digestible crude protein (% DM).
**cDE:** Calf digestible energy (Mcal/kg DM).
**cDM:** Dry matter for calf feeds (% as Fed (AF)).
**cEE:** Calf ether extract (% DM).
**cGE:** Calf gross energy (Mcal/kg DM).
**Cl:** Chlorine (% DM).
**ClBio:** Bioavailability of Cl in a feed (%).
**cMEng:** Calf metabolizable energy (ME) (Mcal/kg).
**cMEovercGE:** cME / cGE which equals the quotient, q, in the calf energy equations.
**cNEg:** Calf net energy for growth (NEg) (Mcal/kg).
**cNEm:** Calf net energy for maintenance (NEm) (Mcal/kg).
**Co:** Cobalt (mg/kg).
**CoBio:** Bioavailability of Co in a feed (%).
**Coat:** Adjustment to insulation due to wetness of coat. Depends on input CoatCond.
**CoatCond:** Input variable describing coat condition. Choices are clean/dry, some mud, wet/matted or covered with snow/mud.
**ColdStr:** Cold stress factor for computing the net energy requirement for maintenance with stress (Mcal/day/$BW^{0.75}$).
**COMP:** Compensation effect for previous plane of nutrition. Used for heifers only.
**CP:** Crude protein (% DM).
**CP():** Crude protein for a specific feed (g/day).
**CPDigest:** Crude protein (CP) digestibility coefficient.
**CPgCalf:** Crude protein required for growth for young calves (g/day).
**CPmCalf:** Maintenance crude protein requirement for young calves (g/day).
**CPPreg:** Crude protein requirement for pregnancy (g/day).
**CP_RDP:** Fraction of crude protein (CP) that is degradable (RDP).
**CP_RUP:** Fraction of crude protein (CP) that is undegradable (RUP).
**CP_Total:** Total crude protein (CP) intake (g/day).
**CS:** Condition score, 1–5 dairy scale.
**CS5EBW:** Empty body weight of animal at condition score 5 (kg).
**CS9:** Condition score, 1–9 scale used internally in the model.
**CS_F(1 To 9):** Factor to calculate reserves for body condition scores 1 to 9.
**Cu:** Copper (mg/kg).
**CuBio:** Bioavailability of Cu in a feed (%).
**CW:** Conceptus weight (kg).
**Cys:** Cysteine (% CP).
**DaysInMilk:** Days in milk.
**DailyMilk:** Daily milk production (kg/day).
**DaysPreg:** Days pregnant (day).
**DaysToChange:** Number of days needed to increase or decrease one condition score (days).
**DE:** Digestible energy (Mcal).
**DE_Total:** Total DE intake (Mcal/day).
**deltaER:** Change in ER needed to increase or decrease one condition score (Mcal).
**DesiredADG:** User-defined target ADG (g/day).
**DietADF:** Fraction of ADF in the animal's ration.
**DietaryNFC:** Total dietary non-fiber carbohydrate (NFC) (g/day).
**DietCP:** Fraction of crude protein (CP) in the diet.
**DietCPCalf:** Dietary CP for young calves (%).
**DietDCPCalf:** Dietary digestible crude protein for calves (%).
**DietFatCalf:** Dietary fat (%).
**DietME:** Quantity of ME in the diet (Mcal/kg).
**DietMECalf:** Dietary metabolizable energy (ME) (Mcal/kg).
**DietNDF:** Fraction of neutral detergent fiber (NDF) in the diet.
**DietNEgCalf:** Dietary NEg for young calves (Mcal/day).
**DietNEmCalf:** Dietary NEm for young calves (Mcal/day).
**DietNEg:** Quantity of NEg in the diet (Mcal/kg).
**DietNEl:** Quantity of NEl in the diet (Mcal/kg).
**DietRUPDigest:** Total RUP digestibility for the diet (weighted average).
**DietTDN:** Fraction of TDN in the diet.
**Dig_ArgFlow:** Flow of digestible arginine to the small intestine (g/day).
**Dig_HisFlow:** Flow of digestible histidine to the small intestine (g/day).
**Dig_IleFlow:** Flow of digestible isoleucine to the small intestine (g/day).

**Dig_LeuFlow:** Flow of digestible leucine to the small intestine (g/day).
**Dig_LysFlow:** Flow of digestible lysine to the small intestine (g/day).
**Dig_MetFlow:** Flow of digestible methionine to the small intestine (g/day).
**Dig_PheFlow:** Flow of digestible phenylalanine to the small intestine (g/day).
**Dig_ThrFlow:** Flow of digestible threonine to the small intestine (g/day).
**Dig_ValFlow:** Flow of digestible valine to the small intestine (g/day).
**DiscDE:** Discounted DE (Mcal/kg).
**Discount:** Factor used to discount energy value to adjust for intake.
**Distance:** Distance traveled between pasture and milking center to calculate activity requirement.
**DivFact:** Factor used to adjust the intake of replacement heifers based on the energy content of the diet.
**DLWReq:** Energy required for daily live weight change.
**DM:** Dry matter (% as Fed (AF)).
**DMFed:** Quantity of a specific feed fed to an animal (dry matter basis, kg).
**DMI():** Dry matter intake of a specific feed (kg/day).
**DMIAvailGrowth**: Dry matter available for growth (kg/day).
**DMIActual:** Actual dry matter intake (kg/day).
**DMIDry:** Dry matter intake of a dry cow (kg/day).
**DMIForGrowth:** Total dry matter intake used for growth (kg/day).
**DMIForMECalf:** Dry matter intake required to meet ME requirement of young calves (Mcal/day).
**DMIForNEmCalf:** Dry matter intake required to meet NEm requirement of young calves (kg/day).
**DMILact:** Dry matter intake of a lactating cow (kg/day).
**DMIMaint:** Dry matter intake required for maintenance (kg DM/day).
**DMIPred:** Predicted dry matter intake (kg/day).
**DMIPreg:** Dry matter intake required for pregnancy (kg DM/day).
**DMIRH_Factor:** An adjustment factor for intake of replacement heifers between 210 and 259 days pregnant.
**DMI_RH:** Dry matter intake of a replacement heifer (kg/day).
**DMI_to_DMIMaint:** Ratio of DMI to DMI required for maintenance.
**DMI_Total:** Total dry matter intake (kg/day).
**DryMatterIntake:** Dry matter intake (kg/day).
**dTotalMCPEndArg:** Contribution of microbial and endogenous protein to the supply of digestible arginine (g/day).
**dTotalMCPEndHis:** Contribution of microbial and endogenous protein to the supply of digestible histidine (g/day).
**dTotalMCPEndIle:** Contribution of microbial and endogenous protein to the supply of digestible isoleucine (g/day).
**dTotalMCPEndLeu:** Contribution of microbial and endogenous protein to the supply of digestible leucine (g/day).
**dTotalMCPEndLys:** Contribution of microbial and endogenous protein to the supply of digestible lysine (g/day).
**dTotalMCPEndMet:** Contribution of microbial and endogenous protein to the supply of digestible methionine (g/day).
**dTotalMCPEndPhe:** Contribution of microbial and endogenous protein to the supply of digestible phenylalanine (g/day).
**dTotalMCPEndThr:** Contribution of microbial and endogenous protein to the supply of digestible threonine (g/day).
**dTotalMCPEndVal:** Contribution of microbial and endogenous protein to the supply of digestible valine (g/day).
**EBG:** Empty body weight gain (kg) equals 0.956 × SWG.
**EBW:** Empty body weight (kg) which equals 0.891 × SBW.
**EBW(1 To 9):** Empty body weight of the animal for specified condition score (1 to 9) (kg).
**EffMEPreg:** Efficiency of use of ME during pregnancy = 0.14.
**EffMP_NPg:** Efficiency of use of MP for NPg.
**EffMPPreg:** Efficiency of use of MP during pregnancy = 0.33.
**EI:** External insulation (Mcal/m$^2$/° C/day).
**EndCP:** Endogenous crude protein (g/day).
**EnergyADGCalf:** Energy allowable average daily gain for young calves (Mcal/day).
**EnergyAllowableMilk:** Amount of milk production possible based on energy available (kg/day).
**EnergyEqClass:** Feed description to select for appropriate routine for energy prediction. Choices are forage, concentrate, and feed from animal sources (i.e., fish meal).
**Energy_TargetDietConc:** Amount of energy needed to meet animal's energy requirement. Expressed as NEl for cows and ME for replacement heifers (Mcal/kg).
**ER(1 To 9):** Energy reserves of the animal at a specified condition score (Mcal).
**EQEBG:** Gain size-scaled to the reference animal (g/day).
**EQEBW:** Equivalent empty body weight (kg) which equals 0.891 × EQSBW.
**EQSBW:** Equivalent shrunk body weight (kg).
**EUN:** Endogenous urinary nitrogen losses used in apparently digested protein calculations for young calves (g/day).

**Fat:** Dietary fat (% DM).
**FatDigest:** Fat digestibility coefficient.
**Fat__Total:** Total fat intake (kg/day).
**FCM:** Fat corrected milk production (kg/day). Corrected to 4 percent fat.
**Fe:** Iron (mg/kg).
**FeBio:** Bioavailability of Fe in a feed (%).
**Fecal:** Fecal endogenous loss of minerals.
**FecalMP:** MP loss in the feces (g/day).
**FeedCategory:** Feed groups. Choices are grass/legume forages, grain crop forages, energy sources, fats, plant protein feeds, animal protein feeds, by-product/other feeds, vitamins and mineral, and calf feeds (milk-based).
**FeedMaint:** Feed required for maintenance (kg DM/day).
**Fetal:** Fetal requirement. Used with minerals.
**FirstCalf:** Age at first calving (months).
**Flat:** A pasture system in which cows move less than 200 m of vertical distance.
**ForageDescrp:** Forage description which is used to predict rate of passage. Choices are wet or dry.
**ForageNDF:** Fraction of forage neutral detergent fiber in the diet.
**Gain1CS:** Energy needed to gain 1 condition score (Mcal).
**Grazing:** Is the animal on pasture? Choices are yes or no.
**Growth:** Growth requirement for minerals.
**HairDepth:** Effective hair depth (cm).
**HeatStr:** Heat stress factor for computing the net energy requirement for maintenance for replacement heifers based on the HeatStress variable. Applies to heifers only.
**HeatStress:** Heat stress description of breathing of heat-stressed animals. Choices are none, rapid/shallow, or open mouth. Applies to heifers only.
**Hilly:** Descriptor for pasture that influences the activity requirement, NEmact.
**His:** Histidine (% CP).
**His__Flow:** Flow of histidine to the small intestine (g/day).
**HisPctMP:** Histidine as a percent of metabolizable protein (%).
**HP:** Heat production (Mcal/m$^2$/day).
I: Iodine (mg/kg).
**IBio:** Bioavailability of I in a feed (%).
**Ile:** Isoleucine (% CP).
**Ile__Flow:** Flow of isoleucine to the small intestine (g/day).
**IlePctMP:** Isoleucine as a percent of metabolizable protein (%).
**INS:** Total insulation (Mcal/m$^2$/° C/day).
**K:** Potassium (% DM).
**KBio:** Bioavailability of potassium in a feed (%).
**Kd:** Protein digestion rate (%/hour).
**Km:** Diet NEl / DietNE is efficiency of use of ME for maintenance.
**LactNum:** Lactation number (integer).
**Lactose:** Lactose content of milk (%).
**Lag:** Week of lactation correction for dry matter intake of cows in early lactation.
**LCT:** Lower critical temperature (° C).
**Leu:** Leucine (% CP).
**Leu__Flow:** Flow of leucine to the small intestine (g/day).
**LeuPctMP:** Leucine as a percent of metabolizable protein (%).
**Lignin:** Lignin (% DM).
**Lose1CS:** Energy needed to lose 1 condition score (Mcal).
**Lys:** Lysine (% CP).
**Lys__Flow:** Flow of lysine to the small intestine (g/day).
**LysPctMP:** Lysine as a percent of metabolizable protein (%).
**Maint:** Sum of the miscellaneous, fecal, urine, and sweat losses for minerals.
**MCP__Total:** Total microbial crude protein (MCP) synthesis (g/day).
**MEAllowGainPreg:** ME allowable gain without pregnancy (kg/day).
**MEAllowGainPreg:** ME allowable gain with pregnancy (kg/day).
**MEcs:** Metabolizable energy required for cold stress (Mcal/day).
**MEFGCalf:** Metabolizable energy for growth for young calves (Mcal/day).
**MEforNEg:** Efficiency of conversion of ME to NEg.
**MEGrowth:** Metabolizable energy for growth. Used for heifers only.
**MEI:** Metabolizable energy intake (Mcal/day).
**MEng():** Metabolizable energy in a specific feed (Mcal/day).
**MEng__Total:** Total ME intake (Mcal/day).
**MEMaint:** Metabolizable energy for maintenance. Used only for heifers (Mcal).
**MEPreg:** Metabolizable energy requirement for pregnancy (Mcal/day).
**Met:** Methionine (% CP).
**Met__Flow:** Flow of methionine to the small intestine (g/day).
**MetPctMP:** Methionine as a percent of metabolizable protein (%).
**MFN:** Metabolic fecal nitrogen. Used in calculations of apparently digested protein (ADP) for young calves (g/day).
**Mg:** Magnesium (% DM).
**MgBio:** Bioavailability of Mg in a feed (%).
**Milk:** Mineral requirement for milk production.

**MilkDMI:** Milk dry matter intake for young calves (kg/day).
**MilkEng:** Energy content of milk (Mcal NEl/kg).
**MilkFat:** Milk fat (%).
**MilkProd:** Milk production (kg).
**MilkTrueProtein:** True protein content of milk (%).
**Misc:** Miscellaneous loss component for minerals.
**Mn:** Manganese (mg/kg).
**MnBio:** Bioavailability of Mn in a feed (%).
**MPAllowableGain:** Gain possible at a given amount of MP without pregnancy (kg/day).
**MPAllowableGainPreg:** Gain possible at a given amount of MP with pregnancy (kg/day).
**MPBact:** Metabolizable protein supplied by microbial protein (g/day).
**MPBalance:** Metabolizable Protein Balance (g/day).
**MPEndo:** Endogenous metabolizable protein (g/day).
**MPEndoReq:** Amount of dietary protein required to supply endogenous protein (g/day).
**MPFeed:** Metabolizable protein supplied by the animal's ration (g/day).
**MPGrowth:** Metabolizable protein required for growth (g/day).
**MPLact:** Metabolizable protein required for lactation (g/day).
**MPMaint:** Metabolizable protein required for maintenance (g/day).
**MPPreg:** Metabolizable protein for pregnancy (g/day).
**MPProvReserves:** MP provided by mobilization of reserves (g/day).
**MPReqReserves:** MP required to replete reserves (g/day).
**MP_TargetDietConc:** Ration density for MP required to meet animal's requirements.
**MSBW:** Mature shrunk body weight (kg).
**MW:** Mature weight (kg).
**MWFromBreed:** Mature weight average for breed (kg).
**Na:** Sodium (% DM).
**NaBio:** Bioavailability of Na in a feed (%).
**NDF:** Neutral detergent fiber (% DM).
**NDF():** Neutral detergent fiber for a specified feed (kg/day).
**NDFDigest:** Neutral detergent fiber (NDF) digestibility coefficient.
**NDFIP:** Neutral detergent insoluble protein (% DM).
**NDF_Total:** Total NDF (g/day).
**NEDietConc:** Concentration of net energy in the diet (kg DM/day).
**NEFGCalf:** Net energy available for growth for young calves (Mcal/day).
**NEFP:** Net energy for production (Mcal/day).
**NEg():** Net energy for growth (Mcal/kg).
**NEg():** Net energy for growth from a specified feed (Mcal/day).
**NEgOverMEng:** NEg_Total / MEng_Total.
**NEGrowth:** Net energy for growth (Mcal/day).
**NEGrowthDiet:** Net energy for growth available in the diet (Mcal/day).
**NEGrowthDietNS:** Net energy for growth available in the diet with no stress (Mcal/day).
**NEg_Total:** Total NEg intake (Mcal/day).
**NEl():** Net energy for lactation (Mcal/kg).
**NEl():** Net energy for lactation from a specified feed (Mcal/day).
**NELact:** Net energy requirement for lactation (Mcal/day).
**NElOverMEng:** Ratio of NEl to ME (NEl_Total / MEng_Total).
**NEPreg:** Net energy for pregnancy (Mcal/day).
**NElReq:** Amount of dietary net energy that will be needed to increase 1 condition score (Mcal).
**NElSub:** Amount of energy retained that will be substituted for dietary NEl in order to lose one condition score (Mcal).
**NEl_Total:** Total NEl intake (Mcal/day).
**NEm:** Net energy for maintenance (Mcal/kg).
**NEm:** Net energy of diet for maintenance (Mcal). This value is assumed to be equal to the net energy value of the diet for lactation (NEl_Total).
**NEmact:** The factor added to the basal maintenance requirement to account for activity (Mcal/day).
**NEMaint:** Net energy required for maintenance for mature dry and lactating cows (Mcal/day).
**NEMaintNS:** Net energy required for maintenance without stress for heifers (Mcal/day).
**NEmCalf:** Net energy required for maintenance for young calves (Mcal/day).
**NEmOverMEng:** Ratio of NEm to ME (NEm_Total / MEng_Total).
**NEm_Total:** Total NEm intake (Mcal/day).
**NEPreg:** Net energy required for pregnancy (Mcal/day).
**NEReserves:** Net energy required for replenishment of reserves or net energy available if reserves are mobilized (Mcal/NEl/day).
**NFCDigest:** Non-fiber carbohydrate (NFC) digestibility coefficient.
**NightCooling:** Factor used to adjust dry matter intake of heat-stressed replacement heifers.
**NonMineralFeeds:** Includes all feeds except for vitamin and mineral mixes that are assumed to contain no energy. Used in energy calculations for young calves.
**NPg:** Net protein requirement for gain (g/day).
**P:** Phosphorus (% DM).
**PAF:** Processing adjustment factor. Used to adjust for effects of processing on the non-fiber carbohydrate (NFC) fraction.
**PBio:** Bioavailability of P in a feed (%).
**PerEAA:** Percent essential amino acids (% RUP).

**Phe:** Phenylalanine (% CP).
**Phe_Flow:** Flow of phenylalanine to the small intestine (g/day).
**PhePctMP:** Phenylalanine as a percent of metabolizable protein (%).
**PredIntake:** Predicted intake (kg).
**PrevTemp:** Previous ambient temperature (° C).
**ProteinAllowableMilk:** Protein allowable milk (kg/day).
**ProteinInGain:** Protein in gain. Used in calculation of protein requirements for growth (g/day).
**ProteinReqCalf:** Protein allowable average daily gain (g/day).
**PrtA:** Fraction A of the crude protein that is non-protein nitrogen and a small amount of soluble true protein. (% CP).
**PrtB:** Fraction B of the crude protein that equals CP–PrtA–Frt C (% CP).
**PrtC:** Fraction C of the crude protein that is completely undegradable (% CP).
**PsgRate():** Predicted passage rate.
**P_TargetDietConc:** Ration density for Phosphorus required to meet animal's requirements.
**RD:** Ration density of a mineral in the animal's ration.
**RDPBal:** RDP balance (RDPReq–RDPSup) (g/day).
**RDPReq:** RDP required (g/day).
**RDPSup:** RDP supplied (g/day).
**RDP_Total:** Total ruminally degraded protein intake (g/day).
**RDP():** Ruminally degraded protein for a specified feed (g/day).
**RDReq:** Ration density of minerals required for young calf rations.
**RE:** Net energy retained (Mcal/day).
**Reserves_WG:** Weight gain due to reserves (kg).
**RUP():** Ruminally undegraded protein for a specific feed (g/day).
**RUPDigest:** Fraction of the rumen undegraded protein (RUP) that is digested (% RUP).
**RUPBal:** RUP balance (RUPReq–RUPSup) (g/day).
**RUPProvReserves:** RUP provided by mobilization of reserves (g/day).
**RUPReq:** RUP required (g/day).
**RUPReqReserves:** RUP required to replete reserves (g/day).
**RUPSup:** RUP supplied (g/day).
**RUP_Total:** Total RUP intake (g/day).
**S:** Sulfur (% DM).
**SBio:** Bioavailability of S in a feed (%).
**SA:** Surface area ($m^2$).
**SBW:** Shrunk body weight (kg) is 96% of full weight.
**ScurfMP:** Scurf MP requirement (g/day).
**Se:** Selenium (mg/kg).
**SeBio:** Bioavailability of Se in a feed (%).
**SRW:** Standard reference weight (kg). For replacement heifers, this number is 478 kg.
**SRW_to_MSBW:** Standard reference weight/mature shrunk body weight (kg).
**StarterDMI:** Young calf intake of starter (kg/day).
**SubFact:** Age-related factor used to adjust intake of replacement heifers.
**Supplied:** Total quantity of a mineral supplied by the animal's diet.
**Sweat:** Sweat loss component for mineral requirements.
**SWG:** Shrunk weight gain (kg).
**T:** Age in days.
**TargetADGwoPreg:** Target ADG without pregnancy (kg/day).
**TargetADGPreg:** Target ADG with pregnancy (kg/day).
**TDN:** Total digestible nutrients (% DM) at 1 X maintenance.
**TDN():** Total digestible nutrients for a specified feed (g/day).
**TDN_Act_Total:** Actual discounted TDN intake (g/day).
**TDN_ActX:** Total digestible nutrients (TDN) adjusted for increment over maintenance intake.
**TDN_Act():** Discounted total digestible nutrients for a specified feed (g/day).
**TDN_Total:** Total 1X-TDN intake (g/day).
**tdNFC:** Truly digestible non-fiber carbohydrate which equals NFCDigest × (100–NDF–CP–Fat–Ash + NDFIP) × PAF.
**Temp:** Current temperature (° C).
**TempFact:** The factor used to adjust the maintenance requirement of cold-stressed replacement heifers.
**TempFactor:** The adjustment to the maintenance requirement for cold-stressed young calves.
**TF(1 To 9):** Total weight of fat at specified condition score (kg).
**Thr:** Threonine (% CP).
**Thr_Flow:** Flow of threonine to the small intestine (g/day).
**ThrPctMP:** Threonine as a percent of metabolizable protein (%).
**TI:** Tissue insulation (° C/Mcal/$m^2$/day).
**Topography:** Description of pasture. Choices are flat or hilly.
**Total:** Total quantity of mineral required.
**TotalDigestedRUP:** Total RUP digestibility for the diet (weighted average).
**TotalDMFed:** Total dry matter fed (kg/day).
**TotalEAA:** Total essential amino acids (g/day).
**TotalMCPEndArgFlow:** Contribution of microbial and endogenous protein to the flow of arginine to the small intestine (g/day).

**TotalMCPEndHisFlow:** Contribution of microbial and endogenous protein to the flow of histidine to the small intestine (g/day).

**TotalMCPEndIleFlow:** Contribution of microbial and endogenous protein to the flow of isoleucine to the small intestine (g/day).

**TotalMCPEndLeuFlow:** Contribution of microbial and endogenous protein to the flow of leucine to the small intestine (g/day).

**TotalMCPEndLysFlow:** Contribution of microbial and endogenous protein to the flow of lysine to the small intestine (g/day).

**TotalMCPEndMetFlow:** Contribution of microbial and endogenous protein to the flow of methionine to the small intestine (g/day).

**TotalMCPEndPheFlow:** Contribution of microbial and endogenous protein to the flow of phenylalanine to the small intestine (g/day).

**TotalMCPEndThrFlow:** Contribution of microbial and endogenous protein to the flow of threonine to the small intestine (g/day).

**TotalMCPEndValFlow:** Contribution of microbial and endogenous protein to the flow of valine to the small intestine (g/day).

**TotalRegDMFed:** Total regular (not milk-based) feed offered (kg/day).

**TotalRUPArgFlow:** Total flow of ruminally undegraded arginine to the small intestine (g/day).

**TotalRUPHisFlow:** Total flow of ruminally undegraded histidine to the small intestine (g/day).

**TotalRUPIleFlow:** Total flow of ruminally undegraded isoleucine to the small intestine (g/day).

**TotalRUPLeuFlow:** Total flow of ruminally undegraded leucine to the small intestine (g/day).

**TotalRUPLysFlow:** Total flow of ruminally undegraded lysine to the small intestine (g/day).

**TotalRUPMetFlow:** Total flow of ruminally undegraded methionine to the small intestine (g/day).

**TotalRUPPheFlow:** Total flow of ruminally undegraded phenylalanine to the small intestine (g/day).

**TotalRUPThrFlow:** Total flow of ruminally undegraded threonine to the small intestine (g/day).

**TotalRUPTrpFlow:** Total flow of ruminally undegraded tryptophan to the small intestine (g/day).

**TotalRUPValFlow:** Total flow of ruminally undegraded valine to the small intestine (g/day).

**TP(1 To 9):** Total weight of protein in the animal at specified condition score (kg).

**Trips:** Number of one-way trips a lactating cow travels between pasture and milking center daily.

**Trp:** Trytophan (% CP).

**UndiscDE_Total:** Total undiscounted DE intake (Mcal/day).

**Urine:** Urine endogenous loss component for minerals.

**UrineMP:** MP requirement for urine (g/day).

**UseTargetADG:** Use target (model-predicted) ADG. Choices are yes or no.

**Val:** Valine (% CP).

**Val_Flow:** Flow of valine to the small intestine (g/day).

**ValPctMP:** Valine as a percent of metabolizable protein (%).

**VitA:** Vitamin A (1000 IU/kg).

**VitD:** Vitamin D (1000 IU/kg).

**VitE:** Vitamin E (IU/kg).

**WG:** Weight gain (kg/day).

**WindSpeed:** Speed of wind (m/s). Maximum windspeed input is 32 kph.

**WOL:** Week of lactation. Used to predict intake in early lactation (week).

**Wt1st:** Weight at first calving (kg).

**Wt1stBred:** Weight at first breeding (kg).

**Wt2nd:** Weight at second calving (kg).

**Wt3rd:** Weight at third calving (kg).

**YEn:** Daily energy secretion in milk (Mcal NEl/day).

**YFatn:** Daily milk fat yield (kg/day).

**YProtn:** Daily milk protein yield (kg/day).

**Zn:** Zinc (mg/kg).

**ZnBio:** Bioavailability of Zn in a feed (%).

# NUTRIENT REQUIREMENTS OF DAIRY CATTLE

## Seventh Revised Edition, 2001

## USER'S GUIDE

National Research Council
Board on Agriculture and Natural Resources
Committee on Animal Nutrition
Subcommittee on Dairy Cattle Nutrition

# Contents

# 1 Introduction

A compact disk containing a self-executable stand-alone program is provided as a companion to the National Research Council (NRC) *Nutrient Requirements of Dairy Cattle, Seventh Revised Edition, 2001*. This computer software allows the user to apply information presented in the report and equations summarized in Chapter 16 to practical situations. The program predicts requirements and allowable production from the dietary ingredients fed. It is a ration evaluator, not a ration balancer, so it does not perform the calculations necessary to develop least-cost rations. In addition, an Excel spread sheet is provided that calculates nutrient requirements for heifers at different weights and rates of gain.

We have attempted to make the software accurate and user friendly. Program help screens and context sensitive help are available in all portions of the software and in this User's Guide. The help material provides information that may assist the user in choosing inputs and in interpreting and applying outputs.

The focus of this User's Guide is to demonstrate features of the software including program operation, default data, input parameters, model structure, and equation documentation. The user is referred to the appropriate chapters for detailed information on the biological basis for equations and assumptions used in the software.

## SYSTEM REQUIREMENTS

The NRC Nutrient Requirements of Dairy Cattle program is designed to run:

- On a Windows 95/98 platform,
- With a minimum of 16 MB of RAM (32 MB recommended), and
- A minimum screen resolution of 600 × 800 pixels

WARNING: The program uses decimal points, not commas, to distinguish whole numbers from decimals. For people whose computers are set to use the comma as the delimiter (primarily, non-U.S. users in Europe and Latin America) settings must be changed in Windows. Before changing the settings uninstall the NRC program using the **Add/Remove Program** option in the **Control Panel** or use the Uninstall routine that comes with the program. Make sure that all parts of the program and the program file are deleted. The **Currency** and **Number** settings can be changed by going to the **Start** icon, then to **Settings**, **Control Panel**, and **Regional Settings.** Both the **Number** and **Currency** settings must be changed.

1. Make the **Number** tab settings look like those in Figure UG-1.
2. Make the **Currency** tab settings like those in Figure UG-2:

## RISK OF USE

Because of the many variables involved and judgments that must be made in choosing inputs, interpreting outputs, and general use of this program, the National Research Council makes no claim for the accuracy of this software and the user is solely responsible for risk of use.

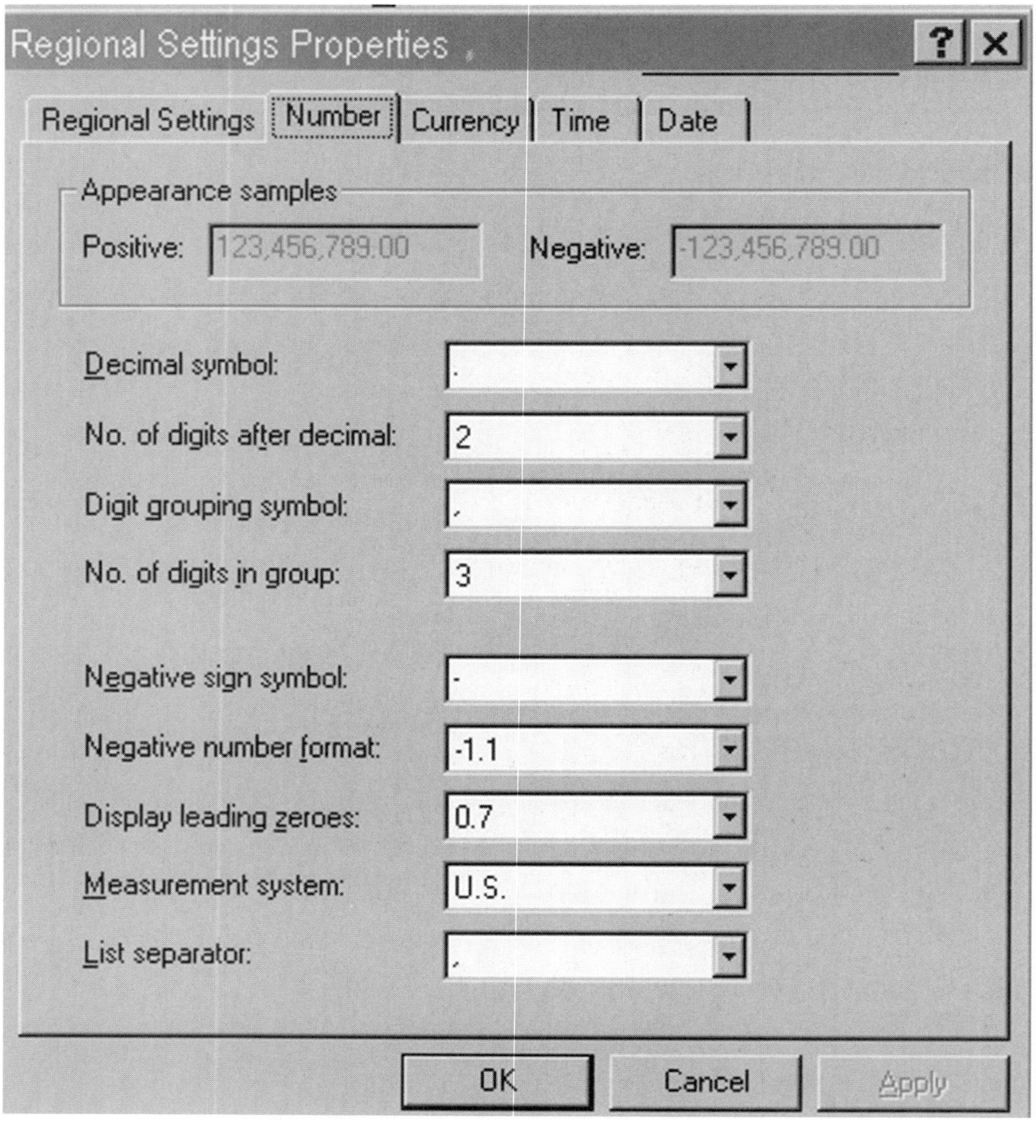


FIGURE UG-1 Settings for number properties.

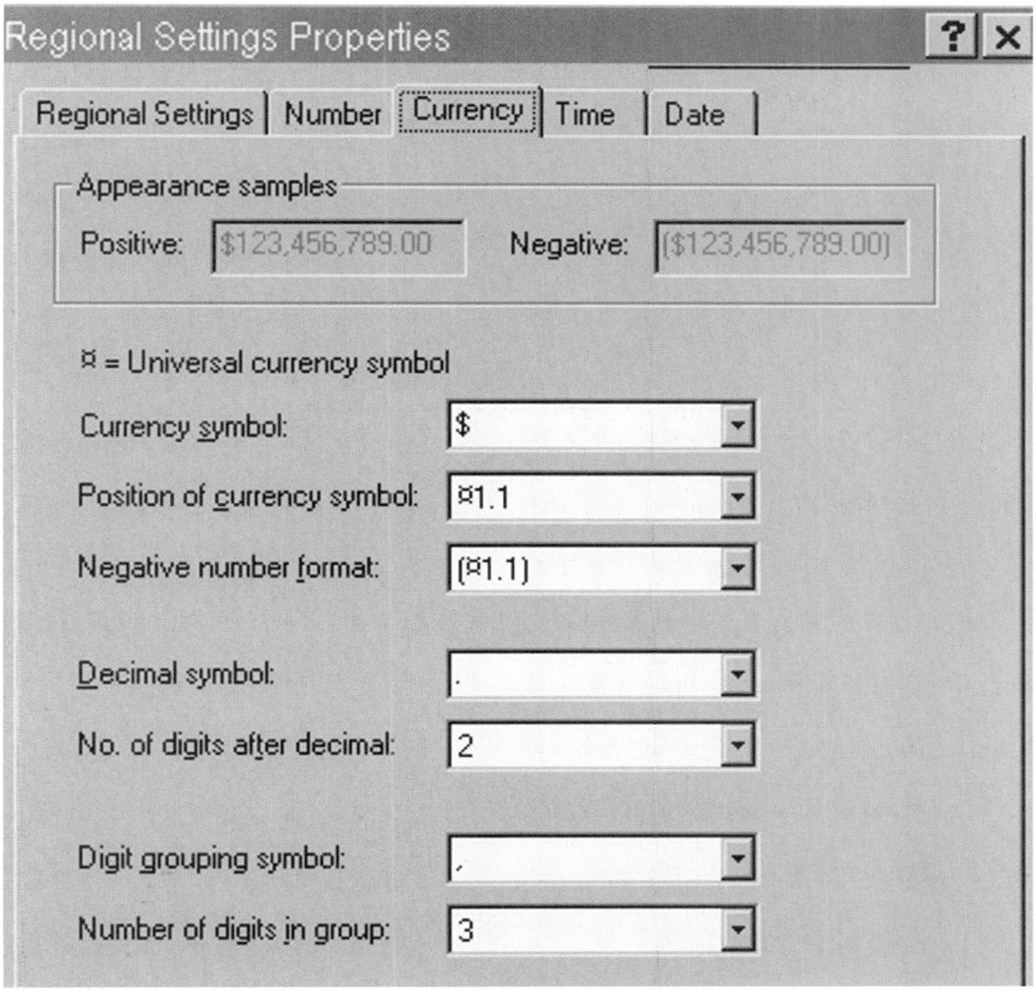


FIGURE UG-2 Settings for Currency.

# 2 Program Operation and Installation

## INSTALLATION

The computer program can be installed from the CD-ROM enclosed with the book by inserting the compact disk into the CD-ROM drive. Before installing the program, other programs should be closed and previous versions of the software should be uninstalled. Failure to properly remove previous versions of the software may result in conflicts and the program may not be stable. During installation, the program will prompt the user for information to complete the installation process.

## OVERVIEW

The program has a menu along the top of the program that includes File, Go To, and Help options (Figure UG-3).

Basic file operations for the program are accessed in the "File" menu.

- *New Simulation*: This command creates a new simulation with no feeds.
- *Load Simulation*: Loads a previously saved simulation data file.
- *Save Simulation*: Saves the current simulation. If the user has already loaded a simulation data file, the current simulation data are saved to that file name. Otherwise, the current data are saved to the Default Simulation Data File.
- *Save Simulation As*: Allows the user to save the current simulation with a new name. This option will permit you to save simulations to a specified directory. Normally simulations are saved to the Simulation Files subdirectory located in the NRC Program directory.
- *Save Current Simulation as Default*: Saves the current simulation data to the default data file. Note that this option is only enabled if the Auto-Save option (see below) is unchecked.
- *Auto-Save Default Data On Exit*: When checked, the program will automatically save the current simulation data to the default data file when the user exits the program. If unchecked, the user must manually save simulation data. It is suggested that you keep this option checked for safety.
- *Exit Program*: Quits the program.

There are two ways to move around the program. The easiest way is to use the toolbar located beneath the menu bar. Click on a button to jump to the corresponding screen.

It is also possible to move through the program by using the menu. Click the "Go To" menu option and select the desired section of the program.

As described above, there are four main screens within the program:

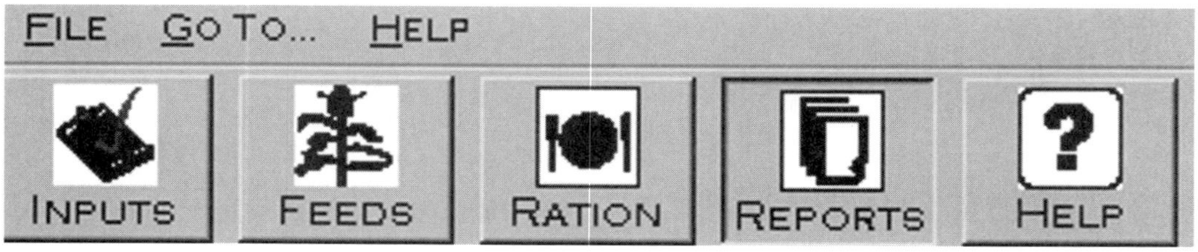


FIGURE UG-3 Program menu bar.

- *Inputs*: Where you enter the general program settings, as well as the animal inputs (e.g., Animal Type, Breed, Body Weight, etc. . . .).
- *Feeds*: Where the feeds in the animal's ration are selected and edited.
- *Ration*: The quantity of each feed in the animal's ration is specified here.
- *Reports*: Go here to view and print output.

## DEFAULT DATA

To permit easy movement within the program, the program must always have reasonable input data defined. Error messages starting with "Run Time Error" indicate that the program is attempting a division by zero. The most common cause of this type of error is failure to enter needed data, especially on feed composition. The program attempts to avoid this type of error by using default data files that are accessed automatically whenever the program is run. There are two types of default data:

*Default Program Settings*: This file stores data that are not specific for a simulation, such as the summary result settings, report headers and footers, and other program settings. It is automatically loaded and saved by the program. If, for whatever reason, this file is lost or corrupted, the program will create new settings for itself.

*Default Simulation Data File*: This file has exactly the same structure as a simulation data file that can be loaded and saved by the user, except that it will automatically be loaded when the program is started up. The user can control how this default file is saved and what data are saved by using the appropriate commands in the "File" menu (see **Program Operation** for more details).

## PROGRAM HELP

In addition to the Help files that are accessed through the menu at the top of the screen, the NRC Dairy Cattle Program also has context-sensitive help for many of its operations.

Context sensitive Help can be accessed in two ways:

- Selecting "What's This?" in the Help menu with the left mouse button. Once this option is selected, the mouse pointer will turn into a pointer with a big question mark next to it. When the question mark is visible, click the input label in question (e.g., "Animal Type") with the left mouse button. If context-sensitive help exists for this label, it will appear.
- Right-clicking the mouse over a label will show a popup menu with "What's This?" as a selection. Left click on the "What's This" help box to view the help message (Figure UG-4). In addition, some labels will have a "Jump to Help Topic" option that will send the user to a specific help topic in this Help section, giving more detailed information concerning the topic.
- Left-clicking on the mouse outside of the help box will cause it to disappear.

Note that when a feed is added to a ration, the program disables the menu system to ensure that the operation is completed before leaving the screen. During this operation the Help system associated with the menus is also disabled.

## INPUTS

The Inputs screen consists of a tabbed dialog box with four different subsections. The first, Program Settings, is shown in Figure UG-5.

- *Units*: Select whether to enter inputs and ration quantities in metric or English units. Although all internal computations are performed in the metric system, output units will be converted as appropriate.
- *Basis*: This determines whether ration quantities will be input on a dry matter or "as-fed" basis. The "As-Fed" basis option uses each feed's dry matter value to compute the dry matter intake from the quantity fed.
- *Report Headers/Footers*: Allows the user to set the output for the report headers/footers. The user can select one of the pre-set options, or can compose his own text.
- *Summary Results*: Allows the user to customize which summary results are presented on the Ration screen. Note that there are summary results specific to Young Calf simulations. These are listed with a "(CALF)" prefix. While it is permissible to have calf summary results mixed with non-calf results, and vice-versa, results that are not applicable will not be shown (e.g., Calf Average Daily Gain will be "N/A" for a Lactating Cow).

The Animal Description tab appears in Figure UG-6.

Most of this screen is self-explanatory, except for Body Condition Score and the Calf Variables. A 1 to 5 scale is used for body condition scoring with 1 for emaciated animals and 5 for obese animals. For animals other than young calves, these variables are disabled (shaded). However, if "Young Calf" is chosen as the Animal Type, then these variables will be enabled, with the others disabled. In addition, since only the program's Calf sub-model only uses these variables, the user will not be able to access the Production and Management tabs if "Young Calf" is the selected Animal Type.

The Production is shown in Figure UG-7.

Items to note on this screen:

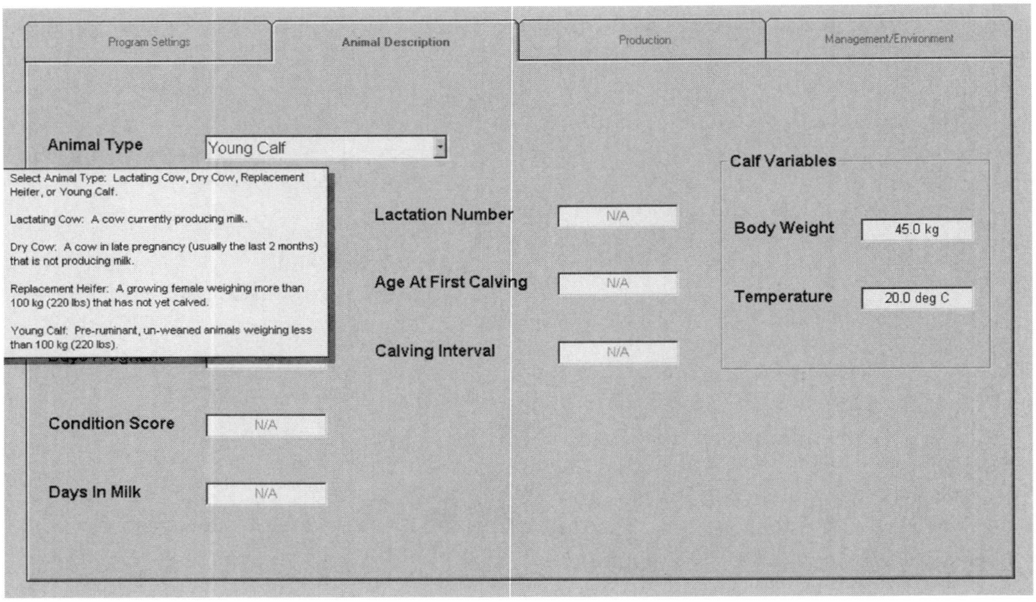


FIGURE UG-4 Help box.

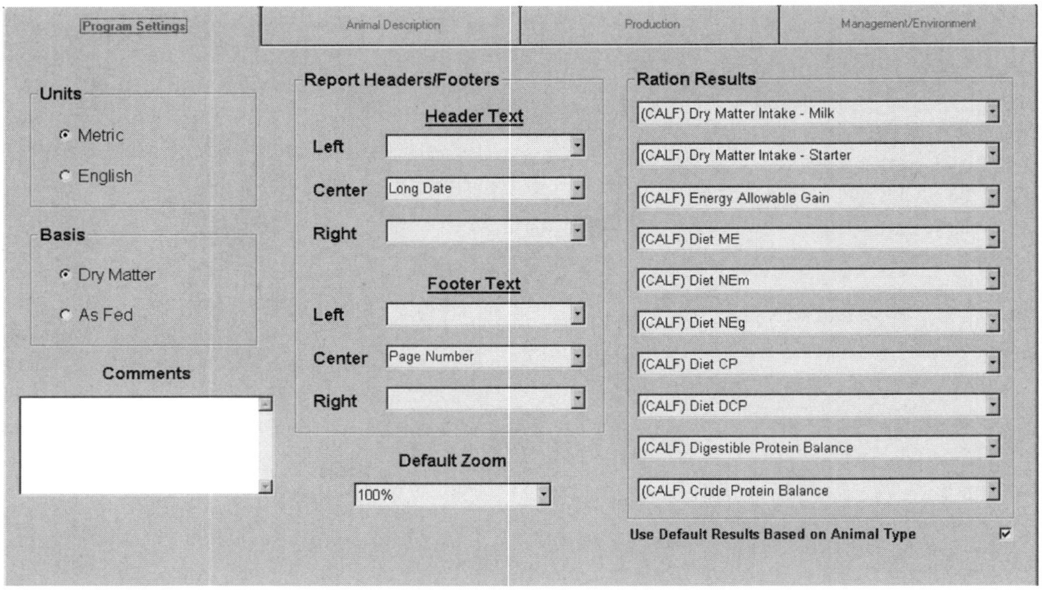


FIGURE UG-5 Program Settings screen.

- If the "Compute Mature Weight from the Breed" option is checked, the mature weight will be set as a function of the selected breed and the user will not be able to change this weight. Likewise, selecting the "Compute Calf Birth Weight from the Mature Weight" option will compute the Calf Birth Weight as a function of the mature weight. These options are recommended if the user does not know the mature weight or calf birth weight of the animals in the herd.
- Whether the Milk Protein is expressed on either a crude or true protein basis can be indicated by selecting the appropriate radio buttons (black dot). True protein equals 0.93 times crude protein.

The Management/Environment screen is shown in Figure UG-8.

- Note that the Previous Temperature, Wind Speed, Coat Condition, Heat Stress, Hair Depth, and Night Cooling variables are only enabled when Replacement Heifer is the chosen Animal Type, since the environmental submodel is only applicable for heifers.

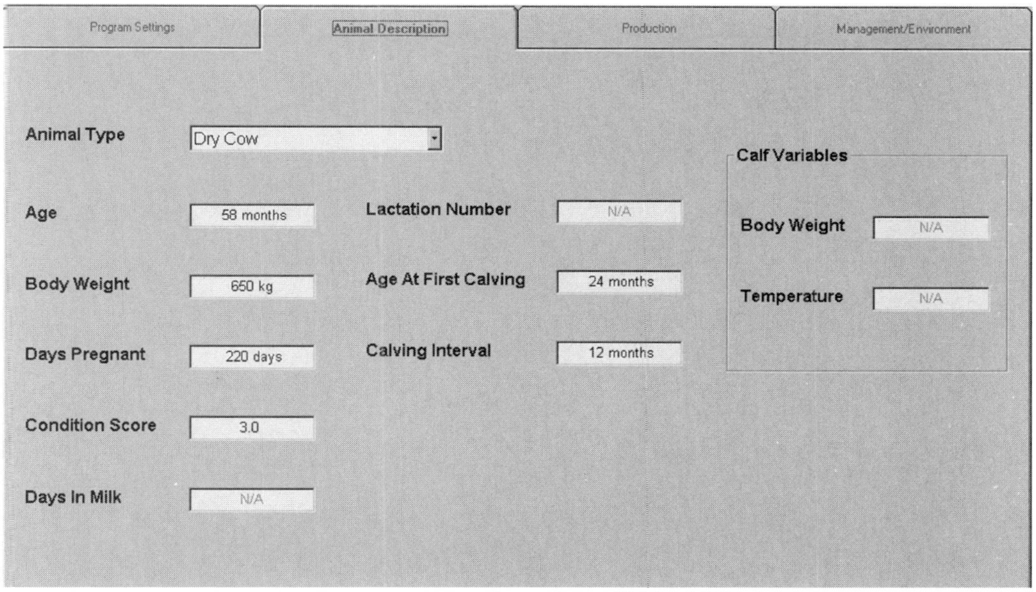


FIGURE UG-6 Animal Description screen.

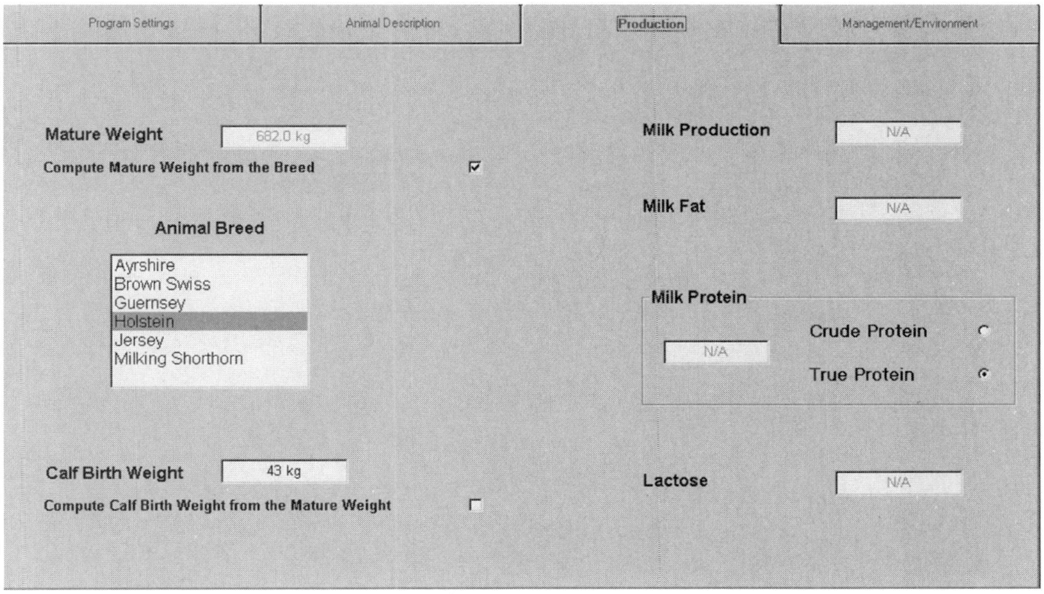


FIGURE UG-7 Production screen.

• If the animal is grazing, then you will have to set the Topography, the Distance Between the Pasture and Milking Center and the Number of One-Way Trips (for Lactating Cows) or the Average Distance Traveled per Day. Distance traveled is measured in either feet or meters.

## FEED

The program handles saving and loading feeds in the following manner: The feeds in the Feed Library that comes with the program cannot be edited or deleted. When a feed is imported into a ration, the program actually makes a copy of the feed data that will be saved with the simulation. This copy can be edited as needed. However, these changes to a feed will only be saved in a specific simulation. The values in the core feed library remain unchanged. To access this edited feed in other simulations, you must save it in the Feed Library (i.e., make a user-created feed). Give the feed a new, unique name and select "Save Feed in Feed Library." To protect the integrity of the Feed Library, it is not possible to save changes to Feeds using names already used in the Feed Library.

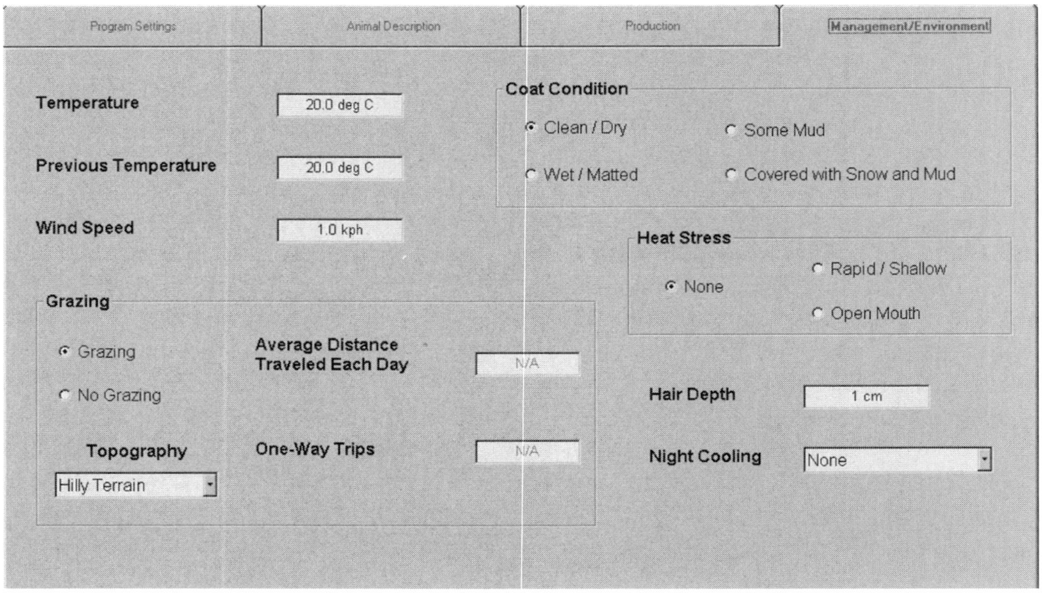


FIGURE UG-8 Management/Environment screen.

• To edit the composition of a feed, enter a new value in the appropriate cell of the Feed Components grid (Figure UG-9). The energy values of feeds, except for milk-based calf feeds, cannot be entered directly. They are computed from the composition of the feeds. In the case of the milk-based calf feeds, energy values can be edited directly but a fixed relationship among the energy values is always maintained. For example, if the ME value of a feed is changed, all of the other energy variables also will change. If fat, ash, or protein of a milk-based calf feed is changed, all energy values also will be recomputed.

• Feeds can be re-ordered in a ration by using the up and down arrows to the right of the Feeds list within the simulation. Select a feed and click on the down arrow to demote the feed to a lower position in the list or click on the up arrow to promote the feed to a higher position in the list.

• The Add Feed(s) button advances the user to another screen where feeds can be selected for the simulation. The

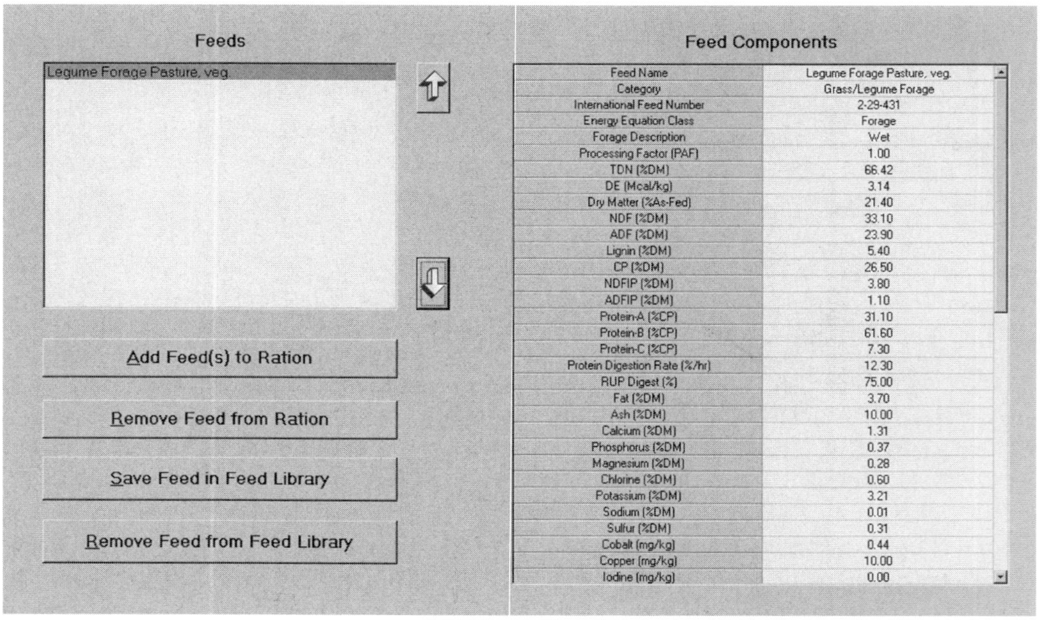


FIGURE UG-9 Feed screen.

feeds in the Feed Library are separated into nine separate categories: Grass/Legume Forages, Grain Crop Forages, Energy Sources, Fats, Plant Protein, Animal Protein, By-Product/Other Feeds, Vitamin and Mineral, and Calf Feeds. As you select feeds in the screen, a grid displaying their component values appears at the bottom of the screen. Also note that user-created feeds are indicated in the different category boxes with a "*" prefix. Multiple feeds can be selected. When the user creates newly defined feeds, it is recommended that the user select a similar feed in the library for editing. This is important for two reasons: 1) if needed information on the new feed is lacking, similar values from the library feed may be used, and 2) the nine boxes to denote feed types also determine which equations are used to predict the energy content of feeds. Mischaracterization of feeds will lead to incorrect energy values.

- The Remove Feed button will remove the selected feed from the ration.
- The Save Feed in Feed Library button will save the current feed in the Feed Library. The program will not allow you to save a feed with a name that matches one of the original feeds in the library. If you want to create and save a user-defined feed in the library, it is recommended that you use a feed that is very similar to the feed that you are entering as a template. Edit the feed as desired but retain feed characterizations such as Category, Energy Equation Class, Forage Description, and Processing Adjustment Factor unless they are patently incorrect. These classifications are used to determine which equations the model uses to predict the energy content of the feed. It is safer to rely on the values in a similar feed than to guess which setting is most appropriate.
- The Remove Feed from Feed Library button allows you to do exactly that. However, only user-created feeds can be removed from the Feed Library.

**Backing Up the Feed Library:** The name of the file containing the Feed Library is NRC Dairy Cattle Program—Feed Library.mdb. This file is a Microsoft Access Database file. This file, including user-defined feeds, can be backed up or shared with other users by copying it into an appropriate location. It is recommended that you make back-up copies of this file, especially if you have entered many user-defined feeds.

**Changing Energy Values of Feeds:** The program predicts the energy content of feeds from chemical composition, and it is not possible to directly adjust the energy value of a feed. If you believe that processing or other conditions have altered the digestibility of fat, NDF or RUP, it is possible to alter the digestibility of these components. These adjustments will affect the energy content of the feed.

## RATION

- On the Ration screen (Figure UG-10), all of the feeds in the simulation are listed, with the amounts fed. The Total Intake entry-box contains the sum of the amounts of all of the feeds included in the ration. This value also can be used to determine the quantities of each feed as a percent of the total intake are also specified.
- Ration quantities can be entered in several ways. First, a quantity can be directly entered in the "Qty" column. When you change a value in this column, the program will recompute the "% Total" using the new quantity fed and the original Total Intake.
- It is possible to enter a ration quantity as a percent of the original total intake and the quantity fed will change to reflect that percentage of the original intake. Finally, you can change the Total Intake. Then the program will recompute all of the quantities of the feeds based on the specified percent of totals for the individual feeds and the new total intake.
- If you change the ration and offer more or less feed than the quantity listed in the "Total Intake" box, the total percent of the "Total Intake" will not equal 100%. Selecting the "Set to 100%" button, the program will re-compute the "% Total" values for all of the feeds based on the individual quantities fed and the total intake, so that the percentages sum to 100% again.
- Clicking the "Estimate" button will cause the program to fill the "Total Intake" box with the model's Predicted Dry Matter Intake.
- Note that the program also displays summary results, which change every time a change is made to the ration. The outputs included in these summary results on the ration page can be customized by making changes on the Program Settings tab of the Inputs screen. The default choices for each Animal Type reflect data most often used in ration evaluation for that class of animal.

## REPORTS

The program's reports are produced in a "Print-Preview" format, where they can be viewed exactly as they will be printed. A typical report screen area is shown in Figure UG-11. Reports are generated on each of the following topics: Summary (of most use to people developing rations), Energy and Protein Supply, Dry Matter Intake, Maintenance Requirements, Growth Requirements, Target Weights and Average Daily Gain, Pregnancy Requirements, Lactation Requirements, and Mineral Requirements.

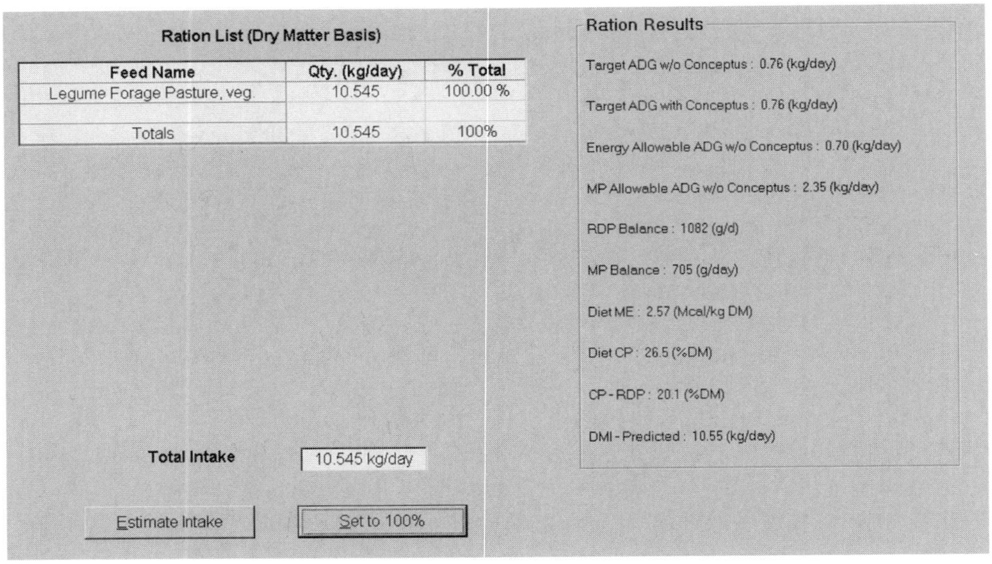


FIGURE UG-10 Ration screen.

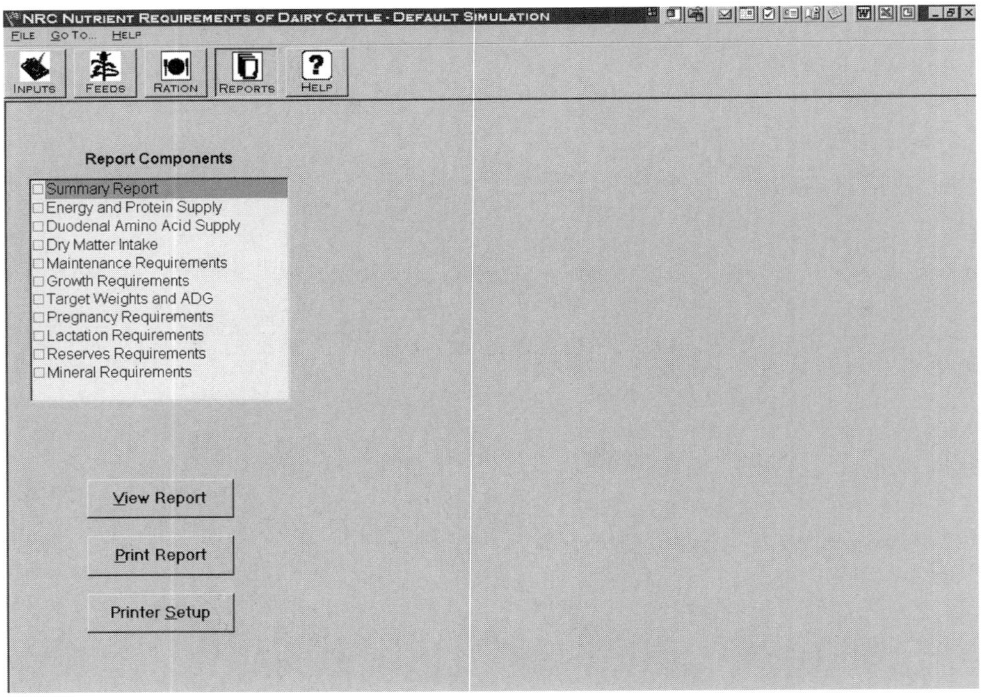


FIGURE UG-11 Reports screen.

• To create a report, select the desired report components by checking the appropriate list-box(es) on the left side of the screen and clicking on the "View Report" button.

• The appearance of the page is set using the "Zoom" list-box, giving you the option of seeing the whole page, thumbnails, two-pages, page-width, and zooms from 25-500%. The default zoom setting can be chosen on the "Default Zoom" box on the Program Settings tab of the Inputs screen. If the "Zoom" box on the Report Screen is adjusted, the change will remain in effect only during that visit to the report screen. Changes made on the Program Settings tab remain in effect until they are changed.

• It is possible to scroll through the pages of the report using the "Page x of y" scrollbar. To move the page up or down in the viewing window, you can use the horizontal and vertical scrollbars. Alternatively, you can click and drag the mouse over the page to move it in any direction you wish. Double-clicking the left mouse button will zoom in, and clicking with the right mouse button will zoom out.

• Reports can be printed out using the "Print Report" button. The page settings such as font type or size or page orientation for the reports can be set by using the "Page Settings" button.

# 3 Tutorials

## GENERAL DESCRIPTION OF THE MODEL STRUCTURE

The model is divided into two major components: prediction of requirements and supply of nutrients. Within this structure, there are sub-models for maintenance, pregnancy, growth, lactation, dry matter intake, minerals, reserves, energy and protein supply, amino acids, and diet evaluation, as well as a young calf sub-model. Chapters 2 and 5 of the accompanying volume describe the biology underlying the equations used in predicting nutrient supply. The equations used in the model are presented in Chapter 16. A glossary of the terms used in the equations is included in this volume. Background information that describes the rationale for choosing the approach and coefficients used in the model is presented in the relevant chapters of the report.

The focus of the tutorials is to demonstrate how to apply the model under various circumstances and conditions. Example lessons are provided for two different situations: one example for mid-lactation cows and one example for heifers.

## MID-LACTATION COW CASE STUDIES

### Case 1: Mid-Lactation Cow

Load Simulation. Click on Inputs. Click on the Program Settings tab.

Program Settings:

| | |
|---|---|
| Units: | Metric |
| Basis: | Dry matter |
| Report: | Header text: important to provide date, page number, and title of document |
| Summary results: | Choose information you are interested in displaying or allow defaults based on animal type |
| Default Zoom: | Set to 75% |

Click on Animal Description tab. Enter the following:

Description:

| | |
|---|---|
| Animal Type: | Lactating cow |
| Age: | 65 months |
| Body Weight: | 680 kg |
| Days Pregnant: | 0 |
| Condition score: | 3.0 |
| Days in Milk: | 90 |
| Lactation Number: | 3 |
| Age at 1st calving | 24 months |
| Calving interval | 12 months |

Click on Production tab. Enter the following:

| | |
|---|---|
| Mature Weight: | 680 kg |
| Breed: | Holstein |
| Calf Birth Weight: | 43 kg |
| Milk Production: | 54.5 kg |
| Milk Fat: | 3.5% |
| Milk True Protein: | 3.0% |
| Lactose: | 4.8% |

Click on Management/Environment tab. Leave default temperature at 20.0 degrees C.

Click on Feeds. Click on Add Feeds to Ration. Select the appropriate categories, highlight the feed and add the following feeds to the ration:

Legume forage hay, immature
Corn silage, normal
Corn grain, steam-flaked
Calcium soaps of fatty acids

Tallow
Cottonseed, whole with lint
Soybean meal, solv. 48% CP
Blood meal, ring dried
Calcium carbonate
Monosodium phosphate (1 H20)
Salt
Vitamin Premix 1

Click on Ration and enter the following diet (as % of DM):

| | |
|---|---|
| Legume forage hay, immature | 18 |
| Corn silage, normal | 40 |
| Corn grain, steam-flaked | 22 |
| Calcium soaps of fatty acids | 1 |
| Tallow | 1 |
| Cottonseed, whole with lint | 7.5 |
| Soybean meal, solv. 48% CP | 8 |
| Blood meal, ring dried | 0.5 |
| Calcium carbonate | 0.1 |
| Monosodium phosphate (1 H20) | 0.2 |
| Salt | 0.5 |
| Vitamin Premix 1 | 1.2 |

Click on Estimate Intake. Note: you cannot enter % of DM until you put an amount (kg/d) in the table, then you can put in %. Of course estimated DMI is not as good as measured DMI.

Click on Reports tab. Check Summary Report and click View Report (Table UG-1).
Click on File. Save As DIET A.

The MP and RUP supplied were short of meeting the required needs for this cow. How can MP supplied be less than required and RDP be more than required? RDP requirements are calculated from TDN. The higher the TDN content of the diet, the higher the RDP requirement.

Go to Ration icon. Change the diet to correct the deficiencies in RUP and MP by increasing the blood meal from 0.5 to 1.7% of ration DM and decreasing the SFC from 22.0% to 20.8% of ration DM. Go to the Reports icon and click on View Report. We have now corrected the deficiencies for MP and RUP. We have, however, increased the total protein in the ration from 15.8 to 16.9%, an additional 330 g CP/d or 226 g of MP/d. The reason that CP increased 330 g but MP only increased 226 g is because the RDP above requirement does not contribute to MP. This additional protein is needed to support this level of milk production. MP allowable milk was 50 kg/d and now it is 55.1 kg/d. Changes in the protein sources used may allow for reduced total protein in the ration.

Click on File. Provide a file name under Save As DIET B.

TABLE UG-1 Summary Report for Diet A

**Summary Report**

Animal Inputs

Animal Type: Lactating Cow
Age: 65 months
Body Weight: 680 kg
Milk Fat: 3.50%
Milk Production: 54.5 (kg/day)
Days Pregnant: 0
Breed: Holstein
Milk True Protein: 3.00%

Diet Nutrient Balances

| Requirements | NE (Mcal/day) | MP (g/day) | Ca (g/day) | P (g/day) | K (g/day) |
|---|---|---|---|---|---|
| Maintenance | 10.7 | 1034 | 22 | 31 | 209 |
| Pregnancy | 0.0 | 0 | 0 | 0 | 0 |
| Lactation | 37.7 | 2440 | 62 | 49 | 76 |
| Growth | 0.0 | 0 | 0 | 0 | 0 |
| **Total Required** | 48.3 | 3474 | 83 | 80 | 285 |
| **Total Supplied** | 47.5 | 3327 | 92* | 80* | 355* |
| **Balance** | −0.8 | −147 | 9 | 0 | 70 |

*Note that these minerals supplied are total *absorbable* supplied.

**Animal Performance**

DMI-Actual: 30.0 (kg/day)
DMI-Predicted: 30.0 (kg/day)

$NE_L$ Allowable Milk: 53.3 (kg/day)
MP Allowable Milk: 51.2 (kg/day)

Milk Production: 54.5 (kg/day)

Days to lose one condition score: 506

Daily Weight Change due to Reserves: −0.2 (kg/day)

**Diet Concentrations**

NDF: 31.2 (%DM)
Forage NDF: 24.5 (%DM)
ADF: 20.6 (%DM)
NFC: 42.4 (%DM)
Undiscounted TDN: 75 (%DM)
ME: 2.48 (Mcal/kg DM)
$NE_L$: 1.58 (Mcal/kg DM)
$NE_G$: 1.19 (Mcal/kg DM)
Ca: 0.6 (%DM)
P: 0.4 (%DM)
Ether Extract: 6.0 (%DM)

**Protein Values**

RDP Required: 2955 (g/d)
RDP Supplied: 3055 (g/d)
RDP Balance: 49 (g/d)

RUP Required: 2046 (g/d)
RUP Supplied: 1871 (g/d)
RUP Balance: −175 (g/d)

MP-Bacterial: 1608 (g/d)
MP-RUP: 1577 (g/d)
MP-Endogenous: 142 (g/d)

CP-Diet: 16.2 (%DM)
CP-RDP: 10.0 (%DM)
CP-RUP: 6.2 (%DM)

**Target Diet Concentration**

$NE_L$: 1.61 (Mcal/kg)
MP: 116 (g/kg)

Ca: 3 (g/kg)
P: 3 (g/kg)

Diet Summary

| Feed Name | kg/day (Dry Matter) | kg/day (As-Fed) |
|---|---|---|
| Legume forage hay, immature | 5.41 | 6.43 |
| Corn silage, normal | 12.02 | 34.25 |
| Corn grain, steam-flaked | 6.61 | 7.50 |
| Calcium soaps of fatty acids | 0.30 | 0.31 |
| Tallow | 0.30 | 0.30 |
| Cottonseed, whole with lint | 2.25 | 2.50 |
| Soybean meal, solv. 48% CP | 2.40 | 2.68 |
| Blood meal, ring-dried | 0.15 | 0.17 |
| Calcium carbonate | 0.03 | 0.03 |
| Monosodium phosphate (1 H2O) | 0.06 | 0.06 |
| Salt | 0.15 | 0.15 |
| Vitamin premix 1 | 0.36 | 0.36 |

Leave this file open.

You can see that this diet is still –0.7 Mcal short of meeting the needs of the cow and $NE_L$ allowable milk is 53.4 kg/d when in fact we hope she will produce 54.4 kg/d.

Go to the Ration icon. Go to the Total Intake frame and type in 30.7 kg. By increasing DMI, $NE_L$ balance is now increased to 0.0 Mcal/d and in the Reports section you will see that $NE_L$ allowable milk is now 54.6 kg/d. Now return to the Ration tab and change the intake by hitting the estimate intake button. It will be 30 kg/d as before. Keep this file open.

### Case 2: Changing True Milk Protein

Click on Inputs. Click on Production. Change True milk protein from 3 to 2.8%. Click on the Reports tab. Check Summary report and then click on View Report. The DMI and the ration are not affected, however, the MP requirement for Lactation decreases from 2440 g to 2278 g/d. The RUP required changes from 2099 g to 1874. RUP requirement is calculated as = ((MP requirement – MP from endogenous – MP from bacterial)/RUP digestibility). MP allowable milk is now 59.1 kg/d.
Click on File and Save this simulation as DIET C.

### Case 3: Changing Days In Milk (90 vs 120 DIM)

Load simulation file DIET B.
Click on File and Save this as a new simulation, DIET D.
Click on the Inputs tab. Click on Programs tab and label this DIET D.
Click on Animal Description. Change DIM from 90 to 120. Click on the Ration icon. You can see under predicted DMI that the intake has increased from 30 kg/d to 30.77. It is very important that you change the intake to reflect the needs of this cow. Click on Estimate Intake. Even though we have not changed anything regarding the diet, some requirements have increased.

As you can see the MP required for maintenance was increased from 1034 grams to 1057 grams/d, which increases the total MP required. As DMI increases the metabolic fecal requirement increases and this represents an important part of the maintenance requirement. The RDP requirement increases because RDP requirement is calculated from TDN and the total TDN has increased. RUP requirement is decreased. The MP from bacteria increased because it is calculated based on TDN. In addition, now we have also increased $NE_L$ from –0.7 Mcal to 0.1 Mcal /d bringing the $NE_L$ allowable milk from 53.5 to 54.7 kg/d.

Click on File and Save this simulation.

### Case 4: Altering Forage Quality

Load file name DIET B.

Click on Feeds. Click on Add Feeds to Ration. Select under Grass/Legumes, Legume Forage Hay, Mature. Click on Add Feed. Click on Ration. Set Legume Hay, immature to 0 % and Legume Hay, Mature to 18%.

There is a message in the right bottom corner: **RDP Limiting-Energy Estimates May be Erroneous.** RDP requirements are calculated from TDN. The higher the TDN content of the diet the higher the RDP requirement. More RDP can be added or the TDN of the ration can lowered or a combination of the two can be used to correct the situation.

Go to the Reports tab.
Highlight Summary Report. Click on View Report. This is a very clear demonstration of how forage quality affects the $NE_L$ and MP allowable milk and puts the cow in greater negative energy and protein balance.

Go to File and Save this simulation as DIET E.

### Case 5: When Only RDP is Limiting

Load DIET B.
Click on Ration. Enter under % Total for Legume forage, immature 17%, corn silage 37.8%, SFC 26%, Tallow to 0%, SBM 6.5%, and Blood meal 2.2%.
Go to Reports and highlight Summary Report. Click on View Report. In this case MP balance is positive and RDP is limiting. RDP may be limiting microbial growth, but the diet contains sufficient RUP such that the MP requirements of the animal are met. Go to File and Save simulation as DIET F.

## REPLACEMENT DAIRY HEIFERS

In the model accompanying *Nutrient Requirements of Dairy Cattle* (2001), energy and protein requirements are computed from the energy and protein contained in the tissue accreted during growth. The gain can be predicted from the current and mature weights of the animal or a desired rate of gain can be entered. After a proposed ration has been entered, the model predicts the energy and protein allowable daily gain. Daily gain is predicted from the net energy available after the requirements for maintenance and pregnancy have been met. The amount of protein required is based on the energy allowable gain. This exercise begins by describing briefly the concepts underlying the heifer growth model, and then simulations demonstrate the theories used to develop this model and evaluate rations of replacement heifers.

### Computing Energy and Protein Requirements of Heifers with Different Mature Weights

The equations used to compute energy and protein requirements for animals at any body weight and any rate of gain were developed from data on body composition of many cattle grown at different growth rates to various mature weights. The energy and protein composition of gain of animals with similar current weights, but different mature weights, differ. To account for the effect of mature weight on chemical composition of gain, a size scaling adjustment using a standard reference animal is used. This adjusted weight is then used to compute the net energy requirement. Table UG-2 compares the net energy and protein requirements of typical and large mature size Holstein heifers, and small Jersey heifers computed with this model.

Table UG-2 shows:

1. Animals with larger mature weights are at an earlier stage of maturity than their peers with smaller mature weights.
2. There is a direct relationship between net energy content of gain and weight as a percentage of mature weight, and an inverse relationship between net protein content of gain and weight as a percentage of mature weight.
3. Efficiency of use of metabolizable protein decreases as weight as a proportion of mature size increases.

Table UG-3 shows the influence of rate of gain on heifer requirements at the same stage of growth for a typical Holstein, a large Holstein, and a Jersey (see Table UG-2). Table UG-3 demonstrates:

1. When the energy and protein content of gain of a typical Holstein, a large Holstein, and a Jersey are the same, the heifer with a largest mature weight will weigh more than the smaller animals.
2. At a given weight, as rate of gain increases, net energy and net protein required increase.
3. At a constant rate of gain, the amount of net energy required increases and net protein required decreases per unit of gain as the animal matures.

TABLE UG-3 Effect of Body Weight and Rate of Gain on Daily Gain

| Mature weight | *Live Body weight (kg) at various stages of growth*[a] | | | | | | |
|---|---|---|---|---|---|---|---|
| 650 kg Holstein | 200 | 250 | 300 | 350 | 400 | 450 | 500 |
| 800 kg Holstein | 246 | 308 | 369 | 431 | 493 | 554 | 616 |
| 400 kg Jersey | 139 | 173 | 208 | 242 | 277 | 312 | 346 |
| Shrunk weight gain, kg/day | *$NE_G$ required, Mcal/d*[b] | | | | | | |
| 0.6 | 1.34 | 1.58 | 1.81 | 2.03 | 2.25 | 2.46 | 2.66 |
| 0.8 | 1.83 | 2.17 | 2.48 | 2.79 | 3.08 | 3.37 | 3.64 |
| 1.0 | 2.34 | 2.77 | 3.17 | 3.56 | 3.94 | 4.30 | 4.65 |
| | *Net protein required for growth, g/d*[c] | | | | | | |
| 0.6 | 122 | 114 | 108 | 101 | 95 | 89 | 83 |
| 0.8 | 161 | 151 | 141 | 132 | 124 | 115 | 107 |
| 1.0 | 199 | 187 | 175 | 163 | 152 | 142 | 131 |
| | *Metabolizable protein required for growth, g/d*[d] | | | | | | |
| 0.6 | 182 | 183 | 185 | 187 | 190 | 194 | 199 |
| 0.8 | 241 | 241 | 243 | 245 | 248 | 253 | 259 |
| 1.0 | 299 | 299 | 300 | 302 | 305 | 310 | 316 |

[a]The body weights are full, not shrunk, body weights. The weights within the same column are at the same stage of growth.

[b]$NE_G$ requirement is computed from Equation 11-2: Retained energy (RE) = $0.0635\ EQEBW^{.75}\ EBG^{1.097}$, where EQEBW is equivalent empty body weight and EBG is 0.956 SWG.

[c]Net protein in the gain is computed from equation 11-3: RP, g/d = SWG × (268 − (29.4 × (RE/SWG))).

[d]Metabolizable protein required is computed from equation 11-4: $MPg = NP_g/(0.83 - (EQSBW \times 0.00114))$; If EQSBW is > 478 kg, then EQSBW = 478 kg.

4. Metabolizable protein is used less efficiently for growth as body weight as a proportion of mature weight increases.

### Target Rates for Herd Replacement Heifers

To compute target weights for replacement heifers, it is assumed that a heifer will weight 55% of mature weight at breeding and 82% of mature weight at first calving. If these targets are reached, the costs of raising replacements will be minimized and first lactation milk production maximized (see Chapter 11). Target weights as a percentage of mature weight (MW) are summarized in Table UG-4 for an average Holstein, a large Holstein, and a Jersey. These target weights are used with current age and weight, age at first calving and calving interval to compute daily gain required to reach the next target weight, as follows.

TABLE UG-2 Net Energy and Protein Requirements of Heifers with Mature Weights of 400, 650, and 800 kg

| | Small Jersey | Typical Holstein | Large Holstein |
|---|---|---|---|
| Mature body weight, kg | 400 | 650 | 800 |
| Current body weight, kg | 313 | 313 | 313 |
| Shrunk body weight (SBW), kg | 300 | 300 | 300 |
| % of mature weight | 75 | 46 | 38 |
| SBW equivalent to standard reference animal, kg | 359 | 221 | 179 |
| Net energy required for 700 grams daily gain, Mcal | 3.09 | 2.15 | 1.83 |
| Net protein required for 700 grams daily gain, g | 97 | 124 | 134 |
| Efficiency of use of metabolizable protein, % | 42.1 | 57.8 | 62.6 |
| Metabolizable protein required for 700 grams daily gain, g | 230 | 215 | 214 |

TABLE UG-4 Target Weights for Dairy Heifers

| Reproductive Stage | Target % of MW | 650 kg MW | 800 kg MW | 400 kg MW |
|---|---|---|---|---|
| 1st breeding | 55% | 358 | 440 | 220 |
| 1st calving (post-parturition) | 82% | 533 | 656 | 328 |
| 2nd calving | 92% | 598 | 736 | 368 |
| 3rd calving | 100% | 650 | 800 | 400 |

For heifers before conception, target daily gain to weight at first breeding is:
((Mature weight × 0.55) − current weight) / ((Age at first breeding − Current age) × 30.4.

For bred heifers, daily gain required is:
((Mature weight × 0.82) − current weight) / (Age at first calving − Current age) × 30.4; the average daily gain of the conceptus is added to get measured weight gain required.

Daily gain required during the first lactation (including the dry period) is:
((Mature weight × 0.92) − current weight) / (calving interval days − days since calving) × 30.4. Daily gain for the second lactation is computed the same way, using 1 to compute the next target weight for the second lactation.

Table UG-5 compares target daily gains for the three mature sizes of replacement heifers. This table shows that daily gain required to reach the target depends on current weight, mature size, and age at first calving.

### Heifer Model Exercise

This exercise is designed to demonstrate how the program can be used to compute requirements for dairy heifers for a desired daily gain, and to compute target and diet allowable daily gains based on animal and dietary information entered in the model. Table UG-6 summarizes the inputs that will be needed for each scenario in this exercise (in order that the variables must be entered). Only changes from the no-stress, open heifer are shown for the other scenarios. Answers are provided in italics in parentheses in the scenarios described below.

TABLE UG-5 Target Daily Gains Post Transition to Pre-Conception for Three Mature Sizes of Dairy Heifers

| | 400 kg mature weight | 650 kg mature weight | 800 kg mature weight |
|---|---|---|---|
| Current age, days[a] | 77 | 77 | 77 |
| Current weight, kg[b] | 52 | 84 | 103 |
| Target bred weight, kg | 220 | 358 | 440 |
| Gain required to conception, kg | 168 | 274 | 337 |
| Days to conception[c] | | | |
| 20 months of age at first calving | 251 | 251 | 251 |
| 24 months of age at first calving | 373 | 373 | 373 |
| 28 months of age at first calving | 494 | 494 | 494 |
| Daily gain required to first conception, g | | | |
| 20 months of age at first calving | 669 | 1092 | 1343 |
| 24 months of age at first calving | 450 | 735 | 903 |
| 28 months of age at first calving | 340 | 555 | 682 |

[a]Weaning at 8 weeks plus 3 weeks transition.
[b]Birth weight at 6.275% of mature weight plus expected weight gain during starting and transition phases.
[c]Age in days at first calving (280 days gestation; 77 days current age).

**Scenario 1.** The effect of age, current body weight, and mature weight on nutrient requirements for the desired daily gain, target daily gain, and diet allowable daily gain.

1. Enter the information for the open heifer with no stress conditions. At the ration screen, note that the target daily gain differs from the desired ADG and the ME allowable ADG. The target ADG exceeds the desired ADG entered. The target is the optimum computed by the model based on the age, current weight, age at first calving, and mature weight. The dietary ME and protein allowable ADGs are what the diet will sustain. In this example, ME and MP allowable ADGs exceed the input desired ADG but are less than the target ADG. This screen also shows that the RDP supply is greater than the RDP required and that the MP balance is positive. Thus, more protein is being fed than is necessary to support the entered desired ADG. Also, note the entered dry matter intake is similar to the model predicted intake. *(Desired ADG = 800 g/d, Target ADG = 930 g/d, Energy allowable ADG = 890 g/d, Protein allowable ADG = 850 g/d, RDP balance = 132 g/d, MP balance = 14 g/d, Actual DMI = 5.99 kg/d, Predicted DMI = 5.99 kg/d).*

2. Next click on the report icon and choose the summary screen. In the balance screen at the top of the report, the energy and protein supplied exceed the requirements. *(MEreq = 13.3 Mcal, MEsupplied = 14.0 Mcal, MPreq = 486 g/d, MPsupplied = 501 g/d).*

3. Now click on the input icon and on the animal description tab. Change the desired ADG to match the target ADG (930 grams). Now click on reports, summary report, and note that the diet now provides less than is needed to attain the target ADG. *(MEreq = 14.3 Mcal, MEsupplied = 14.0 Mcal, MPreq = 522 g/d, MPsupplied = 501 g/d).*

4. Now click on inputs, animal description tab, and change the desired ADG back to 800 grams. Then change the age to 7 months, click on ration, and note the new target ADG is lower. This is because the animal now has more time to reach the target weight. *(Target ADG = 770 g/d).*

5. Next, click on the animal description tab, change the age back to 8 months, and change the body weight to 300 kg. Now click on the ration icon and note that the target ADG and ME allowable ADG decreased. The target ADG decreased because the animal now needs to gain less weight

TABLE UG-6 Inputs for Heifer Growth Exercises

| INPUT ITEM | Open heifer<br>No stress | Cold temperature | Temp. + wet | Temp. + wind | Bred heifer<br>No stress |
|---|---|---|---|---|---|
| Age, months | 8 | | | | 20 |
| Body weight, kg | 240 | | | | 550 |
| Days pregnant | 0 | | | | 220 |
| Condition score | 3 | | | | 3 |
| Age @ first calving | 22 | | | | 22 |
| Calving interval | 13 | | | | 13 |
| Desired ADG, gm | 800 | | | | 800 |
| Mature weight, kg | Breed avg | | | | |
| Breed | Holstein | | | | |
| Previous temperature, C | 20 | 0 | 0 | 0 | |
| Current temperature, C | 20 | 0 | 0 | 0 | |
| Wind speed, kph | 1.6 | | | 16 | |
| Grazing | No | | | | |
| Coat condition | Clean + dry | | Wet + matted | Wet + matted | |
| Heat stress | No | | | | |
| Coat depth, cm | 1 | 2 | 2 | 2 | |
| Night cooling | Yes | | | | |
| Ration (kg/day): | | | | | |
| Legume forage silage, mid maturity | 2.81 | | | | 3.84 |
| Corn silage, normal | 3.08 | | | | 8.67 |
| Corn grain, dry | 0.0 | | | | 0.0 |
| Soybean meal solvent, 48% CP | 0.09 | | | | 0.275 |
| Bloodmeal, ring-dried | 0.0 | | | | 0.0 |
| Calcium phosphate (di-) | 0.01 | | | | 0.012 |
| Calcium carbonate | 0.0 | | | | 0.0 |

to reach the target by the same age. The ME allowable ADG decreased because the animal has a larger body weight to maintain and the energy content of gain is higher as shown in Table UG-2. The predicted DMI increased because intake is a function of body weight and diet energy density. *(Target ADG = 520 g/d, ME allowable gain = 580 g/d, DMIpredicted = 7.08 kg/d).*

6. Click on the animal description tab and change the body weight back to 240 kg. Now change the age at first calving to 24 months, then click on ration. The target ADG is decreased, because the animal has more time to conceive, as shown in Table UG-4. *(Target ADG = 650 g/d).*

7. Click on the animal description tab and change the age at first calving back to 22 months of age. Now click on the animal production tab, click on the choice of using the model mature weight to remove the check, then enter 650 kg. Now click on the ration icon. The target ADG is reduced, because the target weight at breeding was reduced. The target weight at breeding is 55% of mature weight, so reduction in mature weight lowers the weight at breeding (Table UG-3). *(Target ADG = 650 g/d).*

**Scenario 2.** The effect of environment on growth rate.

The effect of environment on heifer daily gain depends on several factors as follows:

- Previous temperature changes metabolic rate; therefore as previous temperature decreases, the maintenance requirement increases, leaving less energy and protein available for growth.
- The combined effects of current temperature, insulation to prevent heat loss (hair coat condition and depth), and wind (affects heat loss due to convective cooling) are used to determine the animal's lower critical temperature. If the lower critical temperature is below the animal's current temperature, more of the diet energy will be required to maintain body temperature, leaving less for growth. Table UG-7 summarizes these effects on maintenance requirements.

1. Click on the environment tab and change the current temperature to -1.1°, -12°, and -23° C. Now click on ration and note the decrease in daily gain. The predicted intake

TABLE UG-7 Maintenance Energy Requirement Multipliers for Various Environmental Conditions[a,b]

| | −1.1°C | | −12°C | | −23°C | |
|---|---|---|---|---|---|---|
| Hair coat code[c] | 1[3] | 3[3] | 1[3] | 3[3] | 1[3] | 3[3] |
| Wind velocity (kph) | | | | | | |
| 1.6 | 1.17 | 1.41 | 1.37 | 1.90 | 1.74 | 2.39 |
| 16 | 1.33 | 1.70 | 1.80 | 2.27 | 2.26 | 2.84 |

[a] Simulations made using the model presented in chapter 11. Temperature values are current temperature ($T_c$).

[b] Values given are net energy maintenance requirements ($NE_M$) required for these conditions divided by the maintenance requirement without stress.

[c] Hair coat code: 1 = dry and clean, 2 = mud on lower body (values not shown), and 3 = wet and matted.

should increase. *(ME allowable gain = 890 g/d, 570 g/d, and 170 g/d when the temperature = -1.1°, -12°, and -23° C respectively.)*

2. Click on the environment tab, and change hair coat to wet and matted. Now click on ration and note the change in daily gain. A wet and dirty hair coat results in the loss of insulation because the hair coat is flattened, losing its insulation value. *(When the temperature = -1.1°, the growth was 450 g/d, and there was no growth for the other 2 temperatures.)*

3. Click on the environment tab, and change wind to 16 kph. Now click on ration, and note the change in daily gain. Wind increases energy loss due to convective cooling. *(When the temperature = -1.1°, the ME allowable ADG was 40 g/d. Weight loss occurred at the two lower temperatures.)*

**Scenario 3.** The effect of pregnancy on heifer requirements.

Once pregnant, the requirements for the growing fetus and fetal membranes (collectively called the conceptus) must be met in addition to those required for maintenance and growth. Because they are relatively small in early pregnancy, requirements for the conceptus are added after 190 days of pregnancy.

1. Enter the information in Table UG-6 for bred heifers. On the ration screen, note that the target ADG is higher when the conceptus is included. The ME and MP allowable ADG exceed the target ADG and desired ADG that was entered (800 grams). *(The ADG with conceptus was 1380 g/d and ADG without conceptus was 750 g/d.)*

2. Click on the report icon, then choose summary report, and view this report to see the pregnancy requirement for ME and MP. Then choose the animal description screen and change days pregnant to 250 days. Now click on the report icon, choose summary report, and view this report. The ME and MP required for pregnancy increased, and the ME and MP balances were reduced. *(The ME required for pregnancy was 4.5 Mcal, and the MP required for pregnancy was 239 g/d. When days pregnant equaled 250 days, the ME required for pregnancy was 5.2 Mcal and the MP required for pregnancy was 299 g/d.)*

3. Next, click on the ration icon to see the increased target ADG required. This is because there are fewer days left to reach the target weight, requiring a higher ADG. *(The target gain with conceptus was 1700 g/d and 1060 g/d without conceptus.)*

4. Click on the animal description screen and change the days pregnant back to 220. Then click on the animal production screen, and increase the birth weight to 50 kg. Now click on the reports icon, choose the summary report, and view this screen. The ME and MP required for pregnancy increased and the ME allowable ADG without and with pregnancy decreased. This occurred because less energy was available for growth because of the increased pregnancy requirement. *(The ME required for pregnancy was 5.3 Mcal and the MP required for pregnancy was 278 g/d. The ME allowable gain without conceptus was 980 g/d and the ME allowable gain with conceptus was 1720 g/d.)*

# About the Authors

**Jimmy H. Clark** (*chair*) is professor of nutrition in the Department of Animal Sciences at the University of Illinois. The focus of his studies is both applied and basic research related to ruminant nutrition and metabolism. He has been awarded numerous honors for his work in research, teaching, and extension. Clark served two consecutive terms (1981–1987) with the National Research Council's Committee on Animal Nutrition and participated in the publication of the 1989 revised edition of *Nutrient Requirements of Dairy Cattle*. He received his undergraduate degree in agriculture from Murray State University in Kentucky and his Ph.D. degree in Animal Nutrition from the University of Tennessee.

**David K. Beede** is professor and C.E. Meadows Endowed Chair for Dairy Nutrition and Management at Michigan State University in the Department of Animal Science. He received his undergraduate degree in animal science from Colorado State University, his master's degree in ruminant nutrition from the University of Nebraska, and his Ph.D. degree from the University of Kentucky in ruminant nutritional physiology and biochemistry. Beede's expertise in nutritional management of dairy herds has led him around the world consulting on six continents.

**Richard A. Erdman** is professor of ruminant nutrition and chair of the Department of Animal and Avian Sciences at the University of Maryland. His research includes work in energy and applied animal nutrition. Erdman pioneered research on the effect of trans fatty acids on milk fat production. At the University of Wisconsin, he received his undergraduate degree in animal science and agronomy. Erdman continued his education at the University of Kentucky, where he received both his master's and Ph.D. degrees in animal science.

**Jesse P. Goff** is Veterinary Medical Officer with the Mineral Metabolism and Mastitis Unit at the National Animal Disease Center at the U.S. Department of Agriculture. His expertise is in diseases of mineral metabolism in domestic animals with special emphasis on milk fever in dairy cows. Goff received his undergraduate degree in microbiology from Cornell University. At Iowa State University he furthered his studies and received his master's degree in veterinary physiology, his doctorate degree in veterinary medicine, and his Ph.D. degree in veterinary physiology and nutritional physiology.

**Ric R. Grummer** is professor at the University of Wisconsin in the Department of Dairy Science. His research interests are in lipid metabolism in dairy cattle, specifically the utilization of supplemental fat in dairy rations, etiology and nutritional prevention of fatty liver and ketosis, and nutrition of the transition cow. Grummer's educational background includes his undergraduate degree received from the University of Wisconsin, his master's degree and his Ph.D. degree received from the University of Illinois, all from the Department of Dairy Science.

**James G. Linn** is professor and extension animal scientist in dairy nutrition at the St. Paul campus of the University of Minnesota's Department of Animal Science and Extension Service. His undergraduate education began at the University of Minnesota where he received his degree in animal science. Linn continued at the University of Minnesota and received his master's and his Ph.D. degrees in Nutrition, with an emphasis in ruminant nutrition for the latter degree. Linn's expertise is a direct result of his 16 years of involvement with the University of Minnesota's Extension Programs.

**Alice N. Pell** is professor at Cornell University in the Department of Animal Sciences. She received her undergraduate degree and a *summa cum laude* on her thesis in architectural science from Radcliffe College at Harvard

University. Her master's degree in education is from Harvard Graduate School of Education; her master's and Ph.D. degrees in animal science from the University of Vermont. Pell's research areas and teaching fields include rumen microbiology and applied nutrition. She has served in numerous advisory capacities including her service on the National Research Council's Committee on Animal Nutrition.

**Charles G. Schwab** is professor in the Department of Animal and Nutritional Sciences at the University of New Hampshire. His interest in dairy science is deeply rooted as he was born and raised on a 200-acre dairy and livestock farm in Wisconsin. Schwab received his undergraduate degree in animal sciences, his master's degree in dairy science nutrition, and his Ph.D. degree in dairy science and nutritional sciences, all from the University of Wisconsin. His research interests include an emphasis in amino acid and protein utilization in dairy cattle nutrition.

**Trevor Tomkins** is President and Chief Operating Officer of Milk Specialties Company. After securing his undergraduate degree in agriculture and animal production, he continued at the University of Reading in England to receive his Ph.D. degree, also in animal production. His primary area of expertise in nutrition and animal health products for the world-wide livestock industry is supplemented by global experience in the animal feed industry and a background in business.

**Gabriella A. Varga** is professor of animal science in the Department on Dairy and Animal Sciences at the Pennsylvania State University. She received her undergraduate degree in biology from Duquesne University, her master's degree in animal science from the University of Rhode Island, and her Ph.D. degree in animal science from the University of Maryland. Varga's research has made major contributions to the area of carbohydrate nutrition.

**William P. Weiss** is professor of dairy science at The Ohio Agricultural Research and Development Center at The Ohio State University. His general research interests include utilization of forages by dairy cattle, feed evaluation, and vitamin E and selenium nutrition. At Purdue University, Weiss studied animal sciences and received both his undergraduate and master's degrees. He received his Ph.D. degree from The Ohio State University in dairy science.

weiss.6@osu.edu

# Index

## C

## D

## F

## G

## I

## M

**R**

## S

## T

## W



## Y



## Z